HANDBUCH DER UROLOGIE

ENCYCLOPEDIA OF UROLOGY

ENCYCLOPÉDIE D'UROLOGIE

HERAUSGEGEBEN VON · EDITED BY
PUBLIÉE SOUS LA DIRECTION DE

C. E. ALKEN
HOMBURG (SAAR)

V. W. DIX
LONDON

H. M. WEYRAUCH
SAN FRANCISCO

E. WILDBOLZ
BERN

II

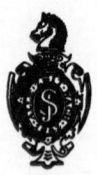

SPRINGER-VERLAG · BERLIN · HEIDELBERG · NEW YORK · 1965

PHYSIOLOGIE UND PATHOLOGISCHE PHYSIOLOGIE
PHYSIOLOGY AND PATHOLOGICAL PHYSIOLOGY
PHYSIOLOGIE NORMALE ET PATHOLOGIQUE

VON / BY / PAR

BERNARD FEY, PARIS · **FELIX HENI,** TÜBINGEN
ALBERT KUNTZ†, ST. LOUIS
D. F. MC DONALD, ROCHESTER · **LOUIS QUÉNU,** PARIS
LAURENCE G. WESSON, JR., PHILADELPHIA
CLIFFORD WILSON, LONDON

MIT 169 ABBILDUNGEN
WITH 169 FIGURES
AVEC 169 FIGURES

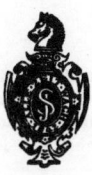

SPRINGER-VERLAG · BERLIN · HEIDELBERG · NEW YORK · 1965

ISBN-13: 978-3-642-46020-3   e-ISBN-13: 978-3-642-46018-0
DOI: 10.1007/978-3-642-46018-0

© by Springer-Verlag · Berlin · Heidelberg · 1965
Softcover reprint of the hardcover 1st edition 1965
Library of Congress Catalog Card Number 58-4788

Titel-Nr. 5874

Inhalt — Contents — Table des matières

XVIII   Inhalt — Contents — Table des matières

Inhalt — Contents — Table des matières **XIX**

Mitarbeiter von Band II — Contributors to volume II
Ont collaboré au volume II

BERNARD FEY, Professeur honoraire a la Faculté de Medicine de Paris, Paris (France.)

FELIX HENI, Direktor der Medizinischen Poliklinik, Tübingen, Liebermeisterstraße 14.

ALBERT KUNTZ †, Dr., St. Louis University, St. Louis, Miss. (USA).

D. F. McDONALD, Professor of Urologic Surgery, University of Rochester, School of Medine, Rochester, New York (USA).

LOUIS QUÉNU, Agrégé d'Urologie à la Faculté de Médicine de Paris, Paris (Frankreich).

LAURENCE G. WESSON, M.D., Professor of Medicine and Director, Division of Renal Diseases and Electrolyte Metabolism, Department of Medicine, Jefferson Medical College, Philadelphia, Penn. (USA).

CLIFFORD WILSON, Professor of Medicine, University of London, Medical Unit, The London Hospital, London E. 1. (England).

Physiology of the kidney

By

LAURENCE G. WESSON, jr.

With 76 figures

A. Historical note

The science of Renal Physiology begins with WILLIAM BOWMAN. Although elements of renal architecture had been described by earlier anatomists, BOWMAN in 1842 was the first to delineate the functional architecture of the nephron as a cluster of capillaries, the glomerulus, dipping into the ostium of a tubule which then leads without interruption to the exterior of the body. Recognition of this simple two component system was for many years sufficient to determine theoretical concepts of mechanism of urine formation. The thin membranes separating blood from tubular lumen in the glomerulus seemed suitable for a filtering process. BOWMAN himself suggested that urinary water and "foreign substances, particularly salts" were filtered through the glomerular capillaries while the remaining components of urine were secreted by the tubules. Within a few years, and apparently quite independently of BOWMAN, KARL LUDWIG (1816—1895) had arrived at similar conclusions. LUDWIG proposed that virtually the entire process of urine formation could be considered that of filtration. To the tubular cells were attributed the property of selective permeability. The cells were permeable to water and substances useful to the body and these substances diffused back into the blood stream under a pressure system analogous to that later described in more detail by STARLING for the extracapillary circulation of plasma water. RUDOLPH HEIDENHAIN (1834—1897), however, strongly influenced by correlations between blood flow and urine formation and by staining of tubular cells by various dyes, believed that the production of urine was entirely compatible with a set of secretory processes similar to those of most exocrine glands. Even the glomerulus was viewed as a secretory organ probably specializing in the transfer of excreted water and salt. The history of renal physiology during the last half of the nineteenth century largely consists of studies, sometimes ingenious, designed to support or refute one or the other of these competing theories. In particular, MORITZ NUSSBAUM'S exploitation of the separate blood supply to the glomeruli and tubules of the amphibian kidney in order to distinguish between glomerular and tubular functions was an important advance during this period. This anatomical characteristic of the fish and amphibian kidney which is retained in varying degrees by reptiles and birds has been the source of an immense literature and constitutes a research tool which is still widely used.

Variation exists with respect to the terminology applied to the kidney structure observed in different orders of vertebrates. Huber, for example, follows the more common anatomical convention of designating the kidney of all amniotes (reptile, bird and mammal) as the *metanephros* while SMITH (1951), emphasizing the significance of the blood supply, has tended to confine the term, metanephros, to the mammalian kidney which has a purely arterial blood supply. SMITH designated as mesonephros the kidney of fish, amphibian, reptile and bird which have a portal venous as well as an arterial blood supply, while HUBER and others restrict that term to the fish and amphibian kidney. More recently, however, SMITH (pers. comm.) has indicated that he is no longer inclined to emphasize the vascular differences to this extent and would agree with the anatomical usage. ROMER, however, points out the considerable artificiality involved in both terms. Apart from a group of nephrons arising from the most anterior somites *(pronephros)* and disappearing early in embryonic life, evolution of the kidney from the fish to bird and mammal has been a fairly uniform process characterized by progressive multiplication of the number of tubules derived from the more posterior somites represented in the nephrogenic ridge and corresponding loss of tubules derived from anterior somites. In reptiles, birds and mammals the tubules are gathered into compact masses (metanephros), but they are identical in origin with the more posterior nephrons of the amphibian and fish kidney. ROMER would abandon the term, mesonephros, as useless in the phylogenetic sense but perhaps appropriate embryologically to designate a group of more anterior nephrons which function for a while in the developing embryo and which later degenerate. ROMER points out that the renal blood supply of cyclostomes is entirely arterial and suggests that the renal portal system is a secondary acquisition necessitated by the circumstance that the pressure of the arterial blood in the fish may be too low, after passing through the gills, to form an adequate volume of glomerular filtrate. Alternatively, the renal portal system might have evolved because the circulatory system of early vertebrates was inadequate to meet steadily mounting demands for both muscle and kidney perfusion. Abandonment of the renal portal system is beginning in reptiles and continuing in birds in that increasing proportions of renal portal blood bypass the kidney (SPERBER 1949). Presumably the rate of loss proceeded faster in that early reptilian branch leading to mammals than in that leading to modern reptiles and birds. All reptilian forms close to the pre-mammalian line are extinct.

The era of controversy between the schools of LUDWIG describing urine formation in hydrodynamic terms and of HEIDENHAIN describing urine formation in terms of secretion was terminated by the monographs of ARTHUR CUSHNY (1917 and 1926). CUSHNY proposed, with LUDWIG, that urine formation commenced with formation of an abundant filtrate containing all materials destined for excretion. He avoided the difficulties created by the concept of mechanical reabsorption in LUDWIG's schema by proposing that the tubular cells reabsorb a fluid containing the constituents of plasma water in the "ideal" proportions. Urine represents the material which could not be present in an ideal fluid. CUSHNY's hypothesis was arbitrary. He offered no new data. He was motivated by a desire for simplicity and by dislike for the apparently infinite complexity of the secretory system proposed by HEIDENHAIN. His choice, however, was a fortunate one and his monograph, appearing when renal physiologists were groping for a new direction to their research, was extremely influential. Within a few years extensive studies on the excretory capacity of the aglomerular tubules of certain marine fish had appeared which supported completely the concepts of HEIDENHAIN. CUSHNY was aware of the excretory function of the aglomerular tubule, but he set this aside as an anomaly. Had he accepted the philosophical threat of the fish nephron to his simplifying concepts, his monograph might never have appeared.

CUSHNY's theory immediately stimulated intense research activity to test or to exploit it. REHBERG, reasoning from CUSHNY's concept that the substance most concentrated in the urine was least likely to have suffered tubular reabsorption, adopted the creatinine clearance as a suitable measure of filtration rate and initiated the concept of definitive and precise analysis of the components of renal function by the use of clearances.

HEIDENHAIN appears to have been the first to employ the clearance concept. Dividing the excretion rate of urea by the plasma concentration, he calculated that a man would need 70 liters of glomerular filtrate in order to excrete urea by filtration alone. Of the 70 liters, nearly all would be reabsorbed to yield the usual urine volumes. These figures, which seemed preposterously large, constituted one of several objections by HEIDENHAIN to the filtration-reabsorption hypothesis. The term, 'clearance', was coined by MÖLLER, McINTOSH and VAN SLYKE.

Other evidence showed that CUSHNY's categorical rejection of tubular secretion was untenable. The excretion of phenol red was shown by MARSHALL (1926, 1931a, 1934) to be incompatible in several ways with any filtration-reabsorption hypothesis. *In vitro* cultures of isolated proximal tubules of chick and man form cysts which accumulate phenol red in their lumina in high concentration (CAMERON and CHAMBERS; CHAMBERS and KEMPTON).

Definitive proof of the correctness of CUSHNY's adaptation of the LUDWIG hypothesis, appropriately modified to allow for tubular secretion of certain substances, was provided by ALFRED N. RICHARDS and his associates. In a long series of papers beginning about 1929 and continuing to the present, they showed by direct puncture of BOWMAN's capsule and the lumina of proximal and distal tubule of frog and NECTURUS with a micropipette and quantitative analysis of withdrawn fluid that an essentially protein-free fluid is formed at the glomerulus containing sodium, chloride, phosphate, urea, uric acid, creatinine, phenol red, glucose, inulin, hydrogen ion and total solute (vapor pressure) in essentially the same concentration as in plasma water (RICHARDS 1934). Slight differences in electrolyte concentration between capsular fluid and plasma water were consistent with a GIBBS-DONNAN distribution. The rate of formation of capsular fluid or glomerular filtrate was of the proper order of magnitude to account for the urinary excretion rate of substances such as phosphate, urea (except frog), and creatinine. Glucose, abundant in the glomerular filtrate, rapidly disappeared from the tubular fluid as it passed down the proximal tubule, whereas creatinine, urea, or glucose following administration of the glucoside phlorhizin, became more concentrated. Reabsorption of sodium chloride, potassium, bicarbonate and water and secretion of acid and ammonia by the nephron were demonstrated. The same methods were applied to mammals, with similar results (WALKER et al. 1941). Of critical importance to future research was the demonstration of equality of concentration of the polyfructoside, inulin, across the glomerular membranes. When this observation was combined with demonstration by RICHARDS, WEST-FALL and BOTT, and by SHANNON and SMITH, and SHANNON (1935a and b) that inulin met the necessary criteria that the clearance of a substance excreted by filtration rate alone must be independent of plasma concentration and urine flow, inulin clearance became the preferred measure of filtration rate. These criteria are not sufficient to prove that some secretion or, in particular, some reabsorption does not occur. In 1938 RICHARDS, BOTT and WESTFALL and SHANNON (1934) reported that they could find no evidence of tubular secretion of inulin by the tubule of the frog, dog or aglomerular fish. With respect to the possibility that inulin might be reabsorbed, SMITH and his associates showed that the clearances of ferrocyanide, of glucose, xylose and sucrose after adminis-tration of phlorhizin, and creatinine and phenol red at high plasma concentration converge upon the same value as the inulin clearance, a circumstance requiring that, if reabsorption of inulin is occurring, then all these substances must be reabsorbed to the same degree. These and other studies were assembled by SMITH (1937) and established inulin clearance as the definitive measurement of glomerular filtration rate in all vertebrates. Creatinine clearance was shown to be an accurate measure of filtration rate in many vertebrates including many mammals, but not in primates including man. At the same time, SMITH established in their present form the concepts of a set of renal functions accessible to precise measurement by clearance techniques. During the next 15 years, renal research was largely occupied by intensive application of these techniques to measurement of renal function in normal, experimental and pathological states of man and animals, and to examination of mechanisms of renal excretion or conservation

1*

of a wide variety of substances. The flowering of this age of inulin, which began about 1937, was disrupted in Europe in its beginning by war and its aftermath, and a decade of what should have been brilliant research was lost. With notable contributions from Sweden and Denmark and a few from England virtually the entire body of definitive studies on renal function in man is written in the North American literature. Only since about 1950 has Europe shown strong signs of reclaiming its ancient heritage of a science second to none.

As this is written, research on the physiology of the kidney is pursuing many promising paths. Among these are the biochemistry at the cellular level of active tubular transport processes; dynamics and distribution of blood flow within the kidney; the significance of the architecture of the renal medulla to excretory function; and, a continuing problem, the role of the kidney in determining the level of arterial blood pressure.

B. Anatomy of the kidney as related to function

Each young adult human kidney contains about 1,000,000 excretory units, or *nephrons*. Each nephron comprises a filtering unit, the *glomerulus*, consisting of a tuft of capillaries by which filtrate virtually free of protein is separated from the blood plasma, and a tubule into which the filtrate passes. The tubule is, in turn, divided into several anatomically and histologically distinct segments, each capable of specific and usually characteristic secretory and reabsorptive operations upon the filtrate, with urine as the final product of all operations.

I. Arteries

The renal artery, on entering the hilum, divides into several branches which pass either anterior or posterior to the pelvis and supply the corresponding portions of the kidney. These vessels then pass peripherally in the renal columns, either directly or after one or two additional branchings, as the *interlobar* arteries. As the interlobar arteries approach the cortico-medullary junction they begin to bend, with much branching, into a course parallel to the capsule and coming to lie in the corticomedullary junction where they are termed *arcuate* or arciform arteries. From the smaller divisions of the arcuate arteries numerous small arteries branch at right angles to pass through the cortex toward the capsule as the *interlobular* arteries, where each supplies from 50 to 150 glomeruli and constitutes the fundamental vascular unit of the kidney (Fig. 1).

II. Vas afferens

A single short, broad *afferent* arteriole (averaging about 167 micra long and 30 micra inner diameter) brings blood from an interlobular artery to the glomerulus (Fig. 2). An afferent arteriole usually supplies one glomerulus but frequently it may supply two or more glomeruli (BOWMAN; BEER; MORE and DUFF).

The original conclusion of BOWMAN, that all blood supplying the renal tubules first passes through the glomeruli, is firmly established. Exceptions to this rule in the normal kidney are distinguished by their scarcity. These are a) small terminal twigs (LUDWIG's arteriole) of the interlobular arteries which contribute some blood to the subcapsular peritubular capillary plexus; and b) vessels in the juxtamedullary region which have the caliber of afferent arterioles but which branch into vasa recta (arteriae rectae verae) without the interposition of a glomerulus (Fig. 3) (VIRCHOW; V. MÖLLENDORFF; MORISON; MORE and DUFF; MACCALLUM; TRUETA et al.; BIALESTOCK).

Considerable controversy exists concerning the origin of these vessels, which sometimes may be numerous. Because they may be more numerous in pathological states (VIRCHOW, TRUETA et al.) and vessels bearing glomerular vestiges can be found in any specimen (MAC-CALLUM, TRUETA et al.), they are generally thought to represent a degenerative process in which all of a juxtamedullary glomerular tuft has disappeared except a single capillary (HUBER 1906). Alternatively, the arteriae rectae verae could represent failures of glomerular development; and their increased frequency in pathological states could be relative to oblitera-

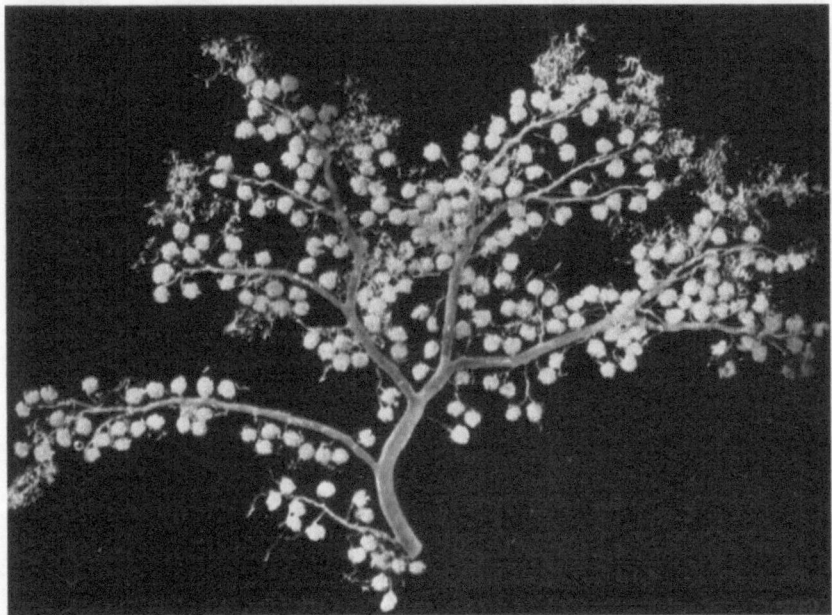

Fig. 1. Neoprene cast of the terminal portion of a human arcuate artery with interlobular arteries and glomeruli. Many of the interlobular arteries terminate in an aglomerular arteriole. After MORE and DUFF. Reproduced by permission of the authors and the American Journal of Pathology

tion of glomeruli and the vessels bearing them. This view is supported by the fact that arteriae rectae verae are easily found in the young of several mammalian species (MACCALLUM, TRUETA et al.) and the fact that all vasa recta arise from a primordial peritubular network which is supplied directly by the arteries. When the glomeruli develop, most of the vasa recta acquire preferential channels to juxtamedullary glomeruli but it seems reasonable to suppose that a few may retain their original direct communication to the arteries (LEWIS 1958 a and b).

Arterioles such as vasa vasorum, the nutrient arterioles to the capsule and pelvis, and the muscular arterioles to the venous "sinusoidal cushions" of KOESTER, LOCKE and SWANN which do not supply the tubules are well recognized.

III. Glomerulus

1. Glomerular capillary tuft

Immediately after entering BOWMAN's capsule, the afferent arteriole divides into 2 to 10 primary branches, each of which quickly subdivides into a variable number of secondary branches, the glomerular capillaries. After intertwining extensively the glomerular capillaries turn inward and back toward their point of origin. In the interior or toward one side of the tuft they recombine to form

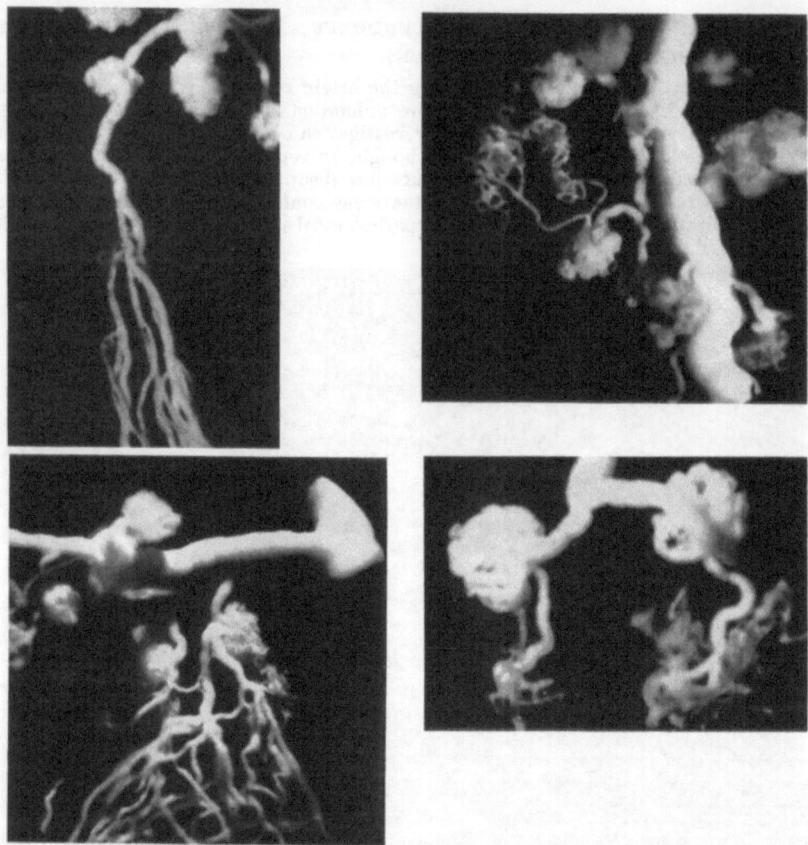

Fig. 2. Casts of human glomeruli with their afferent and efferent arterioles. After TRUETA et al. Reproduced by permission of the authors and Blackwell Scientific Publications, Oxford

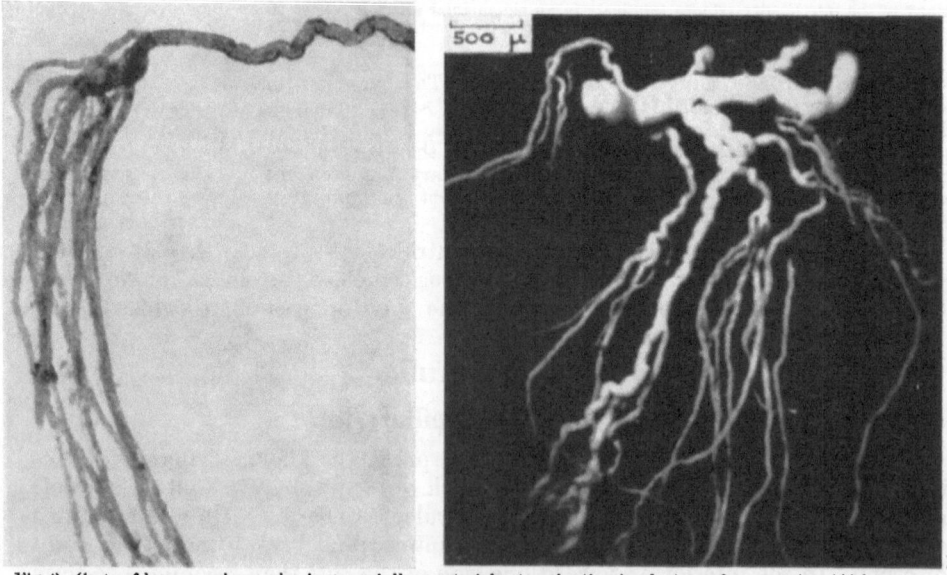

Fig. 3. Casts of human aglomerular juxtamedullary arterioles terminating in clusters of vasa recta. (A) is reproduced by permission of American Journal of Anatomy (MORISON). (B) is reproduced by permission of TRUETA et al. and Blackwell Scientific Publications, Oxford

the *efferent* arteriole which leaves BOWMAN'S capsule close to the afferent arteriole. This arrangement is illustrated schematically in Fig. 4. Although some authors doubt the existence of intercapillary anastomoses (WILMER, VIMTRUP 1928) the available evidence indicates that capillaries interconnect the various secondary

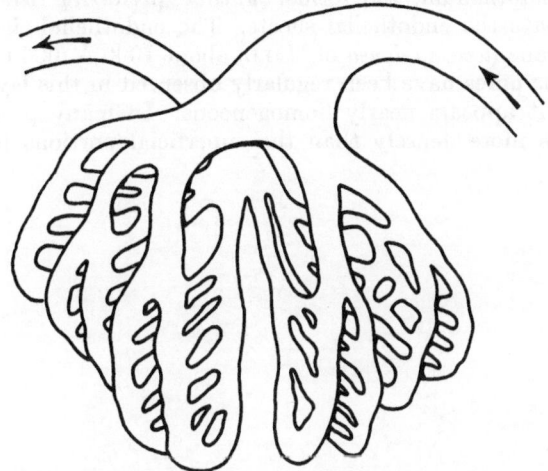

Fig. 4. The intraglomerular circulation (semidiagrammatic). Modified from ELIAS

branches of each primary division of the afferent arteriole in at least man and rat (JOHNSTON; HALL 1955, 1957; BOYER) and may even interconnect the lobules as well, although the evidence here is incomplete (LEWIS 1958b, BOYER). A group of secondary vessels with their anastomoses constitute a lobule of the glomerular tuft (BOWMAN, V. MÖLLENDORFF, JOHNSTON, HALL).

2. Glomerular membranes

The publications of ZIMMERMANN and V. MÖLLENDORFF may be consulted for some of the most complete examinations of glomerular architecture available using light microscopy. In recent years the conclusions of light microscopists have been generally confirmed and extended by use of the electron microscope in studies such as those of OBERLING, GAUTIER and BERNHARD; DALTON; RHODIN 1955; HALL; PEASE 1955a; PEASE and BAKER; RINEHART et al.; YAMADA; BARGMANN, KNOOP and SCHIEBLER; POLICARD, COLLET and GILTAIRE-RALYTE; and MUELLER, MASON and STOUT. The following description represents the available composite picture from both sources. The glomerulus, measured across BOWMAN'S capsule and including the tuft of capillaries and a fluid-filled space (BOWMAN'S space) between capsule and capillaries, averages 200 micra in diameter. Most of the space, perhaps 80 percent, is occupied by the tuft of approximately 50 glomerular capillaries and accessory elements. The membranes forming the wall of the glomerular capillaries and separating the blood from the lumen of BOWMAN'S capsule, consist of three layers: an inner layer of flat, contiguous *endothelial cells*, an acellular *basement membrane* and an outer layer of *epithelial cells*, the "visceral layer" of BOWMAN'S capsule (Fig. 5). Except near the nucleus, the endothelial cells are spread out in thin cytoplasmic sheets about 500—1000 Å (*lamina fenestrata*, or *attenuata*, of HALL) (One micron = 10,000 Angstrom units, Å). In most preparations the endothelial sheet appears to be densely perforated with pores 400 to 1500 Å in diameter. HALL notes, however, that the smallest values are observed in his least dehydrated preparations; REID, RINEHART, and MUELLER, MASON and STOUT suspect that the pores may not exist in life but are derived from cytoplasmic vacuoles or are fixation artefacts. Both HALL and RHODIN (1955) counsel caution in accepting the concept of a gross pore structure of the endothelium, the former author preferring the term *lamina attenuata* to designate the endothelial sheets. The endothelial sheets rest upon a basement membrane (*lamina densa* of HALL) about 1000 Å (600 to 2,500) thick. No fine structure or pores have been regularly observed in this layer with osmic acid staining and it appears nearly homogeneous. In many preparations, the middle third stains more densely than the superficial portions [cement layers

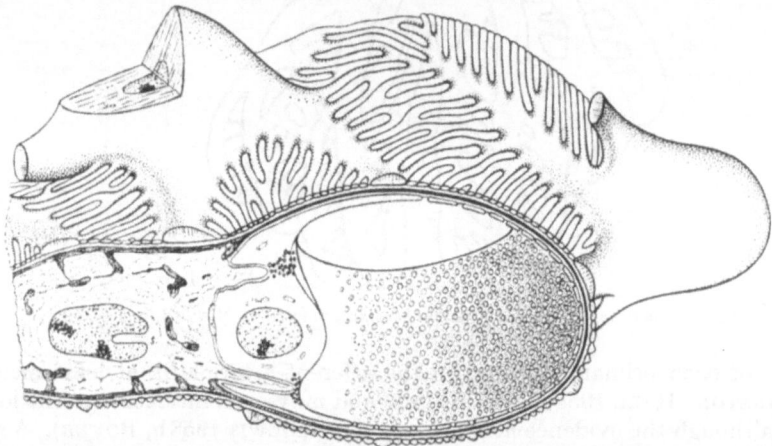

Fig. 5. Cross section of a glomerular capillary of the mouse, reconstructed from electron photomicrographs. The nucleus of an endothelial cell is bulging into the lumen of the capillary while the perforated sheet of cytoplasm of this cell lines the rest of the lumen. Above and outside are two podocytes with their interdigitating processes. The cell body of one podocyte has been cut away to reveal the nucleus. To the left of the endothelial cell is a cell which is considered by some to be endothelial in nature and by others to be a different cell type (mesangial cell). After YAMADA. Reproduced by permission of the author and the Journal of Biophysical and Biochemical Cytology

(PEASE 1955a, PAK POY)]. External to the basement membrane and separating it from BOWMAN's space is the curious array of epithelial cells (*Pericytes*, ZIMMERMANN and others; *Podocytes*, HALL). These are large cells and are about one half to one quarter as numerous as the endothelial cells. From the main body of each cell numerous cytoplasmic processes (*Trabeculae*, HALL) project to the basement membrane and then travel across its surface for as much as 30 micra. The cell body thus does not rest directly upon the basement membrane but is supported at a distance from it by the first portions of the trabeculae. From each trabecula numerous short, narrow processes (*secondary processes*, ZIMMERMANN; *pedicels*, HALL) project at right angles but continue to maintain intimate contact with the basement membrane. Both trabeculae and pedicels are closely interdigitated with other trabeculae and pedicels from the same or adjacent epithelial cells. In many preparations a gap of 200—400 Å appears to separate each pedicel from the other pedicels interdigitating with it (Fig. 5), with the result that gaps ("filtration slits", HALL) allow free communication between BOWMAN's space and the basement membrane (HALL; PEASE 1955; RHODIN 1958; BARGMANN, KNOOP and SCHIEBLER). In other preparations, definite slits between the pedicels have not been visualized (REID, RINEHART) or if present were apparently bridged by a fine membrane extending from one pedicel to its neighbor (YAMADA). The layer of the epithelial cells covering the glomerular capillaries are continuous with the layer of epithelial cells constituting the parietal layer of Bowman's capsule. The disposition of the basement membrane at the vascular pole of the glomerulus is not clear. By some it is thought to be coextensive with the lamina propria of the arterioles (HALL), while others believe it continues as the basement membrane of the parietal layer of Bowman's capsule (YAMADA). It would seem likely that both views are correct and that the basement membranes, proper respectively to the vascular endothelium and to the epithelial cells of Bowman's capsule, fuse where these two layers come together. Existence of a third cell type in the glomerular structure is undecided. YAMADA, POLICARD, COLLET and GILTAIRE-RALYTE and PAK POY believe that a system of cells histologically distinct from the endothelial cells immediately adjoins the latter but while lying more remote from the capillary lumen lies within the basement membrane and serves to bind together endothelial cell groups of adjacent capillaries. This system they feel may be equivalent to the mesangium of ZIMMERMANN or to the "connective tissue cells" of other light microscopists. Other authors have failed to recognize a third cell type but feel that a tendency for the endothelial cells of adjacent loops to lie in bands or bundles could well be mistaken for a specific supporting structure (HALL). v. MÖLLENDORFF, and PEASE (1955a), note a tendency for epithelial cells to lie in the bends of capillary loops. Collagen fibers appear to be absent from the normal glomerulus.

IV. Vas efferens and veins

The efferent arteriole subdivides into a second set of capillaries which invests the tubules and which in turn is gathered into the venous system. Considerable variation is possible in that a glomerulus may have two or more efferent vessels or may drain directly into the peritubular plexus without interposition of muscular arterioles (Fig. 2) (J. F. SMITH). The dimensions of the efferent arterioles, the character and distribution of their capillaries and their venous drainage depend upon whether they arise from cortical or juxtamedullary glomeruli and will be considered with respect to nephron populations.

Pease has described fenestrations in the endothelium of cortical peritubular capillaries and the venae rectae which are about half the diameter and are less numerous than those in the glomerular capillaries. To the extent that these fenestrations are real and signify an increased permeability they are consistent with the observation that exchange of substances between the vascular and extravascular space is rapid (FRIES et al. 1958).

The venous system parallels the arterial, comprising a system of interlobular, arcuate and interlobar veins. In man and in some but not all other mammals an additional network of veins (venae stellatae, or stellate veins) lies in the renal capsule. Venules from the capillary plexus of the outer cortex drain into these veins which join at numerous points (whence the term stellate) and from each junction drain into an interlobular vein.

V. Vascular smooth muscle

The renal artery and its divisions are abundantly supplied with circular smooth muscle fibers among which sympathetic motor nerve fibers end. Scattered among the smooth muscle fibers of the interlobular and afferent arteries are larger, paler, afibrillar "epithelioid" cells. Roughly 50 microns before the glomerulus is reached, the typical smooth muscle cells disappear almost entirely and are replaced by the epithelioid cells which continue to the glomerular surface where they form an expanded cluster (polkissen). The function of these cells is unknown, although diverse regulatory functions have been ascribed to them by various authors (SMITH 1951). The polkissen is best developed in mammals, poorly developed in birds and is absent from other vertebrate orders (EDWARDS 1940). Large, granular cells which occur in this area in the rat are considered by many to be associated with pressor responses and to be homologous with the granulation or vacuolation of epithelioid cells which appears during GOLD-BLATT hypertension in other species (GOORMAGHTIGH 1937; GOORMAGHTIGH and GRIMSON; DUNIHUE and ROBERTSON; HARTROFT; TOBIAN for review).

Smooth muscle is absent from the glomerulus but a few circular fibers occur around the efferent arteriole. In the medulla smooth muscle may be fairly abundant around the descending vasa recta (arteriolae rectae) (EDWARDS 1956). Smooth muscle is nearly if not entirely absent from the smaller veins, including

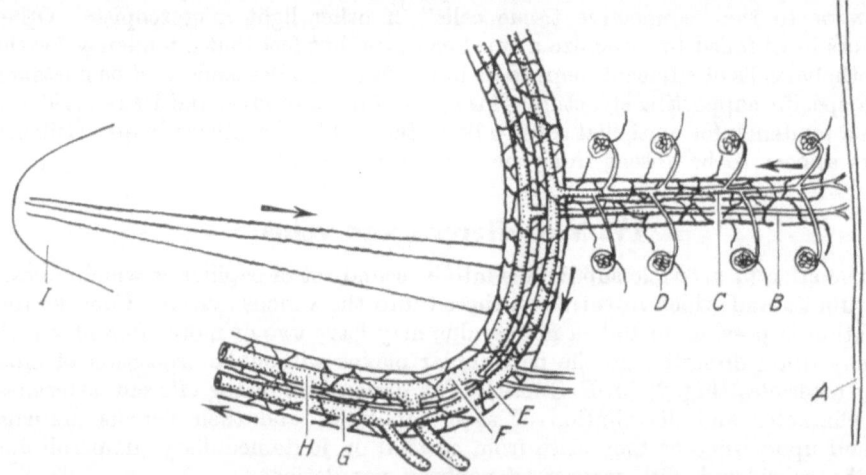

Fig. 6. Lymphatic channels of the human kidney (diagrammatic). Two separate systems are demonstrable. One begins in the cortex and accompanies the interlobular vessels toward the corticomedullary junction; the other starts at the papilla and ascends to join the cortical system at the corticomedullary junction. From there large trunks follow the arcuate and interlobar vessels to leave the kidney at the hilus. Arrows show the probable direction of the lymph flow. The structures shown are: (*A*) tunica fibrosa, (*B*) interlobular vein, (*C*) interlobular artery, (*D*) glomerulus, (*E*) arcuate artery, (*F*) arcuate vein, (*G*) interlobar artery, (*H*) interlobar vein and (*I*) papilla. After RAWSON. Reproduced by permission of the author and Archives of Pathology

the venae rectae and the interlobular veins. It is scarce around the arcuate veins. KOESTER, LOCKE and SWANN have described in dog and human kidney connective tissue diaphragms at the junctions of interlobular and arcuate veins which they have termed "stenoses". A narrow aperture in the diaphragm through which blood flows is surrounded by smooth muscle. These authors also describe small mounds of loose connective tissue, laced with smooth muscle and containing numerous blood sinuses, located usually at the confluence of two arcuate or subarcuate veins. The sinuses of these bodies which they term "sinusoidal cushions" are supplied by a muscular arteriole and considered to be functionally similar to nasal erectile tissue. They believe that the function of both the stenoses and the cushions is regulation of the pressure in the venules. Smooth muscle bundles also occur in the regions of confluence of the capsular stellate veins and where junction is made with an interlobular vein. Longitudinal smooth muscle bundles occur on the medullary aspect of the arcuate veins, a circumstance for which no satisfactory explanation has been forthcoming (v. MÖLLENDORFF). The interlobar and larger venous trunks have a typical musculature.

VI. Interstitial fluid space and lymphatics

An interstitial fluid space lies between the capillaries and the cellular elements of the kidney. Recent studies have cast some doubt on views based on conventional histological methods that this space is relatively small. Experiments designed to fix the tissues before fluid can be reabsorbed by the capillaries suggest that the interstitial fluid space as measured in the mouse may occupy as much as 20 percent of the volume of the cortex (SWANN, FEIST and LOWE), but the conclusions of these authors have not been generally accepted.

An abundant, anastomotic system of lymphatic vessels closely parallels the vascular system at least as far as the interlobular vessels. A second lymphatic plexus lies in the outer, subcapsular cortex. This plexus is large in the dog and it anastomoses freely with the hilar system (SUGARMAN et al.). In man, however, the subcapsular plexus and capsular outflow appear to be insignificant.

The lymphatic capillaries originate for the most part near the outer surface of the glomeruli but have never been observed to enter BOWMAN's space or the glomerular capillary tuft. With respect to the extent of lymphatic drainage from the medulla the evidence is not clear. PEIRCE failed to find evidence of lymphatic drainage from dog or rabbit medulla. In man, however, RAWSON discovered penetration by a lymphatically spreading carcinoma along channels, presumably those of lymphatic capillaries, as far as the mucosa of the papilla (Fig. 6).

VII. Tubular system

The epithelial tube into which BOWMAN's space empties comprises a set of anatomically and histologically distinct regions or segments. The principal subdivisions, beginning from BOWMAN's capsule, are:

proximal segment, subdivided into
    pars convoluta
    pars recta
thin segment
distal segment, subdivided into
    pars recta
    pars convoluta
collecting duct.

Additional histologically distinct subdivisions have been described and will be noted. SJØSTRAND may be consulted for extensive bibliography.

1. Bowman's capsule

Details of the transition at the vascular pole of the glomerulus from the epithelial cells, constituting the visceral layer of BOWMAN's capsule, to the parietal layer are not clear. The parietal capsular cells are thin, clear, with well-defined cell boundaries and with their nuclei bulging into BOWMAN's space. Their permeability characteristics are unknown. The parietal epithelium rests on a homogeneous membrane which is continuous in the one direction with the basement membrane of the proximal segment of the tubular system and in the other with the basement membrane of the glomerular capillaries (at least in part); the basement membrane separates the parietal epithelium from the general interstitial fluid space of the parenchyma.

2. Proximal tubule

The parietal epithelial cells gather, at a point generally opposite the vascular pole of the glomerulus, into a neck or beginning tubule. Almost immediately, however, the tubular epithelium changes from flattened to high cuboidal. The tubule may take its origin in any direction from a glomerulus but irrespective

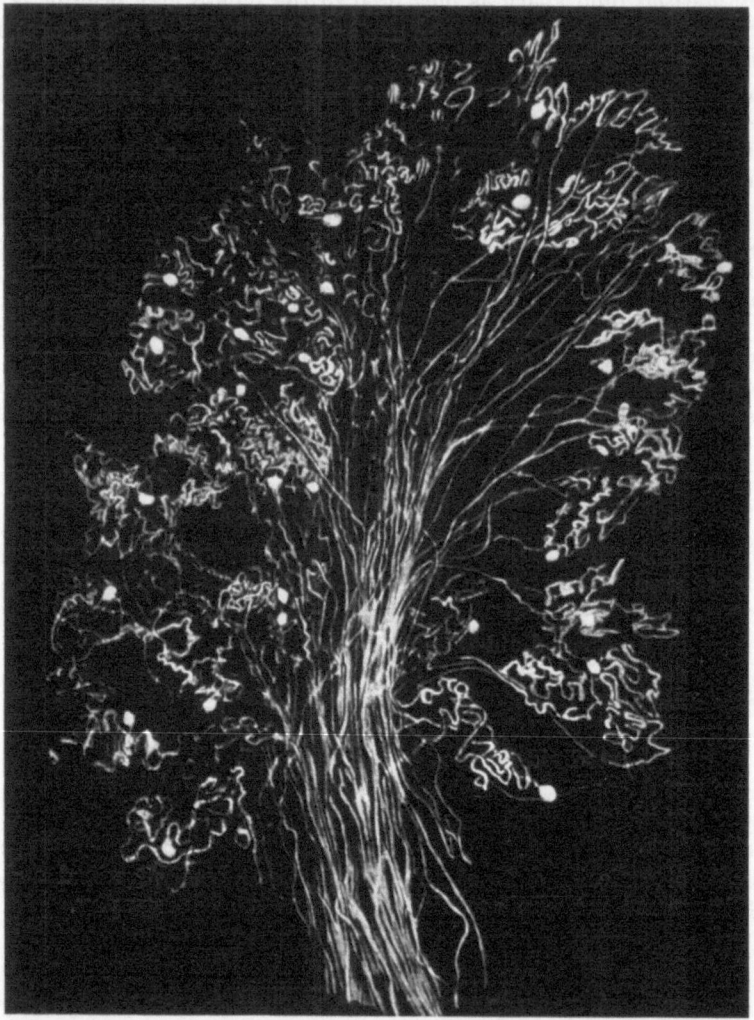

Fig. 7. Nephrons of a lobule of a normal human kidney, teased slightly apart, after Oliver. This figure should be compared with Fig. 1. It represents the nephrons supplied by a single interlobular artery. Reproduced by permission of the author and P. B. Hoeber, Inc., New York

of direction of origin it turns, winding in an irregular spiral for a variable distance toward the capsule (Figs. 7 and 8) (Grafflin 1939). It then reverses, winding back to the general vicinity of its glomerulus whence it continues but now straight *(pars recta)* toward or into the medulla. Groups of such straight portions from adjacent nephrons constitute the *medullary rays*.

The cells of the proximal tubule, as revealed by electron microscopy, are extremely complex and the reader should consult the original literature for details (RUSKA, MOORE and WEINSTOCK; SJÖSTRAND and RHODIN; PEASE 1955c; RHODIN 1958). Some of the details are represented in Fig. 9. Covering the outer aspect of the cells is a smooth, homogeneous basement membrane 0.05 to 0.10 micra thick which is continuous with that of the glomerular capsule and, continuing distally, with that of the entire tubular system. Beneath the basement

membrane the cell surface is not smooth but is interrupted by numerous, deep invaginations forming sinuous slits which wind through the basal half of the cell but always communicate with the extracellular space beneath the basement membrane. Some or most of the invaginations may represent interdigitations of adjacent cells (RHODIN 1958). An enormous cell surface is thus created. At times, the slits appear dilated as though by fluid accumulation (RUSKA, MOORE and WEINSTOCK). Elongate mitochondria are abundant in the invaginated cytoplasm and are constructed of a double-walled membrane enveloping an interior which contains numerous double-walled plates or septa. Details of nucleus, granules, vacuoles and Golgi apparatus as viewed by the electron microscope have been described. The apical (luminal) surface contains numerous straight microvilli 1.0 to 1.5 micra in length and about 750 Å in diameter which project into the lumen of the tubule. Their structure indicates that they are rod-like extensions of cytoplasm covered by a membrane indistinguishable from that covering the rest of the cell. At the base of

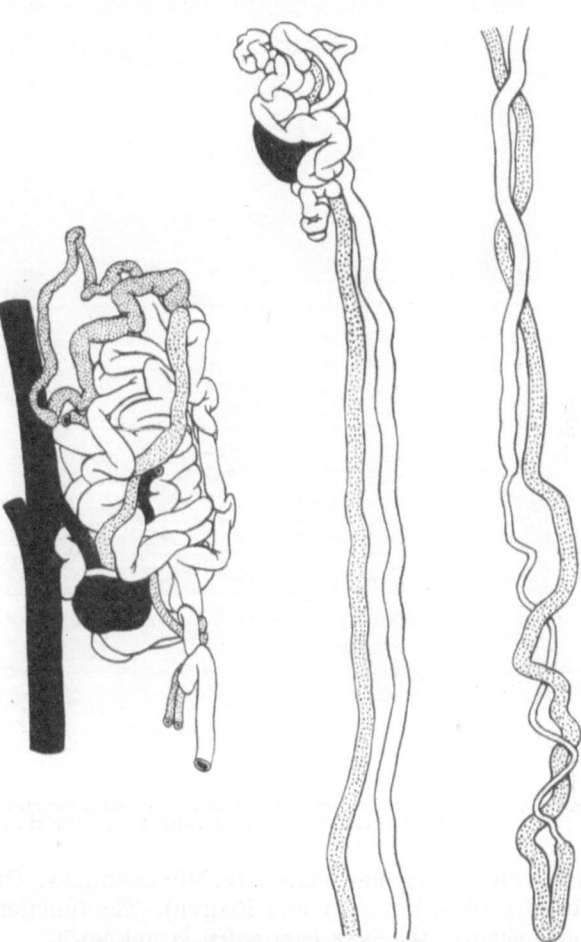

Fig. 8. Scale reconstructions of human nephrons. Left: A cortical nephron with glomerular vessels and proximal and distal convoluted tubules but without the loop of HENLE. Redrawn from PETER. The connecting tubule from another nephron may be seen entering the mass of convoluted tubules near the interlobular artery. It joins behind the nephron with the other connecting tubule to form the collecting duct which appears beside the pars recta of the distal segment. Right: A midcortical nephron without collecting duct or glomerular vessels, after TURLEY. Redrawn from description by GRAFFLIN (1939). The distal convolution in this view is not shown clearly. Reproduced by permission of the author and Archives of Pathology. In these drawings, the interlobular artery and glomerulus and its vessels are black; the proximal tubule, both convoluted and straight portions, are light gray; the thin segment is white; the distal and connecting tubules and collecting duct are light, moderately and heavily stippled, respectively

the microvilli the cell wall is invaginated into numerous pockets or slits. In the nearly collapsed tubule represented in the usual histological section, the microvilli are packed together and constitute the brush border. It is reasonable to suppose that in life, with the tubule distended by fluid, the microvilli are widely separated. As with the basal invaginations, the microvilli greatly increase the cell surface area[1].

Toward the end of the pars recta, the cells become clearer and lower, the brush border less dense, and the type and character of granules, droplets and

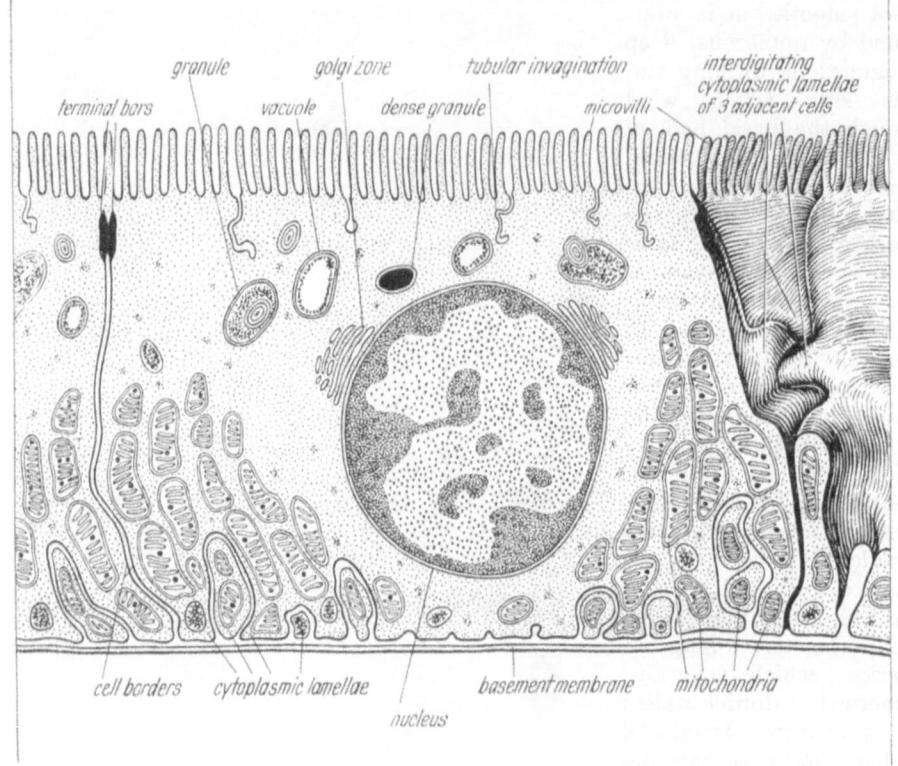

Fig. 9. Cross section of a cell from a mammalian proximal convoluted tubule as reconstructed from electron photomicrographs. Prepared under the direction of Dr. Johannes Rhodin

intracellular enzymes change (v. Möllendorff, Grafflin 1942, Oliver 1944, Rhodin 1958, Longley and Fisher). The functional significance of this structural change, the *pars terminalis*, is unknown.

3. Thin segment

At some point in its descent to or toward the medulla, the epithelium changes rather abruptly to a flattened type composed of a clear cytoplasm with few mitochondria. The brush border has disappeared and only a few short microvilli project into the tubular lumen (Fig. 10) (Zimmermann, Rhodin 1958). This portion of the nephron, the *thin segment*, is highly variable in length. In all nephrons of the human kidney except those arising close to the medulla, the thin segment is fairly short. It continues a short distance toward or into the medulla, then the epithelium shifts rapidly to a low cuboidal type which, as the *pars recta* of the *distal tubule*, soon doubles sharply back toward the cortex. In juxta-

_____

[1] Very similar cells have been described from the excrttory organ of the crustacean, Cambarus (Anderson and Beams).

medullary nephrons, the thin segment is much longer although variably so. In these nephrons the thin segment itself at some point deep in the medulla doubles back toward the cortex before the epithelium changes to that of the distal tubule. The sequence of segments passing toward the medulla then returning to the cortex and composed of pars recta of the proximal tubule, the thin segment and the pars recta of the distal tubule constitutes collectively the loop of HENLE. An important role in the formation of hypertonic urine is attributed to one or more portions of the loop of HENLE.

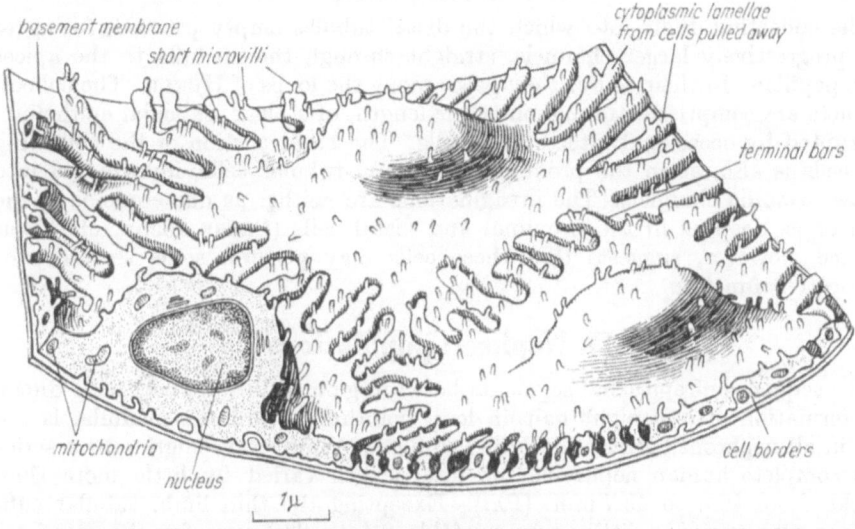

Fig. 10. Epithelium of the thin segment of the mouse nephron viewed from the luminal aspect, reconstructed from electron photomicrographs. After RHODIN (1958). Reproduced by permission of the author and the American Journal of Medicine

4. Distal tubule

The pars recta of the distal tubule passes nearly straight toward the cortex until it reaches the vascular pole of its glomerulus where it becomes closely appressed against the afferent arteriole. Here the cells are taller and also narrower so that more nuclei are seen in a given area of a section. This area has been termed the *macula densa* by ZIMMERMANN. Its function is unknown. It is absent from the fish nephron, present but poorly developed in the frog, best developed in bird and mammal (EDWARDS 1940). The extraordinary constancy of this association together with the functional capabilities of the apposed parts suggest that the macula densa may assist in maintaining glomerulotubular balance (OLIVER 1944), particularly with respect to electrolyte excretion.

From the vicinity of the afferent arteriole, the distal tubule twists as the *pars convoluta*, generally following a somewhat lateral course until, joining with one or more other distal tubules, it enters the first portion of the collecting duct system. The extensive infolding of the basilar surface of the proximal tubular cells is present and even more extensive in the distal tubule (PEASE 1955a and c, RHODIN 1958). Microvilli are absent. Several histologically distinguishable subdivisions are attributed to the distal convoluted tubule but no single system of nomenclature has been widely accepted and the subdivisions vary greatly in character and extent from one mammalian group or species to another (v. MÖLLEN-DORFF). The most frequently noted of these subdivisions are, proceeding distally from the region of or just prior to the macula densa, a short section with clearer cytoplasm and cuboidal cells similar to the pars recta, a section with taller, granular cells, a section with clear cuboidal cells similar to those of the collecting ducts but containing numerous large, granular, specifically staining cells (intercalated cells) and finally the epithelium of the collecting ducts. Small diverticula are frequently observed in the last two thirds of the pars convoluta. The functions of these various regions are unknown.

5. Collecting ducts

The collecting ducts into which the distal tubules empty proceed, fusing to form progressively larger channels, straight through the medulla to the apices of the papillae. In their course they pass among the loops of HENLE. The collecting ducts are comprised, throughout their length, of a clear, cuboidal epithelium interrupted by occasional intercalated cells. The basal portion of the collecting duct cells is also, as in the proximal and distal tubular cells, invaginated into narrow, winding channels. The invaginations are neither as numerous as in the distal or as deep as in the proximal and distal cells (PEASE 1955a, c). Their presence, however, suggests that these cells may perform some secretory or reabsorptive function.

VIII. Nephron populations

The sequence of epithelial segments between glomerulus and collecting ducts, with formation of a straight hairpin loop pointing toward the medulla, is the same in all nephrons. Also remarkably similar is the overall length. In a series of 10 complete human nephrons, the total length varied by little more than twofold, from 19.8 to 43.7 mm. (PAI). Excepting the thin limb, tubular subdivisions also varied a little over twofold: 8.4 to 23.1 mm. for the proximal tubule; 6.1 to 15 for the pars recta of the distal tubule; 2.3 to 4.2 for the pars convoluta of the distal tubule. Badly needed, however, are studies on a statistically representative sample of human nephrons. The size limits may well be substantially beyond these cited; and no measure of the distribution of dimensions among the nephron population is available.

Tubular outer diameters vary from about 30 to 80 micra, but the available studies have little functional significance since they are made on tubules in various degrees of collapse following drainage of their contents. It seems probable, for example, that the proximal convoluted tubule is normally dilated and its epithelium low cuboidal or flattened. No reliable estimates of tubular resistance to flow or of reabsorptive surface area can be made.

Qualitative studies show, however, that the nephrons can be divided into two main groups, the *cortical* and the *juxtamedullary* nephron groups (Fig. 11) according to location, character of the thin segment and character of the post-glomerular blood flow.

1. Cortical nephrons

In the human, all nephrons arising in the outer two thirds of the cortex are of this type and represent 80 to 90 percent of all nephrons (PETER). The thin segment is very short or is absent altogether (PETER, PAI, GRAFFLIN 1939, TRUETA et al.). With little contribution from the thin segment, the shortened loop of HENLE is composed principally of the pars recta of the distal tubule which also forms the bend of the loop. The efferent arterioles of the cortical nephrons are one to two glomerular diameters long. They terminate in a dense capillary plexus which interanastomose freely with the plexus from adjacent nephrons before being gathered into the interlobular veins. According to LUDWIG, a few capillaries, slightly larger than the rest, turn toward the medullary rays to follow the loops of HENLE in a manner similar to that observed in the medulla. Toward the corticomedullary junction the number and caliber of these "vasa recta" increases and the number of twigs joining the plexus among the convoluted tubules progressively diminishes. Further details of the postglomerular capillary plexus are unknown. The plexus supplies blood to all portions of the cortex including much of the loops of the cortical nephrons and the proximal and distal convoluted portions of the juxtamedullary nephrons.

2. Juxtamedullary nephrons

The corticomedullary junction is marked by the abrupt disappearance of convoluted tubules and glomeruli, which are wholly restricted to the cortex together with their anastomotic capillary system. The junction also contains the numerous arcuate arteries, veins and lymphatics. On the medullary side of the junction, the tissue mass is composed wholly of parallel tubes: blood vessels, loops of HENLE, collecting ducts and lymphatics. Although loops from glomeruli of the cortical group usually penetrate into the outer zone of the medulla, the medullary loops for practical purposes arise exclusively from the juxtamedullary nephrons. These nephrons in man arise from the inner third of the cortex, or perhaps from an even narrower zone, and they comprise an estimated 10 to 20 percent of all nephrons[1].

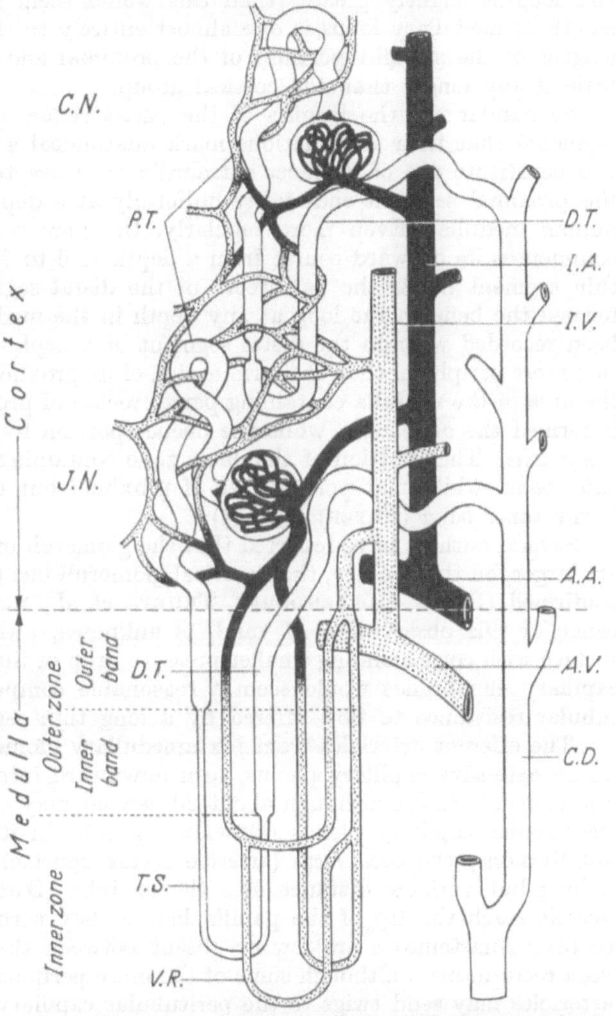

Fig. 11. Diagram of a cortical and a juxtamedullary nephron. Apart from location, significant differences between the two nephrons lie principally in the loop of HENLE and in the postglomerular blood flow. Association between the loop of HENLE of cortical nephrons and the proximal convolutions of juxtamedullary convolutions is not as close as illustrated in the figure although the postglomerular capillary plexus are intercommunicating. *C.N.* and *J.N.* cortical and juxtamedullary nephrons; *P.T.* and *D.T.* proximal and distal tubules; *T.S.* thin segment; *I.A.* and *I.V.* interlobular artery and vein; *A.A.* and *A.V.* arcuate artery and vein; *V.R.* vasa recta; *C.D.* collecting duct

---

[1] Information is not sufficient to determine the significance of any particular numerical partition between cortical and juxtamedullary nephrons. According to SPERBER (1944), herbivores tend to have predominantly cortical nephrons while carnivores and rodents have predominantly medullary nephrons.

The thin segments are long but, since they are variably so, the loop of HENLE may descend to any depth of the medulla. The longest human thin segment measured by PAI was 5.6 mm. but lengths up to 10 mm. are recorded by PETER and lengths slightly greater than this would seem reasonable. Variability in length of medullary loops is due almost entirely to thin segment variation, the lengths of the straight portions of the proximal and distal segments averaging little if any longer than the cortical group.

So regular are the lengths of the *partes rectae* of the proximal and distal segments that their terminations mark anatomical subdivisions of the medulla and constitute one of its most extraordinary characteristics. The pars recta of the proximal segment ends fairly uniformly at a depth of about 2 mm. in the human medulla. Even more regularly, the pars recta of the distal segment commences its outward course from a depth of 6 to 7 mm. in the medulla. The thin segment meets the pars recta of the distal segment in its ascent having formed the bend in the loop at any depth in the medulla. No instance has yet been recorded wherein the distal segment of a nephron originated from a position more peripheral than the termination of its proximal segment. Anatomically, the area of the medulla containing partes rectae of proximal and distal segments is termed the *outer zone*, while the deeper portion free of these segments is the *inner zone*. That portion of the outer zone containing proximal segments is the *outer band*, while that portion free of proximal but containing distal segments is the *inner band* (PETER) (Fig. 11).

Several authors have reported that the glomeruli of juxtamedullary nephrons are larger, on the average, than cortical glomeruli but this has not been generally confirmed (PAI, v. MÖLLENDORFF, TRUETA et al., DE CARVALHO). The significance of this observation, if valid, is unknown, although a greater filtration surface with corresponding smaller pressure drop of filtrate across the glomerular capillary membranes would seem a reasonable compensation for the increased tubular resistance to flow offered by a long thin segment.

The efferent arterioles from juxtamedullary glomeruli, instead of giving rise to an extensive capillary plexus, turn downward into the medulla parallel with the loops of HENLE although about 20 percent may supply blood to the cortical peritubular capillary plexus (EDWARDS 1956). In its passage it forms several subdivisions, the *vasa recta* (arteriae rectae spuriae), each of which may pass a long but variable distance into the medulla (HUBER 1906). Some of these vessels reach the tip of the papilla before they turn sharply back toward the cortex. Anastomoses are few or absent between the efferent arterioles or the vasa recta in man, although some of the more peripheral juxtamedullary efferent arterioles may send twigs to the peritubular capillary plexus (MORE and DUFF; TRUETA et al.). As the vasa recta return toward the cortex they fuse with the ascending limbs of vessels which have turned back in more superficial areas of the medulla, the common channels thus formed draining finally into the arcuate or lower portions of the interlobular veins. The outflow path of the juxtamedullary arterioles therefore comprises a smaller number of very long channels which may be 10 to 20 times the length of capillaries in the cortex. The excessively high resistance to blood flow which would otherwise be created by these circumstances is offset by a large diameter. The diameters of both the efferent arteriole and the vasa recta are equal to or greater than that of the afferent arteriole (Fig. 2) (EDWARDS 1956).

In the outer zone of the medulla the vasa recta, both the descending and ascending channels, tend to lie grouped together in bundles (vascular tufts). The loops of HENLE surround the vascular bundles while the collecting ducts are outside of these. In the inner zone, however, vasa recta, thin segments and collecting ducts are more uniformly intermingled (v. MÖLLENDORFF).

3. Glomerulotubular balance

No technique is currently available to determine whether the anatomically distinguishable groups of cortical and juxtamedullary nephrons also differ functionally. The available evidence suggests, however, that apart from such functions as may be attributed to the thin segment, the two groups are functionally alike. Analysis of the nephron populations on the basis of proximal and distal tubular functions therefore is probably descriptive of a single population, with a similar functional distribution curve in both the cortical and the juxtamedullary group. As pointed out by SMITH et al. (1943), the actual distributions of rates of glomerular filtration or of maximal rates of tubular transport capacity among the nephron population are not measurable nor are they of particular significance. Much more significant, and also available for measurement under certain circumstances, is the ratio in a nephron of either its rate of filtration or its peritubular blood supply to its maximal transport capacity (reabsorptive or secretory) for any specific substance. The ratio of filtration rate to a reabsorptive capacity is the more generally useful measurement and is termed "glomerulotubular balance" or "glomerular activity". Dividing this figure in any group of nephrons by the corresponding ratio for the entire population (one or both kidneys) measures the extent to which glomerulotubular balance of that group differs from that of the entire population. In spite of variation in the lengths of various segments and in size of glomeruli, the rate of filtration and rate of blood flow to the convoluted tubules seem nicely adjusted to the transport capacity of each nephron. In the case of the ratio of glomerular filtration to tubular transport capacity for glucose and sulfate in the dog, the number of nephrons with a glomerular activity measurably different from the group mean is too small to measure, and the population appears homogeneous (SHANNON and FISHER; LOTSPEICH). In man, however, more variation in glomerular activity is evident although the population is still remarkably homogeneous. Glomerular activity with respect to glucose transport lies within ± 40 percent of the mean in 95 percent of the nephrons (SMITH et al. 1943). The nephron population has also been examined for variation by the time required for a filtered substance to appear in the renal pelvis or the bladder (BRADLEY, NICKEL and LEIFER; BRADLEY, LEIFER and NICKEL). It is assumed that material which appears late following injection has come from the longest nephrons, or more generally, from nephrons with the lowest ratio of filtration rate to nephron length. Unfortunately, further assumptions, which materially restrict the significance of the conclusions, are necessary to these studies. Among these are the assumption of uniform tube diameter, the assumption that axial flow (the tendency for the center of a stream to move more rapidly than the peripheral portions) is insignificant, and the assumption that water reabsorption is proportional either to filtration rate or to total tubular length. A critical analysis of experimental methods designed to measure heterogeneity of the nephron population has been published by BRADLEY and WHEELER.

4. Medulla as an accumulating unit

In recent years, physiologists have become aware that many hitherto perplexing observations concerning the chemical composition of the medulla are in fact intimately related to its structure. The medullary pyramids and particularly their papillary portions are composed, as noted above, of a dense bundle of U-shaped tubes, whose outflow channels lie close to the inflow channels. Only the collecting ducts and the lymph capillaries pass in one direction through the medullary substance. Suppose now that a change is produced in the fluids of the medulla such that a concentration difference exists between cortex and medulla, or between the blood and the medulla. Such a concentration difference would generally be the result of cell activity and could refer equally to lowering of concentration by consumption of a nutrient or to raising of a concentration by production of a metabolite or by transport of a substance from the tubular lumina into the medullary interstitial fluid. Once a concentration gradient has been established, it can be dissipated or abolished by diffusion or by convection. Diffusion is inconsequential since diffusion is blocked laterally by the calyceal walls and the diffusion path from medulla to cortex is relatively long. Alternatively, medullary fluid could equilibrate with a flowing stream of blood which would abolish the concentration gradient by convection. In unidirectional capillary networks this is extremely effective. In the U-shaped capillaries of

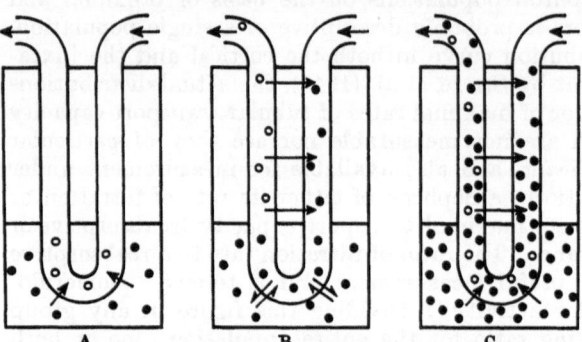

Fig. 12. Diagram illustrating mechanism by which countercurrent exchange promotes medullary accumulation (or depletion). A Initial state. Accumulating metabolite molecules (dots) diffuse from parenchyma into capillary lumen (circles) at tip of loop. B Intermediate state. Molecules in ascending limb of capillary (circles) diffuse into descending limb (dots) until concentration is subequal in the two limbs. Since capillary fluid entering the tip now contains metabolite molecules, further movement from parenchyma into tip of the loop is arrested (two-way arrows). C Final state. Metabolite molecules accumulate in the parenchyma until diffusion into the capillary lumen is again possible (circles). Accumulation continues until rate of acquisition of metabolite molecules equals rate of escape from the top of the ascending limb of the capillary loop

the medulla, however, the outflowing stream of blood transfers to the parallel inflowing stream much of the solute excess or deficit which it has acquired in the medulla. The result of this exchange, which is a well known principle in heat engineering, is that the inflowing stream reaches the depths of the medulla with a composition already similar to that of the latter so that further exchange between blood and interstitial fluid is small (Fig. 12). Isolation of medulla from extramedullary area cannot be complete since the inflowing and outflowing streams do not have the same composition. Ultimately a steady state is reached with respect to the intramedullary concentration of an accumulated or depleted substance when net inflow or outflow equals the rate of medullary utilization or production.

The steady state concentration is given by

$$Cm = Co + \frac{M}{V} + \frac{\alpha\,ML}{V^n}$$

where Cm is the equilibrium concentration in the medulla; Co is the concentration of the substance in the entering blood; M is the rate of accumulation (M is negative if the substance is depleted); V is the rate of blood flow; α is the efficiency of equilibration between the inflow and outflow channels; and L is the length of the capillary loops. n has a theoretical value of 2. If, however, M depends in part on Cm, then the equation can be approximately corrected by setting n equal to some value between 1 and 2 (Berliner et al. 1958). If M also has a significant degree of osmotic activity, then water as well as M will equilibrate between the limbs of the loop and the equation becomes more complex.

The high intramedullary concentrations of urea, sodium, chloride and total solute concentration (ULLRICH and JARAUSCH; BERLINER et al. 1958; LJUNG-BERG 1947; WIRZ 1953; APPELBOOM and BRODSKY), the slow rate of penetration of radiokrypton into the medulla as well as the low oxygen tension (RENNIE, REEVES and PAPPENHEIMER) and high osmotic concentration of the urine (BERLINER et al. 1958) appear to depend to a considerable extent upon the conserving capacity of countercurrent exchange in the vasa recta.

IX. Renal nerves

The mammalian kidney receives an abundant motor nerve supply derived almost if not entirely from the sympathetic division of the autonomic nervous system. In man, the nerve plexus around the renal arteries communicates freely with preaortic ganglia, the splanchnic nerves, and directly with the paravertebral sympathetic chain. Ganglion cells occur abundantly around the renal arteries and well into the hilum of the kidney but are absent in the parenchyma. The nerve fibers terminate almost entirely in the walls of the blood vessels: arteries, afferent and efferent arterioles and veins. Fibers have been described in the epithelium of the proximal tubules and the glomerular tuft but the existence of these remains in doubt. Fibers have also been described as ending on BOWMAN's capsule and the juxtaglomerular apparatus. In some of these latter circumstances the fibers may be sensory (HARMAN and DAVIES). A few vagal fibers may enter the renal nerves but it is not clear whether these are motor or sensory and no effect on renal function either of stimulating or sectioning the vagi has been clearly demonstrated (KUNTZ). Nerves are absent from the medulla (DE MUYLDER).

In acute experiments on anesthetized animals, section of the renal or splanchnic nerves quite regularly is followed by an increase in urine flow and sodium excretion. The hemodynamic functions of filtration rate and renal blood flow also increase indicating that active vasoconstrictor fibers have been interrupted by section. Although some investigators feel that the increase in sodium excretion is greater than can be explained as a simple consequence of the hemodynamic changes, data adequate to establish a specific effect of the nerves on tubular functions have not been published (WESSON 1957). In the trained, unanesthetized dog, functions of a unilaterally, chronically denervated kidney are indistinguishable from the normal contralateral organ (WESSON 1957, BRICKER et al. 1958) and blocking or cutting the nerves of an explanted kidney causes no detectable changes in renal blood flow or urea clearance (RHOADS et al.). The totally denervated kidney in both dog and man is capable of adjusting sodium excretion to intake in a near if not entirely normal fashion (DEMPSTER and JOEKES; BRICKER et al. 1956). The principal function of the renal nerves appears to be production of an acute, transitory reduction of renal blood flow by vasoconstriction as part of a general set of body vasomotor responses to stress (KUNTZ; MITCHELL; GRUBER; HAMBURGER; SMITH 1939; PAGE and McCUBBIN; DE MUYLDER).

C. Renal hemodynamics

In this and the following sections it will be assumed that the various methods for the measurement of renal blood flow and glomerular filtration rate are valid and that the interpretation of the methods is unquestioned. The methods themselves will be examined more closely in a later section. In general, therefore, the particular method employed to obtain a given datum will be noted only if it is relatively unique. The interested reader should refer to the original literature for further details pertinent to a particular study.

I. Renal blood flow

The blood flow through the two normal human kidneys is about a liter per minute or 20 to 25 percent of the resting cardiac output. The perfusion per unit weight, 3 to 4 ml./min./gram, is therefore as great or greater than that of any other organ of the body. This figure may be compared with about 0.1 ml. for the entire body, 0.7 for the brain, 1.0 for liver and 1.5 ml./min./gm. for the thyroid gland (MYANT, POCHIN and GOLDIE). Only the posterior pituitary gland has a comparable rate of perfusion (GOLDMAN and SAPIRSTEIN). The relatively high renal blood flow per gram indicates that the resistance to flow is correspondingly low. In most tissues, the resistance lies preponderantly in the arterioles. The resistance offered by capillaries, venules and smaller arteries is relatively small and, unless they are extreme, variations in the resistance of these vessels does not play a significant role in total resistance. In the normal kidney not only is the total resistance low but the fraction of the total contributed by the arterioles is relatively smaller. Consequently, the resistances of other elements of the renal vascular tree are relatively larger than in other tissues and variations in them can represent significant changes in the total resistance and hence in the blood flow through the organ. The fact that significant changes in the total resistance can occur at many points unquestionably contributes to the complexity of the renal vascular responses and may well be the source of some of the anomalous properties of the renal circulation. Probably correlated with a low renal resistance is a large intrarenal blood volume.

One of the most extraordinary properties of the renal circulation is that the blood flow under most conditions is almost completely independent of the arterial pressure within the physiological range: the higher is the arterial pressure, the higher is the resistance, the latter cancelling nearly all of the tendency of the increased pressure to enhance flow. Although blood flow in the isolated kidney is quite constant, renal blood flow in the intact organism exhibits large changes under a great variety of physiological and pathological conditions. Both the afferent and efferent arterioles are densely innervated and respond to incoming nerve impulses by constriction with consequent reduction in flow. This presents the paradox that a capacity for great flexibility is superimposed upon an intrinsic stability. Decreases in flow are observed acutely during emotional, traumatic, anesthetic and other stress states and are probably caused by nerve impulses via the renal nerves. Circulating epinephrine and various other sympathomimetic drugs also cause decreases and in the intact organism endogenous epinephrine probably augments the action of the renal nerves. Flow decreases during exercise probably as the result of nervous activity or epinephrine release, although the exercise changes differ slightly from those of epinephrine administration. Fluid loading, pyrogens and anoxia result in acute increases in flow. Decreases in flow are observed chronically in hypertension, congestive heart failure, decompensated hepatic cirrhosis, adrenal and anterior pituitary inadequacy, toxemia of pregnancy and severe disease states generally. Sustained increases in flow are observed in adrenocortical, anterior pituitary and thyroid hyperfunction, in normal pregnancy, and on a high protein diet. The mechanisms involved in most of these persistent changes are not clear.

1. Intrarenal pressures

Knowledge of pressures in the renal vascular system and in the tubules is essential for calculation of the resistance offered by various portions of the blood flow path and for discussion of aspects of filtration and tubular reabsorption. Information of varying reliability is available, however, for pressures only in the following areas: glomeruli, interstitial fluid, interlobular vein, and proximal and distal convoluted tubules.

a) Glomerular capillary pressure

Pressures in the afferent arterioles and glomerular capillaries have been measured directly only in the frog (HAYMAN). When aortic pressure varied from 16 to 47 mm. Hg, afferent arterial and glomerular capillary pressures varied from 11.5 to 43 and from 3 to 40 mm. Hg, respectively. Glomerular capillary pressure averaged about 54 percent of the aortic pressure.

Various indirect approaches to the measurement of the pressures in the glomerular capillaries of mammals have been reviewed by WINTON (1937, 1951) and by SMITH (1951). The minimum arterial pressure consistent with continued urine formation is generally about 75 mm. Hg in the absence of diuretics. In the presence of diuretic measures such as osmotic loading, cyanide administration, or cooling, the arterial pressure may decrease to values as low as 30 to 40 mm. Hg before urine formation ceases. The difference between these two figures, as suggested by WINTON (1937), is probably attributable to differences in tubular reabsorption in the two circumstances. In the normal kidney the greater fraction of each solute present in quantitatively significant amounts in the filtrate is reabsorbed by the tubules. Even urea, quantitatively one of the most important urinary constituents, is reabsorbed to the extent of 60 or 70 percent in the absence of diuresis. Hence a 30 to 50 percent decrease in volume of filtrate can suffice to permit virtually complete absorption of all major urinary constituents, and urine formation must cease. During osmotic loading with urea or sodium sulfate, however, even a small volume of glomerular filtrate may contain more solutes than can be reabsorbed. In the latter circumstance urine formation will cease, for practical purposes, only when glomerular filtration ceases. WINTON (1937) appears correct therefore in concluding that the minimum arterial pressure consistent with urine formation cannot measure the normal glomerular capillary pressure.

Somewhat similar objections can be registered in many studies against use of the maximum ureteral pressure required to stop urine flow as a measure of filtration pressure. At the reduced level of glomerular filtration effected by a relatively small increase in ureteral pressure, reabsorption of solutes may equal their rate of filtration. Therefore urine flow ceases, although filtration is continuing. When, however, the tubules are unable to reabsorb the filtered solute, as with urea loading (WINTON 1934b) or cooling (WINTON 1934a, b) or cyanide (STARLING and VERNEY), the maximum ureteral pressure is much higher and approximates 70 mm. Hg at arterial blood pressures of 120 mm. Hg. This figure probably represents a valid approximation to the 'effective' filtration pressure. Adding to this 'effective' filtration pressure a value of about 25 mm. Hg for the colloid osmotic pressure of the blood plasma yields a glomerular capillary pressure in the dog of 95 mm. Hg or about 80 percent of the arterial pressure under the conditions of the experiments.

WINTON (1931a, b, d) and EGGLETON, PAPPENHEIMER and WINTON (1940b) observed that when urine flow was reduced by a fixed amount either by elevation of ureteral pressure or elevation of renal venous pressure the composition of the resulting urine was the same with either procedure. Furthermore, a greater increase of venous than of ureteral pressure was necessary to effect an equal reduction in urine flow (Fig. 13). From the first observation they concluded that the principal effects on urine flow of both pressure changes was mediated through changes in glomerular filtration which in turn were presumed to result from changes in the pressure gradient across the glomerular capillaries. Two additional assumptions permitted them to calculate the glomerular capillary pressure. The first assumption is that the difference between the venous and ureteral pressure increments which effect the same decrease in urine flow represents the amount by which the venous pressure increment has elevated glomerular capillary pressure. The second assumption is that the fraction of venous pressure rise transmitted back to the glomerular capillaries is equal to the fraction of the total pressure drop from artery to vein represented by the pressure drop from artery to glomerulus. Combining these assumptions yields the relationship: glomerular capillary pressure equals arterial pressure times the ratio of ureteral to venous pressure increments which yield equal reductions in urine flow. Unfortunately, however, the ureteral and venous pressure increments which effect an equal reduction in urine flow do not effect equal reductions in creatinine clearance, relatively greater ureteral pressure being required for the latter. Assuming that creatinine clearance constitutes the better index of filtration rate under the conditions of their experiments (the dog heart-lung-kidney preparation) EGGLETON, PAPPENHEIMER and WINTON calculated a glomerular capillary pressure averaging 64 percent of the arterial pressure. Data applicable to the relatively untraumatized dog are not available.

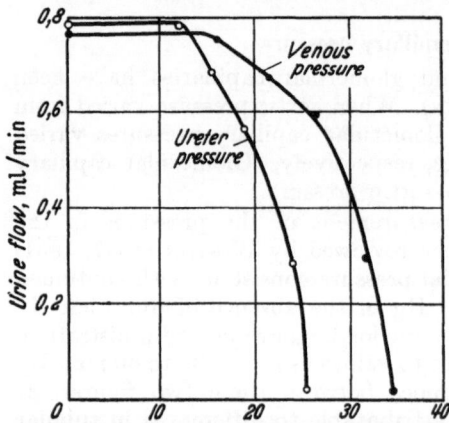

Fig. 13. Effects of ureteral and venous pressure increases, applied one at a time, on the urine flow of the isolated dog kidney. Relatively greater venous than ureteral pressure is required to produce the same reduction in urine flow. Increasing ureteral or venous pressure does not affect urine flow until a certain value (here, about 12 mm. Hg) is reached which is about the same for both; after WINTON (1951). Reproduced by permission of the author and Academic Press, Inc., New York

b) Interlobular and arcuate venous pressure

SWANN et al. observed an abrupt rise in venous pressure from 7 to about 23 mm. Hg as they passed a catheter up the venous system in the dog. The rise generally occurred in the region of the junction of the arcuate and inter-lobular veins, a region where they found muscular or fibrous tissue elements capable of obstructing the flow of venous blood. They interpreted the pressure of 25 mm. to represent that of the venous system above the obstructive "stenoses" or "sinusoidal cushions". It is possible, however, they may have been measuring "wedged" pressures which, by damming back the blood, would measure the pressure attained in some area where collateral circulation is possible. WAUGH and HAMILTON also measured a large drop in pressure (9 to 24 mm. Hg) in oil-perfused kidneys between the arcuate and the main renal vein, but attributed this drop to compression of the veins by the relatively high interstitial pressure, and questioned the need to consider organic stenoses to explain their data.

BRUN et al. obtained "wedged" venous pressures averaging 18 mm. Hg in 9 normal human subjects and 20 mm. in 4 patients with acute renal failure. They believe that the "wedging" occurred at the level of the interlobar veins (MUNCK).

c) Renal interstitial pressure

The pressure of the fluid in the interstitial spaces of the kidney has been measured by both indirect and direct means. From several lines of evidence, WINTON (1937, 1951) concluded that the interstitial pressure equals the ureteral or venous pressure required to effect a just perceptible decrease in urine flow (Fig. 13). In kidneys not subjected to diuretic agents, this averaged about 10 mm. Hg or a little more. GOTTSCHALK, using microneedles and a manometer, obtained interstitial fluid pressures averaging 10 mm. Hg in rats, guinea pigs, rabbits and cats, and 16 mm. in dogs. WINTON (1956) has suggested that values of intrarenal pressure of 20 to 25 mm. Hg, measured through relatively large 25 gauge needles inserted into the parenchyma (SWANN and PRINE) probably are falsely high because of rupture of tubules and blood vessels and impaired flow of manometer fluid from the puncture site. In other studies, GOTTSCHALK and MYLLE (1956) and WIRZ (1955b) found the pressure in the peritubular capillaries of the rat to be 14 to 19 and 17.4 ± 2.6 mm. Hg, respectively.

Ureteral, venous and interstitial fluid pressures are partially interdependent. Ureteral and venous pressures have no effect upon interstitial pressure as long as they are low. As ureteral and venous pressure increase, interstitial pressure does not change until its resting value, 10—20 mm. Hg, is exceeded. Thereafter, all three pressures, together with the peritubular capillary pressure, increase equally (WINTON 1933; GOTTSCHALK 1950, 1952; GOTTSCHALK and MYLLE 1956; SWANN, MONTGOMERY and LOWRY).

Renal interstitial pressure also increases to 30 mm. Hg or more during diuresis from causes related to decreased reabsorption of water (WINTON 1933; MILES and DE WARDENER 1954; GOTTSCHALK and MYLLE 1956, 1957). Since the diuretic agent (chilling; cyanide administration; urea, mannitol, saline, or sulfate loading) does not usually increase blood flow or filtration rate and, by diminishing tubular reabsorption, actually lessens the fluid volume entering the interstitium, the pressure rise is probably caused by swelling of the tubules whose lumina can be observed to dilate (BRODIE and MACKENZIE; GOTTSCHALK and MYLLE 1957). This view receives further support from the observation that interstitial pressure generally returns toward control values during sustained diuresis.

Variations in arterial pressure have little effect on interstitial pressure over a range of 40 to 140 mm. Hg, indicating that very little of the arterial pressure changes within this range are transmitted past the afferent and efferent arterioles. Below 40 mm. Hg, arterial and interstitial pressures vary more or less proportionately. Even when increased arterial pressure causes a diuresis, the increase in interstitial pressure is half or less than that observed at the same volume of diuresis caused by chilling or urea-loading. Further study is needed to explain this anomalous behavior (WINTON 1933, 1936; GOTTSCHALK 1952). Resistance of interstitial pressure to arterial pressure change is probably correlated with the phenomenon of autoregulation, since interstitial pressure rises with arterial pressure when renal blood flow also increases (SCHER 1959). Hemorrhage is associated with a decrease in interstitial (intrarenal) pressure probably because of intrarenal arteriolar constriction (MILES and DE WARDENER 1954).

Acute changes in interstitial pressure are reflected qualitatively in parallel changes in renal capsular tension and renal size.

d) Intratubular pressures

Pressure in the *proximal convoluted tubule* of the rat lies between the interstitial fluid and the peritubular capillary pressure. In two studies during non-diuretic conditions it averaged 12.5 and 14.8—15.5 mm. Hg, respectively (GOTT-SCHALK and MYLLE 1957; WIRZ 1955b). Concurrent capillary pressures in the latter studies averaged 17.4 mm.

Intratubular pressure increases parallel with interstitial pressure during osmotic diuresis or following venous or ureteral pressure elevation. Proximal tubular pressure exhibits little variation between various points, although the puncture sites necessarily vary considerably in their distance from the glomerulus. This indicates that the pressure drop along the proximal tubule is small and that the pressure in BOWMAN'S capsule is probably no more than 5 mm. Hg above the interstitial pressure.

Intratubular pressure decreases markedly between the proximal and the distal convoluted tubules. In the rat kidney during antidiuresis, distal pressure may vary from nearly zero to 7 mm. Hg. During osmotic diuresis (urea, mannitol or saline loading), distal tubular pressure approaches that of the proximal tubule at a time when the latter is increasing. During water diuresis, distal pressure rises toward that of the proximal tubule, but the latter does not change (GOTT-SCHALK and MYLLE 1957; WIRZ 1955a). WIRZ attributes to the thin segment the property of establishing the proximal-distal tubular pressure gradient. Presumably because of its thin walls, the thin segment should be the first tubular area to collapse when interstitial pressure exceeds intratubular pressure. No urine will pass from the proximal segment until pressure in the latter is sufficient to force open the collapsed thin segment. Whether this mechanical property of the thin segment has functional importance is unknown. *A priori*, it would seem that stabilization of the proximal tubular pressure and its adjacent intra-capsular pressure would constitute a significant element in the stabilization of glomerular filtration.

2. Renal vascular resistance

The volume of blood which flows through an organ depends upon the blood pressure and viscosity, and upon the size, number and arrangement of the blood vessels. Of particular importance is the radius of a vessel, the resistance increasing rapidly as the radius diminishes. A decrease in radius of approximately 10 percent is sufficient to double the resistance. Although the resistance of a small vessel, such as a capillary, may be extremely high, the resistance can be offset by multiplying the number of vessels available for flow. For example, the afferent arteriole, on entering the glomerulus, divides into vessels no more than twice its length and about half its diameter. If only one such vessels were available, the resistance to flow would be 30 to 50 times that of the afferent arteriole. With 50 glomerular capillaries, however, the resistance should approximately equal that of the afferent arteriole and be substantially less than that of the smaller efferent arteriole. Generally, the fraction of the total resistance offered by any segment of the renal vascular tree will equal the fraction of the total pressure drop which takes place over that segment. Assuming that the data in the preceding section, obtained mostly from dog and rat, can be extended to normal man, we have pressures of 90, 60, 25 and 10 mm. Hg in renal artery, glomerulus, peritubular capillaries and renal vein. Hence, 37 percent of the total resistance is offered by the arterial system between renal artery and glomeruli; 44 percent is offered by the efferent arterioles; and 19 percent by the venous system. Although these resistances are termed the afferent, efferent and venular resistances, respectively, they should not be identified with discrete anatomical entities. The afferent resistance, in particular, should not be identified with the vasa afferentia. From anatomical considerations, each interlobular artery probably offers nearly as much resistance as does the group of afferent arterioles which branch from it. Similarly, the afferent resistance includes a portion of that of the glomerular capillaries since no means is available to measure the pressures at the beginning and end of these. The efferent resistance includes the efferent arterioles, the most important fraction, and also portions of the resistances offered by the glomerular and postglomerular capillary nets. The venular resistance comprises that of the venous system together with the resistance of an indeterminate fraction of the postglomerular capillaries. GOMEZ has devised more elaborate calculations of the renal resistances in which provision is made for fluid which by filtration and reabsorption bypasses the efferent arterioles and part of the peritubular capillaries. From his calculations he obtained a relatively higher value (27 to 31 percent) for the venular resistance. The low resistance (5—7 dyne sec. cm^{-5}) offered by the two human kidneys can arise only from the large number of glomerular circuits containing relatively large diameter arterioles.

In the foregoing discussion it has been assumed that the resistances offered by different fractions of the vascular path arise from the size and numbers of their components. This may not be strictly true, since not only is it probable that the viscosity of the blood is different in different parts of the path but it is possible that the pattern of variation in blood viscosity within the kidney may change in various physiological and pathological states.

The vast bulk of experimental studies of renal hemodynamics comprise paired observations on two variables: renal blood or plasma flow, and glomerular filtration rate. To interpret these data the renal resistance can be divided into only two useful fractions: the *afferent* resistance, arising from the flow path prior to the glomeruli, and the *efferent* resistance arising from all of the flow path subsequent to the glomeruli. An example will serve to indicate how these terms are employed in most studies. In essential hypertension, arterial blood pressure is increased while renal blood flow is moderately and glomerular filtration rate is slightly decreased. A decreased renal blood flow at an increased pressure indicates a large increase in renal resistance. Assuming that changes in filtration rate constitute a measure of changes in filtration pressure in essential hypertension, relative constancy of filtration rate indicates that little change has occurred in the pressure in the glomerular capillaries. Some increase in colloid osmotic pressure (plasma protein concentration) in the glomeruli resulting from abstracting a fixed volume of filtrate from a diminished volume of plasma does not substantially alter this conclusion. Since a smaller volume of blood is flowing at a constant pressure gradient from glomeruli into the veins, the efferent resistance has increased in proportion to the decrease in blood flow. On the afferent side, however, resistance has increased both in proportion to decrease in flow and in proportion to increase in pressure gradient from artery to glomerulus. Hence, afferent resistance has increased more than on the efferent side. The proportions of the change in total resistance assigned to the afferent and efferent resistances depend ultimately, however, upon the specific value assigned to glomerular capillary pressure.

3. Blood viscosity, intrarenal hematocrit, blood volume and transit times

a) Viscosity

The viscosity of a homogeneous fluid such as water, saline or even plasma can be considered as a constant, subject only to certain limitations such as constancy of temperature. When red cells are added to plasma, which has a viscosity about 1.5 times that of water, not only is the viscosity increased but the viscosity of the resulting heterogeneous fluid becomes quite variable. In particular, the viscosity of the blood varies with the diameter of the tube through which it is flowing and also with the velocity with which it flows. Since viscosity is not constant but depends upon characteristics of the system through which it is flowing, Whittaker and Winton have proposed the term "apparent viscosity" to designate the viscosity of blood under the conditions of observation. In large tubes, the viscosity is relatively independent of velocity (except at very low flows) and of tube diameter, averaging 4 to 5 times that of water. In small tubes, particularly below 0.3 mm., and at high velocity, viscosity decreases rapidly, approaching that of plasma. The explanation of this phenomenon, supported by direct observation of blood vessels, is that the red cells move to the center of the flowing stream where they form a column moving much more rapidly than the generally peripheral plasma. The hematocrit of the blood within such a small tube will then be lower than that of the blood entering the tube in proportion as the average velocity of the red cells exceeds the average velocity of the plasma. Since flowing blood within a small tube is mostly plasma, it follows that the viscosity also should be very nearly that of plasma. In the hind limb of the dog, the apparent viscosity of blood with an hematocrit of 40 percent is no more than 50 percent greater than that of plasma, a fact presumably indicative of a high degree of axial streaming of the red cells in the arterioles wherein lies most of the resistance of the limb. Over an arterial blood pressure range of 40 to 140 mm. Hg, apparent viscosity shows little change and separation is virtually complete. Below 40 mm. Hg, viscosity increases rapidly, indicating that insufficient kinetic energy of flow is available to separate red cells from plasma in the small vessels (Whittaker and Winton).

b) Renal blood volume

The volume of the dog kidney which is occupied by blood has been consistently estimated at 20 to 25 percent of the organ by a variety of methods (Swann, Feist and Lowe; Julian; Lilienfield 1957 et al.; Pappenheimer and Kinter; Lochner and Ochwadt; Kramer and Ullrich). Of this volume two thirds is estimated to lie on the venous side (Julian; Weaver, McCarver and Swann). Renal blood volume either does not change significantly with arterial blood pressure over the physiological range, or, in the isolated kidney, may show a slight tendency to *decrease* with increasing pressure. Poisoning with KCN is associated with a slight decrease in blood volume (Lochner and Ochwadt).

c) Transit times of red cells and plasma

The *minimum* transit times of red cells and plasma through the kidney of anesthetized dogs averaged 1.9 and 2.1 seconds, respectively, in separate studies (Kramer, Saxton and Timmons; Lochner and Ochwadt). The values for red cells obtained by Kramer, which were based on oxyhemoglobin measurements, are probably low since oxygen, which may diffuse from interlobular arteries

to the parallel interlobular veins, appears about
1.25 seconds earlier than
methemoglobin-labelled
red cells (LEVY and
SAUCEDA). *Mean* tran-
sit times of cells and
plasma average 6.4 and
7.6 seconds (LILIEN-
FIELD et al. 1957). The
difference (1.2 seconds)
would seem to be quali-
tatively compatible with
axial streaming of the
red cells and not require
postulation of special,
short anatomical chan-
nels for the red cells.
Transit times for red
cells are shortened in
hypoxia (5—7 percent
oxygen) and lengthened
after epinephrine injec-
tion (KRAMER, SAXTON
and TIMMONS). Inter-
pretation of transit time
is complicated by the
observations in cat and
dog that passage of
thorotrast (measuring
plasma) is about twice
as rapid through cortex
as through medulla
(DANIEL, PEABODY and
PRICHARD 1950) and
that the transit time

Table 1. *Hematocrits of the kidney and some other tissues*

Tissue	Hematocrit (percent)	Reference
Measured by single passage methods		
Whole dog kidney . .	{ 89	LILIENFIELD et al. (1957)
	{ 90	OCHWADT (1957)
Measured by steady state methods		
Whole dog kidney . .	49	ALLEN and REEVES[1]
Whole cat kidney . .	48	PAPPENHEIMER and KINTER[2]
Whole rat kidney . .	73	LEWIS, GOODMAN and SCHUCK[3]
"Small and medium vessels", dog kidney	{ 37	GIBSON et al.[4]
	{ 34	DUNN et al.[4]
"Small vessels", dog kidney	25—35	GOODYER and GLENN[5]
Cat cortex	57	PAPPENHEIMER and KINTER[6]
Outer cortex, dog . .	43	LILIENFIELD et al. (1958)[7]
Inner cortex, dog . .	50	LILIENFIELD et al. (1958)[7]
Outer medulla, dog .	56	LILIENFIELD et al. (1958)[7]
Inner medulla, dog .	34	LILIENFIELD et al. (1958)[7]
Outer papilla, dog . .	20	LILIENFIELD et al. (1958)[7]
Inner papilla, dog . .	18	LILIENFIELD et al. (1958)[7]
Papilla, rat	22	LONGLEY, LASSEN and LILIENFIELD[5]
Dog liver	{ 31	ALLEN and REEVES
	{ 102	GIBSON et al.
	{ 42	DUNN et al.
Rat liver	87	LEWIS, GOODMAN and SCHUCK
Dog intestine	{ 42	GIBSON et al.
	{ 10	DUNN et al.
Dog brain	45	GIBSON et al.
Dog muscle	{ 52	GIBSON et al.
	{ 66	DUNN et al.
Dog heart	{ 55	GIBSON et al.
	{ 64	DUNN et al.
Dog skin	42	DUNN et al.

Renal hematocrit values, measured as percent of large vessel hematocrit, which have
been reported by various authors. Hematocrits of some other tissues are listed for comparison.

In the "single passage" methods, known amounts of isotopically labelled red cells and
albumin are injected into a renal artery. Hematocrit is then calculated either from transit
times or from relative dilutions of the isotopes during passage through the kidney.

In the "steady state" methods, hematocrit is calculated from relative intrarenal red cell
and plasma spaces after continuous perfusion for some time by blood containing labelled
red cells and plasma in constant concentration. The superscript numerals in the table refer
to specific methods, as follows:

[1] T-1824 and radio-P labelling; clamp renal pedicle.
[2] Radio-I-labelling and acid hematin; clamp pedicle.
[3] T-1824-labelling and acid hematin; clamp pedicle.
[4] Isotopically labelled red cells and albumin; indeterminate drainage from vessels.
[5] Isotopically labelled red cells and albumin; 5 minute drainage of large vessels.
[6] Surface radiation from isotopically labelled red cells and albumin.
[7] Frozen sections after perfusion with isotopically labelled red cells and albumin; clamp
pedicle.

through the capillaries of the medulla is about 12 times that through the cortical capillaries, with times of 30 and 2.5 seconds, respectively (THURAU et al.).

d) Renal hematocrit

From the behavior of blood flowing through small tubes, and from the difference between the transit times of cells and plasma, it can be predicted that the functioning kidney contains more plasma than cells relative to the ratio in the large vessels of the body. That is, the renal hematocrit should be lower than the large vessel hematocrit. This prediction has been confirmed, and the magnitude of the relative depression of the renal hematocrit under various experimental conditions has been extensively investigated. Intrarenal red cell mass is measured by radioisotope-labelled red cells or by hemoglobin content; renal plasma content is measured by radioiodine- or dye-labelled albumin.

Reported hematocrit values for the entire kidney, for cortex and medulla, and for the "small vessels" (those from which blood does not drain freely after excision of the organ) are listed in Table 1. Hematocrit values for some other tissues are listed for comparison. Although much of the variation in the renal hematocrits probably arises from differences in analytical methods and handling of the animals prior to analysis, the large difference between the renal hematocrit values measured by single transit of an indicator (LILIENFIELD et al. and OCH-WADT, Table 1) and that measured by analysis of kidney contents after time has been allowed for intrarenal equilibration of an indicator can to a very large extent be attributed to inclusion of an extravascular albumin pool in the hematocrit calculations from the steady-state type of experiments. Several tentative conclusions may be drawn, however. There is no evidence of an increase in hematocrit in cortex compared with whole kidney, or in outer cortex compared with inner cortex, such as might be predicted by the "plasma skimming" hypothesis (see below); whole kidney hematocrits are not sufficiently lower than those of other organs to suggest the existence of a qualitatively different blood flow pattern; a quantitatively significant difference exists, however, between the cortical and medullary hematocrits. The reasons for the low medullary hematocrits are not clear, but three possibilities may be considered: the measured albumin space may be larger than the intravascular plasma volume by including exchangeable extravascular albumin; diversionary channels may exist by which red cells are shunted away from the medulla; the inner medulla and papillary hematocrits may be exceptionally low because they are devoid of large vessels, and contain only straight small vessels (vasa recta) presenting a favorable situation for axial streaming of red cells. The renal hematocrit in the dog and cat has been reported to increase with decreasing blood pressure. In the cat the renal hematocrit averaged 80 percent of the perfusing blood at a perfusion pressure of 50 mm. Hg compared with an hematocrit of 50 percent at 140 mm. pressure (PAPPENHEIMER 1958; PAPPENHEIMER and KINTER). Changes in hematocrit with blood pressure in the dog could not be confirmed (OCHWADT 1957). Renal hematocrit is reported to decrease after hemorrhage at constant blood pressure (GOODYER and GLENN).

4. Blood pressure-flow relationships and autoregulation

If a kidney is supplied with blood under circumstances such that the blood pressure can be controlled and influences from the sympathetic nervous system can be stabilized a curious phenomenon is observed: Over a wide range of arterial pressures between 90 and 200 mm. Hg, renal blood flow hardly changes (Fig. 14).

In the isolated kidney, blood flow seldom increases more than 50 percent with this change in pressure and frequently exhibits no discernible rise at all. In hemodynamic terms, renal resistance has increased parallel with the increase in perfusion pressure. In the hindlimb or the ileum of the dog, on the other hand, blood flow not only varies essentially linearly with pressure but also increases or decreases to a slightly greater extent than does the perfusion pressure. The limb pressure-flow relationships are essentially those predictable in a simple system of small tubes which are capable of dilating slightly with increasing pressure (WHITTAKER and WINTON; PAPPENHEIMER and

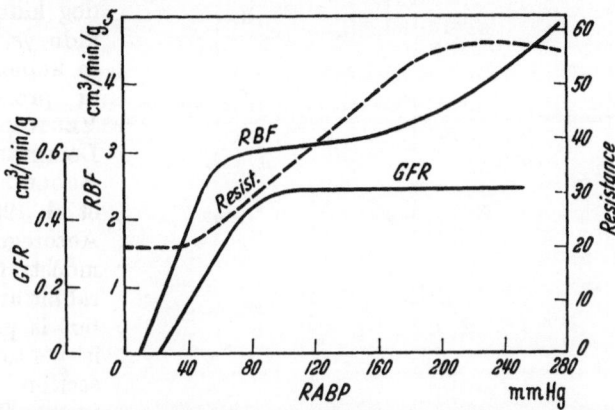

Fig. 14. Renal blood flow (*RBF*) and resistance and glomerular filtration rate (*GFR*) as related to renal arterial blood pressure (*RABP*) in the isolated dog kidney, after SELKURT (1955). Over a wide range of pressures in the physiological range, blood flow and filtration rate are relatively constant, while resistance exhibits large variation. Reproduced by permission of the author

MAES; GREEN et al. 1944; SELKURT, SCIBETTA and CULL). The difference between the limb and the kidney in the response of their flow resistance to arterial pressure change is illustrated in Fig. 15.

The phenomenon of flow-stability in the presence of changing blood pressure in the kidney is usually termed "autoregulation". Autoregulation is not unique to the kidney, being exhibited also by the intact cerebral circulation, but it is not demonstrable in most organs and tissues of the body. It is primarily a function of the cortex (which receives 90 percent of the renal blood) and is probably absent from the medulla (THURAU et al. 1960). Renal autoregulation rapidly disappears at pressures below 80 or above 180 mm. Hg. Within this range, however, it is one of the most consistently demonstrable of all renal vascular phenomena having been observed repeatedly under a great variety of experimental circumstances (WINTON 1937, and SMITH 1939, may be consulted for summaries of the

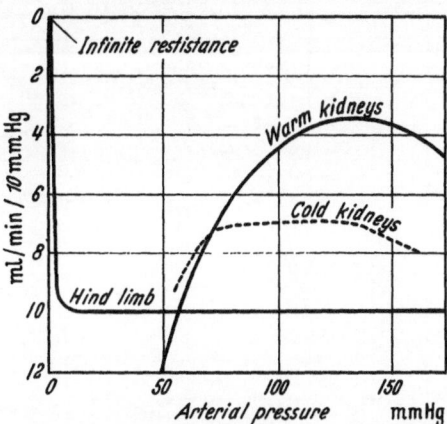

Fig. 15. Relationship of resistance to flow (measured as change in blood flow per 10 mm. Hg change in pressure) to arterial pressure in isolated kidneys and isolated hind limbs of the dog. Above a certain minimum pressure, resistance of the hind limb is quite constant while that of the kidneys increases, tending to decrease again only at high pressures (compare Fig. 14); after WINTON (1951). Reproduced by permission of the author and Academic Press, Inc., New York

earlier literature); in recent years it has been described by LOCHNER and OCHWADT (1954), SELKURT (1946), MILES, VENTOM and DE WARDENER, KINTER and PAPPENHEIMER (1956b), FORSTER and MAES, THOMPSON et al. (1957), HADDY et al. (1958a, b), WAUGH (1958a, b) and others. It has been demonstrated in dog, cat and rabbit. It is assumed to exist in man. In studies in which autoregulation could not be demonstrated in healthy kidneys (LANGSTON, GUYTON and GILLESPIE

1959, 1960), the absence of autoregulation has been attributed to passage of perfused blood through nonrenal (e.g. lumbar) arteries (HARDIN, SCOTT and HADDY). Autoregulation in the dog kidney disappears in killed kidneys, oil-perfused kidneys and in kidneys subjected to cyanide or procaine (Fig. 16) (MILES, VENTOM and DE WARDENER; LOCHNER and OCHWADT 1956; BRULL and LOUIS-BAR; HADDY et al. 1958a, b; WAUGH 1958b). Autoregulation may not be demonstrable in the kidney of the rabbit anesthetized with ethanol, but is present if the anesthetic is pentobarbital or spinal cord section (ROSENFELD and SELLERS). The effects on autoregulation of sympatholytic and autonomic ganglion-blocking drugs are contradictory (OCHWADT 1956; BRULL and LOUIS-BAR; BRULL, LOUIS-BAR and LYBECK; HADDY et al.).

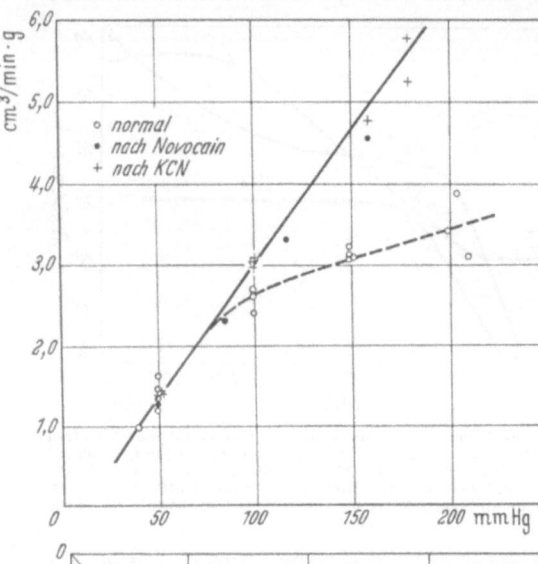

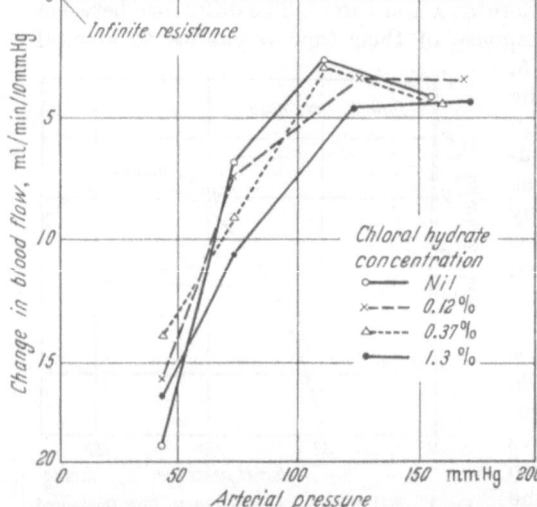

Four theories have been proposed to explain autoregulation: intraglomerular viscosity; plasma-red cell separation; intrinsic arteriolar adjustment; and interstitial fluid pressure effects. WINTON (1937) and SELKURT (1946) suggested that the increased resistance to flow offered by the kidney when blood pressure is increased could be explained if increased filtration of plasma water at higher blood pressures produced a rise in viscosity and hence in resistance to flow within the glomeruli. This theory was rendered unlikely, however, by the demonstrations that the fraction of intraglomerular water converted to filtrate (filtration fraction), and hence the viscosity, is quite constant over a wide range of blood pressure (SELKURT, HALL and SPENCER 1949b;

Fig. 16. Effects of various agents on autoregulation in the isolated dog kidney. (above) Blood flow in kidneys perfused with cyanide (+) or, procaine (●) compared with the normal (○); after LOCHNER and OCHWADT (1955). Autoregulation is present only in the normal kidneys. Reproduced by permission of the authors (below). Resistance of kidneys perfused with chloral hydrate 0.12% (×), 0.37% (△) or 1.3% (●), compared with the normal (○). Autoregulation is not evidently affected by chloral hydrate. This figure may be compared with Fig. 15 which illustrates some persistence of autoregulation in cold kidneys. After WINTON. Reproduced by permission of the author and Academic Press, Inc., New York

KINTER and PAPPENHEIMER 1956b; THOMPSON et al. 1957) and that the amount of filtrate formed in kidneys exhibiting autoregulation was insufficient to produce the necessary increase in viscosity (WINTON 1951).

PAPPENHEIMER (1958) proposed that autoregulation could be explained by the notion of "plasma skimming" (KROGH). As applied to the kidney, red cells will tend to move toward the center of the vessel while blood is flowing through the interlobular arteries, leaving relatively more plasma at the periphery to flow into the laterally-branching afferent arterioles. "Skimming" of plasma will leave the blood progressively richer in red cells as it moves to the ends of the interlobular arteries. After the blood passes through the glomeruli, cell-plasma separation continues in such a fashion that the cells are diverted through short, "preferential" channels while the plasma flows through the usual peritubular capillary plexus. Autoregulation is achieved in the following manner. At higher blood pressures, more energy is imparted to the blood, with the result that separation of cells from plasma in the interlobular arteries is more complete and the hematocrit of the blood reaching the outer cortical glomeruli increases. Since viscosity rises steeply at high hematocrits, but decreases slowly at low hematocrits, the increased resistance in the cortical area will be greater than the concomitant decrease in resistance in juxtamedullary nephrons. Hence, resistance of the whole kidney will increase with increasing blood pressure. PAPPENHEIMER has extended the cell-plasma separation hypothesis to explain autoregulation of glomerular filtration rate (at higher pressure, increased filtration in juxtamedullary nephrons is offset by decreased filtration in cortical nephrons since less plasma from which to form filtrate is flowing through the latter). Decreased extraction of the secreted substances, diodrast and p-aminohippurate, at low blood hematocrits can be explained by the supposition that at low hematocrit plasma instead of red cells can traverse the postglomerular "preferential" channel, thus avoiding exposure to the tubules where the substances can be removed. Finally, "plasma skimming" can explain the increasing renal hematocrit at low blood pressures, since less energy is available to separate cells from plasma in the flowing blood, and the large rate of change in renal blood flow with change in hematocrit at low plasma hematocrit, since cells must be present to create high hematocrit-high resistance areas in the cortex. Although plasma skimming explained the experimental observations of PAPPENHEIMER and KINTER, such as loss of autoregulation and decrease in PAH extraction at low hematocrits, and increase in hematocrit, decrease in resistance and decrease in PAH extraction at low blood pressures, a number of objections have been raised to the plasma-skimming hypothesis of autoregulation. Loss of autoregulation could not be confirmed in the dog by THOMPSON et al. (1957) or by WAUGH (1958b) at hematocrits of 4 to 10 percent although these workers confirmed the decrease in PAH extraction. SELKURT (1946) and HADDY et al. (1958a) agree with PAPPENHEIMER that autoregulation may disappear when dog kidneys are perfused with pectin or dextran solutions, but persistence of autoregulation was observed in the dextran-perfused dog kidney by HINSHAW et al. (1959); and WEISS, PASSOW and ROTHSTEIN observed autoregulation in the dextran-perfused rat kidney when the perfusion rate was high. KESSLER, HEIDENREICH and PITTS, and REUBI (1958) were unable to detect evidence of premature loading of cortical nephrons during glucose titration at low hematocrits in the dog, or in man, such as is predicted by the cell-separation theory; and PHILLIPS et al. and THOMPSON et al. observed no change in PAH extraction with variation in blood pressure. Values for the cortical hematocrit in the cat reported by PAPPENHEIMER and KINTER are half those of large vessel hematocrit and fail to indicate an accumulation of red cells in the cortex; and LILIENFIELD, ROSE and LASSEN were unable to detect a higher hematocrit in the outer cortex compared with the inner cortex or outer medulla of the dog. Oxygen saturation of cortical capillary blood does not differ significantly from that of renal venous blood, an observation difficult to explain if red cells follow a preferential path between artery and vein (KRAMER and ULLRICH 1957). "Preferential" paths bypassing the peritubular capillary plexus and physically capable of conducting highly viscous masses of red cells have not been found by injection studies nor is there evidence that plasma is moving by such preferential paths in the anemic rabbit (REUBI 1958). Finally, it is not clear that the small increase in velocity of blood flow through the interlobular arteries which attends a rise in blood pressure is sufficient to effect a significant increase in axial streaming of red cells.

The third notion concerning the nature of autoregulation is that diameters of some portion of the preglomerular vessels decrease with increasing blood pressure. A response of this nature is assumed, but not proven, to require some element dependent upon tissue viability which can sense a deformation resulting from a pressure change and convert this information into a signal affecting vascular diameters. The weakness of this concept is that neither the location nor nature of the mechanism is known. It is supported mostly in the negative sense by doubtful aspects of the alternative concepts (WINTON 1956). As noted above, autoregulation is abolished by cyanide or procaine (dog) and by ethanol anesthesia (rabbit). This suggests that some cellular activity responsible for autoregulation has been inhibited. On the other hand, chloral hydrate, in a concentration (1.3 percent) many times that sufficient to completely paralyse most smooth muscle and also cooling to 3^0 C fail to abolish autoregulation (Fig. 15 and 16) (WINTON 1956; BICKFORD and WINTON). Studies of vasomotor influences on autoregulation are conflicting. Autoregulation was generally absent from denervated kidneys but could be demonstrated in innervated kidneys in the experiments of HADDY et al. (1958b) and of BRULL, LOUIS-BAR and LYBECK. However, in the acute experiments of these workers it may be assumed that intense vasomotor tone was present in most if not all of their innervated kidneys so that appearance of autoregulation within their experimental parameters could be attributed as well to the altered vascular geometry of the vasoconstricted kidney as to the action of a reflex arc dependent upon intact extrinsic nerves. UNNA, however, observed persistence of autoregulation during epinephrine or histamine infusion and HARTMAN, ØRSKOV and REIN found no effect on autoregulation from section of the vagi or renal nerves. In studies of de WARDENER and MILES, autoregulation was present before but disappeared following hemorrhage in the dog.

According to the fourth theory, regulation arises from the same mechanism proposed to explain increasing renal vascular resistance associated with increasing venous pressure, namely, that interstitial fluid pressure changes parallel with changes in perfusion pressure (SCHER 1959; HINSHAW, DAY and CARLSON). Most studies, however, fail to demonstrate any dependence of interstitial fluid pressure or of filtration rate on perfusion pressure within the pressure range over which autoregulation is observed, and tissue pressure change is least if autoregulation is present (SCHER 1959).

An interesting observation which may or may not be related to the mechanism of autoregulation is that of KOROBKOW. He noted that if the isolated, cooled (25^0 C), LOCKE's-perfused dog kidney is subjected for a few minutes to a pulsatile perfusion pressure, a self-perpetuating rhythmic renal volume change could be induced with a frequency of 15 to 30 cycles per minute and which might last several hours.

An increase in vascular resistance also appears when renal venous pressure is raised (WINTON 1951; SELKURT, HALL and SPENCER 1949a; OCHWADT 1956;

HADDY et al. 1958a; WAUGH 1958b) although evidence is conflicting whether
the increase in resistance persists if arterial pressure is raised sufficient to maintain constant blood flow (OCHWADT 1956, HADDY et al.). Elevation of renal
venous pressure does not abolish autoregulation provided the arteriovenous
pressure difference is large or exceeds 90 mm. Hg (GRUPP; SEMPLE and DE WAR-
DENER). If pressure equal to that of the venous pressure be applied externally
to the kidney, then the expected rise in resistance attending venous pressure
increase does not occur (OCHWADT 1956). It appears unlikely that the same
mechanism operates to change resistance with venous as with arterial pressure
changes and most workers believe that a rising venous pressure, by lowering
the hydrostatic pressure difference across arteriolar walls permits the latter to
contract with consequent increase in resistance, and that this constitutes a
passive mechanism of resistance adjustment separate from an active process
associated with arterial pressure changes. Beyond this, experimental evidence
does not yet permit us to go.

5. Intrarenal shunts

Many otherwise perplexing aspects of renal blood flow could be readily
explained if alternate flow paths, or shunts, through the kidney were available,
and careful search has been made for them. Proposed shunts fall into two classes:
flow paths by which blood may bypass the glomeruli; and flow paths by which
portions of the conventional flow path through the glomeruli may be utilized
preferentially.

As noted in the preceding section, several glomerular bypasses are recognized
by anatomists, but neither their number nor dimensions support the belief that
more than a very small fraction of the renal blood flow moves by these channels.
Direct arteriovenous connections have been described by SPANNER and by
LAMMERS and SMITHIUS but their conclusions have not been generally confirmed;
and little if any blood, as estimated by the glass bead technique, passes through
such channels (PIIPER and SCHÜRMEYER). Of the second or preferential-channel
concept, the red cell diversion and the juxtamedullary shunts have received
the most attention. PAPPENHEIMER, and LILIENFIELD, ROSE and PORFIDO, in
order to explain the faster transit times of red cells than plasma, the low renal
hematocrit, and the decrease in PAH extraction with decreasing hematocrit
have suggested that red cells follow a path through the post-glomerular capillary
bed which is faster and shorter than that followed by plasma. Although a preferential channel for red cells successfully explains their observations, it is not
essential to the explaining of them and further studies are needed before a shunt
of this nature can be considered probable (BRADLEY 1957).

A juxtamedullary shunt has been described by TRUETA et al. These authors
observed that when rabbits were injected with epinephrine, or the peripheral
end of the splanchnic nerves were stimulated, or the animals were subjected to
severe stress, the renal cortex became ischemic while blood flow persisted through
the juxtamedullary glomeruli. They proposed that such an absolute or relative
diversion of blood from the cortical to the juxtamedullary nephrons, with the
further consequence that most of the postglomerular blood perfuses the loops
of HENLE in the medulla rather than proximal or distal convoluted tubules,
could occur also in man and, in a variety of circumstances, account for various
physiological and pathological phenomena. Thus, juxtamedullary shunting was
suggested to play a role in essential hypertension, water diuresis, degenerative
renal disease and acute renal failure as well as to constitute the probable pattern

3*

of renal blood flow in hypotensive states and shock. A vast body of experimental study has, however, failed to demonstrate any evidence in man consistent with a measurable degree of juxtamedullary shunting, although the phenomenon has been repeatedly demonstrated in rabbits, less often in cat, rat and dog, as an acute, transitory response to sympathetic excitation, renal nerve stimulation or administration of vasoconstrictor drugs. Smith (1951) should be consulted for a detailed analysis of the implications of the Trueta shunt and experimental studies which bear on it. Other observations may contribute significantly to understanding of juxtamedullary shunting. Scher (1951), using small thermocouples implanted in cortex and medulla, observed that decreases and increases in renal blood flow, caused by sympathomimetic amines or acetylcholine, were divided approximately equiproportionally between cortex and medulla; Lilienfield, Maganzini and Bauer (1960a, b), and Thurau et al. have reported that medullary flow is normally about 10 percent of cortical flow; and Thurau et al. observed that autoregulation, an important property of the entire kidney, does not occur in the medulla.

In retrospect, it appears that the two major vascular areas of the kidney, the juxtamedullary-medullary and the outer cortical, may differ in their responsiveness to vasomotor influences, the cortical being much the more responsive in rabbit, dog, cat, sheep and monkey (Goodwin, Sloan and Scott; Daniel, Peabody and Prichard 1952). The reason for this difference is not clear. It could result from a greater sensitivity or intensity of innervation of the cortical vessels or from the circumstance that the long interlobular arteries and narrow efferent arterioles of the cortical circuits offer areas geometrically more suitable for effecting a resistance change. No data are available to indicate that shunting occurs in the sense that erstwhile cortical blood is diverted through juxtaglomerular circuits.

6. Summary of factors influencing the renal blood flow in the isolated or semiisolated kidney

a) Pressures

Effects on renal blood flow of arterial, venous, ureteral and interstitial pressure changes have been referred to frequently in the preceding section. Blood flow begins at a pressure of 10 to 20 mm. Hg, rises rapidly until pressure reaches 80—90 mm. Hg, rises slowly but definitely between 90 and 160 mm. Hg, then more rapidly again at still higher pressures (Winton 1956; Shipley and Study). Blood flow does not change as between a pulsatile and nonpulsatile arterial pressure (Winton 1937; Selkurt 1951; Goodyer and Glenn; Ritter). Increases in venous pressure cause a decrease in renal blood flow somewhat more than the decrease in arterio-venous pressure difference, a reflection of the effect of venous pressure on renal vascular resistance noted earlier.

When ureteral pressure is acutely increased in the dog, no renal function change occurs until the pressure reaches 10 to 15 mm. Hg (Fig. 13). Below this pressure all intrarenal pressures exceed ureteral pressure and dynamics are unaffected by changes in the latter. Above 15 mm. Hg, which represents the approximate magnitude of the pressure in the large veins, interstitial fluid and proximal tubular fluid, an increase in ureteral pressure is associated with increase in size of the kidney, decrease in urine flow and decrease in glomerular filtration rate as the increased pressure is transmitted to the glomerulus (Winton 1931a, c, 1933, 1934b). Still considering studies on the dog, GFR and RPF decrease about 15 and 5 percent, respectively, at 30—40 mm. Hg (Share; Selkurt,

BRANDFONBRENNER and GELLER) with RPF tending to return with time to the control values (SHARE). The exact point at which filtration ceases is not clear since filtration cannot be measured in the absence of urine formation and the ureteral pressure at which urine formation ceases (maximum ureteral pressure) depends upon the control rate of urine flow. At low urine flows, flow may cease at 30—40 mm. Hg while at high flows caused by urea loading flow may not cease until ureteral pressure attains 60 percent or so of arterial pressure (EGGLETON, PAPPENHEIMER and WINTON 1940b). The difference between the maximum ureteral pressures at low and high flows is probably attributable more to differences in tubular reabsorption than to changes in glomerular dynamics. Ureteral obstruction sufficient to prevent urine flow is associated with a small decrease in blood flow in the isolated kidney perfused at constant arterial pressure (WINTON 1931a) although ureteral obstruction during osmotic diuresis, which results in higher intrapelvic pressures, may be associated with greater decreases (30 percent) in blood flow (BRODSKY, KAIM and CARRASQUER). These decreases are attributed to compression of the veins by the dilated tubules. At high ureteral pressure, blood flow may be moderately depressed: 31 percent at 100 mm. Hg in the studies of LINDEMANN.

b) Temperature

When the isolated kidney is cooled to 3—12° C, renal blood flow is approximately half that at 37°. The change is largely attributable to the increase in blood viscosity which occurs at the lower temperature (BICKFORD and WINTON).

c) Hematocrit

Renal blood flow increases rapidly at hematocrits below 30 percent. At hematocrits below 10 percent, flow may be 2 to 4 times that observed at normal hematocrits (PAPPENHEIMER and KINTER; THOMPSON et al. 1957). At hematocrits between 30 to 60 percent, flow does not change significantly (PAPPENHEIMER and KINTER; SPENCER 1951, 1954).

d) Renal nerves

Section or block of the renal nerves in the unanesthetized, untraumatized dog or man is followed by no detectable change in blood flow although stimulation of the nerves is followed by large decreases in flow (AVERBECK, MEITNER and SCHNEIDER). In the anesthetized or traumatized animal, however, section of the nerves is followed by an increase in flow (SMITH 1939) and flow in a denervated kidney decreases less than in an intact kidney during acute hypotension (CORCORAN, TAYLOR and PAGE 1943). This and related evidence indicates that the renal nerves are wholly vasoconstrictor and that blood flow changes on cutting the nerves depends on whether impulses were entering the kidney at the moment of cutting. Because renal blood flow decreases relatively more than filtration rate during renal nerve stimulation, it has been concluded that constriction occurs principally in the efferent arterioles. Reflex renal vasoconstriction can arise from a great number of stimuli, mostly of a painful or stressful nature. Of particular interest are stimuli arising from the general circulation, and stimuli arising from the urinary tract. Pinching, obstruction, manipulation, or distension of the ureter is generally associated with vasoconstriction (BIETER 1929; HIX). The actions of the renal nerves can be mimicked by many sympathomimetic amines. The vasoconstrictor effects of both renal nerve stimulation and sympathomimetic amine injection can be blocked by sympatholytic drugs such as ergotamines and dibenamine (SMITH 1939; WINTON

1931c, 1951; BROD, FEJFAR and FEJFAROVA; HANDLEY and MOYER 1954a, b; MOYER and HANDLEY; MOYER, HANDLEY and HUGGINS; BERNE et al.).

II. Glomerular filtration

1. Evidence supporting the theory of filtration

Approximately 2,000,000 glomeruli, constituting nearly one square meter of capillary surface area (BOOK) filter approximately 130 ml. of fluid per minute. For two reasons physiologists no longer doubt that filtration is a purely physical process in the sense that the cells of the filtering surface perform no work on the filtrate or any component of it. These reasons are: 1. below a certain size, consistent with pore dimensions and subject to the GIBBS-DONNAN distribution in the case of electrolytes, all substances occur in the glomerular filtrate in the same concentration as they occur in the plasma water; 2. the known physical forces and membrane dimensions are sufficient to account quantitatively for observed volume of filtrate without invoking supplementary agencies.

Proof that glomerular filtrate is consistent in composition with an ultrafiltrate of plasma water rests upon the studies of RICHARDS and his associates. They compared plasma with fluid drawn through a microneedle from the lumen of BOWMAN's capsule. After correcting for volume occupied by, and binding capacity of, plasma proteins and, in the case of electrolytes, for the GIBBS-DONNAN distribution produced by the proteins, they found concentrations of plasma and filtrate to be identical, within the limits of their methods, for glucose (WALKER and REISINGER), urea, uric acid (BORDLEY and RICHARDS), creatinine (BORDLEY, HENDRIX and RICHARDS), phenol red and indigo carmine (RICHARDS and WALKER 1930), inorganic phosphate (WALKER 1933), inulin (HENDRIX, WESTFALL and RICHARDS), chloride (WESTFALL, FINDLEY and RICHARDS; EKEHORN), sodium (BOTT 1943), potassium (BOTT 1955), pH (MONT-GOMERY; PIERCE and MONTGOMERY), total electrolyte as conductivity (BAYLISS and WALKER) and total solute as vapor pressure (WALKER 1930). Of particular importance are the studies on proteins. Below a molecular weight of 14,500, proteins appear freely in the filtrate while above 70,000 they are virtually absent (BOTT and RICHARDS). Because of the easy accessibility of their glomeruli almost all of these studies were performed on amphibia. A few studies of glomerular filtrate of the guinea pig accord completely with those of amphibia. They show that the concentrations of glucose, creatinine, inulin, pH, and total solute equal those of plasma and that the filtrate is virtually free of plasma proteins (WALKER et al. 1941).

2. The glomerular membranes

The character of the glomerular membrane through which filtration takes place represents the least understood aspect of filtration. The endothelium is 0.05 to 0.1 micron thick. If the pores, roughly 0.1 micron in diameter and comprising roughly half of the surface area, exist in life, then the endothelium offers no serious barrier to filtration and is incapable of retaining proteins. The next layer, the basement membrane, is somewhat thicker (0.06—0.25 micra). Pores having a diameter slightly less than that of the smallest molecule which does not enter the filtrate are postulated to exist in this layer but they have not yet been clearly visualized. The nature of filtration through the epithelial cell layer of the capillary wall is even less clear. Anatomists have proposed that filtration occurs in the narrow gaps between the terminal processes of the epithelial cells. Since the surface area represented by these "filtration slits" constitutes perhaps 5 and certainly no more than 10 percent of the total capillary surface area, the actual filtering surface can be only a small fraction of the theoretically possible area of 0.8 M². An additional problem arises from electron microscopic studies of glomeruli from children with nephrosis. In these glomeruli, the "trabeculae" and "pedicels" of the epithelial cells are thickened and fused into a uniform mass with obliteration of the "filtration slits" (FARQUHAR, VERNIER and GOOD; FOLLI et al.). Since filtration is normal or sometimes increased in volume in nephrosis, the question arises how the filtrate passes through the epithelial cells and why the same process cannot operate in the normal glomerulus.

3. Theoretical descriptions of filtration

A different approach to the mechanism of filtration is to assume its passive nature and then calculate the extent to which known quantitative data such as the rate of formation of filtrate, the dimensions of the membranes, the physical forces, and the rates of excretion of various-sized macromolecules are consistent with specific hypotheses. PAPPENHEIMER, RENKIN and BORRERO, and PAPPENHEIMER (1955) have treated filtration on the assumption that all components of the filtrate leave the plasma through pores. All molecules can pass freely through the pores provided their radii are small compared to the pore radius. When the molecular radius exceeds about 25 percent of the pore radius, the molecules experience significant difficulty in entering the pore (steric hindrance) and tend to be restrained somewhat (molecular sieving) (Fig. 17). A sieving effect on the larger molecules tends to establish a concentration gradient between filtrate and plasma which will have two effects: First, the colloid osmotic pressure created

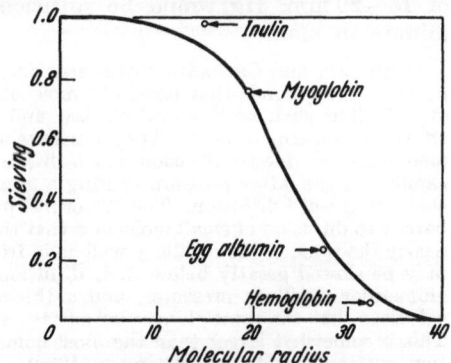

Fig. 17. Theoretical relationship between molecular size (calculated as apparent spherical radius) to sieving effect of pores with radius of 40 Å. The experimentally measured sieving of various macromolecules in the dog illustrates the generally satisfactory fit of the curve. Sieving is measured as the ratio of concentration in glomerular filtrate to that of the plasma (see text). The apparent molecular radius is calculated from diffusion data. After PAPPENHEIMER (1955)

by the restrained molecules will tend to decelerate filtration of water; second, the concentration difference will favor diffusion of the larger molecules through the pores into the filtrate in addition to their passage by bulk flow. For the smaller of the large molecules, such as inulin, diffusion is effective in dissipating nearly all of the concentration difference created by sieving. For the larger molecules with low diffusion coefficients, diffusion is unimportant. PAPPENHEIMER et al. develop their theory from the standpoint either of round or rectangular pores and of uniform or nonuniform pore dimensions but the experimental evidence does not permit a choice to be made among these various possibilities. The upper limit of pore size, determined by the smallest molecules which enter the filtrate in no more than traces, has a radius of 35 to 40 Å for round pores. Very similar curves are described by the excretion of dextrans of varying molecular weights (WALLENIUS; GIEBISCH; LAUSON and PITTS) and of polyvinylpyrrolidone (HECHT and SCHOLTAN).

Sieving of a macromolecule is measured as the concentration of the molecule in the glomerular filtrate divided by its concentration in the plasma. This ratio is equal to the clearance of the molecule divided by glomerular filtration rate (inulin clearance) provided appropriate correction is made for tubular reabsorption of the molecule. From an expression relating the net sieving (i.e. hindrance less diffusion) to glomerular filtration rate and the diffusion coefficients of a macromolecule in pores of 35 to 50 Å radius in free solution, PAPPENHEIMER (1955) calculates that the ratio of total pore area to the pore length in the glomerular membranes lies between 11 and 21×10^4 cm./gm. of kidney. Pore length is an unknown variable. Assuming pore length to equal the thickness of the basement membrane (0.1 micron or 10^{-4} cm.), and multiplying pore length by the area-length ratio gives a pore area of 11—21 cm.^{2}/gm. of kidney or, in 2 kidneys totalling 260 gm., 2,840 to 5,160 cm.^{2}, representing 3.5 to 6.5 percent of an assumed total area of 0.8 M^2. From total area and single pore diameter, the total number of pores can be easily calculated. This number multiplied by the rate of flow of water through a pore 80 Å in diameter and 1000 Å long, as calculated from POISEULLE's law, yields a filtration rate of 3.1 ml./min./mm. Hg filtration pressure/100 grams of kidney. A very reasonable filtration pressure of 15—20 mm. Hg would be sufficient to form 100 to 150 ml. of filtrate per minute in man.

CHINARD, and CHINARD, VOSBURGH and ENNS reject the concept of bulk flow through pores on the grounds that pores of "molecular dimensions" cannot be held to obey the laws of bulk flow such as POISEULLE's law and that larger pores have not been visualized by electronmicroscopic studies. They attribute movement of all molecules through the glomerular membranes as due to diffusion which draws its energy from the hydrostatic pressure in the capillaries, the latter pressure causing a greater outward diffusion than the plasma proteins cause an inward diffusion. The structural proteins are postulated to offer a sufficiently low barrier to diffusion of small molecules that the diffusion of water, salts, etc. can be considered nearly the same in the capillary wall as in free solution while the diffusion of larger molecules may be slowed greatly below their diffusion in free solution. Assuming the usual range of glomerular capillary pressures, and a thickness of 0.1 micron for the capillary wall, they calculate that the total glomerular surface area needed for diffusion would be about 2.1 M^2. This is somewhat larger than the most commonly accepted upper limit to glomerular filtration surface, 1.6 M^2, by VIMTRUP (1928). If any considerable fraction of the glomerular capillaries is 0.2 or 0.3 micra thick, as the anatomical evidence indicates is likely, then the total surface area necessary for filtration according to this theory becomes impossibly large. Besides predicting a too large surface area, a weakness of the diffusion hypothesis is that it has not yet developed a rigorous theory applicable to macromolecular diffusion except in the general sense that by a suitable assignment of diffusion coefficients to each molecular species within the glomerular membrane, a filtrate of any composition can be produced. CHINARD et al. have rightly noted that osmotic pressure values, as figures which should be subtracted from the hydrostatic pressure to give the net outward force available for effecting bulk flow, should be employed with care, but this does not mean that osmotic gradients cannot importantly influence the net outward movement of water in a bulk-flow system; and the high rates of exchange of water across the peritubular capillaries, which they believe is best described by a diffusion system, does not indicate that this is the preferable description for net water transport through the highly specialized glomerular capillaries (GARBY). As between these two theoretical concepts, the weight of the evidence favors the filtration-diffusion hypothesis as against the purely diffusion hypothesis.

Further strong support to the pore theory comes from the studies of LAMBERT, GREGOIRE and HEINZELEIN DE BRAUCOURT and LAMBERT et al. (1957) which shows that the rise in the hemoglobin-creatinine clearance ratio (sieving) when creatinine clearance decreases in the dog is almost exactly that predicted by the formulation of PAPPENHEIMER. An additional advantage to the pore theory is that very little of the total surface is needed for filtration. Weaknesses are that pores have yet to be visualized (perhaps only a question of technique) and if filtration is restricted to the area of the filtration slits, which constitute about the same fraction of the total area as is represented by the pores, then the basement membrane underlying the slits must consist almost entirely of a freely permeable material.

4. Colloid osmotic pressure

In normal plasma equilibrated against saline, the osmotic pressure of the plasma proteins (colloid osmotic pressure or COP) amounts to about 24 mm. Hg. As plasma is concentrated, by removal of 20 percent of its volume as glomerular filtrate, the more concentrated proteins should exert a pressure of about 30 mm. Hg. For purposes of evaluating glomerular dynamics it is appropriate to use the average of these two values. Direct measurement of the effect of COP on filtration pressure and filtration rate has proven as difficult to obtain as that of the glomerular hydrostatic pressures.

WHITE (1929), on the basis of direct measurements of the forces operating across the glomerular membranes of NECTURI, concluded that filtration was continuing in the apparent absence of a filtration pressure. That is, filtrate was formed when COP and intracapsular pressures exceeded the capillary hydrostatic pressure. Elimination of COP from the equation restored a positive filtration pressure. From the data of HAYMAN it seems possible that WHITE's difficulty could arise from the criteria employed to signify attainment of capillary pressure.

In theory, rate of filtration should increase or decrease in an inverse fashion with changes in COP. If a kidney is perfused by saline, which offers no colloid pressure, the kidney swells, vascular perfusate flow decreases after a momentary rise and urine flow ceases, presumably because of renal edema (WINTON 1937). A decrease in COP which results from saline loading in either anesthetized or unanesthetized dog is usually accompanied by an increase in filtration. However, renal blood flow also increases rendering interpretation difficult. Infusion of 2 liters of saline in man at rates less than 50 ml./min. is rarely accompanied by more than very small increases in filtration rate although the resulting 10 to 25 percent decrease in COP would be predicted to yield a roughly 10 percent rise in filtration pressure and hence in filtration rate. In the isolated and semiisolated dog kidney in which arterial pressure, intrarenal pressure and blood flow are stabilized it is possible that filtration may change in response to changes in COP not only sensitively but even to an exaggerated degree. For example, ureteral pressure must be increased about 18 mm. Hg in the isolated and about 45 mm. in the semiisolated kidney[1] in order to prevent a rise in urine flow associated with a 3 mm. Hg decrease in COP (EGGLETON, PAPPENHEIMER and WINTON 1940a). Both the difference in response between the two types of kidney preparation and also some of the disparity in magnitude between the colloid and ureteral pressure effects on urine flow may be attributable to changes in tubular reabsorption after the blood has been diluted by saline. Lack of direct measurement of filtration rate is a serious weakness in the experiments. Nevertheless, the authors suggest that the contribution of plasma proteins to determining filtration pressure may be incompletely described by the usual theoretical formulation described above. That is, representation of filtration pressure as the algebraic sum of colloid pressure and trans-membrane hydrostatic pressures, and application of this filtration pressure to POISEUILLE's equation to calculate rate of filtrate formation through a system of pores, may be strictly applicable only to steady or reversible states in which no more than infinitesimal quantities of filtrate are being formed. When, however, filtrate is being formed at a finite rate two additional factors could appear, both of which should increase roughly in proportion to the filtration rate. First, the current of fluid entering the pores will tend to carry protein molecules with it and increase the probability that

---

[1] The isolated kidney is disconnected from the animal and perfused by a pump-lung or pump-oxygenator machine. The semiisolated kidney remains in situ, and is perfused by the animal's own circulation with only renal arterial and venous pressures controlled.

flow into each pore will be partially obstructed for a finite period of time (pore-clogging effect); second (not specifically developed by EGGLETON et al.), abstraction of protein-free fluid by filtrate formation will cause the layer of plasma lying next to the filtering membrane to have a greater protein concentration and hence a greater colloid pressure than the bulk of the plasma. Both of these factors would cause the plasma proteins to limit the rate of filtrate formation more than predicted from the steady-state equations. Whether this theoretical increase in relative importance of proteins during filtrate formation is in agreement with the observations of EGGLETON et al. is unknown.

5. Filtration pressure

Although the hydrostatic pressures across the glomerular membrane are not known, their possible upper and lower limits are sufficiently well established that reasonably satisfactory approximations can be made. From the data in Section C1a, the glomerular capillary pressure probably lies between 70 and 85 mm. Hg. As a fraction of the arterial blood pressure, however, the figure must be quite variable, since autoregulation requires that the fraction increase with falling and decrease with rising blood pressure. The pressure in BOWMAN's capsule must at least equal the hydrostatic pressure of 10—15 mm. Hg in order to avoid collapse. In addition, a slight excess of pressure, giving a total intra-capsular pressure of perhaps 15—20 mm. Hg, is necessary to force fluid through the nephron.

The theory that the force driving fluid down the tubules arises from alternate expansion and contraction of the glomerular tuft under the influence of the pulse pressure (BRODIE) is disproven by the circumstance that urine flow and filtration rate are unaffected by elimination of pulse pressure (SELKURT 1951; GOODYER and GLENN).

Subtracting the opposing capsular and the colloid osmotic pressures (18 and 27 mm. Hg) from the intracapillary pressure yields a net pressure of 25—40 mm. Hg which is available to force water from plasma. This pressure, which will be termed 'filtration pressure', is more than twice the magnitude necessary for the normal rate of filtration according to the calculations of PAPPENHEIMER.

6. Autoregulation of filtration

Autoregulation of glomerular filtration rate, although less intensively studied because of more recent acquisition of methods of measuring filtration, is fully as remarkable a feature of renal hemodynamics as is autoregulation of blood flow. It seems probable, in fact, that autoregulation of blood flow is subsidiary to the more central need to regulate filtration since water and electrolyte balance in the mammal are acutely sensitive to even small variations in this function. Constancy of filtration rate does not seem to represent the operation of an intrinsic property of the glomerular capillaries but rather is the consequence of the operation of at least three extraglomerular mechanisms. Each of these mechanisms has the common property of tending to keep the filtration pressure constant. The first and least understood of these is autoregulation of the renal blood flow. In the semi-isolated or isolated dog kidney, filtration rate is fully as constant as blood flow in the presence of wide variations in arterial pressure changes within the physiological range (SELKURT, HALL and SPENCER 1949b). This is illustrated semidiagrammatically in Fig. 15. In data kindly furnished by Dr. SELKURT, a change of 10 mm. Hg in mean blood pressure in the auto-regulated range was associated with about 1.5 percent change in filtration rate. According to the vasoconstrictor theory of autoregulation (see Section C I 4) a rise in blood pressure by an unknown mechanism causes some portion of the preglomerular vessels, presumably the afferent arterioles, to constrict. The increased pressure drop, approximately equalling the rise in arterial pressure, across the constricted vessels causes the intraglomerular pressure to remain constant. Conversely, a pressure decrease results in arteriolar dilation. Only when arterial pressure decreases to within approximately 10 to 15 mm. Hg of normal glomerular pressure will compensation fail and glomerular pressure and filtration fall. According to the cell-separation theory of autoregulation, a rise in blood pressure will cause peripheral cortical glomeruli to receive a fluid containing mostly cells. Even though filtration pressure has risen with blood pressure, these glomeruli have a decreased volume of plasma available from which to form filtrate, with the result that their filtration may fall. Decreased filtration from these glomeruli is offset by increased filtration from juxtamedullary glomeruli with the result that overall filtration is constant. In the experiments of KINTER and PAPPENHEIMER autoregulation of filtration rate was lost at low hematocrits, but these findings could not be confirmed by THOMPSON et al. (1957). In addition, changes in glucose titration splay, such as might by expected to occur with changes in filtration rate within limited groups of nephrons, could not be detected (KESSLER, HEIDENREICH and PITTS). The intrinsic vasomotor theory, therefore, seems the more plausible explanation at present in spite of its vagueness and will be adopted for purposes of subsequent discussion. The second mechanism governing filtration rate is the relative reactivity of the smooth muscle of the afferent and efferent blood vessels to various acute stimuli, such as stimulation of the renal nerves. Reactivity is here used in the sense of the total resistance change occurring in the pre- or postglomerular circulations and does not indicate that the muscle cells necessarily have a quantitatively different sensitivity to these agents. In general, either constrictor or dilator resistance changes such as occur in response to renal nerve stimulation or injection of epinephrine or pyrogenic substances, are about twice as great in the efferent as in the afferent vessels provided, of course, that blood pressure does not change much. Since about two thirds of the resistance in the normal kidney lies on the efferent side, the reactivity ratio may signify only that the change in resistance of each portion of the vascular tree is proportional to its normal resistance. The consequence of an equiproportional change in resistance is that glomerular pressure either is constant in the presence of moderate changes in blood flow or it changes comparatively little in the presence of large changes in blood flow. If blood pressure rises or falls in the presence of epinephrine (vasoconstrictor) or pyrogen (vasodilator) then the autoregulatory mechanism discussed above specifically adds or subtracts an element of resistance to the afferent portion. For example, an increase in blood pressure during epinephrine administration may result in an equal or greater increase in resistance in the afferent than the efferent vessels, but again, with constancy of glomerular filtration. Numerous examples of these variable resistance changes will be observed in the following sections. The third mechanism tending to maintain constancy of filtration is the valve action of the loop of HENLE, as suggested by WIRZ (1955b). If fluid pressure in the loop tends to drop below interstitial pressure, the thin segment will collapse, preventing further escape of fluid. If pressure rises, the loop will dilate. The result is that pressure in the proximal tubule and hence in BOWMAN's capsule will always remain slightly greater than interstitial fluid pressure and will remain constant to the extent that interstitial fluid pressure remains constant. The tubular valve must be considered in any description of glomerular dynamics although its contribution to the efficiency of body control

of glomerular filtration cannot be assessed. A possible *fourth* and highly significant mechanism has been proposed by GOORMAGHTIGH (1937) and was suggested
by the invariable close approximation of a specialized area of the distal tubule,
the macula densa, to the vascular pole and particularly the afferent vessel of
the glomerulus. GOORMAGHTIGH proposed that the macula densa responds to
the state of fullness within the nephron as a pressure-sensitive device and
stimulates the afferent arteriole to constrict, causing filtration rate to decrease
if the nephron is too full, or to relax if the nephron is empty. By a slight modification of this view, the macula densa could be considered a chemo instead of
a baroceptor and could stimulate afferent relaxation if the concentration of
some substance, sodium ion, for example, should fall below a critical concentration at the macula densa. Should such a mechanism involving the individual
adjustment of each nephron exist, it would be of critical importance to adjusting
the filtration of each glomerulus to the reabsorptive capacity of its subjoined
tubule and to the maintenance of glomerulo-tubular balance generally.

7. Variation in filtration

Filtration rate has been considered thus far as a stabilized function. It is
apparent, however, that to function normally filtration must respond to body
needs. Since salt is the most important of excreted substances which is highly
dependent on the rate of filtration, it is not surprising that variations in filtration
are closely associated with needs to maintain body fluid (salt and water) balance
and, conversely, that changes in balance are closely associated with changes
in filtration. Observed changes in filtration rate generally fall into three categories. The first is a rise or fall in filtration associated with increases or decreases
in the amount of salt which the body must excrete. The second is a rise or fall
in filtration associated with changes in tubular function. It is evident that,
should tubular function change as the consequence, for example, of an endo-
crinopathy or nephrotoxin, changes in salt excretion would occur leading to
dehydration or edema unless appropriate changes occurred also in filtration rate.
The third category is a rise or fall in filtration rate associated with large, acute
changes in blood flow. When changes in blood flow are moderate, the autoregulatory mechanisms efficiently protect filtration from change. When flow
changes are extreme, compensation is incomplete and filtration rate changes
occur in the same direction as, but generally to a lesser degree than, the changes
in blood flow. Regulation also fails when arterial blood pressure falls below
filtration pressure, when ureteral pressure exceeds interstitial fluid pressure and
when the filtering membranes are damaged by disease.

It was noted earlier (Section B VIII 3) that rate of filtration in each glomerulus
is nearly proportional to the reabsorptive capacity of its subjoined tubule. Before
concluding this discussion of glomerular filtration it is appropriate to reconsider
the question of distribution of glomerular function among the population of
glomeruli. Alternative to the view that all glomeruli are functioning at all times
at a rate roughly proportional to the transport capacity of their tubules is the
view that filtration may be minimal or absent in a certain fraction of the glomeruli
(glomerular reserve) while filtration is proceeding actively in the remainder.
A glomerular reserve could exist in several hypothetic forms: individual glomeruli
could remain inactive (unperfused) for prolonged periods; glomeruli could become
inactive at random and for short periods (glomerular intermittence); perfusion
could continue in all glomeruli but under such low pressure in certain glomeruli
that filtration ceases. The available evidence indicates, however, that all

glomeruli are open and functioning in undisturbed, nondehydrated mammals and amphibians. A glomerular reserve therefore does not exist in the sense of glomeruli and nephrons which normally are nonfunctioning but which can become functional if excretory demands increase. Mammal and amphibian appear to differ, however, in their glomerular response to stress.

When the kidney of a frog is observed under a microscope, variable numbers of glomeruli may be observed to be inactive at any given moment. The fraction may vary from nearly zero to 30 percent in an animal in fairly good condition (RICHARDS and SCHMIDT; BIETER 1929) and fractions of inactive glomeruli as high as 90 percent have been reported (EKEHORN). During observation, closed glomeruli open and open glomeruli close in an apparently random fashion although over a short interval a glomerulus frequently appears successively to open and close in rhythm of its own; and some glomeruli may exhibit no periods of closure. Inactive periods vary from a few seconds to several minutes. If the sympathetic or splanchnic nerves are cut, closed glomeruli become rare indicating that intermittence depends on the extrinsic nerves (RICHARDS and SCHMIDT; BIETER 1929). Injection of frog blood or saline to replace fluid lost as a result of the operation, meticulous attention to the care of the animal, and also caffeine results in opening of virtually all glomeruli (RICHARDS and SCHMIDT; GRAFFLIN and BAGLEY). Conversely, stimulation of the sympathetic or splanchnic nerves, irritation of the ureter, stimulation of the sciatic nerve, epinephrine injection or dehydration results in an increased number of intermittently inactive glomeruli (RICHARDS and SCHMIDT; BIETER 1929). RICHARDS and SCHMIDT point out, however, that absence of red cells in a glomerulus, the usual criterion for inactivity, may be deceptive in the frog since some glomerular capillaries were observed to admit small sheep red cells but not frog cells which are 3 to 4 times larger. The preponderant opinion is that intermittence is present in the frog only when renal vasoconstrictor tone is present (RICHARDS 1925; GRAFFLIN and BAGLEY).

In the mammal, confirmation of the existence and nature of glomerular inactivity by direct observation has not been possible. WALKER and OLIVER watched 6 glomeruli on the surface of guinea pig kidneys for periods up to 5 minutes each, and although none of these became inactive, the surface glomeruli must be considered atypical since their capsular space was completely filled by capillaries whereas that of deeper glomeruli was not completely filled, suggesting the existence of differing hydrostatic pressures. Another experimental approach has been that of injecting a recognizable substance such as Janus Green or India Ink intravenously into a renal artery, then removing the kidney and examining the glomeruli for the presence of the test substance. The results have been exceedingly variable and inconclusive. Generally, those experiments in which most of the glomeruli have been injected appear more reliable than those experiments in which injection has been incomplete or irregular (WHITE 1939). More convincing and somewhat more consistent are experiments relating glucose transport capacity of the renal tubules to filtration rate. A tubule cannot transport glucose unless glucose is first filtered into its lumen. Hence, an increase or decrease in transport capacity suggests the possibility that a number of glomeruli are opening or closing. When an increase in filtration rate is effected by fluid loading, or theophylline or pyrogen injection in man, rabbit or dog glucose transport capacity is unaffected (SHANNON and FISHER; HARE and HARE; KRUHØFFER; SMITH et al. 1940; MILLER). This indicates that additional glucose transport capacity has not appeared as a result of the rise in filtration rate, such as would have to be the case if filtration rate increased primarily by the opening of previously inactive glomeruli. Likewise, small decreases in filtration rate are unaccompanied by changes in glucose transport capacity, again indicating that decreased filtration occurs as a result of small changes in all glomeruli rather than large changes in a few (Smith et al. 1940). A point is reached, however, where further decrease in filtration rate is accompanied by somewhat less than proportional decreases in glucose transport capacity. This point is reached at a filtration rate of 8 to 10 ml./min. for a 2—3 kg. rabbit (Kruhøffer) and 50 to 60 percent of resting, postabsorptive filtration rate in the dog (Shannon and Fisher; Thompson, Barrett and Pitts) while corresponding studies on man are not available.

It should be noted that a number of authors have reported results which are contrary to the view that filtration rate can decrease while reabsorptive capacity remains constant. For example, Handley, Sigafoos and La Forge, Handley and Keller (1950a, b), and Houck (1951) in dogs, and Dicker and Heller, and Forster (1947) in rabbits observed that filtration rate and glucose reabsorptive capacity could vary equiproportionally, a relationship described also for the frog by Forster (1942) at filtration rate values where other authors observed a constant transport capacity. The reason for these divergent observations is unknown, although it should be noted that the commoner sources of experimental error are likely to produce an apparent correlation of this form.

It is apparent that at the decompensation point a further decrease in glomerular filtration is carried disproportionately by a relatively small number of glomeruli. In circumstances associated with low arterial blood pressure, such as in the experiments of Thompson, Barrett and Pitts and Shannon and Fisher in the dog, this may represent for the most part an insufficient filtration pressure in glomeruli lying in areas of relatively high afferent resistance. In neurogenic vasoconstriction in the rabbit, as in the studies of Trueta et al., perfusion of cortical glomeruli fails progressively, beginning in the outer cortex, as the result of intense constriction of interlobular and afferent vessels. The nature of glomerular decompensation during intense vasoconstrictor activity in man is unknown.

8. Filtration fraction

Filtration fraction (FF) is the ratio of filtration rate to effective renal plasma flow and in the normal human is about 0.20. As a first approximation, it represents the fraction of plasma in the glomeruli which is extruded through the glomerular membranes as filtrate. The exact fraction of plasma which is filtered is unknown, however, for the reason that it is impossible to be certain how much of either the total or effective renal plasma flow has actually passed through the glomeruli. To the extent that some plasma may enter the peritubular capillary net by Ludwig's arterioles and anastomoses with arteriae rectae verae, ERPF may be too high. To the extent that some of the measuring substance (PAH) which traverses the glomeruli may not be entirely removed because of diffusion limitations from either red cells or plasma, ERPF may be too low. However, the uncertainty in FF which is introduced by these factors is probably not much more than 5 percent. The significance of the absolute magnitude of FF to renal function is unknown and may well be of little importance. FF varies from species to species, ranging among common laboratory animals from about 0.17 in the rabbit to 0.32 in the dog (Smith 1951). Rather characteristic changes in FF occur in certain physiological and pathological states, but without reference to the simultaneous magnitudes of filtration, blood flow and blood pressure changes no inference can be made from FF concerning renal resistance changes. FF may range from as low as 0.10 to 0.12 in pyrogenic reactions or acute glomerulonephritis (Earle, Taggart and Shannon) to as high as 0.5 to 0.6 in chronic congestive heart failure. Values of FF as high as these latter are generally viewed sceptically as reflecting either cumulative errors or failures of extraction. Since variability of random measurements in the normal is relatively small, and impaired extraction has not yet been demonstrated in heart failure, the possibility remains that at least some of these high figures are correct.

III. Lymph flow

In the dog, flow from the various hilar lymphatic trunks was found to be highly variable. An upper limit of 0.5 ml./min. per kidney to dog renal lymph flow was estimated by multiplying maximal observed flow per channel (0.05 ml./min.) by maximum observed number of channels (SUGARMAN et al.). Total flow from one kidney ranged from 0.03 to 0.30 ml./min. but the normal value is probably closer to the upper figure since the studies were performed on partially eviscerated animals, in whom renal function was frequently depressed (SCHMIDT and HAYMAN). Saline, osmotic and xanthine diuretics, epinephrine and renal vein and ureteral occlusion caused lymph flow to increase, but never to exceed 0.6 ml./min. (KATZ; KATZ and COCKETT; MURPHY et al.). All of these agents cause swelling of the kidney usually with, but occasionally without (epinephrine; venous occlusion) increase in urine flow and renal blood flow. On the other hand, lymph flow was unchanged during blood flow increase resulting from a rise in blood pressure (HADDY et al. 1958a). In retrospect, it seems probable that the increased lymph flow observed in many if not all of these acute experiments is caused by rising renal interstitial pressure. Whether increased lymph flow is sustained is not known, but would probably depend upon whether factors causing increased pressure are also such as to promote increased interstitial fluid formation. With respect to interstitial fluid, at least, pressure is not sustained following initiation of a diuresis, but, following an initial rise, reverts slowly to the control value (WINTON 1956). In less traumatic but also less concise experiments, changes in thoracic duct lymph flow were measured in anesthetized dogs when both ureters were clamped or diuresis produced by hypertonic glucose injection. Both of these procedures resulted in increases of 2 to 4 ml./min. in thoracic duct flow, but the data are uninterpretable (GOODWIN and KAUFMAN 1956b). Lymph flow has not been measured in man. GOODWIN and KAUFMAN may be consulted for bibliography.

The average urea concentration of hilar lymph samples was 55 percent greater while that of 3 capsular samples was 34 percent greater than that of venous plasma concentration (SUGARMAN et al.). Lymph glucose concentration averages 7 to 10 percent less than that of plasma while the concentration of inulin in renal lymph averaged 32 percent below that of arterial plasma (KAPLAN, FRIEDMAN and KRUGER; LEBRIE and MAYERSON). However, assuming a 30 percent extraction of inulin, it seems likely that the ratio of lymphatic to renal venous inulin concentrations would probably be close to unity. Sodium and chloride concentrations in dog renal capsular lymph are higher (11 and 27 percent, respectively) than those in plasma (LEBRIE and MAYERSON) but whole renal lymph sodium concentration does not differ significantly from plasma (KATZ and COCKETT). Protein content of dog hilar lymph varied between 0.40 and 4.0 g. percent (SUGARMAN et al.; BABICS and RENYI-VAMOS; DRINKER and YOFFEY; HADDY et al. 1958a), the concentration varying inversely with rate of lymph flow (SUGARMAN et al.). Electrophoretic fractionation of dog hilar lymph protein showed that the relative percentages of the major serum protein fractions were not particularly different from fractions observed in lymph from other organs (BABICS and RENYI-VAMOS).

IV. Renal hemodynamics in physiological states

1. Terminology and measurement

Renal plasma flow (RPF) in man is regularly measured by the clearance of p-aminohippurate (PAH) or diodrast. Frequently, these clearances are termed the "effective" renal plasma flow (ERPF) to signify that they cannot represent blood which, for one reason or another, was not "cleared" of the test substances. The total renal plasma flow (TRPF) can be measured if a sample of renal venous blood is obtained so that the extraction (E) of PAH or diodrast can be computed. Extraction is the renal arteriovenous concentration difference, A—V, divided by the arterial concentration, A. Dividing the clearance as conventionally measured by E yields TRPF. In the dog, flows so calculated agree well, under stable conditions, with direct measurements of the outflow from a renal vein (Phillips et al.; Study and Shipley; Sellwood and Verney). Except in certain circumstances which will be noted, E does not differ greatly from 0.9 in man so that effective renal plasma flow is generally a fair approximation of the total.

Renal blood flow (RBF), except under artificial circumstances wherein output or input can be measured directly, is calculated by dividing renal plasma flow by the fraction of plasma in blood. The plasma fraction is measured by one minus the hematocrit (1—Ht). Thus, dividing ERPF by 1—Ht yields the *effective renal blood flow*; and dividing TRPF by 1—Ht yields *total renal blood flow*. Since the clearance of PAH or diodrast constitutes, in all cases, the primary datum, it is usually considered sufficient to report that value alone, and to report the derivative blood flow values only when hematocrit deviates significantly from normal.

Filtration rate (GFR) is measured by the clearance of inulin. The clearances of creatinine, mannitol or thiosulfate have at times been used as alternatives to inulin but careful studies, particularly in man, have shown that these substances frequently fail to agree with the inulin clearance and sometimes may deviate widely from it. From this and other evidence, measurements of GFR by clearances other than inulin are considered unreliable and suitable only as approximation values.

2. Basal values

Effective renal plasma flow (ERPF) in man varies with respect to body size, sex, age, time of day, diet, metabolic rate and degree of hydration as well as many other physiological and pathological factors. Unless otherwise noted, function measurements are generally made in the forenoon with the subject recumbent, postabsorptive and moderately hydrated with 500 to 1000 ml. water. The effects of size variation are minimized by correcting all measurements to $1.73\ M^2$ or, less often, to $1.0\ M^2$. Under these conditions the mean effective renal plasma flow of young adult men and women is 655 and 600 ml./min./$1.73\ M^2$, respectively. These figures were compiled by Smith (1951) from various sources in the literature representing measurements on 179 men and 57 women whose ages for the most part lie between 20 and 40 years. The distribution (sigma) of the population is not readily available from these data. In a group of 18 men between 24 and 39 years old studied by Davies and Shock sigma averaged 96 ml./min. or 15 percent of the mean of their measurements. A figure close to this 15 percent distribution is observed so frequently in human renal function studies that it may be assumed to describe the population to a first approximation.

Total renal plasma flow, calculated by dividing ERPF by the average extraction ratio in man, 0.92 (BRADLEY 1947; MAXWELL, BREED and SMITH; SMITH 1951), is 720 and 660 ml./min./1.73 M² for men and women, respectively, while total renal blood flows, assuming average hematocrits of 45 and 40 percent, are 1,300 and 1,100 ml./min./1.73 M².

Filtration rate (GFR) measured under the same conditions of rest and hydration averaged about 130 and 120 ml./min.1.73 M² in men and women, respectively, between 20 and 40 years old. Sigma is about 18 percent for men and 14 percent for women in the data from which these figures were compiled (WESSON 1957). Filtration fraction (FF) measured as the ratio of GFR and ERPF is virtually identical in the two sexes, averaging 0.198 in men and 0.200 in women.

3. Effects of age

Effective renal plasma flow and filtration rate, equated to 1.73 M², are low in infancy, averaging about 20 and 70 ml./min., respectively, in infants less than 10 days old. Marked variability, probably related to changes in bodily hydration, is observed and the standard deviation is about 50 percent of the mean (BARNETT; McCANCE and YOUNG; YOUNG and McCANCE; BARNETT, PERLEY and McGINNIS; BARNETT et al. 1948, 1949; DEAN and McCANCE 1947; TUDVAD and VESTERDAL). Very premature infants (less than 2 kg. birth weight) have slightly lower filtration rate and blood flow per 1.73 M² than do full term or heavier premature infants (TUDVAD and VESTERDAL; VESTERDAL and TUDVAD). Essentially adult values per unit surface area are attained by about one year of age (WEST, SMITH

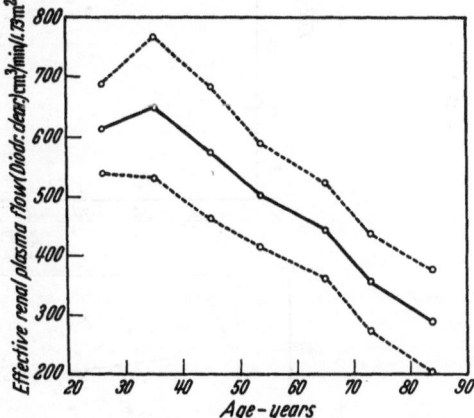

Fig. 18. Renal plasma flows per 1.73 M² as related to age in a group of 70 normal men, after DAVIES and SHOCK

and CHASIS; RUBIN, BRUCK and RAPOPORT; RANNEY and McCUNE; FRIEDERISZICK) and are maintained without a clear separation of the values for the separate sexes through late childhood (PEREZ-STABLE, FRIEDERISZICK). Function studies during adolescence have not been reported. The adult values are well maintained to about 40 years of age, after which, in men, plasma flow declines at the rate of about 70 ml./min. and filtration rate declines at about 13 ml./min. per decade (Fig. 18 and 19) (DAVIES and SHOCK; WESSON 1957). Information on women in the later decades of life is not available.

Filtration fraction remains constant at about 0.20 from 20 to 50 years. Thereafter, it rises slowly reaching about 0.23 in the age range 70 to 90 (DAVIES and SHOCK; McDONALD, SOLOMON and SHOCK). Extraction of PAH remains constant throughout life (BRADLEY 1947; MILLER, McDONALD and SHOCK 1951).

4. Diurnal variation

Normal filtration rate varies during the diurnal cycle. It is lowest at night during sleep and highest in the late morning. In three studies, the ratio of the nighttime to the daytime values averaged 0.92, 0.96 and 0.91 in 4, 16 and

3 subjects, respectively (Jones, MacDonald and Last; Sirota, Baldwin and Villarreal; Stanbury and Thomson 1951). These studies were not designed

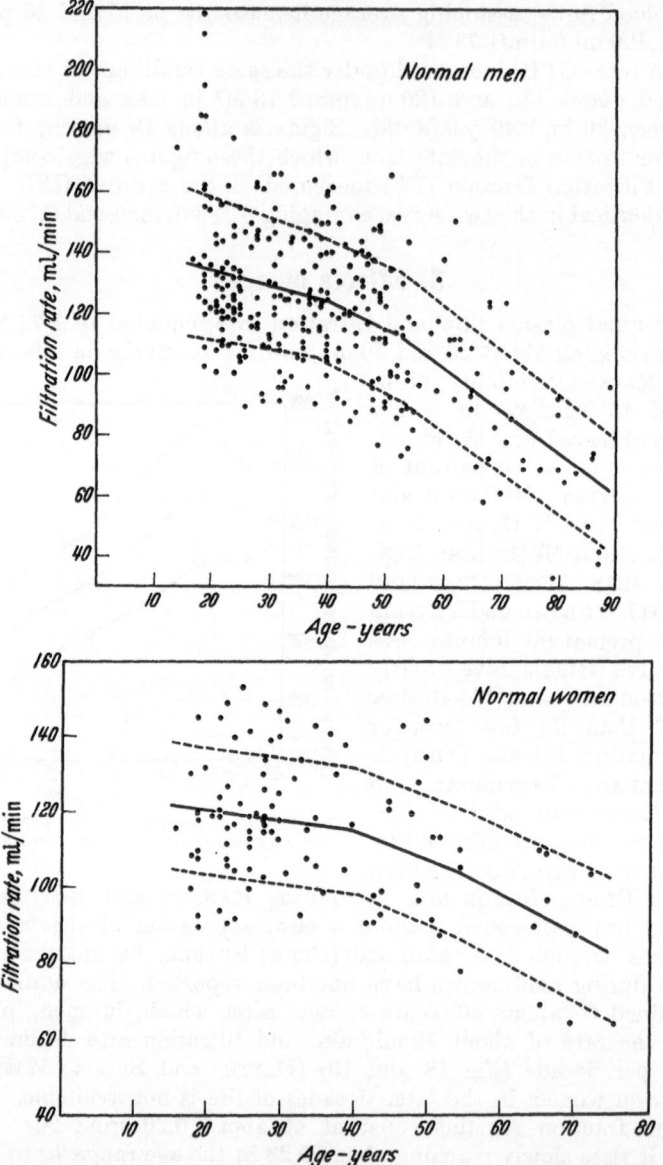

Fig. 19. Filtration (inulin clearance) per 1.73 M² in normal men and women. The data are taken from the sources listed in Table 2 and selected as described in the text. Reproduced by permission of the Williams and Wilkins Co., Baltimore

to detect the maximum and minimum values, so that the complete extent of the diurnal variation is probably greater than that indicated by the night/day ratios (see, for example, Fig. 72). This diurnal variation in filtration, although not large as a percentage, is sufficient to account for many observed parallel diurnal variations in excretion.

In several studies on resting subjects renal plasma flow exhibited surprisingly little variation as between day and night. In 10 patients studied by SIROTA, BALDWIN and VILLARREAL, the ratio of night to day values averaged 98 percent.

Table 2. *Sources of the glomerular filtration rate data (inulin clearance) plotted in Fig. 19*

Source	No.	Men Age span	No.	Women Age span
AAS and BLEGEN (1949) .	3	25—49	4	26—43
BARCLAY et al. (1947) . .	11	17—20	1	19 (approx.)
BARNETT et al. (1950) ..	5	22—32	—	—
BERGER et al. (1947) . .	8	31—48	—	—
BRICKER (pers. comm.) .	19	20—65	—	—
BROD and FEJFAR . . .	2	29—37	7	18—28
BRUN et al. (1947b) . .	13	21—27	10	19—27
BRUN et al. (1947c) . .	4	22—25	—	—
DAVIES and SHOCK . . .	70	24—89	—	—
DIGNAM et al. (1958) . .	—	—	11	55—76
EDELMAN et al.	6	19—40	4	28—48
FISHMAN et al. (1951) . .	3	21—61	—	—
FOA et al. (1942)	6	22—56	—	—
FRIEDMAN et al. (1941) .	4	22—47	5	25—40
GOLDRING et al. (1940) .	40	17—68	11	22—51
LADD	19	21—65	—	—
MAXWELL and BREED . .	11	20—63	—	—
MILLER et al. (1940) . .	5	21—44	1	36
NICKEL et al. (1954) . .	8	17—48	10	24—55
SIROTA et al. (1950) . . .	16	18—74	—	—
SMITH et al. (1943) . . .	24	28—60	10	16—55
STEINITZ	6	19—40	—	—
TALBOTT et al. (1942) . .	4	18—54	2	23—32
WESTON et al.	20	19—65	18	18—52
WIGGINS et al.	3	14—43	1	49
WILKINS et al. (pers. comm.)	4	26—45	8	19—44

In five subjects studied by JONES, McDONALD and LAST, the night/day ratio averaged 104 percent. This stability is in contrast to GFR and excretion measurements in these same studies in which day values generally considerably exceed night values in the normal subject. BROD and FENCL, however, report that RPF generally decreased at night in 9 normal subjects, and WESSON and LAULER (unpubl.) found that ERPF at night frequently attained values 20 to 30 percent below the daytime maximum in 2 subjects.

The diurnal cycle can be altered in some human pathological states. In patients with congestive heart failure or with cirrhosis and ascites GFR may be greater during the night than the day (BALDWIN, SIROTA and VILLARREAL; JONES, McDONALD and LAST), a circumstance possibly contributing to the nocturia frequently observed in these states. BURNETT, SELDIN and WALSER report that inulin clearance was greater during the day than the night in a patient with ADDISON's disease but they give no data.

5. Diet

The protein content of the diet markedly influences renal blood flow and filtration rate in the dog in which flow may nearly double either following a high protein meal or after several days on a high protein diet (MOUSTGAARD). Corresponding dietary effects in man are smaller. Following a meal high in protein, no change in RPF or GFR could be observed; but RPF increased 18 and GFR increased 31 percent in one subject after one week on a diet containing 220 grams of protein daily (WHITE and ROLF 1948). BANG and NIELSEN observed an average decrease of 2 percent in RPF of 8 young women on a low protein (27 gram daily) diet for 10 to 15 days while GFR in the same subjects decreased 7 percent. PULLMAN et al. report that GFR/RPF in 20 normal young adults, of whom 15 were men, averaged 117/640 on a diet containing 2.3—3.0 g. protein/kg./day and 95/538 ml./min. on a diet containing 0.1—0.4 g. The diets generally had

Table 3. *Effects of exercise on renal plasma flow and glomerular filtration rate.* RPF and GFR are measured in periods during or immediately following exercise as percent of preexercise control periods

Reference	Exercise	RPF	GFR
		(percent of control)	
BARCLAY et al. (1947) .	Run 0.4 km. as fast as possible	61	53
WHITE and ROLF (1948)	Running 6.4—11.3 km.;/hr. for 10—15 min.	54	58
MERRILL and CARGILL .	Step-climbing for 12 minutes	72	82
	Foot-pedalling aginst 10 kg. weights 12 minutes, while recumbent	84	87
AAS and BLEGEN . . .	Stair-climbing, 20—25 min.		
	Not exhausting to 1 man	63	94
	Exhausting to 2 women	30	38
FREEMAN et al.	Foot-pedalling against 4.5 kg. weights "as vigorously as possible" about 8 min.	91	98
CHAPMAN et al.	Walking 4.8 km.;/hr. at zero grade for 32 minutes	85	—
	Walking 4.8 km./hr. at 5 percent grade for 32 minutes	73	—
	Walking 5.6 km./hr. at 10 percent grade for 32 minutes	63	—
CHAPMAN, HENSCHEL and FORSGREN . . .	Walking 4.8 km./hr. at 5 percent grade for 3 hours	73	—
RADIGAN and ROBINSON	Walking 4.8 km/hr. at 5 percent grade (duration unstated) at 21° C	58	100
	at 50° C	64	83
BUCHT et al. (1953) . .	Foot-pedalling, recumbent, O_2 consumption 0.95—1.0 L./min.	79	86
RAISZ et al. (1959 a) . .	Stair-climbing, for 30 min.	—	70
	Step-climbing for 30 min. during osmotic diuresis	—	98

the same salt and calory content. Intermediate values were obtained by a diet of 1.0—1.4 g./kg. In studies on 11 subjects by MURDAUGH et al. GFR averaged 6 percent less on a 4 gram percent protein diet than on a 25 percent diet. CHASIS et al. observed no significant change in the RPF or GFR of 5 women after 1 to 2 weeks on a rice diet to which 10 grams of salt had been added. On rice diets without added salt, however, RPF and GFR may be variably decreased, averaging, in the case of RPF, 4.5 percent below control values on mixed ward diet in 9 women and 1 man studied by CHASIS et al. and 28 percent below the control in 7 women and 2 men studied by WESTON et al. (1950). Much greater changes than in normals were reported in nephrotic children. Farr observed that creatinine clearance (offering a rough measure of filtration rate) and also urea clearance were more than twice as great on a 4 as compared with an 0.5 g./kg./day protein diet. The effects on renal function of prolonged consumption of specific diets or of various vitamin deficiencies is not known. ERPF and GFR of two nonedematous female starvelings, aged 25 and 21, was 240 and 578 and 106 and 118 ml./min./1.73 M², while both RPF and GFR of 1 to 3 year old severely malnourished infants averaged about 2/5 normal (MOLLISON; GORDILLO et al.).

6. Exercise

Renal plasma flow and filtration rate regularly decrease during exercise, the amount of the decrease being related generally to the degree of exhaustion of the individual. In exercise which is sufficient to exhaust the individual in 5 to 15 minutes, flow is frequently reduced by half and occasionally to one third of the resting value (Table 3). The actual measurements in severe exercise, however, can indicate only the order of magnitude of the hemodynamic changes since clearance methods are unreliable during or immediately following rapid changes in renal function such as accompany severe exercise. An indication of the influence of abrupt changes in urine flow is suggested by the studies of RAISZ, AU and SCHEER (1959a). In 3 subjects, apparent GFR decreased 30 percent during exercise when they were nondiuretic and did not change significantly (decreased in two and increased in one) when they exercised during an osmotic (mannitol)

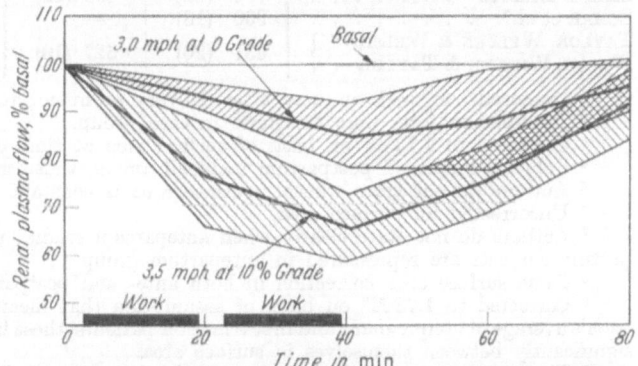

Fig. 20. Effect of exercise on renal plasma flow in man, after CHAPMAN, HENSCHEL, MINCKLER, FORSGREN and KEYS. Heavy lines indicate mean changes in flow and the shaded areas represent standard deviations. Reproduced by permission of the authors and the Journal of Clinical Investigation

diuresis. The nondiuretic urine flow decreased about 50 percent while the diuretic urine flow decreased about 10 percent during exercise. Unfortunately, it is not certain that the exercise was equally strenuous in the two situations.

Perhaps the quantitatively most reliable values of RPF during exercise are those of CHAPMAN and coworkers who employed less strenuous exercise for longer periods (Fig. 20). At exercise levels corresponding to average consumption rates of 419, 612 and 1070 ml. oxygen/min./M², RPF decreased to 85, 73 and 63 percent of control values during the second of two 16 minute periods. The minimum value during moderate, sustained exercise is reached after 45 minutes. At the termination of exercise, approximately an hour is required to recover the preexercise values.

Filtration fraction shows relatively little change during exercise, differing in that respect from most other vasoconstrictor phenomena. This is consistent with a proportionally greater increase in afferent than efferent resistance. Extraction of PAH is unchanged, indicating that no intrarenal blood is diverted away from excretory tissue (BUCHT et al. 1953).

7. Pregnancy

Renal plasma flow and filtration rate are increased in pregnancy. Although this is evident from a general inspection of Table 4, much of the data is difficult to interpret because of uncertainty in surface area adjustments. Probably the most complete studies are those of BUCHT (1951), DIGNAM, TITUS and ASSALI,

Table 4. *Renal plasma flow and glomerular filtration rate in the last trimester of pregnancy.*
Numbers in parentheses are number of subjects measured

	Renal plasma flow		Filtration rate	
	Antepartum	Postpartum[1]	Antepartum	Postpartum[1]
Assali et al.[3]	708 (4)	—	110 (5)[11]	—
Bonsnes & Lange[2, 3]	—	—	183 (13)	119 (8)
Bucht (1951)[2]	571 (13)[3]	557 (23)	156[3]	122
	639[9]	—	170[9]	—
Chesley & Chesley[2, 3]	610 (8)	518 (8)	—	—
Dignam et al.[8]	800 (9)	550 (9)	153 (9)	99 (9)
Dill et al. (1942a)[4, 5]	637 (8)	630 (8)	116 (7)	136 (7)
Dill et al. 1942b)[4, 6, 10]	500 (6)	394 (6)	84 (6)	98 (6)
Kariher & George[5, 7]	754 (8)	653 (2)	150 (8)	141 (2)
Sims & Krantz[8]	700 (12)	450 (12)	155 (12)	90 (12)
Sohar et al.[3]	900 (18)	—	180 (18)	
Taylor, Wellen & Welsh[4, 8] } Welsh, Wellen & Taylor . }	631 (20)	527 (10)	124 (20)	116 (10)

[1] Measured one week or more after delivery or in normals.
[2] Different subjects were measured in each group.
[3] Corrected to 1.73 M² on basis of surface area at time of measurement.
[4] Subjects measured postpartum included among those measured antepartum.
[5] Authors do not state whether surface area is constant ante and postpartum.
[6] Uncorrected for surface area.
[7] Authors do not state clearly when antepartum studies were made or whether postpartum subjects are represented in antepartum group.
[8] Same surface area correction in both ante- and postpartum studies.
[9] Corrected to 1.73 M² on basis of assumption that mean surface area in pregnancy equals average of nonpregnant and first trimester patients, these latter two groups not differing significantly between themselves in surface area.
[10] These patients were eclamptic or pre-eclamptic in an earlier pregnancy but apparently normal when studied.
[11] Measured as the mannitol clearance.

and Sims and Krantz and the following description is derived largely from their works. Renal plasma flow has probably attained its maximum increase, about 25 percent over nonpregnant values, by the end of the first trimester. The increase in renal blood flow is much smaller because of the decrease in hematocrit in pregnancy. In the studies of Chesley and Chesley, for example, hematocrit averaged 30.5 percent in pregnant compared to 37.9 percent in nonpregnant women. The difference caused the renal blood flow in their studies to be virtually unchanged. ERPF maintains its elevated value until near the middle of the third trimester, when it begins to decline, reaching normal levels near term (Sims and Krantz). This explains the failure of some studies to detect much elevation of RPF antepartum (Table 4). Postpartum, ERPF continues to decline to levels about 20 percent below the average nonpregnant value. It remains at the depressed level for several months, then slowly returns to normal (Sims and Krantz). Apparently, neither the extent and duration of lactation, nor the menstrual cycle affect RPF.

Filtration rate, like RPF, rises rapidly early in pregnancy and attains a value about 20 to 30 percent above the nonpregnant level before the end of the first trimester. FF is unchanged or increased slightly. Unlike RPF, elevation of GFR is sustained virtually to term, so that FF rises to 0.25 during the last half of the third trimester. Near term, GFR begins to decline and returns rapidly to normal values postpartum without passing through a clear hyponormal phase (Sims and Krantz; Bonsnes and Lange; Sohar, Scadron and Levitt).

Extraction of PAH does not change in pregnancy (Bucht 1951).

8. Emotional stress and pain

SMITH (1939) showed in classic studies that the renal circulation of man is profoundly affected by fear. In a subject exposed to alarming information, RPF decreased to 50 percent of control values and returned only slowly toward normal after assurance that the alarm was false (Fig. 21). WOLF et al. measured RPF and GFR in various subjects during psychiatric interviews intentionally designed to elicit emotional responses. In 20 hypertensive subjects, blood pressure invariably rose and RPF usually but not always decreased. In non-hypertensive subjects blood pressure response was less marked and RPF showed little change. Following sympathectomy, RPF decreased less during the stressful interview although the pressor response remained. Unfortunately, the complete data are not presented. CHALMERS et al. report no consistent RPF response to stressful interview in 21 presumably normotensive subjects, but they give no data.

Pain, as head pressure, caused RPF to decrease as much as 70 percent (G. A. WOLF) but holding a hand, arm or foot in ice water until pain becomes severe causes little change or small decreases in RBF. The greatest decreases reported (foot immersion) averaged 21 percent (G.A. WOLF; WHITE and ROLF 1948; TALSO, CROSLEY and CLARKE).

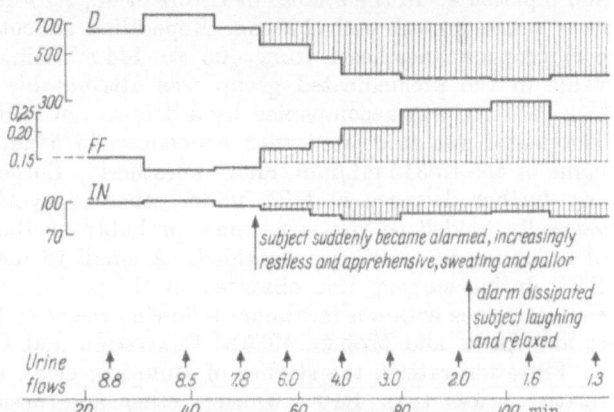

Fig. 21. Effect of fear on renal hemodynamics in a normal man, after SMITH (1939). Diadrast clearance (*D*), filtration fraction (*FF*), inulin clearance (*IN*), and urine flow (*V*). Reproduced by permission of the author and the Academic Press

In these studies filtration rate shows little change if RPF decrease is small and a small decrease if RPF decrease is large. As a consequence, FF quite regularly rises. This pattern of hemodynamic changes in pain or fear closely resembles that following epinephrine administration to man or renal nerve stimulation in experimental animals, and was partially or entirely suppressed in sympathectomized subjects. These considerations make it appear likely that a major function of the renal nerves, perhaps reinforced by epinephrine release, is to depress renal blood flow, probably simultaneous with vasoconstriction in the general splanchnic area at times of stress.

MILES, DE WARDENER and McSWINEY and MILES and DE WARDENER have described increases in GFR and RPF during experimental studies in both normotensive and hypertensive "emotionally labile" women. Their observations are as consistent with withdrawal of intense vasoconstrictor tone, caused, perhaps, by apprehension preceding the experiment, as with the appearance of a specific vasodilator action.

V. Renal hemodynamics in pathological states

1. Effects of anesthesia

General anesthesia by any agent is usually but not always associated with a decrease in RPF and in GFR. REES and IOB, and COLLER et al., observed no significant change in average RPF in 8 patients anesthetized with ether and in 4 patients anesthetized with cyclopropane, although one patient in each group exhibited a profound decrease. GFR, however, decreased to 74 and 45 percent of the control values with ether and cyclopropane so that FF decreased. However, a generally profound reduction in RPF was observed during anesthesia in most studies. In studies by Miles et al. GFR/RPF decreased by 24/32 percent in light and 51/63 percent in deep ether or cyclopropane anesthesia with no further change in RPF observed when hypotension was induced during anesthesia by pentamethonium infusion. In studies by Burnett et al. and by Habif et al. RPF decreased from preanesthetic control values of 569 and 495 to 349 and 230 ml./min. under ether anesthesia in 8 and 6 patients, respectively. Under cyclopropane, RPF decreased from 593 and 536 to 282 and 130 ml./min. in 7 and 5 patients. In the studies of Habif et al., RPF in a group of 6 patients who were premedicated with 100 mg. Meperidine subcutaneously decreased during cyclopropane anesthesia from 406 to 144 ml./min. The lower preanesthetic value in the premedicated group was attributable to the Meperidine which, in 8 patients, was accompanied by a decrease in RPF from 520 to 367 ml./min. Thiopental was associated with a decrease in 5 patients from a preanesthetic value of 455 to 315 ml./min. under anesthesia. Surgery was not associated with any further decrease in RPF under ether or cyclopropane, but rather RPF generally tended to rise somewhat, probably as the effects of the excitement of induction of anesthesia subsided. A small to moderate further decrease in RPF during surgery was observed in thiopental anesthesia. RPF returns to control values within a few hours following recovery from the anesthesia (Habif et al.; Ariel and Miller 1950b; Crawford and Gaudino; Papper).

Filtration rate in the studies of Burnett et al. and Habif et al. decreased relatively less than RPF. During ether anesthesia GFR decreased 21 and 40 percent compared with decreases of 39 and 54 percent for RBF. During cyclopropane, GFR decreased 31 and 45 percent compared with 52 and 65 percent for RBF. Thiopental was associated with a 33 percent decrease in GFR. As a consequence, FF regularly increased. Apart from the studies of Coller et al., and consistent with other changes observed during anesthesia, the renal hemodynamic alterations are consistent with variable degrees of sympathetic excitation and epinephrine release.

No change in renal plasma flow occurs during spinal anesthesia provided blood pressure does not fall (Smith et al. 1939; Assali et al. 1951; Mokotoff and Ross).

2. Effects of various drugs

Any substance can, under suitable circumstances such as severe intoxication, cause changes in renal blood flow and filtration rate. In this section we shall consider a few better known substances which affect the renal circulation in a rather direct manner and which have been studied in man.

a) Sympathomimetic amines

Epinephrine and norepinephrine affect the human renal circulation almost indistinguishably (Table 5). They depress RPF to an extent roughly proportional to the dose. When the effect on RPF is less than 20 percent GFR shows little change, or may increase slightly, suggesting a slight relative preponderance of efferent vasoconstriction. Findings which agree qualitatively with those in Table 5 are reported by Ranges and Bradley for epinephrine, ephedrine (70 to 75 mg. subcutaneously) and paredrinol (paredrine; hydroxyamphetamine).

Table 5. *Effects of sympathomimetic amines on renal plasma flow and glomerular filtration rate in normal, hypertensive, sympathectomized and anesthetized subjects*

Reference	Substance, quantity and method of administration	ERPF	GFR
		mean percent change	
BARCLAY, COOKE & KENNEY (1947)	Adrenalin { 0.5—0.8 mg. i.m.	−44	−24
	0.5—10 µgm./min. i.v.	−44	−15
MAXWELL et al. . .	Epinephrine { 1.0—1.5 mg., half i.m., half s.c.	−45	− 9
	3—10 µgm./min. i.v.	−33	−15
SMITH (1939) . . .	Adrenalin 1 mg. s.c.	−38	− 4
SMITH et al. (1943) .	Adrenalin 1 mg. half i.m., half s.c.	−28	+ 4
CHASIS et al. (1938).	Adrenalin 1 mg. s.c.	−45	− 1
DUPRE and COXON .	Epinephrine 0.013—0.015 mg./kg. s.c.	−23	− 7
SMYTHE, NICKEL & BRADLEY . . .	Epinephrine (USP) } 2—46 µgm./min. i.v.	−15	+ 6
	l-epinephrine } rate adjusted to sustain	−22	0
	l-norepinephrine } 25—50 mm. Hg B.P. rise	−28	− 3
NICKEL et al. . . .	l-norepinephrine } rate adjusted to sustain	−21	− 5
	ephedrine } 25—50 mm. Hg B.P. rise	+ 6	+ 1
PULLMAN & Mc-CLURE (1954) . .	l-norepinephrine { 2—4 µgm./min. i.v.	−20	0
	10—40 µgm./min. i.v.	−50	−5 to −20
BARNETT et al. (1950)	l-norepinephrine 20—30 µgm./min. i.v.	−28	− 5
KOZA, KOTTKE & OLSON	Epinephrine { 100 µgm./hr. i.v. in normals	−21	+ 5
	300 µgm./hr. i.v. in normals	−30	+ 4
	100 µgm./hr. i.v. in hypertensives (av. B.P. 189/116)	−18	+ 1
	100 µgm./hr. i.v. in sympathecto-mized (av. B.P. 189/114)	−23	− 9
WERKO et al. (1951)	l-norepinephrine 12—40 µgm./min. i.v.	−23	− 3
	Epinephrine 14—40 µgm./min. i.v.	−16	+ 2
JACOBSON, HAMMAR-STEN & HELLER .	Epinephrine 10—18 µgm./min. i.v.	−41	−15
MILLS, MOYER & SKELTON . . .	Norepinephrine 0.16—0.50 µg./kg./min. i.v.	−40	− 6
CHURCHILL-DAVID-SON & WYLIE . .	Epinephrine } Patients anesthetized with	−15	+ 1
	Norepinephrine } ether or cyclopropane	−18	+ 2
	Deoxyephedrine }	+19	+30

MAXWELL, MORALES and CROWDER, and NICKEL et al., however, were unable to detect a significant depressant effect of ephedrine (Table 5). Decreases in RPF greater than 20 percent, however, are accompanied by relatively smaller decreases in GFR. Filtration fraction regularly rises, but at doses of epinephrine or norepinephrine considered safe to employ acutely in man, FF has never approached the values seen in chronic congestive heart failure. That the vaso-constrictor effect is a general one, not limited to particular areas and not asso-ciated with diversion of blood through shunts, is indicated by the circumstances that both the maximal tubular transport rate of PAH and the extraction of PAH are unchanged (MILLS, MOYER and SKELTON; WERKO et al. 1951; REUBI and SCHROEDER; MAXWELL, BREED and SMITH). Mean transit time of labelled albumin in the dog is increased by norepinephrine so that intrarenal vascular volume is unchanged or increased somewhat (MEHRIZI and HAMILTON). An increase in vascular volume recalls the earlier observations by RICHARDS and PLANT that small quantities of adrenalin and pituitrin cause the kidneys of rabbit, dog and cat to swell ('adrenalin paradox').

Hypertensive, hypertensive-splanchnicectomized, and anesthetized subjects respond qualitatively as do normals (KOZA, KOTTKE and OLSEN; CHURCHILL-DAVIDSON and WYLIE). On the other hand, the low RPF and GFR of patients in shock frequently rises to near normal levels on administration of these amines presumably because increase of blood pressure from shock levels favors renal perfusion more than increased arteriolar tone opposes it (MOYER, MORRIS and BEAZLEY). The response is different in the maximally vasodilated kidney. Minute quantities of epinephrine (0.05 microgram/kg.) causes a profound vasoconstriction in the dog kidney in which renal arterial pressure, lowered by partial occlusion of the renal artery, has previously evoked maximal vasodilation through the autoregulatory mechanism (SCHROEDER and STEELE). All sympathomimetic amines do not cause increased renal resistance, as indicated by the fact that deoxyephedrine, contrary to epinephrine, caused both RPF and GFR to increase in anesthetized subjects (CHURCHILL-DAVIDSON and WYLIE).

The denervated kidney of the dog appears to be hypersensitive to circulating epinephrine. Epinephrine sufficient to elevate the diastolic blood pressure 25 mm. Hg was associated with little change in innervated kidney but was associated with a 40 to 50 percent decrease in RBF and GFR in the denervated kidney (KUBICEK, HARVEY and KOTTKE).

b) Renin and angiotensin

In both dog and man the renal pressor agents, renin and angiotensin (hypertensin, angiotonin), cause a rise in blood pressure, decrease in RPF and a smaller decrease in GFR with a rise in FF, thus resembling epinephrine (CORCORAN and PAGE 1939, 1940, 1941c; CORCORAN, KOHLSTAEDT and PAGE; WHITNEY et al.; NICKEL et al.). Unlike epinephrine, however, angiotensin failed acutely to cause a significant vasoconstriction in the dog kidney which was maximally vasodilated because of partial renal artery constriction (SCHROEDER and STEELE). In two studies, angiotensin infused into normal human subjects at a rate sufficient to elevate the diastolic blood pressure 20 to 50 mm. Hg caused GFR/RBF to decrease from 110/590 and 122/587 to 75/268 and 93/333 ml./min. Correspondingly, FF increased from 0.17 and 0.21 to 0.28 and 0.28 (CORCORAN, BROWNING and PAGE; NICKEL et al.). Angiotensin restored RPF and GFR to normal when these functions were depressed in a patient during orthostatic hypotension but did not affect hemodynamics when they were normal but with the patient orthostatic (CORCORAN, BROWNING and PAGE).

c) Depressor drugs

Ganglioplegic and sympatholytic drugs cause no consistent changes in renal hemodynamics. If hypotension occurs, RPF and GFR decrease but the pattern is nonspecific. If renal vasoconstrictor tone is present, the effect of these drugs may be similar to acute renal denervation and result in variable increases in RPF and GFR.

Dibenamine and dihydroergotamine (which block the action of sympathomimetic amines on smooth muscle) caused no change in two normal, resting subjects. RPF increased in two normal subjects exhibiting marked anxiety, and also in 11 of 15 subjects with congestive heart failure. GFR increased relatively less than RPF so that FF declined (BROD, FEJFAR and FEJFAROVA). Massive doses of dibenamine cause no significant change in GFR in the dog (WANG and NICKERSON).

Hexamethonium (which blocks nerve impulse transmission through autonomic ganglia) causes little change in normal subjects unless blood pressure decrease is profound. In patients with impaired renal function, however, RPF following a pressure drop due to hexamethonium frequently failed to return rapidly to control values (KIRKENDALL and CULBERTSON; MILLS and MOYER; FORD, MOYER and SPURR; FREIS et al. 1953). A moderate decrease in blood pressure in patients with essential hypertension is associated with a temporary decrease in RPF and GFR, both of which generally return to control levels in 30 to 60 minutes. Small or absent decreases in pressure are associated with no change or slight increases in RPF and little change in GFR, with a tendency for FF to decrease. Similar observations are reported with mecamylamine (MOYER et al.; FORD, MADISON and MOYER), with Pendiomide (MOYER and McCONN) and with tetraethylammonium (LYONS et al.). Prolonged depression of renal blood flow and filtration rate in hypertensives treated with pentapyrrolidinium is reported by STOVER, GRIFFIN and FORD.

Hydrazinophthalazine (hydralazine) causes variable but significant increases in RBF in normals and patients with hypertension or heart disease (rheumatic valvular disease) unless a profound decrease in blood pressure occurs. A small increase in GFR occurs if the increase in RPF is large. The mechanism of the action of hydralazine is unknown but the drug is presumed to act as a direct relaxant of afferent and efferent arteriolar smooth muscle (WILKINSON, BACKMAN and HECHT; WERKO et al. 1954b; GJORUP and HILDEN; JUDSON, HOLLANDER and WILKINS; CROSLEY, ROWE and CRUMPTON; DUSTAN et al.). Extraction of PAH may decrease variably (CROSLEY, ROWE and CRUMPTON).

d) Reserpine

Intravenous injection of 0.02—0.05 mg./kg. of reserpine to hypertensive subjects is associated with variable and generally insignificant changes in GFR and RPF. In two studies, the average change was a 5 to 10 percent decrease in both functions which tended to be correlated with decreases in blood pressure (MOYER, HUGHES and HUGGINS; KROGSGAARD). Intravenous doses of 5 to 7.5 mg. of reserpine in 6 subjects, some of whom were normotensive, yielded similar results in that RPF generally decreased acutely only when blood pressure also decreased. Relatively large quantities of reserpine (0.35 mg./kg.) did not cause any acute changes in GFR or RPF in pentobarbitalized dogs (DE FELICE). Extraction of PAH was not affected by this quantity of reserpine (REUBI, MÜLLER and STUCKI). Reserpine did not block the renal vasoconstrictor effects of norepinephrine. Daily administration of 3—5 mg. of reserpine for 3 months was associated with a statistically insignificant decrease in GFR of 5 percent and increase in RPF of 2 percent (MOYER, HUGHES and HUGGINS).

e) Pyrogens

The principal effect of pyrogens is vasodilation with consequent increase in RPF. GFR increases significantly if the increase in RPF is very large, but shows little change if RPF increases moderately. FF regularly decreases. These hemodynamic changes appear to consist principally of dilation of the efferent arterioles with some relaxation also of the preglomerular vessels. The changes thus represent the hemodynamic opposite of the effects of epinephrine. The first observations were those of SMITH (1939) and SMITH et al. (1943). They reported increases of 24 to 79 percent (average, 47) in RBF following injections of a pyrogenic inulin preparation. Changes in GFR in the same studies were random and smaller, ranging from a decrease of 19 percent to an increase of 13 percent, with an average change of less than 1 percent decrease. In other studies, in which intravenous injections of 50 to 75 million typhoid bacilli have been used as the pyrogen, GFR and RPF increased 15 and 62 percent (CHASIS et al. 1938), 2 and 50 percent (LATHEM 1956), and 27 and 136 percent (MAXWELL et al.). MAC-DONALD, SOLOMON and SHOCK observed average increases in RBF of 71, 86 and 91 percent in subjects grouped into 3 age ranges: 20 to 49; 50 to 69 and 70 to 85 years of age. The average control RPF in these 3 groups was 603, 449 and 277 ml./min. Since GFR did not change perceptibly FF decreased from 0.19, 0.21 and 0.23 to 0.12 in all groups during the peak of the pyrogenic reaction. The renal effect usually begins about an hour after injection of the pyrogen and when the chill is subsiding. The renal effect is not caused by rise in body temperature, however, since the hemodynamic changes were unaffected when temperature rise was prevented by aminopyrine (SMITH 1939, LATHEM 1956) nor, in the dog, is the pyrogenic response affected by renal denervation (HIATT 1942). A pyrogenic hyperemia could not be elicited in the rabbit (W. W. SMITH). Extraction of PAH is unchanged during pyrogenic renal hyperemia (MAXWELL et al.).

f) Xanthines

Studies of the effects of xanthines on human renal hemodynamics are confined almost exclusively to theophylline (dimethylxanthine) usually combined with ethylenediamine as Aminophylline or Euphyllin. The effects of intravenous administration of 0.3 to 0.5 gm. of these preparations are apparently unique. Theophylline administration to normal subjects is followed by a rise in creatinine or inulin clearance of 10 to 20 percent or more which may be sustained for an hour or longer (HERRMANN, STONE and SCHWAB; HERRMANN and DECHERD; CHASIS et al. 1938; GUKELBERGER; DAVIS and SHOCK; EK and JOSEPHSON 1953a; MILLER 1953b). With the exception of the first clearance period immediately following injection of the drug in which both inulin and PAH clearances may exhibit large and in part probably artefactual increases, renal plasma flow does not change significantly or may even decrease. As a result, FF increases after theophylline (DAVIS and SHOCK; EK and JOSEPHSON 1953a). The effects of theophylline are variable in patients with congestive heart failure. If the failure is of mild to moderate severity, little or no change in either GFR or RPF is observed following injection of the drug (BLUMGART et al. 1932; SINCLAIR-SMITH et al.; EARLE et al. 1949). In severely decompensated cardiac patients and in patients with adrenocortical or anterior pituitary deficiency, however, GFR usually increases and by amounts sometimes as great as 30 percent (SINCLAIR-SMITH et al.; WESTON et al. 1952; KLEEMAN, MAXWELL and ROCKNEY 1958). The effect of theophylline on RPF in these latter groups is not clear but it seems likely that the drug causes a rise in RPF to which the rise in GFR is secondary. The effects of caffeine (1 to 2 gm. given half i.m. and half i.v. as caffeine-sodium benzoate) on the renal circulation of normal subjects are qualitatively similar to those of theophylline. CHASIS et al. (1938) and SMITH et al. (1943) observed increases in filtration rate ranging from 4 to 38 percent and averaging 15 percent in 6 experiments. RPF, measured in 2 experiments on one subject, increased 16 and 13 percent.

The stimulating effects of theophylline on GFR can be added to those produced by rapid hydration (EK) and are independent of renal nerves as indicated by elicitation of the usual response (a 20 percent rise in GFR with no change in RPF) in a kidney which had been grafted from one to the other of identical twin men (BRICKER et al. 1956).

g) Histamine, serotonin, atropine

In limited studies, these substances exert variable effects upon renal hemodynamics.

Histamine (0.3 to 0.5 mg. subcutaneously) was followed in both normotensive and hypertensive subjects by a 10 to 15 percent decrease in RPF and much smaller changes (usually a small decrease in the normotensives) in GFR. As a consequence, FF increased (REUBI and FUTCHER). Larger quantities (1.0 mg. subcutaneously) were associated with 10 to 50 percent decreases in creatinine clearance and variable decreases in blood pressure (BJERING 1937). The changes are similar to the effects of renal nerve stimulation and they may to that extent be nonspecific. In the dog, both GFR and RPF increased moderately although urine flow decreased (BLACKMORE, WILSON and SHERROD).

Serotonin (5-hydroxytryptamine) given intravenously at the rate of 0.01 to 0.02 mg./kg./min. or of 0.25—2.0 mg. in divided doses resulted in a decrease in RPF and a lesser decrease in GFR with a consequent increase in FF (HOLLANDER, MICHELSON and WILKINS; SCHNECKLOTH, PAGE and CORCORAN). Similar hemodynamic changes were observed in 2 patients with carcinoid tumors who were excreting 25 and 239 mg. of 5-hydroxyindoleacetic acid daily. In these patients, mannitol and PAH clearances were 65 and 87 and 263 and 198 ml./min. respectively, with filtration fractions (after correcting mannitol clearance for an average mannitol-inulin clearance ratio of 0.9) of 0.275 and 0.49. In 5 subjects studied by NOTTER, GFR (thiosulfate clearance) decreased about 10 percent while RPF was unchanged following 5 mg. intramuscularly or subcutaneously. CORA, ABRIGNANI and DEBIASI, on the other hand, were unable to detect any change in GFR (thiosulfate clearance) or in RPF in four normotensive and one hypertensive subjects following injection of 5 mg. intravenously. Daily injection of 5 mg. for 13 and 17 days in 2 subjects was associated with a roughly 25 percent increase in both functions.

In the dog infusion of serotonin at 0.005 to 0.025 mg./kg./min. is associated with a small decrease in GFR and an increase in RPF while larger doses are associated with a decrease in both functions (SPINAZZOLA and SHERROD; BLACKMORE 1958). Similar depressant effects are reported in the rat and in the isolated dog kidney (see PAGE 1958, for review).

Serotonin appears to act directly upon the renal vessels (EMANUEL et al.). The renal effects could not be blocked by regitine, hexamethonium, atropine, benadryl or phantolamine (HOLLANDER, MICHELSON and WILKINS; EMANUEL et al.). Serotonin antagonists (1 benzyl-2,5 dimethyl serotonine and bromolysergic acid diethylamide) also generally failed to block the renal effects of serotonin or resulted in a further decrease in RPF (HOLLANDER, MICHELSON and WILKINS; SCHNECKLOTH et al.).

It has been suggested that serotonin is a hormone specifically responsible for control of the renal circulation (ERSPAMER and OTTOLENGHI) but the evidence in support of this view is inadequate.

Atropine administration to dogs during an infusion of Pitressin was attended by an increase in GFR and little change in RPF in one study (CORCORAN and

Page 1939) and by a decrease in GFR in another study (Solomon, Davis and Boone). Studies on man are not available.

h) Vasopressin and oxytocin

Large quantities of posterior pituitary principles affect renal function but small quantities have no detectable effect.

Quantities of Pituitrin or Pitressin or pituitary extract sufficiently large to exert pressor effects may produce transitory decreases in renal blood flow in the dog (Wakim et al.) associated with some swelling of the kidney (Richards and Plant). Filtration rate sometimes may be elevated (Shannon 1942b). Smaller quantities (50—5,000 milliunits per hour intravenously) in man had no detectable effect on GFR, RPF or extraction of PAH (Maxwell and Breed). No effects were observed of Pituitrin on RBF in dog or rabbit (Walker et al. 1937a) or of Pitressin or Pitocin (each at 20 milliunits per hour) on GFR in the dog (Anslow and Wesson 1955b).

Relatively large quantities (150 milliunits intravenously as a single injection) of pure oxytocin are reported to cause both GFR and RPF to increase in the dog, an effect which is prevented by 2 milliunits of arginine vasopressin (Ali 1958).

3. Acute and chronic fluid loading and depletion

Renal hemodynamics exhibit significant and frequently profound alteration in association with changes in body hydration and presumably constitute part of the defenses of the body against hypohydration or hyperhydration. The evidence suggests that the kidneys respond primarily to a change in the volume of some portion of the extracellular rather than the intracellular compartment and that the portion of the extracellular compartment which is most sensitive to change is in or closely related to one or more portions of the vascular system. Understanding of the renal responses to hydration changes is complicated by the circumstance that several different mechanisms appear to be involved. In acute blood sequestration, both GFR and RPF decrease, the latter to a relatively greater extent so that FF rises. This pattern is similar to that observed following renal nerve stimulation or epinephrine infusion and presumably is the direct result of activity of the sympathetic nervous system when the body is stressed by impairment of the circulatory system. In the dog, the acute renal hemodynamic responses to hemorrhage or to impeded venous return are smaller in a denervated than an innervated kidney (Goodyer and Jaeger; Farber and Baxter, pers. comm.; Wesson 1957). During blood sequestration by a tourniquet in dogs, GFR was unchanged in the denervated but depressed in the contralateral innervated kidney (Chait and Camponovo). On the other hand, a denervated kidney frequently exhibits at least half and sometimes fully as much response to cardiovascular impairment as an innervated kidney (Berne and Levy; Goodyer and Jaeger). The response of the denervated kidney may be attributed in part to epinephrine and norepinephrine liberated from the adrenal medulla or from extrarenal sympathetic vasomotor nerves. This possibility is strengthened by the report that the denervated kidney of the dog is more sensitive to epinephrine than the innervated kidney (Kubicek, Harvey and Kottke). Injection of dibenzyline into one renal artery of hypotensive dogs caused RBF and GFR to be less depressed than on the uninjected side, but the blood pressure of 60 mm. Hg resulting from the hemorrhage is sufficient to lower these functions moderately in the isolated kidney (Handley and Moyer 1954b). After prolonged or repeated hemorrhage in the dog, RBF and GFR tended to remain depressed following restoration of blood pressure by retransfusion and the persistent vasoconstriction signified by the depressed functions could not be relieved by a sympatholytic agent, piperoxan (933 F). Hence, the accumulation of nonsympathetic vasoconstrictors (e.g. angiotensin) was postulated (CORCORAN and PAGE 1943b).

During *acute* overhydration the hemodynamic pattern observed during blood sequestration or cardiovascular embarrassment is reversed. Both GFR and RPF increase but RPF generally increases more than GFR so that FF decreases. The response pattern thus resembles that following pyrogen administration and the mechanism affecting the response is equally unknown. Also like the pyrogenic response, extraction of PAH decreases to a moderate extent. The increases cannot be explained by a release of vasoconstrictor tone since no such tone exists in the normal resting state as measured by renal denervation or injections of sympatholytic or ganglioplegic drugs, and activity of vasodilator fibers cannot be invoked since the acute response to fluid administration, in the dog at least, is only slightly affected by renal denervation (SELLWOOD and VERNEY; BRICKER et al. 1958). After considering the magnitudes involved, SELLWOOD and VERNEY discounted a decrease in viscosity as significantly contributing to the increased RPF during saline loading in the dog. This and the circumstance that both RPF and GFR may increase in both dog and man following injection of colloidal (dextran, albumin or plasma) solutions virtually eliminate viscosity as an important variable in most fluid loading studies, although it may play a subsidiary role in some experiments.

The rate of fluid administration is an important factor in the responses to acute overhydration. Generally, if fluid (water or saline) is taken orally or infused intravenously in normal subjects at a rate less than 25 ml./min., increases in RPF are small and increases in GFR are barely detectable. If fluid is administered faster than 50 ml./min., which must be accomplished by intravenous infusion, GFR and RPF increase by large amounts. Smaller infusion rates of hypertonic saline are required to produce significant increases than are required of iso- or hypotonic infusions.

The renal hemodynamic response to chronic changes in body hydration are opposite to those observed during acute changes and suggest that different mechanisms are active. In chronic water or salt depletion, GFR decreases at least as much as, and frequently more than RPF so that FF is either unchanged or decreases. Conversely, GFR tends to increase relatively more than RPF during chronic hyperhydration. Little additional information is available. The findings suggest variations in the level of humoral factors specifically controlling GFR, presumably by altering the tone of the afferent glomerular vessels.

The response of patients in various pathological states differs from the normal although the basis for the different hemodynamic response is frequently obvious. The patient with congestive heart failure, for example, may respond to fluid depletion with an increase in GFR and RPF and a decrease in FF while a dehydrated patient responds to fluid loading by a return of GFR and RPF toward normal.

More precise quantitative descriptions of the hemodynamic responses to body fluid changes are not possible since amount, composition and rate of change of body fluid volume and duration of observation, selection and preparation of the subjects, and the renal functions examined differ extensively from one to another experimental study.

Sources of data on the effects of fluid balance changes in normal and in various pathological states are listed in Table 6.

Table 6. *Sources of experimental data on the effects of acute or chronic fluid loading or depletion in normal and pathological states.* Abbreviations: IN, inulin clearance; PAH, p-amino-hippurate clearance; DI, Diodone, Diodrast or Perabrodil clearance; CR, endogenous crea-tinine clearance; TH, thiosulfate clearance; MAN, mannitol clearance

Clinical condition	Acute loading with plasma, albumin or Dextran	Acute loading with protein-free fluids	Chronic loading with water or salt	Acute blood sequestration: orthostasis, phlebotomy, venostasis	Chronic depletion: salt or water deprivation
Normal	CARGILL (IN, PAH) BRICKER et al. (CR) GOODYER et al. (MAN) PETERSDORF & WELT (CR) WELT and OR-LOFF (CR) WILSON & HAR-RISON (CR, PAH) MICHIE (IN, PAH) BARKER et al. (PAH)	BRICKER (CR) BLACK et al. (1950) (IN) BIRCHALL et al. (IN, PAH) BUCHT et al. (IN, PAH) BIRCHARD & STRAUSS (CR) CRAWFORD & LUDEMANN (IN, PAH) LADD (IN) DEAN & Mc-CANCE (IN) EK (IN, PAH) MOKOTOFF et al. (IN) PAPPER et al. (CR) STRAUSS et al. (1951) (CR) STRAUSS et al. (1952) (CR) WIGGINS et al. (IN, PAH) BLACK & LITCH-FIELD (IN, PAH)	LEAF et al. (IN, PAH) MARKLEY et al. (IN, PAH) BIRCHARD et al. (CR)	BRICKER (CR) BRUN (1945) (IN, DI) EPSTEIN (MAN, IN) FARBER et al. (1953) (IN, PAH) FITZHUGH et al. (1953) (IN, PAH) LEVITT et al. (1952) (IN) SUBTSHIN & WHITE (CR) WILKINS et al. (IN, PAH) WERKO et al. (IN, PAH) SMITH (1939) (IN, DI) BLACK et al. (IN, DI)	BLACK et al. (1942) (IN, DI) BLACK et al. (1950) (IN) McCANCE & WIDDOWSON (IN) WIGGINS et al. (IN, PAH)
ADDISON'S disease		ROSENBAUM et al. (CR)	BURNETT et al. (IN)	ROSENBAUM et al. (CR)	LIPSETT & PEARSON (CR
BRIGHT'S disease (chronic nephritis)	CARGILL (IN, PAH)	BLACK & LITCH-FIELD (IN, DI)		LATHEM et al. (IN, PAH)	NICKEL et al. (IN, PAH)
Cirrhosis	PATEK et al. (IN, PAH)				
Congestive heart failure		BUCHT et al. (IN, PAH)		JUDSON et al. (1955) (IN, PAH)	BLACK & LITCH FIELD (IN, DI)
CUSHING'S disease		BIRCHALL et al. (IN, PAH)			
Diabetes insipidus	PETERSDORF et al. (CR)	BIRCHALL et al. (IN, PAH)			
Hypertension	CARGILL (IN, PAH) WESTON et al. (1950) (IN, PAH)	BIRCHALL et al. (IN, PAH) EK (IN, PAH) WESTON et al. (1950) IN, PAH) COTTIER et al. (1958) (IN, PAH)		WILKINS et al. (IN, PAH)	CHASIS et al. (1954) (IN, PAH) WESTON et al. (1950) (IN, PAH)

Table 6. (Continuation)

Clinical condition	Acute loading with plasma, albumin or Dextran	Acute loading with protein-free fluids	Chronic loading with water or salt	Acute blood sequestration: orthostasis, phlebotomy, venostasis	Chronic depletion: salt or water deprivation
Nephrosis	CARGILL (IN, PAH) ORLOFF et al. (1950) (CR) JAMES et al. (IN, PAH) LUETSCHER et al. (IN)				
Postsympath- ctomy in hyper- tension				WILKINS et al. (IN, PAH)	
Toxemia of pregnancy	ORLOFF et al. (1950) (CR)				

a) Acute loading with colloidal solutions (plasma, albumin etc.)

Infusions of 100 to 400 ml. of 25 percent human albumin at 3 to 10 ml./min. produced no detectable change in mannitol or endogenous creatinine clearance during or immediately following the infusion in normal subjects (GOODYER, PETERSON and RELMAN; BRICKER et al. 1956) or in 2 patients with diabetes insipidus (PETERSDORF and WELT). More rapid infusions are attended or immediately followed by increases in blood flow and filtration rate. Infusion of 300 ml. of 25 percent human albumin at 12 to 30 ml. per minute was followed in 5 subjects by average increases in GFR/RPF from 135/711 to 146/931 ml./min. (CARGILL 1948) and in 2 subjects from 103/467 to 119/529 (MICHIE et al.). Qualitatively similar changes were observed by BARKER et al. FF decreased in these studies from 0.19 to 0.16 in the first and was unchanged in the second study (BARKER et al. 1948). Infusion of 900 to 1955 ml. of plasma into 10 subjects at 33 to 164 ml./min. was associated with changes in creatinine clearance and RPF from 161 and 594 ml./min. before the infusion to average maxima of 244 and 1107 ml./min. immediately afterward. The postinfusion figures represent an increase of 51 percent for creatinine clearance (assumed to change nearly proportionally to filtration rate) and 77 percent for RPF. Three hypertensive patients responded to rapid plasma infusion approximately as did normals. GFR and RPF increased from 82 and 354 ml./min. before to 85 and 446 ml./min. afterward with a decline in FF from 0.24 to 0.21 (CARGILL 1948). Infusion of 1100 ml. of salt-poor 5 percent human albumin at 12 ml./min. in a patient with hypertension was followed by a very small, transitory increase in GFR and a greater, sustained rise in RPF so that FF decreased from 0.190 to 0.146 (WESTON et al. 1950).

Patients with nephrosis appear to exhibit greater response to albumin or plasma infusions than do normals. Following infusions of 100—400 ml. of 25 percent albumin at less than 10 ml./min., average endogenous creatinine clearance was slightly and inulin clearance moderately elevated but the data exhibit so great variation that quantitative statements are not meaningful (ORLOFF, WELT and STOWE; LUETSCHER, HALL and KREMER). RPF increased 34 to 217 percent with a median value of 50 percent in 7 nephrotic children infused at 2—4 ml./min. with 300 to 400 ml. of 12 percent Dextran per M^2 of surface area. Thiosulfate clearance (inulin could not be measured in the presence of the Dextran) increased in 3 of 4 children in which it was measured, but in no instance to the same extent as RPF. Consequently, FF decreased from 0.27 before to an average of 0.18 after the Dextran infusion (JAMES, GORDILLO and METCOFF). Two nephrotic subjects infused rapidly with plasma exhibited profound increases in both GFR (from 71 to 120) and in RPF (from 471 to 799 ml./min.) with no significant change in FF.

Patients with cirrhosis appear to resemble nephrotics in exhibiting a greater hemodynamic response to albumin infusion than do normals. One to three hours following infusion of 200 ml. of 25 percent albumin at 4 to 6 ml./min., average GFR/RPF in 3 patients with cirrhosis increased from 135/581 to 177/1141 ml./min. with a decrease in FF from 0.23 to 0.16 (PATEK et al.).

In the studies of CARGILL (1948) of MICHIE et al. and of BARKER et al. (1949) extraction of PAH regularly decreased following plasma or albumin infusion both in the normal and pathological subjects indicating that total plasma and blood flow increased relatively more than was measured by p-aminohippurate clearance (ERPF) alone. The average values for PAH extraction before and after plasma infusion are 84.7 and 70.2 in the normals, 76 and 64 in the 3 hypertensives, 64 and 45 in the patient with chronic nephritis, and 90 and 75 percent in the two nephrotics (CARGILL 1948). Following infusion of 75 g. of salt-poor albumin in 2 subjects, extraction of PAH decreased from 92 to 52 and to 46 percent, respectively (MICHIE et al.).

b) Acute loading with colloid-free fluids

Infusion of 1—3 L. of isotonic or somewhat hypotonic (0.1 M.) saline solutions at 10 to 50 ml./min. is accompanied or followed by little change in GFR. In several studies, the average values of inulin or endogenous creatinine clearance after infusion are unchanged, slightly decreased or are elevated no more than 5 percent above the controls (CRAWFORD and LUDEMANN; BRICKER et al. 1956; WIGGINS et al.; BLACK and LITCHFIELD; PAPPER et al.; BIRCHARD and STRAUSS; STRAUSS et al. 1951, 1952). RPF, however, when measured in these studies, has tended to increase 5 to 10 percent with the result that average FF decreases slightly (CRAWFORD and LUDEMANN; WIGGINS et al.). More rapid isotonic saline infusion (3 L. at 150 ml./min.) consistently evoked a well-sustained increase in inulin clearance averaging 55 percent in nonprehydrated subjects and 22 percent in subjects hydrated 12 hours previously by 2 L. water (LADD 1951b). RPF was not measured.

Glucose solution appears to exert a more profound effect on renal hemodynamics than does isotonic saline. 2.2 to 3.3 L. of a 3—5 percent solution infused at 28 ml./min. was attended or followed by a 17 to 24 percent increase in GFR and a 9 to 15 percent increase in RPF (EK). Ladd has reported that GFR increased about 23 percent in 4 of 5 subjects after drinking 2 L. of water.

In contrast to the comparatively small effect on hemodynamics of all save massive infusion rates of isotonic saline, hypertonic saline infused at slower rates and representing a no greater total quantity of sodium usually exerts significant acute effects on blood flow and filtration. GFR and RPF increased 37 and 33 percent in a subject infused with approximately 800 ml. of 0.4 M. saline at about 18 ml./min. (BIRCHALL et al.). Average GFR increased 3 and 20 percent after infusion of 400—500 ml. of 0.85 M. saline at 5 and 24 to 39 ml./min., respectively (PAPPER et al.; CRAWFORD and LUDEMANN). RPF in the latter study is stated to have increased between 11 and 90 percent in five of the six subjects suggesting a tendency for FF to decrease. GFR increased 27 and 230 percent after infusing 300—600 ml. of 1,7 M. saline at 10 ml./min. (MOKOTOFF, ROSS and LEITER; DEAN and McCANCE 1949). GFR decreased 10 and 15 percent in 2 subjects following infusion of 200 ml. of 0.85 M. saline at 8.3 and 10 ml./min. (BLACK, PLATT and STANBURY).

Patients with various pathological conditions frequently exhibit greater responsiveness than normal subjects to saline or water loading just as they do with plasma or albumin loading. In a salt-depleted patient with heart failure GFR and RPF increased 48 and 36 percent 30 minutes after infusing 1.8 L. of isotonic saline at 45 ml./min. (BLACK and LITCHFIELD). In 7 patients with mitral stenosis, GFR and RPF increased 44 and 62 percent respectively, with a decrease in FF from 0.23 to 0.21 following infusion of about 3 L. of 3 to 5 percent glucose solution at 28 ml./min. (BUCHT et al. 1956). Twelve hypertensive patients responded to the same protocol with increases of 36 and 51 percent in GFR and RPF and a decrease in FF from 0.20 to 0.18 (EK). The large effects of loading with glucose solution in the patients with hypertension and mitral stenosis may be compared with the smaller effects of the same fluid loading procedure on normal subjects noted above. In single experiments on a hypertensive patient (BIRCHALL et al.) a hypertensive patient on a low salt (rice) diet (WESTON et al. 1950) a patient with diabetes insipidus and a patient with CUSHING's disease (BIRCHALL et al.) hypertonic saline infusions were associated with increases in GFR varying from none to 32 percent. RPF regularly decreased less or increased more than GFR with the result that FF decreased. In 8 hypertensive subjects, FF decreased from 0.24 to 0.20 following loading by 300 ml. of 5 percent NaCl. Following several months of treatment by depressor drugs, the response to loading was virtually unchanged (HOLLANDER and JUDSON 1958). Generally similar findings were obtained by COTTIER, WELLER and HOOBLER (1958a). They compared the hemodynamic responses to loading with 500 ml. of 2.5 percent NaCl of 4 groups, each of 5 individuals, of normal, mild, moderate or severely hypertensive patients. Filtration rate increased an average of 7 ml./min. in the group of normals and changed apparently randomly within a narrow range in the other groups. Filtration fraction which did not change significantly in the normal or mildly hypertensive groups, decreased significantly in the moderately and severely hypertensive groups (from

0.22 and 0.24 prior to loading to 0.20 and 0.23 immediately after). Three patients with ADDISON's disease maintained on corticosteroids responded to infusion of 2 L. hypotonic saline with a small rise in endogenous creatinine clearance (ROSENBAUM, PAPPER and ASHLEY). Relatively small hypertonic saline infusions (200 ml. of 1.7 M. NaCl at 8 ml./min.) in salt-depleted normal subjects was associated with relatively large (30 percent) increases in GFR (BLACK, PLATT and STANBURY).

E-pah decreases during colloid-free fluid loading, at least in the glucose solution-loading studies of BUCHT et al. (1956) and EK. E decreased from 91.5 to 87.5 percent in 2 normals and from 89 to 83 percent in 2 hypertensive subjects.

c) Chronic fluid loading

The chronic effects of fluid loading, as distinguished from the effects observed within a few hours of loading, have not been extensively studied. Eighteen hours following infusion of 40 ml./kg. of 0.9 percent saline, endogenous creatinine clearance averaged 10 percent above preloading control values (BIRCHARD and STRAUSS). After gradual loading over a 21 hour period by 100 ml./kg. of isotonic saline GFR and RPF increased 31 and 7 percent, respectively, with a rise in FF from 0.175 to 0.217 (MARKLEY et al.). Oral administration of 1.0 to 1.66 moles of $NaHCO_3$ daily for 20 days to 3 patients with peptic ulcer was associated with increases in inulin clearance of zero, 25 and 55 percent (SANDERSON 1954). Endogenous creatinine or inulin clearances had increased 20, 27 and 38 percent in three subjects after 2 or 3 days of a sustained increase in body water content produced by combined water drinking and injections of Pitressin tannate (LEAF et al. 1953). In a patient with ADDISON's disease GFR was not increased (as measured, it was lower) on a high (30 g.) as compared with a moderate (10 g.) salt diet, but salt excretion rates during the filtration rate measurements were not reported (BURNETT, SELDIN and WALSER).

d) Acute blood sequestration

A variety of procedures have in common the circumstance that they exclude from free circulation a fraction of the blood volume. Although differences may exist in some physiological responses as between one and another of these procedures, little or no difference is evident in the renal hemodynamic changes. Thus, whether blood is removed from free circulation by holding it in a limb by venous tourniquets, by obstructing its return to the heart through a major vein, by orthostatic pooling of blood in the veins of the lower portion of the body or by bleeding, the renal changes are generally the same. An important consideration is whether or not acute hypotension occurs, with or without syncope. With hypotension, pressure becomes insufficient for filtration, urine formation slows, and, in human subjects, reliable measurements of blood flow cannot be made. In the absence of hypotension, GFR decreases by a small to moderate amount, generally in the range of 10 to 30 percent, while RPF decreases to a proportionally much greater extent so that FF regularly increases. Extraction of PAH, as with epinephrine administration, is not changed.

In tilt-table (orthostasis) studies, no change in renal function was oberved during one hour's tilting at 20 degrees from horizontal. Changes were evident, however, at 40 and 60 degree tilt. Considering a limited group of 5 experiments in the 40—60 degree tilt in which both RPF and GFR were measured and in which oliguria was absent, GFR decreased from 126 to 114 (9 percent) while RPF decreased from 628 to 502 (20 percent) with consequent increase in FF from 0.20 to 0.227 (BRUN, KNUDSEN and RAASCHOU 1945a). In an orthostasis experiment reported by SMITH (1939) GFR decreased 39 percent from 140 to 85 ml./min. during 70 degree tilt while RPF decreased 50 percent from 650 to 325 ml./min. FF consequently increased from 0.215 to 0.25. E-pah was unchanged during tilt (WERKO, BUCHT and JOSEPHSON). Effects of blood sequestration have been examined by application of venous tourniquets to the legs, by obstructing inferior or superior caval flow by inflating a balloon carried on an intravenous catheter, or by phlebotomy. Percentage decreases in GFR/RPF in several studies are 24/33 (WILKINS et al.), 15/30 (FITZHUGH et al.), 17/25 during obstruction of the inferior vena cava above the renal veins, 11/25 during caval obstruction below the renal veins and 3/8 percent during obstruction of the superior vena cava (FARBER, BECKER and EICHNA). In one study, however, GFR decreased during orthostasis (quiet standing) relatively more than RPF, 15 percent in the former compared with 11 percent in the latter (EPSTEIN et al. 1951). In other studies, endogenous creatinine clearance decreased 5 percent during standing as compared to values observed during recumbency (SURTSHIN and WHITE), and inulin clearance decreased about 8 percent during sequestration of an estimated 10 to 20 percent of the blood volume by venous tourniquets (LEVITT, TURNER and SWEET). FF was elevated immediately following gastric hemorrhage, as compared to later values following recovery, in three patients of whom two were hypotensive at the time of the first measurement (BLACK, POWELL and SMITH). The decreases in GFR and RPF are not attributable to the antidiuresis observed with these procedures since decreases of the same order of magnitude as in the preceding studies are observed when urine flow is sustained by mannitol infusion (DE WARDENER and McSWINEY).

In various pathological states, blood sequestration by venous tourniquets was associated with decreases in GFR and RPF of 20 and 12 percent in 3 hypertensive patients, 29 and 30 percent in 5 hypertensive patients after sympathectomy, and 9 and 13 percent respectively in patients with congestive heart failure. Following phlebotomy of 450 to 600 ml. blood in 3 patients with congestive heart failure, neither GFR nor RPF changed significantly (WILKINS et al.; JUDSON et al. 1955c). Many of the patients with heart failure, however, exhibited small increases in GFR and RPF during tourniquet application. GFR and RPF decreased 43 and 45 percent, respectively, in a group of patients with chronic nephritis (LATHEM et al.) but the nearly proportional decrease in glucose reabsorptive capacity indicated that depression of filtration, at least, was accomplished in part by nearly complete cessation of filtration in a restricted group of nephrons. Creatinine clearance did not change in a patient with ADDISON's disease (ROSENBAUM, PAPPER and ASHLEY) during tourniquet application. Decreases in GFR and RPF caused by blood sequestration (quiet standing, or leg tourniquets) are particularly marked in pregnant women (DIGNAM, ASSALI and DASGUPTA).

e) Chronic fluid depletion

A decrease in body weight occurs in salt depletion, as well as in water deprivation, indicating that water is lost as well as salt. In either circumstance, a decrease in GFR is the most prominent change in renal function. RPF decreases no more than, and generally less than GFR so that FF frequently falls.

GFR decreased from 114 to 90 ml./min. in 3 normal subjects after 5 to 6 days on a low salt (rice) diet (BLACK, PLATT and STANBURY) and from 141 to 106 ml./min. in 3 subjects on a low salt diet combined with additional salt loss by sweating (McCANCE and WIDDOWSON 1937). In two subjects, GFR was 117 and 121 ml./min. on a low (0.5 g./day) salt diet compared with 158 and 123 ml./min. on an increased (10 g./day) salt diet (LEAF and COUTER). In 4 subjects deprived of water but not salt for 3 to 4 days, average GFR decreased from 124 to 108 while RPF increased from 546 to 610, representing a decrease in FF from 0.227 to 0.177. GFR decreased slightly less than RPF in a group of 5 normal subjects depleted of salt and water by a mercurial diuretic so that they lost an average of 3.6 kg. GFR and RPF in these subjects decreased 3 and 7 percent respectively (WIGGINS et al.).

Extensive studies have been reported on the effects of low salt diets on renal hemodynamics in hypertensive patients. In one series of 10 patients GFR decreased 21 percent and RPF decreased 5 after one or more weeks on a rice diet. Average FF decreased from 0.218 to 0.180. When salt was added to the rice diet of 5 hypertensive subjects, average GFR, RPF and FF increased from 69 to 92, 474 to 494 and from 0.146 to 0.187, respectively (CHASIS et al. 1950). In another series (WESTON et al. 1950) GFR and RPF decreased 22 and 5 percent on a low salt diet (20—35 mM. per day) and 38 and 28 percent on a rice diet. Filtration fraction was 0.189 and 0.200 on the two low salt diets as compared with a control average of 0.233. In other studies, chronic sodium depletion was associated with approximately equiproportional decreases in GFR and RPF of about 45 percent. In a 72 year old patient with congestive heart failure, GFR and RPF were depressed 40 and 26 percent by moderate salt depletion resulting from low salt diet combined with vigorous employment of mercurial diuretics (BLACK and LITCHFIELD).

GFR (estimated as the endogenous creatinine clearance) also decreases on a low salt diet in patients with ADDISON's disease who are maintained on a constant dosage of cortisone (LIPSETT and PEARSON).

4. Congestive heart failure

Renal plasma flow is regularly decreased in chronic congestive heart failure, frequently to extremely low values. In the data summarized in Table 7 representing classes III and IV of functional impairment, average RPF of the

various studies was 250 ml./min. or less than half normal. Values less than
100 ml./min. are observed frequently. No evidence is available that the measured

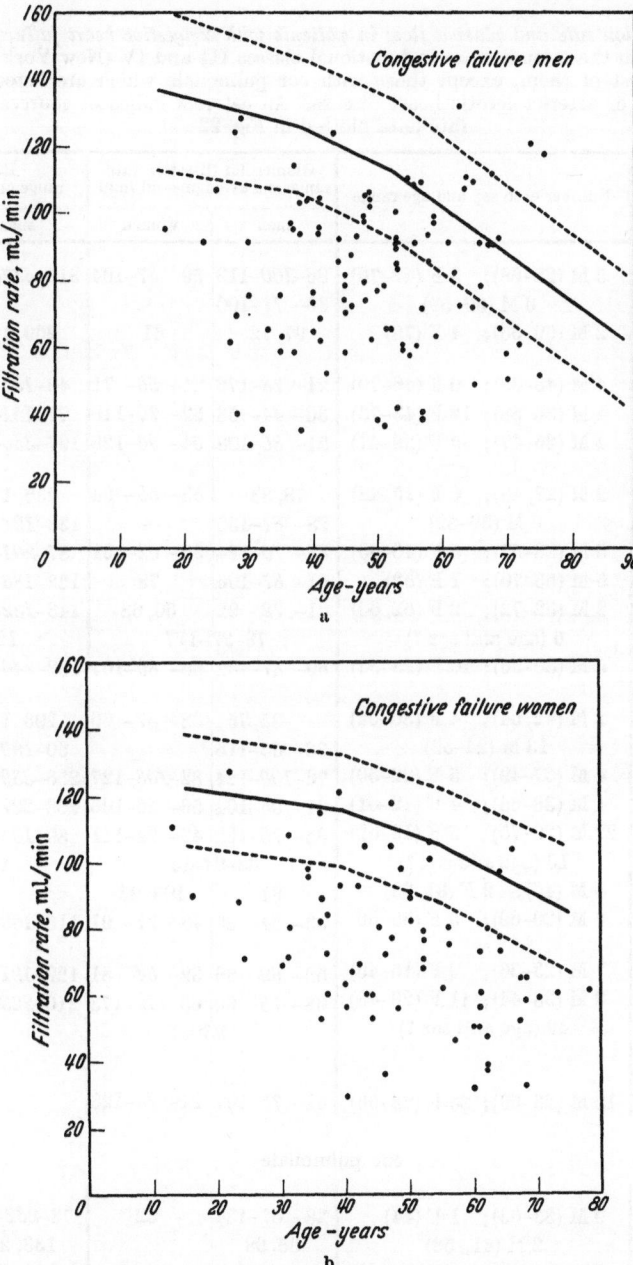

Fig. 22 a and b. Filtration rate per 1.73 M² in men and women with congestive heart failure. The data are taken
from those sources listed in Table 7 which are marked by an asterisk. A few mannitol clearance values
were multiplied by 1.1, the mean inulin-mannitol clearance ratio

plasma flow values are too low because of failure to extract PAH. In 5 patients
with rheumatic heart disease and 2 with cor pulmonale, studied by DAVIES and

Kilpatrick, the lowest extraction observed was 0.81 (normal, 0.91). Extraction in one patient with RPF of 78 ml./min. was 0.87.

Table 7. *Filtration rate and plasma flow in patients with congestive heart failure.* Nearly all of the patients in these studies are in functional classes III and IV (New York Heart Association) and most of them, except those with cor pulmonale which are listed separately, have rheumatic or arteriosclerotic heart disease. An asterisk indicates sources of filtration rate data plotted in Fig. 22

Reference	Number each sex and age range	Glomerular filtration rate range and average — ml./min.		Renal plasma flow range and average — ml./min.	
		men	women	men	women
*Aas & Blegen	5 M (28–68); 3 F (42–70)	86-*100*-113	59- *87*-104	319-*437*-538	335-*390*-495
*Baldwin et al. (1950)	6 M (39–59)	36- *77*-100			
*Blegen[2]	2 M (59, 65); 1 F (78)	97, 72	61	269, 170	203
Brod, Fejfar & Fejfarova[1]	4 M (48–69); 6 F (46–70)	21- *78*-172	21- *56*- 71	49-*157*-339	53-*160*-314
*Brod & Fejfar	4 M (36–58); 12 F (43–73)	36- *44*- 58	32- *70*-118	77-*151*-212	80-*234*-421
Bucht et al. (1956)	4 M (26–47); 5 F (29–47)	51- *86*-108	64- *96*-125	197-*356*-419	331-*401*-512
Davies & Kilpatrick	2 M (27, 48); 6 F (15–48)	78, 83	53- *66*- 94	236, 112	152-*234*-300
*Davis & Shock (1949)	6 M (39–82)	28- *81*-135	—	133-*194*-282	—
*Edelmann et al.	5 M (28–57); 5 F (40–60)	31- *70*-124	32- *62*- 91	87-*201*-316	137-*175*-270
*Eichna et al. (1953)	5 M (53–70); 1 F (52)	61- *87*-106	78	122-*186*-237	151
Farber et al.[1]	8 M (52–72); 2 F (52, 60)	41- *72*- 92	50, 68	143-*182*-235	130, 132
Freeman et al.[1]	6 (age and sex ?)	79-*97*-117		126-*286*-431	
Grossman et al.	5 M (30–56); 10 F (23–55)	59- *87*-102	66- *89*-107	132-*246*-391	220-*292*-434
Hammond & Whittaker[1]	2 M (42, 54); 4 F (36–54)	85, 75	32- *57*- 69	296, 112	85-*195*-282
Heller & Jacobson[4]	13 M (24–59)	38- *83*-115		90-*190*-439	
Judson et al. (1955a)	4 M (37–49); 5 F (22–50)	76-*100*-124	82-*108*-127	256-*339*-451	206-*376*-589
*Judson et al. (1955b)	4 M (38–66); 4 F (42–61)	91- *95*-104	56- *86*-106	206-*227*-279	143-*244*-350
*Merrill	22 M (29–75); 15 F (13–62)	35- *78*-162	47- *74*-111	89-*183*-345	115-*222*-448
Merrill & Cargill	10 (age and sex ?)	65-*94*-143		114-*312*-665	
*Miller et al.	1 M (45); 2 F (31, 39)	81	108, 93		
Mokotoff & Ross[3]	5 M (20–60); 3 F (35–50)	33- *64*- 85	48- *71*- 91	116-*169*-234	88-*204*-280
*Mokotoff, Ross & Leiter	7 M (23–56); 9 F (16–46)	52- *69*- 86	32- *64*- 81	129-*191*-315	138-*191*-266
Werko et al. (1952)	3 M (38–44); 11 F (26–48)	68- *75*- 80	65-*112*-173	210-*229*-244	188-*363*-548
Werko et al. (1955)[1]	49 (age and sex ?)	*93*		*290*	
*Weston Grossman and Leiter, pers. com.	18 M (23–59); 25 F (23–56)	41- *78*-107	24- *75*-128		

cor pulmonale

Davies & Kilpatrick[1]	9 M (33–63); 1 F (44)	28- *67*-134	62	78-*262*-479	261
Eichna et al. (1953)	2 M (41, 56)	96, 98		133, 253	
Fishman et al.	2 M (55, 52); 2 F (64, 56)	58, 80	57, 69	196, 189	210, 280

[1] Not corrected to 1.73 M².
[2] Patients also reported in series of Aas and Blegen are excluded.
[3] Patients also reported in series of Mokotoff, Ross and Leiter are excluded.
[4] Mannitol clearance data are corrected to probable inulin clearance values by multiplying by 1.1.

Filtration rate is also reduced but invariably to a lesser degree than RPF and to an extent which is related to age (Fig. 22). In men and women with heart failure and less than 50 years old, GFR is significantly depressed. In men older than 60, however, GFR has essentially normal values. The reason for this age difference is unknown. That the decrease in filtration rate is uniformly distributed among all nephrons is suggested by the observation that maximal rate of tubular glucose transport is essentially normal (328 mg./min.) in patients with congestive heart failure in whom GFR averaged 89 ml./min. or 25 percent below mean normal for the age of the patients (average, 38 years) (GROSSMAN et al. 1950). If the decrease in GFR had resulted from complete or nearly complete cessation of function in a small block of nephrons, glucose transport should be depressed proportionally to GFR and average about 250 mg./min.

Because of the large decrease in RPF compared with GFR, FF is increased. Average FF of all studies listed in Table 7 is 0.32 which is greater than that observed in any other clinical or experimental condition. Filtration fractions as high as 0.60 are observed too frequently to be attributable to experimental error. In the studies of MERRILL, for example, FF exceeded 0.50 in 10 of 61 measurements. Hemodynamic values return to or toward normal in patients who respond to treatment to the extent that they can tolerate an increase in dietary salt (DAVIES 1951; EICHNA et al. 1953).

Patients with cor pulmonale in congestive heart failure exhibit a hemodynamic pattern similar to that seen with other heart disease (Table 7).

Since GFR necessarily is always lower than ERPF, it is apparent that depression of the former becomes obligatory as RPF drops significantly below 200 ml./min. The extreme rise in FF is evidence, however, of the efficiency with which the effect on GFR of extreme depression in RPF is minimized. A relative maintenance of GFR theoretically could be accomplished by the same mechanisms operative in renal nerve stimulation or epinephrine injection. The effects of large increase in viscosity (FF) on resistance to flow through the efferent arterioles presumably would be exactly cancelled by the corresponding decrease in volume of flow. To what extent the renal nerves or unidentified humoral factors bring about the hemodynamic changes in congestive heart failure is uncertain. MOKOTOFF and ROSS observed no change in average RPF during high spinal anesthesia in a group of 14 heart failure patients, but ephedrine, which they used to sustain blood pressure, might have tended to block a rise in flow. BROD, FEJFAR and FEJFAROVA, however, observed increases in GFR and RPF in most of their patients with congestive failure to whom they gave dibenamine or dihydroergotamine and similar evidence indicating the existence of increased vasomotor activity over the renal nerves has been obtained in dogs with heart failure (BARGER, LIEBOWITZ and MULDOWNEY). Studies of the vasoconstrictor substances renin or renal vasoexcitor material of SHORR and coworkers (1951) indicate that the concentration of each in renal venous blood is increased in congestive heart failure but since volume flow is reduced to nearly $^1/_5$ normal, the total output from the kidney does not appear to be increased (MERRILL, MORRISON and BRANNAN; EDELMAN et al.).

Renal hemodynamic changes during exercise in patients with heart failure are qualitatively similar to those seen in normal subjects but, as might be predicted, appear with smaller work loads (MERRILL and CARGILL; AAS and BLEGEN; WERKÖ et al. 1954a; SINCLAIR-SMITH et al.; FREEMAN et al.; HOLLANDER and JUDSON 1956).

5. Anoxia

The effects of anoxia on human hemodynamics are not clear but the available evidence suggests a tendency for RPF to increase. Neither RPF nor GFR showed any significant change in 8 experiments on 2 healthy subjects during 5 to 17 minute periods of breathing 9.3 to 13 percent oxygen in the studies of Cald-well, Rolf and White. Berger, Galdston and Horowitz, however, observed an increase in GFR and RPF averaging 2.5 and 8.4 percent in 7 normal subjects after 45 to 60 minutes breathing a gas mixture sufficient to lower arterial O_2 tension to about 50 mm. Hg. Larger changes in RPF are observed in patients with emphysema sufficiently severe to interfere with oxygenation of the blood. When emphesematous patients who had been breathing oxygen were returned to room air, average GFR and RPF increased acutely 15 and 29 percent (Berger, Galdston and Horowitz). In 13 emphysematous patients with cor pulmonale of varying severity RPF and GFR averaged 329 and 94 ml./min. while breathing 30 percent O_2 and 374 and 96 ml./min. while breathing 16 percent O_2. This represents an increase of 14 percent in RPF and no significant change in GFR at the lower O_2 tension (Fishman et al. 1951). Neither extraction nor maximal rate of tubular transport of PAH was affected by acute changes in blood oxygenation in either normal or emphysematous subjects (Fishman et al. 1951). Exposure of normal subjects to simulated altitudes of 10,000—18,000 feet for 4 to 6 hours daily for 4 to 6 weeks produced no evident change in RPF or GFR (Alving et al., quoted from Smith 1951), while GFR and RPF in Peruvian Indians acclimatized to 15,000 feet (4,600 M) elevation averaged 11 and 52 percent below and hematocrit 44 percent greater than mean values reported for North Americans and Europeans (Becker, Schilling and Harvey).

6. Anemia and polycythemia

Renal functions are generally elevated in anemic children and reduced in reported studies on chronic anemia in adults. In children with sickle cell, nutritional, Mediterranean (thalassemia) and hemolytic anemias, GFR and ERPF range from average to twice average normal (Bruck; McCrory, Goren and Gornfeld; Heinemann and Cheung). In a group of 12 sicklemic children aged 4 to 11, GFR (mannitol clearance) ranged from 126 to 219, averaging 169, and ERPF ranged from 722 to 1,321 averaging 1,309 ml./min./1.73 M^2. Blood flow was also elevated in spite of the low hematocrit (6.5 to 9 gm./100), ranging from 1,105 to 1,833 ml./min. (Ettledorf, Tuttle and Clayton). Although extraction data are not reported, it seems unlikely that E could be markedly depressed in view of the high value for ERPF.

As the individual with sicklemia ages, GFR declines relative to the normal level for the age. Four women and one man 32 to 37 years old had an average value for GFR of 74 ml./min./1.73 M^2 (range, 59 to 122) compared with 137 (range, 116—150) for 3 women and one man aged 16 to 20. ERPF also declines in roughly the same proportion so that no clear age trend in FF is evident in the sicklemic (Ettledorf et al.).

Bradley and Bradley (1947a) studied 15 adult patients of whom 8 had pernicious anemia and the rest had paroxysmal nocturnal hemoglobinuria, chronic blood loss, iron deficiency or lymphatic leukemia. Hematocrits varied from 13 to 28 percent of blood volume. Since diagnosis showed little correlation with renal function measurements, it will be sufficient to note the overall averages. Renal plasma flow averaged 522 in the 8 male and 534 in the 7 female patients, representing decreases of 20 and 10 percent, respectively, below the mean normal values. In the same groups, GFR was 32 and 11 percent below mean normal. Because of the low hematocrit, however, blood flow was decreased by 28 and 44 percent, respectively. Since extraction ratio of PAH is normal (WARREN, BRANNON and MERRILL) the decrease in RBF is real and cannot represent failure of the kidney to remove the test substance, PAH. RPF and GFR in 5 patients with pernicious anemia averaged 419 and 73 ml./min. and in 6 patients with sickle cell anemia averaged 398 and 60 ml./min. RBF averaged 617 ml./min. in the first group but hematocrits are not reported for the sicklemics (LEVIN, GREGORY and BENNETT). In two female and one male anemic patients reported by AAS and BLEGEN, however, GFR/RPF averaged 121 and 607 ml./min. respectively at an average hematocrit of 19 volumes percent. GFR in four male and three female patients, aged 27 to 68 and with average hemoglobin of 8 gm. percent, averaged 113 ml./min. and does not differ significantly from normal (HEINEMANN and CHEUNG). Renal function changes in chronic anemia are slowly if at all reversible. Transfusion of the two female patients to hematocrits of 43 and 40 percent were accompanied by small decreases in function of questionable significance. Also in the studies of BRADLEY and BRADLEY (1947a), increased hematocrit as the result of therapy was associated in 7 subjects with an average increase of 3.5 ml./min. in GFR and a decrease of 35 ml./min. in RPF. In a patient with pernicious anemia reported by REUBI (1958), filtration rate (thiosulfate clearance) and plasma flow were 126 and 625 ml./min. before treatment with an hematocrit of 0.15, and 110 and 639 ml./per min. after treatment when hematocrit was 0.43. These changes have no statistical significance. Diodrast Tm which averaged 38 and 33 mg. I/min. in the men and the women and is to be compared with mean normal values of 52 and 43, also showed little significant response to therapy. The differences between subacute anemia in dogs and chronic anemia in man must be stressed. In the dog, RPF and GFR increase and extraction decreases. In man, RPF and GFR, while elevated in children, are variably depressed and associated with a normal extraction when these functions are measured in the adult.

The most frequently reported hemodynamic pattern in *polycythemia*, whether primary (vera) or secondary to heart disease, consists of normal or occasionally somewhat depressed filtration rate, moderately to markedly depressed renal plasma flow, and a generally elevated renal blood flow. Average GFR/RPF in 5 patients with polycythemia vera, aged 34 to 64 (average 56) and with hematocrits of 63 to 85 percent was 77.4/300. After the hematocrits had been lowered by phlebotomy, the average values were 82.8/474 (DE WARDENER, MCSWINEY and MILES; REUBI 1952). GFR/RPF in a 54 year old man with a red cell count of 8.2 millions was 184/581 ml./min./1.73 M^2 (CHIARINI). In a group of 19 patients aged 5 to 45 years with cyanotic heart disease and with hematocrits of 60 to 88 percent, FF varied from 0.20 to 0.55, averaging 0.31. Low values of ERPF do not represent failure of extraction of PAH since extraction in 7 patients (omitting two technically doubtful determinations) averaged 87.1 percent (SCOTT and ELLIOTT). Entirely normal hemodynamic values, however, are reported on 5 patients aged 35 to 69 with polycythemia secondary to chronic lung disease. The hematocrits of these subjects was 47 to 65, averaging 56 percent (LEWIS et al. 1952). In 4 men and one woman aged 50 to 62 years and with hematocrits of 44 to 75 percent, GFR was normal in two and depressed (45, 53 and 70 ml./min.)

in three. ERPF, however, was elevated relative to GFR so that FF was 0.112 to 0.176, averaging 0.142 (Bradley et al. 1950).

7. Hypertension

The characteristic renal hemodynamic change in essential hypertension is a large increase in renal vascular resistance, particularly in the preglomerular vessels. According to the calculations of Gomez, afferent resistance, which constitutes 32 percent of the total renal resistance in a group of 22 normal subjects with mean blood pressure 91 mm. Hg, represents 65 percent of the total resistance in a group of 16 subjects with mean blood pressure 145 mm. Hg. RPF is usually slightly reduced but GFR is normal. Filtration fraction therefore is slightly increased, from a normal value of about 20 percent, to 22—32 and averaging about 26 percent (Foa et al. 1942; Friedman, Selzer and Rosenblum 1941b; Goldring et al. 1941; Goldring and Chasis; Gregory et al.; Watkin et al.; Cargill 1949; Weston et al. 1950; Hollander and Judson 1957, 1958; Cottier, Weller and Hoobler 1958a). Tubular function as measured by the maximal tubular capacity to excrete diodrast (Tm-D) tends to be depressed while capacity to reabsorb glucose (Tm-G) is within the normal range. As nephrosclerosis with destruction of renal tissue progresses, Tm-D, GFR and RPF decrease nearly proportionally but with a significant tendency for GFR to decrease relatively less rapidly and RPF relatively more rapidly than tubular function. With decreasing function extraction of PAH also slowly declines, attaining values of 0.6 to 0.7 compared to the normal of 0.9 when filtration rate is 25 to 30 percent of normal (Cargill 1949). These relationships also mark a tendency for FF to increase with decreasing total renal function (Goldring et al. 1941; Talbott et al. 1943; Findley et al.), from 20 to 24 percent when function is good, to 30 to 35 percent when function is poor. Depressed values of Tm-D in hypertensives are not attributable to insufficient renal perfusion, since the values fail to increase during pyrogen hyperemia (Goldring et al. 1941). Tm-D as well as GFR and RPF are depressed to an equal extent in both kidneys (Chasis and Redish).

Measures designed to lower the blood pressure in hypertensives regularly fail to cause an increase in RPF. Specifically, high spinal anesthesia (Page et al. 1944; Corcoran, Taylor and Page 1947; Gregory et al.), splanchnicectomy or sympathectomy (Adams et al.; Corcoran and Page 1941b; Foa et al. 1943; Goldring and Chasis), low salt diets (Watkin et al.; Weston et al. 1950), dibenamine (Weston et al. 1950) and reserpine with or without supplementary or alternative hydralazine or hexamethonium (Hughes, Dennis and Moyer; Hollander and Judson 1957; Unger et al.) failed to cause more than a very small rise in RBF in patients in whom blood pressure decreased significantly following therapy. Gjorup and Hilden, however, reported a rise in RBF and decrease in FF in hypertensive patients provided the decrease in blood pressure was not large. GFR responded variably to these various therapeutic regimes. It decreased on the low salt diets and increased slightly following splanchnicectomy in the data of Foa et al. 1943. In contrast to the negative results of spinal anesthesia in essential hypertension, RPF increased in 8 patients with neurogenic hypertension (Page et al. 1944). Pregnancy does not alter the general pattern of renal function in hypertensive women. In 10 pregnant hypertensive women, GFR and RPF averaged 93 and 435 ml./min. respectively (Robinson et al. 1942).

These studies indicate that no significant amount of the increase in vascular resistance in essential hypertension is attributable to vasoconstrictor activity mediated by way of the renal nerves. They suggest that a large and unknown part of the increase in afferent resistance is attributable to autoregulatory adjustment which, in hypertensive patients, may be more sensitive than in the normal. In experimental renal hypertension produced in the dog by perinephritis or renal artery constriction, GFR and RPF are normal. Only when the hypertension is very severe in these animals are decreases in function observed (CORCORAN and PAGE 1942).

In patients with brachial artery hypertension associated with coartation of the aorta, filtration rate is within normal limits. RPF, however, is variably decreased, probably in relation to the severity of the disease, to values which may be 30 percent below the mean normal. In several studies representing 45 patients, FF varies from 0.21 to 0.29 with an overall average of about 0.23 (FRIEDMAN, SELZER and ROSENBLUM 1941a; GENEST et al. 1948; HARRIS, SEALY and DeMARIA; WERKO et al. 1956; KIRKENDALL, CULBERTSON and ECKSTEIN). Following surgical correction of the coarctation, RPF returns to essentially normal values (GENEST et al. 1948).

Table 8. *Renal hemodynamics in toxemia of pregnancy and essential hypertension during pregnancy* [1], [2], [3]

Reference	GFR[4]			RPF		
	normal pregnant	pre-eclamptic toxemia	hypertension in pregnancy	normal pregnant	pre-eclamptic toxemia	hypertension in pregnancy
ASSALI et al. (1953)[5]	121 (7)	86 (9)	88 (4)	699	557	422
CHESLEY et al. (1939, 1940)[6]				610 (8)	579 (21)	
CHESLEY & WILLIAMS[7]	131 (10)	95 (10)				
CORCORAN & PAGE (1941)[8]		108 (4)	62 (1)		534	276
DILL et al. (1942)	116 (8)	84 (10)	87 (10)	637	680	515
KARIBER & GEORGE	150 (8)	112 (14)	145 (8)	754	555	613
TAYLOR et al.	124 (20)	102 (7)	111 (6)	631	663 (5)	430

[1] A few patients with overt eclampsia have been omitted.
[2] Patients are designated as having essential hypertension if blood pressure was known to be elevated before pregnancy or remained elevated after delivery.
[3] All figures corrected to 1.73 M² surface area at time of measurement except those of CHESLEY and WILLIAMS.
[4] The figures in parentheses are the number of subjects in each group.
[5] The mannitol clearance data in this study have been multiplied by 1.1, the mean inulin-mannitol clearance ratio.
[6] Average RPF of 6 eclamptic patients was 526 ml./min.
[7] Corrected to 1.73 M² SA nonpregnant.
[8] Average RPF and GFR of 5 eclamptic patients was 525 and 99 ml./min.

8. Toxemia of pregnancy

Data on renal hemodynamics in pregnant women with preeclamptic toxemia are summarized in Table 8. RPF averages slightly below that expected in normally pregnant women and GFR is reduced relatively more than RPF with the result that FF is lowered. Postpartum, RPF in the preeclamptic patient decreases slightly as does that in the normal, while GFR rises, with the result that FF returns to normal. For unexplained reasons, however, renal function in preeclamptic patients averages less than normal for an indefinite period postpartum (Dill et al. 1942b). Renal function data in pregnant women with essential hypertension are included in Table 8 for comparison. The tendency for FF to be slightly elevated in hypertensive subjects persists in pregnancy.

9. Cirrhosis

The renal hemodynamic changes in Laennec's cirrhosis are unique in certain respects (Table 9). In patients who are less severely ill and who have no history of ascites formation, both GFR and RPF are increased, GFR particularly so. Filtration fraction is increased, averaging 26.5 percent in these studies. In patients with progressively more advanced disease, RPF and GFR are lower.

In patients forming ascites relatively slowly, all functions are within normal limits, while in the most severely ill group GFR and RPF are in the lower limits of the normal range.

Table 9. *Renal plasma flow and filtration rate in patients with cirrhosis.* Figures in parentheses refer to the number of patients in each group

	GFR	RPF	FF
No ascites			
Leslie et al. . .	213 (6)	805	26.5
Slow ascites			
Leslie et al. . .	107 (6)	592	18.1
Patek et al. . .	132 (3)	581	22.7
Jones et al. . .	104 (8)	562	18.5
Rapid ascites			
Leslie et al. . .	88 (7)	517	17.0
Normal	115	575	20

10. Nephrosis

Renal hemodynamic measurements in the nephrotic syndrome are difficult to interpret for several reasons. Most of the observations are on children in whom the normal values are less well established than in adults. Moreover, it is difficult to determine the extent to which glomerular or vascular damage may have affected the observed hemodynamic values. The factors which operate to change renal function in nephrosis are probably diverse both in their origin and in their effects so that the final pattern in any patient will be determined by the extent to which one or another factor predominates. In Table 10 are summarized data on untreated nephrotic patients with minimal hypertension, hematuria and azotemia. The variability is so large that averages have little significance. Low values are attributable for the most part to disorganization and degeneration of the parenchyma, particularly the glomeruli. In addition, some depression of function probably occurs in response to loss of fluid from the blood into extravascular spaces during edema formation. The mechanisms responsible for producing supranormal renal function values with considerable frequency are nor clear. Emerson, Futcher and Farr and Emerson and Dole drew attention to nephrotic children with GFR and RPF exceeding 200 and 800 ml./min./1.73 M^2 and equally high values may be observed in other studies (Table 10). The supranormal hemodynamic values appear to be part of a general increase in renal function probably secondary to nutritional or endocrine influences since tubular transport capacity for glucose and PAH also tend to be elevated above normal and frequently to a greater degree than GFR (Eder et al.; Galan; Bruck, Rapoport and Rubin; Metcoff, Nakasone and Rance; Metcoff, Kelsey and Janeway). Renal hemodynamics in nephrosis are consistent in two respects: FF is usually decreased in untreated patients averaging approximately 0.17 with values as low as 0.10 frequently observed; and GFR increases markedly during treatment with ACTH, corticosteroids of human serum albumin so that FF averages about 0.24. Changes in RPF are irregular following treatment but increasing about 10 percent in the overall averages (James, Gordillo and

METCOFF; LUETSCHER, HALL and KREMER; METCOFF, KELSEY and JANEWAY; METCOFF, NAKASONE and RANCE; BARNETT et al. 1951; LAUSON et al. 1954; EDER et al.). In the four nephrotic children with hypernormal function reported by EMERSON and DOLE, however, FF was elevated, varying from 0.21 to 0.32, as the result of a relatively greater increase above normal in filtration rate than in plasma flow. In 4 adult glomerulonephritic nephrotics, GFR was markedly while RPF was only slightly depressed, Table 10 (BRADLEY et al. 1950).

In a patient with syphilitic nephrosis, GFR, RPF and FF were 76 and 456 ml./min. and 0.17. Thirty-nine and 80 days following penicillin therapy all

Table 10. *Renal plasma flow and glomerular filtration rate in nephrosis.* All data adjusted to 1.73 M². Average values are italicized

Reference	Number, sex and age	GFR	RPF
METCOFF et al. .	4 F (2–6)	49– *81*–117	465–*510*– 800
METCOFF et al. .	8 M, 12 F (1–14)	7– *64*–160	35–*404* 841
BRUCK et al. . .	11 M, 9 F (1–11)	19–*139*–258	103–*745*–1907
BARNETT et al. .	5 M, 3 F (3– 4)	24– *80*–147	215–*462*– 695
JAMES et al. . .	1 M, 2 F (3–12)	43– *63*– 99	460–*526*– 570
GALAN	7 M, 2 F (2–10)	91–*143*–208	
LAUSON et al. . .	6 M, 3 F (2– 7)	18– *70*–149	82–*397*– 783
EMERSON & DOLE[1]	1 M, 3 F (3–10)	178–*205*–243[1]	622–*852*–1138[1]
BRADLEY et al. .	3 M, 1 F (17–36)	43– *49*– 58	321–*490*– 684
FRIEDERISZICK .	4 M, 1 F (3–10)	22– *45*– 74	170–*341*– 698

[1] Selected patients with high renal function.

signs of nephrosis and renal involvement were absent and these values changed to 121 and 152 ml./min. for GFR and 418 and 494 ml./min. for RPF. Tubular transport of PAH, also depressed during the nephrotic phase, had returned to normal levels (FURMAN et al.).

11. Hyper- and hypothyroidism

Both GFR and RPF are reduced in human hypothyroid states. Surprisingly, however, these functions are frequently increased comparatively little in hyperthyroidism. No clear trends in FF are evident, since RPF may decrease relatively either more or less than GFR in myxedema or increase either more or less than GFR in hyperthyroidism. GFR and RPF of 14 *myxedematous* patients averaged 65 and 347 ml./min./1.73 M² with a filtration fraction of 0.188 (CORCORAN and PAGE 1947; HLAD and BRICKER; YOUNT and LITTLE). GFR/RPF of 6 female myxedematous patients studied by DAVIES, MACKINNON and PLATTS averaged 68/495 ml./min. while that of a 26 year old woman studied by LUFT and SJÖGREN (1950) was 59/316. In 8 *hyperthyroid* patients, on the other hand, GFR was approximately normal, but RPF was relatively increased, the values averaging 129 and 740 ml./min./1.73 M² respectively, with FF averaging 0.174 (CORCORAN and PAGE 1947; AAS and BLEGEN; HLAD and BRICKER). In 6 hyperthyroid women studied by BRADLEY (1955) mannitol clearance was significantly elevated, averaging 139 ml./min./1.73 M². Since mannitol tends to give a slightly low estimate of GFR, the true values may well have been 10 percent greater, ranging from 133 to 178 ml./min. Values of RPF tended to be increased to the extent reported by others, ranging from 525 to 1,080 and averaging 780 ml./min./1.73 M². The apparently random correlation between GFR and RPF changes is illustrated by values for FF ranging from 0.12 to 0.27. Thyroid function is not specifically reported on the 7 myxedematous patients of YOUNT and LITTLE or the hyperthyroid patients of BRADLEY (1955). Thyroid function is measured by basal metabolic rate in the myxedematous and hyperthyroid patients of CORCORAN and PAGE (1947), DAVIES, MacKINNON and PLATTS, and LUFT and SJÖGREN (1950) and the 2 hyperthyroid patients of AAS and BLEGEN, and is measured by radioactive iodine uptake in the 4 hyperthyroid and 5 myxedematous patients of HLAD and BRICKER. In the hyperthyroid patients, BMR averaged plus 70 (CORCORAN and PAGE 1947) and plus 123 (AAS and BLEGEN) percent and radioiodine uptake in 24 hours averaged 65 percent. Tubular transport capacity measured by diodrast or PAH is consistently below normal in the myxedematous and above normal in the hyperthyroid patients (CORCORAN and PAGE 1947; HLAD and BRICKER). Functions revert to or toward normal following treatment.

In dogs, thyroidectomy results in a decrease in GFR, RPF and tubular transport, while thyroid or thyroxine feeding results in an increase in these functions (HEINBECKER, ROLF and WHITE; HARE et al. 1944; EILER, ALTHAUSEN and STOCKHOLM 1944a; WHITE, HEINBECKER and ROLF 1947).

12. Adrenal cortex and anterior pituitary

These endocrine organs exert very different effects upon the kidney in experimental animals. Their inclusion here under a single heading reflects the paucity of information in man.

The principal effect of adrenalectomy in the dog is dehydration resulting from unremitting sodium chloride loss. Although the salt loss results from a quantitatively small change in overall tubular function, the cumulative effects on the animal are devastating and GFR and RPF may decrease to very low values. If efforts are made to prevent salt depletion the changes in GFR and RPF are less remarkable although still significant, and decreases in these functions in different experimental situations range from 6 to 77 percent and average about 40 percent. Various tubular functions decrease about 20 to 30 percent. Whole adrenal extract is more effective than desoxycorticosterone in restoring function to or nearly to normal in the adrenalectomized dog.

Removal of either the anterior or the entire pituitary in dogs is followed by decreases in GFR and RPF to about 60 percent of normal but some tubular functions such as glucose transport may be reduced to extremely low values, 10 to 30 percent of normal. In addition, dehydration does not occur. Since adrenocorticotropin (ACTH) is an important member of the several principles elaborated by the anterior hypophysis, the effects of ACTH administration to hypophysectomized dogs have been examined. ACTH results in significant improvement in hemodynamic and tubular functions but the improvement is usually to about $2/3$ of the normal levels. The somatotrophic principle of the anterior pituitary, however, causes large increases in all renal functions and to levels frequently twice normal. This is the circumstance whether somatotropin is given to normal or, in conjunction with ACTH, to hypophysectomized dogs. Conclusions as to the effects of ACTH and somatotropin should not be accepted uncritically since it is felt that each of the purified preparations remains contaminated with small, unknown, but functionally significant quantities of the other principles (WHITE, HEINBECKER and ROLF 1941, 1942, 1949a, b; GAUDINO and LEVITT; SURTSHIN, ROLF and WHITE; EARLE et al. 1953; GERSHBERG, HODLER and GASCH; HOWELL, DAVIS and LAQUER; GERSHBERG and GASCH; LITTLE, KELSEY and YOUNT).

Renal functions are generally depressed in adrenocortical and adenohypophyseal hypofunction in man. Average GFR in 8 men and 2 women with ADDISON's disease controlled by a high salt diet and averaging 42 years old (range, 21 to 57) was 87.4 ml./min./1.73 M² (TALBOTT et al. 1942). RPF measured in 7 subjects averaged 516 ml./min. and tubular transport capacity was also decreased. FF at times of simultaneous RPF and GFR determinations was low, averaging 14.7. In other studies values of 84/485 and 70/390 ml./min./1.73 M² are reported for GFR/RPF in 2 female Addisonians aged 36 and 39 (WATERHOUSE and KEUTMANN) and 63/457 ml./min. in a 51 year old female patient with combined ADDISON's disease and diabetes insipidus (SKILLERN, CORCORAN and SCHERBEL). The mannitol clearance data in these two studies has been multiplied by 1.1, the average inulin-mannitol clearance ratio, to yield the above figures. In 7 other patients (3 female, 4 male; average age 46) under treatment with desoxycorticosterone and with or without supplementary salt, GFR and RPF were not significantly different from the non-desoxycorticosterone treated patients, averaging 67 and 342 ml./min. GFR/RPF in 8 patients studied by LUFT and SJÖGREN (1949b, c) and averaging 32 years old was 70/365 ml./min. before treatment. During treatment with 10—20 mg. desoxycorticosterone and 5—10 g. sodium chloride daily, the values were 105/368. WATERHOUSE and KEUTMANN also found some decrease in tubular transport capacity of PAH in their patients.

In normal man, both acute and chronic administration of cortisone and hydrocortisone are associated with increases in glomerular filtration rate, although the mechanisms are probably somewhat different in the acute as compared with the chronic circumstance. Acutely, small to moderate increases in GFR are observed in most subjects when these steroids are administered intravenously at the rate of 50 mg. or more per hour. Smaller quantities intravenously, or oral or intramuscular administration, are not clearly associated with changes in filtration (LAIDLAW et al. 1955; HUFFMAN et al. 1956; RAISZ et al.; DINGMAN et al.). Chronic administration of adrenocorticotropin, cortisone, hydrocortisone and prednisone is associated with large increases in GFR. The increase is gradual, attaining in 5 to 10 days values which may be nearly double the control (INGBAR et al. 1950, 1951; BURNETT; ALEXANDER et al.; RAISZ et al.; FROESCH et al.). The hemodynamic effects are similar to those associated with chronic salt or water loading in that RBF increases relatively less than GFR or may not change significantly. The changes are probably caused for the most part by the tendency of these steroids to cause varying degrees of salt and water retention. A 30 percent rise in GFR is reported also in subjects on a salt-poor diet who are receiving cortisone. This is presumably explained by an expansion of the extracellular fluid volume, the latter resulting from internal shifts of salt and water and serving as a stimulus to filtration (LEVITT and BADER). The effects of acute administration of steroids on RPF have not been described. In patients with ADDISON's disease, relatively small (1—10 mg. per hr. intravenously) quantities of hydrocortisone may cause significant increases in GFR (LAIDLAW et al. 1955; DINGMAN et al.).

In a total of 12 patients with panhypopituitarism (9 men and 3 women aged 18 to 70, average 44) GFR averaged 72 ml./min./1.73 M². RPF and FF, measured in 8 subjects, averaged 339 ml./min. and 0.23. Tubular transport capacity of PAH was greatly diminished in 7 of 9 subjects studied (WATERHOUSE and KEUTMANN; HLAD and BRICKER). GFR/RPF averaged 40/185 in 3 women aged 28, 39 and 52 years old studied by LUFT and SJÖGREN (1949a, 1950). In 3 patients with panhypopituitarism reported by BURSTON and GARROD GFR averaged about 47 ml./min. but age, sex and size are not given. Luft and Sjögren (1949a, 1950) studied the effects of hormonal treatment on 2 patients. Thyroxine administered in amounts sufficient to restore metabolic rate to normal was associated with a 50 and 100 percent increase in ERPF although the values (331 and 290 ml./min.) were still below normal. GFR increased relatively much less, about 30 percent. Desoxycorticosterone either alone or combined with thyroxine was associated with no significant change in RPF but was associated with a 30 percent increase in GFR. ACTH (25 mg. daily) alone, in one patient, was associated with little change in function.

GFR/RPF of five male and seven female acromegalic patients aged 23 to 54 years old studied by Ikkos, Ljunggren and Luft averaged 152/800 and 135/634 ml./min./1.73 M^2. These figures are compared with average values in their laboratory of 108/573 and 106/490 for normal men and women of approximately the same age range. In an earlier study by Luft and Sjögren (1950), GFR/RPF (uncorrected for surface area) in 5 male and 3 female acromegalic patients averaging 44 and 36 years old was 142/507 and 155/493, respectively. They do not evaluate the degree of clinical activity of the disease. In three male patients with active acromegaly studied by Gershberg, Heinemann and Stumpf, Dustan (pers. comm.) and Fishman (pers. comm. to Gershberg et al.) GFR was 237, 320 and 178 ml./min./1.73 M^2. RPF was 1063 ml./min./1.73 M^2 and FF 0.30 in Corcoran's patient, and 653 and 844 ml./min./1.73 M^2 on two occasions in the patient of Fishman. Tubular transport capacity for PAH, glucose and sulfate was greatly increased. Increases in function are reported by Heller, Smith and Lubin.

13. Gondal hormones: testosterone and estradiol

Neither testosterone propionate (25—100 mg./day) nor estradiol benzoate (4—6 mg./day) causes significant changes in filtration rate or renal blood flow in man (Lattimer; Klopp, Young and Taylor 1945; Dean, Abels and Taylor; Langeron, Nolf and Liefooghe; Dignam, Voskian and Assali). Similar lacks of effect are observed in the dog (Lattimer; Welsh et al.; Richardson and Houck). Testosterone has, however, been reported to increase levels of both hemodynamic and diodrast transport functions during compensatory hypertrophy following unilateral nephrectomy in rat, dog and man (Lattimer).

14. Ureteral and abdominal pressure

Acute elevation in ureteral pressure causes a roughly proportional decrease in filtration rate but little change in blood flow until pressures equal to or higher than those following complete ureteral obstruction are applied (Section C I 6a).

Sustained ureteral occlusion is associated with rapid deterioration of function, the mechanism of which in the earliest stages is unknown. Filtration rate, as measured an hour after release of a ureter which had been occluded for one week, averaged 27 percent of the control value and recovery over one to three weeks after release was incomplete (Kerr 1954, 1956).

When intrabdominal pressure is raised the pressure change can probably be viewed as being transmitted in a roughly equal manner to the entire renal contents. Of the pressure changes thus effected, the most important is the arterio-venous pressure difference, the gradients between vein and interstitial fluid and between tubule and interstitial fluid being largely unaffected. Hemodynamically, the effects should be roughly equivalent to those which would follow a simple lowering of the renal arterial pressure by an amount equal to the intrabdominal pressure rise. In the dog ERPF and GFR decreased with increasing abdominal pressure between 10 mm. Hg, representing the control level of intrarenal pressure, and 50 mm. Hg at which urine formation and hence measurable clearances ceased (FRENCH, MOLANO and BOOKER). In man, increasing intrabdominal pressure to 20 mm. Hg was associated with decreases in RPF and GFR of about 24 and 28 percent, respectively, while glucose transport capacity was decreased roughly in proportion to filtration rate (BRADLEY and BRADLEY 1947 b). Blood pressures are not reported in these studies, however.

15. Effect of temperature

Renal blood flow tends to rise with increasing temperature and fall with decreasing body temperature. The mechanisms involved are not clear. Changes in blood viscosity and in renal oxygen consumption with changing temperature undoubtedly affect blood flow but their importance in the intact organism has not been evaluated. Hyperemia associated with fever resulting from pyrogens is complicated by the fact that the pyrogenic substances which have been employed cause renal hyperemia even when fever is prevented by antipyretics (Section CV2e).

When the body is cooled all renal functions decrease. In two subjects whose body temperature (rectal) was lowered to 27—30° C, GFR/RPF decreased from 120/650 to 70/230 (TALBOTT 1951). The rise in FF from 18.5 to 30.5 with cooling is probably genuine and not caused by failure of extraction, since a similar rise in FF was observed in the dog in which extraction remained constant over the observable range of body cooling (PAGE 1955). In the studies of PAGE and also of BLATTEIS and HORVATH on the dog, GFR and RPF decreased about 5 and 8 percent of the control values, respectively, per degree of decrease in temperature. These values agree closely with those observed by TALBOTT in man.

D. Tubular transport

I. Classification of transport processes

1. Energetics

The corollary of the filtration hypothesis of renal function in mammals is that large quantities of materials in the glomerular filtrate are returned to the blood stream so that the urine represents only a small amount of the total quantities of material filtered. The operation of returning constituents of the filtrate to the blood is termed *tubular reabsorption*. In addition, certain substances may appear in the urine in amounts greater than the amounts filtered, indicating that *tubular secretion* has occurred. Both reabsorption and secretion are termed, generally, *tubular transport*, irrespective of mechanisms involved.

Transport always depends ultimately upon an energy supply. It is convenient, however, to classify the tubular transport of various substances according to the source of the energy which is utilized in the transfer process. If energy is supplied by the cell directly to the transported substance with the result that the substance either can or does move from a lower to a higher chemical potential the process may usually be termed *active transport*. Alternatively, a substance may traverse the epithelium because of a concentration gradient which has been created in other ways as by active transport of other substances. This process may be termed *passive transport* or *diffusion*. It should be noted, however, that energy was required to create the initial concentration gradient and the diffusing substance never moves to a higher concentration.

Biochemists are not in agreement on a classification of the various theoretical mechanisms by which a substance can traverse a set of one or more cell membranes. For representative discussions of the problems of classification and differing usage USSING, ROSENBERG, TOSTESON, and JARDETZKY may be consulted. The views of these and other researchers may be found in symposia such as Electrolytes in Biological Systems, Waverly Press, Baltimore, 1955; Metabolic Aspects of Transport Across Cell Membranes, University of Wisconsin Press, Madison, 1957; and Active Transport and Secretion, Academic Press, New York, 1954. The most widely recognized mechanisms of transport are as follows:

a) **Energy of transport of the substrate is derived or could be derived solely from its electrochemical potential gradient across the membranes.** Electrochemical potential includes all sources of energy in a solution, such as temperature, pressure, electrical potential, as well as concentration or activity which could drive a diffusion process.

α) *No chemical interaction with elements of the membrane is demonstrable during passage through the membrane.* This has been termed 'diffusion' or 'free diffusion'. When concentration difference is the principal energy source the process for non-electrolytes can generally be described in a satisfactory way by FICK's diffusion law. Diffusion may be fast or slow, but the rate of passage (flux) is directly proportional to the electrochemical potential difference. Unfortunately for any simple categorization, however, the permeability constant, such as the fraction of the surface area of the cell available for free diffusion, could be subject to cellular control or even could vary with the chemical potential difference.

β) *The substrate interacts at least once with one or more elements of the membrane as a requisite to passage.* Various processes of this nature have been termed 'exchange diffusion', and 'facilitated diffusion' depending upon details of kinetics and the point of view of the author. Consider, for example, a substance, S, which cannot freely traverse a membrane but which can react with equal velocity from either side of the membrane with an element, M, in the membrane to form SM. Consider further that SM can dissociate to yield S and M but that the rate of dissociation is equal on both sides of the membrane. In this circumstance, energy of transport is derived from the chemical potential gradient, but, if the rate of dissociation of SM is slow compared with the rate of reaction S and M, then transport will not increase as a linear function of the potential gradient but may seem to approach limiting values (WILBRANDT 1956). If, however, rate of dissociation of SM is very large, then any limitation to transport due to reaction with S may not be detectable and the mechanism cannot be distinguished from free diffusion. Furthermore, the velocity constants of the reactions involving S and M may be subject to cellular control or may be a function of the electrochemical potential gradient of S.

γ) A current of water may carry small solute molecules with it as it traverses a pore in a membrane. This process, termed 'solvent drag' or bulk flow can theoretically move solute molecules against their concentration gradient and includes the process of glomerular filtration.

b) **Energy of transport of the substrate across the membranes is derived partly from metabolic energy of the cell.** Reaction of the substrate with one or more elements in the membranes is implicit. This process has regularly been included under the term 'active transport'. In the simplest example, which probably does not exist in nature but which may serve as an example, we may refer to the model described above. The cell may supply energy in such a way that the rate of dissociation of SM is greater, or else the rate of reaction of S and M is lower, in one direction from the membrane than in the opposite direction. If the rate of dissociation in one direction becomes zero, then this model reduces to that of SHANNON (1939). The number of variations within this system are so large that further classification has little to offer here. Energy derived from the electrochemical potential gradient may be either added to or subtracted from the energy supplied by the cell. Cellular energy potentials may be large or small relative to possible electrochemical potential differences across the membrane. Either free or restricted exchange diffusion may proceed concomitantly with energized transport. Among all of these theoretically possible transport systems the only system which can be unquestionably recognized experimentally is that in which net transport proceeds or can proceed against the existing chemical potential gradient. Transport may be termed 'passive' if without, or 'active' if with energy contributions from cell metabolism. Active transport is broadened to include any cellular transport process for which evidence exists that it is energized irrespective of whether or not an adverse chemical potential exists at a given moment. Classification of the renal transport of many substances must, however, be very tentative.

For example, removal of solutes in the proximal segment of the nephron leaves intratubular water hypoosmotic to blood (concentration gradient of water) with the result that energy is available to transport water. Removal of water together with many solutes from tubular fluid creates a concentration gradient between tubular lumen and blood for other substances such as dissolved carbon dioxide, acetone, and urea, so that these cell-permeable substances may now cross the epithelium. Nearly all renal passive transport processes are dependent for their energy supply on one or the other of two active processes. One of these is the bulk removal of solutes and, secondarily, water as in the above example, which creates high intratubular concentrations of some filtered substances. The other active transport process which results in concentration gradients is the creation of a hydrogen ion (p_H) gradient across the membrane

Table 11. *Classification of substances transported across the tubular epithelium according to whether transport is "active" or "passive"*

Active		Passive	
Reabsorption	Secretion	Reabsorption	Secretion
		(secondary to solute reabsorption)	
Sugars (pentoses and hexoses)	Certain organic bases	Water	None
		Acetone	
Amino acids	Certain aromatic	Ethanol	
Ascorbic acid	acids	Carbon dioxide	
Certain organic acids (as lactic etc.)	Hydrogen	Urea	
	Potassium	(secondary to p_H difference)	
Phosphate	Ammonium	Bicarbonate in	Ammonia
Sulfate	Creatinine	part (?)	Weak acids in alkaline urine (?)
Potassium		Weak acids in acid	
Sodium (and chloride ?)		urine	Weak bases in acid
Urate		Weak bases in alkaline urine (?)	urine (?)
Bicarbonate in part (?)			
Calcium			
Magnesium			

by the secretion of hydrogen ions. Substances whose transport may be governed entirely or in part by transepithelial p_H differences are some weak acids and weak bases. These substances exist in solutions partly in an ionized and partly in a nonionized phase, the relative proportions of the 2 phases being dependent mostly upon the p_H of the solution and upon the pK of the substance. Since the permeability of the epithelium is rarely the same toward each of the two phases, the substance will tend to accumulate in that solution in which, as a result of a p_H difference, the less permeative of the two phases is present in relatively greater abundance.

In Table 11 various substances are listed according to whether they are believed to be actively or passively transported by the tubules. Some substances are transported by more than one system. Potassium, for example, is both actively secreted and actively reabsorbed. Ammonia excretion is determined by rate of cell synthesis and by hydrogen ion secretion. With the possible exceptions of the highly diffusible ethanol and acetone, serious deficiencies exist in our knowledge of all tubular transport processes.

Theoretically, quantitative limits to any active transport process exist. In defining these limits it is necessary first to postulate the existence of some form of carrier system.

6*

Unfortunately, the details of no cellular carrier system have yet been discovered. The general types of carrier which have been suggested are the migrating complex (e.g. see Thomas), the 'energy ladder' and the membrane transport (Wilbrandt 1954). In the 'migrating complex' system the substrate to be secreted reacts with a carrier molecule at one pole of the cell; the complex then moves to the opposite pole where energy sufficient to break the bond between substrate and carrier is received and the substrate is released. In the 'energy ladder', the substrate reacts at one pole with the first of a series of specific reactive sites which extend across the cell. Each successive binding site from blood to luminal surface has a higher bonding energy and therefore can take a substrate molecule from a preceding site. At the opposite pole, energy is supplied which breaks the last bond, releasing the substrate molecule. In the membrane transport system, active transport of the substrate takes place only at one or both surfaces of the cell while passage of the substrate across the cell is by diffusion. The membrane carrier is a special case of the first two systems in that either a migrating complex or energy chain is presumed to extend no more than through the thickness of the membrane instead of through the full length of the cell.

Quantitative limit to the rate of transport of a specific transported substance may occur from any of four general causes: 1. The rate of access of the substance to the first portion of the carrier system may be limited. Effective renal blood flow, blood concentration, binding by plasma proteins, and various barriers to diffusion can limit the supply to the cell of the transported substance. In addition, molecular configuration, such as the presence of side chains near the reactive pole of the molecule and also molecular size could interfere in varying degrees with penetration of the cell surface. 2. The number of reactive sites on the carrier system is limited; that is, the system can be transporting a certain limited number of molecules at a given moment. 3. The cell energy which is available to the carrier system can be limited. With respect to possibilities 2 and 3, clear experimental distinction can seldom be made between the physical size of the carrier system and the rapidity of its use or the number of reactive sites which become available for transport per unit time. This last measures the rate of energy utilization by the system and is in turn substantially dependent on the energy supply. This complex limit to transport in which several variables are interdependent is an extremely important one in renal physiology and constitutes the *"tubular transport maximum"*, or *Tm*, of renal function measurements[1]. 4. The concentration gradient of the substance between blood and tubular lumen can be limiting. When substrate supply is adequate, transport is limited by product of energy supply and size of the carrier system. Concentration gradient presumably becomes a particularly important limiting factor in *in vitro* studies where no glomerular filtration is available to remove transported substance from the luminal surface of the tubule and thus prevent the luminal concentration from reaching such high values that further transport ceases. Cessation of transport could occur either because each of the reactions involved in active transport might be reversible, or because an alternate pathway for retrograde movement, as by diffusional processes, might exist. In either circumstance movements of substrate in each direction would approach equality as concentration difference increased.

One of the more widely applicable of biochemical descriptions of tubular active transport processes is that implicit in the Michaelis-Menten equation. When the variables are represented in terms applicable to renal function, this equation takes the form, $T = \dfrac{P \times Tm}{P + K}$ where T is observed rate of transport, Tm is maximal rate of transport as described above, P is plasma concentration of

---

[1] The abbreviation, *Tm*, was first applied by Smith, Goldring and Chasis to the term, "tubular mass". Since the methods of measurement and basic concepts are the same, the functional term, "transport maximum", will be substituted for the somewhat restrictive term, "tubular mass", and *Tm* can be applied to either.

the substrate and K is an affinity constant. It can be seen that as P increases, T approaches Tm as a limiting value, but that the rate that T approaches Tm is determined by the affinity constant, K. This particular equation is a valid description of the relation of transport to substrate concentration only within the context of the following conditions and assumptions: 1. Within the transport system, which can be complex, one reaction is substantially slower than the others and therefore represents the principal limiting reaction in the overall transport process; 2. This limiting reaction can be described by the MICHAELIS-MENTEN equation, which is a general description of certain first-order reactions between an enzyme and its substrate. 3. The concentration of the substrate, as related to the limiting reaction, is a constant fraction of the plasma concentration; 4. Transport can be considered to be independent of substrate concentration at the outflux surface of the cell (predicted for a first order reaction); 5. Alternative metabolic pathways by which the substrate as a function of its concentration can variably affect the limiting reaction do not exist; and 6. All other terms are constant. The load-transport relationship of all known active transport processes is asymptotic in character (in the sense that as substrate concentration indefinitely increases, transport rate approaches a fixed, constant value) and therefore can be fitted, at least roughly, to the MICHAELIS-MENTEN equation. An analogous mathematical description of transport kinetics has been framed by SHANNON (1939). Since most asymptotic equations fit renal transport data about equally well, a fit of neither the MICHAELIS-MENTEN nor SHANNON'S equation constitutes, alone, good evidence that the transport process is of a nature which these equations were designed to describe.

2. Titration curves

A concentration-transport relationship as represented in the MICHAELIS-MENTEN equation can seldom be examined directly in the intact kidney. Instead, the volume of the medium which contains the substrate constitutes an additional limiting variable. The product of volume and concentration, that is, the quantity or load of substrate available to the epithelium for transport, is generally employed as an alternative to concentration. In secretory transport processes, load equals plasma concentration times volume of postglomerular blood flow (ERPF-GFR). In reabsorptive processes, load equals filtrate concentration times rate of glomerular filtration. Transport as related to load is a complex entity and volume and concentration are not interchangeable. An additional complicating factor in evaluating tubular transport is that load is not necessarily distributed uniformly with relation to transport capacity. Two nephrons of equal capacity may have different glomerular filtration rates or may be perfused by different volumes of blood flow. Since concentration may be assumed to be uniform at any moment, asymmetry in distribution of load is actually asymmetry in distribution of volume. Generally, as noted earlier with respect to nephron populations, filtration rate tends to be nearly proportional to reabsorptive capacity in the instances where this problem has been studied. A similar tendency to equiproportionality appears to exist with respect to secretion and tubular blood supply.

The rate of transport, T, of a substrate by the tubules is measured as the difference between observed urinary excretion rate and the quantity of substrate admitted to the tubules in the glomerular filtrate. When T is plotted against load, L, as L is caused to increase from low to high values by varying plasma concentration, T is observed to increase rapidly at low values of L, then rise more slowly and finally attain a fixed value, Tm, at high values of L. The asymptotic curve so generated has been termed a tubular titration curve by SMITH et al. (1943). A titration curve is composed of three sections (Fig. 23): a first section at low concentrations in which T and L increase proportionally and almost equally ($dT/dL = $ a constant, approximately 1.0); a third section at high loads in which T is constant and any change in L is accompanied by an equal change in excretion ($dT/dL = 0$); and an intermediate section in which the effect of L on T is rapidly decreasing ($dT/dL < 1, > 0$). Interest centers principally on the intermediate section, which has been termed the 'titration splay' (SMITH 1943). As can be seen from the foregoing description, the titration splay may represent a complex combination of two elements: a chemical process and an anatomical structure. The chemical process represents the progressive saturation of the transport system as the substrate concentration in the ambient medium rises, such as might be described by the MICHAELIS-MENTEN or SHANNON equations. The anatomical element represents the progressive saturation first of those nephrons which receive the largest load of substrate in relation to their transport capacity, and lastly of those nephrons which receive the smallest load of substrate in

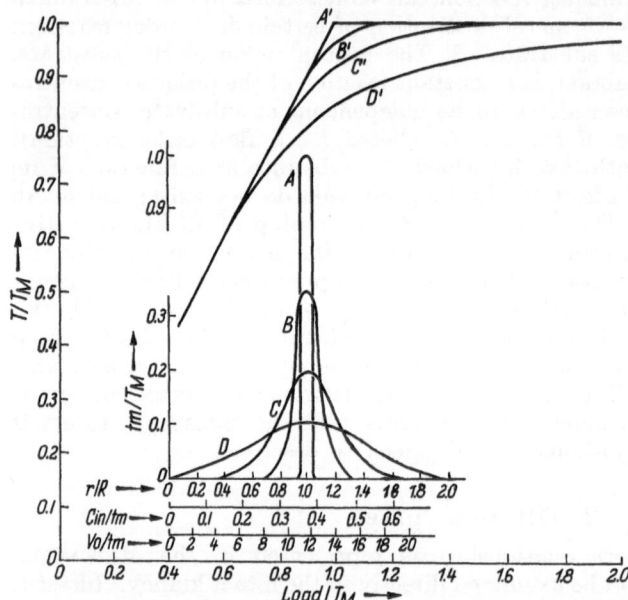

Fig. 23. Theoretical titration curves for an actively transported substance assuming that the major variable determining the titration splay is variation within the nephron population of the ratio (R) of load of substrate presented for transport to transport capacity. Since plasma concentration is considered as uniform throughout, the term which distinguishes the substrate load presented to one nephron from that presented to another is inulin clearance C_{in} in the case of reabsorptive transport and postglomerular blood flow (Vo) in the case of secretory transport. R and r are the load-transport ratios (C_{in}/Tm and Vo/Tm for reabsorption and secretion) for the entire kidney (R) and for fraction of the nephron population with a ratio (r) different from that of the entire kidney. Curves A, B, C and D (lower graph) represent hypothetical nephron populations with increasing degrees of dispersion about the mean of the ratio r/R. A is an extremely homogeneous and D a heterogeneous population. In the upper graph, the curves A', B', C' and D' represent the titration curves which would be observed during loading experiments on kidneys composed of the corresponding nephron populations. From SMITH, GOLDRING, CHASIS, RANGES and BRADLEY. Reproduced by courtesy of the authors and Journal of the Mt. Sinai Hospital

relation to their transport capacity. In the case of reabsorptive systems, when one nephron is saturated, the excess substrate cannot be made available to another, unsaturated nephron, but, instead, is delivered into the urine. The titration splay thus represents an upper limit to both processes. When the titration splay is very small or narrow, as is the case, for example, with glucose and PAH transport, it indicates both that the slowest reaction in the transport system is nearly complete at very low plasma concentrations and also that nearly all nephrons have approximately the same ratio of fluid delivery to transport capacity. When the titration splay is increased or 'widened', however, as in certain renal glycosurias or in urate transport, it is usually difficult to determine to which factor to attribute the widening.

If, as seems reasonable with respect to certain transport systems, we can assume that most of the titration splay arises from the anatomical term, then *the slope of the titration curve at a given load equals the fraction of the nephrons which are unsaturated at that load* (SMITH 1943). The rate of change of this fraction as a function of the load can be expressed in terms of the fraction of nephrons with a load/transport ratio (load expressed as volume flow carrying a substrate) different from the mean ratio for the entire population of nephrons. Examples of distribution curves within the nephron population of the function, filtration/transport in the case of tubular reabsorption or of blood flow/transport in the case of tubular secretion, as calculated from hypothetical titration curves, are illustrated in the lower portion of Fig. 23.

II. Anatomical location of transport processes

The belief that the histologically distinct cell types of the nephron would be discovered to perform correspondingly unique operations upon the urine has been amply confirmed by experiment. Among the earliest studies are those of HEIDENHAIN who observed that injected dyes tended to be localized in proximal tubular cells. Subsequent studies designed to locate transport processes by histochemical methods yielded ambiguous results partly because no theoretical basis was available to evaluate the role of glomerular filtration and partly because the rapidity of postmortem diffusion changes was not fully appreciated. Definitive assignment of transport functions to specific segments or regions of the nephron was made by RICHARDS and his associates. After establishing the character of the glomerular filtrate as an ultrafiltrate of plasma they analysed samples of fluid aspirated through a microneedle from the lumen of various regions of the nephron in amphibians (frog and *Necturus*) and mammals (rat, guinea pig and opossum) (RICHARDS and WALKER 1937; WALKER and OLIVER). Reabsorption was demonstrated for substances which disappeared from the tubular fluid within a given segment. Initially, RICHARDS could not determine whether substances which increased in concentration in the nephron were secreted or whether they were concentrated by reabsorption of water. When, however, the approximate equality of the urinary-plasma concentration ratios for inulin, creatinine, and glucose (after phlorhizin administration) established a measure of water reabsorption then secretion could likewise be recognized. In this way were located the loci for transport of glucose (WHITE and SCHMITT; WALKER and HUDSON 1937a; WOOD; WALKER et al. 1941), sodium and chloride and water in part (WALKER et al. 1937b, 1941; GIEBISCH 1956; BOTT 1958), potassium in part (WIRZ and BOTT), hydrogen ion (MONTGOMERY and PIERCE), ammonia (WALKER 1940) and phenolsulphonphthalein (EDWARDS and MARSHALL). Subsequently, information concerning anatomical loci of transport has been expanded by the technique of stopped-flow analysis (MALVIN, WILDE and SULLIVAN 1958a; WILDE and MALVIN 1958).

In this procedure, a ureter is clamped for several minutes during a diuresis produced, for example, by osmotic loading. While the ureter is clamped, some inulin and perhaps some PAH are injected. The ureter is unclamped, and the urine discharged during the ensuing few minutes is collected serially at intervals of roughly 1 second. Analysis of the successive samples obtained after unclamping is compared with the urine composition before or much later following the period of ureteral clamping. The appearance in the urine of filtrate formed after release of the clamp is recognized by the presence of the inulin injected after flow had been stopped. The validity of the method rests on the assumptions that: 1. the fluid in each portion of the nephron during the period of stopped flow will assume an exaggerated composition in relation to the transport characteristics of that segment of the nephron within which it has remained in prolonged contact; thus, fluid in the proximal tubule might be expected to become glucose-free during stopped flow although the bladder urine during free flow might have contained glucose; 2. fluid coming from the same segment in all the nephrons will reach the renal pelvis and ureter at roughly the same time. If, therefore, the maximal concentration change in two substances (whether rising or falling concentration) occurs in the same serial fractions collected after ureteral release, then the transport processes of the two substances responsible for the respective concentration change are presumed to lie in the same segment of the nephron. Stopped-flow analysis could never yield more than a set of functional relationships without correlation with the direct anatomical studies of Richards and others. Thus, glucose and sodium reabsorption, shown to occur in the proximal and distal segments, respectively, can serve as reference points in the serialized urine samples collected following stopped flow. Substances whose maximal concentration change occurs simultaneously with that of glucose or sodium are therefore transported by the proximal or the distal segments and in the same portions of these segments. If a substance is displaced from these reference substances in the urine, then the transport area is presumed to be correspondingly displaced, anatomically, in the nephron.

Stopped-flow analysis has confirmed the regions of PAH secretion (Malvin, Wilde and Sullivan 1958a), potassium secretion (Sullivan et al.; Hierholzer et al.) and phosphate reabsorption (Pitts et al. 1958a; Malvin et al. 1958a, b); confirmed the areas of sodium reabsorption (Malvin et al. 1958a, b); and located the tubular regions affected by various diuretics (Hierholzer et al.; Kessler, Hierholzer and Pitts; Vander et al. 1958b, 1959). Information obtained from both micropuncture and stopped flow studies is summarized in Table 12.

Table 12. *Anatomical location of tubular transport processes*

Proximal segment	Distal segment and collecting ducts
bicarbonate (in part)	ammonium
glucose	hydrogen
phenolsulphonphthalein and PAH	potassium
phosphate	sodium and chloride (in part)
potassium	water (in part)
sodium and chloride (in part)	
water (in part)	

III. Tubular secretion of acids and bases

1. Transport of aromatic acids

a) General properties

Grouped in what appears to be a single class of substances are an enormous number of organic acids. Many of them, for example phthaleins and diazo compounds, are highly colored; and for this reason study of their excretion has figured prominently in the development of renal physiology and has resulted in an enormous literature. The theories of Heidenhain rested, for the most part, on his studies of cellular and tubular accumulation of indigo carmine. The phenolsulfonphthalein excretion test, introduced into clinical medicine by Rowntree and Geraghty, is even now one of the most widely used of all renal function tests. The capacity of the tubules to transport these acids from blood to the tubular lumen is the most universal of all known renal functions. The tubules of the pronephros of the fish *(Fundulus)* or the frog embryo secrete indigo carmine and phenolsulphonphthalein as soon as capillaries develop around them and before glomeruli have appeared (Armstrong; Jaffee). Secretion is actively performed by the mesonephric tubule of the chick embryo (Chambers and Kempton 1933). No vertebrate of any class has yet been studied whose kidney, glomerular or aglomerular, does not actively secrete some or all of these substances. In addition to the possession of this secretory system by all classes of vertebrates is the circumstance that the qualitative selectivity of the system (that is, the acceptance

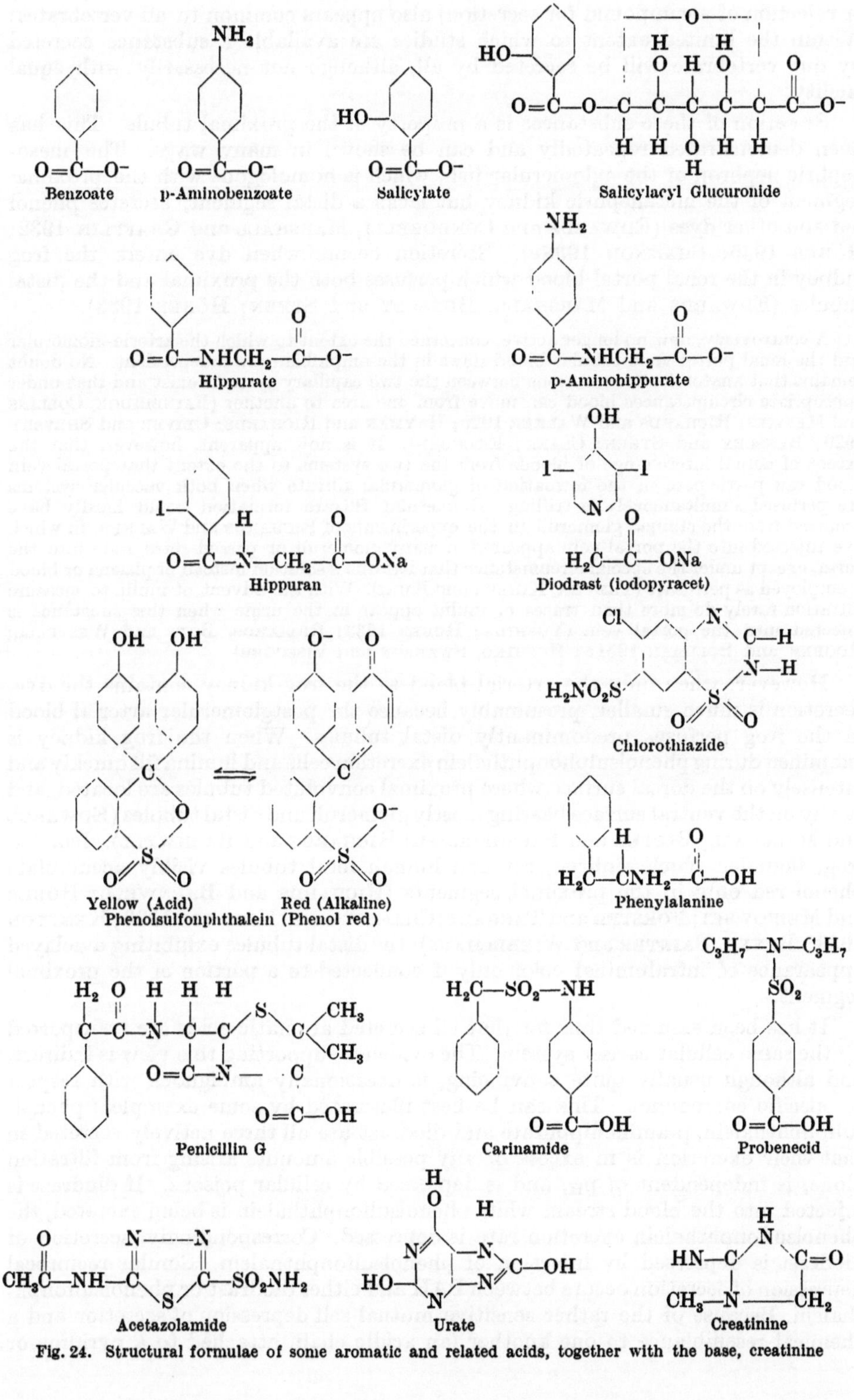

Fig. 24. Structural formulae of some aromatic and related acids, together with the base, creatinine

or rejection of a compound for secretion) also appears common to all vertebrates: Within the limited extent to which studies are available a substance secreted by one vertebrate will be secreted by all, although not necessarily with equal facility.

Secretion of these substances is a property of the proximal tubule. This has been demonstrated repeatedly and can be shown in many ways. The meso-nephric nephron of the aglomerular fish, which is homologous with the proximal segment of the metanephric kidney but lacks a distal segment, secretes phenol red and other dyes (Edwards and Condorelli; Marshall and Grafflin 1932; Höber 1935; Shannon 1938e). Secretion occurs when dye enters the frog kidney in the renal portal blood which perfuses both the proximal and the distal tubules (Edwards and Marshall; Bensley and Steen; Höber 1933).

A controversy, now no longer active, concerned the extent to which the arterio-glomerular and the renal portal veno-tubular blood flows in the amphibian are independent. No doubt remains that anatomical connections between the two capillary systems exist and that under appropriate circumstances blood can move from one area to another (Bainbridge, Collins and Menzies; Richards and Walker 1926; Hayman and Richards; Oliver and Shevsky 1929; Bensley and Steen; Clark; Ekehorn). It is now apparent, however, that the extent of actual interchange of bloods from the two systems to the extent that portal vein blood can participate in the formation of glomerular filtrate when both vascular systems are perfused simultaneously is trifling. Glomerular filtrate formation could hardly have occurred from the stained glomeruli in the experiments of Richards and Walker, in which dye injected into the portal vein appeared in many glomeruli or passed retrograde into the aorta, except under the special circumstance that Ringer's solution instead of plasma or blood is employed as perfusate (Tamura, Kihara and Kuki). With the advent of inulin to measure filtration rarely do more than traces of inulin appear in the urine when this substance is injected into the portal vein (Yoshida; Höber 1933; Richards, Bott and Westfall; Hogben and Bollman 1951a; Hoshiko, Swanson and Visscher).

However, when only the arterial blood to the frog kidney contains the dye, secretion is much smaller, presumably because the postglomerular arterial blood in the frog perfuses predominantly distal tubules. When the frog kidney is examined during phenolsulphonphthalein excretion cells and lumina fill quickly and intensely on the dorsal surface where proximal convoluted tubules are located, and slowly on the ventral surface bearing mostly glomeruli and distal tubules (Edwards and Marshall; Bieter and Hirshfelder; Richards and Barnwell). Isolated frog, flounder, chick embryo, rat and human fetal tubules visibly accumulate phenol red only in the proximal segments (Richards and Barnwell; Höber and Meirowski; Forster and Taggart; Chambers and Kempton 1933; Kempton 1939; Beyer, Painter and Wiebelhaus), the distal tubules exhibiting a delayed appearance of intraluminal color only if connected to a portion of the proximal segment.

It has been assumed thus far that all secreted aromatic acids are transported by the same cellular carrier system. The evidence supporting this view is indirect, and although usually quite convincing, is occasionally ambiguous with respect to specific compounds. This can be best illustrated by some examples: phenol-sulfonphthalein, p-aminohippurate and diodrast are all three actively secreted in that their excretion is in excess of any possible amounts arising from filtration alone, is independent of p_H, and is depressed by cellular poisons. If diodrast is injected into the blood stream while phenolsulfonphthalein is being excreted, the phenolsulfonphthalein excretion rate is depressed. Correspondingly, secretion of diodrast is depressed by injection of phenolsulfonphthalein. Similar reciprocal depression of secretion occurs between PAH and either diodrast or phenolsulfonph-thalein. Because of the rather sensitive mutual self depression of secretion and a chemical resemblance to one another (an acidic chain attached to a pyridine or benzene ring), it is postulated that both PAH and diodrast are transported by a single carrier system which, when presented with both molecules, carries both but carries each in an amount less than would be transported were it present alone. In the case of phenolsulfonphthalein, the chemical resemblance to the two other compounds, diodrast and p-aminohippurate, is more remote, having only an acidic group and a ring structure in common. Between any two transported aromatic acids, no matter how dissimilar chemically, it is possible, however, to construct a series of intermediate compounds, each differing structurally only slightly from the next, yet each being secreted by the tubular epithelium. For this reason it has been suggested that all these acids are secreted by the same transport system. Uric acid, creatinine and urea, on the other hand, are examples of puzzling situations. In the mammal uric acid is reabsorbed by the nephron from the glomerular filtrate but in the chicken and elsewhere this substance is secreted by the epithelium into the urine. Similarly, creatinine which is chemically a weak base, appears to be secreted in the primates, birds and other species and urea is secreted by the frog tubule. In the case of all three substances secretion can be depressed, apparently competitively, by aromatic acids. Moreover, aromatic acids such as diodrast, which can inhibit urate secretion in the chicken, can also inhibit urate reabsorption in mammals where urate and diodrast are moving in opposite directions across the epithelium.

Studies of the renal excretion of aromatic acids are immensely complicated by the circumstance that for certain acids a tubular reabsorptive system also exists. Measurable degrees of tubular reabsorption have been noted particularly with respect to benzoic acid derivatives. Benzoic acid itself has not been clearly detected in the urine of man after oral ingestion of sodium benzoate (BORG-STRÖM, SCHACHTER) and p-aminobenzoate is largely reabsorbed from glomerular filtrate (FISHER et al.; SMITH et al. 1945; BEYER et al. 1945a, 1952). Reports of high excretion rates of p-aminobenzoate (LUNDQUIST) have not distinguished excretion of the free substance from that of its conjugate, p-aminohippurate. Carinamide, probenecid, salicylate and, perhaps, even urate may be reabsorbed in varying degrees in addition to being secreted. The dynamics of this aromatic acid reabsorptive system are among the least understood of all renal tubular transport functions.

A departure from the general pattern has been described for the amphibian, *Necturus*, and the cat. In *Necturus* both p-aminohippurate and diodrast are reabsorbed. Simultaneous administration of both substances, however, results in a net secretion of diodrast suggesting that the p-aminohippurate has competitively blocked the reabsorptive component of a double system composed of both reabsorptive and secretory pathways (KINTER). In the cat both PAH and diodrast may exhibit a net reabsorption at plasma concentrations of 1 mM./L. These findings are suggestive of the renal handling of urate and of benzoic acid analogs and indicate that bidirectionality may be a common phenomenon.

b) Metabolism of aromatic acid transport

The conclusion that the movement of aromatic acids from blood to proximal tubular lumen is an active process is supported by the observations, first, that a high concentration is attainable in the lumen relative to that in the blood (or in the medium in the case of isolated tubules); second, that intraluminal accumulation is independent of pH (CHAMBERS and KEMPTON 1933; KEMPTON 1939); third, that accumulation is prevented by inhibitors of cell metabolism; fourth, that rate of transport becomes essentially constant when the concentration at the blood surface exceeds a certain value, and does not rise even if blood concentration exceeds that of the urine (SHANNON 1938e).

Properties of the system which transports these acids have been studied in three ways which generally complement each other nicely: The effect of various agents on excretion rate can be studied in the intact organism; the rate of uptake of a secreted substance by slices of kidney in a suitable nutrient medium can be measured under various conditions (CROSS and TAGGART); the appearance and approximate concentration of a visible dye in the lumina of isolated fish or amphibian tubules can be observed under the microscope (RICHARDS and BARNWELL; FORSTER 1948). The first method is limited to circumstances which are tolerable to the animal and which do not greatly disturb the blood supply to the kidney. The second method permits examination and precise quantitation of the effects of a great number of variables, but cannot clearly distinguish accumulation of substrate within the cells from accumulation within the tubular lumina. The third method differs from the second in that luminal accumulation of substrate can be distinguished from intracellular accumulation, but quantitation is less precise.

Accumulation of aromatic acids by kidney tissue is depressed by many metabolic inhibitors. Accumulation of phenolsulfonphthalein (PSP) is nearly or entirely abolished in chick mesonephros and frog kidney slices by cooling to 3—6°C (CHAMBERS and KEMPTON 1933; FORSTER and HONG). The temperature coefficient for the transport of diodrast in man (GOLDRING et al. 1940; TALBOTT 1951) and of PAH in fish (FORSTER 1953) is approximately 2.0 at temperatures not too distant from those normal for the species[1]. This is a figure commonly observed for many enzymatically catalysed biochemical processes. PAGE (1955) obtained a value of 3.6 for PAH transport in the dog but considered that the large decrease in renal blood flow with cooling (8.2 percent per degree C) observed in his studies might also have impaired transport and thus yielded a high coefficient. Accumulation of PAH or PSP by slices or isolated tubules is dependent on oxygen and is abolished by nitrogen (CHAMBERS, BECK and BELKIN; CROSS and TAGGART; BEYER, PAINTER and WIEBELHAUS), although mild hypoxia produced by breathing 6.3 or 9.4 percent oxygen does not depress PAH transport in dog or man (AXELROD and PITTS 1952b) and exposure of dogs to simulated altitude of 18,000 or 24,000 feet (5,500 or 7,300 meters) was associated with an increase rather than a decrease in PAH transport. Cyanide, which blocks respiratory enzymes, depresses accumulation and transport of PAH and PSP at 10^{-3} M. concentration (RICHARDS and BARNWELL; NICHOLSON 1949; CHAMBERS, BECK and BELKIN; CROSS and TAGGART; BEYER, PAINTER and WIEBELHAUS; WHITE 1957). Accumulation and transport are strongly inhibited by various substituted phenols, particularly 2,4-dinitrophenol. Most of these inhibitory phenols also block the formation of energy-rich phosphate bonds without interfering with, or even with stimulation of, oxygen uptake (uncoupling of phosphorylation). 2,4,6-trinitrophenol also reversibly inhibits accumulation of PAH but this substance does not prevent formation of energy-rich phosphate bonds and the mechanism of the inhibition is unknown.

Barbiturates, at blood concentrations obtained during surgical anesthesia, inhibit PAH uptake by slices (STØREN 1958b), depress oxygen consumption (STØREN 1958b, WHITE 1957) and block phosphorylation (BRODY and BAIN). Phlorhizin which interferes with many cellular enzymatic processes including phosphorylation (BECK; KALCKAR 1937; BEYER, PAINTER and WIEBELHAUS; LOTSPEICH and KELLER) also impedes PAH and PSP accumulation and diodrast transport at 5×10^{-3} M. concentration (WHITE 1940b; CROSS and TAGGART; BEYER, PAINTER and WIEBELHAUS). Other inhibitors of various cellular enzyme systems, such as mercuric ion, azide, fluoride, arsenite, iodoacetate, phenylhydrazine and quinone also block accumula-

---

[1] In this temperature range, a temperature coefficient of 2.0 indicates that a 10 degree centigrade rise or fall in temperature results in a doubling or a halving of the transport rate.

tion (CHAMBERS, BECK and BELKIN; BECK and CHAMBERS; CROSS and TAGGART; BEYER, PAINTER and WIEBELHAUS; KUWABARA; KOISHI 1959b). Theophyllin ethylenediamine (aminophyllin) at 2×10^{-5} M. inhibits PAH accumulation by slices (HUANG, KING and GENAZZONI) but not in the intact kidney. Acetate, pyruvate and lactate at moderate concentrations and succinate and ketoglutarate at low concentrations potentiate accumulation by slices (KUWABARA, KOISHI 1959a). Acetate was particularly effective but acetate stimulation was not observed if serum instead of saline was used as the incubation medium (KUWABARA). Glucose, hexosediphosphate, citrate and isocitrate, formate, acetoacetate and other substances did not affect uptake in this in vitro system. Ketoglutarate, succinate, fumarate, malate, dehydroacetate, fluoroacetate, caprylate and caprate were generally inhibitory at moderate concentrations (CROSS and TAGGART; FARAH and RENNICK; FARAH) while acetate, pyruvate and lactate become inhibitory at higher concentrations (KOISHI 1959a). In the intact dog kidney, PAH transport is enhanced by acetate and lactate and depressed by succinate, fumarate (MUDGE and TAGGART 1950a; SCHACHTER and FREINKEL; STØREN 1958a), dehydroacetate, malonate (SHIDEMAN and RENE) and maleate (BERLINER, KENNEDY and HILTON 1950a). The mechanism of action of maleate is not clear. Acetate also partially or completely reverses, depending on the quantities of the various agents employed, depression in PAH, PSP or p-acetylaminohippurate accumulation or transport produced by dehydroacetic acid, 2,4-dinitrophenol and carinamide (SHIDEMAN, RATHBUN and STONEMAN). Acetate fails to reverse barbiturate depression of PAH uptake (WHITE 1957, STØREN 1958b) and it fails to enhance PAH Tm in rabbit or cat (JOSEPHSON et al.).

SCHACHTER, MANIS and TAGGART observed that kidney slices condense various aliphatic (as well as aromatic) acids with amino acids. Some of these condensation products inhibit PAH accumulation, perhaps by reacting with portions of the carrier system, while others do not. Thus, laurylglycine, and acylglycines longer than 5 carbon atoms, inhibit accumulation while acetylglycine does not. They attribute the enhancement by acetate of PAH transport to the ability of acetate to obligate the kidney cells in the direction of synthesizing a maximum quantity of noninhibitory acetylglycine. Similarly, in their view, the depressing of PAH accumulation by l-alanine is due to formation of acylalanines which act much as do long chain acylglycines, while the stimulating effect of d-alanine in the rabbit is due to its oxidation to acetate. SCHACHTER et al. note finally in support of their concepts that, with the possible exception of the rat in which the effects are ambiguous, acetate stimulates PAH accumulation only in kidney slices from those species whose kidneys synthesize acylglycines.

Energy utilization by the kidney for the synthesis of PAH from p-aminobenzoate and glycine apparently does not interfere detectably with the PAH transport system (MCINTOSH, KNOEFEL and SCHARFF) although synthesis may involve components of the transport system (SCHACHTER and TAGGART). Benzoate, which is synthesized to hippurate, interferes with PAH uptake, possibly because of competitive inhibition from the hippurate formed (SCHACHTER, MANIS and TAGGART) and possibly also because of actions such as preemption of coenzyme A (BEYER 1957). SCHACHTER and FREINKEL observed that high blood concentrations of PAH in the dog were occasionally associated with depression in PAH transport. This depression, when it occurred, could be reversed with acetate.

These studies indicate that transport of aromatic acids is dependent in some fashion on a supply of high-energy phosphate bonds and that transport can be depressed by agents which interfere with high energy phosphate formation, presumably with formation of adenosine triphosphate (CROSS and TAGGART; TAGGART and FORSTER; MUDGE and TAGGART 1950a; BEYER, PAINTER and WIEBELHAUS; MENDELSOHN; COPENHAVER and FORSTER). The fraction of cellular oxidative energy used in aromatic acid transport is too small to measure, since oxygen utilization does not change detectably when transport is inhibited by probenecid (FORSTER and COPENHAVER). In addition to oxidative phosphorylation, transport is also dependent upon a suitable electrolyte environment. Calcium in the bathing fluids is necessary for PSP transport (Richards and Barnwell). The defect due to calcium deficiency seems to be at the luminal surface of the cell since in a calcium-free medium PSP enters and deeply colors the cells but fails to enter the lumen of the tubule. Addition of calcium permits rapid movement of dye into the lumen (Puck, Wasserman and Fishman[1]). Potassium ion also is necessary for transport (Taggart, Silverman and Trayner). In a potassium-deficient medium the defect appears to be at the contraluminal or blood surface of the epithelium since not only does transport fail but dye also fails to appear in the cell even when the concentration in the medium is high (Puck, Wasserman and Fishman). Because of the selective effects of these electrolytes and from studies of their effects on accumulation of chlorphenol in or loss from tubular lumina in the presence of metabolic inhibitors such as cyanide or dinitrophenol it is concluded that transport of acid dyes in the flounder occurs in two steps, one at each surface of the cell, and that each step is energy-dependent (Hong and Forster). Whether a two step transport system exists in the mammalian nephron is unknown. An accumulation relative to the cells of PSP in some tubular lumina of mammalian cortex slices has been reported (Beyer, Painter and Wiebelhaus) but their findings could not be confirmed (Forster and Copenhaver). Josephson and Kallas (1953b) concluded that diodrast is more concentrated in the lumina of rabbit kidney but that massive quantities can cause a relative intracellular accumulation of diodrast (Engström and Josephson). Carinamide may inhibit transport at both the blood and luminal surface of the epithelium (Josephson and Kallas 1953b). An intermediate position is taken by Foulkes and Miller based on studies of the dynamics of penetration of PAH into rabbit cortex slices. They postulate that the first step in transport consists of movement with little change in concentration across the plasma surface of the cell into a fraction of the cell which exchanges rapidly with the medium. PAH next enters another, slowly exchanging fraction of the cell at high concentration and in this fraction traverses the cell. Entry into either cell fraction can be inhibited or stimulated either by direct competition (diodrast) or by altering the energy supply. They postulate no specific transport step at the luminal surface.

Manganese, magnesium and cobalt do not affect transport at concentrations up to 10 mEq./L. (Taggart, Silverman and Trayner) but hypertonic sodium chloride (0.25 M.) depresses PSP accumulation by chick mesonephros (Chambers, Beck and Belkin). PAH accumulation is generally lower when the anions of the medium are other than chloride, the relative degree of depression correlating with the Hofmeister series (Taggart, Silverman and Trayner).

The chemical properties which must be present in order that an acid should be secreted are unknown. Aliphatic acids such as amino acids, and acetic, lactic and other acids are reabsorbed. However, the aromatic amino acids tryptophane and phenylalanine also are reabsorbed. Correspondingly, benzoate and p-aminobenzoate are reabsorbed, while their glycine conjugates, hippurate and p-aminohippurate, are among the most vigorously secreted of all acids. In general, an aromatic nucleus should be present for rapid secretory transport to occur and for this reason we have chosen to designate this the aromatic acid transport system. Within the limited group of aromatic carboxylic acids an unobstructed

---

[1] High concentrations of phenol red also caused the dye to accumulate in the cells of flounder tubules in artificial media, and blocked movement into the lumen (Wasserman, Becker and Fishman). This "self depression" is probably caused by binding of calcium ions by the excess PSP molecules.

benzamido group must be present and at not too great a distance from the carboxyl for vigorous secretion to occur (KNOEFEL and HUANG 1959). The importance of obstruction of the benzamido group lies in the circumstance that reactive groups in the ortho position on the benzene ring can react, as by hydrogen bonding, with the benzamido group and thereby impede secretion. Although carboxyl or sulfonate groups are present on most secreted acids, these groups do not seem to be essential for secretion (cf. chlorothiazide, acetazoleamide, N^1-acetylsulfanilamide, urate, creatinine). When secreted acids are arranged in the order of decreasing maximal transport rates several interesting regularities emerge. Those which have the highest Tm appear the most quickly in the tubular lumen or the urine (SPERBER 1954); they accumulate within the cell in the lowest concentration; their transport is the most easily depressed by cold or metabolic inhibitors; they diffuse from the tubular lumen the most rapidly after transport has been arrested. Conversely, those acids with a low transport rate appear later in the urine following injection; are less sensitive to metabolic inhibitors; tend to accumulate in the cell in high concentrations; and diffuse from the tubular lumen slowly after inhibition of transport. They may accumulate in the cell in the cold indicating that uptake to this extent is independent of cell energy. The slowly-transported, cell-accumulated acids strongly inhibit transport of the more rapidly transported acids, while the latter are rather ineffective as inhibitors of the slowly-transported members (FORSTER, SPERBER and TAGGART; FORSTER and HONG; JOSEPHSON; JOSEPHSON et al.).

Reciprocal depression of transport by two substances which appear very similar chemically is usually termed *competitive inhibition* of transport. Substances such as metabolic inhibitors which interfere with some aspect of the functioning of the transport system or which destroy part of the transport system and whose effect cannot be reversed by adding more substrate, are said to be *noncompetitive inhibitors*. Situations which are not easily classifiable are those such as the inhibitory effects of diodrast on uric acid transport in the chicken or mammal or of PAH and probenecid on urea transport in the frog (FORSTER 1954). Until contrary information is available, it seems reasonable to assume that both of these interactions represent examples of competitive inhibition. In the case of diodrast-inhibition of PSP transport it is assumed that each substance is competing with the other for some highly specific site of attachment in the carrier system; in the case of PAH inhibition of urea transport, on the other hand, the mechanism is ambiguous. It is apparent that viewing tubular transport systems as a set of independent machines, each specializing in the transport of a single family of chemically related compounds which can be separated one from another by presence or absence of competitive inhibitions, is an oversimplification. Nevertheless, the concept of discrete transport processes and the two terms, *competitive* and *noncompetitive* inhibition, are useful simplifications in that they can categorize certain observed types of interactions between transported substances and can relate them to current concepts of active transport. It must be emphasized, however, that precise meaning is impossible as long as the carrier systems to which these terms refer are, themselves, hypothetical (SPERBER 1948).

Carinamide and probenecid, which are members of this family of aromatic acids, are representative of the slowly transported group. In addition to having a very low Tm they are accumulated in the cells and block the transport of other aromatic acids. These differences in aromatic acids have been attributed by FORSTER and HONG to variation in the affinity or binding capacity of the acid for cellular constituents, particularly those constituting the transport apparatus. Occupation of reaction sites by firmly bound molecules could effectively block transport of less reactive molecules. In addition, transport could be slowed by the low rate of dissociation of the protein-acid complexes. The degrees of coloration of tubular cells observed during the transport of various dyes thus are attributable both to the degree of intracellular adsorption of the dye and to the relative velocities of transport of the dye molecules at the two poles of the cell as affected, for example, by Ca and K concentrations. Other chemical factors which affect transport are poorly understood. The molecule must be reasonably small (Oliver and Shevky 1930; Schulten; Höber 1935). It should contain no strong basic group and all acid radicals, if more than one are present, should be at the same end of the molecule (Orzechowski; Höber and Briscoe-Woolley 1939, 1940a, b; Höber et al.). The presence of negative charges at both ends of the molecule is presumed to interfere with approach of the molecule to the cell surface. The acid need not be lipid-soluble although lipid-soluble molecules are thought to be more readily transported by the isolated frog kidney than are lipid-insoluble ones (Liang; Höber 1930a; Höber and Meirowsky). The nature of the reactions between the aromatic acid and the transport system is unknown. The present evidence suggests that binding of substrate to carrier is more probably of an electrostatic than a covalent type (Taggart 1956).

c) Normal values of diodrast and PAH transport in man

The average maximal tubular transport rate (Tm) of diodrast in young men is 50 and in young women 40 to 44 mg. I/min/1.73 M² of body surface area (Smith 1951). In various studies, the values for men vary from 39 to 53 (Goldring

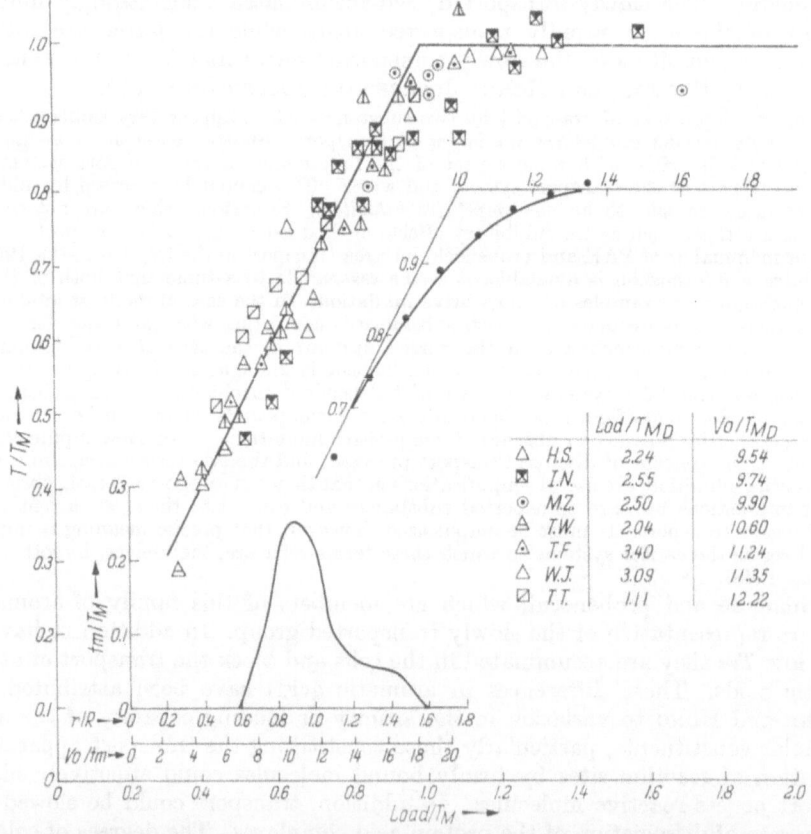

Fig. 25. Diodrast titration curve for normal subjects, from Smith, Goldring, Chasis, Ranges and Bradley. Upper curve: transport-load data for 7 subjects; middle curve: graph of the averaged data from these subjects; lower curve: frequency distribution in the nephron populations of glomerular activity, r, (perfusion rate, vo, divided by transport capacity, tm_D) as related to mean glomerular activity, $R(Vo/Tm_D)$ of the entire kidney, calculated as illustrated in Fig. 23. The tabular data are the values for each of the subjects for the load at which saturation was attained (L/Tm) and the ratio of postglomerular blood flow to Tm (Vo/Tm). Reproduced by permission of the authors and Journal of the Mt. Sinai Hospital

et al. 1940; WHITE, FINDLEY and EDWARDS; BRUN, HILDEN and RAASCHOU 1947b; DAVIES and SHOCK; FOA et al. 1942). The Tm of PAH lies between 65 and 78 mg./min. with no discernible sex difference (SMITH 1951; CHASIS et al. 1945; BRUN, HILDEN and RAASCHOU 1947c, d). PAH is transported about twice or somewhat more than twice as rapidly as diodrast when measured as moles per minute (CHASIS et al. 1945; BRUN, HILDEN and RAASCHOU 1947c, d). The ratio of the Tms of the two substances is quite constant in the presence of wide variation in their absolute magnitudes (STOLOFF, WATKIN and SHOCK) and a PAH-diodrast Tm ratio similar to man is reported for the rabbit (JOSEPHSON et al.). Children attain the adult value of Tm-PAH per unit surface area between 6 months and one year of age, although considerable variation is observed in children under 2 years of age (WEST, SMITH and CHASIS; RUBIN, BRUCK and RAPOPORT). Diodrast Tm in 2 children aged 8 and 10 years averaged 64 and 43 mg. I/min./ 1.73 M² (GALAN et al.). Like GFR and RPF, diodrast Tm declines in older people. From a value of about 55 in the third decade, Tm decreased to about 31 mg. I/min. in the 9th decade. The rate of decline is the same as for filtration rate so that the ratio, GFR/Tm-D, remains constant with aging (DAVIES and SHOCK).

A PAH titration curve obtained from studies on 10 normal adults by SMITH and his coworkers is represented in Fig. 25. In order to compare one subject with another, or to portray all subjects with the same curve, all values of T and L for each individual are divided by the measured value of Tm for that individual. The very small titration splay indicates that virtually all nephrons become saturated simultaneously. Since a similar small titration splay is observed in chronic pyelonephritis in which widespread damage both to tubules and to their blood supply has occurred (RAASCHOU), it seems likely that local intrarenal adjustment of load to transport capacity is attainable by extensive diffusion of PAH through interstitial fluid spaces.

d) Metabolic and other influences on PAH and diodrast transport in the intact kidney

Changes in diodrast or PAH Tm in various physiological or pathological states in man are summarized in Table 13.

Variations in blood oxygen tension produced by breathing 16 or 30 percent oxygen in patients with emphysema caused no detectable change in PAH Tm (FISHMAN et al. 1951). Exposure of dogs to simulated high altitude was associated with an actual increase in transport of PAH (KELLEY and McDONALD). This paradoxical effect may have resulted from an increase in the blood of some energy-supplying metabolite, such as acetate or lactate. Acetate infused at 0.08 to 0.19 mM./kg./min. or injection of 100 mM. of lactate followed by a sustaining infusion of 2 mM./min. was associated with a 23 and a 30 percent increase, respectively, in Tm-PAH in normal subjects (BALDWIN and McLEAN; McDONALD, SHOCK and YIENGST). These effects are similar to, but less marked than the effects of acetate or lactate infusion in the dog (MUDGE and TAGGART 1950b) but are greater than those in cat or rabbit (JOSEPHSON et al.). The increased amount of tubular work involved in loading the kidneys with diodrast or PAH does not detectably increase oxygen consumption (BUCHT, WERKO and JOSEPHSON; CLARK and BARKER).

PAH and diodrast Tm is decreased acutely by mercury (mercurophylline or mersalyl) in man (BRUN, HILDEN and RAASCHOU 1947a; McDONALD and MILLER; BERLINER, KENNEDY and HILTON) but not in the dog (BERLINER, KENNEDY and HILTON 1948; SHIDEMAN and RENE) although some decrease

Table 13. *Changes in p-aminohippurate (PAH) or Diodrast (D) maximal transport rate (Tm) in human physiological and pathological states*

Condition	Reference
Tm unchanged	
Anoxia (emphysema)	Fishman et al. (PAH)
(heart disease)	Scott and Elliott (PAH)
Drugs	
aminophyllin . . .	Miller (PAH)
epinephrin	Mills et al. (PAH)
hexamethonium . .	Ford et al. (PAH); Moyer and Mills (PAH)
Gout (early)	Gutman and Yü (1957) (PAH)
Hypercorticism	
(cortisone)	Burnett (PAH)
Pregnancy	Welsh et al. (D); Sohar et al. (PAH)
Toxemia of pregnancy	Wellen et al. (D)
Tm unchanged or somewhat decreased	
Anemia (adults) . . .	Bradley and Bradley (D); Ettledorf et al. (1955) (PAH)
Glomerular nephritis	
(acute)	Earle et al. (1944, 1951) (D)
Heart failure (chronic)	Hilden (D); Grossman et al. (PAH); Fishman et al. (PAH)
Starvation (chronic) .	Mollison (D)
Tm decreased	
Addison's disease . .	Sanderson (D); Talbott et al. (D); Waterhouse et al. (PAH)
Anemia (adults) . . .	Bradley and Bradley (D)
Fanconi syndrome . .	Sirota and Hamerman (PAH)
Glomerular nephritis	
and nephrosis . . .	Bradley et al. (PAH)
Gout (late)	Gutman and Yü (1957) (PAH)
Hypertension	Foa et al. (D); Chasis et al. (1950) (D); Watkin et al. (PAH); Goldring et al. (1941) (D); Findley et al. (D)
Hypothermia	Talbott (D)
Hypothyroidism . . .	Hlad and Bricker (PAH)
Protein deficiency . .	Weston et al. (PAH); Chasis et al. (1950) (PAH); Watkin et al. (PAH)
Nephrotic syndrome .	Bradley et al. (1950) (D); Metcoff et al. (PAH); Furman et al. (PAH)
Myelomatosis	Myhre and Brodwall (PAH)
Tm increased	
Anemia (children) . .	Ettledorf et al. (PAH); Bruck (PAH)
Cirrhosis (nonascitic).	Leslie et al. (PAH)
Hyperpituitarism . .	Gershberg et al. (PAH)
Hyperthermia (fever)	Goldring et al. (1940) (D)
Hyperthyroidism . .	Corcoran and Page (1947) (D); Bradley (D)
Nephrosis ("pure") .	Bruck et al. (PAH); Eder et al. (PAH); Metcoff et al. (PAH); Earle (PAH)
Vitamin A	
administration . .	Taylor et al. (D)

in Tm is reported by others (Handley, Chapman and Moyer). In addition to depressing Tm, mersalyl (2 ml.) caused extensive widening of titration splay (Brun, Hilden and Raaschou 1947a). Transport is also depressed by uranyl salts in the dog (Wills and Main), phenylbutazone and pyrazinamide in man (Yü, Sirota and Gutman; Yü et al. 1957) and by hypertonic sodium chloride in the dog (Levy and Ankeny). Transport is depressed, presumably competitively, by carinamide and probenecid in the dog and probably in man (Beyer 1947; Beyer et al. 1947b, 1951; Earle and Brodie). Transport is unaffected immediately by pentobarbital anesthesia in the dog (Corcoran and Page 1943a) but may decrease slowly by 16 to 26 percent over several hours of pentobarbital anesthesia (Glauser and Selkurt; Støren 1958a). The slow onset of barbiturate depression suggests that the capacity of barbiturates to depress phosphorylation *in vitro* is relatively unimportant in the intact kidney.

Transport is unaffected by renal denervation in the dog (Berne), by mannitol diuresis in the dog (Levy and Ankeny), by aminophylline in man (Miller 1953b), by

pyrogen hyperemia in man (GOLDRING et al. 1941), by acute fluid loading in man
(MICHIE et al.; BARKER et al. 1949) or by 5,000 to 50,000 units of vitamin A daily
in dogs. Transport increased in dogs which received 200,000 units daily (BING) and
probably increased slightly in a group of 14 hypertensive patients who received
100,000 to 400,000 units daily (TAYLOR et al. 1943). Diodrast clearance also
increased in most of these patients. Some confusion exists concerning the effects of
hyperglycemia on PAH transport. Hyperglycemia has been reported by some
authors to depress PAH transport in both dog and man (KLOPP, YOUNG and
TAYLOR 1944; HOUCK 1946; GRIMELLI et al.) but in other studies no depression
was observed in the dog (SELKURT 1944) or man (MICHIE etal.). Moreover, diodrast
transport is unaffected by glucose loading in dog or man (EILER, ALTHAUSEN and
STOCKHOLM 1944a; SMITH et al. 1943). The apparent depression in PAH transport
has been attributed to formation of a poorly or non-secreted complex between
PAH and glucose (BALDWIN et al. 1950). Transport is depressed chronically 9
to 14 percent in man by a low protein (rice) diet (WESTON et al. 1950; CHASIS
et al. 1950; WATKIN et al.) and by severe general starvation in two subjects
(MOLLISON). Transport is moderately depressed (44 percent) in the dog by acute,
severe acidosis (JENSEN et al.).

Transport is profoundly affected by changes in adrenocortical, thyroid, and
pituitary function and variously by androgens, estrogens and dietary factors.
In men and women 90 to 300 mg. testosterone for 8 to 29 days or 4 to 6 mg.
estradiol for 9 to 12 days caused no detectable change in transport (DEAN,
ABELS and TAYLOR). In the dog the effects of these steroids are not clear: In
one study, 100 mg. testosterone daily to females caused a marked increase
(nearly a doubling) in diodrast Tm (WELSH et al. 1942a); while in another
study testosterone in 3—6 mg. and estradiol in 0.013—0.33 mg./kg. daily caused
no change and a decrease, respectively, in PAH Tm (RICHARDSON and HOUCK).

Diodrast and PAH Tm are decreased to 20 to 50 percent of normal 5 to
10 days after hypophysectomy in dogs (WHITE and HEINBECKER 1940; WHITE,
HEINBECKER and ROLF 1941, 1942, 1949a). Tm can be restored to normal or
increased to 65 or 84 percent above normal by anterior pituitary growth hormone
(WHITE, HEINBECKER and ROLF 1949b, 1951). The effects of anterior pituitary
principles on renal function are complicated by possible effects from the neurohypophysis. PAH Tm decreased to about 50 percent of the control value
following section of the pituitary stalk in 7 dogs. Pituitrin and oxytocic principle (Pitocin) were associated, acutely, with a rise in Tm to 77 and 63 percent
of control levels, respectively, for the two preparations (DEMUNBRUN et al.).
Administration of 10 units of Pitocin 6 times daily for 7 days has been reported
to elevate PAH Tm from 64 to 92 mg./min. in patients with panhypopituitarism
(SPURR and FORD).

Diodrast Tm is affected by thyroid activity but not as markedly as by
anterior pituitary. Thyroidectomy in the dog is followed by a decrease of
diodrast Tm to 71 and 76 percent of normal while large doses of dessicated
thyroid (5 to 7 gm. per day for 5 to 38 days) to normal dogs was associated
with an increase in Tm of 48 to 115 percent (WHITE, HEINBECKER and ROLF
1947; HEINBECKER, ROLF and WHITE; EILER, ALTHAUSEN and STOCKHOLM
1944a).

The effects of adrenocortical hormones on diodrast and PAH Tm are not
wholly clear. Tm decreases in adrenalectomized dogs (9 and 33 percent) and
the decrease can be prevented or reversed by desoxycorticosterone (DOC) (WHITE,
HEINBECKER and ROLF 1947; GAUDINO and LEVITT). On the other hand, 20
to 30 mg. DOC daily to normal dogs was associated with a 16 and 24 percent

decrease in PAH Tm although GFR and RPF increased. Adrenocortical extract had no effect on diodrast Tm in normal or hypophysectomized dogs in the studies of WHITE et al. but PAH Tm was associated with increases of 11 and 43 percent in normal dogs studied by GAUDINO and LEVITT. In studies on patients with ADDISON's disease, diodrast Tm averaged 35 and 32 mg. I/min. (TALBOTT et al. 1942; SANDERSON 1948) and PAH Tm in a 36 year old woman was 53 mg./min. (WATERHOUSE and KEUTMANN). Treatment with DOC was associated with only a small increase in diodrast Tm (SANDERSON 1948). In limited studies on 4 normal subjects, 70 to 600 mg. of ACTH daily for 7 days is reported to have resulted in an increase in PAH Tm while 200 mg. of cortisone daily for the same period had no effect. Renotropic factors other than corticotropin may have been present in the ACTH preparation (INGBAR et al. 1950; BURNETT). Diodrast Tm was moderately depressed in 5 patients with CUSHING's disease, although not to the same extent as the concomitant depression in RBF and GFR (CORCORAN, TAYLOR and PAGE 1948).

PAH and diodrast Tm are normal or elevated in children or adults with "pure" lipid nephrosis, that is, when the disease process is relatively uncomplicated by present or past findings of hypertension, hematuria or azotemia (BRUCK, RAPOPORT and RUBIN; EARLE 1950; EDER et al.). Transport is depressed, however, when the nephrotic syndrome is present as a complication of another or more general disease (BRADLEY et al. 1950; METCOFF, KELSEY and JANEWAY; FURMAN et al.). PAH Tm may frequently be increased in the early stages of LAENNEC's cirrhosis (LESLIE, JOHNSTON and RALLI).

In view of the known sensitive dependence of diodrast and PAH transport on processes of oxidative phosphorylation, energy sources such as blood acetate level, competition from other aromatic acids claiming excretion and the probable existence of important undiscovered variables, the mechanism of action of various nutritional and endocrine factors is impossible to surmise.

e) Excretion of specific aromatic acids

Most of the individual members of the family of aromatic acids are of little interest. Because of various technical advantages which they possess, transport of diodrast or PAH has been extensively employed as an arbitrary measure of the capacity of this tubular transport system in various physiological and pathological states. Many members of the family, however, are important in physiology and medicine and should be described individually. Some of these are: phenolsulfonphthalein, penicillin, detoxication products, iodinated compounds, probenecid, and chlorothiazide.

α) Phenolsulfonphthalein (PSP, phenol red)

This compound (Fig. 24) is representative of a large group of acid dyes. Interest in PSP lies in the circumstance that it was selected and studied by ROWNTREE and GERAGHTY in 1910 as a measure of renal function in man. These authors selected PSP because of its rapid rate of excretion, low toxicity, lack of irritation if injected subcutaneously, ease of absorption from the gastrointestinal tract, high solubility, and intense color in alkali. Widespread clinical use of the compound stimulated intensive studies of the properties of its secretion by intact and isolated tubules of a great variety of vertebrates although for most physiological studies it is not discernibly superior to many other colored acids. PSP is a weak tribasic acid since the phenolic hydroxyl groups as well as the sulfonic group are capable of forming salts. At the p_H of blood it exists partially in a nonionized state (yellow) and partially as a salt (red). Conversion of the yellow to the red form occurs in the presence of alkali by opening of the —S—O—C— bond followed by dehydration to form the colored quinone group. It is not clear whether the yellow or the red is the actively transported form or whether, as is entirely possible, both forms are transported. Color is generally indetectable within cells which are actively transporting PSP, but since the intracellular p_H is in the range (6.8) at which a red color is just becoming detectable, colorlessness is hardly surprising (CHAMBERS and CAMERON). In a high potassium or low calcium medium PSP may occur intracellularly in high concentration in the red form (WASSERMAN, BECKER and FISHMAN).

The Tm of PSP measured in one normal subject, was about 36 mg. or 0.1 mM./min. (SMITH, GOLDRING and CHASIS). This may be compared with about 0.4 mM./min. for PAH. At low plasma concentrations, PSP should be completely removed from the blood perfusing the proximal convoluted tubules, but this has not proven to be the case. The clearance of PSP at plasma concentrations of 0.1 to 1.0 mg. per 100 ml. averages about 390 ml./min. (GOLDRING, CLARKE and SMITH), a figure which is about 60 percent of the diodrast clearance (SMITH, GOLDRING and CHASIS). The low clearance of PSP may be partly attributable to the high degree of binding of this substance to plasma proteins, particularly albumin (GROLLMAN 1925). At plasma concentrations of the order of 1 mg./100 ml., approximately 80 percent of the dye is bound to plasma proteins (GOLDRING, CLARKE and SMITH; SMITH and SMITH) so that the tubular cells will be presented with a concentration of not more than 0.2 mg./100 ml. Low concentration of free PSP together with slow dissociation of the dye-protein complex constitute in effect a diffusion barrier to excretion. This view is supported in part by the observations that when renal blood flow decreases as after epinephrin, PSP clearance approaches that of diodrast, while with augmented flow as following pyrogen administration the PSP-diodrast clearance ratio decreases (CHASIS et al. 1938). Moreover, much but not all of the difference between the clearances of PSP and diodrast disappears in dog kidney which is perfused by Dextran instead of plasma (OCHWADT and PITTS 1956a).

Since roughly 20 percent of the PSP in blood is free and diffusible in the plasma water and 20 percent of the plasma water is converted into glomerular filtrate, it follows that only about 4 percent (0.2×0.2) of excreted dye is derived from the process of filtration.

β) Penicillin

The penicillins are carboxylic acids (Fig. 24). At low plasma concentrations such as those usually encountered in therapy the clearance of most of the penicillins (Δ^2-pentenyl-(F, I), benzyl-(G, II) and p-hydroxybenzyl-(X, III) but not n-heptyl-(K)) is very high and of the same magnitude as that of diodrast and PAH (RAMMELKAMP and BRADLEY; RANTZ and KIRBY; JENSEN, MOLLER and OVERGAARD; EAGLE and NEWMAN). Indeed, the clearance of penicillin has been suggested as a measure of the renal plasma flow (BRYNER, RANDALL and RANTZ 1948a, b) but analytical methods are not sufficiently precise to justify adoption of penicillin for this purpose. Penicillin clearances are equally high in infants and children (BARNETT et al. 1949) but values somewhat lower than those consistent with renal plasma flow have been reported in elderly patients (MATHIESEN, ØRNSHOLT and TROLLE-LASSEN). The reason for the relatively low extraction of penicillin K is not entirely clear but may be attributable at least in part to the high degree of binding of this penicillin to plasma proteins), 91 percent as compared with the 50 percent plasma protein binding of other penicillins (Thompsett et al.). Penicillin K resembles PSP in this respect. The Tm of penicillin G in man is roughly 30 mg., or 0.1 mM./min. (Bryner et al.).

As could be predicted, excretion of penicillin can be depressed by other aromatic acids such as diodrast (Rammelkamp and Bradley) and PAH (Beyer et al. 1944a, b, c, 1945b; Loewe et al.) and the general property of competitive inhibition among members of this family was quickly put to practical use. During the first years following recognition of the value of penicillin in combatting infections the supply was very limited. Extravagant renal excretion of a drug which was both expensive and in limited supply was intolerable. A search for more effective competitive inhibitors of penicillin transport led to the discovery first of carinamide and then of probenecid (Beyer 1947).

γ) Iodinated compounds

Introduction of heavy iodine atoms into aromatic acid molecules permits radiopaque material to be concentrated in the urinary system for roentgenography (Fig. 24). Although iodine is not necessary in the molecule for tubular secretion, the quantitative effects of iodination (or halogenation generally) on maximal transport rate are not clear. Mono-, di- and triiodobenzoates are reabsorbed in the dog kidney just as is benzoate itself, but the maximal transport rates of the iodinated forms are lower (Knoefel and Huang 1956). Introduction of 2 iodine atoms into the aromatic nucleus of tyrosine converts this amino acid from a compound which is actively reabsorbed to a compound (3,5-diiodotyrosine) which is actively secreted. Diiodotyrosine has in the dog a Tm approximating that of p-aminohippurate, with which it competes for secretion, and various derivatives of diiodotyrosine are also actively secreted (Huang and Knoefel). The effects on tyrosine of iodination can be duplicated by introduction of bromo or nitro groups into the same position, and the conversion from a reabsorbed to a secreted substance is attributed in this case to alteration of the steric arrangement of the active groups (Huang).

Diodrast, hippuran and iopax at low concentrations are extracted almost completely from the renal plasma so that their clearances constitute an accurate measure of renal plasma flow. No evidence has been discovered that passage of these or the various hippurates into or out of red cells occurs in man to an extent sufficient to affect their clearances (Smith et al. 1945). In the dog, however, diodrast can traverse the red cell membrane at a significant rate. During passage of blood through the dog kidney, outward diffusion of red cell diodrast permits not only plasma but some of the red cell water to be cleared (White 1940a; Corcoran, Smith and Page). The tubular transport maxima of diodrast, hippuran and iopax in man are about 0.3, 0.6 and 0.2 mM./min., respectively. Neoiopax, a dicarboxylic acid, is poorly extracted and has a low Tm (0.1 mM./min. or less) (Smith and Ranges). Skiodan contains no aromatic nucleus and is not evidently secreted (Elsom, Bott and Shiels; Smith and Ranges).

δ) Conjugates

Many organic molecules of either exogenous or endogenous origin are conjugated in the body with glycine, glucuronate or sulfate. The conjugation processes occur almost if not entirely in the liver and kidneys and generally result in a stronger acid than the parent compound (Quick 1932b).

Marked species differences exist as between the relative rates of formation of the different conjugates in liver and kidney. In the dog, the kidney is virtually the sole locus of hippurate and other 'urate' (glycine conjugate) formation, while in man liver is equal to and sometimes somewhat more active than kidney (BUNGE and SCHMIEDEBERG; SNAPPER and LAQUER; QUICK 1932a; BORSOOK and DUBNOFF; BÉNARD and GAJDOS). Glucuronide and ethereal sulfate formation generally occur more rapidly in the liver (LIPSCHITZ and BUEDING; BÉNARD and GAJDOS). On the other hand, the o- and m-hydroxybenzoates are excreted predominantly as glucuronides (mostly the diglucuronide) in the dog and as the 'urates' in man (QUICK 1932b).

Glycine is conjugated more frequently with carboxylic and alcoholic groups of an acid while glucuronate and sulfate form esters with carboxylic or phenolic hydroxyl groups. Frequently, the acid or phenol which is conjugated is rather toxic. The conjugates tend to be not only less toxic than the primary compounds but they are also rapidly excreted by the aromatic acid transport system. For these reasons, conjugation has been termed 'detoxication' and the conjugates 'detoxication products'. It is the elimination of these substances which may well be the primary function of the acid secretory transport system (SPERBER 1946). The operation of this system can be illustrated by an example. Many fruits, such as cranberries and plums, contain large quantities of quinic acid. Quinic acid is metabolized to benzoic acid which is rapidly conjugated with glycine in the kidney and liver to yield hippuric acid. Some benzoylglucuronate may be formed by liver, kidney or both (BORGSTÖM). The hippurate, accounting for about 90 percent or more of the benzoic acid, is rapidly excreted (QUICK 1931). The excretion rate of the glucuronate, although unknown, is probably rapid also and accounts for most if not all of the remaining benzoate (SCHACHTER 1957) while no more than traces of benzoic acid, itself, appears in the urine at tolerable doses in man. Similarly, p-aminobenzoate is conjugated to yield the well-studied p-aminohippurate and many other hippurates such as o-iodohippurate (Hippuran), m-aminohippurate and m- and p-hydroxyhippurates are actively transported. In the chicken, selected for study because substances can be injected into the renal portal blood stream going to a single kidney thus permitting tubular secretion to be evaluated as the difference in the excretion rates of the separate kidneys, glucuronate and sulfate esters of phenol, menthol and resorcinol are actively secreted (SPERBER 1946). In man, conjugates of salicylic acid (salicylurate and salicylglucuronides, Fig. 24) and glucuronides of various 17-keto- and hydroxysteroids are secreted (SCHACHTER and MANIS; BONGIOVANNI and EBERLEIN; SAYERS et al.).

ε) Probenecid and carinamide

The rapid renal excretion of the acid, penicillin, stimulated a search for substances which could depress excretion by competing for the same tubular transport system. In addition to competing for transport, such a blocking agent also needs other qualities such as nontoxicity, stability, absorbability from the intestinal tract, and effectiveness in reasonably low doses in order to be useful (BEYER 1954). Carinamide (Fig. 24) was the first such compound developed which was clinically suitable although earlier it had been shown that penicillin excretion could be retarded by PAH and diodrast. Carinamide is an aromatic acid and its transport is fundamentally similar to that of other members of the family. Suitable doses of carinamide were capable of depressing penicillin G excretion by nearly 90 percent (SHAW et al.; EARLE and BRODIE; BEYER et al. 1947a; BOGER and FLIPPIN). Carinamide was not entirely satisfactory because its relatively high excretion rate required doses of at least 10 grams per day to maintain an effective competitive block of penicillin excretion. Continued search led to the discovery of the more potent probenecid (Fig. 24) which can effectively block penicillin secretion at a dose of 2 grams per day (Boger, Gallagher and Pitts). Probenecid incorporates to a high degree the apparently correlated properties of intense binding with cellular components and slow transport rate, the latter being so low that it cannot be clearly measured (Beyer et al. 1947b, 1950b, 1951). Complicating measurements of the tubular secretion of carinamide and probenecid is the circumstance that carinamide may be reabsorbed to a small extent and probenecid is certainly reabsorbed to a large extent (Beyer 1951). The reabsorptive transport mechanism is unknown but may well be the same as that which reabsorbs benzoic and p-aminobenzoic acid.

The effects of probenecid and carinamide on the transport of many substances has been extensively studied and it will be convenient to describe them together. They inhibit the tubular secretion of other aromatic acids such as p-aminohippurate, phenolsulfonphthalein, androsteronglucuronide, chlorothiazide and salicylic acid as well as penicillin (Beyer et al. 1947b; Bongiovanni and Eberlein; Schachter and Manis). They also depress the tubular secretion of exogenous creatinine in man and in sheep and goat (Brod and Sirota; Bucht 1949; Ladd et al.), thiosulfate in man (Bucht 1949), urea in the frog (Forster 1954) and phlorhizin in the dog (Braun, Whittaker and Lotspeich). A natriuretic effect from probenecid has been described in patients with congestive heart failure (Bronsky, Dubin and Kushner), but this is not clearly attributable to inhibition of tubular transport and no natri- or chloruretic effect has been observed in the dog or in healthy human subjects. In addition to inhibiting the excretion of other organic acids, probenecid also inhibits conjugation of benzoic acid derivatives such as p-aminobenzoate and salicylate, with glycine. The effect is highly specific in that probenecid blocks the utilization of oxidative energy by way of adenosine triphosphate (ATP) for the conjugation reactions without blocking the use of ATP for other metabolic processes such as phosphorylation of glucose (Beyer et al. 1950c).

Probenecid and carinamide do not affect the transport of glucose, arginine, organic bases, sodium, chloride, potassium or phosphate (Beyer et al. 1947b, 1950a, 1951; Sirota, Yü and Gutman; Despopoulos 1958; Spurr, Ford and Moyer), secretion of divalent inorganic anions and cations by aglomerular fish Berglund and Forster), reabsorption of urea by the elasmobranch, *Squalus acanthias* (Forster and Berglund), the clearances in man of urea, or endogenous creatinine (Beyer et al. 1947b, 1951), inulin or p-aminohippurate (Spurr, Ford and Moyer) or the excretion of thiopental in mice (Goldbaum and Hubbard). A depressant effect of probenecid on the elevated plasma phosphate concentrations observed in human hypo- and pseudohypoparathyroidism has been reported (Hoffman, Pascale and Dubin; Jackson et al.; Beidelman) and attributed by some to an increase in excretion. Although examination of the data shows that the increase in excretion is undramatic, and could not be detected by some (Jackson et al.), it is clear that kinetics of renal tubular phosphate reabsorption have been altered to permit sustained excretion at a lower plasma concentration. An acute increase in phosphate excretion with probenecid has been reported in gouty subjects (Bronsky, Kushner and Dubin) but no effects have been observed in the dog or in healthy human subjects (Beyer et al. 1951; Spurr, Ford and Moyer; Beidelman).

The general capacity of aromatic acids to inhibit urate transport, whether this is secretory as in birds or reabsorptive as in mammals, finds great clinical usefulness in the uricosuric properties of probenecid. Probenecid markedly depresses urate reabsorption in both normal and gouty subjects so that urate clearance may triple (SIROTA, YÜ and GUTMAN; GUTMAN; PASCALE; CRONE and LASSEN 1955a). If reabsorption of urate is low, however, (urate/inulin clearance ratio near 1.0) probenecid has no effect (SIROTA and HAMERMAN).

ζ) Chlorothiazide

Although the nature of its acidic groups is not yet clear, the diuretic agent chlorothiazide (Fig. 24) has the properties of a dibasic acid with pK values of 6.8 and 9.4 (SPRAGUE). It appears to be secreted by the tubules with considerable facility since it is accumulated by kidney slices *in vitro* (TAGGART 1958) and the clearance approaches that of PAH even though 50 percent or more of the substance is bound to plasma proteins at low plasma concentrations (BEYER 1958; BAER et al. 1958, 1959). In the dog, chlorothiazide depresses the clearance of penicillin while probenecid depresses that of chlorothiazide (BAER et al. 1959). *Tm* values have not been reported, however.

2. Transport of uric acid

Uric acid (Fig. 24) has long attracted considerable attention both because of its importance as an end product in purine metabolism and because of its role in causing gout. At the same time, the excretion of this substance is extremely complex and the mechanisms are still unclear. Uric acid is actively secreted by the renal tubules of most vertebrates including amphibian (LUEKEN; BORDLEY and RICHARDS), reptile (MARSHALL 1931b; BORDLEY and RICHARDS) and bird (MARSHALL 1931b; SHANNON 1938d; BERGER, YÜ and GUTMAN). Urate is accumulated by rabbit kidney slices (PLATTS and MUDGE) and it inhibits the accumulation of PAH without depressing tissue metabolism (DESPOPOULOS 1959). For these reasons urate transport is classified here with tubular secretory processes. Uric acid is slightly concentrated over plasma in the urine from the aglomerular tubules of the fish, *Lophius*, but these studies need amplification (MARSHALL and GRAFFLIN 1928). In mammals, on the other hand, net tubular reabsorption appears to be the rule, although significant exceptions have been reported. POULSEN and PRAETORIUS report that net tubular secretion occurs in the rabbit during urate loading; and in the Dalmatian dog urate reabsorption appears to be absent and a small secretory transport appears to be present at normal plasma urate concentrations which, in this animal, are very low (FRIEDMAN and BYERS 1948; BEYER 1954). Stopped flow studies suggest that both the secretion of urate in Dalmatian and reabsorption of urate in nondalmatian dogs occurs in the nephron segment coextensive with p-aminohippurate secretion (KESSLER, HIERHOLZER and GURD). PRAETORIUS and KIRK discovered a pattern of urate excretion similar to the Dalmatian in a healthy, otherwise normal human. In this 28 year old male, urate/inulin clearance ratio averaged 1.46 with a plasma urate concentration of 0.2 to 0.6 mg. percent. Plasma 'oxypurine precursors', however, averaged higher than normal.

In the human, the clearance of urate is much lower than that of the glomerular filtration rate. Although early studies suggested that the low and variable urate clearance might be attributable, at least in part, to an incomplete and variable filterability of plasma urate (WOLFSON et al.), detailed analysis has not borne out this possibility and all plasma urate is believed to be freely filterable both in normal and gouty subjects nor is the filterability affected by uricosuric agents (SMITH 1951 for review; YÜ and GUTMAN 1953; SIROTA, YÜ and GUTMAN). The low clearance combined with free filterability indicates that most of the filtered urate is reabsorbed. At normal plasma urate concentrations,

the urate/inulin clearance ratio ranges between 5 and 10 percent, indicative
of 90 to 95 percent reabsorption of filtered urate (TALBOTT 1943; COOMBS et al.;
GUTMAN and YÜ 1957).

When blood urate concentration is elevated acutely in healthy normal subjects by urate infusion, rate of urate reabsorption rises slowly as filtered load
increases, attaining finally a Tm value of 13.5 to 19.5 mg./min./1.73 M² at a
load/Tm ratio of about 1.5 or a plasma urate concentration of about 20 mg.
percent (Fig. 26) (BERLINER et al. 1950). The wide splay in the urate titration
curve describes how normal man remains in urate balance at low filtered loads
and at plasma urate concentrations of 3 to 5 mg. percent, values which are far
below those necessary to attain saturation of the tubular transport system.

Urate reabsorption is depressed by a wide variety of agents, collectively
termed 'uricosurics'. Of particular interest are aromatic acids: phenolsulfonphthalein, diodrast (TALBOTT 1943; BONSNES, DILL and DANA), carinamide, probenecid
(WOLFSON et al.; PASCALE; SIROTA, YÜ and GUTMAN; GUTMAN; CRONE and
LASSEN 1955a), salicylate (QUICK; CRONE and LASSEN 1955b, c; GUTMAN and

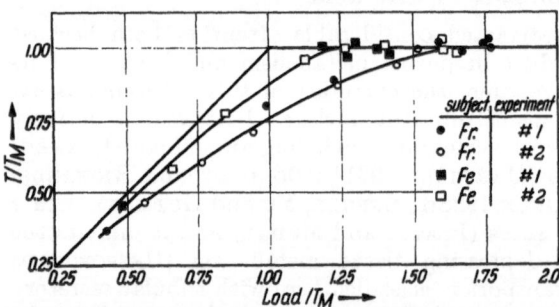

Fig. 26. Urate titration curve for 2 normal subjects, after BERLINER
et al. (1950). See Chapter D I 2 for method of calculation. Reproduced by permission of the authors and the Journal of Clinical
Investigation

YÜ 1955), cinchophen (TAL-
BOTT 1943; COOMBS et al.)
and other acids (SMITH 1951)
can in appropriate quantities
cause urate clearance to increase by 2 to 5 times with
associated decrease in plasma
urate concentration (CRONE
and LASSEN 1955a, b). Other
agents reported to increase
uric acid excretion are o-
amino-benzoate (MARTIN),
phenacetin (MARTIN), organomercurials (COOMBS et al.;
FERRANINI and FONTANA;

FERRANINI and CASTORIA; GROSSMAN et al. 1950a), phenylbutazone and some
of its derivatives (YÜ, SIROTA and GUTMAN; YÜ et al. 1956; BURNS et al.),
the xanthines caffeine and theophylline (MARTIN), sorbitol in dogs (GRABFIELD
and SWANSON), hyperglycemia or glucosuria in man (TALBOTT 1943; BONSNES
and DANA; CHRISTENSEN and STEENSTRUP), and adrenocorticotropin and
cortisone (SPRAGUE et al.; INGBAR et al. 1950, 1951; GUTMAN and YÜ 1950).
Adrenocorticotropin effects acutely a 10 to 100 percent increase in urate clearance but generally is inferior to other agents in the treatment of gout. An
osmotic diuresis due to mannitol is ineffective (TALBOTT 1943). In the chicken,
in which urate is eliminated almost entirely by secretion, human uricosuric
agents are either ineffective (salicylate) or depress urate excretion (PAH,
probenecid, phenyl butazone) (BERGER, YÜ and GUTMAN).

Certain substances depress urate excretion. Among these are lactate which,
in a group of normal subjects, nearly suppressed urate excretion. Urate clearance
decreased from an average of 10.4 to 1.4 ml./min. (YÜ et al. 1957b). In addition,
lactate abolished the uricosuria resulting from salicylate or probenecid administration. Other substances which in small quantities inhibit urate excretion enhance
excretion at higher blood concentrations. Salicylate, phenylbutazone and its
p-hydroxy and p-nitro derivatives and probenecid at low blood concentrations
enhance urate reabsorption and depress its clearance. Not until higher blood
levels are attained do the uricosuric effects appear (QUICK 1933; KLEMPERER

and BAUER; GUTMAN and YÜ 1955; YÜ and GUTMAN 1955; YÜ et al. 1959). Relatively high blood levels of phenylbutazone (10 mg. percent) must be attained before uricosuria appears. In the case of salicylate, a minimum of 1 gram must be taken to obtain uricosuria (QUICK 1933). The 4-phenylthioethyl analog of phenylbutazone, however, appears uricosuric at all blood levels and exhibits no clear antiuricosuric phase (YÜ et al. 1956). Other compounds exhibit a predominantly antiuricosuric effect. Orthochlorobenzoate (QUICK 1933), pyrazin-amide and pyrazinoic acid (YÜ et al. 1957a; AMINI et al.), acetazoleamide (YÜ and GUTMAN 1959) and chlorothiazide (OREN, RICH and BELLE) are examples of these. Presumably, urate excretion is depressed by these agents in the same way that it is depressed by salicylate et al. at low blood concentrations. Interesting observations, the significance of which is not clear, are the interactions between uricosuric agents. Salicylate is not additive to but interferes with the uricosuric effect of probenecid (PASCALE; GUTMAN). Glycine, which in 5 gm. doses has little uricosuric activity of its own is reported to enhance the uricosuric effect of appropriate doses of salicylate in man (QUICK 1933) but not in the rat (FRIEDMAN 1948). Larger (25 gm.) doses of glycine may be uricosuric as well as a stimulant of increased urate production (FRIEDMAN 1947b). The antiuricosuric effects of smaller doses (0.5—1.5 g.) of salicylate are inhibited by glycine (ELLIOTT and MURDAUGH). Urate clearance is affected slightly by urine p_H. In alkaline urine, the urate/inulin clearance ratio may average 20 percent higher than that observed in acidosis (YÜ and GUTMAN 1959), but the changes observed are not yet clearly attributable to the effects of p_H on a passively-diffusing acid.

The complex and frequently paradoxical effect of various substances on urate excretion lead QUICK (1933) to suggest that salicylate has both an inhibitory and stimulatory effect on salicylate excretion. With the evolution of the filtration-reabsorption hypothesis of renal function, QUICK's hypothesis has been restated by YÜ and GUTMAN (1958, 1959) in terms of a dual transport system for urate. These authors suggest that the ancient vertebrate capacity to secrete urate persists in mammals in a variably weakened or rudimentary form and that a reabsorptive system, which may well be the same as that which reabsorbs benzoic and related acids, has been acquired. Various substances can affect either the secretory, or the reabsorptive system primarily, or else they can affect both processes, as in the instance of salicylate (o-hydroxybenzoate) and phenyl-butazone. Administration of the uricosuric agent, sulfinpyrazone, to either normal or gouty subjects during urate infusion causes the urate/inulin clearance ratio to exceed 1.0, indicative of tubular secretion (GUTMAN, YÜ and BERGER). Unmasking of a slow secretory system by nearly complete suppression of reabsorption appears more probable than stimulation of secretion. In the Dalmatian dog, which appears to lack a detectable urate reabsorptive system, salicylate or probenecid act only as depressants of excretion (FRIEDMAN and BYERS 1948; BEYER 1954). Urate excretion in this animal appears to be enhanced by renin (SCHAFFER, DILL and STANDER).

Few if any extensive studies have been made on urate transport in human physiological or pathological states so that changes in urate Tm and titration splay are unknown. All studies relate to urate clearance and urate/inulin clearance ratios at spontaneously occurring filtration rates and plasma urate concentrations. In *pregnancy* urate clearance is elevated, averaging 32 ml./min. in 12 women in the last trimester and is related chiefly to an increase in excretion. Urate clearance is somewhat lower, 22 ml./min., in preeclamptic patients with corresponding increase in average plasma urate concentration (5.3 mg. percent compared with 3.8 in the normal pregnant). The urate/inulin clearance ratio is also elevated in pregnancy but is increased relatively less than is the urate clearance alone, and the ratio is subequal as between nonpregnant and preeclamptic women. The decreased clearance in the preeclamptics seems partially attributable to decreased filtration rate observed in this group (SCHAFFER, DILL and CADDEN; CHRISTENSEN and STEENSTRUP) but increased blood lactate in the toxemic patients is cited as an additional factor which could enhance tubular reabsorption of urate (HANDLER).

In primary gout uric acid is produced in increased amounts (FRIEDMAN and BYERS 1950; GUTMAN and YÜ 1957). Increased urate production is not the sole abnormality in this disease since the high frequency of acute gouty arthritis in men as compared with women with primary gout or with patients with secondary hyperuricemia at equivalent blood urate concentrations is unexplained. Whether or not a primary renal dysfunction exists in gout prior to the onset of gouty nephritis is unknown. The urate clearance and urate/inulin clearance ratio is statistically the same in normals and young gouty subjects early in the disease in spite of marked differences in plasma urate concentration (COOMBS et al.; FRIEDMAN and BYERS 1950; SIROTA, YÜ and GUTMAN; GUTMAN and YÜ 1957). On the other hand, urate clearance in normals is *increased* at either acutely or chronically elevated plasma urate concentrations (BERLINER et al. 1950; NUGENT and TYLER). In the two subjects on whom complete titration curves were obtained by BERLINER et al., urate clearance increased from 16 and 15 ml./min. at low plasma concentrations to 27 and 41 ml./min. at plasma urate concentrations of 9 and 10 mg. percent. As gouty nephropathy progresses with associated decrease in filtration rate, urate clearance remains essentially constant so that an ever increasing fraction of the filtered urate is excreted (COOMBS et al.). In certain instances of tubular dysfunction such as the *Fanconi syndrome*, urate transport capacity may be absent, and urate/inulin clearance ratio is 1.0 (SIROTA and HAMERMAN).

3. Transport of creatinine

Creatinine (Fig. 24) is a weak base with a pK' of about 4.8. It is actively secreted by the renal tubules in most orders of vertebrates, but the capacity to transport this substance has been lost by certain groups, particularly among mammals. Thus, creatinine is actively secreted by both glomerular and aglomerular fish (MARSHALL and GRAFFLIN 1928, 1932; EDWARDS and CONDORELLI; CLARKE and SMITH; SHANNON 1933, 1940; PITTS 1935), chicken (SHANNON 1938c; LAMBERT) and probably turtle[1] but is excreted by filtration alone in the amphibian, *Necturus* (KINTER). In the bullfrog, *Rana catesbiana*, the creatinine/inulin clearance ratio has been variously reported as 0.996 (FORSTER 1938a, b) and 1.27 (SWANSON; HOGBEN and BOLLMAN 1951a). The latter value would be consistent with creatinine secretion.

Among mammals, creatinine is actively secreted by the tubules of man (SHANNON 1935c; SHANNON and RANGES; SMITH, FINKELSTEIN and SMITH; CRAWFORD; BUCHT 1949) and other primates including orangutan, chimpanzee, gibbon, baboon and monkey (SMITH and CLARKE; GAGNON and CLARKE). Creatinine secretion is very low, however, in the monkey and is not clearly detectable

---

[1] Creatinine/inulin clearance ratios of 1.0 are reported for the fresh-water turtle, *Pseudemys elegans* (FRIEDLICH, HOLMAN and FORSTER) but internal evidence from the effects of phlorhizin suggests that the inulin clearance values are about 20 percent too high and that creatinine is, in fact, secreted.

in the human infant (DEAN and McCANCE 1947). The mechanisms of excretion in ruminants are not clear. In experiments on one sheep, SHANNON (1937) observed an average creatinine/inulin clearance ratio of 1.03. LADD et al., however, reported that creatinine clearance exceeded that of inulin at low plasma concentrations in sheep and goats but fell below that of inulin as plasma creatinine concentration was progressively elevated, while SPERBER and SPERBER concluded from studies on four goats and a sheep that creatinine has a typical secretory Tm and its clearance is regularly greater than that of inulin. Creatinine is not clearly secreted or reabsorbed, however, by the kidney of the dog (RICHARDS, WESTFALL and BOTT 1934; SHANNON 1935b; VAN SLYKE, HILLER and MILLER), cat (GAMMELTOFT and KJERULF-JENSEN), rabbit (KAPLAN and SMITH; JOSEPHSON and KALLAS 1953a; EFFERSØE 1949), seal, *Phoca vitulina*, (SMITH 1936), and probably in the rat (FRIEDMAN 1947a; CORCORAN et al.; LIPPMAN; GRIBETZ, VAN LOON and CRAWFORD) although other studies in this animal suggest secretion (STONER and DEXTER). Its clearance is therefore equal to that of inulin in many of these latter species and it provides an accurate measure of glomerular filtration rate.

In those species in which creatinine is actively secreted, creatinine is unique in that, as a base, its secretory component is depressed by aromatic acids, the latter causing creatinine clearance to decline to, or occasionally below, inulin clearance. Thus, creatinine secretion in the chicken is depressed by hippuran (LAMBERT), in sheep and goat by PAH and probenecid (LADD et al.), in the chimpanzee by PAH (GAGNON and CLARKE) and in man by diodrast (CRAWFORD; SMITH, FINKELSTEIN and SMITH), PAH (CRAWFORD; BROD and SIROTA) and caronamide (BUCHT 1949; BROD and SIROTA; MATTAR et al.). In view of this evidence, creatinine, like uric acid, may possibly be transported by the aromatic acid transport system, but more studies are needed. The effects of phlorhizin on creatinine secretion are not clear. In chicken and man phlorhizin is reported to reduce the creatinine/inulin clearance ratio to 1.0 (SHANNON 1935c, 1938c) although in older studies no significant effect of phlorhizin on the creatinine/ xylose clearance ratio in man was observed (CHASIS, JOLLIFFE and SMITH) and LADD et al. observed no effect of phlorhizin on creatinine excretion in sheep or goat. Hypothermia in man reduces the creatinine/inulin clearance ratio to 1.0 (TALBOTT 1951).

Although creatinine in the dog generally appears to be excreted by filtration alone, it fails to agree with inulin clearance under certain circumstances. RICHARDS, WESTFALL and BOTT (1936) observed that the creatinine/inulin clearance ratio decreased to about 0.87 in the dog kidney poisoned with uranyl salts. Clearance ratios significantly less than 1.0 were also observed in both isolated and intact dog kidney and in the kidney of sheep and goat when the arterial or perfusion pressures were low (SHANNON and WINTON; LADD, LIDDLE and GAGNON; LADD et al.). In rabbits, the creatinine/inulin clearance ratio which is usually 1.0 may decrease to 0.80—0.85 following oral administration of 0.5—1.0 gm. of sodium benzoate (EFFERSØE 1949). These findings indicate that tubular reabsorption of creatinine may occur under certain circumstances but the mechanisms which are involved are unknown and have not been shown to represent an active process.

A clear description of creatinine excretion in man is not available. This is attributable in part to technical difficulties in the measurement of the normal concentrations of this substance in the blood plasma and in part to a complex excretion pattern. Normally, 15 to 40 percent of the substance reacting with nitrophenols (usually picric acid) in alkali to yield a red color (total creatinine chromogen) is not true creatinine chromogen. The latter must be measured either following adsorption and elution from Fuller's earth (Lloyd's reagent) or calculated by difference after removal of true creatinine by creatininase. Both procedures involve uncertainties. In addition, color development may be capricious and recovery from plasma protein precipitation may be incomplete (Lauson; Owen et al.; Smith, Finkelstein and Smith). These problems would not be serious were it not for the circumstance that the cumulative systematic error should be less than 10 percent. Although the results of various researchers do not agree closely, probably because of variation in their methods, most studies show that the endogenous true creatinine clearance is distinctly greater than inulin clearance in normal subjects. This indicates that some creatinine is being actively secreted by the human kidney at all times (Miller and Winkler 1938; Barclay and Kenney). When plasma creatinine concentration rises either because of administration of exogenous creatinine or because of kidney disease, the creatinine/inulin clearance ratio increases further and may attain values as high as 2.0 (Steinitz and Turkand; Shannon 1935c; Miller and Winkler 1938; Brod and Sirota; Mattar et al.). This rise in clearance ratio results from reduction in the significance of the noncreatinine chromogen in the plasma, an actual suppression by creatinine of chromogenicity of noncreatinine substances (Lauson) and perhaps by an actual increase in tubular transport. When plasma creatinine concentration is acutely elevated, creatinine clearance rises abruptly to values which may be 1.3 to 1.6 times that of inulin. Over a period of an hour or more, creatinine/inulin clearance ratio may then decrease to lower values indicating that tubular transport is decreasing and illustrating the difficulty in defining a constant Tm (Shannon and Ranges; Miller and Winkler 1938; Winkler and Parra 1957a). Transport does not cease entirely, however, unless a competitor such as diodrast, PAH or caronamide is administered *(vida supra)*. In patients with renal disease in whom plasma creatinine concentration is elevated, a decrease in clearance following acute loading with exogenous creatinine is not observed (Winkler and Parra 1937b). While the clearance of creatinine either at normal or elevated plasma concentrations distinctly exceeds that of inulin, the 'clearance' of the non-creatinine chromogen is much less, averaging roughly 25 percent of that of inulin. The total chromogen clearance, which represents the combination of one clearance which is greater and one which is less than that of inulin, is therefore intermediate and, by reason of the relative proportions of true creatinine to total chromogen, coincidentally approximates closely to that of inulin (Brod and Sirota; Steinitz and Turkand; Blegen, Haugen and Aas; Baldwin, Sirota and Villarreal). The term, 'endogenous creatinine clearance', usually refers to the clearance of total chromogen. With possible changes both in rate of secretion as well as in the relative proportions of true creatinine to total chromogen in the plasma, 'endogenous creatinine' clearance seldom mirrors changes in filtration rate precisely (Ingbar et al. 1950; Burnett; Patalano and Vivone; Dodge and Daeschner; Talbott 1951; Barnett et al. 1951). In species such as dog and rat, in which no significant rate of tubular secretion is evident, the endogenous total chromogen clearance is distinctly less than that of inulin (Lippmann; Davenport et al.) while endogenous true creatinine clearance coincides as closely to that of inulin as the methods permit (Shannon 1935b). Alternatively, by adding creatinine exogenously to the plasma in such species the noncreatinine chromogen can be reduced to relatively insignificant proportions and the total chromogen clearance brought to equality with that of inulin (GFR).

4. Transport of organic bases

Certain organic bases are actively secreted from the blood into the urine. This is indicated by their excretion in amounts greater than can be accounted for by filtration alone. Although this tubular transport system has been studied much less than that which transports aromatic acids, available evidence indicates that it resembles the acid transport system in many respects. It is present in many and perhaps all orders of vertebrates, having been demonstrated in birds (SPERBER 1954; RENNICK et al. 1954) and the aglomerular fish (FORSTER, BERGLUND and RENNICK) as well as in mammals. It is located in the proximal segment of the nephron (RENNICK, EVANS and MOE).

Two organic bases have been extensively studied. These are the quaternary ammonium bases tetraethylammonium and N'-methylnicotinamide (Fig. 27). At low plasma concentrations, nearly all of both of these substances is completely removed from the plasma, so that their clearances approximate the effective renal plasma flow (RENNICK et al. 1947; BEYER et al. 1950a). Clearances decrease

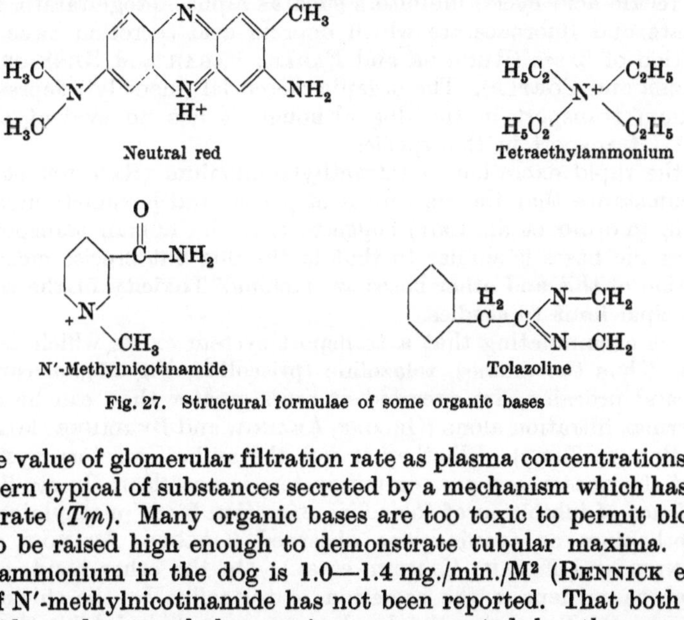

Fig. 27. Structural formulae of some organic bases

toward the value of glomerular filtration rate as plasma concentrations rise, which is the pattern typical of substances secreted by a mechanism which has a maximal transport rate (Tm). Many organic bases are too toxic to permit blood concentrations to be raised high enough to demonstrate tubular maxima. The Tm of tetraethylammonium in the dog is 1.0—1.4 mg./min./M^2 (RENNICK et al. 1954). The Tm of N'-methylnicotinamide has not been reported. That both N'-methylnicotinamide and tetraethylammonium are excreted by the same transport system is indicated by the fact that these substances interfere with the excretion of each other but have no effect upon the excretion of aromatic acids such as PAH (KANDEL and PETERS). Other strong bases, some of considerable physiological importance, are also secreted by this system and exhibit cross inhibition with other bases. Some of these are tetraalkylammonium compounds as a class (GREEN et al. 1959), mepiperphenidol (DARSTINE) and other piperidinium derivatives (BEYER et al. 1953; VOLLE et al.); methylguanidine, guanidine, piperidine, choline and thiamine by the chicken (SPERBER 1949b; RENNICK; FARAH, RENNICK and FRAZER) and trimethylamine oxide which is secreted as a normal metabolite by the aglomerular fish[1] (FORSTER, BERGLUND and RENNICK). In-

---

[1] Surprisingly, bases which inhibit the secretion of trimethylamine oxide by the aglomerular tubules of *Lophius* do not inhibit the reabsorption of trimethylamine oxide by the glomerular tubules of *Squalus* (FORSTER, BERGLUND and RENNICK).

hibitory interactions on the chicken kidney between tetraalkylammonium and N'-methylnicotinamide decrease with increasing methyl substitution. Tetramethylammonium exhibits little inhibitory effect and is not significantly secreted (Green and Peters; Farah, Rennick and Frazer). Small quantities of the organic cyanine bases, on the other hand, strongly inhibit the transport of bases in a fashion quite analogous to inhibition of aromatic acid secretion by probenecid (Farah, Frazer and Porter). Also like probenecid, cyanine 863, the most potent inhibitor among the cyanines examined, is strongly bound to cell proteins, particularly mitochondria, and is itself excreted slowly. Cyanine has no effect on transport of PAH or glucose (Peters et al.; Rennick, Kandel and Peters) while carinamide and probenecid have no effect on secretion of bases (Beyer et al. 1950a, 1951; Sperber 1954; Rennick and Farah; Rennick, Kandel and Peters).

Transport of tetraethylammonium like that of the aromatic acids is depressed in the dog by 2,4-dinitrophenol (which uncouples oxidation from phosphorylation), fluoride, cyanide, azide and iodoacetate. On the other hand, various Krebs-cycle (citric acid cycle) inhibitors such as alpha ketoglutarate, malonate, dehydroacetate and fluoroacetate which depress acid secretion have no effect on the secretion of bases (Rennick and Farah; Farah and Rennick; Farah; Farah, Frazer and Porter). The organic mercurial (mersalyl) depresses tetraethylammonium transport in the dog although it has no evident depressant effect on PAH transport in this species.

In man the rapid excretion of tetraethylammonium (Rennick et al. 1947) and the circumstance that the clearances of penta- and hexamethonium exceed that of inulin (Young et al. 1951) suggests that the human transport system for strong organic bases is similar to that in the dog but precise measurements of the excretion of this and other bases are lacking. Toxicity of the compounds sets the principal limit to studies.

Evidence is accumulating that a transport system exists which can excrete amine bases. Thus the amines, tolazoline (priscoline, Fig. 27), mecamylamine, epinephrine and procaine, are excreted at rates greater than can be accounted for by glomerular filtration alone (Orloff, Aranow and Berliner; Milne et al.; Jones and Blake; Terp). Whether or not the amine secretory system is independent of the quaternary ammonium system is not clear. In studies on the dog, no evidence of inhibition of tolazoline excretion by N'-methylnicotinamide, tetraethylmethonium or cyanine was observed (Orloff, Aranow and Berliner; Rennick and Farah; Kandel et al.). On the other hand, cyanine as well as other bases depress the secretion of tolazoline by the chicken kidney (Volle, Green and Peters) and tolazoline can reversibly inhibit the secretion of N'-methylnicotinamide and tetraethylammonium in both chicken and dog (Kandel et al.; Farah). Excretion of mecamylamine and tolazoline as well as members of the quaternary ammonium group was enhanced by potassium loading in the dog (Kandel and Domer; Domer). Until clear evidence is available that they are distinct, the transport processes for both groups of organic bases may be treated as a single system.

5. Excretion of tissue permeable weak acids and bases
a) General considerations

When the epithelium of the nephron is nearly or quite impermeable to an excreted substance, excretion can be described in reasonably simple terms as the quantity present in glomerular filtrate which may be increased or decreased by an active secretory or reabsorptive process. Many other substances may be filtered and for which, also, active processes may exist, but to which the epithelium is permeable in varying degrees. As a rule, the tubules are permeable to substances which are capable of diffusing across the membranes of body cells generally. For convenience of description, tissue permeable substances may be grouped into 1. various lipid-soluble, nonionized substances such as oxygen, carbon dioxide, ethanol and others which pass easily across cell membranes; 2. urea, which is a small molecular weight substance to which the tubular epithelium is slightly permeable; and 3. certain weak acids and weak bases. The first two groups will be described in Section D VI. The excretion of weak acids and bases will be described here.

As related to excretion an acid or base is considered to be weak if it is incompletely dissociated at the pH of body fluids (4.5 to 8.0). When it is partially dissociated, such a substance exists in two forms: the dissociated or ionized

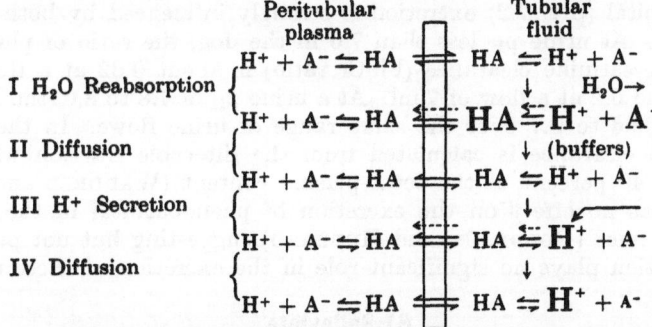

Fig. 28. Hypothetical steps in the reabsorption of a weak acid. The relative sizes of the symbols indicate relative concentrations. I. A weak acid, HA, is filtered with its salt, A⁻, at the glomerulus. Since the same concentrations are present in peritubular blood and filtrate, HA is not lost from the filtrate although it can penetrate epithelium. All fractions of the filtrate are concentrated by reabsorption of water, so that some HA can diffuse into the blood. II. Buffers supply hydrogen ion, permitting the equilibrium to shift to the left. The final concentrations of HA and A⁻ return toward those of the blood. III. In a distal region of the nephron, H⁺ is secreted in amounts capable of raising the concentration up to 800 times that of the blood. The equilibrium is shifted strongly from A⁻ to HA. Because of the high concentration gradient, large amounts of HA diffuse into the blood. IV. HA has attained diffusion equilibrium. Because of the high H⁺ which drives the reaction toward HA, A⁻ may be much less concentrated than in the original filtrate

form, and the undissociated or nonionized form. Generally, cells, including those of the renal tubules, are not freely permeable to ions but may be permeable to the nonionized moiety. In the latter circumstance excretion will be determined not only by filtration, with or without active transport, but also by the extent to which the nonionized fraction of the weak acid or base diffuses in either direction between tubular fluid and blood. The rate of diffusion will depend upon the concentration difference between tubular fluid and blood and upon the permeability of the nephron which may be assumed to vary from segment to segment. The concentration difference will depend on the quantity filtered, on the extent of water reabsorption by the nephron, on the pK of the weak acid or base, and, in particular, on the pH of the fluid in each segment of the nephron. Some of these variables, such as the pK of the substance, are known; other variables, such as the degree of water reabsorption and the pH in each segment of the nephron, can be estimated; while permeability factors are quite unknown. Another important variable determining the concentration difference is the concentration of the weak acid or base in the peritubular blood or tissue fluid. In the cortex this is undoubtedly close to that of the glomerular filtrate but in the medulla the peritubular concentration may be much greater because of the

accumulating properties of the loops of the vasa recta (Section B VIII 4). It
is not surprising, therefore, that excretion of these weak acids and bases has
not yet been described in quantitative terms although the effects of changes
in urine flow and p_H can be predicted qualitatively. These are illustrated for
a weak acid in Fig. 28. A similar process in which the effects of p_H are reversed
will exist for weak bases. Milne, Scribner and Crawford should be consulted
for a discussion of quantitative aspects of the excretion of tissue-permeable weak
electrolytes.

The corollary of these predicted effects of water reabsorption and p_H change
is that any weak acid or base which exhibits such effects is presumed to be
handled by the kidney in the manner illustrated in Fig. 28.

b) Tissue-permeable weak acids

α) Barbiturates

Phenobarbital (pK, 7.2) excretion is strongly influenced by both urine flow
and urine p_H. At urine p_H less than 7.0 in the dog, the ratio of phenobarbital
clearance to creatinine clearance (Ph/Cr ratio) is about 0.02 at a flow of 1 ml.
per minute and 0.2 at a flow of 7 ml. At a urine p_H of 7.8 to 8.0, the Ph/Cr ratio
varied from 0.06 to 0.7 over the same range of urine flows. In these studies,
phenobarbital clearance is calculated from the filterable fraction which represented about 40 percent of the total plasma content (Waddell and Butler).
Probenecid has no effect on the excretion of phenobarbital in the dog or on
thiopental in mice (Goldbaum and Hubbard) suggesting but not proving that
tubular secretion plays no significant role in the excretion of these acids.

β) Salicylate

The excretion of salicylic acid (o-hydroxybenzoic acid, Fig. 24) is complex.
Some of the salicylate absorbed into the body is conjugated with glycine at the
carboxyl group by kidney and liver in man to form salicylurate, just as benzoate
is conjugated to form hippurate. Additional salicylate is conjugated with glucuronic acid at either the carboxyl or the phenolic group or at both (probably
in the liver) to form salicylacylglucuronate (Fig. 24) and salicylphenolic glucuronate (Quick 1932b; Kapp and Coburn; Bjørneboe, Dalgaard-Mikkelsen
and Raaschou; Dalgaard-Mikkelsen; Galimard; Schachter and Manis).
Salicylurate and the salicylglucuronates are extracted efficiently from the renal
blood by the aromatic acid active transport system just as are conjugates in
general (Schachter). At low plasma concentrations, their clearance in man
approximates that of the effective renal plasma flow and appears to be independent of urine flow and p_H (Schachter and Manis). Although a dependence of
salicylurate excretion on p_H has been reported in one study, (Bjørneboe, Dalgaard-Mikkelsen and Raaschou), this seems contrary to the general pattern
of conjugate excretion. In the studies of Schachter and Manis, about 64 percent of the total conjugate was excreted as salicylurate, 23 percent as the acyl-
glucuronate and 13 percent as the phenolic glucuronate. The remainder of the
salicylate is excreted unconjugated, or free.

Free salicylic acid has a pK of about 3.0. Therefore, in weakly acid urine
(p_H 6.0), 0.1 percent of the free salicylate will exist as salicylic acid. At the p_H
of blood (7.3) the fraction existing as salicylic acid will be less than 10 percent
of the urine value so that at least a 10 fold gradient for undissociated salicylic
acid exists between urine and blood even before introducing an additional effect
on the concentration gradient by water reabsorption. Theoretically (assuming

no effects from the medullary interstitial fluid) undissociated salicylic acid should continue to diffuse into the blood from a urine of pH 6 until the urine concentration of salicyl ion, which constitutes 99 percent or more of the free salicylate, is 10 percent of that in the blood. Actual excretion rates are somewhat greater than predicted, probably because of inexactness of the assumptions.

In man as little as 1 percent of filtered free salicylate is excreted at a urine pH of 5. Between pH 5 and 6, 5 to 15 percent is excreted. As the urine pH approaches that of blood, the excreted fraction of filtered salicylate rises rapidly, approaching 100 percent at a urine pH of 7.2—7.5, and exceeding 100 percent by a significant amount at urine pH of 7.8—8.0 In strongly alkaline urines, more than twice as much free salicylic acid may be excreted than can be accounted for in the filtrate (P. K. SMITH et al.; WILLIAMS and LEONARDS; BJØRNEBOE, DALGAARD-MIKKELSEN and RAASCHOU; GUTMAN, YÜ and SIROTA; DAVIS and SMITH; SCHACHTER and MANIS). Salicylate clearance also varies with urine flow, increasing approximately 5 times as urine flow increases from 1 to 15 ml./min. at constant pH (MACPHERSON, MILNE and EVANS).

Free salicylate clearance in man may be described empirically by the following equations (MACPHERSON, MILNE and EVANS):

$$\log C = 0.52 \, \text{pH} - 2.0$$
$$\log C/C_{4.5} = 0.55 \log V - 0.36$$

where C is salicylate clearance and $C_{4.5}$ is mean salicylate clearance at a urine flow of 4.5 ml./min.

That the free salicylate in alkaline urine in excess of the quantity filtered is probably secreted by the aromatic acid transport system, is evidenced by the fact that probenecid depressed excretion without causing the urine to become more acid (GUTMAN, YÜ and SIROTA; SCHACHTER and MANIS) while salicylate itself depresses the excretion of PAH in both acid and alkaline urine (FRANKLIN et al.). Similarly, in the dog, high salicylate excretion in alkaline urine can be depressed by probenecid, acetazolamide, p-aminohippurate and other acids (WEINER, WASHINGTON and MUDGE). Probably because of the preponderant role of diffusion forces, tubular secretion and its depression by probenecid cannot be detected in acid urine.

γ) p-aminosalicylic acid

The success of carinamide and probenecid in retarding the excretion of penicillin prompted research to determine whether excretion of p-aminosalicylic acid (PAS), employed in the treatment of tuberculosis and other conditions, could be similarly retarded. Studies of HORNE and WILSON, BOGER, PITTS and GALLAGHER, and BOGER et al. indicated that this was indeed the case. A PAS clearance which averaged 1.31 times that of the inulin clearance (after correction for plasma binding of PAS) decreased to 0.56 after carinamide (HORNE and WILSON). However, the effect of probenecid on PAS plasma level does not become evident for several hours after ingestion of a single 4 gram dose of probenecid (BOGER et al.) and probenecid has no effect on PAS clearance in acute studies in the dog (BUCKLEY, VIDT and SAPIRSTEIN). However, clearance of conjugates of PAS in the rabbit which averaged 2.66 times that of inulin (after correction for binding) decreased to approximately 1.0 following carinamide administration (RAGAZ). It seems probable, therefore, that PAS, like salicylic acid, is conjugated in kidney and liver and that probenecid and carinamide may inhibit the tubular secretion of the conjugates but have little effect on the excretion of the unconjugated compound under the experimental conditions employed. In one experiment in man, for example, WAY et al. found only 18 percent of a 2.5 gram dose of PAS excreted unaltered. Thirteen percent was excreted as the 'urate' (glycine conjugate) and 59 percent as acetylated PAS. As with salicylic acid, excretion of free PAS is greatly depressed by acidosis in the rabbit (RAGAZ). The effect of urine volume on PAS excretion has not been reported.

δ) Acetazoleamide

The carbonic anhydrase inhibitor, acetazoleamide (Fig. 24), like chlorothiazide, is a dibasic acid (pK 7.4 and 9.0) although it has no carboxyl or sulfonate group (SPRAGUE). Its excretory pattern resembles that of salicylate. The acetazoleamide-inulin or creatinine clearance ratio (after correcting for binding to plasma proteins) is less than 1.0 at low urine flows and in acid urines, but increases with increasing urine flow (at constant filtration rate) or with increasing urinary p_H and becomes greater than 1.0 in both man and dog in alkaline urine and diuresis (WEINER, WASHINGTON and MUDGE; MAREN). In alkaline urine, acetazoleamide inhibits the excretion of salicylate, while the excretion of acetazoleamide is, itself, inhibited by probenecid causing clearance ratios to creatinine to decrease from 1.2—1.5 to 0.3—0.6 indicating the presence of an active secretory component. From stopped-flow studies, secretion probably occurs in the proximal convoluted segment and is accomplished by the aromatic acid transport system (WASHINGTON, WEINER and MUDGE; WEINER, WASHINGTON and MUDGE).

c) Tissue-permeable weak bases

As distinct from weak acids, tissue-permeable weak bases should be excreted most rapidly in acid urines and most slowly in alkaline urines. Some of the weak bases whose excretion exhibits this dependence on urinary p_H are neutral red, mecamylamine, procaine, nicotine, and quinine alkaloids.

Neutral red (Fig. 27) is the first weak electrolyte whose excretion was proven to be dependent on the p_H difference between blood and urine. When fluid containing neutral red was perfused through the peritubular renal portal venous system of the frog, the concentration of neutral red was high in acid urine and was very low in alkaline urine. The p_H of the urine could be controlled through the acidity of the arterial perfusate. Poisoning the tubular cells with cyanide, ethyl urethane or caffeine failed to affect the excretion of this base unless the urinary p_H changed (CHAMBERS and KEMPTON 1937; KEMPTON 1939; FORSTER and HONG). Neutral red remains the classic example of passive transport which is dependent on p_H changes in the urine.

Mecamylamine (3-methylaminoisocamphane) is an amine base with pK about 11.3. The ratio of the mecamylamine clearance to that of creatinine in the dog is 3.0 to 4.0 at urine p_H between 5.0 and 6.0 and may exceed somewhat the simultaneous clearance of p-aminohippurate. This indicates that mecamylamine is almost completely removed from the renal blood. At urine p_H of 7.3—7.5 and 8.0, the mecamylamine-creatinine clearance ratio is 0.8 and 0.3 to 0.4 (BAER et al. 1956; MILNE et al.; SCRIBNER, CRAWFORD and DEMPSTER). Provisional evidence indicates that mecamylamine is transported by the common organic base secretory system since it inhibits tubular secretion of N'-methyl-nicotinamide in the chicken (VOLLE and PETERS). Mecamylamine probably enters the tubular fluid by glomerular filtration and tubular secretion. If the tubular fluid is acid, mecamylamine is retained and excreted quantitatively. If the tubular fluid is alkaline, variable quantities of the base return to the blood by diffusion.

The base, 3-aminoisocamphane behaves similarly. At urinary pH of 5.4—5.6 and 6.7—7.2 the clearance of the base is 61 and 25 percent, respectively, of the simultaneous p-aminohippurate clearance (SCRIBNER, CRAWFORD and DEMPSTER). Urine flow affects the excretion of mecamylamine in a fashion similar to the effect on salicylate clearance. In the pH range of 4.7—5.8, an increase in urine flow from 2.8 to 8.6 ml./min. was associated with a 70 percent increase in the base-PAH clearance ratio: from 0.7 to 1.2. In the pH range 6.0—6.7, a roughly similar increase in urine flow (mannitol diuresis) from 3.2 to 12.6 ml./min. was associated with increase in the base-PAH clearance ratio from 0.9 to 1.2 (SCRIBNER, CRAWFORD and DEMPSTER).

The ratio of *procaine* clearance to creatinine clearance is about 4.0 at urine pH below 7.0 in dog and rabbit and 1.5 at pH of 7.8 in the dog and 0.1 to 0.2 at pH 8.6 in the rabbit (TERP). Transport studies have not been reported. Analogy with other bases suggests that excretion is the result of active tubular secretion followed by variable degrees of back-diffusion from urine to blood in alkaline urine.

The ratio of *pentamethylpiperidine* clearance to p-aminohippurate clearance in the dog is 1.42 at urine pH 6.3—6.7 and 0.66 at pH 7.8—7.9 (SCRIBNER, CRAWFORD and DEMPSTER).

Nicotine, a quaternary ammonium base with pK about 8.1, is excreted three to four times more rapidly in man in urine of pH 4.9 to 5.5 than in urine of pH 7.1 to 7.3 (HAAG and LARSON).

Quinine alkaloids (quinine, quinacrine, chloroquine, santoquine and perhaps all members of the family) are weak bases (pK of quinine, 8.3) which are excreted 2 to 10 times more rapidly in acid than in alkaline urine in man and dog (ANDREWS and CORNATZER; TRAGER and HUTCHINSON; JAILER, ROSENFELD and SHANNON; HAAG, LARSON and SCHWARTZ; ORLOFF and BERLINER). Quinine inhibits tubular secretion of N'-methylnicotinamide in the chicken (VOLLE and PETERS) suggesting that tubular transport of quinine is possible, but definitive evidence that these bases are secreted in mammals is lacking.

IV. Tubular reabsorption of organic compounds

1. Sugars

a) Glucose

α) General considerations

Glucose is freely filtered at the glomeruli, being present in glomerular filtrate in the same concentration as in the plasma water (WEARN; WALKER and REISINGER; WALKER et al. 1941). A highly efficient reabsorptive transport system, restricted to the proximal segment of the nephron of those amphibia and mammals in which the locus of reabsorption has been sought, removes glucose from the tubular fluid and returns it to the peritubular blood (WALKER and HUDSON 1937a; SOLOMON et al.; WALKER et al. 1941; WOOD; MALVIN, WILDE and SULLIVAN 1958a; WILDE and MALVIN 1958). If glucose concentration in the filtrate is not increased, glucose is reabsorbed more rapidly than water so that the tubular glucose concentration decreases rapidly below that of blood and may attain unmeasurably low values (WALKER and HUDSON 1937a; WALKER et al. 1941). No evidence of permeability of the nephron to glucose in an outward (blood to lumen) direction has been detected. This is shown in several ways. Urine of the aglomerular fish subjected to glucose loading is glucose-free (BIETER 1931; MARSHALL and GRAFFLIN 1932). When the frog kidney is perfused by the portal vein, which supplies the peritubular capillaries, the urine is glucose-free, whereas perfusing the renal arteries with glucose-rich fluid evokes an abundant glucosuria (CLARK; AKKINSON, CLARK and MENZIES). Radioactive carbon-tagged glucose does not pass from blood to urine in measurable amounts in the dog (CHINARD et al. 1957, 1959). Although transport against a concentration gradient denotes an active process, the mechanics of glucose transport are even less well known than are those of aromatic acid secretion. This may be due in large measure to the circumstance that no suitable *in vitro* system is available to study glucose transport, and available information has been derived almost entirely from studies on intact kidneys. From studies on other cell systems it seems probable that the first step in transport is reaction with a highly specific element in the membrane (LEFEVRE and MARSHALL). This reaction and the subsequent release of glucose in the cell need not be energized but may be an exchange diffusion. In Ehrlich tumor cells, for example, such an exchange diffusion may have a very high temperature coefficient and be rate-limiting with respect to external concentration changes, characteristics which are often attributed to energized processes (CRANE, FIELD and CORI). NI and REHBERG (1930) proposed that rate of glucose transport was determined ultimately by a maximum attainable blood-urine concentration gradient which they estimated to be about 500 mg. percent in the dog. This concept, certain aspects of which remain valid theoretically, has not been found to play an important role within the limits of measurable and attainable plasma or urine glucose concentrations in the intact animal. In separate perfusion of the renal arterial and portal venous circulations in the frog no difference in reabsorption rate of glucose could be detected in the proximal tubule of Necturus when portal venous concentrations were varied threefold, from 50 to 143 mg. percent (WOOD). (In earlier experiments of CLARK, urinary glucose concentration increased during portal perfusion with 400 to 500 mg. percent glucose solution, but this author was unable to correct for the possible urinary concentrating effect of the hyperosmotic peritubular blood.) Rate of glucose transport in the dog may remain unchanged when the urine-plasma concentration difference varies widely in relation to changes in glomerular filtration rate (SHANNON and FISHER.) BURGEN showed that known glucose titration curves can be derived from theoretical considerations, among the more important of which are: 1. the rate-limiting step in glucose transport can be described by the Michaelis-Menten equation; 2. water is reabsorbed in the proximal segment of the nephron at a linear and constant rate; 3. reabsorptive capacity has a Gaussian (normal) distribution in the nephron population. Mean transit time of glucose molecules across the epithelium of the dog nephron has been estimated to require about 10 seconds and is accomplished without rupture of the carbon chain (CHINARD et al. 1957, 1959).

The source of transport energy and how it is linked to glucose transport are unknown. Unlike the secretion of aromatic acids and organic bases neither generation of high energy phosphate bonds, nor oxidative energy from the citric acid (KREBS) cycle are critical elements in glucose transport. Whether or not transport energy is derived from another, coenzyme II-specific oxidative pathway (DICKENS and GLOCK) is unknown. 2,4-dinitrophenol, which uncouples phosphorylation from oxidation, does not affect glucose transport in the dog at concentrations which suppress aromatic acid transport (MUDGE and TAGGART 1950a). Citric acid (KREBS) cycle inhibitors, dehydroacetate and malonate, in quantities which depress PAH transport 70 to 100 percent cause no more than 11 percent decrease in glucose transport (SHIDEMAN and RENE). Glucose transport is not remarkably sensitive to cyanide in the dog. Cyanide concentrations of about 1.7 mM./L. in renal blood evoke a modest increase (10 to 20 times) in glucose excretion, but a sharp decrease in urea clearance suggests the possibility of alterations in epithelial permeability (NICHOLSON 1949). In the pump-lung-kidney preparation, glucose/creatinine clearance ratio increases slowly, attaining finally a value of 1.0 when general renal function is deteriorating rapidly (BAYLISS and LUNDSGAARD). Cooling to 20 degrees C virtually suppresses glucose transport in the dog (SEGAR). The changes with cooling appear to consist primarily of a progressive widening of the titration splay, but the process cannot be measured accurately because of the simultaneous large decrease in GFR (KANTER). In two patients who ingested cyanide, glucose Tm was essentially normal but glucosuria was observed at low plasma glucose concentrations after all cyanide has been neutralized by sodium thiosulfate injection (LAMBERT et al. 1950), again suggesting that the effects of cyanide on glucose transport are indirect. This system also is difficult to inhibit by mercury. Mercuzanthin (2 ml.) did not significantly affect glucose transport in man, while PAH transport was depressed 40 percent in the same studies (McDONALD and MILLER). In the dog 5 mg. of mercury/kg. as mercuhydrin effected no significant change in glucose Tm unless filtration rate decreased more than 40 percent (THOMPSON, BARRETT and PITTS).

Contrary results in the dog are reported by HANDLEY, CHAPMAN and MOYER, who observed a decrease in both glucose and p-aminohippurate transport after injection of mercury. Neither effect has been confirmed by other researchers and the reason for their divergent results is not clear, but probably are hemodynamic in origin.

Glucose transport is specifically and sensitively blocked by the glucoside, phlorhizin, some of its derivatives, and some other glucosides. In spite of intensive research, the mechanism of phlorhizin glucosuria is still not clearly understood. From fragmentary and largely indirect evidence the principal action of phlorhizin appears to be competitive inhibition of the reaction of glucose with an initial group-specific step in transport from tubular lumen into the cell. In the Ehrlich tumor cell, which may be employed again as an example, and in renal cortex slices phlorhizin at concentrations less than 1 mM./L. markedly inhibits passage of glucose and other sugars through the cell membrane without being, itself, transported (CRANE, FIELD and CORI; LOTSPEICH and WORONKOW; KRANE and CRANE). Reciprocal competitive inhibition exists between sugars and phlorhizin as well as its aglycone, phloretin, for penetration into erythrocytes (LEFEVRE; WILBRANDT 1954). Some properties of phlorhizin will be considered in a later section.

β) Normal values of glucose transport in man

Glucose excretion by healthy subjects is very low, ranging from about 25 to 50 mg./24 hours during fasting to about 130 mg./24 hours on random diets (HARDING, NICHOLSON and ARCHIBALD; DATE). This is consistent with tubular reabsorption of 99.95 percent of filtered glucose. When the quantity of glucose in the glomerular filtrate is progressively elevated, usually by increasing the blood glucose concentration, reabsorption rises at a rate equal, at first, to the increase in filtered load so that the urine remains glucose-free. With increasing load of filtered glucose, reabsorption of each increment in load becomes progressively less complete so that glucosuria appears. The blood glucose concentration at the time of first glucosuria is termed the "minimum threshold" or simply the "threshold". Finally, all of each increment of filtered load is excreted and reabsorption has attained a maximal, or Tm, value. The curve so generated from 10 normal subjects is illustrated in Fig. 29. On the assumption that saturation of the cellular transport system is attained at low intratubular concentrations of glucose the titration splay can be attributed to diversity within the nephron population of the glomerular activity (ratio of filtration rate to glucose Tm). The frequency distribution within the nephron population of different values of this ratio is indicated in the lower curve of Fig. 29.

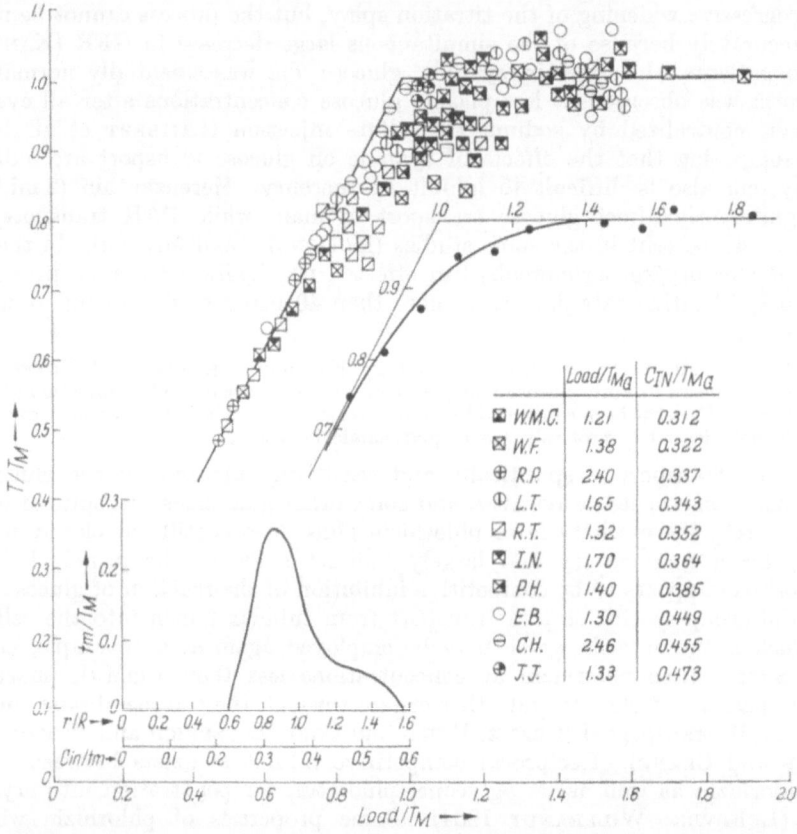

	Load/T_{Ma}	C_{IN}/T_{Ma}
W.M.C.	1.21	0.312
W.F.	1.38	0.322
R.P.	2.40	0.337
L.T.	1.65	0.343
R.T.	1.32	0.352
I.N.	1.70	0.364
P.H.	1.40	0.385
E.B.	1.30	0.449
C.H.	2.46	0.455
J.J.	1.33	0.473

Fig. 29. Glucose titration curve for normal subjects, from Smith, Goldring, Chasis, Ranges and Bradley. Upper curve: transport-load data for 10 subjects; middle curve: graph of the averaged data of the 10 subjects; lower curve: frequency distribution of glomerular activity, r (filtration rate, c_{in}, divided by transport capacity, tm_G) plotted as absolute units or as related to mean glomerular activity, R (C_{in}/Tm_G) of the entire kidney, calculated as illustrated in Fig. 23. Reproduced by permission of the authors and Journal of the Mt. Sinai Hospital

The maximal tubular transport rate (Tm) of glucose in healthy male subjects in the third and fourth decades is about 365 mg./min. Average values of 375 mg./min. in 24 men averaging 41 years old and of 359 mg./min. in 3 men in the third decade are reported by Smith et al. (1943) and Miller, McDonald and Shock (1952). Studies on women are less extensive but are sufficient to demonstrate a significant sex difference. The mean value in 11 women averaging 35 years of age was 303 mg./min. (Smith et al. 1943). The standard deviation (sigma) of the adult male population is about 55 mg./min. (Miller, McDonald and Shock 1952). These values are corrected to 1.73 M². Somewhat lower mean values, 312 and 266 mg./min. (uncorrected for surface area), are reported by Lambert (1954) for 26 men and 35 women.

Like other renal functions such as filtration rate, blood flow and PAH Tm, glucose Tm varies with age. Tm is low, 30—80 mg./min./1.73 M^2 in the newborn and older premature infants. It rises rapidly, however, attaining about 50 percent of the adult value in the first month (TUDVAD). The development of glucose transport capacity during childhood and adolescence is obscure. GALAN et al. observed values of 353 to 620 and averaging 527 mg./min./1.73 M^2 in 6 children aged 2 to 11 and averaging 8.5 years. This figure which is about 50 percent greater than the adult value may, if confirmed, reflect the action of anterior pituitary somatotropin or other factors. Glucose Tm decreases uniformly throughout adult life at the rate of about 7 percent per decade, attaining in males a value of about 225 mg./min. at age 80 (MILLER, McDONALD and SHOCK 1952). Studies of changes with aging in women are lacking.

γ) Metabolic and other influences on glucose Tm

Directional changes in various physiological and pathological states in man are summarized in Table 14. Of particular importance to theory of renal function are the relative lack of effects of acute or chronic changes in renal blood flow and glomerular filtration rate on glucose Tm. For example, Tm in man is not significantly changed following adrenalin, pyrogen (SMITH et al. 1943), albumin infusion (MICHIE et al.), caffeine (SMITH et al. 1943) or aminophylline (MILLER 1953 b) which cause variable acute decreases or increases in renal blood flow and to a lesser degree in filtration rate; and Tm is not significantly decreased in congestive heart failure of moderate severity in which filtration rate and blood flow are chronically decreased (GROSSMAN et al. 1950 b). Similar results are observed in the dog which appears to exhibit marked stability of Tm in the presence both of large increases in glomerular filtration rate caused by saline infusion or a meat meal and of small decreases (not more than 40 percent) caused by hemorrhage or decreased aortic blood pressure (Fig. 30) (SHANNON and FISHER; SHANNON, FARBER and TROAST; HARE and HARE; MOUSTGAARD; LEVY and ANKENY; THOMPSON, BARRETT and PITTS; THOMPSON and BARRETT 1952). Other workers, on the other hand, have concluded that glucose Tm in the dog varied directly with filtration rate (HANDLEY, SIGAFOOS and LaFORGE; HANDLEY and KELLER; MOYER and HANDLEY). The degree of stability of glucose Tm in the rabbit is not clear, a situation which is not surprising in view of the marked vasomotor lability in this animal. FORSTER (1947) concluded that filtration rate and glucose Tm varied in an almost constant ratio while LAAKE and KRUHØFFER found that Tm is constant at filtration rates above about 3 ml./min./kg.

Glucose Tm is not affected by mercurial diuretics in the dog (HANDLEY, TELFORD and LaFORGE; THOMPSON, BARRETT and PITTS), although the effect of mercury in man is undecided (McDONALD and MILLER; WESTON et al. 1949).

Table 14. *Changes in glucose Tm in human physiological and pathological states*

Condition	Reference
Tm little or not changed	
Anemia	BRADLEY and BRADLEY
Heart failure (mod. severe) .	GROSSMAN et al.
Hypertension (early) . . .	SMITH et al. (1943)
Pregnancy	CHRISTENSEN; WELSH and SIMS
Tm decreased	
ADDISON's disease	TALBOTT et al.
Diabetes mellitus (late) . . .	LUNDBAEK and PETERSEN
Hypertension (late)	SMITH et al. (1943)
Tm increased	
Acromegaly	GERSHBERG et al. (1957)
Diabetes mellitus (early) . .	FARBER, BERGER and EARLE
Nephrosis (pure, 'lipoid') . .	GALAN; EDER et al.

Tm is not affected by carinamide or probenecid (BEYER et al. 1947b, 1951), renal denervation in the dog (BERNE) unless filtration rate is acutely depressed or by severe acute metabolic acidosis (blood pH 7.01) in the dog (JENSEN et al.). The effect of anoxia is not clear. In dog and man, no effect on Tm was observed while breathing 6.3 or 9.4 percent oxygen (AXELROD and PITTS 1952b) but a decrease in Tm was reported in dogs during exposure to simulated 18,000 feet (5,500 meters) altitude (KELLEY and McDONALD). Data are also lacking on the effects of diet. In the dog, a high protein meal caused no acute change in glucose Tm (MOUSTGAARD) while SHANNON, FARBER and TROAST observed that Tm was about 15 percent greater in two dogs on a high than on a low protein diet. In dogs on a vitamin B-deficient diet, glucose Tm is increased at the same time that titration splay is widened (HAMAR). Tm is unaffected by potassium depletion in the dog (BESKIND and MUDGE).

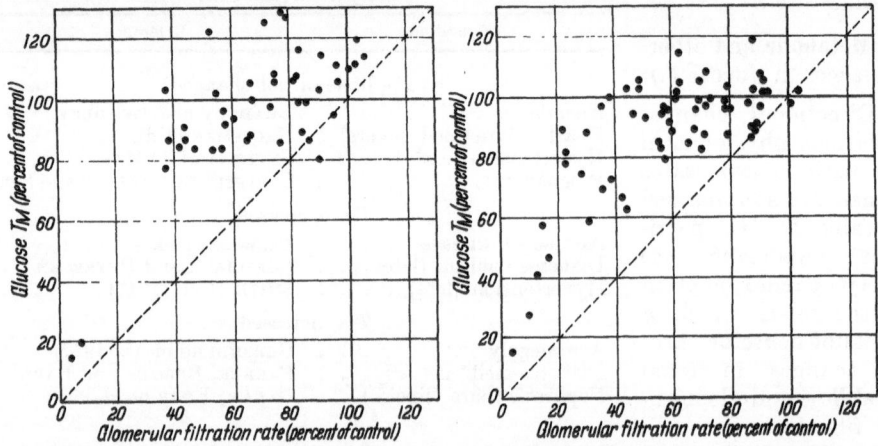

Fig. 30. Relationship between glomerular filtration rate and glucose Tm in the dog. Left: filtration rate was reduced by inflating a balloon catheter in the abdominal aorta above the renal arteries. Right: filtration rate was reduced by controlled hemorrhage. After THOMPSON, BARRETT and PITTS. Reproduced by permission of the authors and the American Journal of Physiology

Glucose Tm is depressed in the presence of severe reductions in filtration rate in the dog and particularly in man [THOMPSON, BARRETT and PITTS; THOMPSON and BARRETT 1952 (Fig. 30); KRUHØFFER 1950; HOUCK 1951; HANDLEY and KELLER 1950; CRAIG, VISSCHER and HOUCK; PITESKY and LAST; DEMPSTER, EGGLETON and SHUSTER; BRADLEY and BRADLEY 1947b; LATHEM et al.]. In the same circumstances diodrast or PAH Tm are usually normal or no more than slightly depressed, supporting the view that filtration may virtually cease in some nephrons while blood flow continues. Acute elevation of ureteral pressure in the dog is associated with nearly an equiproportional decrease in filtration rate and glucose Tm (SELKURT, BRANDFONBRENNER and GELLER). P-aminohippurate loading has been reported to increase (KLOPP, YOUNG and TAYLOR 1944) decrease (HOUCK 1946) or to have no effect (SELKURT 1944; MICHIE et al.) on glucose Tm. The latter seems the more probable circumstance since no other aromatic acids, including probenecid, have been observed to affect glucose transport, and complex formation between p-aminohippurate and glucose when these are mixed in priming or infusion solutions can account for many vagaries (BALDWIN et al. 1950).

Of particular interest is the effect of hypernatremia. Glucose Tm is depressed in the dog by 15 to 25 percent and in the rabbit by 30 percent during loading with hypertonic sodium chloride (KRUHØFFER 1950; LEVY and ANKENY) or sodium sulfate (SCHOU 1944a). The effects of saline could not be reproduced by mannitol loading (LEVY and ANKENY; THOMPSON and BARRETT 1952).

Glucosuria in rabbits as the result of injections of various sodium salts has been reported (see, for example, McDANELL and UNDERHILL) but effects of possible filtration rate changes could not be evaluated by these authors. A decrease in glucose Tm during mannitol loading in the dog reported by DEMPSTER, EGGLETON and SHUSTER is probably correlated with large decreases in filtration rate in their experiments.

Effects of endocrine function changes on glucose transport in man are fragmentary so that extensive reference must be made to animal studies. Large quantities of thyroxine (20 mg.) or dessicated thyroid (5 gm.) daily resulted in about 50 percent increase in glucose Tm (EILER, ALTHAUSEN and STOCKHOLM 1944a; HARE et al. 1944) in normal dogs. Glucose Tm which was 219 mg./min. before, decreased to the extremely low value of 17 mg. after hypophysectomy in one dog and was restored to 162 mg. by somatotropin (EARLE et al. 1957). Less marked (10 to 20 percent) increases in Tm were observed in 2 dogs given somatotropin for 3 days (GERSHBERG and SAWYER pers. comm.). In the chronic state of human acromegaly, however, glucose Tm was 780 mg./min./1.73 M² (GERSHBERG, HEINEMANN and STUMPF). The anterior pituitary, whether in excess or deficiency, constitutes an extraordinarily potent influence on glucose transport. Much smaller changes are observed in relation to adrenocortical function changes. In two male patients with ADDISON's disease, glucose Tm was 143, and 220 mg./min./1.73 M² (TALBOTT et al. 1942). Adrenocorticotropin (ACTH) acutely or in quantities of 75 to 200 mg. daily for 4 to 22 days in 10 subjects was associated with no significant change in glucose Tm or in titration splay, although a small decrease in Tm was observed on cessation of ACTH administration in 3 subjects (EARLE et al. 1951a; ALEXANDER et al.; FROESCH et al.; LAMBERT, TAGNON and CORVILAIN; LAMBERT et al. 1951). Testosterone or testosterone propionate, 90—300 mg. daily for 8 to 29 days, caused no significant change in glucose Tm (KLOPP, YOUNG and TAYLOR 1945).

Few interrelationships between the transport of glucose and of other substances have been examined. The phosphorylation theory of glucose transport (LUNDSGAARD) suggested that glucose and phosphate might share a common mechanism. This received some support from the observations that glucose loading depresses phosphate Tm (PITTS and ALEXANDER 1944; COHEN, BERGLUND and LOTSPEICH 1956, 1957). In addition to phosphate, sulfate and ascorbate Tm are markedly depressed and acetoacetate Tm and urate excretion (q.v.) are slightly to moderately depressed (COHEN, BERGLUND and LOTSPEICH 1956, 1957; SELKURT 1944). Depression of ascorbate and acetoacetate tends to be temporary, however, and considerable recovery of transport occurs during sustained glucose loading. Small quantities of phlorhizin tend to reverse glucose depression of phosphate, sulfate and acetoacetate transport.

In uncomplicated diabetes mellitus, renal glucose transport is essentially normal. Titration splay is not widened, while Tm is, if anything, somewhat elevated, particularly if appropriate corrections are made for the age of the subjects (STEINITZ 1940a; NIELSEN; FARBER, BERGER and EARLE). This observation offers one line of support to the older view that glucose 'threshold' may be increased in diabetes. Late in the disease, however, after glomerular and arteriolar sclerosis has resulted in extensive destruction of renal parenchyma, glucose Tm is reduced together with other renal functions (LUNDBAEK and PETERSEN). An increase in glucose Tm is reasonably attributable to a decrease in circulating insulin. Twenty units of insulin resulted in a decrease of glucose Tm from 424 to 379 mg./min. in 12 diabetics (FARBER, CONAN and EARLE;

Farber, Berger and Earle) and from 275 to 235 mg./min. in 12 normals (Miller 1953a). Carbutamide may possibly effect a slight decrease in glucose Tm in the dog (Lee, Anderson and Chen).

Glucose Tm is well maintained in essential hypertension when filtration rate is moderately and blood flow and diodrast Tm are markedly reduced. Glucose titration curves suggest, however, that filtration rate depression may be far from uniformly distributed and that in a large fraction of the nephron population, the ratio of filtration rate to glucose reabsorptive capacity may be significantly below both the mean of the entire kidney of the hypertensive patient or the mean of the normal kidney (Smith et al. 1943).

δ) Renal glucosuria

Renal glucosuria refers to appearance of glucose in the urine at a time when blood glucose concentration is less than the maximum value usually associated with glucose-free urine in normal subjects. This can occur either as the result of an increase in volume of glomerular filtrate so that filtered load is increased in spite of a relatively low glucose concentration in the filtrate, or as the result of a decrease in tubular transport. Glucosuria as the result of an increase in filtration rate is observed in pregnancy and in association with adrenocortico-tropin administration (Christensen; Welsh and Sims; Froesch et al.). In most of those instances which are referred to as renal glucosuria (or renal diabetes), however, glucosuria occurs as the result of a deficiency of transport. This deficiency can be of two general types: Tm can be decreased; or titration splay can be widened. Both types of deficiencies have been described. In about half of approximately 25 collected cases, glucose Tm was within normal limits (250 mg./min. or above) but excretion began or was present at low filtered loads, and relatively high load/Tm ratios (above 1.4) were necessary to attain full saturation of the transport system. In the other cases, Tm was low, ranging from 45 to 200 mg./min. Titration splay was not measured in all of these, but in six it was essentially normal (Friedman et al.; Castex, Biasotti and Pata-lano; Nielsen; Govaerts and Lambert; Reubi 1951, 1954; Froesch, Wine-grad and Renold). The disease (or diseases) is presumably hereditary with different genes probably involved in different cases (Harris 1956). The heredi-tary basis is particularly convincing with respect to many of the subjects with low Tm while some or most of the subjects with normal Tm and widened splay may represent acquired defects (Govaerts 1952). Heijkenskjold and Sand-berg have reported an increased excretion of other sugars in the urine of two renal glucosurics, but the type of transport defect in their subjects is unknown. A glucosuria which is seldom massive, perhaps because of decreased glomerular filtration, occurs frequently in association with other specific renal tubular diseases such as the aminoacidurias and phosphaturias. Measurements of glucose transport have been reported in a few of these cases. Glucose Tm in a 30 year old male patient with childhood type of De Toni-Debré-Fanconi syndrome was 30 mg./min. This value is low even as related to the depressed GFR of 53 ml./min. in the patient (Froesch, Winegrad and Renold). In another patient, however, a 44 year old woman with the same or similar syndrome, glucose Tm and GFR were 530 mg/min./1.73 M^2 and 137 percent of normal, respectively (Anderson,. Miller and Kenny). Inasmuch as hypernormality of GFR has seldom been reported in the aminoacidurias, the hypernormal Tm-G, which requires GFR data in the calculation, should be accepted with reservations. Cyanide poisoning causes titration splay to be greatly widened but Tm is not notably depressed.

In two cases of poisoning studied by LAMBERT et al. Tm were 238 and 347 mg./min. at normal GFR. Titration splay was immensely widened so that these subjects were excreting glucose at plasma glucose concentrations less than 100 mg./100 ml.

ε) Phlorhizin

This substance is a glycoside with the structural formula shown in Fig. 31. Although phlorhizin was discovered by de KONINCK in 1835 and used medicinally, its glucosuric properties were not clearly recognized until 1888 when they were

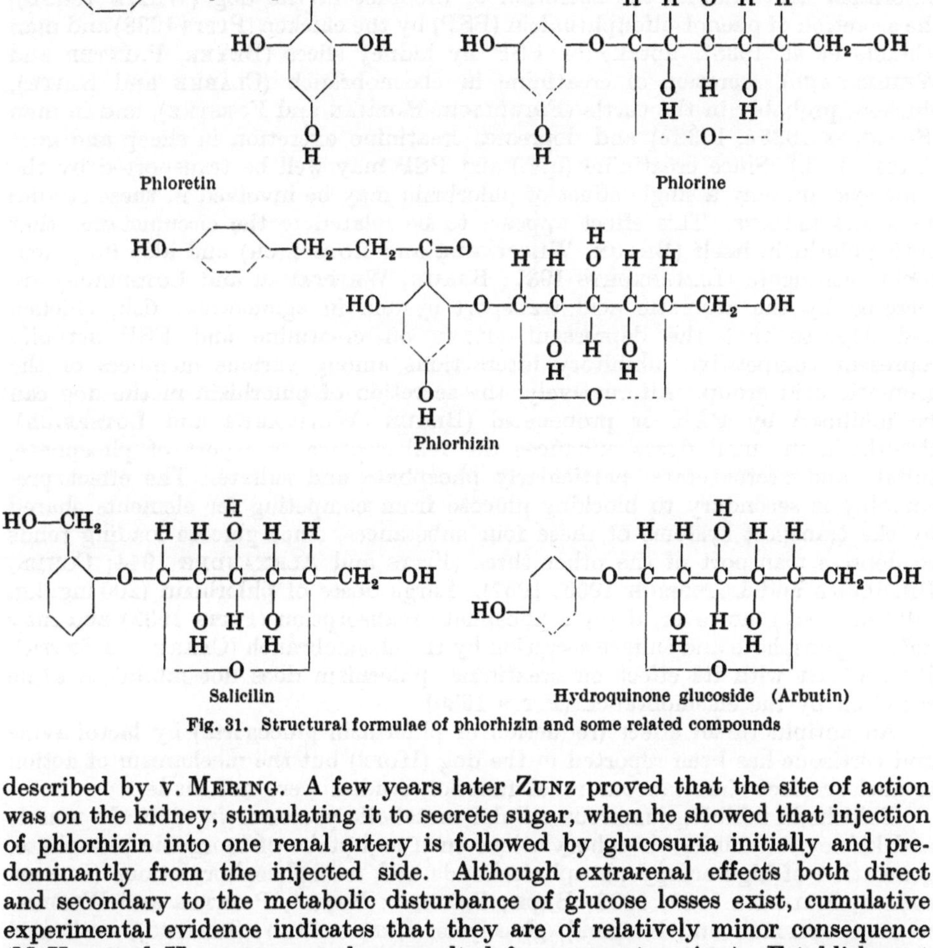

Phloretin

Phlorine

Phlorhizin

Salicilin

Hydroquinone glucoside (Arbutin)

Fig. 31. Structural formulae of phlorhizin and some related compounds

described by v. MERING. A few years later ZUNZ proved that the site of action was on the kidney, stimulating it to secrete sugar, when he showed that injection of phlorhizin into one renal artery is followed by glucosuria initially and predominantly from the injected side. Although extrarenal effects both direct and secondary to the metabolic disturbance of glucose losses exist, cumulative experimental evidence indicates that they are of relatively minor consequence (McKEE and HAWKINS may be consulted for a recent review). Establishment of the filtration-reabsorption hypothesis of renal function recast the renal role of phlorhizin as that of a nearly specific inhibitor of the glucose reabsorptive transport system. Inhibition of glucose transport has been demonstrated in all glomerular vertebrates examined: elasmobranch (CLARKE and SMITH; SHANNON 1933, 1934), teleost (PITTS 1935), frog (WALKER and HUDSON 1937a; HÖBER 1933), chicken (PITTS 1938), rat and guinea pig (WALKER et al. 1941), rabbit (WHITE 1923; POULSSON) and dog (WHITE and MONAGHAN; GOVAERTS and

CAMBIER; SHANNON 1935a) as well as man. Only in the aglomerular fish
(MARSHALL; MARSHALL and GRAFFLIN 1932) or in the frog whose portal vein,
alone, is perfused with glucose-containing fluid (HÖBER 1933) does phlorhizin
fail to evoke a glucosuria. In adequate quantities (200 mg./kg. intravenously
in mammals) inhibition of glucose reabsorption becomes virtually complete.
Within the limits of measurement, all filtered glucose is excreted and glucose
clearance becomes identical with inulin clearance (SHANNON 1935a). Smaller
quantities or oral instead of intravenous administration of phlorhizin bring the
glucose-inulin clearance ratio in man to 0.8 to 0.9 (SHANNON and SMITH; GOLD-
RING; CHASIS, JOLLIFFE and SMITH). In addition to its effect on glucose,
phlorhizin also inhibits the secretion of diodrast in the dog (WHITE 1940b),
the secretion of phenolsulfonphthalein (PSP) by the chicken (PITTS 1938) and man
(CHASIS et al. 1938), uptake of PSP by kidney slices (BEYER, PAINTER and
WEIBELHAUS), secretion of creatinine in elasmobranch (CLARKE and SMITH),
chicken, probably in the turtle (FRIEDLICH, HOLMAN and FORSTER), and in man
(SHANNON 1935c, 1938c) and depresses creatinine excretion in sheep and goat
(LADD et al.). Since creatinine (q.v.) and PSP may well be transported by the
same system, only a single effect of phlorhizin may be involved in these studies
on intact kidneys. This effect appears to be related to the circumstance that
both phlorhizin itself (BRAUN, WHITTAKER and LOTSPEICH) and also its glucuronide conjugate (LAMBRECHTS 1937; BRAUN, WHITTAKER and LOTSPEICH) are
secreted by the aromatic acid transport system in aglomerular fish, chicken
and dog, so that the depressant effects on creatinine and PSP actually
represent competitive inhibitory interactions among various members of the
aromatic acid group. Alternatively, the secretion of phlorhizin in the dog can
be inhibited by PAH or probenecid (BRAUN, WHITTAKER and LOTSPEICH).
Phlorhizin in small doses enhances the reabsorptive transport of phosphate,
sulfate and acetoacetate, particularly phosphate and sulfate. The effect presumably is secondary to blocking glucose from competing for elements shared
by the transport systems of these four substances, since glucose loading tends
to depress transport of the other three (PITTS and ALEXANDER 1944; COHEN,
BERGLUND and LOTSPEICH 1956, 1957). Large doses of phlorhizin (200 mg./kg.
intravenously), however, depress phosphate reabsorption (PITTS 1933) and may
depress phosphate and sulfate secretion by the elasmobranch (CARKE and SMITH).
By contrast with its effect on creatinine, phlorhizin does not inhibit creatine
secretion by the elasmobranch (PITTS 1939).

An antiphlorhizin effect (reduction of phlorhizin glucosuria) by lactoflavine
and cortisone has been reported in the dog (HOFF) but the mechanism of action
is unclear since simultaneous renal function studies were not made.

Phlorhizin inhibits numerous cellular metabolic processes *in vitro*. In muscle
and kidney it inhibits phosphorylations such as uptake of inorganic phosphate,
generation of high-energy phosphate bonds and transphosphorylations (LUNDS-
GAARD; KALCKAR 1937, 1939; BECK; SHAPIRO; BEYER, PAINTER and WEIBEL-
HAUS; LOTSPEICH and KELLER), glycolysis (LUNDSGAARD; SHAPIRO), both acid
and alkaline phosphatase activity (LUNDSGAARD; BECK; MARSH and DRABKIN)
and oxidation of pyruvate, citrate and possibly other acids of the citric acid cycle
(SHAPIRO; BEYER, PAINTER and WEIBELHAUS; LOTSPEICH and KELLER; LOT-
SPEICH and WORONKOW). Respiration is depressed moderately but respiratory
quotient is unaffected (SHORR, LOEBEL and RICHARDSON; KALCKAR 1937). The
intriguing hypothesis of LUNDSGAARD that interference with phosphorylation
of glucose, as the first step in glucose transport, constituted the specific biochemical lesion of phlorhizin diabetes has encountered serious objections. Most

of the *in vitro* studies have employed much higher concentrations of phlorhizin (regularly greater than 1.0 and usually greater than 5.0 mM./L.) than occur in the intact animal during submaximal or maximal inhibition of glucose transport. BECK has noted that inhibition of phosphorylation at concentrations comparable to those attained in the intact animal requires a p_H more acid than body fluids, and that at greater dilutions phlorhizin may even enhance phosphorylation. Many of the *in vitro* effects are attributable to the nonglucosuric portion of the molecule. For example, the aglucone, phloretin, which is nearly devoid of glucosuric potency *in vivo* is subequal to phlorhizin in inhibiting phosphorylation and phosphatase activity in kidney cortex (KALCKAR 1937; LAMBRECHTS 1937) or zymin (acetone-extracted yeast) fermentation of glucose (DANN and QUASTEL) and is more active than phlorhizin in inhibiting phosphate uptake by or glucose loss from erythrocytes (HARRIS and PRANKERD; ROSENBERG and WILBRANDT). Finally, phlorhizin in glucosuric quantities *in vivo* fails to affect activity of blood phosphatase (LAMBRECHTS 1937) or rate of turnover of radioactive phosphate or of various organic phosphate fractions with the possible exceptions of pyrophosphate and phosphoglycerate (RAPOPORT et al. 1941; WEISSBERGER; DRATZ and HANDLER; DICZFALUSY). Studies designed to demonstrate presence or absence of kidney phosphatase inhibition by phlorhizin *in vivo* are inconclusive (KRITZLER and GUTMAN; MARSH and DRABKIN).

The glucosuric properties of the phlorhizin molecule depend upon its glucoside structure. The aglucone, phloretin, is virtually devoid of activity, and such small glucosuric activity as it possesses (about 0.4 percent of that of phlorhizin in the dog) is attributed to resynthesis of phlorhizin (LAMBRECHTS 1936). The glucoside, phlorine, however, which is generated by removing the p-hydroxy-phenylpropionate portion of the molecule (Fig. 31), is very active (LAMBRECHTS 1937). Other but not all glucosides are glucosuric. The glucosides of resorcinol and hydroquinone (Arbutin) (MICHEL; LAMBRECHTS 1937) in the dog and desoxycorticosterone glucoside in man and dog (LAMBERT, LEBRUN and DE BRAUCOURT 1948, 1949; GREEN et al. 1950; DESPOPOULOS and KAUFMAN; MATTAR et al.) are strongly glucosuric. Desoxycorticosterone glucoside is of particular interest since it has nearly 10 times the glucosuric potency of phlorhizin. The aglucone, desoxycorticosterone, like phloretin, is inactive (LAMBERT, LEBRUN and DE BRAUCOURT 1948, 1949). Apparently, a phenolic hydroxyl group must also be present since methylation of the three phenolic hydroxyl groups of the phlorhizin molecule or the single phenolic hydroxyl of hydroquinone glucoside (Fig. 31) abolishes activity. Introducing other groups into the phloretin moiety of the molecule, providing the phenolic hydroxyl are intact, generally does not destroy glucosuric activity (LAMBRECHTS 1937). The glucosides amygdalin and salicylin (Fig. 31), which also lack phenolic hydroxyl groups, are inactive although they possess the capacity to inhibit cell respiration (MICHEL).

b) Other sugars: fructose, galactose, xylose, sucrose, raffinose

The dynamics of tubular transport of sugars other than glucose are poorly understood. All are excreted freely at low plasma concentrations. Urine/plasma concentration ratios of fructose and galactose less than 1.0, indicating efficient conservation, may be obtained in man but not in rabbit, cat or dog at plasma concentrations less than 15 mg. percent.

Fructose attains an apparent Tm in man of about 40 mg./min. and a Tm seems to be demonstrable in rabbit and dog. The titration splay is extremely wide, and load/Tm ratios of 3 to 5 or more are necessary to attain saturation of the reabsorptive system. A clear Tm has not been demonstrated in the cat. Glucose-loading has a small but variable tendency to depress fructose reabsorption in cat and man but no evident effect in rabbit and dog. The effect of glucose is greatest in man: a glycemia of 193 to 272 mg. percent being associated with a doubling of the fructose/creatinine clearance ratio (HANSEN, JACOBSEN and PETERSEN; GAMMELTOFT and KJERULF-JENSEN; LEVINE and HUDDLESTUN). Phlorhizin depresses fructose reabsorption whether at Tm or less than Tm loads in rabbit and dog but the effect is less than is the case with glucose. Phlorhizin does not clearly depress fructose reabsorption in the cat (GAMMELTOFT and KJERULF-JENSEN). These observations suggest that fructose is reabsorbed by a tubular transport system largely distinct from that which reabsorbs glucose.

Galactose appears to have a Tm in man of about 30 mg./min., but no clear Tm has been discerned in cat or dog (GAMMELTOFT and KJERULF-JENSEN; EILER, ALTHAUSEN and STOCKHOLM 1944b). Both phlorhizin and glucose-loading have a small depressant effect on galactose reabsorption in cat, dog and rabbit.

Xylose, sucrose and *raffinose* are reabsorbed to a small extent from the glomerular filtrate. Reabsorption of xylose represents about 10 to 35 percent of the filtered load in many animals, including man, dog, rabbit and elasmobranch *(Squalus)* (JOLLIFFE, SHANNON and SMITH; PITTS 1933; SHANNON 1934, 1935a, 1938a; KAPLAN and SMITH). The fraction of sucrose and raffinose reabsorbed by the dog nephron is about the same as that of xylose (JOLLIFFE, SHANNON and SMITH). Reabsorption of xylose varies in a nearly but not quite exactly linear ratio with filtered load, so that reabsorption as a fraction of load tends to rise at low loads and decrease at high loads (SHANNON 1938a). That xylose and perhaps also sucrose and raffinose, are transported slowly by the glucose transport system is suggested by the circumstance that glucose loading suppresses xylose reabsorption in the dog (SHANNON 1938a); and xylose, sucrose and raffinose reabsorption in the dog and xylose reabsorption in man, rabbit and elasmobranch are easily depressed by phlorhizin causing the clearance ratios of these sugars to one another to approach unity (JOLLIFFE, SHANNON and SMITH; SHANNON, JOLLIFFE and SMITH 1932b; PITTS 1933; SHANNON 1934, 1935a; SHANNON and SMITH; COPE).

2. Amino acids

Although small, variable quantities of all alpha amino acids known to be present in dietary proteins or to circulate in the blood plasma may be detected in the urine by appropriate microbiological or chromatographic methods (FRANKL and DUNN; WOODSON et al.; DUSTIN; EVERED), reabsorption of filtered amino acids as estimated from plasma concentrations (IYER) is nearly complete. In healthy individuals on usual diets, clearances (which in man roughly approximates the percent of the filtered load which is excreted) of the naturally occurring, or levo-, isomers are less than 1.0 ml./min. for alanine, arginine, glutamine, isoleucine, leucine, lysine, methionine, phenylalanine, proline, threonine and valine; clearances are 1.0 to 2.0 for serine, tryptophane, and tyrosine, 2.0 to 4.0 for cystine (DENT, SENIOR and WALSHE) and 4.0 to 7.0 for glycine and histidine (DOOLAN et al.). These clearance values and urinary excretion rates supply little information concerning the physiological properties of the tubular transport systems but are useful clinically as standards of reference for the recognition of disorders of tubular reabsorption of amino acids.

Studies of interactions between various amino acids and including creatine suggest that, in the dog, amino acids are reabsorbed by at least three and possibly more distinct reabsorptive systems. Glycine, alanine and glutamate, but not other amino acids, depress the reabsorption of creatine, although creatine does not clearly increase aminoacid excretion at usual blood levels of these (PITTS 1943, 1944a). Hence, glycine, alanine, glutamate and creatine may be tentatively assigned to a single reabsorptive system. Similarly, lysine, arginine, cystine, ornithine and histidine mutually depress the reabsorption of one another but not that of members of the first group in both dog and man (BEYER et al. 1947c; KAMIN and HANDLER; ROBSON and ROSE). A third group comprises leucine and isoleucine (BEYER et al. 1947c). Maximal transport rates have been found for glycine, alanine, glutamate (PITTS 1944a), arginine (PITTS 1944a; WRIGHT et al.), lysine (WRIGHT et al.), leucine, isoleucine and valine (EATON, FERGUSON and BYER) but not for histidine (WRIGHT et al.; DOTY), methionine (WRIGHT et al.; FERGUSON, EATON and ASHMAN), tryptophane (BEYER et al. 1946b), tyrosine (DOTY), threonine and phenylalanine (RUSSO et al.). In the latter category, plasma concentrations sufficient to saturate the tubular transport system could not be attained either because of insolubility of the amino acid or because of the toxicity of high blood concentrations. The l-isomer was employed in most of these studies although the d, l compound was employed in a few instances. Available but limited evidence indicates that the d-isomer is reabsorbed in a manner quite different from that of the l-isomer. Thus, the clearances of d-cystine and d-methionine are much greater than those of the l-form; and in the case of d-methionine, at least, a partial dependence of clearance on urine flow suggests that reabsorption may be passive (DENT, SENIOR and WALSHE; DOOLAN et al.). Amides such as glutamine and asparagine may be reabsorbed by a distinct amino acid transport system (KAMIN and HANDLER 1951a).

Transport of arginine is unaffected by carinamide; the effects of mercury and other inhibiting agents are unknown. Glycine is reported to depress the reabsorption (or enhance the secretion) of urate in man and rat (FRIEDMAN 1947), and glycine, alanine and arginine depress sulfate Tm in the dog (BERGLUND and LOTSPEICH). Tubular transport of one or more groups of amino acids (frequently in concert with other tubular transport systems) is depressed in certain metabolic disorders such as WILSON's disease (COOPER et al.; STEIN, BEARN and MOORE) and galactosemia (HOLZEL, KOMROWER and SCHWARZ) but the mechanisms involved are unknown. The tubular transport system for an amino acid group may be deficient or entirely absent on a congenital basis, the best known of these congenital defects being that of the cystine-lysine-arginine-ornithine group (cystinuria) (DENT; HARRIS 1956, 1957; ARROW and WESTALL).

3. Aliphatic acids: ascorbic, acetoacetic, citric, hydroxybutyric, lactic, malic

These acids, important to the intermediary metabolism of the body, have in common only the circumstance that they are actively reabsorbed from the glomerular filtrate. Comparatively little information is available concerning them, and they are grouped together here for convenience.

a) Ascorbic acid (vitamin C)

The general description of the renal tubular handling of ascorbic acid closely resembles that of glucose. At plasma concentrations below 1 mg. percent the urine contains distinct but small amounts of ascorbate (less than 0.07 mg./min.)

indicating moderately efficient reabsorption. During either acute or chronic loading, substantial excretion begins at plasma concentrations slightly greater than 1.0 mg. percent (threshold) while above 2.0 mg. percent any further increment in filtered load is completely excreted in the urine (RALLI, FRIEDMAN and RUBIN; FRIEDMAN, SHERRY and RALLI; LEWIS, STORVICK and HAUCK; KLOSTERMAN et al.; AHLBORG). The maximal transport rate, attained at blood concentrations above 2.0 mg. percent is 2.1—2.2 mg./min. (RALLI, FRIEDMAN and RUBIN; FRIEDMAN, SHERRY and RALLI; AHLBORG). The titration splay is somewhat greater than that of glucose. A titration curve similar to that in man is observed in the dog, the dog differing from man principally in excreting relatively more ascorbate at low plasma concentrations (SHERRY et al.; SELKURT, TALBOT and HOUCK).

Ascorbate reabsorption is markedly depressed during acute loading with glucose, p-aminohippurate (PAH) (SELKURT 1944), and hypertonic sodium or potassium chloride (SELKURT and HOUCK) in the dog. Mannitol loading, however, is without effect. A partial recovery of transport occurs during sustained loading with glucose or PAH, but not during one or two hours observation with the salts. Ascorbate loading, however, does not affect sodium or potassium excretion (STAMLER). Ascorbate reabsorption is depressed by phlorhizin in guinea pigs (PIANTONI). Contrary to observations on the dog, glucose loading did not affect ascorbate transport in man (RALLI, FRIEDMAN and RUBIN).

No change in the clearance of ascorbic acid was observed through the menstrual cycle of women (HAUCK). In the dog, however, administration of estrogens (estradiol benzoate) increased the clearance and lowered the resting blood concentrations, but did not lower Tm (SELKURT, TALBOT and HOUCK). This estrogenic effect is equivalent to a widening of the titration splay.

b) Acetoacetic acid

Definitive studies on the tubular transport of this acid in man are not available. In the dog, reabsorption is active, with a fixed Tm and moderate titration splay. The Tm shows an apparent tendency to decrease somewhat under heavy loads (SCHWAB and LOTSPEICH). Acetoacetate Tm, together with that of sulfate and phosphate is depressed by glucose loading while phlorhizin increases the Tm COHEN, BERGLUND and LOTSPEICH 1956, 1957). These observations are consistent with acetoacetate and glucose having some portion of their reabsorptive ystems in common.

c) Citric acid

The generally low clearance of citric acid in the dog suggests that it is probably reabsorbed actively by the tubules (HERRIN and LARDINOIS). Little additional information is available concerning the tubular transport of this acid. Excretion is not affected by ascorbate loading (HERRIN and LARDINOIS). Marked changes in citrate excretion are observed in relation to certain acid-base changes. Urinary citrate excretion in man and rat is decreased during metabolic acidosis caused by ammonium chloride or acetazoleamide (carbonic anhydrase inhibitor) administration and increased by sodium bicarbonate, the excretion of other organic acids being little affected (CLARKE et al.; EVANS et al. 1957; HARRISON and HARRISON 1955). Potassium depletion is also associated with decreased citrate excretion although the urine may not become strongly acid (FOURMAN and ROBINSON; EVANS et al. 1954). Intracellular acidosis, the factor common to ammonium chloride acidosis and potassium depletion, led CLARKE et al. to postulate an effect of pH on tissue synthesis of citrate. A decrease in cellular pH would lead, sequentially, to decreased citrate formation, low blood concentration and lower urinary excretion. In the studies of HERRIN and LARDINOIS, however, citrate clearance increased during alkalosis caused by sodium bicarbonate without significant change in blood concentration or filtered load, while an intracellular alkalosis caused by potassium administration was, acutely at least, without effect.

SHORR, BERNHEIM and TAUSSKY have described variation in citrate excretion through the menstrual cycle. Excretion is maximal at midcycle and minimal during the menses. The cycle could be reproduced in amenorrheic women by estradiol administration.

d) Hydroxybutyric acid

The blood threshold for the appearance of significant amounts of beta-hydroxybutyrate in man is in excess of 20 mg. percent (MARTIN and WICK). Limited studies in the dog suggest that this substance has a true reabsorptive Tm (VISSCHER).

e) Lactic acid

Small amounts of lactate are present in normal human urine, having a clearance of 1—2 ml./min. Both excretion and clearance begin to increase rapidly when blood concentration exceeds 60 mg. percent (threshold) as during severe exercise (MILLER and MILLER). Studies in the dog indicate that when a racemic mixture is infused at less than Tm loads the l-isomer is absorbed by the tubules approximately 1.5 times as rapidly as the d-isomer. The Tm, however, is constant and independent of the proportions of the two isomers which are present (CRAIG).

f) Malic acid

L-malate is normally reabsorbed almost completely from the glomerular filtrate in the dog. Reabsorption is enhanced by fumarate and depressed by citrate. Infusion of succinate or alpha-ketoglutarate, however, results in excretion of malate in excess of the quantity filtered. The source of the excess malate is not clear, but may arise from increased synthesis of malate in the presence of succinate since renal venous concentration of malate may exceed arterial during succinate infusion. Malonate blocks the effects of succinate and alpha-ketoglutarate but does not evidently affect the actions of fumarate and citrate (CRAIG et al.; VISHWAKARMA). Similar effects of succinate and malonate on malate excretion are observed in the chicken (VISHWAKARMA and LOTSPEICH 1960a). D-malate (unlike the levo isomer) is actively secreted by the chicken kidney but the secretion exhibits no evidence of competitive inhibition by aromatic acids such as probenecid or by bases such as cyanine (VISHWAKARMA and LOTSPEICH 1960b).

4. Benzoic acid and analogues

It was noted in a previous section (DIII 1a) that certain aromatic acids are usually reabsorbed from the glomerular filtrate either in addition to or instead of being secreted. It should be recalled, however, that certain of the organic acids which are normally secreted may be reabsorbed by certain species. Examples of these are reabsorption of urate by mammals, and of diodrast by *Necturus* (KINTER) and the cat (JOSEPHSON et al.). Evidence that reabsorption is active and, further, that any of these substances share a common reabsorptive transport system is so inadequate that the grouping of them together here is wholly arbitrary. The most important of these acids are benzoic and p-aminobenzoic acid and the sulfonamides.

a) Benzoic and p-aminobenzoic acid

Following oral ingestion of 10—15 g. of sodium benzoate in man, or of quantities less than 500 mg./kg. in the rat, no more than traces of free benzoate appear in the urine. With quantities greater than 500 mg./kg., however, excretion in the rat may be substantial (Neuberg; Borgstöm; Schachter). A tendency for benzoate excretion to vary directly with rate of urine flow suggests that some transport across the epithelium may occur passively (Machella, Helm and Chornock). In the dog, about 25 percent of filtered benzoate is excreted at filtered loads of 30 micromols/min./kg. The titration splay suggests that a maximal transport rate might be observed at a load of 70 micromols which would require blood benzoate concentrations close to the LD-50 in the dog (Knoefel and Huang 1956).

Somewhat more information is available concerning p-aminobenzoate. The clearance of this substance is less than that of creatinine in the dog at all concentrations studied (Smith et al. 1945; Beyer et al. 1952). Even at concentrations as high as 40 mg. percent, the p-aminobenzoate-creatinine clearance ratio is no greater than about 0.16 (Beyer et al. 1945a). Since approximately 93 percent of plasma p-aminobenzoate is filterable (Fisher et al.), extensive tubular reabsorption is demonstrated. The effects of p_H or of urine flow on p-aminobenzoate clearance are unknown.

b) Sulfonamides

Although the sulfonamides and allied compounds have usually been studied as a group, the mechanisms of renal excretion of the individual members are heterogeneous. With most of them, the net result of tubular transport operations is that of reabsorption.

Others, however, are manifestly secreted and undoubtedly by the aromatic acid secretory system. In examining excretion by the dog kidney of a large group of sulfonamides, those members which are acidic and which have a pronounced hydrophilic-hydrophobic configuration to the molecule were usually secreted while those members which are alkaline or are weakly polar in the above sense were reabsorbed. Exceptions to this rule were the acidic p-aminobenzoate and sulfanilate which were reabsorbed and a few weakly polar compounds such as acetylaminosulfanilamide which were secreted (Fisher et al.).

Excretion is further complicated by the circumstance that in man extensive but variable acetylation of the p-amino group occurs, a process which appears to be largely a hepatic function. Clearance of the acetylated form generally exceeds that of the free form by factors of 2 to 6 times in both man and dog (Frisk; Reinhold et al.; Beyer et al. 1946a). In addition, all of the sulfonamides are bound to plasma proteins to highly varying extents. Degree of plasma binding differs as between man and dog, and presumably other species would differ from these. Although the degree of plasma binding is roughly equal as between the free and acetylated forms of sulfamerazine, sulfadiazine and sulfathiazole in human plasma, substantial differences in the degree of binding of the two forms is evident in dog plasma. With sulfamerazine, the free/acetylated percentages bound at a plasma concentration of 5 mg. percent are 78/80 for man and 36/45 for dog; with sulfadiazine the free/acetylated percentages bound are 45/49 for man and 16/29 for dog; for sulfathiazole, the percentages are 71/76 for man and 53/80 for dog (BEYER et al. 1946a).

The dynamics of transport in the conventional sense — tubular maximum, titration curve, competitive interactions — have not been measured for any sulfonamide whether secreted or reabsorbed. Effects of variation in urine flow and p_H on sulfonamide excretion are not clear. LOOMIS, KOEPF and HUBBARD observed no significant changes in sulfanilamide or acetylsulfanilamide excretion in man when urine flow varies between 1 and 12 ml./min. Clearance of the filterable fractions of both free and acetyl sulfathiazole, however, approximately doubles in the rabbit during brisk sulfate osmotic diuresis sufficient to cause urine flow to increase from 0.03—0.2 to 10—16 ml./min. (BECKER-CHRISTENSEN and SCHOU). A net reabsorption (correcting for plasma binding) of the free and a moderate net secretion of 0.1—3.0 times the amount filtered of the acetylated during the control periods becomes during diuresis a net secretion of 0.5—3.0 for the free and 6—10 times the amount filtered for the acetylated. However, the filterable fraction of the sulfonamide was assumed to be constant throughout

Table 15

Compound	Formula[1]	Clearance ratio[2,3]		Plasma binding, percent[4]
		Free	Acetylated	
Sulfanilamide	R—H	0.24[5,7,9] 0.2 —0.3[5,7,18] 0.22—0.55[6,8,10] 0.41[6,8,12] 0.45[6,8,15]	0.5—1.3[6,8,10] 0.41[6,8,12] 1.03[6,8,15]	10[7,9] 12[8,14]
Sulfadiazine	R—	0.33[5,7,9] 0.31[5,8,16] 0.3[5,7,17] 0.35[5,8,19]	0.9—1.1[5,7,17] 0.87[5,8,16]	20[7,10] 16[7,17] 45[8,17] 32[8,19]
Sulfathiazole	R—	1.0[5,7,9] 0.24—0.54[6,8,10] 1.0[5,8] 0.4[6,8,12] 0.87[5,8,16] 0.6[5,7,17]	0.4—0.8[6,8,10] 0.2[6,8,12] 1.5—2.7[5,7,17] 2.76[5,8,16]	60[7,10] 60—80[8,13] 70[8,14] 53[7,17] 71[8,17]
Sulfamerazine	R—	0.20[5,8,16] 0.16[5,7,17] 0.15[5,8,19]	1.0[5,7,17] 1.1—6.4[5,8,16] 2.4[5,8,19]	36[7,17] 78[8,17] 63[8,19]
Sulfapyridine	R—	0.55[5,7,9] 0.10—0.20[6,8,10] 0.22[6,8,12] 0.28[5,8,16]	0.20—0.74[6,8,10] 0.30[6,8,12] 0.26[5,8,16]	30[7,9] 30[8,14]

[1] R in these formulae is p-$H_2N(C_6H_4)SO_2HN$—.

[2] Ratio of sulfonamide clearance to creatinine clearance in the dog and to endogenous creatinine or inulin clearance in man.

[3] Plasma concentrations, where reported, generally ranged between 3 and 6 mg. percent.

[4] Free form, only.

[5] Corrected for plasma binding.

[6] Uncorrected for plasma binding.

[7] Dog data.

[8] Human data.

[9-19] Sources: [9] FISHER, TROAST, WATERHOUSE and SHANNON; [10] FRISK; [11] CHAPMAN and PEOPLES; [12] LINDAHL and JOSEPHSON; [13] ANDERSEN, MILLER and SIMESEN; [14] ANDERSEN; [15] LOOMIS, KOEPF and HUBBARD; [16] REINHOLD, FLIPPIN, DOMM, ZIMMERMAN and SCHWARTZ; [17] BEYER, RUSSO, PATCH, PETERS and SPRAGUE; [18] MARSHALL, EMERSON and CUTTING; [19] EARLE (1944).

the diuresis, and hypertonic sodium salts are known to depress other transport systems such as those of ascorbate and glucose. BEYER et al. (1946a) observed increases in acetylsulfonamide-creatinine clearance ratios in the dog with both increasing urine flow and increasing pH. The effects of flow and acidity, although significant, were small compared with those observed for salicylate. The greatest change in clearance was less than twofold for sulfamerazine, sulfadiazine, sulfamethazine and sulfathiazole, and an increase of 1.0 pH units enhanced clearance to roughly the same extent as a 10 fold increase in urine flow. These observations suggest that a small but significant permeability of the tubules to passive transport is superimposed upon active secretory or reabsorptive processes.

Among the more studied of the clinically important sulfonamides, extensive reabsorption of the free forms of sulfanilamide, sulfadiazine, sulfapyridine and sulfamerazine occur (Table 15). Sulfathiazole, however, is not reabsorbed to any significant extent, rapid excretion of this drug being prevented by extensive plasma binding. Among the acetylated forms of this group, net secretion has been clearly demonstrated only for sulfathiazole.

V. Tubular transport of electrolytes

1. Sodium chloride

a) General description

With the possible exception of water, the excretion of no substance has attracted as much research effort as that of sodium and chloride. Salts of sodium account, in molar terms, for 85 percent of the plasma solutes, and, because they are almost completely dissociated, they account for 90 percent of the osmotic activity of plasma. About 75 percent of plasma sodium salts is sodium chloride. Because sodium and chloride are bound to plasma proteins in no more than trace amounts, they pass freely through the glomerular membranes and represent in the glomerular filtrate a quantitative importance similar to that in plasma. In the average normal pair of human kidneys, approximately 14 mM. of sodium chloride is filtered per minute, representing in a 24 hour period nearly 1.2 kilograms of salt. Of this amount, more than 99 percent, or about 14 mM./min., is normally reabsorbed. Nor is 14 mM./min. the maximum rate of salt reabsorption of which the kidney is capable, for in states associated with increased glomerular filtration, reabsorption usually increases also and may attain values of 20 mM./min. or more. The values for tubular transport of sodium chloride may be compared with that of glucose, quantitatively the most important nonelectrolyte transported by the tubules in either direction, which moves at 2.0 mM./min. (10 to 15 percent of the sodium chloride value) when transported at its Tm rate. These considerations represent the important properties of *efficiency* and *massiveness* of the tubular transport of sodium chloride: great quantities of salt can be reabsorbed with often no more than traces appearing in the urine.

It is of interest that the vertebrate kidney nowhere appears to have acquired the capacity to secrete sodium chloride. Salt in the urine of aglomerular fish is regularly small in amount and less than blood concentration. Where salt secretion has appeared, this excretory function has been performed by organs other than the kidney, as in the supraorbital salt-glands of marine birds and marine lizards, the cloacal salt gland of elasmobranchs, and the gills of teleosts.

Knowledge of the nature of the sodium chloride transport system begins with the micropuncture studies of A. N. RICHARDS and his associates. From the studies of WALKER, of BOTT, of WIRZ and of GOTTSCHALK on the composition of tubular fluid; of PITTS and associates on the excretion of acid; of BERLINER and associates on the excretion of potassium and ammonium, and of many others in these and related fields, the following composite description of sodium and chloride transport has emerged (Fig. 32). The abundant glomerular filtrate has the electrolyte composition of an ultrafiltrate of plasma (BAYLISS and WALKER; WALKER 1930, 1933; WESTFALL, FINDLEY and RICHARDS; MONTGOMERY; WALKER et al. 1937, 1941; BOTT 1943, 1955), differing slightly from the latter as a result of the space-occupying and the electrical charges of plasma proteins which are prevented by the glomerular membranes from entering the filtrate. The space-occupying effect and the effect of the negative electrical charge on the protein molecules tend to cancel each other in the case of cations and to be additive in the case of anions. Sodium and potassium concentrations in glomerular filtrate therefore are approximately equal to those in plasma, while filtrate concentrations of chloride and bicarbonate are about 10 percent greater than in plasma. Reabsorption of sodium and chloride from tubular fluid occurs in two stages. The first stage, or proximal transport system, is located in the proximal convoluted tubule. This system transports large quantities of sodium and chloride but, because of free permeability of this segment to water, transport occurs against a relatively small concentration gradient and net transport ceases if the concentration gradient becomes significant.

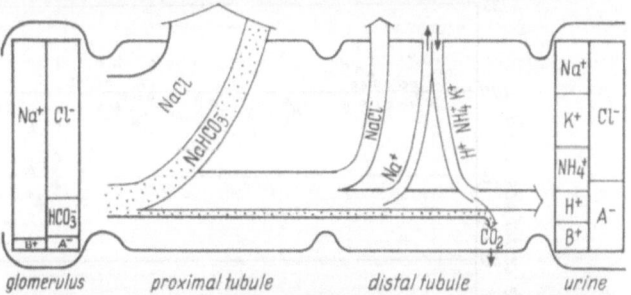

Fig. 32. Processes of sodium reabsorption in the nephron. NaCl and NaHCO₃ are reabsorbed in the proximal tubule, the latter perhaps largely secondary to a hydrogen secretory process. Additional NaCl is reabsorbed in the distal tubule, while some of the Na remaining from this process may be reabsorbed on an ion exchange basis for K⁺, H⁺ and NH₄⁺. Electrolyte compositions of glomerular filtrate and a typical urine are represented in the graphs at the left and right

As the result of this last property, transport in this segment is at all times incomplete and substantial quantities of salt and water pass into the distal segment. The second stage or distal transport system is located in the pars recta of the distal segment of the nephron (broad, ascending segment of the loop of HENLE). This system transports smaller quantities of sodium chloride than the proximal system. Since this portion of the nephron is relatively impermeable to water, the tubular concentration of sodium chloride declines as transport proceeds. Consequently, transport occurs against a significant concentration gradient and, depending upon the quantities escaping proximal reabsorption and constituting the distal load of salt, the distal system may effect very low intratubular sodium chloride concentrations. The kinetics of transport of the distal system probably resemble those of glucose, sulfate and phosphate in that reabsorption is very nearly complete until a fixed Tm is approached. The proximal system has the function of contracting the bulk of the glomerular filtrate but large amounts of salt can be transported with the available energy only if the concentration gradient against which transport occurs is small. The distal system, capable of transporting less salt but against a large concentration gradient, can render the urine salt-free and therefore is ultimately responsible for efficient salt conservation. Sodium salts, including that sodium chloride which escapes the distal transport system, pass to a third stage which involves sodium but not chloride. Tubular sodium ions are exchanged in the distal convoluted tubule or the collecting ducts on an equimolar basis for hydrogen, ammonium and potassium ions. The quantity of sodium exchanged depends upon the concentration of sodium available and also upon the magnitude of various forces driving the exchange reactions. Chloride together with sodium remaining from the cationic exchange systems pass into the urine as excreted salt.

b) Proximal tubular transport of sodium chloride

Proximal tubular reabsorption is measured by comparing concentration of sodium or chloride in tubular fluid with rate of water removal. Micropuncture studies on the amphibian, *Necturus*, and rat and guinea pig showed that chloride

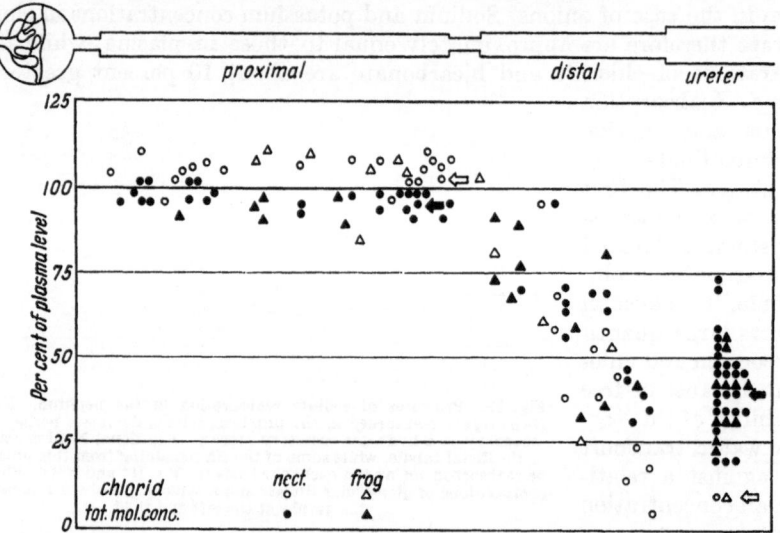

Fig. 33. Chloride and total molecular (osmotic) concentrations in the proximal and distal tubules of Amphibia (*Necturus* and frog). After WALKER, HUDSON, FINDLEY and RICHARDS. Reproduced by permission of the American Journal of Physiology

concentration of tubular fluid remains approximately equal to that of plasma throughout the length of the proximal segment in the amphibian and to half or a little more of the distance down the proximal convoluted tubule in the mammals (Figs. 33 and 34) (WALKER, HUDSON, FINDLEY and RICHARDS; WALKER, BOTT, OLIVER and MacDOWELL; GIEBISCH 1956; SOLOMON et al.; BOTT 1958). The terminal third to half of this segment, lying deep in the parenchyma in mammals, is not reached by the microneedle. Early studies on rat and guinea pig which showed a tubular chloride concentration 25 percent greater than that in plasma (Fig. 34) have not been confirmed (GIEBISCH 1956). Measurements of intratubular creatinine, glucose (after phlorhizin) or inulin concentrations show a continually rising concentration as related to that in plasma or glomerular filtrate (U/P ratio) as the distance from the glomerulus increases (Fig. 35). Since these substances are secreted comparatively little (as with creatinine) or not at all, a rising U/P ratio can occur only by abstraction of water from the glomerular filtrate. If sodium and chloride concentrations throughout the proximal convolution remain equal to those in the filtrate, it follows that the fraction of filtered salt reabsorbed is approximately equal to the fraction of filtered water. In *Necturus*, U/P ratios of creatinine, phlorhizinized glucose and inulin attain values of 1.5—2.0 at the end of the proximal segment, indicating absorption of 30 to 50 percent of filtered salt and water. In rat and guinea pig, U/P ratios are much higher, averaging about 2.5 at the midpoint of the proximal convoluted tubule and indicating absorption of 60 percent of filtered salt and water (Fig. 35). Since rate of rise of creatinine concentration is showing no evidence of decreasing at this point, extrapolation suggests that 75 to 90 percent of salt and water might be reabsorbed at the end of the proximal segment. These figures serve to illustrate the general magnitude of the proximal process. They cannot be applied directly to the intact animal since they are obtained from superficial nephrons, which may not be representative of the population of nephrons, and in animals which were both saline-loaded to sustain urine formation and also subjected to the severe trauma involved in exposure of the surface of the kidney for micropuncture. The micropuncture estimates agree well, however, with the amount of salt calculated to be reabsorbed proximally on the hypothesis that the solute-free water of a maximal water diuresis, free-water clearance (Section D VI 4 e), constitutes an approximate measure of distal salt reabsorption. Subtracting distal reabsorption and urinary excretion of salt from the filtered

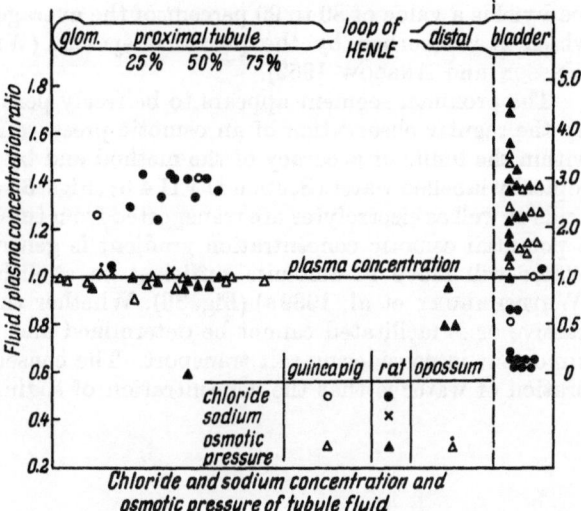

Fig. 34. Sodium, chloride and osmotic concentrations in the proximal tubule of mammals, after WALKER, BOTT, OLIVER and MACDOWELL. Reproduced by permission of the American Journal of Physiology

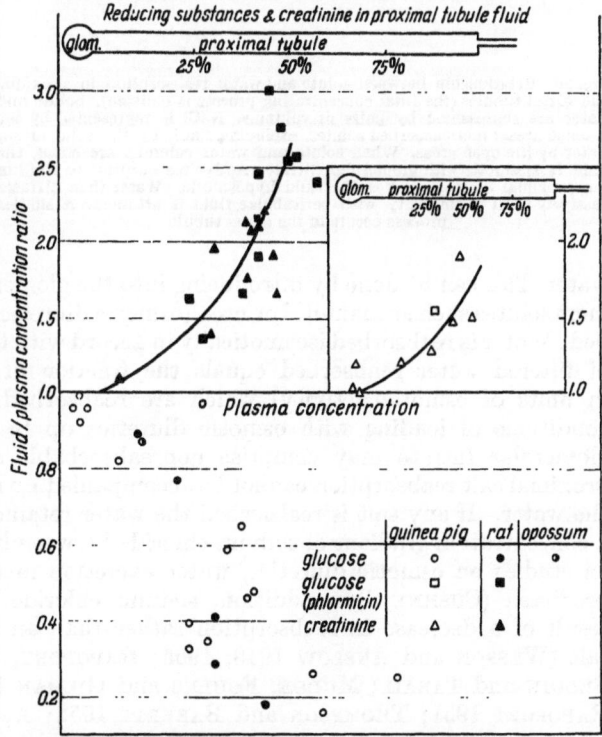

Fig. 35. Fluid/plasma concentration ratios of glucose, glucose after phlorhizin, and creatinine in the proximal tubule of mammals. By the midpoint (50 percent) of the proximal tubule, creatinine and glucose (phlorhizin) have attained a fluid/plasma ratio of 2.5 consistent with reabsorption of 60 percent of the filtered water. After WALKER, BOTT, OLIVER and MACDOWELL. Reproduced by permission of the American Journal of Physiology

load yields a value of 80 to 90 percent of the average filtered load in man and dog which is reabsorbed by the proximal system (WESSON, ANSLOW and SMITH; WESSON and ANSLOW 1952).

The proximal segment appears to be freely permeable to water, as evidenced by the regular observation of an osmotic pressure identical with that of plasma within the limits of accuracy of the method and by the rates of exchange of iso-topically labelled water (Section D VII 4 b) (Figs. 33 and 34). As sugars and amino acids as well as electrolytes are transported from tubular lumen to interstitial fluid, a potential osmotic concentration gradient is generated which can move water. Water will move in amounts sufficient to abolish the concentration gradient (WHITTEMBURY et al. 1939a) (Fig. 36). Whether the water movement is wholly passive or is facilitated cannot be determined and the question has not become important in considering salt transport. The consequence of free osmotic equili-bration of water is that the concentration of sodium in the tubular lumen need not fall significantly below that of plasma, and, in the micropunc-ture studies of WALKER and coworkers, no con-centration gradient could be clearly demon-strated. Without a measurable concentra-tion gradient and with other forces not elimina-ted as transporting agents, active transport cannot be clearly affir-med. The question can be answered by restric-ting the reabsorption of

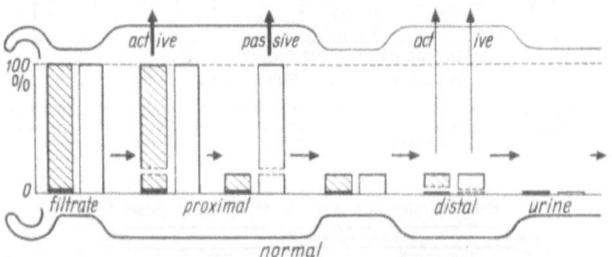

Fig. 36. Relationship between solute and water reabsorption in proximal and distal tubules (the final concentrating process is omitted). Solute and water are represented by pairs of columns. NaCl is represented by the hatched areas; nonreabsorbed solutes, excluding NaCl, by the solid areas; water by the open areas. When solute and water columns are equal, the fluid is isosmotic with glomerular filtrate. Active reabsorption of NaCl in the proximal segment leaves the fluid hyposmotic. Water then diffuses passively until isosmoticity with peritubular fluid is attained. A similar process occurs in the distal tubule

water. This can be done by introducing into the glomerular filtrate from the blood inert solutes such as mannitol or urea (osmotic diuretics) which are poorly reabsor-bed. Water is reabsorbed isosmotically in accord with the relationship: the fraction of filtered water reabsorbed equals the fraction of filtered solutes (measured in units of osmotic activity) which are reabsorbed. Since under appropriate conditions of loading with osmotic diuretics up to half of the solutes of the glomerular filtrate may comprise nonreabsorbable substances, it follows that proximal salt reabsorption cannot be accompanied by movement of more than half the water. If any salt is reabsorbed the water retained in the lumen must cause a concentration gradient of sodium chloride between lumen and blood to develop. In studies on osmotic diuretics, water excretion increases (osmotic diuresis) as predicted (CUSHNY). In addition, sodium chloride excretion increases as the result of a decrease in reabsorption rather than an increase in filtered load of salt (WESSON and ANSLOW 1948, 1955; RAPOPORT, WEST and BRODSKY 1949; SELDIN and TARAIL; MUDGE, FOULKS and GILMAN 1949; KAPLAN, FOMON and RAPOPORT 1951; THOMPSON and BARRETT 1952; ANSLOW and WESSON 1955a; LAUSON and THOMPSON). The fact that maximal free-water clearance, or more exactly the osmotic equivalent of the free-water clearance (Section D VII 4 e) is not significantly changed under simultaneous water and urea loading indicates that the distal transport process is relatively unaffected and that it is proximal transport which is depressed during solute loading (WESSON and ANSLOW 1952).

Although proximal reabsorption is depressed during osmotic diuresis, a small but significant tubule to blood concentration gradient appears which is consistent with active transport. Calculations from clearance studies during osmotic diuresis (data of WESSON and ANSLOW 1948, 1952; and ANSLOW and WESSON 1955a) in which both distal reabsorption and urinary excretion of salt and water are subtracted from the filtered loads indicate that the sodium and chloride concentrations at the end of the proximal transport area are 15 to 25 and 2 to 8 mM./L., respectively, below that of the blood. These figures agree reasonably well with direct analyses of proximal tubular fluid obtained by micropuncture during mannitol osmotic diuresis in the rat sufficient to produce an average creatinine U/P ratio of 5 in the bladder urine (WINDHAGER and GIEBISCH 1959). Sodium concentrations 2 to 38 (av., 20) and chloride concentrations 2 to 19 (av., 9.0) mM./L. below those of plasma were observed. In these same studies, proximal NaCl transport has virtually ceased by the midpoint of the tubule since no significant difference is observed in either creatinine or chloride U/P ratios (averaging approximately 2.0 and 0.89, respectively) between the second and third quarters of the tubule. The difference between sodium and chloride concentration gradients is illustrated also by studies in which proximal tubules of *Necturus* were perfused with NaCl solutions of various concentrations. Isosmolarity was achieved in each solution by adding appropriate quantities of mannitol. Concentrations of sodium and chloride in serum water, assuming an average protein concentration of 2 percent, averaged about 100 and 68 mM./L., respectively (SHIPP et al.). Net outward transport of NaCl ceased when intratubular concentration was 62 to 65 mM./L., or 36 below plasma sodium and 3 to 5 mM./L. below plasma chloride concentration (WINDHAGER et al.; WHITTEMBURY et al. 1959a). That the transport system is apparently incapable of transporting salt against a gradient greater than this is indicated, first, by the fact that the calculated terminal proximal tubular salt concentration gradient is independent of filtered load as the latter is varied by filtration rate change alone and, second, by the fact that fluid which was static for several minutes in the proximal tubules during acute ureteral occlusion (stopped-flow analysis) has a concentration not significantly different from that observed during free flow (WILDE and MALVIN 1958; MALVIN, WILDE and SULLIVAN 1958a; MALVIN et al. 1958a, b; SKULAN, WILLIAMSON and SHIDEMAN; MURDAUGH, GALLOWAY and HAYES). It therefore may be concluded that during osmotic diuresis a net transport of salt has ceased by the time the end of the proximal segment has been reached, and that the greater the fraction of nonreabsorbable solute in the glomerular filtrate, the earlier in the proximal segment will the point of concentration equilibrium and transport arrest be reached. Whether the same limiting concentration gradient and transport arrest are attained in the absence of exogenous osmotic loading is unknown, but no information is yet available to indicate that the unloaded state should be considered as different from a small, chronic osmotic diuresis (WEST and BAYLESS).

Proximal transport of sodium chloride has referred to net transport. When rate of passage of sodium and chloride ions across the tubular epithelium is measured by means of radioactive ions introduced into the fluid at the luminal or the blood surface of the cells, rate of both sodium and chloride ion passage is much greater than that of net salt movement. In *Necturus* kidney, outward passage of sodium and chloride ions is only about 25 percent greater than inward passage, that is, for every 5 ions which move out 4 ions move in (GIEBISCH and WINDHAGER; OKEN et al.). A high rate of blood to lumen movement of sodium ions (influx) has been observed in frog and dog (HOSHIKO, SWANSON and

VISSCHER; WILDE and MALVIN 1959; MOREL and FALBRIARD), indicating at least a qualitative similarity of these species to *Necturus*. The high radiosodium influx in the dog is observed during stopped flow studies under osmotic loading, the same conditions which are associated with depressed net transport and with attainment of proximal concentration equilibrium. Under these conditions it follows that a high influx is being exactly balanced by a high outflux. A relatively high permeability of the epithelium to sodium and chloride ions may be assumed as essential to having a large transport rate. When concentration gradient is zero, no significant quantity of salt can return to the tubular lumen by passive diffusion. If a concentration gradient develops as with restriction of water movement during osmotic diuresis, passive back diffusion appears, increasing in magnitude as concentration gradient increases. Finally, a concentration gradient is attained where influx equals outflux and net transport ceases. Although the above hypothesis of a dual path (one, active; the other, passive) for sodium and chloride ions through the epithelium suffices to explain the available data it is by no means essential. An alternative concept is that each step in an active outward transport process is reversible permitting at a given moment a substantial fraction of the ions in the transport system to be moving opposite to the principal direction of travel.

Thus far, limiting concentration gradients of sodium and chloride have been considered as though they were constant and more or less interchangeable. It is evident, however, that this cannot be true in electrolyte systems except in certain limiting cases. Both active and passive transport of sodium and chloride are closely interdependent and net transport of one ion cannot occur unless transport of the counter ion occurs also. Movement of sodium will depend, therefore, not only upon the concentration gradient of sodium but upon that of chloride also, and the diffusion potential of the sodium chloride ion pair will depend more closely upon the product of the concentrations of sodium and chlorides (ion product) than upon the concentrations of each ion considered separately. Instead of referring to limiting concentration gradients of sodium or chloride between tubular fluid and blood a closer approximation to a theoretically valid description of proximal tubular transport is afforded by referring to a limiting difference between the ion products in tubular fluid and blood. A limiting 'ion product difference' between plasma and proximal tubular fluid offers a simple explanation of occurrence of tubular chloride concentrations which equal or exceed plasma and also an explanation of the low chloruretic efficacy of many ionic osmotic diuretics such as sodium sulfate (RAPOPORT and WEST).

Proximal reabsorption of sodium chloride varies directly with rate of glomerular filtration. This observation has been clearly established only in the dog (LOTSPEICH, SWAN and PITTS; GREEN and FARAH; WESSON et al.; KRUHØFFER 1950; SELKURT and POST; WESSON and ANSLOW 1955) but no reason is known to believe that other vertebrates and particularly mammals differ in any but minor quantitative details. The dependence upon glomerular filtration exists not only under saline loading but also under loading with osmotic diuretics (mannitol, urea) in which reabsorption is depressed (WESSON and ANSLOW 1955). Variation of proximal reabsorption with filtration finds a ready explanation in the concept that a constant ion product difference between plasma and tubular fluid is regularly attained in the proximal segment. Assuming that plasma concentrations of sodium chloride and of osmotic diuretics are constant and ignoring effects on water movement of the transport of sugars and other solutes, proximal sodium chloride reabsorption necessarily must vary linearly with glomerular filtration rate.

In the light of available data is seems simpler to postulate separate transport system for sodium and for the various anions rather than a single system for sodium chloride. Whether the transport system for both cations and anions is active, or whether the transport of one or more ions is passive, transport being effected by the electrochemical gradient established by the prior active transport of ions of opposite sign, cannot be clearly resolved (Section D I 1). Microelectrodes inserted into the lumen of proximal tubules establish the existence of an electrical potential difference of 10 to 20 and as high as 30 millivolts between lumen and interstitial fluid in *Necturus* (WILBRANDT 1938; GIEBISCH 1958) and 19 to 39 millivolts in the rat (SOLOMON). Since lumen was negative to interstitium, this potential is a force capable of moving anions, but against which sodium and other cations must be transported. Whether the negative intraluminal potential is generated by transport of sodium ions or other cations, as would seem reasonable, or whether the negative potential represents the difference between a stronger active transport system for sodium and a set of weaker active transport systems for anions cannot be resolved by available data.

The most extensively studied electrolyte-transporting epithelium is that of frog skin, which transports sodium chloride from outside the body into the interstitial fluid and blood. The hypothetical mechanism by which this system operates is as follows (KOEFOED-JOHNSEN and USSING). The external or outward-facing surface of the epithelium has a high permeability to sodium and a low permeability to potassium while the internal or inward-facing surface has a relatively high permeability to potassium and a low permeability to sodium. An energy-dependent carrier at the inner surface of the cells transports sodium ions from cell into interstitial fluid in exchange for potassium ions which are transported into the cell. Sodium from the external solution diffuses passively down its concentration gradient into the cells which have a low intracellular concentration as a result of the exchange activities at the inner surface. Diffusion of sodium creates a potential difference which drags chloride or other small anions to which the cell surface is permeable. Potassium which has been actively transported into the cell diffuses passively out into the interstitial fluid dragging with it, electrostatically, the chloride which has entered through the external surface. The result is a net transport of sodium chloride.

In the case of the anions, phosphate, sulfate and various organic acids, the demonstration of tubular transport maxima and titration curves similar to those for glucose and aromatic acids supports the view that transport is "active" even though most or all movement of these acids from lumen to blood is from higher to lower electrochemical potential. A more complex situation exists with respect to bicarbonate anion. Limited studies indicated that hydrogen ions can be secreted into the lumen of the proximal tubule of frog and rat and dog (ELLINGER 1940a, b; NICHOLSON 1957a; GOTTSCHALK, MYLLE and LASSITER; WINDHAGER and GIEBISCH 1960), although in *Necturus* any proximal hydrion secretion is too slow to be easily detectable (MONTGOMERY; GIEBISCH 1956). Secreted hydrogen ions can react with bicarbonate and result in the liberation of water and carbon dioxide. The latter, diffusing rapidly across cell membranes, moves from lumen to blood and constitutes in effect a transport of bicarbonate. Although hydrogen secretion might represent a specific hydrogen-sodium exchange system, it seems simpler for the present to consider hydrogen movement as dependent on sodium only to the extent that the negative potential generated or contributed to by sodium movement constitutes a force which can facilitate either the active or passive movement of hydrogen into the tubular lumen (PITTS 1958).

The question remains open concerning the extent to which the chloride transport system can be more generally termed a transport system for monovalent inorganic anions which is capable of effecting the active or passive transport of fluoride, bromide, iodide, nitrate, bicarbonate and other small monovalent anions as well as chloride. The marked influence of changes in bicarbonate excretion on chloride reabsorption suggests that bicarbonate, as a monovalent anion, is also to a limited extent competitive with chloride (Hilton et al. 1956; Wesson and Anslow 1955; Toussaint, Telerman and Vereerstraeten 1958).

It was noted above that proximal sodium chloride reabsorption changes in proportion to glomerular filtration rate. Assuming that this relationship can be explained by the hypothesis of a limiting tubule-blood concentration gradient, a somewhat similar relationship would be predicted to exist between reabsorption and filtrate chloride concentration. The evidence indicates, however, that the relationship is quite different. When filtered load of sodium chloride in the dog is increased by increasing the filtrate chloride concentration through injec-

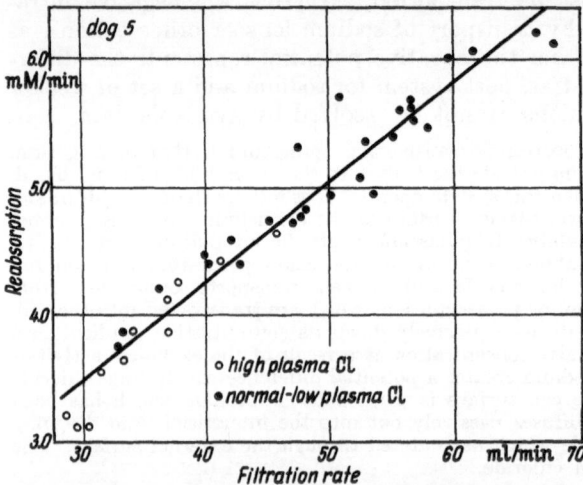

tion of hypertonic sodium chloride solution, excretion increases rapidly. When reabsorption (the difference between filtered load and excretion rate) is measured at constant glomerular filtration rate, it is observed to be quite constant and essentially equal at both normal and elevated plasma sodium chloride concentrations (Fig. 37) (Selkurt and Post; Kruhøffer 1950; Wesson and Anslow 1955). Reabsorption behaves, in effect, as though it were limited by a fixed maximal rate of transport, a circumstance which is incompatible with a constant, limiting tubule-blood concentration gradient in

Fig. 37. Tubular chloride reabsorption in the dog at normal (110—120 mM./L.) and elevated (140—160 mM./L.) plasma chloride concentrations as related to glomerular filtration rate. Two other animals were similar while in a fourth reabsorption was lower at the normal concentrations (Wesson and Anslow 1955). Reproduced by permission of the American Journal of Physiology

the proximal tubule combined with a fixed rate of distal tubular transport. The difficulties can be resolved provisionally, however, by the suggestion of Kruhøffer who, noting that hypertonic saline infusion depresses proximal tubular transport of various substances such as glucose (Levy and Ankeny; Kruhøffer 1950), ascorbic acid (Selkurt and Houck) and p-aminohippurate (Levy and Ankeny), suggested that sodium transport might itself be self-depressed by hypernatremia. In terms of the concept of a limiting concentration gradient, it could be postulated that the effect of hypertonic saline is to decrease the limiting gradient, presumably by decreasing the rate of outward transport of sodium or chloride. This concept of the effect of changing plasma concentration finds further support in two observations that otherwise cannot be easily explained. First, in the rabbit, unlike the dog, the increment in sodium chloride excretion at constant filtration rate during hypertonic saline infusion exceeds the increment in filtered load (Kruhøffer 1950), compatible with depression of reabsorption and suggesting that the apparently fixed chloride Tm in the dog may reflect no more than the circumstance that the limiting concentration gradient changes in an approximate inverse ratio to the change in plasma sodium chloride concentration. Second, NaCl excretion in the dog remains elevated following a decrease in plasma NaCl concentration from elevated to normal levels, for longer than can be explained on the basis of intratubular fluid transit times (Fig. 38), suggesting that NaCl transport requires at least 45 minutes to recover from its depression (SELKURT and POST;WESSON 1959).

The hypothetical description of proximal sodium reabsorption set forth above can be summarized as follows. Sodium is transported rapidly through a membrane highly permeable to sodium, chloride and probably other ions. Electroneutrality of tubular fluid is maintained by inward migration of considerable amounts of positively charged hydrogen ion and by outward migration of anions, the sum of hydrion and anion transfer equalling sodium movement. Anions are transported by a set of partially or entirely independent processes, most of which, but constituting in sum only a small portion of the total ionic charge, are transported actively. Monovalent anions represented by chloride, probably by other halogens, and possibly by bicarbonate in part are transported by a process which has not been proven to be active. Net outward transport of both sodium and chloride represents the difference between a massive efflux and an only slightly smaller influx. As intratubular concentration of

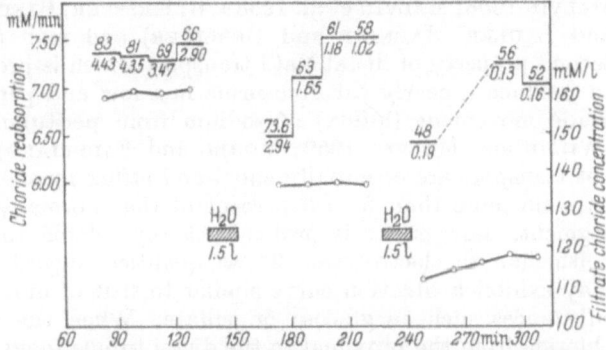

Fig. 38. Depression in tubular chloride reabsorption following intravenous injection of 1.5 L. of water. Reabsorption in each period has been corrected to a filtration rate of 65 ml./min. The figures above and below the graph representing reabsorption are the measured filtration and excretion rates in the clearance periods. Open circles represent filtrate chloride concentration. Nearly an hour elapses from completion of the water infusion before reabsorption has returned to control levels (WESSON 1958). Reproduced by permission of the American Journal of Physiology

either sodium or chloride decreases progressively below that of peritubular fluid, influx increases until influx and efflux are equal and net transport ceases; the ion product difference at which this occurs lies in the range of 3,000 to 3,500 (measured in mM./L.) or at a mean NaCl concentration gradient of 15 to 25 mM./L. and is probably attained under both normal and abnormal conditions well before the fluid reaches the end of the proximal convoluted tubule.

c) Distal tubular transport of sodium chloride

Proof of the existence of a sodium chloride transport system in the distal tubule was obtained from micropuncture studies. These showed that the chloride concentration of fluid obtained from progressively more distal sites in the distal tubule of frog and *Necturus* decreased rapidly to that of bladder urine (Fig. 33). That this was due to the subtraction of salt rather than to the addition of water was indicated by the fact that other substances did not also become dilute (WALKER et al. 1937b). The most active transport area in *Necturus* lies in the first 40 percent of the segment (BOTT 1958). In mammals (rat) fluid in the first portion of the distal convoluted tubule and issuing from the loop of HENLE has lower chloride or total salt concentrations (as deduced from osmotic pressure measurements) than plasma or proximal tubular fluid and by the midpoint of the distal convoluted tubule the concentrations may be very low (WALKER et al. 1941; WIRZ 1956; GOTTSCHALK and MYLLE 1959; WINDHAGER and GIEBISCH, pers. comm.). Considerable salt transport presumably occurs in the pars recta of the distal tubule (broad ascending segment of the loop of HENLE). These observations also establish the first important difference between proximal and distal NaCl transport systems in that the latter is capable of establishing, and transporting against, a large tubule-blood concentration gradient. Confirmation of this property is obtained by stopped-flow studies in which the sodium or chloride concentration of urine collected in serial samples following acute ureteral obstruction drops to very low values in a region proximal to that of ammonium and potassium secretion but distal to that of p-aminohippurate and glucose transport. A region producing low urinary Na or Cl values has been thus demonstrated for rabbit (O'CONNOR and CONWAY), rat (SKULAN, WILLIAMSON and SHIDEMAN), dog (MALVIN, WILDE and SULLIVAN 1958a, b; WILDE and MALVIN 1958; MALVIN et al. 1958a, b; KESSLER, HIERHOLZER and PITTS; WESSON and LAULER; JAENIKE and BERLINER) and man (LAULER, pers. comm.). A second property of distal NaCl transport which is probably critical to the ability to produce a nearly salt-free urine is a low and perhaps inconsequential retrograde movement (influx) of sodium from peritubular fluid to tubular lumen (WILDE and MALVIN 1959; MOREL and FALBRIARD). Hence, distal efflux and net transport are essentially equal and efflux must be vastly less than and perhaps no more than 2 to 3 percent of that normally occurring in the proximal segment. Low efflux is probable closely related to a low permeability of the epithelium to electrolytes. These qualities suggest that distal NaCl transport may exhibit a titration curve similar to that of most other actively transported substances such as glucose or sulfate. When the rate of delivery of sodium chloride from the proximal to the distal tubule (distal salt load) is large, a fixed, maximal rate of transport, Tm_{Cl}^{d} should be attained which should not change with further increases in distal load. When distal load is substantially less then Tm_{Cl}^{d}, all except traces of this salt will be reabsorbed and virtually salt-free urine will result. Between the two areas should lie a region of titration splay. Indirect evidence of the existence and approximate magnitude of distal NaCl Tm has come from two sources. On the assumption that the free-water clearance (see section D VI 4 e) during maximal water diuresis results from distal NaCl transport (WESSON, ANSLOW and SMITH), constancy of this term during variable, massive chloruresis suggests that Tm is constant, and Tm_{Cl}^{d} should be not less than one-half the osmotic equivalent of this free-water clearance. In four 16 to 19 kilo dogs, Tm_{Cl}^{d} so calculated ranged from 1.3 to 1.7 mM./min. (WESSON and ANSLOW 1952). Similar calculations applied to man, assuming a *maximal* free-water clearance of 20 to 30 ml./min., give an estimated Tm_{Cl}^{d} of 3 to 4 mM./min. The second source of evidence lies in chloride excretion data. Chloride rather than sodium must be employed in this calculation since sodium escaping distal salt transport may be variably diminished by involvement in acid or potassium exchange while chloride escaping distal transport is probably excreted without further alteration. On the assumption that proximal NaCl reabsorption varies linearly with filtration rate and that Tm^{d} is constant, then a graph of total salt transport (filtered load minus excretion) against filtration rate should yield a straight line under conditions of full tubular salt loading. When this line is extrapolated to zero filtration rate, the intercept on the reabsorption axis should measure Tm^{d}. Distal Tm measured in this way in the dog is higher and more variable than that estimated from the osmotic equivalent. In the same dogs whose Tm_{Cl}^{d} was estimated from the osmotic equivalent as 1.3 to 1.7 mM./min., Tm^{d} estimated from the intercept at zero filtration varied from 1.6 to 4.2 In 11 animals the average was 0.13 mM./min./kg. (WESSON and ANSLOW 1955). In view of the circumstances that osmotic equivalent measures a least rather than an average estimate of Tm_{Cl}^d, that extrapolation introduces large percentage errors in the intercept, and that considerable uncertainty exists concerning the effects of variation in plasma NaCl on proximal reabsorption, the agreement is reasonable. Titration splay cannot be measured since no acceptable means is available to measure the distal salt load. For purposes of discussion, however, titration splay of distal NaCl transport in man will be assumed to resemble that of glucose.

Whether both sodium and chloride or whether only sodium is actively transported by the distal system is not known. Electrical potentials in which the lumen is negative to interstitial fluid and which are significantly greater than those in the proximal tubule have been recordedfrom the distal tubule. These potentials average 40 millivolts in *Necturus* (GIEBISCH 1958) and 34—70 millivolts in the rat (SOLOMON). This constitutes a force capable of moving anions passively. A hypothetical transport mechanism is illustrated in Fig. 49 (p. 166).

In summary, the distal NaCl transport system may be described tentatively as differing from the proximal system in being simpler and restricted to sodium and chloride transport with other monovalent anions possibly being competitive with the latter. Also unlike the proximal process it can produce a chloride-free urine and has a fixed, maximal transport rate.

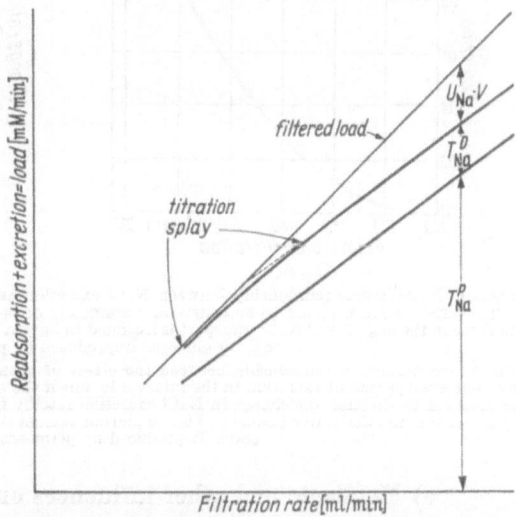

Fig. 39. Graphical representation of NaCl excretion as related to filtration rate and proximal and distal reabsorption. Proximal reabsorption, T_{Na}^P, linearly related to filtration rate, is represented by the lower line. Addition or a smaller but filtration rate-independent distal transport process, T_{Na}^d, to proximal transport gives total reabsorption, represented by the middle line. The distance between total reabsorption and filtered load (upper line) represents excretion, $U_{Na}V$. If titration splay were absent, reabsorption would follow the extrapolation (broken line) to the left and excretion would cease where this intersects the load line. With titration splay present, significant excretion continues at much lower values of filtration rate

d) Total tubular transport of sodium chloride

The foregoing descriptions of the proximal and distal transport processes for NaCl permit a quantitative theoretical description of the overall process. The proximal process is assumed to be a linear function of filtration rate (provided other variables such as concentrations of nonreabsorbable solutes are constant) and independent, to a first approximation, of plasma concentration. The distal process is assumed to be adequately described by a glucose-like titration curve. Addition of the two processes gives total transport rate. Subtracting this from the filtered load gives the NaCl excretion rate. This is illustrated graphically in Fig. 39. In this combined system the factors of particular importance are filtration rate and the titration splay of the distal process. Assuming that the latter in man has the same configuration as that for glucose and assuming quantitative values for proximal and distal transport compatible with known human studies or taken from the dog data, the relationship between filtration rate and salt excretion rate can be illustrated in Figs. 40 and 41. Of particular interest is the circumstance that salt excretion in normal persons on diets containing less than 30 to 40 grams of salt daily occurs under conditions such that the distal transport process is not fully saturated, and in persons on average diets containing 2 to 8 grams of salt daily, the distal tubular load is less than Tm^d. Salt excretion in man must occur almost entirely in the region of distal tubular titration splay.

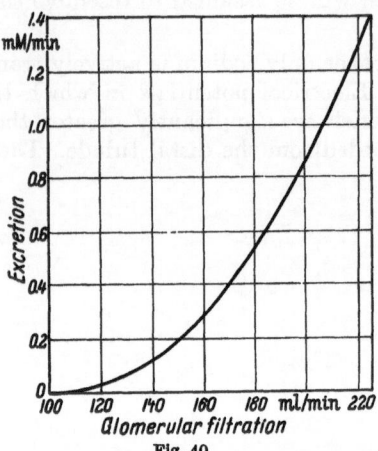
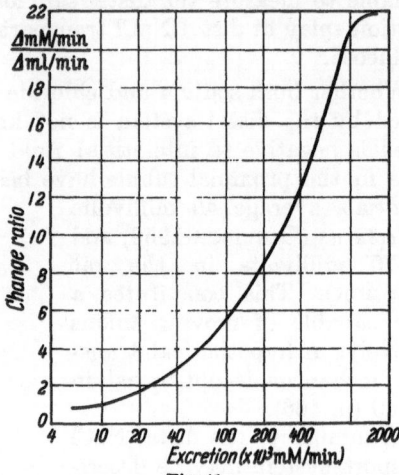

Fig. 40   Fig. 41

Fig. 40. Hypothetical relationship between NaCl excretion and filtration rate in an average young man. All other variables are assumed to be constant. Parameters of proximal NaCl transport are assumed to be similar to those in the dog. Distal NaCl transport is assumed to have a Tm of 4.0 mM./min. and a titration splay similar to that for glucose. Reproduced by permission of Medicine

Fig. 41. Hypothetical relationship between the effect of change in filtration rate on excretion (change ratio) and the average rate of excretion in the interval in which the change in filtration rate occurs. The change ratio is obtained by dividing the change in NaCl excretion rate by the change in filtration rate. In essence, this is a graph of the first derivative (slope) of Fig. 40 plotted against the ordinate. Excretion is plotted on a logarithmic scale. Reproduced by permission of Medicine

e) Metabolic and other influences on sodium chloride transport
α) General description

Tubular transport of NaCl is affected by many agents, most of which are depressant. When the depressant action of a substance is sufficiently intense and specific for NaCl transport systems, the substance may become clinically useful as a chloruretic to remove excessive accumulations of sodium chloride from the body.

NaCl transport is depressed by cyanide in the kidney of frog (Hoshiko, Swanson and Visscher) and dog (Bayliss and Lundsgaard; Nicholson 1949); by azide in the frog kidney (Hoshiko, Swanson and Visscher); and by dinitrophenol in the kidney of frog (Hoshiko, Swanson and Visscher) and Necturus (Schatzmann, Windhager and Solomon). For the most part, no information is available which distinguishes proximal from distal tubular effects or which distinguishes the effects on proximal NaCl transport of depression in reabsorption of other substances such as glucose from direct depression of the NaCl transport system. In the isolated Necturus nephron perfused by fluid containing 100 mM. NaCl and 2 mM./L. glucose, dinitrophenol in a concentration of 0.2 mM./L. resulted in a decrease in the fraction of water reabsorbed from the perfusate from 27 to 10 percent (Schatzmann, Windhager and Solomon).

β) Temperature

Sodium chloride reabsorption is decreased with decreased temperature in both frog and mammal. Although David in early studies concluded from urine concentration and perfusion rate data that temperature had no direct effect on the reabsorption in the frog, HOSHIKO measuring reabsorption in the frog concluded that the overall process, both proximal and distal, had an ARRHENIUS' activation constant of about 20 Cal./mol. In the dog, cooling from 37 to 22—25 deg. C results in an increase in NaCl excretion and a decrease in concentration of the glomerular filtrate. At the lower temperature 15 to 25 percent of filtered salt and water may be excreted (compared with 1 to 8 percent at normal temperature), although filtration rate may decrease to 10 percent of the values at normal body temperature. At the same temperature, glucose transport is completely inhibited but phosphate and amino acid transport are only partially inhibited (SEGAR; SEGAR, RILEY and BARILA; BOYLAN and HONG). Stop-flow experiments in the dog indicate that the distal process can effect a low urinary NaCl concentration at 25 deg. but yield no information concerning depression of distal Tm (HONG and BOYLAN).

γ) Mercury

It has long been known that compounds of mercury cause an increase in renal excretion of sodium chloride. Although it was postulated at one time that the chloruresis might be of extrarenal origin and due to changes in blood chloride concentration[1] or "mobilization" of tissue chlorides subsequent studies demonstrated conclusively that the chloruresis resulted from the action of mercury on the kidney. GOVAERTS showed that the kidney of dogs undergoing a mercurial diuresis continued to excrete chloride abundantly after transplantation to another animal while the kidney of an uninjected dog failed to diurese when transplanted to the neck of a mercurialized animal. CHRISTIAN and BARTRAM, and BARTRAM showed that mercury injected into one renal artery elicited chloruresis only from the injected organ. With acceptance of the filtration-reabsorption hypothesis of renal function, numerous studies showed that mercurial diuresis was not accompanied by an increase in glomerular filtration rate. The initial conclusions from the less precise creatinine and urea clearances in man were confirmed in later studies by inulin clearances in man and creatinine clearances in the dog (CHROMETZKA and UNGER; GAVAZZENI; HERRMANN, STONE and SCHWAB; SCHMITZ; BLUMGART et al. 1932, 1934; PAGE 1933; HERRMANN and DECHERD; GUKELBERGER; FARNSWORTH; BERLINER, KENNEDY and HILTON 1948; DUGGAN and PITTS; PITTS and DUGGAN; DALE and SANDERSON; GROSSMAN et al. 1950a; KLEEMAN, MAXWELL and ROCKNEY 1958). Only in the rat has an increase in inulin clearance following injection of an organic mercurial been reported (DICKER 1946). Mercury therefore acts by depressing the renal tubular transport of NaCl. Depression in NaCl transport although constituting the justification for the employment of mercury clinically is by no means the only depressant effect of small quantities of mercurial compounds. Organic mercurials (2 ml. of Mersalyl, Mercuxanthin, Salyrgan) depress PAH and Diodrast Tm in man with widening of titration splay of Diodrast (BRUN, HILDEN and RAASCHOU 1947a; BERLINER, KENNEDY and HILTON 1948; McDONALD and MILLER) and inhibit uptake of diodrast by rabbit kidney (JOSEPHSON) but do not affect PAH Tm in the dog (BERLINER, KENNEDY and HILTON 1948; HANDLEY, TELFORD and

---

[1] Changes in plasma chloride concentration during mercurial diuresis are small, irregular and may be dependent as much upon rates of water ingestion and absorption as upon salt and water excretion. Some studies are those of HANSEN, FOSDICK and DRAGSTEDT (no change in the dog); BLUMGART et al. (1932) (no change); HERMANN, STONE and SCHWAB (slight fall then a rise); FULTON et al. (no change or a slight fall); BOUYOUCOS (rise if initially low, fall if initially high); DECOURT, FISCHER and GUILLEMIN (slight rise then a fall).

LaForge). They depress potassium secretion in the dog (MUDGE et al. 1950; BERLINER, KENNEDY and ORLOFF 1951; McBRIDE, WEINER and MUDGE) and increase excretion, presumably by depressing reabsorption, of magnesium (W. O. SMITH et al.), calcium (BLUMGART et al. 1934), 11-oxy and 17-keto steroids (LASCHE, PERLOFF and DURANT) and urate. Other transport processes are relatively unaffected. No effect on glucose Tm was observed with mercuxanthin in man (McDONALD and MILLER; LETTERI and WESSON, unpub.) or with Salyrgan or mercuhydrin in the dog (HANDLEY, TELFORD and LaFORGE) although a de-

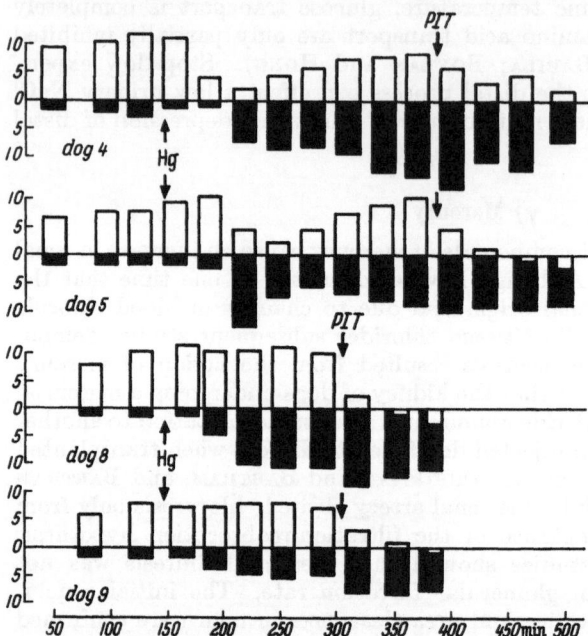

pression of 40 percent or more in glucose Tm in man has been reported (WESTON et al. 1949). Phosphate excretion or clearance is unaffected in man by Merbaphen or mercupurin (BLUMGART et al. 1934; DALE and SANDERSON) and titratable acidity and ammonia production are not affected by mercaptomerin (HILTON 1951; WESTON, GROSSMAN and LEITER 1951). Both respiration and ammonia formation by kidney slices from rabbits injected with $HgCl_2$ are unaffected unless histologically evident lesions are present (STEIGER and STREHLER).

Of the two NaCl transport systems in the nephron, that in the proximal tubule appears to be the one principally affected by organic mercurials. The question has long been a controversial one, and many arguments advanced to

Fig. 42. The effect of mercury (10 mg. Hg/kg. as mercurin intravenously) on maximal free water clearance in the dog. Free water clearance is measured by open columns and osmolar clearance by solid columns. Free water clearance is positive if above and negative if below the zero line. Increase in osmolar clearance after mercury represents increase in NaCl excretion. Pitressin (10 milliunits intravenously plus 40—80 milliunits per hour by infusion) caused free water clearance to decrease and to become negative (hypertonic urine) in 3 of the 4 experiments. Cysteine hydrochloride (8 mg./kg.) was given together with the mercurin. After WESSON and ANSLOW 1952). Reproduced by permission of the American Journal of Physiology

support the view that one another other site is primarily affected are unconvincing. Among such arguments, the greater intensity of pathological lesions in the proximal tubule resulting from toxic quantities of mercury (EDWARDS 1942), and the effect of mercury on aromatic acid transport, a known proximal tubular function, have been offered in support of a proximal locus of the chloruretic action while the relatively small fraction of filtered chloride which is excreted under the usual experimental conditions following administration of relatively large quantities of organic mercurials has been offered in support of a distal locus. Current belief that the action of organic mercurials is primarily on proximal NaCl transport rests mostly upon inability to obtain evidence of marked interference with concentration or dilution of urine during mercurial chloruresis. During water diuresis in the dog, mercurin (10 mg. Hg/kg.) caused no decrease in free water clearance (Fig. 42) (WESSON and ANSLOW 1952; BLACKMORE 1959) and mercaptomerin did not cause a decrease in free-water clearance in diabetes insipidus dogs (MILLER and RIGGS). In man, similarly, meralluride was not associated with a decrease in free water clearance in water-diuresing normal subjects (LARAGH) or patients with diabetes insipidus (HEINEMANN and BECKER). In other studies, however, variable decreases in free water clearance have been reported in man after mercaptomerin (LADD 1952), mercurin (CAPPS et al.) or mersalyl (DALE and SANDERSON) and in dogs after mercurin (CAPPS et al.). The decreases in free water clearance observed by these last researchers may have been similar in origin to transient decreases observed occasionally by others (WESSON and ANSLOW 1952) (Fig. 42). During hydropenia or administration of antidiuretic hormone (Pitressin) the maximal negative free water clearance after meralluride in the dog (BRODSKY and GRAUBARTH 1953b) or after mercaptomerin in man (LADD 1952; WELT et al. 1953) has been variously reported as not significantly less than that observed during mannitol or saline diuresis or as being significantly less by as much as 36 to 48 percent than during mannitol or urea loading (GROSSMAN et al. 1955; AU and RAISZ; HAUSER, POLIMEROS and LEVITT). If the hypothesis that distal NaCl transport generates the positive free water clearance of antidiuretic hormone withdrawal (water diuresis) is accepted, then absence of change in the free water clearances implies that little disturbance in distal NaCl transport has occurred and relegates the major site of mercurial chloruretic action to the proximal segment. Additional evidence in support of a proximal locus for mercurial action are the observations that under appropriate experimental conditions of saline or osmotic diuretic loading, the increment in sodium excretion resulting from the action of mercury may greatly exceed that to be expected from total suppression of distal transport in man (WESTON, GROSSMAN and LEITER 1951) or dog (FARAH, COBBEY and MOOK; WESSON and ANSLOW 1952), and the observations that the minimum sodium concentration attained in the distal region during stopped flow is unaffected by chlormerodrin (KESSLER, HIERHOLZER and PITTS; VANDER et al. 1958b). The stopped flow procedure could not, of course, detect a possible change in distal Tm caused by mercury. Attribution of a depressant effect from mercury solely to the proximal process may well prove to be an oversimplification. In particular, it is possible that compounds of mercury may differ among themselves with respect to their relative capacity to depress different transport systems.

No evidence has been obtained which would indicate that mercury primarily affects sodium transport or affects an active or passive chloride transport system. The composition of the urine would be the same in either event provided hydrogen secretion is unimpaired. Increased entry of radioisotopic sodium into proximal tubular fluid during stopped flow in dogs undergoing mercurial diuresis suggests that mercurial diuretics may increase retrograde movement of Na ions thus, in effect, lowering the limiting concentration gradient (BISNO et al.). Additional evidence might be obtained from transepithelial potential measurements.

Compounds of mercury which have significant chloruretic effects and which have been extensively studied belong to two principal groups: Inorganic mercuric salts such as $HgCl_2$ and $Hg(NO_3)_2$ which ionize to yield Hg^{++}, and organomercurials with the general formula R—CH_2—$CH(OY)$—CH_2—Hg—X in which the terms R, X and Y are variables (Fig. 43). Both Hg^{++} and the organomercurials react strongly with thiols. When injected or absorbed into the body of man, dog, rat, amphibian, fish, reptile and bird the highest concentration of mercury is regularly found in the kidney which has several times the concentration of the liver, the organ with the next highest concentration (AIKAWA and FITZ; BORGHGRAEF and PITTS; GIEBISCH and DORMAN). The distribution is appar-

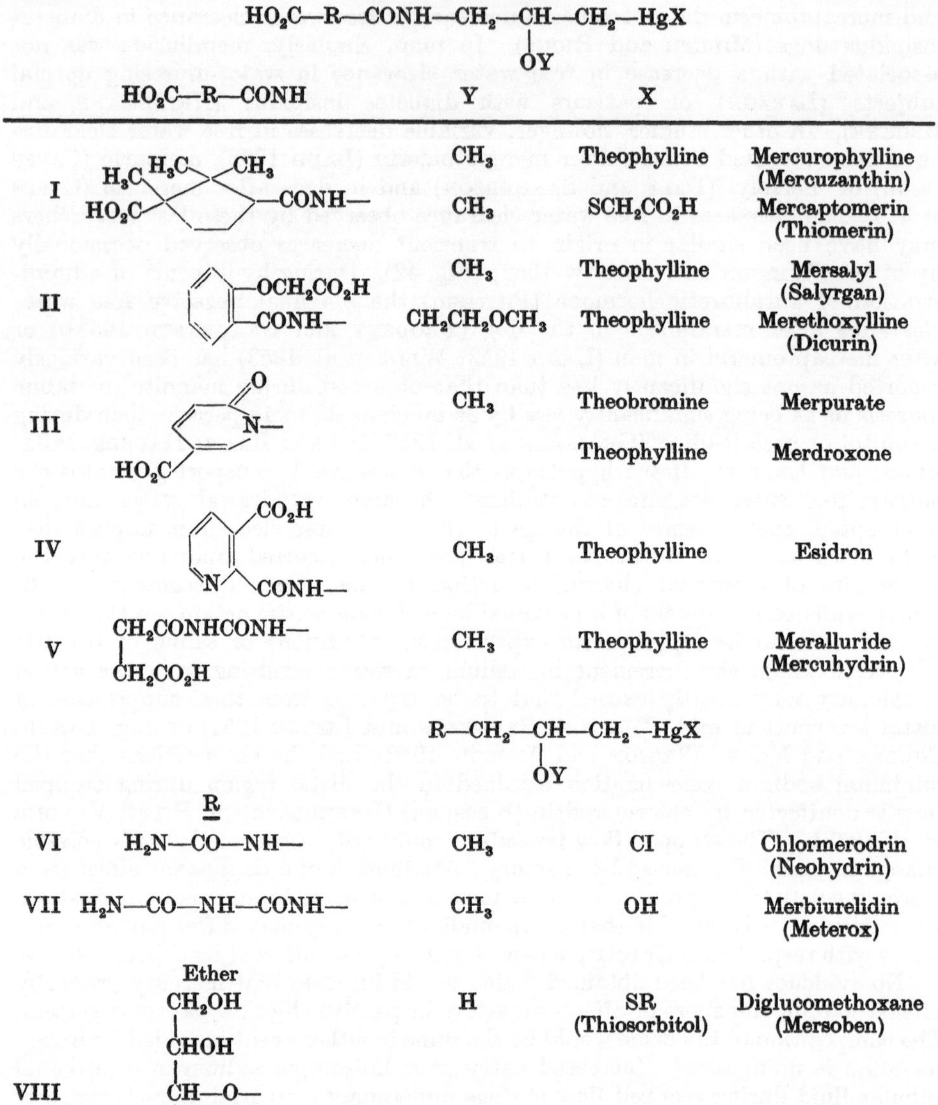

$$HO_2C—R—CONH—CH_2—CH—CH_2—HgX$$
$$\underset{OY}{|}$$

$$HO_2C—R—CONH \qquad\qquad Y \qquad\qquad X$$

	$HO_2C—R—CONH$	Y	X	
I	H₃C, H₃C, CH₃ / HO₂C —CONH—	CH₃	Theophylline	Mercurophylline (Mercuzanthin)
		CH₃	SCH₂CO₂H	Mercaptomerin (Thiomerin)
II	—OCH₂CO₂H / —CONH—	CH₃	Theophylline	Mersalyl (Salyrgan)
		CH₂CH₂OCH₃	Theophylline	Merethoxylline (Dicurin)
III	O ‖ N— / HO₂C	CH₃	Theobromine	Merpurate
			Theophylline	Merdroxone
IV	CO₂H / N CONH—	CH₃	Theophylline	Esidron
V	CH₂CONHCONH— / CH₂CO₂H	CH₃	Theophylline	Meralluride (Mercuhydrin)

$$R—CH_2—CH—CH_2—HgX$$
$$\underset{OY}{|}$$

	R	Y	X	
VI	H₂N—CO—NH—	CH₃	Cl	Chlormerodrin (Neohydrin)
VII	H₂N—CO—NH—CONH—	CH₃	OH	Merbiurelidin (Meterox)
VIII	Ether / CH₂OH / CHOH / CH—O— / (CHOH)₂ / CH₂OH	H	SR (Thiosorbitol)	Diglucomethoxane (Mersoben)
IX	Carbon-Carbon Linkage / O ‖ HO₂C O	CH₃	Theophylline	Mercumatilin (Cumertilin)

Fig. 43. Structural formulae of some diuretic, organomercurials. In the general formulae (top and middle of the figure), R, X and Y are variables. After SPRAGUE. Reproduced by permission of the author and the New York Academy of Sciences

ently determined in part by blood flow but mostly by tissue-binding capacity as, for example, to —SH groups. Small differences in the relative degree of renal accumulation of organomercurials may also be related in part to differences in rate of excretion. Both mercuric ions and organomercurials react readily with cysteine, and when they enter the blood stream probably circulate in combination with this and other thiols (HUGHES). The affinity of organomercurials for cysteine is less than for renal cellular enzymes related to chloride transport so that cysteine is unable to interfere with mercurial diuresis. 2,3-dithiopropanol (BAL), however, has a greater affinity for mercury than either cysteine or tissue binding sites and will abolish or prevent mercurial diuresis (HANDLEY and LaFORGE; FARAH and MARESH; EARLE and BERLINER 1947) and depress the high rate of renal accumulation (BORGHGRAEF and PITTS). Ethylenediamine-tetraacetate (versene) can inhibit Mersalyl diuresis in the rat, presumably by preferential binding as with dithiopropanol (FILOMENI; FILOMENI and PALUMBI). Although mercuric cysteine is, itself, a diuretic (MUDGE and WEINER) it is not known whether the cysteine remains attached to the mercuric ion while the latter is exerting a chloruretic effect. Nondiuretic mercurials such as p-chloro-mercuribenzoate can prevent or abolish the effect of diuretic mercurials such as mersalyl or mercuric glutathione, perhaps by preferential binding (MILLER and FARAH). The highest concentrations of radioactive mercury, administered as chlormerodrin, are found in the proximal tubules of *Necturus* (GIEBISCH and DORMAN) and in the cortex, presumably the proximal convoluted tubules, of rat and dog (GREIF et al.; YAGI and WHITE). Mersalyl containing radioisotopic mersury and administered in relatively small quantities in the rat was concentrated principally in the distal portion of the proximal tubule (DARMADY and STRANACK). In sucrose homogenates of cortex, most of the mercury was present in the soluble fraction although significant amounts were firmly bound to sedimentable particles (GREIF et al.; SURTSHIN and YAGI).

An interesting aspect of intracellular distribution of mercury is the changes observed in association with body protein depletion. Rats which are protein-depleted either by experimental toxic nephrosis or by feeding a protein-free diet survive quantities of $HgCl_2$ which are fatal to nondepleted rats. The rate of excretion of mercury and the content of mercury in the renal cortex of the protein-depleted is as great or greater than in the controls (SURTSHIN and PARELMAN; SURTSHIN and YAGI; YAGI and WHITE; SHORE and SHORE). The difference between the depleted and nondepleted animals is attributed to an increase in the sulfhydryl content of the soluble fraction of renal cells in the depleted animals and a corresponding increase in mercury bound in the soluble fraction. A corresponding decrease in the mercury bound to the particulate (nuclei, mitochondria, etc.) fraction (SURTSHIN and YAGI; YAGI and WHITE) may be associated with a decreased depression in the tricarboxylic acid (KREBS) cycle in the depleted. Extent of Hg depression of alkaline phosphatase, cathepsin and beta glucuronidase was not affected by protein depletion (SHORE and SHORE).

Organic mercurials inhibit numerous enzyme systems *in vitro* which probably depend for their activity on free —SH groups while many other enzymes are unaffected. Among enzymes involved in carbohydrate metabolism, p-chloro-mercuribenzoate inhibits pyruvate oxidase, carboxylase, alpha ketoglutaric oxidase, malic oxidase, adenosinetriphosphatase and the dehydrogenase of the succinoxidase system (BARRON and SINGER). *In vivo*, mersalyl and $HgCl_2$ have been reported to depress the concentration of free sulfhydryl groups in the loop of HENLE and collecting ducts of rat and dog (medulla) while dithiopropanol but not cysteine blocks the depression (FARAH, CAFRUNY and DI-STEFANO; CAFRUNY and FARAH; FARAH et al.). The depression in sulhydryl is less in alkalosis (FARAH et al.). DE METRY and AIKAWA, however, report a 35 percent depression in sulfhydryl concentration in rabbit cortex using larger quantities of mercury (14—30 mg. Hg/kg.) as mercaptomerin. Meralluride in relatively

large quantities is variably reported to inhibit succinic dehydrogenase activity
in either the proximal convoluted segment (MUSTAKALLIO and TELKKA; TELKKA
and MUSTAKALLIO) or loop of HENLE (BAHN and LONGLEY) in the rat. Mercurophylline was observed to differ from meralluride in affecting primarily the
succinic dehydrogenase activity of the pars recta of the distal segment (TELKKA
and MUSTAKALLIO). Toxic doses of mercurials are necessary to produce a significant depression of enzyme activity (BICKERS and BRESLER) and no significant
depression of this enzyme was observed with fully chloruretic doses of 4 mg.
Hg/kg. (FAWAZ and FAWAZ; BAHN and LONGLEY) while those mercurials which
react most strongly with —SH groups or are the most potent inhibitors of
succinic dehydrogenase may have little chloruretic activity (HANDLEY and
LAVIK; KESSLER, LOZANO and PITTS 1957b). Concentrations of chlormerodrin
consistent with those observed to be bound to isolated renal cortical mitochondria do not depress mitochondrial oxidative phosphorylation, although
depression of phosphorylation can be observed with higher concentrations
(GREIF and JACOBS). Renal binding of meralluride but not of $HgCl_2$ is decreased
by 2,4-dinitrophenol although this substance has little evident effect on the
excretion of mercury (CAFRUNY and ROSS).

Chloruretic efficacy of mercurial compounds is determined by filtered load
of salt as related to tubular reabsorptive capacity (Load-Tm ratio) and by the
extent of mercurial depression of transport capacity. Factors which determine
the importance of filtered load can be appreciated when it is recognized that
load may be so low that NaCl may continue to be almost entirely reabsorbed by
the tubular transport system after it has been depressed by a mercurial compound.
A mercurial diuresis can be suppressed or restored by appropriate increases
or decreases in GFR or plasma NaCl concentrations (PITTS and DUGGAN; STOCK,
MUDGE and NURNBERG; WESTON et al. 1952). Factors which determine the
relative ability of mercurial compounds to depress NaCl transport are not clear.
No correlation is evident between diuretic potency and rate of excretion or
extent of concentration in renal tissues (LEHMAN, KING and TAUBE; KESSLER,
LOZANO and PITTS 1957b). Mercurials with little diuretic potency are as avidly
bound by sulfhydryl groups and as intensely concentrated in the kidney as
potent diuretics. In a group of organomercurials, the only property which
appeared to be common to those which were significantly diuretic was occurrence of a hydrophilic group at least three carbon atoms distant from the mercury
(KESSLER, LOZANO and PITTS 1957a). A possible small tubular depressant
effect from the apparently inactive organomercurial, p-chloromercuribenzoate,
(KESSLER, LOZANO and PITTS 1957a; WEINER, LEVY and MUDGE) may have
been masked, however, by depression in filtration rate (KESSLER, LOZANO and
PITTS 1957b; VARGAS and CAFRUNY). Administration of acidifying salts to
produce an acidosis results in enhancement of the diuretic effect of subsequently
administered organomercurials (KEITH and WHELAN; HARRIS, RUBIN and
LAWRENCE; ETHRIDGE, MEYERS and FULTON). Although the effects of the
acidifying salt, ammonium chloride, have been attributed to elevation in plasma
chloride concentration (KEITH and WHELAN; AXELROD and PITTS 1952a) acidosis itself is a major factor as shown by a similar potentiating effect from
ammonium nitrate and phosphoric acid (ETHRIDGE, MEYERS and FULTON) by
continued existence of marked potentiation in chronic acidosis after renal compensation has restored plasma chloride and bicarbonate concentrations virtually
to normal levels (HILTON 1951), by failure to obtain a chloruresis in the presence
of hyperchloremia and alkalosis (MUDGE and WEINER; LEVY, WEINER and
MUDGE), and by blocking mercurial diuresis by prior administration of the

carbonic anhydrase inhibitor, acetazolamide, which causes the excretion of an alkaline urine without lowering plasma chloride or elevating plasma bicarbonate (AXELROD and PITTS 1952a; RIGGS and BERKSON). Since inorganic mercurials such as mercuric cysteine are chloruretic during both aciduria and alkaluria, while organomercurials are generally effective only during aciduria, it has been frequently suggested that acid urine is essential to convert organomercurials to inorganic, active mercuric ions. This view finds support both from the observation noted above that the chloruretic action of inorganic mercuric ions is relatively independent of urinary pH and also from the observation that most organomercurials are acid labile and that acid lability is markedly increased by binding of the organomercurial to cysteine and perhaps to thiols generally (MUDGE and WEINER). Opposed to this view, however, are the observations that no clear correlation can be observed between either the ionizability (breaking the —Hg—X bond) or the dissociability (breaking the —C—Hg bond, Fig. 43) of organomercurials (H. FRIEDMAN). Some potent diuretics may not be significantly dissociated at the pH of urine even in the presence of cysteine, and generally no more than traces are excreted in any form other than the parent compound. MUDGE and WEINER argue, however, that dissociation of no more than a trace of an organomercurial should, if selectively distributed, depress NaCl reabsorption. In the dog, acidosis attendant upon respiring 12 percent carbon dioxide does not significantly potentiate organomercurial diuresis (AXELROD and PITTS 1952a) nor does extracellular alkalosis resulting from potassium depletion inhibit diuresis (MUDGE and HARDIN). These observations indicate the unlikelihood of blood pH affecting mercurial potency from the plasma surface of the epithelium but leaves open the question whether pH within the proximal segment has been significantly altered. Although alkaluria, by whatever means produced, can block an organomercurial chloruresis, alkaluria is ineffective in suppressing chloruresis if induced after the latter has commenced (AXELROD and PITTS 1952a; PITTS 1958). In summary of the relationship of urine pH to mercurial diuresis, it would appear that an acid pH within the lumen of the proximal segment of the nephron is important for completion of an early step in a series of events leading to reaction of an organomercurial with the critical cellular elements involved in NaCl transport and that inorganic mercuric ions (or mercuric cysteine) either do not require this first step or an acid pH is not required in their case. Although hydrolysis of the organomercurial is a plausible first step, this may not be the critical one. More likely, elements in the cell membrane require an acid pH in order to assume a configuration permitting them to react with organomercurials (monovalent mercuric ions) of the proper configuration, while such a configuration of membrane elements is not essential to react with inorganic (divalent) ions. The distinct delay in the onset of chloruresis following injection of an organomercurial, amounting to about 20 minutes in the dog (for example, see Fig. 42) and 15 minutes following unilateral injection into the renal portal system of the chicken (CAMPBELL 1957), although excretion of mercury begins immediately and profusely (GROSSMAN et al. 1955; PITTS 1958) and urate clearance is increased immediately (GROSSMAN et al. 1950a), is unexplained.

The organomercurials are excreted rapidly and for the most part unchanged. Fifty to sixty percent of parenterally administered meralluride or mercaptomerin is excreted in 3 to 6 hours (GROSSMANN et al. 1951; MOYER, HANDLEY and SEIBERT). Excretion may be somewhat faster by the dog than by man (MOYER, HANDLEY and SEIBERT) while excretion of chlormerodrin by the rat is substantially slower than in the dog: 24 hours to excrete 50 percent by the dog

(BORGHGRAEF and PITTS; BORGHGRAEF, KESSLER and PITTS). More than 95 percent of injected meralluride and mersalyl are excreted as such in the urine of both dog and man (MOYER, HANDLEY and SEIBERT; WEINER and MÜLLER; MÜLLER and WEINER). In the urine they are bound to thiols, perhaps mostly to cysteine, as is probably also the case in the blood (WEINER and MÜLLER; WEINER, LEVY and MUDGE). Excretion of mercurials is unaffected by desoxycorticosterone (GROSSMAN et al. 1951) or by acidosis or alkalosis (WEINER, LEVY and MUDGE) but is increased somewhat by aminophylline, presumably by means of the stimulating effect of this xanthine on the renal circulation (GROSSMAN et al. 1951). In patients with severe congestive heart failure, excretion of meralluride is significantly slower than in normals and the fraction of injected organomercurial excreted in an altered or degraded form may increase to 11 percent (MOYER, HANDLEY and SEIBERT). The rapid excretion of many organomercurials is explained in part by tubular secretion. Mercaptomerin and Diurgin were excreted rapidly; mersalyl, meralluride and Esidron were secreted to a moderate extent; and chlormerodrin was secreted slightly by the ipsilateral chicken kidney when injected into one iliac vein. Mercumatilin and Oradon were not evidently secreted (CAMPBELL 1957; WEINER, BURNETT and RENNICK). Chloruresis was essentially unilateral with mercumatilin and Oradon. Probenecid and bromcresol green blocked both the secretion of the mercurials and also, if given prior to injection of the mercurial, the diuretic effect (CAMPBELL 1957, 1959).

Dimercaptopropanol (dimercaprol, BAL) affects excretion and renal content of mercury in different ways according to the mercurial preparation administered. Excretion of mersalyl is affected relatively little by dimercaprol. Excretion of chlormerodrin, which is accumulated by the kidney to a greater degree than mersalyl, is increased by dimercaprol at the expense, primarily, of the intrarenal content. Renal content of inorganic mercury (mercuric cysteine) is also lowered by dimercaprol but the disposition of the mercury appears to depend extensively on the p_H of the urine: when the urine is alkaline, intrarenal mercury enters the urine whereas it passes to unknown sites in the rest of the body when the urine is acid (WEINER et al.).

δ) Xanthines

Administration of the methylated xanthines, caffeine, theobromine and theophylline to man or animals generally is attended by an increase in sodium chloride excretion. Of the three, the most potent chloruretic is theophylline which may be either free or as a salt with ethylenediamine (aminophylline).

The mechanism of the diuretic effect is far less clear than is that of mercury. Although some researchers have failed to detect a significant increase in filtration rate in man (GAVAZZENI; BLUMGART et al. 1932, 1934; EARLE et al. 1949), others have concluded that an increase in filtration rate occurs either usually or regularly following the acute administration of xanthines to normal subjects (GUKELBERGER; KLEEMAN, MAXWELL and ROCKNEY 1958); patients with congestive heart failure (HERRMANN, STONE and SCHWAB; HERRMANN and DECHERD; SINCLAIR-SMITH et al.; WESTON et al. 1952) and dogs (SCHMITZ). The most extensive studies are those of DAVIS and SHOCK. These researchers observed that following injection of 0.48—0.96 g. of aminophylline GFR increased an average of 10 ml./min. in 25 normal subjects and 1 ml./min. in 6 patients with congestive heart failure. Sodium excretion increased from 0.3 to 0.8—1.0 mM./min. in the normals and by about 0.34 mM./min. in the cardiacs. Since both of these increments in sodium excretion are larger than reasonably attributable to the increase in filtration rate (Fig. 44) it must be concluded that a substantial although possibly a highly variable fraction of the chloruretic effect of xantines arises from a depression in tubular transport capacity.

Nothing is known concerning the intrarenal mechanisms or site of action of xanthines. Intact renal nerves are not necessary for xanthine effects (BRICKER et al. 1956). Combined with mercury or chlorothiazide they cause an enhanced chloruresis which may, however, be attributable to their ability to increase GFR (HERRMANN and DECHERD; GOODMAN, CORSARO and STACY; WESTON et al. 1952; NECHAY). Bicarbonate, calcium and potassium as well as sodium and chloride excretion may increase during xanthine diuresis (BLUMGART et al. 1934) and the urine is usually less acid than during a mercurial diuresis. Potassium secretion is unaffected (MUDGE et al.) but other transport systems have not been studied. When injected into one renal artery, an approximately equal chloruretic effect appears from both kidneys indicating minimal fixation of the drug by the tissues of the injected kidney (BARTRAM).

ε) Chlorothiazide

Chlorothiazide and hydro-chlorothiazide are potent natri- and chloruretic agents which are related chemically to the sulfonamides (SPRAGUE). The chloruretic effect is not correlated with increase in GFR or RPF in man or dog (MOYER, FORD and SPURR) and, if injected into one renal artery of the dog, it evokes a chloruresis on the injected side without evident change in GFR (LAVENDER and PULL-MAN). When injected intra-venously, filtration rate may

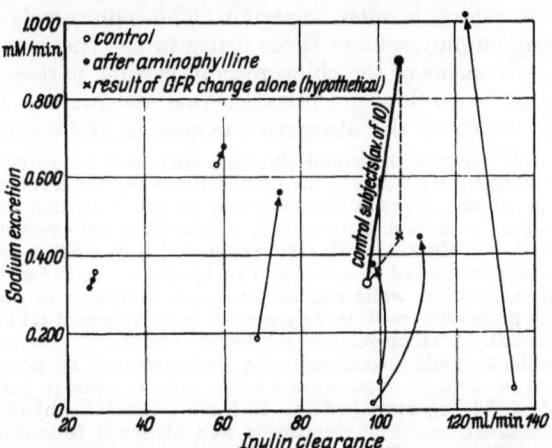

Fig. 44. Effect of aminophylline on sodium excretion and glomerular filtration rate in normal subjects and in subjects with congestive heart failure (DAVIS and SHOCK). Natriuresis generally exceeds that hypothetically attributable to a rise in GFR. Xanthine depression of sodium reabsorption is therefore inferred

be unchanged (BERGSTRÖM, BUCHT and EK) or depressed about 15 percent (JANUSZEWICZ et al.). These observations indicate that the drug acts by depressing sodium transport. Preliminary studies suggest that the site of action is predominantly within the proximal segment. This is indicated by the observations that maximal free water clearance during water diuresis is not significantly changed during chlorothiazide and hydrochlorothiazide natriuresis (LARAGH, HEINEMANN and DEMARTINI; JANUSZEWICZ et al.; BLACKMORE 1959), and that electrolyte concentrations attained in the distal area of the nephron during stopped-flow are unaffected (HIERHOLZER et al.; VANDER et al. 1959). Chlorothiazide and its derivatives are weak carbonic anhydrase inhibitors and significant quantities of bicarbonate as well as chloride may appear with sodium in the urine. Among derivatives of chlorothiazide, the chloruretic efficacy is not correlated with the carbonic anhydrase inhibitory activity (HWANG et al.). Potassium secretion is unaffected (MOYER, FORD and SPURR; PITTS et al. 1958b). Studies of the effects of chlorothiazide on other renal transport systems have not been reported. When given with or shortly after injection of a mercurial diuretic or aminophylline, natriuresis is greater than with either alone (BAYLISS et al.; PITTS et al 1958b; NECHAY).

Chlorothiazide is an acid which is secreted by the tubules (BEYER 1958; BAER et al. 1959). This aspect of the molecule may account for its ability when taken orally to depress urate clearance, presumably by interfering with a secretory component of urate excretion or, in large intravenous doses, to enhance urate excretion by interference with urate reabsorption. Hydrochlorothiazide, which attains maximal chloruretic effect at much smaller doses ($1/10$—$1/20$ those of chlorothiazide) has little effect on urate excretion (LARAGH, HEINEMANN and DEMARTINI; JANUSZEWICZ et al.). Probenecid, while blocking chlorothiazide secretion, does not abort the chloruretic effect (BAER et al. 1958).

ζ) Digitalis glycosides

Administration of digitalis leaf or various purified digitalis glycosides to patients with cardiac edema is regularly followed by an increase in NaCl excretion which is often massive. This chloruresis is an important reason for the long employment of these drugs in the therapy of congestive heart failure. The mechanisms of the chloruresis in cardiac patients are not clear, however, because renal blood flow and filtration rate also increase to an extent sufficient to account for much of the observed increase in NaCl excretion.

Exogenous creatinine clearance increased following Digalen in all three cardiac patients studied by HERRMANN, STONE and SCHWAB. GFR increased 6 to 19 (av., 12) ml./min. following 1.5 mg. Digoxin intravenously in all 5 cardiac patients studied by DAVIES, although sodium excretion increased by relatively small amounts (0.004—0.017 mM./min.). FARBER et al. and EICHNA et al. (1951) observed that GFR increased in 9 of 10 cardiac patients from average values of 68 before to 76 ml./min. in one to two hours following 1.0 to 1.5 mg. Digoxin intravenously, while sodium excretion increased in all by 0.10 to 0.20 mM./min. Because the patients were 50 to 70 years old these values of GFR are only moderately decreased below normal. A chloruretic effect which was much smaller than that observed in the cardiac patients could occasionally be demonstrated in noncardiac subjects. Chloride excretion increased in 17 of 20 normal subjects from average values of 0.117 before to 0.187 one hour after the Digoxin injection. In 5 other normal subjects in whom GFR and RPF were being measured, no clear chloruresis was observed following Digoxin. Small increases in NaCl excretion were observed after Digoxin in 5 cirrhotics and two nephrotics, and relatively large increases (0.022, 0.13 and 0.271 mM./min.) in three normal subjects rendered edematous by administration of a high salt diet and desoxycorticosterone (FARBER et al.). GFR and RPF were not measured in the cirrhotics, nephrotics or edematous normal subjects, however. Results similar to those of FARBER et al. were obtained by HAMMOND and WHITAKER. They gave 1 to 1.5 mg. Digoxin intravenously to 6 patients with congestive heart failure and to 7 patients with mitral valvular disease but without failure. Filtration rate increased in 7, decreased in 4 and was unchanged in 2. The changes in sodium excretion correlated positively (that is, changed in the same direction as filtration rate) in 7, was indeterminate in 3 and correlated negatively in 3. The effect of digitalis glycosides can be extremely rapid since an increase in GFR, RPF and sodium excretion was observed within 10 minutes after intravenous injection of lanatoside C (WERKO et al. 1956a). GREVE et al. observed no clear natriuresis in healthy subjects given 0.2 mg. Digitoxin orally, but since cardiac output and creatinine clearance appeared to decline, a possible natriuretic effect might have been blocked by decreasing GFR. Dogs with congestive heart failure caused by pulmonary artery constriction respond similarly to man, with an increase in both GFR and sodium excretion in most of the animals following injection of 1.0 to 1.2 mg. Digoxin (DAVIS, HOWELL and HYATT 1955).

These drugs may have a small depressant effect directly upon the tubular NaCl transport systems. The latter possibility is supported by the studies of HYMAN, JAQUES and HYMAN who observed that injection of 0.125 mg. of Digoxin into one renal artery of the dog is followed by the slow onset of a relative natriuresis from the injected kidney without an evident increase in creatinine excretion. Similar natriuretic effects from strophanthidin and other active digitalis glycosides following renal arterial injection in the dog have been reported by others (CADE, SHALHOUB and CANESSA; STRICKLER, KESSLER and PITTS). That the natriuresis could arise from depression of proximal NaCl transport is suggested by the observation that Ouabain at concentration of 0.14 mM./L. in the perfusate decreases water reabsorption by perfused proximal tubules of *Necturus* from 27 to 10 percent (SCHATZMANN, WINDHAGER and SOLOMON).

η) Adrenocortical and related steroids

Loss of the adrenal glands in man or experimental animals is followed by numerous metabolic changes. Among the most important of these are an unremitting, moderate to large rate of sodium chloride excretion (LOEB, ATCHLEY and STAHL). Unlike in a normal individual the urine fails to become salt-free at the low rates of glomerular filtration which are frequently present in Addisonian patients (Section C V 12). Salt loss persists in the presence of hypotension, dehydration and hyponatremia. Administration of any of a large number of natural or synthetic steroids is followed by a decrease in sodium chloride excretion. Since the decrease in excretion is not accompanied by any corresponding decrease in filtered sodium load, it must be concluded that tubular reabsorption has increased.

Incomplete evidence indicates that the principal tubular reabsorptive function which is subject to the influence of these steroids is the titration splay of the distal transport process. When adrenalectomized dogs are saline-loaded, so that as the result of increasing filtration rate they are excreting large amounts of salt, overall rate of tubular NaCl reabsorption is not measurably lower than in

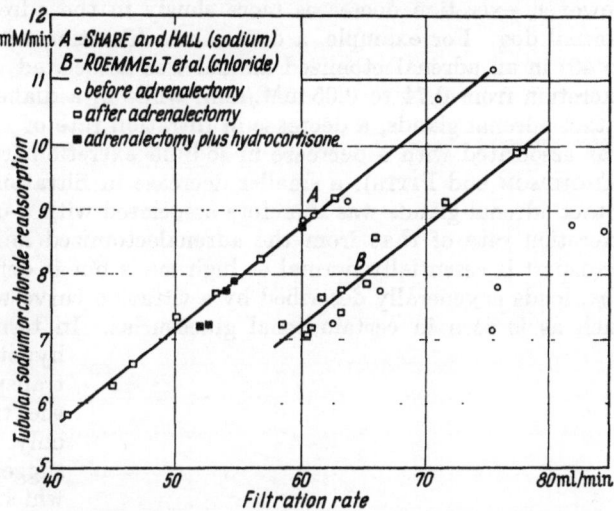

Fig. 45. Tubular transport rate of sodium or chloride in normal and adrenalectomized dogs, plotted from data of SHARE and HALL (*A*) and ROEMMELT, SARTORIUS and PITTS (*B*). In the data of ROEMMELT at al., chloride reabsorption was greater after adrenalectomy. Reproduced by permission of Medicine

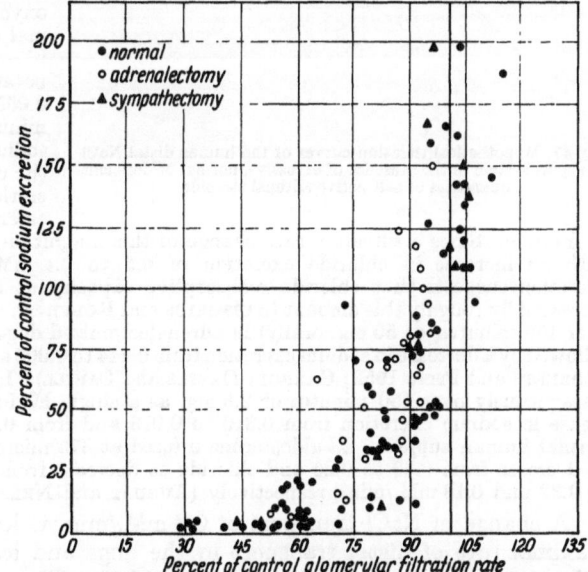

Fig. 46. Relationship between changes in sodium excretion and filtration rate in adrenalectomized and sympathectomized dogs compared with normal dogs. Both excretion and filtration are expressed as percentage of control rates. Adrenalectomized or sympathectomized animals are not markedly different from normals. Modified from THOMPSON and PITTS

normal dogs (Figs. 45 and 46) (Roemmelt, Sartorius and Pitts; Thompson and Pitts; Share and Hall). As filtration rate and filtered salt load are reduced, however, excretion decreases more slowly in the adrenalectomized than in the normal dog. For example, a decrease in filtration rate of 24 ml./min. (from 67 to 43) in an adrenalectomized animal was associated with a decrease in sodium excretion from 0.74 to 0.05 mM./min. while in a diabetes insipidus animal with intact adrenal glands, a decrease in filtration rate of 17 ml./min. (from 81 to 64) was associated with a decrease in sodium excretion from 0.74 to 0.02 mM./min. (Thompson and Pitts); a smaller decrease in filtration rate in the animal with intact adrenal glands was therefore associated with a urine with half the sodium excretion rate of that from the adrenalectomized animal. A system in which transport is essentially normal at high loads but is deficient at low, or less than Tm, loads is generally described by a titration curve with a wide titration splay such as is seen in certain renal glucosurias. In terms of the two-component hypothesis of tubular NaCl transport, such a widening of the titration splay can occur only in the distal system and suggests this system as the one which is most sensitive to the steroids. Whether distal Tm is also affected is not clear but seems probable.

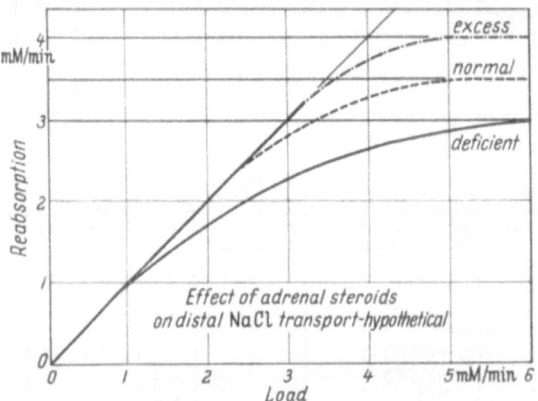

Fig. 47. Hypothetical titration curves of the human distal NaCl transport system in the presence of excessive, normal or deficient quantities of salt-active adrenal steroids

Injection of 0.08 mg./kg. of desoxycorticosterone (DOC) into a normal dog was followed by a decrease in sodium excretion (chloride and potassium were not measured) from 0.055 to 0.005 mM./min. By 210 minutes following the injection, sodium excretion has returned to the control rate but this rise in excretion was associated with an increase in filtration rate from 50 to 56 ml./min. Since a filtration rate change of this magnitude might normally be associated with an increase in chloride excretion of 0.3 to 0.4 mM./min., failure to obtain this excretion suggests that chloride reabsorptive capacity at that level of filtered load was increased by roughly this amount (Sartorius and Roberts). Cortisone (20 mg. intravenously over 150 minutes, or 50 mg. orally) in adrenalectomized dogs at constant filtration rate was followed by a decrease in sodium excretion from 0.144 to 0.005 and from 0.125 to 0.075 mM./min. (Roberts and Pitts 1952; Garrod, Davies and Cahill). In the same studies, DOC (1 mg. intravenously over 150 minutes or 2.5 mg. as a single IV injection) was followed by a decrease in sodium excretion from 0.340 to 0.013 and from 0.125 to 0.010. In saline-loaded normal human subjects, d,l-aldosterone infused at 375 micrograms per hour caused sodium to decrease from 0.58 to 0.26 and chloride to decrease from 0.58 to 0.40 mM./min., changes of 0.32 and 0.18 mM./min., respectively (August and Nelson 1959a).

A change in NaCl transport of 0.3 mM./min. is less than $1/5$ of the estimated maximal rate of distal transport in the dogs and less than $1/10$ of that in man (Wesson and Anslow 1955; Wesson 1957). The effects of steroids on distal NaCl transport in man are illustrated hypothetically in Fig. 47. Both Tm and titration splay are assumed to be affected. Since the load of salt passing from the proximal to the distal system is usually much less than distal Tm, the changes in the titration splay are the more important in body salt balance.

Studies designed to locate the site of action of steroids directly are conflicting. Stopped-flow studies in the dog indicate that during arrest of urine in the distal tubule following acute ureteral obstruction the final urine concentration in adrenalectomized animals is much higher than in normals and appears to be determined by a limiting concentration gradient between blood and urine. Aldosterone caused distal sodium concentration during arrest to decrease nearly to zero as in normal animals. The apparent increase in limiting distal tubular concentration did not, as distinguished from the proximal transport system, appear to result from an increase in sodium diffusion from blood to distal tubular fluid (VANDER et al. 1958a; VANDER, WILDE and MALVIN). Similar studies in the rat, however, failed to show any change in distal tubular concentration (WILLIAMSON, SKULAN and SHIDEMAN) and attempts to differentially poison the proximal tubule and distal tubule by intraarterial injection of tartrate and ureteral injection of $HgCl_2$, respectively, showed that response to DOC was absent in the "proximally" damaged but present from the "distally" damaged kidney (NICHOLSON 1957b). The effects of these poisons are too complex and unpredictable, however, to permit any simple interpretation.

The steroids stimulating NaCl transport which have been the most intensively studied are the synthetic desoxycorticosterone (which also occurs in traces in the adrenal gland) and aldosterone which is currently believed to be the adrenal hormone physiologically important in control of electrolyte balance. Fluoro-hydrocortisone is a potent synthetic sodium-retaining steroid while cortisone, hydrocortisone and progesterone and many other steroids possess significant sodium-retaining properties in addition to influences in other metabolic systems. Preliminary studies suggest that various steroids can compete with one another for attachment to NaCl-transporting cells. Thus, various synthetic steroids (LIDDLE), progesterone and testosterone (LANDAU and LUGEBIHL; LANDAU et al. 1955, 1957; KAGAWA; KAGAWA and JACOBS) depress the sodium-retaining effects of aldosterone and DOC in man and rat.

When aldosterone is injected into one renal artery, electrolyte excretion changes appear from both kidneys and at about the same time, indicating that little of the steroid is extracted from blood on a single circulation (BARGER, BERLIN and TULENKO; GANONG and MULROW). A significant time lapse is required before the effects of the steroids on either Na reabsorption or K secretion become evident. In the adrenalectomized dog this interval is 5 to 60 minutes, averaging 30 minutes, after injection into the renal artery. In Addisonian and normal subjects two hours elapsed following commencement of aldosterone infusion intravenously before changes in electrolyte excretion were observed (ROSS et al.; AUGUST and NELSON 1959b). Although salt-active steroids usually cause a decrease in NaCl excretion acutely, they are generally unable to cause a a positive sodium balance indefinitely in the intact organism. In the dog, desoxy-corticosterone is unable to depress the chloruretic effect of mannitol significantly although restriction of dietary sodium exerts a markedly depressant effect. Similarly, desoxycorticosterone is unable to block natriuresis from mercurial diuretics in the adrenalectomized animal (GOODKIND, HYATT and DAVIS) or from chronic water loading (CHEEK and WEST). Sodium excretion, which in normal man may be depressed to low levels acutely, ultimately increases to or above control rates in spite of continued administration of large quantities of DOC, hydrocortisone, aldosterone or fluorohydrocortisone (ZIERLER and LILIEN-THAL; DINGMAN et al.; AUGUST, NELSON and THORN 1958a; RELMAN and SCHWARTZ 1951; COLE; AUGUST and NELSON 1959b). An increase in filtration rate (which has been measured and found elevated in a few studies) appears to be a reasonable cause of the secondary rise in salt excretion (ZIERLER and LILIENTHAL; DINGMAN et al.).

In addition to their effect on NaCl reabsorption, the same steroids stimulate other tubular transport processes involving sodium ion. In particular they stimulate the exchange of sodium for potassium and hydrogen. These effects will be described in subsequent sections. The salt-active steroids have little significant influence on other transport systems although other steroids, such as cortisone, can affect the transport of urate and probably aromatic acids as a group.

9) Renal nerves and sympathomimetic amines

Nerves to the renal tubular epithelium are rare and most anatomists have doubted their existence (Section B IX). Nevertheless, alteration in activity of the renal nerves may frequently exert profound influences on the excretion of sodium chloride and sometimes of other substances. Stimulation of the nervous pathways to the kidney generally causes a decrease in NaCl excretion while cutting or locally anesthetizing the nerves frequently causes an increase in excretion. These observations have caused intensive and repeated attempts to demonstrate that the renal nerves stimulate the tubular epithelium to reabsorb greater amounts of sodium chloride. It is fair to summarize these efforts by concluding that virtually all studies have failed to demonstrate changes in NaCl excretion resulting from changes in renal nerve activity which are not reasonably attributable to renal vascular effects and particularly to effects on glomerular filtration rate (see, for example, Fig. 46).

Early studies of the functions of the autonomic nervous system showed that interruption of the sympathetic pathways to the kidney in anesthetized animals, whether by thoracolumbar sympathectomy, splanchnicectomy or stripping or cocainization of the renal pedicle, resulted in an increase in urine flow and NaCl excretion. Parasympathetic pathways have not been established. These studies were reviewed by Smith (1939) who emphasized the intense sympathetic activity which generally occurs during anesthesia, the marked vasoconstrictor effects which occur in the kidney and the release of the sympathetic vasoconstrictor effect by interrupting the nerves. Subsequent studies, recognizing the potential significance of hemodynamic effects, have been designed to determine whether changes in NaCl excretion are greater than can be reasonably attributed to simultaneously occurring changes in glomerular filtration or whether NaCl excretion changes under conditions such that filtration fails to change. Unfortunately, experiments of the first type require quantitative knowledge of the effects of filtration rate on excretion during the special conditions existing during the experiment. Since such knowledge is not available, we can only conclude for the present that the relationship between filtration and excretion changes as related to renal nerves and adrenergic drugs is reasonably in accord with current general hypotheses. In human studies, high spinal anesthesia was generally correlated with decreases in both sodium excretion and mannitol clearance (GFR) in pregnant women (Assali et al. 1951). In hypertensive subjects, splanchnicectomy did not significantly affect the pattern of GFR and excretion responses to blood sequestration (Wilkins et al.). Hexamethonium, an autonomic ganglion blocking drug, was associated with well-correlated changes in both filtration rate and sodium excretion (Moyer and Mills, Fig. 48 B) while filtration rate and sodium excretion were correlated positively in 5 of 8 patients with minimal heart failure and in 7 of 8 patients with severe congestive heart failure during dibenamine infusion (Brod and Fejfar 1954). Functions tended to decrease in the less and to increase in the more severely decompensated groups. The excretion-filtration change ratios are 0.009 and 0.005 mM./min./ml./min. at mean sodium excretion rates of about 0.13 and 0.08 mM./min. These change ratios are a little greater than but in fair agreement with predicted values, Fig. 41. A kidney completely denervated by transplantation from one to the other of identical twins, remained indistinguishable from the contralateral innervated organ in its responses to various stimuli (BRICKER et al. 1956).

Epinephrine and norepinephrine, which mimic the effects of activity of adrenergic sympathetic nerves, may or may not cause small changes in glomerular filtration rate (see section C-V-2a). Changes (usually decreases) in sodium

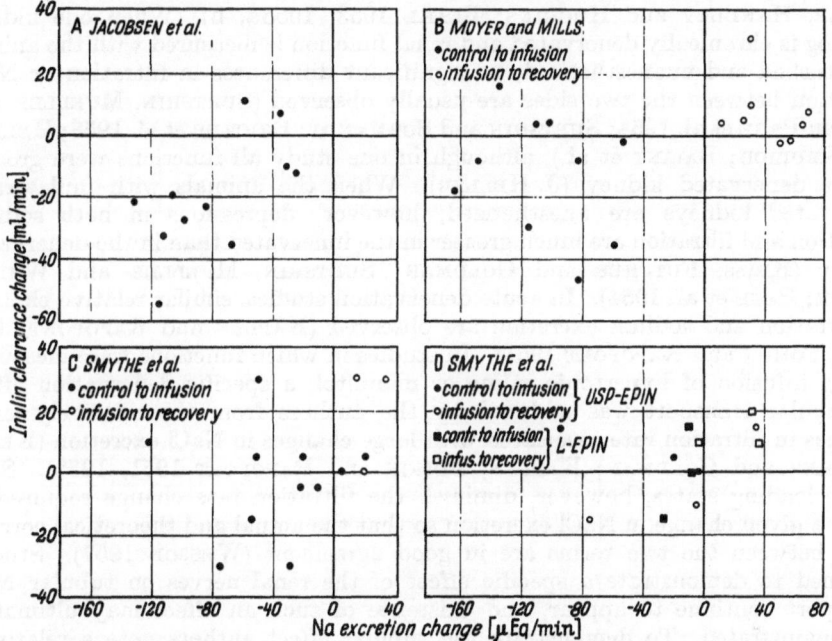

Fig. 48. Correlation between filtration rate and sodium excretion changes during infusion of autonomic drugs in man. *A* Effects of epinephrine (plotted from data of JACOBSON, HAMMARSTEN and HELLER). *B* Effects of hexamethonium (plotted from data of MOYER and MILLS). *C* Effects of *l*-norepinephrine (plotted from data of SMYTHE, NICKEL and BRADLEY). Closed circles represent changes between control periods and infusion of the drug; open circles represent changes between infusion of the drug and recovery periods. *D* Effects of USP epinephrine (circles) and L-epinephrine (squares) (plotted from data of SMYTHE et al.). Closed points represent changes between control periods and infusion of the drugs; open points represent changes between infusion of the drugs and recovery periods. Reproduced by permission of Medicine

excretion are correlated within the limits of error of measurement with changes in filtration rate (Fig. 48A). The mean excretion-filtration change ratio for sodium is about 0.004 mM./min./ml./min. which, at an average excretion rate of 0.10 to 0.12 mM./min., is in good agreement with theoretical values illustrated in Fig. 41 (JACOBSON, HAMMARSTEN and HELLER; SMYTHE, NICKEL and BRADLEY; NICKEL et al.). When filtration rate showed little change with norepinephrine infusion, changes in sodium excretion were small and appeared to be random (PULLMAN and MCCLURE 1952). The variable but significant, acute rise in blood pressure associated with infusion of epinephrine and norepinephrine is probably of critical importance to the response. Autoregulation is not absolute, and a small but significant change in RPF and GFR occurs in relation to a change in mean blood pressure (SELKURT 1951; PITTS and DUGGAN; THOMPSON and PITTS). The final response of filtration rate and of the excretion of substances dependent on filtration following injection of sympathomimetic amines will be the algebraic sum of an intrarenal effect depressing filtration and an extrarenal, pressor effect increasing filtration.

In the dog, injection of the adrenergic drugs, epinephrine and norepinephrine, as well as adrenergic blocking drugs such as hydergine or dibenzyline have regularly failed to evoke a statistically significant dissociation between sodium excretion and filtration rate change although the data are frequently difficult to evaluate because measurements are made while functions are changing rapidly, and may be reported as percentage changes instead of absolute values (KAPLAN, FOMON and RAPOPORT 1952; BERNE et al.; HANDLEY and MOYER 1954a, b; MOYER, HANDLEY and HUGGINS; BLAKE 1953, 1955a, b). When one kidney of a dog is chronically denervated and renal function is measured with the animal undisturbed and unanesthetized, no significant differences in filtration or NaCl excretion between the two sides are usually observed (SURTSHIN, MUELLER and WHITE; PAGE et al. 1954; SURTSHIN and SCHMANDT; BRICKER et al. 1958; HELLER and KRULICH; BALINT et al.), although in one study all functions were greater in the denervated kidney (J. HELLER). When the animals with unilaterally denervated kidneys are anesthetized, however, depressions in both sodium excretion and filtration are much greater in the innervated than in the denervated kidney (KRISS, FUTCHER and GOLDMAN; SURTSHIN, MUELLER and WHITE; BERNE; PAGE et al. 1954). In acute denervation studies, similar relative changes in filtration and sodium excretion are observed (KAPLAN and RAPOPORT; KAPLAN, FOMON and RAPOPORT 1951). In studies in which functions were measured during infusion of hypertonic saline or mannitol, a specific denervation effect on tubular transport was adduced by the authors from the relatively small changes in filtration rate associated with large changes in NaCl excretion (KRISS, FUTCHER and GOLDMAN; KAPLAN, FOMON and RAPOPORT 1951, 1952). Such solute loading states, however, diminish the filtration rate change required to cause a given change in NaCl excretion so that the actual and theoretical correlations between the two terms are in good agreement (WESSON 1957). Studies designed to demonstrate a specific effect of the renal nerves on tubular NaCl transport continue to appear, and existence of such an effect may ultimately be demonstrated. To demonstrate the tubular effect authors note a relatively greater excretion rate of NaCl in the denervated dog kidney when filtration rates in innervated and denervated kidneys are apparently equal or have changed to the same extent (BALINT, FEKETE and SZALAY; BALINT; BALINT et al. 1956; FISCHER, TAKACS and VARGA). Interpretation of their data is, however, subject to much the same difficulties as those besetting earlier work. In spite of as yet inconclusive experimental evidence, the renal nerves should be predicted to influence tubular transport through their control of renal blood flow, where the latter is significant both with respect to supply of nutrients and with respect to intrarenal temperature (GRUPP 1957).

SARTORIUS and BURLINGTON report that the denervated dog kidney subjected to high perfusion pressures excretes a significantly greater fraction of filtered sodium than the innervated organ. This interesting observation is unexplained.

ι) Anterior pituitary and thyroid

Filtration rate is increased in hyperthyroidism and by administration of thyroxine or dissicated thyroid; and in acromegaly and by administration of somatotropin. Decreases in filtration are observed in hypothyroidism and hypopituitarism (see Sections C—V 11 and 12). Departures from normal are particularly marked in the presence of anterior pituitary changes. It seems probable that tubular NaCl reabsorptive capacity in these circumstances has changed in the same direction as filtration rate but not to quite the same degree since salt excretion rate tends to increase or decrease in proportion to changes in total body metabolism. Studies designed to measure reabsorption under conditions of salt excretion equal to those of normal populations have not been made.

ϰ) Posterior pituitary

The effects of extracts of the neurohypophysis on NaCl excretion are unclear. According to the conclusions of most researchers, the pressor-antidiuretic fraction of the neurohypophysis (vasopressin) is both antidiuretic and chloruretic in dog and rat but doubtfully chloruretic in man. The oxytocic fraction (oxytocin) is slightly antidiuretic and usually is not chloruretic. A chloruretic effect from small quantities of vasopressin usually cannot be recognized during antidiuresis. Large doses of vasopressin may be chloruretic during antidiuresis. In nearly all to these studies, however, potentially significant variables such as glomerular filtration rate, plasma NaCl concentrations and control rate of NaCl excretion have either not been measured or not controlled. In studies lasting more than a few hours, NaCl excretion may be responding to changes in body fluid balance.

In man, a small chloruresis following Pituitrin or partially purified vasopressin (Pitressin) has been reported by several researchers (SMITH and MACKAY; ANDERSON and MURLIN; LITTLE et al.; CRUTCHFIELD and WOOD). Conversely, a decrease in chloride excretion during the onset of a water or water-type (ethanol) diuresis has been reported (CRUTCHFIELD and WOOD; WELT and NELSON; RUBINI, KLEEMAN and LAMDIN). Others, however, have observed no clear chloruretic effect of vasopressin (PASQUALINI and ETALA; TARAIL and MATEER; CHALMERS, LEWIS and PAWAN; WHITE, RUBIN and LEITER 1951; MURPHY and STEAD) or oxytocin (Pitocin) (CHALMERS, LEWIS and PAWAN; BRUNNER et al.) on chloride or sodium excretion; or else chloruresis has been reported only with chronic administration (MANCHESTER 1931). Small quantities of vasopressin (intravenous infusion at 50—100 milliunits/hour) had no detectable effect on GFR or RPF although quantities above 500 milliunits resulted in decreases in both or these and which were relatively greater in RPF (MURPHY and STEAD; MAXWELL and BREED). Patients with diabetes insipidus may (ANDERSON and MURLIN) or may not (PASQUALINI and ETALA) exhibit a chloruresis in relation to acute vasopressin administration.

In the dog, small quantities of vasopressin (Pituitrin or Pitressin) given to water-loaded or water-diuresing animals generally results in an increase in NaCl excretion (UNNA and WALLERSKIRCHEN; SHANNON 1942; SARTORIUS and ROBERTS; ROEMMELT, SARTORIUS and PITTS; ANSLOW and WESSON 1955b; BROOKS and PICKFORD), although no increase in sodium excretion was observed during infusion of Pitressin into one renal artery during water diuresis (BARGER, BERLIN and TULENKO). The chloruresis with these quantities is independent of changes in glomerular filtration rate or plasma composition (ANSLOW and WESSON 1955b) and is related to control rate of chloride excretion, being small or absent if the latter is low (UNNA and WALLERSKIRCHEN; ANSLOW and WESSON 1955b). In water-diuresing animals, chloruresis also attends the endogenous liberation of antidiuretic hormone which follows morphine injection. Larger quantities (e.g. 1—2 ml. of Pituitrin) usually evoked chloruresis in antidiuretic animals (FROMHERZ; STEHLE and BOURNE) but filtration rate is frequently elevated by such quantities (SHANNON 1942). In the dog heart-lung-kidney preparation,

Pituitrin in relatively large quantities evoked a chloruresis although renal blood flow decreased (Bayliss and Fee). In more prolonged studies, effects of vaso-pressin (Pitressin tannate) are uninterpretable without filtration rate measurements (Spingarn, Mulinos and Maculla).

Oxytocin (Pitocin but not Pituitrin) is a potent stimulant to glomerular filtration in the hypophysectomized dog (Demunbrun et al.). Injected intra-venously in small doses in the normal, water-diuresing dog it has little influence either on GFR or NaCl excretion (Anslow and Wesson 1955b; Brooks and Pickford), but RPF may be increased (Brooks and Pickford; Ali). Intra-venous and particularly intracarotid injections of oxytocin in the oliguric dog, however, is associated with an increase in NaCl excretion without clear changes in GFR and RPF. Similarly, a chloruretic effect of oxytocin in the diabetes insipidus dog is particularly marked if the animals are also given vasopressin (Brooks and Pickford).

The normal and diabetes insipidus rat responds to small quantities of poste-rior pituitary extract or vasopressin with a chloruresis during water diuresis or to larger doses during antidiuresis (Fromherz; Nelson and Woods; Sil-vette 1940a, b; Corey and Britton; Ham 1943; Croxatto, Rosas and Bar-nafi; Morel 1955a; Brunner, Kuschinsky and Peters 1956a; Croxatto and Zamorano; Barnafi et al.; Alexander). Five milliunits intravenously is significantly chloruretic while one milliunit, although capable of completely abolishing a water diuresis, is not evidently chloruretic (Morel 1955a; Jacobson and Kellogg). On a low salt diet, no significant chloruretic effect may be elicitable (Croxatto and Zamorano). Oxytocin (Pitocin, Postlobin-O), also may be markedly chloruretic (Kuschinsky and Bundschuh; Fraser; Dicker and Heller; Brunner et al.; Brunner, Kuschinsky and Peters 1956b; Jacobson and Kellogg; Croxatto, Rosas and Barnafi; Peters 1959). Inter-pretation of rat data is complicated by reports of increases in GFR following both vasopressin and oxytocin administration (Dicker and Heller) although others have observed no effect of either polypeptide on creatinine clearance (Brunner et al.). Moreover, vasopressin and oxytocin when injected simul-taneously in appropriate proportions are able either to cancel partially or else to enhance the chloruretic affects of each other (Croxatto, Rosas and Barnafi; Brunner, Kuschinsky and Peters 1956b). For example, natriuresis is minimal if vasopressin and oxytocin are given in subequal quantities while vasopressin in quantities $1/2$ to $1/4$ that of oxytocin enhances the chloruretic effect of the latter (Brunner, Kuschinsky and Peters 1956b). Chloruretic effects of oxy-tocin are depressed by adrenalectomy and restored or enhanced by cortisone.

2. Potassium
a) General description

The mechanisms of renal potassium excretion bear little resemblance to those of sodium chloride. Potassium is excreted largely if not entirely by se-cretion in the distal tubule or collecting duct. Thus, unlike the filtration-reab-sorption system of sodium, the factors governing potassium excretion are largely enzymatic or chemical and difficult to describe quantitatively. The relatively simple mechanical process of filtration plays no more than a subordinate role.

Proof that potassium could be secreted came from the observations that, under certain conditions, the potassium-creatinine clearance ratio exceeds 1.0 and may attain values as high as 2.0 or more (Berliner and Kennedy; Mudge, Foulkes and Gilman 1948). If all filtered potassium were excreted without modification by reabsorptive or secretory processes, the clearance ratio should by exactly 1.0. If the clearance ratio exceeds 1.0, accepting identity of exogenous creatinine clearance with filtration rate in the dog, the excess potassium necessarily has been secreted. Tubular secretion has thus been demonstrated in rabbit (KRUHØFFER 1950), chicken (ORLOFF and DAVIDSON), and frog (LIANG; VOGEL, KRÄMER and HEYM) as well as dog. Secretion does not evidently occur in the aglomerular fish (EDWARDS and CONDORELLI; MARSHALL and GRAFFLIN 1928). In man, secretion has been observed in chronic uremia (KEITH, OSTERBERG and KING; KEITH, KING and OSTERBERG; LEAF and CAMARA; ELKINTON, TARAIL and PETERS; WHITE and RUBIN; PLATT), acute renal failure (SIROTA and KROOP), nephrosis following PAH infusion (METCOFF, GORDILLO and AUTONOWICZ) and in normals following intravenous acetazolamide (GORDON et al. 1959). The extent to which excreted potassium arises from secreted or filtered potassium moieties, irrespective of the potassium-inulin clearance ratio required micropuncture examinations of tubular fluid to which was added evidence obtained from stopped-flow experiments (Section D II). Plasma potassium is freely filterable at the glomerulus (BOTT 1955). In the proximal segment of *Necturus*, fluid potassium concentration remains close to or somewhat less than the plasma concentration (BOTT 1953, 1957). By the midpoint of the proximal segment in the rat, potassium concentration of tubular fluid averaged somewhat less (74 percent) than the concentration in the plasma (WIRZ and BOTT). In view of the negative potential within the lumen of the tubule, even a fluid/plasma concentration ratio of 1.0 represents a considerable transport potential for potassium (BERLINER 1960). Since approximately 60 percent of the filtered water has been reabsorbed by this point (Fig. 35), approximately 70 percent of the filtered potassium has also been reabsorbed. The fate of the remaining 30 percent is unknown. Presumably, much if not most of this is reabsorbed in the distal half of the proximal segment as suggested by *Necturus* data, but whether proximal reabsorption is complete or is subject to significant variation is unknown. Within the distal segment of *Necturus*, potassium concentrations are highly variable, but low values indicate that reabsorption can occur in portions of the nephron below the proximal convoluted segment, and potassium U/P ratios less than 1.0 have been recorded from 'early distal' areas during stopped flow studies on potassium-loaded dogs (MURDAUGH and ROBINSON). Clear evidence of entry of potassium into tubular fluid in 'late distal' areas comes from stopped flow experiments. During arrest of urine flow, potassium concentration rises markedly, yielding potassium/creatinine clearance ratios substantially greater than 1.0, in an area which is distal to the area of minimal sodium concentration (PITTS et al. 1958a; SULLIVAN et al.; VANDER et al. 1959); WESSON and LAULER; AUGUST et al.; WILLIAMSON, SKULAN and SHIDEMAN; SULLIVAN, WILDE and MALVIN; JAENIKE and BERLINER). Corroborative evidence of distal secretion is obtained by injection of radioisotopic potassium in tracer quantities during stopped flow. These show marked entry of activity in distal fluid samples and little activity in proximal samples (MOREL and FALBRIARD; REES et al.). Lack of radioactivity in proximal areas indicates either a highly unidirectional process as with distal sodium reabsorption (MOREL and FALBRIARD) or a nearly complete proximal reabsorption. The high specific activity of urine potassium following injection of radioisotope indicates that most of the secretion occurs in cortical areas of the distal segment (BRADLEY, NICKEL and LEIFER; BLACK et al.; MOREL 1955b; MOREL and GUINNEBAULT). The potassium content of medullary blood is insufficient to supply all of the excess potassium excreted at high excretion rates, even assuming no reabsorption of filtered potassium (Berliner 1960). No significant K secretion is observed in the intramedullary portions of the collecting ducts in the hamster (Hilger, Klumper and Ullrich) and in stopped-flow studies maximum potassium entry occurs proximal to the area of maximal urine osmotic concentration (Jaenike and Berliner).

Potassium, as a strong cation, cannot be secreted as such. To preserve electrical neutrality, each secreted potassium ion either must be accompanied by an anion or must be exchanged for another cation which enters the cell as the potassium leaves. The available evidence indicates that the former process does not occur. Secretion (potassium/inulin clearance ratios exceeding 1.0) could be demonstrated in the dog during infusion of potassium ferrocyanide under conditions such that ferrocyanide is virtually the sole urinary anion (Berliner, Kennedy and Hilton 1950b). Since ferrocyanide enters the urine solely by filtration and since other anions were electrically inadequate to cover the excess potassium, it was evident, by exclusion, that the major portion and probably all of the secreted potassium entered the urine by a process of mole-for-mole exchange of potassium ions within the tubular cells for some other cation within the tubular lumen. Sodium is the only cation present in amounts sufficient for the exchange. Variation in the supply of sodium to the potassium secretory area therefore constitutes the only important link between filtration rate and potassium excretion. If precaution is taken, as by use of diuretics, to assure an abundant supply of urinary sodium, then potassium excretion becomes independent of wide variations in filtration rate (Davidson, Levinsky and Berliner). In common with the partially related process of hydrogen ion secretion, potassium secretion is termed a 'cation exchange' process. A hypothetical model of the potassium secretory system is illustrated in Fig. 49.

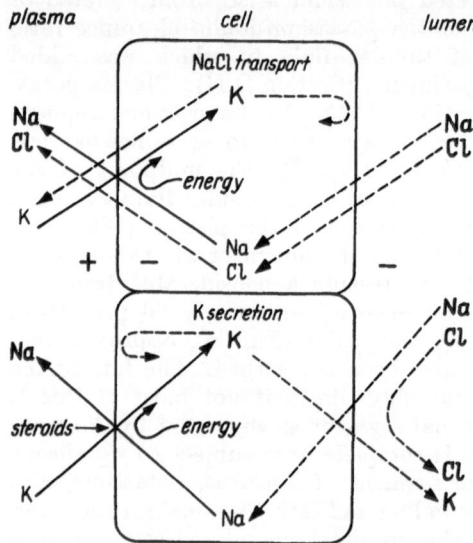

Fig. 49. Hypothetical model of the potassium secretory mechanism compared with an analogous model of the distal NaCl transport mechanism. The NaCl mechanism is based on the frog skin model. Solid lines indicate active transport; dotted lines indicate passive, or diffusional, transport

The major drive to K secretion is plasma K concentration. This drive probably acts through its effect on intracellular K concentration. Since the latter cannot be measured, its role is hypothetical but supported inferentially by analogy with other cellular electrolyte systems. In this view, the immediate drive for potassium secretion is the intracellular K concentration where the latter is determined by plasma K concentration, intracellular H ion concentration (p_H) and plasma Na concentration, the latter relatively unimportant. Hydrogen ions are viewed as significant competitors with K for a limited intracellular cation content. Intracellular K concentration will therefore be greatest, and offer the greatest drive to the K-Na exchange system, when plasma K is high and hydrogen ion concentration is low (high p_H). Although considerable uncertainty exists concerning precise relationship of the factors determining intracellular pH it is probably determined by a combination of plasma pH and plasma carbon dioxide tension. The role of salt-active steroids appears to be largely that of catalysing the K-Na exchange reaction. The plurality of actions in the body of substances such as steroids and drugs and of changes in acid-base balance indicates that each of these factors has the possibility of affecting K excretion in several ways which may either oppose or reinforce one another. For example, steroids tend to facilitate K secretion. On the other hand, by also stimulating NaCl reabsorption, steroids may so depress the supply of Na available for exchange in far distal regions that K excretion actually decreases. It is hardly surprising, therefore, that studies of potassium excretion are confusing and frequently contradictory. When, as is often the case, insufficient information concerning blood and urine chemistry is available, attempts to interpret potassium excretion changes are futile.

b) Variables affecting potassium excretion

α) Plasma potassium concentration

Plasma K closely reflects body K balance. The relationship between concentration and body content is non-linear, the effects of balance changes tending to be exaggerated in the plasma. Plasma K is low in K depletion states, occasionally going as low as 1 mM./L., and is high in conditions of K excess. Nevertheless, roughly 90 percent of most gains and losses of body K come from the intracellular compartment. Following acutely administered loads of 1 mM./kg. of potassium bicarbonate to healthy subjects, plasma K concentration increased about 10 percent and K excretion rate doubled (KEITH). In subjects on K-deficient diets, both plasma K and K excretion rate decrease (EVANS et al. 1954; WOMERSLEY and DARRAGH). Excretion may decrease to 10 mM. per 24 hours or less, with urine/plasma potassium concentration ratios as low as 0.5 (FOURMAN); the decrease in excretion is gradual and values as low as these are not attained until the body potassium deficit exceeds 250 mM. A maximum rate of K-excretion is not clearly recognized because secretion is affected by so many significant variables. Within any given set of experimental conditions, however, an apparent limiting excretion rate as related to plasma K concentration can frequently be discerned. For example, WOLF (1947) in man and ORLOFF and DAVIDSON in the chicken observed an apparently limiting excretion rate of secretion during progressive, acute infusion of KCl or K_2SO_4 solutions, but these values have little significance outside of the experimental circumstances within which they were measured. Complicating analysis of the effects of plasma K on secretion are direct effects of changes in plasma K on body acid-base balance and on sodium chloride excretion. When additional K ions enter the body, hydrogen ion is displaced from the intracellular into the extracellular compartment (ROBERTS, MAGIDA and PITTS; ORLOFF, KENNEDY and BERLINER) and the urine becomes more alkaline. Both immediate and delayed consequences of the increased body K are, therefore, a tendency to extracellular acidosis which becomes apparent if the K is given as KCl but which is suppressed if given as bicarbonate, citrate or acetate. Since acidosis is inhibitory (intracellular hydrogen ion effect?) excretion will be greater at a given plasma K concentration with alkaline salts than with KCl.

The mechanisms of the potassium effect on NaCl excretion is unknown. When K is given either as the chloride or as an alkaline salt the excretion not only of K but also of Na bicarbonate (variably) and chloride is enhanced in dog and man (BALDWIN, KAHANA and CLARKE). The effect is not attributable to increase in plasma concentration of Na or Cl and, in the absence of any evidence that filtration rate is elevated, probably represents a direct depression of tubular reabsorption. The chloruretic effect is sufficiently intense to reverse or abolish the NaCl retention following surgery (Le Quesne and Lewis) or adrenocorticotropin administration (Liddle, Bennett and Forsham), although other variables are also operative in these states. The K-induced chloruresis has two important, indirect but brief consequences with respect to K excretion: the quantity of Na delivered to the K-secretory area is increased; and body NaCl depletion stimulates secretion of aldosterone (Falbriard et al.; Luetscher 1956). Such a depressant action of K on NaCl reabsorption may account in part for the ability of the Na-depleted dog to excrete a large K load (Anderson and Laragh).

The converse effects are observed in K depletion: NaCl is retained (Black and Milne; Blahd and Bassett; Womersley and Darragh; Vermet, Duckert and Muller; Johnson, Leiberman and Mulrow); extracellular alkalosis appears; and aldosterone excretion decreases (Vermet, Duckert and Muller; Muller, Manning and Riondel 1958a).

β) Distal sodium load

When Na excretion rate is relatively low (less than 0.2 mM./min., in man), Na and K excretion frequently vary in the same direction. According to the cation exchange hypothesis, such a correlation in excretion of the two ions is inevitable whenever the rate of delivery of sodium to the exchange system becomes so low, as indicated by Na excretion, that Na supply is rate-limiting to K secretion. Table 16 is a partial list of such situations which illustrates the ubiquity of the phenomenon. This dependence of K upon Na supply at low excretion rates must always be kept in mind when possible influences upon the K-Na exchange system, itself, are being considered.

Of particular interest is the large kaliuretic effect of Na salts of non-reabsorbable anions in conditions favoring Na retention. When Na salts of p-aminohippurate, sulfate or thiosulfate are administered, they are rapidly excreted by filtration, with or without supplementary secretion, and with negligible reabsorption. A large amount of electrolyte, probably as the Na salt, is delivered to distal areas where, presumably, the anions cannot be reabsorbed and only cation exchanges can transpire. In normals, no more than a small increase in K excretion may be observed, and most of the anion will be excreted with Na, indicating that Na was not severely rate-limiting to cation exchanges. In either acute or chronic sodium retaining states such as nephrosis (Metcoff, Nakasone and Rance; Metcoff, Gordillo and Antonowicz), cirrhosis (Wesson, Sunshine and Epstein), sodium depletion (Schwartz, Jensen and Relman) or orthostasis (Epstein et al. 1956), little and sometimes none of the anion will be excreted with Na and nearly all will be excreted with K. In addition, the exchange reaction with hydrogen ion is facilitated so that the urine becomes more acid and more concentrated in ammonium as well as in K. The parallel increase in K and hydrogen excretion is quite opposite to the reciprocal relationship between K and H excretion observed during acute blood acid-base changes (see below) and indicates that the cation-exchange systems of these two ions are not wholly interdependent. The extraordinary magnitude of the kaliuretic and acidification response in Na-retaining states, frequently yielding potassium-inulin clearance ratios above 1.0, is probably related to increase in aldosterone secretion in those states.

Table 16. *Some conditions associated with parallel changes in sodium and potassium excretion*
I or D indicate increase or decrease in excretion

Abdominal compression, man[1] . . . . . D	Fluid or salt loading
Alcohol diuresis, man[2] . . . . D	sodium p-aminohippurate
Altitude, man[3] I	nephrosis[23] I
Aminophylline	premature infants[24] I
dog[4] I	sodium sulfate
man[5] I	cirrhosis[25] I
Anesthesia	sodium-depleted man[26] I
dog[6] . . . . D	urea solution
man[7] . . . . D	dog[37, 38] I
Blood sequestration, man	man[36] I
orthostasis[8, 9] . . . . D	sodium thiosulfate, nephrosis[27] I
supine position, pregnancy[10] . . . . . D	water-loading and diuresis
venous obstruction[11, 12] . . . . D	dog[4, 28] . . . . D
Exercise[13] . . . . D	man[29] . . . . D
Fluid or salt loading	Mercurial diuretics I
calcium chloride to alkalotic infants[14] . I	Pendiomide, man[30] . . . . D
colloidal solutions, dog[15] I	Posterior pituitary principles I
glucose solution, man[16, 17, 36] I	Probenecid, man, heart failure[31] I
sodium chloride	Pyrogens, dog[32] I
dog[18, 19, 20] I	Reserpine, dog[33, 34] I
man[21, 22] I	Serotonin, man[35] . . . . D

[1] BRADLEY et al. 1955; [2] RUBINI, KLEEMAN and LAMDIN; [3] BURRILL, FREEMAN and IVY 1945; [4] MUDGE et al. 1950; [5] BLUMGART et al. 1934; [6] SURTSHIN, MUELLER and WHITE; [7] HABIF et al. 1951; [8] PEARCE and NEWMAN; [9] HOLLAND and STEAD; [10] PRITCHARD, BARNES and BRIGHT; [11] FARBER, BECKER and EICHNA; [12] WILKINS et al. 1953; [13] JUDSON et al. 1955b; [14] GAMBLE, ROSS and TISDALL; [15] RAISZ; [16] EK 1955; [17] BUCHT 1956; [18] MUDGE, FOULKS and GILMAN 1950; [19] WESSON et al.; [20] KOCH, BRAZEAU and GILMAN; [21] DARRAGH et al. 1953; [22] PAPPER et al. 1956; [23] METCOFF, GORDILLO and ANTONOWICZ 1955; [24] MCNAMARA and BARNETT; [25] WESSON, SUNSHINE and EPSTEIN; 26 SCHWARTZ, JENSEN and RELMAN; [27] METCOFF, NAKASONE and RANCE; [28] ANSLOW and WESSON 1955b; [29] URBACH et al. 1953; [30] MOYER and MCCONN 1956; [31] BRONSKY, DUBIN and KUSHNER; [32] BRANDT et al.; [33] DROVANTI, CEI and STRADA 1954; [34] MOYER, HUGHES and HUGGINS; [35] HOLLANDER, MICHELSON and WILKINSON 1957; [36] SELDIN and TARAIL; [37] MUDGE, FOULKS and GILMAN 1949; [38] ANSLOW and WESSON 1955a.

γ) Steroids

The corticosteroids exert a marked influence on cellular electrolyte exchanges involving sodium and potassium. They affect both the intracellular contents of these ions and the rates of transport across epithelium, although the fundamental mechanisms involved in intra-extracellular distribution ratios and in transepithelial transport are probably the same. In saliva, colonic secretion, sweat and urine, the effect of steroids is a decrease in Na content and an increase in K content which is attributable to acceleration of Na-K exchange across the secretory surface of the epithelium. The cumulative effect in the body is Na conservation and K elimination. Although all of the corticosteroids catalyse Na-K exchange, marked variation exists from one to another with respect to the ability to stimulate electrolyte transport as compared with the ability to affect other aspects of body metabolism. Among naturally-occurring steroids, only aldosterone has a relatively large electrolyte-stimulating capacity (mineralocorticoid). Desoxycorticosterone is present in amounts too small to be biologically significant (FARRELL, RAUSCHKOLB and ROYCE) and is probably a metabolic intermediate in steroid synthesis. Numerous synthetic steroids also possess the property of stimulating electrolyte transport, among the more potent being desoxycorticosterone and 9-alphafluorohydrocortisone. The mineralocorticoids are generally not specifically necessary for satisfactory maintenance of the adrenoprival man or animal, since the residual electrolyte-catalysing properties of those steroids with relatively greater effect on body metabolism (glucocorticoids) is sufficient for electrolyte balance under all except extreme conditions of sodium deprivation.

When salt-active steroids are administered to adrenoprival animals or men by injection or continuous infusion, a significant delay occurs before an increase in potassium and decrease in sodium excretion are observed. This delay is about 30 minutes following intravenous injection of desoxycorticosterone, aldosterone or hydrocortisone in dog and man (GANONG and MULROW; BARGER, BERLIN and TULENKO; SARTORIUS and ROBERTS; DINGMAN et al.; BRICKER et al. 1956; Ross et al.) and a marked change is usually not evident until two hours following injection. The delay cannot be appreciably shortened by increasing the quantity. The increase in K excretion may occur slightly earlier (SARTORIUS and ROBERTS) or essentially simultaneous with the decrease in Na excretion (BARGER, BERLIN and TULENKO). In normal dogs, however, no decrease in sodium excretion was observed during several hours of aldosterone infusion although potassium excretion increased (BARGER, BERLIN and TULENKO).

When Na excretion is initially low, or else decreases markedly following steroid administration, an acute increase in K excretion may fail to occur (WOMERSLEY, THORUP and WELT 1953; ROBERTS and RANDALL; GRIBOFF et al.; MULLER, MACH and NAEGELI; HUFFMAN et al. 1956; AUGUST, NELSON and THORN 1958a) or K excretion may actually decrease (ROBERTS and PITTS 1952). This is presumably attributable to depression of the supply of Na available for K-Na exchange. When, however, supply of Na to the distal segment is increased following activation of the Na excretory system by excess Na retention, prior saline loading (AUGUST and NELSON 1959a) or by direct stimulation of glomerular filtration (DINGMAN et al.), K excretion invariably increases. The increase in excretion is not sustained unless intake is also increased to equal the increase in excretion, since negative K balance results in progressive depletion of body K and decrease in plasma K concentration. As the latter declines, so also does excretion rate until output comes into balance with intake, but at a new plasma K concentration (LUFT and SJOGREN 1951). A factor complicating the interpretation of the acute effects of some steroids on K excretion is the increase in plasma K concentration following their injection. Acute increases in plasma K concentration are reported in normal subjects following aldosterone (BECK et al. 1955) or hydrocortisone (KNIGHT et al.) and decreases in hypoadrenal patients during aldosterone infusion (Ross et al.). These concentration changes probably result from steroid-induced shifts of body water and electrolyte.

Gamma lactones of certain steroids, e.g. 3-(3-oxo, 17 beta-hydroxy-4 androstenly-alpha-yl) propionic acid-gamma lactone, appear to block the catalytic effect of mineralocorticoids on K-Na exchanges as well as that on NaCl reabsorption. Na excretion increased moderately and potassium excretion decreased slightly following administration of these steroid lactones in edematous subjects or in a hypoadrenal subject under treatment with desoxycorticosterone, while no changes were observed in normal subjects on a high salt diet (aldosterone secretion suppressed) or in the hypoadrenal subject when untreated (LIDDLE). The small decrease in K excretion is highly significant since the normal response to a purely natriuretic agent in edematous patients is an increase in K-excretion.

δ) Acidosis and alkalosis

A profound inverse correlation exists between excretion of potassium and excretion of hydrogen ions (pH and titratable acidity). When any of several methods are employed to lower the acidity of the urine, potassium excretion increases. Thus, potassium excretion increases during the alkaluria which results from sodium bicarbonate ingestion or infusion (BURNETT, BURROWS and COMMONS), hyperventilation (BARKER et al. 1957; McCANCE and WIDDOWSON 1936; TAYMOR, MINOR and FRIEDBERG) or administration of the carbonic anhydrase inhibitor, acetazolamide (BERLINER, KENNEDY and ORLOFF 1951; ROBERTS, MAGIDA and PITTS). Conversely, respiratory acidosis caused by carbon dioxide inhalation is associated with a decrease in potassium excretion provided the urine is not acid prior to the CO_2 breathing (BARKER et al. 1957; TAYMOR, MINOR and FRIEDBERG) and injection of acetic acid into the renal portal circulation of the chicken is followed by a rapid, marked decrease in K excretion (ORLOFF and DAVIDSON). The effects on potassium excretion of changes in acid-base balance are, to a considerable extent, the reciprocal of the effects on acid or base excretion of changes in potassium balance. Acute potassium administration causes an acid urine to become alkaline (BRIGGS; WINKLER and SMITH; WOLF 1947). The reciprocal relationships between hydrogen and potassium ions in the urine are probably homologous with those observed in the blood as the result of shifts between the intra- and the extracellular spaces and are consistent with the hypothesis that K, H and Na compete for shares of a relatively fixed intracellular cation space (GARDNER, MacLACHLAN and BERMAN; HUTH, SQUIRES and ELKINTON). BERLINER, KENNEDY and ORLOFF (1951, 1954) have proposed that hydrogen ion is secreted by cation exchange by the same cells which secrete potassium. Provided an ample supply of intratubular sodium substrate is available, both H and K ions will be secreted in accord with the intracellular potential of each. The effect of acidosis is to increase the intracellular supply or concentration of H, the latter displacing potassium from the cell, or more specifically, from elements of the transport system, and inhibiting its secretion. Alkalosis and carbonic anhydrase inhibitors decrease the supply of intracellular H, permitting increased entry of K into the cell or into the transport system. This concept appears to describe adequately the cortical distal ion exchange system but is clearly not applicable to the medullary acid-secretory area in rodents.

The quantitative changes in potassium excretion in various forms of acidosis and alkalosis are not clearly understood. Metabolic alkalosis caused by sodium bicarbonate administration causes a relatively small increase in potassium excretion compared with that caused by acetazolamide (see below) or respiratory alkalosis (ROBERTS, MAGIDA and PITTS; TAYMOR, MINOR and FRIEDBERG). The massive kaliuresis associated with bicarbonate administration to sodium-retaining subjects (JEANNERET, ESSELLIER and HOLTMEIER) is probably the result for the most part of increased distal delivery of exchangeable sodium. Prolonged administration of sodium bicarbonate to non-sodium-retaining subjects is associated with no more than a small degree of K depletion (SANDERSON 1954), but suppression of aldosterone secretion in these circumstances probably facilitates K conservation.

ε) Acetazolamide

Acetazolamide is the most intensively studied of substances with the property of inhibiting carbonic anhydrase (Section D V 4 b γ). When administered acutely both to normal and to sodium-retaining animals and men, acetazolamide causes an acute increase in potassium and bicarbonate excretion and in urine p_H (BERLINER, KENNEDY and ORLOFF 1951; BERLINER and ORLOFF; COUNIHAN, EVANS and MILNE; MAREN et al.; METCOFF, GORDILLO and ANTONOWICZ; MAREN; PERLMUTT and OLEWINE; GORDON et al. 1959). According to the concepts of

BERLINER and coworkers (above), acetazolamide interferes with generation of hydrogen ions for secretion by the renal tubules by blocking the catalytic action of carbonic anhydrase on the formation of bicarbonate from carbon dioxide, water and hydroxyl ions.

The pattern of electrolyte excretion in the alligator appears to be nearly the reverse of that obtaining in mammals. Excretion is largely as ammonium, potassium and sodium bicarbonates (COULSON and HERNANDEZ 1955). It is of interest, therefore, that acetazolamide in the alligator is associated with a decrease in bicarbonate excretion with little change or perhaps a slight increase in potassium excretion (COULSON and HERNANDEZ 1957).

The stimulating effect of acetazolamide on K secretion is observed only in that distal tubular area which is usually associated with K secretion (PITTS et al. 1958a) and is additive to the effect of administration of potassium salts (FALBRIARD et al.; ORLOFF and DAVIDSON). During prolonged administration of acetazolamide, K excretion steadily decreases (MAREN) probably because of decreasing cell K and increasing cell H concentrations caused by hypokalemia and acidosis.

ζ) Lithium

Infusion of lithium salt in the dog causes urine acidity to decrease and potassium excretion to increase (FOULKS, MUDGE and GILMAN; ORLOFF and KENNEDY 1952). The mechanism is unknown.

η) Chlorothiazide

Chlorothiazide administration is associated with an increase in K excretion both in normal and Na-deficient man and animals (MOYER, FORD and SPURR; LARAGH, HEINEMANN and DEMARTINI; LARAGH; SHERLOCK et al.; BERGSTRÖM, BUCHT and EK). In normal subjects, the kaliuresis is probably due largely to the carbonic anhydrase activity of this substance, while in sodium-retaining subjects the effect probably is largely attributable to its delivery of an increased supply of sodium salts to the distal tubule.

ϑ) Plasma sodium concentration

No significant difference in K excretion was observed as between 0.9 percent and 5 percent saline infusion in healthy subjects (PAPPER et al.) but the difference in plasma sodium concentration following the two solutions averaged no more than about 6 mM./L. In the dog, massive, hypertonic saline infusion is reported to increase K excretion significantly above that observed with isotonic saline (BALDWIN, KAHANA and CLARKE; MUDGE, FOULKS and GILMAN 1950). The mechanism of the sodium concentration effect is unknown, but it may represent the converse of the apparent effect of potassium concentration on NaCl reabsorption.

ι) Magnesium

The effects of magnesium on K excretion are small and variable. In the dog, $MgCl_2$ (and $CaCl_2$) infusion may be associated with an increase in K excretion to a potassium/creatinine clearance ratio of 1.3 (SAMIY, BROWN and GLOBUS). In normal man, infusion of magnesium salts is associated acutely with little change or a decrease in K excretion in spite of the concomitant chloruresis (HELLER, HAMMARSTEN and STUTZMAN; CHESLEY and TEPPER). In nephritic patients, no change in excretion was observed (HAMMARSTEN, ALLGOOD and SMITH). The magnesium infusions caused no detectable change in plasma potassium concentration.

ϰ) Mercury

Mercurial diuretics offer an apparent paradox in both increasing and decreasing potassium excretion. In sodium-retaining patients (congestive heart failure, etc.), and also in normals if their potassium excretion rate is low, mercurial diuretics are associated with a small to moderate increase in potassium excretion (KEITH and WHELAN; BLUMGART et al. 1934; GRIGGS and JOHNS; STOCK, MUDGE and NURNBERG; HILTON 1952; LESSER et al.). Alternatively, mercurial diuretics depress potassium excretion when the latter is large as the result of potassium, acetazolamide or hypertonic saline administration (MUDGE, FOULKS and GILMAN 1950; MUDGE et al.; BERLINER, KENNEDY and ORLOFF 1951; ORLOFF and DAVIDSON). Mercurial compounds which depress K secretion are those which also are chloruretic, and nonchloruretic mercurials do not depress K secretion (McBRIDE, WEINER and MUDGE). The antikaliuresis, like the chloruresis, can be inhibited by dimercaptopropanol (BAL) (MUDGE et al.; ORLOFF and DAVIDSON). Unlike mercurial chloruresis, the antikaliuretic effect is observed in alkaline urine and with very low doses of mercury, suggesting that formation of mercuric ions is not necessary for antikaliuresis (McBRIDE, WEINER and MUDGE). Although K excretion is very sensitive to small quantities of mercurials when excretion is high, excretion is insensitive to mercury at lower although still significant K excretion rates during isotonic saline loading in the dog (MUDGE, FOULKS and GILMAN 1950). Hydrogen excretion is unaffected by mercury.

λ) Digitalis glycosides

Effects of members of the digitalis family on K excretion are not clear. They appear to resemble mercury, at least superficially. In sodium-retaining patients (congestive heart failure or nephrosis), digoxin is associated with an increase in K as well as Na and Cl excretion. On the other hand, injection of digoxin into one renal artery of the dog was associated with a small increase in NaCl but no change in K excretion (HYMAN, JACQUES and HYMAN). Since the normal response to natriuresis is an increase in K excretion, the effect can be interpreted as inhibitory. Injection of strophanthidin into the renal portal circulation of the chicken caused K excretion to decrease during K-loading but caused little change at low K excretion rates (BURG and ORLOFF). Strophanthidin at 0.03 mM. concentration caused potassium to leave and sodium to enter slices of rabbit kidney cortex *in vitro* (BURG and ORLOFF).

μ) Posterior pituitary

Whether posterior pituitary principles, vasopressin and oxytocin, exert specific influences on K excretion is unknown. K excretion may be unchanged, or may increase or decrease in relation to administration of these substances but the changes are almost always parallel to those of NaCl excretion and therefore attributable to some extent to the general sodium supply effect (STEHLE 1926; SMITH and MacKAY; WHITE, RUBIN and LEITER; MURPHY and STEAD; ANSLOW and WESSON 1955b; CROXATTO, ROSAS and BARNAFI; BRUNNER, KUSCHINSKY and PETERS 1956a; BRUNNER et al.; ALEXANDER). Oxytocin is reported to be associated with a relatively greater increase in potassium excretion per unit change in sodium in the rat than is vasopressin (BARNAFI et al.). Dissociation between changes in Na and K excretion have been seldom reported and are contradictory; both a decrease in K in a patient with diabetes insipidus (ANDERSON and MURLIN) and an increase in K in Na-loaded, normal subjects (MURPHY and STEAD) have been reported following Pitressin administration.

ν) Epinephrine and norepinephrine

These sympathomimetic amines significantly inhibit K secretion in both man and dog. This is demonstrated by either no change or a decrease in excretion when sodium excretion increases or a decrease in excretion when sodium excretion is unchanged (DUNCAN et al.; EVERSOLE, GIERE and ROCK; GIERE; BLAKE 1955b; BLAKE and DAVIDSON; PULLMAN and McCLURE 1952; NICKEL et al.). In a few studies, excretion changes of the two cations, Na and K, are parallel, probably reflecting the Na-dependence effect on K (SMYTHE, NICKEL and BRADLEY; ERANKO et al.; BLAKE 1955b; O'CONNOR 1958b). No qualitative difference is evident between epinephrine and norepinephrine, and the effect can be blocked with the sympatholytic drug, hydergine (BLAKE and DAVIDSON). The antikaliuretic effect of these amines has been attributed to intrarenal vasoconstriction (NICKEL et al.).

ξ) Urea

The effect of urea on K excretion is unclear. Marked kaliuresis has been reported at high plasma urea concentrations in the dog (MUDGE, FOULKS and GILMAN 1948; ANSLOW and WESSON 1955a). At urea concentrations above 80 mM./L., definitive secretion of K (potassium-creatinine clearance ratio above 1.0) was observed regularly in the absence of alkalosis or hypernatremia (ANLOW and WESSON 1955a). At less elevated plasma urea concentrations in man, the kaliuretic effect of urea did not differ from that of mannitol (SELDIN and TARAIL).

c) Factors associated with decreased potassium excretion

The effects of hypokalemia, antinatriuresis, steroid withdrawal, steroid lactones, acidosis, mercury, magnesium, and epinephrine as factors depressing potassium excretion have been described above. Other circumstances in which a specific decrease in K excretion has been described is following administration of triazine derivatives in the rat (WILLIAMSON, SHIDEMAN, and LeSHER), administration of organic bases such as mecamylamine and N'-nicotinamide to the dog (KANDEL and DOMER), injection of pyrogen (typhoid) in man (LATHEM 1956); ureteral occlusion for 1—2 hours in the dog (HASHIMOTO); beer drinking in man (EK and JOSEPHSON 1953b); and vasopressin-sustained water loading in man (WRONG 1956).

Cooling to 20° C in the dog abolishes all evidence of active transport, and urine K concentration becomes the same as that of plasma (SEGAR, RILEY and BARILA).

d) Factors not associated with change in potassium excretion

The potassium transport system is not affected by loading with members of the group of secreted aromatic acids (p-aminohippurate, diodrast, carinamide), cinchoninic acid, tetrathionate, sulfanilamide, ascorbate, amino acids or aminophylline (MUDGE et al.; STAMLER). It is unaffected by the metabolic inhibitors phlorhizin, azide, dinitrophenol and barbiturates (CHEN and NEUMANN 1955b; MUDGE et al.). Excretion does not change following renal denervation (SURTSHIN, MUELLER and WHITE; J. HELLER) or during mild exercise (KATTUS et al.).

e) Posttraumatic kaliuresis

Following injury or surgery, K excretion increases significantly for one or two days (CASEY, BICKEL and ZIMMERMANN). Sodium is retained at the same time, but the period of sodium retention usually is longer than the period of K loss and the time of maximum Na retention may occur one or two days later than the time of maximal K excretion (FEYEL and VARANGOT; LE QUESNE and LEWIS). The kaliuresis might reasonably be attributable to increased adrenal secretion were it not for the circumstance that an indistinguishable posttraumatic kaliuresis occurs in steroid-sustained, adrenoprival man and in the saline-sustained adrenoprival rat (MASON; ROBSON et al. 1955; SHARE and STADLER). In the rat, excreted K comes from healthy as well as injured tissues (SHARE and STADLER). The mechanism is unknown.

f) Diurnal variation

Like sodium, potassium exhibits a characteristic diurnal excretory rhythm. A minimum excretion rate occurs during the early hours of the morning and about midway through the normal sleeping period (MANCHESTER 1931, 1933; LEVY, POWER and KEPLER; NORN; BARBOUR et al.; AZERAD et al.) and a maximum a few hours after awakening. The minimum usually coincides approximately with the minimum rate of sodium excretion, but the maximum may occur somewhat earlier (STANBURY and THOMSON 1951; LEWIS and LOBBAN 1957b; WESSON and LAULER unpubl.). The maximum is generally 3 to 5 times the minimum excretion rate. The diurnal cycle of K excretion is independent of, although affected by, eating, sleeping and activity (NORN; ROSENBAUM et al.; MILLS and STANBURY; STANBURY and THOMSON 1951). Potassium adheres more rigidly than sodium to a 24 hour cycle after adoption by experimental subjects of a 22 or 27 hour 'day' (LEWIS and LOBBAN 1956, 1957a, b). The cycle becomes reversed, however, in individuals (night watchman) with a reversed living pattern (NORN). Also unlike sodium, the potassium cycle is closely correlated with adrenocortical activity. Excretion is partially correlated with 17-hydroxy-corticoid excretion and blood concentrations (DOE, FLINK and GOODSELL; DOE, VENNES and FLINK), is frequently absent in hypoadrenal patients (LEVY, POWER and KEPLER), and is suppressed or reversed in normal subjects by cortisone administration (ROSENBAUM et al.). When a cycle is present in untreated hypoadrenal patients, it appears to be more closely correlated with that of sodium (DOE, VENNES and FLINK). The cycle is not correlated with aldosterone secretion (Section E II 3).

g) Control of body potassium balance

No clear evidence is available indicating existence of an extrarenal feed-back system, as with sodium, which controls body potassium balance or plasma potassium concentration. Although aldosterone excretion increases with potassium excess and decreases with potassium deficit, the changes in aldosterone excretion are relatively small and are attributable in part to alterations in body sodium chloride balance (Section E II 3). The effects of changes in plasma Na/K ratios on adrenocortical secretion (ROSENFELD et al.; DENTON, GODING and WRIGHT 1959a) are much less significant than the direct effects on the renal tubules of vastly smaller changes in plasma K concentration. No method is available to test for the existence of an intrarenal or intracellular feed-back system. Available information concerning the control mechanism is consistent, in general, with a simple steady-state system (Section E I).

h) Potassium depletion

Potassium depletion occurs frequently in various pathological states in man and can be produced experimentally both in man and animals (Table 17). Characteristically, plasma K is low, much Na and some Cl is retained, K content of cells is decreased and their contents of Na and H ions is increased. Transfer of H from extracellular fluid into cells results in an intracellular acidosis and an increase in bicarbonate concentration and pH of plasma. These changes are in agreement with the general concept of intra-extracellular cation equilibria. Theoretically, the intracellular acidosis should cause the urine to become more acid and excretion of acid to increase. Acutely, this is seen, and excessive acid excretion probably contributes to accumulation of plasma bicarbonate (Klee-man et al. 1955; Mudge). In chronic depletion, however, the urine is seldom strongly acid and frequently is alkaline. Histological changes appear in the cells of all segments of the nephron (Relman and Schwartz 1956; Fourman, McCance and Parker; Milne, Muehrcke and Heard; Welt, Hollander and Blythe). In man and dog these changes are inconspicuous or are more prominent in the proximal segment. In rodents, changes are particularly prominent in the collecting ducts and are correlated with increased activity of numerous enzyme systems in the same region (Wachstein and Meisel). It seems probable that K depletion impairs numerous transport systems and particularly acid-secretory mechanisms of the proximal and distal convoluted segments. Such a deficiency impairment is supported by the observation that in chronic K depletion the urine may become 'paradoxically' acid during the phase of K repletion (Eales and Linder; Muehrcke and Milne). Deficiency in excretion of acid is compensated by increased excretion of ammonium ion (Milne, Muehrcke and Heard), the response of the latter to intracellular acidosis being apparently less affected by the K deficiency. Theoretically, if the metabolic disturbances resulting from K depletion should extend to the ammonia-synthesizing system, acid-base compensation would fail and the indivi-

Table 17. *Potassium deficiency states*

A. Potassium deficiency with metabolic alkalosis: 'pure' K deficiency.
   1. Deficient intake (low K diet)[1-7].
   2. Excessive gastrointestinal losses (vomiting, drainage, diarrhea)[8-11].
   3. Excessive renal excretion.
      a) Excess of salt-active steroids.
         1. Exogenous excess (usually experimental: dog, rat, man)[12-16].
         2. Endogenous excess.
            Cushing's disease[17,18].
            Primary aldosteronism[19-28].
      b) Kaliuretic drugs (e.g. chlorothiazide)[29].
      c) Primary renal hypersecretion (?)[30].
B. Potassium deficiency with metabolic acidosis[11,31-35]: a group of etiologically distinct and poorly understood entities which include many patients with 'renal tubular acidosis'. The following subdivisions are conjectural and no method is available to prove them or to distinguish between them.
   1. Primary potassium deficiency leading to pathological impairment of acid excretion.
   2. Metabolic disturbance of acid excretion 'obligating' excessive potassium excretion (cf. carbonic anhydrase inhibitors).

[1] Black and Milne; [2] Blahd and Bassett; [3] Evans et al. 1954; [4] Clarke et al.; [5] Womersley and Darragh; [6] Squires and Huth; [7] Huth, Squires and Elkinton; [8] Schwartz and Relman 1953; [9] Vermet, Duckert and Muller; [10] Relman and Schwartz 1956; [11] Relman and Schwartz 1958 (review); [12] Relman and Schwartz 1951; [13] Davis and Howell 1953b; [14] Howell and Davis; [15] Roberts and Randall; [16] Seldin, Welt and Cort; [17] McQuarrie, Johnson and Ziegler; [18] Teabeaut, Engel and Taylor; [19] Mader and Iseri; [20] Foye and Feichtmeir; [21] Conn and Louis; [22] Dustan, Corcoran and Page; [23] Eales and Linder; [24] Milne, Muehrcke and Aird; [25] Hewlett et al.; [26] Goldsmith et al.; [27] Bartter and Biglieri; [28] Hilton et al. 1959; [29] Laragh, Heinemann and Demartini; [30] Earle et al. 1951c; [31] Milne, Stanbury and Thomson; [32] Siebenmann; [33] Fitzgerald and Fourman; [34] Mahler and Stanbury; [35] Owen and Verner.

dual would develop a secondary metabolic acidosis indistinguishable from a "renal tubular acidosis". In addition, ability to concentrate the urine is lost (RUBINI) so that patients with chronic K deficiency are characteristically polyuric, and magnesium conservation is impaired (MADER and ISERI; RELMAN and SCHWARTZ 1956; MILNE, MUEHRCKE and AIRD; MILLER, FALOON and LLOYD). Interpretation of mechanisms is complicated by the frequent occurrence of pyelonephritis, apparently the result of increased vulnerability to infection of the K-deficient kidney (MILNE, MUEHRCKE and AIRD; STANBURY 1958a; RELMAN and SCHWARTZ 1956; KLEEMAN and MAXWELL 1959).

3. Lithium and rubidium

Little is known about the mechanisms of excretion of these alkali metals.

Lithium is excreted more rapidly than sodium, the Li-creatinine clearance ratio in the dog being about 0.3 and independent of plasma concentrations up to 22 mM./L. (FOULKS, MUDGE and GILMAN). The toxicity of Li in man is such that excretion cannot be studied at concentrations above 3 to 4 mM./L. (TRAUTNER et al.). Mutual interference in reabsorption between Na and Li is suggested by the increase in Na excretion which accompanies Li ingestion or infusion (FOULKS, MUDGE and GILMAN; TRAUTNER et al.) and the increase in Li excretion which accompanies the natriuresis resulting from sodium thiosulfate infusion. In the latter circumstance, the Li-creatinine clearance ratio may rise to 0.57 without significant change in filtration rate (FOULKS, MUDGE and GILMAN). Li depresses tubular secretion of acid and potassium (ORLOFF and KENNEDY; FOULKS, MUDGE and GILMAN) but neither K loading nor mercurial diuretics affect Li excretion (FOULKS, MUDGE and GILMAN).

The distribution, biological properties and excretion of *rubidium* are very similar to those of potassium. Rb can effectively relieve a metabolic alkalosis resulting from K depletion (RELMAN, ROY and SCHWARTZ). Rb is secreted together with K when perfused through the portal circulation of the frog (LIANG). In man, radioactive tracer Rb is excreted a little over half as rapidly as that of K although the relative distribution of the two ions in cells is approximately equal (THREEFOOT, BURCH and RAY; TYOR and ELDRIDGE). In the dog, Rb is excreted about 90 percent as rapidly as K, and tubular secretion of Rb is demonstrable under the same conditions as is K (KUNIN et al.). Also, as with K, high rates of Rb excretion are depressed by mercury.

4. Bicarbonate, acid and ammonia

a) General description

Glomerular filtrate is a weakly alkaline solution of salts which has very nearly the composition of plasma water (C II 1). The sodium salts of chloride and bicarbonate at concentrations in man of about 110 and 30 mM./L., respectively, comprise over 90 percent of the saline content. It is evident that the first stage in renal regulation of acid and base excretion lies with the reabsorption of bicarbonate. If reabsorption of bicarbonate is incomplete, with the result that bicarbonate appears in the urine, the urine will be neutral or alkaline causing the body fluids from which the urine was formed to become more acid. The body has no known defense against alkalosis other than incomplete reabsorption of filtered bicarbonate. Alternatively, complete tubular reabsorption of filtered bicarbonate leaves the urine more acid than the body fluids (plasma water) from which it was formed and the body fluids become more alkaline.

If the quantity of acid which must be excreted in order to maintain the body fluids in a steady state is small, simple reabsorption of filtered bicarbonate is sufficient to maintain balance. However, further acidification of the urine can be achieved by two supplementary devices: secretion of hydrogen ions and secretion of ammonia. By means of these two processes, 1,000 or more mM. of acid can be excreted daily, an amount which is roughly 20 times the average daily requirement for excretion. The mechanism of neither process, hydrogen secretion or ammonia secretion, has been clearly established. Both bicarbonate reabsorption and acid secretion can, theoretically, be accomplished by a single mechanism and concepts of acid and base excretion have usually been erected on the premise that only one general type of mechanism is operative: when the filtered load of bicarbonate is large or when the reabsorptive rate is low, the urine is alkaline; when filtered load of bicarbonate is small or when reabsorption is rapid, the urine is acid.

Acidification occurs in both proximal and distal segments of the nephron and, in rodents, in the collecting ducts also. In *Necturus*, fractional rate of reabsorption of bicarbonate is about equal to that of water, chloride and other components of the glomerular filtrate so that the p_H of the intratubular fluid remains about equal to that of plasma (MONTGOMERY and PIERCE; GIEBISCH 1956). In the elasmobranch (KEMPTON 1943), rat (ELLINGER 1940a, b; GOTTSCHALK, LASSITER and MYLLE; WINDHAGER and GIEBISCH 1960), dog (NICHOLSON 1957a), human fetal metanephros (CAMERON and CHAMBERS) and occasionally in the frog (ELLINGER 1940a, b) proximal tubular fluid becomes significantly more acid than plasma or extratubular fluid indicating (with the assumption of approximate uniformity of carbon dioxide tension) that a high concentration gradient of bicarbonate is established and maintained across the epithelium. No further change in p_H occurs in the loop of HENLE (LASSITER, GOTTSCHALK and MYLLE). In all species, including *Necturus*, a further decrease in p_H occurs in the distal segment so that acidification of the urine, like excretion of chloride and of potassium, represents the sum of two or more tubular processes. In *Necturus* the distal acidifying process is located near the middle of the distal convoluted tubule and occupies about $1/4$ of the total length (MONTGOMERY and PIERCE) but its exact location in mammals is not clear. In rodents (hamster, rat) a decrease in p_H averaging 1.0 unit occurs in the medullary collecting ducts (ULLRICH et al.; WINDHAGER and GIEBISCH 1960). In view of the buffering capacity of urine, this p_H change signifies a rather substantial acid secretion. The relative acidities of the fluids in the proximal and distal segments are maintained when the urine becomes weakly acid or alkaline, and the blood-to-tubular fluid p_H gradient disappears first in the proximal segment (NICHOLSON 1957a).

Two mechanisms have been proposed which account for variable rates of bicarbonate reabsorption and acid secretion. They may be termed the hydrogen secretion and the bicarbonate reabsorption hypotheses. They are illustrated for comparison in Fig. 50. Of these two hypotheses, the hydrogen secretion hypothesis is the simpler, requires the introduction of fewer assumptions and is in better agreement with information concerning acid or alkali secretion by other tissues (BERLINER 1957).

According to the theory of acid secretion (SMITH 1937) hydrogen ion derived from intracellular carbonic acid is exchanged for intraluminal sodium. The hydrogen ion reacts with bicarbonate to form carbonic acid, the latter decomposing to yield water and carbon dioxide. Carbon dioxide, a substance soluble in both water and lipids, returns rapidly to the blood stream by diffusion. According to the theory of bicarbonate reabsorption (PITTS 1945; BRODSKY et al. 1958), both sodium and bicarbonate are reabsorbed by parallel, active processes. Carbonic acid, whose supply is sustained by continuous diffusion of carbon dioxide from blood to tubular lumen, reacts with other buffer salts in the tubular lumen to yield buffer acids plus reabsorbable bicarbonate. The importance of sodium ion was established by PITTS and his coworkers (PITTS and ALEXANDER 1945; PITTS et al. 1948; SCHIESS et al.) who showed in dog and man during metabolic acidosis that hydrogen (titratable acidity) could be excreted in amounts greatly exceeding that attainable if the acid phase of all filtered buffers were excreted quantitatively while the alkaline (salt) phase were reabsorbed quantitatively. Both hypotheses must account for the depression of acid excretion and bicarbonate reabsorption following administration of carbonic anhydrase inhibitors (see below). In the hydrogen secretion hypothesis, carbonic anhydrase can assure continuous removal of intracellular alkali by catalysing the relatively slow reaction between carbon dioxide and water to yield carbonic acid. Inhibition of carbonic anhydrase may depress the rate of formation of carbonic acid to the point where the supply of the latter becomes rate-limiting to the overall process of hydrogen secretion. In the bicarbonate reabsorption hypothesis, carbonic anhydrase must contribute in some way to the reabsorption of bicarbonate and may also catalyse hydration of carbon dioxide. The hypothesis that acid excretion results from the preferential reabsorption of carbonate or hydroxyl ions (MENAKER), while quantitatively feasible, is unlikely from kinetic considerations because of the minute concentrations of both ions in neutral and acid solution.

Without prejudice to the theoretical validity of the bicarbonate reabsorption hypothesis, the sodium-hydrogen exchange theory (Fig. 50 A) will be assumed to describe best the renal mechanisms involved. Although both the proximal and the distal processes of acid secretion are probably similar in being

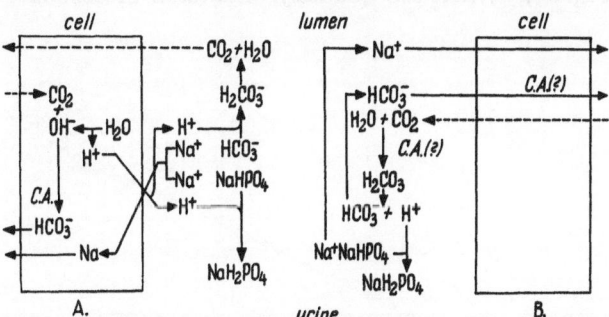

Fig. 50. Hypothetical mechanisms for reabsorption of bicarbonate and secretion of acid. A. Primary secretion of acid. B. Primary reabsorption of bicarbonate. With both systems, a neutral or alkaline tubular fluid containing sodium bicarbonate and disodium phosphate is converted into an acid urine containing monosodium phosphate. C.A. is carbonic anhydrase. Broken lines indicate diffusion

hydrogen secretory systems, partially dependent on carbonic anhydrase and sensitive to changes in carbon dioxide tension and potassium concentration, it is equally probable that they differ in important respects. The feebleness of the proximal compared with the distal system in *Necturus* has been noted. Indeed, it remains to be demonstrated that a hydrogen secretory system exists in the proximal segment of this species. Little quantitative information is available concerning the two processes separately in other species. Analogy with the division of function between proximal and distal segments in other areas would suggest that such flexibility in tubular response to body p_H changes as may exist is more likely to lie with the distal system.

Ammonia, like hydrogen ions, is a secretory product of the tubular epithelium and is formed from substances containing amino groups, but not from urea. Whether ammonia is formed as such and diffuses from the cells into the tubular lumen, or whether it is secreted as ammonium ion by a cation exchange system is uncertain, with some evidence in favor of both views. The ammonia secreting and the hydrogen secreting systems complement each other nicely in elimination of acid from the body (PITTS 1945, 1948, 1950, 1952). The hydrogen system utilizes waste buffer salts as vehicles to carry acid from the body without drawing upon nutrients. Also, it responds rapidly to changes in acid base balance. The ammonia system permits the body to excrete acid under all circumstances, is independent of quantity or kind of buffer salts, but requires amino acids as source material and responds slowly to changes in acid-base balance.

b) Bicarbonate

α) Relationships to chloride transport

Under usual circumstances of acid urine production, filtered bicarbonate is almost completely reabsorbed in the proximal segment (Ellinger 1940b; Nicholson 1957a; Gottschalk, Lassiter and Mylle). When plasma bicarbonate concentration is progressively elevated, bicarbonate appears rather abruptly in the urine at a plasma concentration ("threshold") which is characteristic of each species. In dog, the concentration is about 24 and in man about 28 mM./L. Any further increment in filtered load resulting from increase in plasma bicarbonate concentration is excreted more or less quantitatively (Pitts and Lotspeich 1946a; Pitts, Ayer and Schiess) so that bicarbonate reabsorption appears to be governed by a fixed, maximal rate or Tm similar to glucose (Fig. 51). When the quantity of filtered bicarbonate is increased by increasing

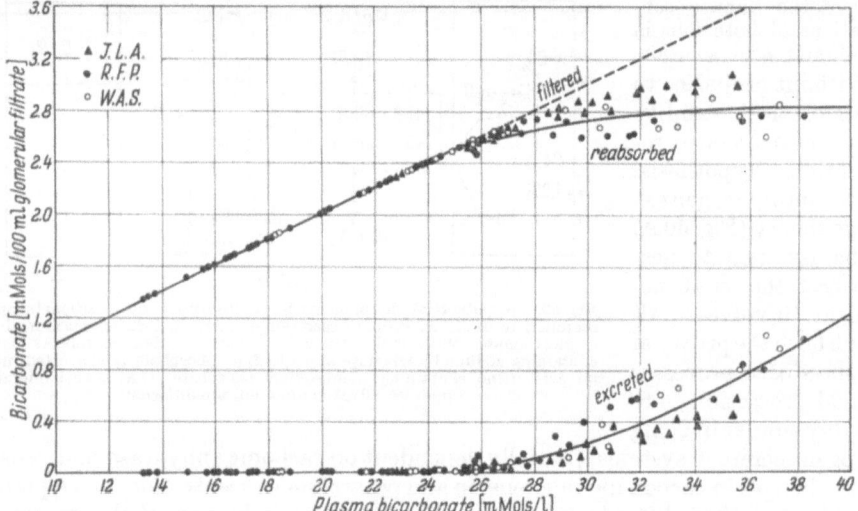

Fig. 51. Bicarbonate reabsorption and excretion in man as related to plasma bicarbonate concentration. Reabsorption and excretion are corrected to 100 ml. of glomerular filtrate. From Pitts, Ayer and Schiess. Reproduced by permission of the authors and the Journal of Clinical Investigation

filtration rate, no such maximal transport rate is evident and bicarbonate reabsorption increases as a linear function of filtration rate (Thompson and Barrett 1954a). In this respect therefore, bicarbonate, more closely resembles chloride than glucose. The resemblance between chloride and bicarbonate reabsorption may be partly superficial since plasma pH may remain constant during variation in filtration rate but usually changes during variation in plasma bicarbonate concentration.

Other studies, however, indicate that the relationships between chloride and bicarbonate reabsorption may extend beyond a similarity in their reabsorption patterns. During bicarbonate loading in dogs, chloride excretion regularly increases although filtration rate may be unchanged and plasma chloride concentration has decreased (Pitts and Lotspeich 1946; Pitts, Ayer and Schiess; Wesson and Anslow 1955; Wesson 1959). Respiratory acidosis, induced by breathing 10 percent carbon dioxide gas mixture, reverses the bicarbonate-induced chloruresis in proportion to the decrease in bicarbonate excretion, although plasma sodium and chloride concentrations and filtration rate are unchanged (WESSON 1959). The antichloruretic effect of the respiratory acidosis is probably not a direct one upon the chloride reabsorptive system since chloride excretion does not change significantly in respiratory acidosis if the urine is already acid (BARKER et al. 1957; WESSON 1959). A similar chloruresis in relation to increased bicarbonate excretion may be observed when the latter is effected by acetazolamide (GORDON et al. 1959; WESSON, unpublished observations) or respiratory alkalosis (BARKER et al. 1957). The chloruretic effect of bicarbonate excretion could be attributed to an osmotic diuretic action (D V 1 b) were it not for two further observations. First, the chloruretic effect of bicarbonate is substantially greater than is reasonably attributable to a simple osmotic diuretic (WESSON 1959). Second, chloride markedly affects bicarbonate reabsorption: chloruresis resulting from isotonic saline loading with increased filtration rate (WESSON et al.), hypertonic saline loading with or without change in filtration (PITTS and LOTSPEICH 1946a; HILTON et al. 1956; WESSON, unpub.), or osmotic loading by urea or mannitol (MUDGE, FOULKS and GILMAN 1949; WESSON and ANSLOW 1948; ANSLOW and WESSON 1955a) is regularly accompanied by a significant decrease in reabsorption and increase in excretion of bicarbonate. In studies of PITTS and LOTSPEICH in the dog, for example, an increase in plasma chloride concentration from 103 to 140 mM./L. resulting from infusion of 5 percent NaCl solution caused bicarbonate reabsorption to decrease nearly 30 percent. Increments in bicarbonate excretion as a fraction of the filtered load are generally less, however, than the concomitant fractional increments in chloride excretion. Conversely, hypochloremia is associated with an increase in bicarbonate reabsorption, requiring, at a given filtration rate, that a higher plasma bicarbonate concentration be attained before significant excretion occurs than is required at normal chloride concentrations (TOUSSAINT, TELERMAN and VEREERSTRAETEN 1958). In studies such as these, plasma p_H, carbon dioxide tension and potassium concentration have not changed significantly or have varied randomly. They have suggested strongly, but without final proof, that chloride shares with some of the bicarbonate, and probably with other small monovalent anions as well, a common reabsorptive pathway within which each competes with all others.

β) Plasma carbon dioxide tension

Rate of tubular reabsorption of bicarbonate is profoundly influenced by the carbon dioxide tension of plasma. In man, when carbon dioxide tension is lowered by hyperventilation, the urine becomes alkaline and bicarbonate excretion increases (DAVIES, HALDANE and KENNAWAY; BRASSFIELD and BEHRMANN; OCHWADT 1950; STANBURY and THOMSON 1952; BARKER et al. 1957). The increase in bicarbonate excretion occurs in spite of the fact that plasma bicarbonate is regularly and filtration rate is frequently decreased (STANBURY and THOMSON 1952). Correspondingly, an increase in carbon dioxide tension caused by breathing 5 to 10 percent carbon dioxide is associated with an increase in bicarbonate reabsorption (BARKER et al. 1951). The same dependence of bicarbonate reabsorption on carbon dioxide tension can be observed in dogs under more rigorous experimental conditions (Fig. 52). Bicarbonate reabsorption varies as a nearly linear function of arterial carbon dioxide tension between 25 and 100 mm. Hg. Under the conditions of the experiments, reabsorption changes at the rate of 0.15—0.38 mM./liter of glomerular filtrate/mm. Hg change in CO_2 tension, averaging 0.20. The relationship does not suggest that reabsorption would be zero at zero tension. Rather, linear extrapolation to zero tension (which, however, is theoretically unwarranted) indicates that reabsorption could be as high as 13 to 22 mM./L. of filtrate. Changes in arterial pH caused by altering plasma bicarbonate concentration failed to alter rate of reabsorption (Brazeau and Gilman; Relman, Etsten and Schwartz; Dorman, Sullivan and Pitts 1954a; Toussaint, Telerman and Vereerstraeten 1959b). Dependence of bicarbonate reabsorption on pCO₂ is in good agreement with the general principle that intracellular pH is very sensitive to changes in extracellular pCO₂ but relatively insensitive to changes in extracellular pH. An increase in CO₂ tension, therefore, probably accelerates hydrogen secretion in 2 ways: first, increasing the hydrion concentration gradient between cell and tubular lumen may accelerate each step in the transport process; second, the uncatalysed reaction between CO₂ and alkaline products to form bicarbonate should be accelerated. The latter effect should be quantitatively important only when carbonic an-

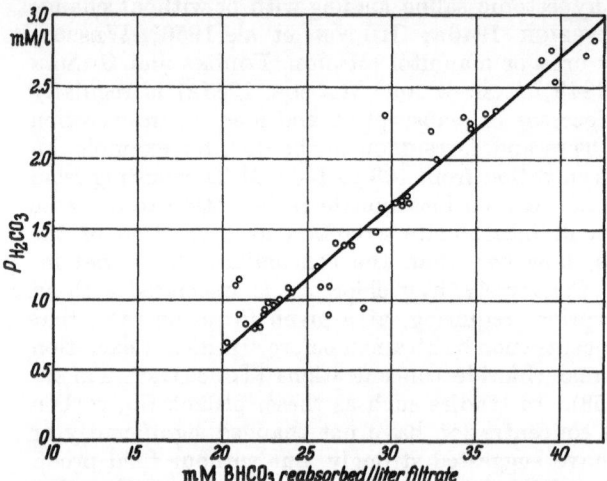

hydrase is almost completely inhibited. The bicarbonate titration curve as a function of plasma bicarbonate concentration (adjusted to constant filtration rate) exhibits in the dog a marked widening of the titration splay together with an increase in Tm during respiratory acidosis (plasma CO₂ tension, 100 mm. Hg) and a decrease in Tm with narrowing of the titration splay during respiratory alkalosis. Acetazolamide administration is associated with a decrease in Tm together with a widening of the titration splay (Schwartz, Falbriard and Lemieux; Schwartz,

Fig. 52. Bicarbonate reabsorption in the dog as related to carbonic acid concentration. Reabsorption is expressed as mM. per liter of glomerular filtrate. Carbonic acid concentration is directly proportional to carbon dioxide tension. After Brazeau and Gilman. Reproduced by permission of the authors and the American Jornal of Physiology

Lemieux and Falbriard; Schwartz, Falbriard and Relman). The authors interpret their results in terms of two rate-limiting reactions: Na-H exchange, dependent upon pCO₂, which becomes rate-limiting during respiratory acidosis and carbonic anhydrase inhibition; and carbonic anhydrase function which becomes rate-limiting during respiratory alkalosis. Maintenance of a constant plasma pH by parallel changes in plasma CO₂ tension (determining rate of reabsorption) and bicarbonate concentration (determining filtered load) results in increased urine acidity when tension and concentration are decreased and decreased acidity when these are increased (Simmons, Assali and Avedon). With respect to the effects of extracellular pH change, it should be emphasized that in most studies in which bicarbonate reabsorption has been measured during changing bicarbonate concentration, precautions have generally not been taken to prevent change in plasma chloride. In view of the known interactions between chloride and bicarbonate it seems probable that a small but significant (up to 10 percent) decrease in bicarbonate reabsorption might be observed in metabolic alkalosis at constant plasma chloride concentration.

In experimental chronic respiratory acidosis, induced by continuous exposure of dogs to atmospheres containing about 10 percent carbon dioxide for several days, bicarbonate reabsorption may considerably exceed that observed at the same CO_2 tension in acute respiratory acidosis (SULLIVAN and DORMAN). The response of the bicarbonate reabsorptive system to further acute CO_2 changes is unimpaired, and a further immediate rise in reabsorption results from an acute increment to the chronically elevated CO_2 tension (TOUSSAINT, TELERMAN and VEREERSTRAETEN 1959b). Since total inhibition of carbonic anhydrase results in depression of reabsorptive capacity by no more than 25 to 50 percent, the uninhibited enzyme is far from being rate-limiting and, in fact, no significant increase in the enzyme occurs during chronic respiratory acidosis (CARTER, SELDIN and TENG). An explanation which at least partially explains the enhanced bicarbonate reabsorption during chronic respiratory acidosis has been offered by TOUSSAINT, TELERMAN and VEREERSTRAETEN (1959b) who noted that plasma chloride is significantly lower during chronic than acute acidosis and that the same increase in bicarbonate reabsorption can be induced in acute respiratory acidosis by a simultaneous hypochloremia.

The effects on bicarbonate reabsorption of changes in CO_2 tension are directionally but not necessarily quantitatively additive to those of carbonic anhydrase inhibitors and potassium salts.

γ) Carbonic anhydrase inhibitors

Carbonic anhydrase catalyses the reversible reactions between carbon dioxide and water that yield carbonic acid or bicarbonate ion. The enzyme is widely but far from universally distributed in the body. It is usually present in moderate to high concentration in tissues associated with electrolyte exchange or transport such as gastric mucosa, intestine, pancreas, salivary glands, liver, eye and red cells, and is usually absent from nonsecretory tissues such as most muscle, the adrenal glands and lungs (DAVENPORT, review). In the kidney it is abundant in the cortex but absent from the medulla (DAVENPORT and WILHELMI). The exact function of carbonic anhydrase in secretion is not clear but by inference from *in vitro* behavior it is assumed to assist in supplying carbonic acid to neutralize base (hydroxyl) remaining from acid secretion, or else to catalyse the direct reaction of carbon dioxide and hydroxyl (DAVIES 1948; DAVIES and LONGMUIR; BERLINER and ORLOFF, review). That carbonic anhydrase is not essential for acid secretion is shown by the fact that it is absent from the kidney of the elasmobranch, *Squalus*, although the latter secretes strongly acid urine (HODLER et al.), and may prove to be deficient in the acid-secreting collecting ducts of rodents.

A large group of compounds, characterized by possession of an unsubstituted sulfonamide (—SO_2NH_2) group, possess the property of inhibiting the catalytic effect of carbonic anhydrase on the reaction of carbon dioxide and water (MANN and KEILIN; LOCKE, MAIN and MELLON). The inhibition appears to be noncompetitive in type (LEIBMAN and ALFORD). Although sulfanilamide was the first member of the group to be investigated, most studies have been made on the far more potent acetazolamide (Fig. 24). Other sulfonamides have been studied relatively little. The effect of all members of the group on carbonic anhydrase-dependent systems is qualitatively similar and consists of interference with the formation of secretions whose pH differs from that of blood. The fundamental activity of the affected secreting cells is always the same and consists of extrusion of hydrogen from one pole and extrusion of bicarbonate from the opposite pole of the cell. The glandular secretion is acid or alkaline according to the orientation of the poles. Carbonic anhydrase inhibitors act in such secretory systems presumably by inhibiting the function of carbonic anhydrase in facilitating base removal from the cell. Secretion by gastric and duodenal mucosa and by the pancreas, and production of aqueous humor and cerebrospinal fluid are decreased (BERLINER and ORLOFF, review).

Oral or parenteral administration of carbonic anhydrase inhibitor (sulfanilamide, acetazolamide, etc.) causes the urine of most vertebrates such as frog (HOBER 1942), chicken (WOLBACH; ORLOFF and DAVIDSON) and dog (PITTS and ALEXANDER 1945) to become less acid or causes bicarbonate excretion to increase. Apparent exceptions to this rule are consistent with the theoretical function of carbonic anhydrase in the excretion of acid: acetazolamide does not affect acid excretion by the elasmobranch kidney, which lacks carbonic anhydrase (HODLER et al.), and bicarbonate secretion by the alligator kidney is decreased causing the urine of this animal to become more acid (COULSON and HERNANDEZ 1957). The full effect of acetazolamide on bicarbonate reabsorption is attained in dogs by 5 to 10 mg./kg. injected intravenously. Between doses of 10 and 50—100 mg./kg., little further change in excretion is observed, suggesting that renal carbonic anhydrase activity is completely suppressed at the lower figure (MAREN et al.; BERLINER and ORLOFF). Above 100 mg./kg., and particularly at quantities of 400—500 mg./kg., bicarbonate and particularly chloride excretion increase markedly (SCHWARTZ and RELMAN 1954; HANLEY et al.; WESSON, unpublished). Twenty to 40 percent of filtered chloride together with 60 to 90 percent of the filtered bicarbonate may be excreted, suggesting that acetazolamide possesses to a significant degree the chloruretic property of the allied chlorothiazide. Under usual circumstances, administration of a full dose of acetazolamide lowers bicarbonate reabsorptive capacity by 8—10 mM./L. of filtrate in the dog (BRAZEAU and GILMAN) and evokes excretion of about 25 percent of the filtered load in dog and man (MAREN; COUNIHAN, EVANS and MILNE; HANLEY et al.). Alternatively, the same dose fails to elicit significant bicarbonate excretion when plasma bicarbonate lies below 12 mM./L. in the dog (normal, 20—22) (MAREN) and about 15—20 mM./L. in man (FRIEDBERG, HALPERN and TAYMOR; BUHLMANN et al.; FALBRIARD; COUNIHAN, EVANS and MILNE; SELDIN et al.). Analysis of dose response curves suggests that hydrogen ion secretion uncatalysed by carbonic anhydrase can account for at least half of the total normal bicarbonate reabsorption (SCHWARTZ, FALBRIARD and RELMAN; HANLEY et al.). No particular significance should be attached to these exact figures, however, because they are subject to numerous other variables. For example, the effect of acetazolamide can be enhanced by respiratory alkalosis (decreased CO_2 tension) or partially or completely cancelled by respiratory acidosis (increased CO_2 tension), although the net contribution of the inhibitor to the algebraic sum of all actions does not appear to be influenced by the level of CO_2 tension (BRAZEAU and GILMAN; DORMAN, SULLIVAN and PITTS 1954a; TAYMOR, MINOR and FRIEDBERG; SULLIVAN and DORMAN; VANAMEE et al.; BRODSKY and SATRAN). In chronic respiratory acidosis in man, the high rate of bicarbonate reabsorption is frequently susceptible to sufficient depression by acetazolamide to allow a marked diuresis to ensue (SCHWARTZ, RELMAN and LEAF). In chronic respiratory acidosis in dogs, the rise in arterial pCO_2 following acetazolamide administration and resulting from interference with erythrocyte contribution to pulmonary gas exchange may stimulate bicarbonate reabsorption sufficiently to completely cancel the depressant effect of carbonic anhydrase inhibition (CARTER, SELDIN and TENG). Conversely, simultaneous respiratory alkalosis and carbonic anhydrase inhibitor administration (with or without potassium loading) may elicit excretion of over 90 percent of filtered bicarbonate (VANAMEE et al.; ROBERTS et al. 1956; SELDIN et al.). In hypokalemic alkalosis, however, the response to acetazoleamide is depressed although plasma bicarbonate contentration is elevated (MAREN, SORSDAHL and DICKHAUS). The effects of variations in plasma chloride concentration have been noted above. Hydration as well as other variables contributes importantly to the apparent effects of carbonic anhydrase inhibitor and probably acts through changes both in filtration rate and in plasma chloride. Saline-loading, with increased filtration rate, in the dog may cause 50 percent of filtered bicarbonate to be excreted after acetazolamide (BERLINER 1952), while no significant effect may be observed in patients with severe congestive heart failure who presumably have a depressed filtration rate (FRIEDBERG, HALPERN and TAYMOR; RELMAN, LEAF and SCHWARTZ; COUNIHAN, EVANS and MILNE). Similarly, depression of filtration rate by lowering blood pressure in the abdominal aorta in the dog requires that plasma bicarbonate attain high concentrations (threshold) before bicarbonate excretion appears (THOMPSON and BARRETT 1954).

Carbonic anhydrase inhibitors, particularly the extensively studied acetazolamide, have other renal effects, some of which are unclear. Potassium excretion rises as the urine becomes more alkaline (D V 2 b ε) presumably as a result of a rise in pH in hydrion-secreting cells following suppression of the alkali-removing function of carbonic anhydrase. The changes in potassium excretion apparently occur largely if not entirely in the distal area, there being no evidence of a decrease in proximal potassium reabsorption (PITTS et al. 1958a). Potassium excretion also rises in sodium-retaining subjects who do not excrete bicarbonate, but how much of this is attributable to the usual kaliuresis associated with increased distal electrolyte loads (D V 2 b β) is unknown. Phosphate reabsorption is depressed but to no greater extent than may result from the equivalent rate of bicarbonate excretion induced by sodium bicarbonate administration (MALVIN and LOTSPEICH). Acetazolamide may competitively interfere with secretion of other aromatic acids (Section D III 1 e ζ).

Chlorothiazide, although predominantly chloruretic, is frequently associated with a significant increase in bicarbonate and potassium excretion. These effects are attributable to a weak carbonic anhydrase-inhibitory property of the molecule (BEYER 1958; MOYER, FORD and SPURR; PITTS et al. 1958b).

δ) Potassium

Acute administration of any potassium salt, such as KCl, is associated with a decrease in urine acidity, frequently to the point of a large excretion of bicarbonate. If the potassium is administered during alkaluria resulting from sodium bicarbonate administration, bicarbonate reabsorption is decreased. In the dog, reabsorption is decreased to about half the control value in relation to a 10 mM./L. increase in plasma potassium concentration (LOEB et al.; KEITH, OSTERBERG and BINGER; WOLF 1947; ROBERTS, MAGIDA and PITTS; FULLER, MACLEOD and PITTS; ROBERTS et al. 1955). Alternatively, reabsorption is increased in potassium depletion (Section D V 2 h). The relationships are compatible with the general concept that potassium is competitive with hydrion (and also sodium) intracellularly. Elevation of plasma potassium causes potassium to shift into cells, but the potassium can be accepted to a considerable extent only by displacement of hydrion extracellularly. Thus, potassium loading may be presumed to produce an intracellular alkalosis, the latter, in turn, depressing the rate of hydrogen secretion. Rubidium, which accumulates in cells more readily than potassium, may produce a chronic block of acid excretion and a severe acidosis (LAMBIE, RELMAN and SCHWARTZ).

As with changes in carbon dioxide tension and carbonic anhydrase inhibitors, the effects of potassium loading or deficiency are directionally, although not necessarily quantitatively, additive. Thus, potassium loading can block or reverse the rise in bicarbonate reabsorption expected in respiratory acidosis (ROBERTS et al. 1955; TOUSSAINT, TELERMAN and VEREERSTRAETEN 1959a). Steroid administration in the dog produces no changes in bicarbonate transport which are not attributable to potassium depletion (GIEBISCH, MACLEOD and PITTS).

ε) Relationships to phosphate transport

Bicarbonate exhibits toward phosphate reabsorption an inverse relationship similar in some respects to that toward chloride. Infusion of orthophosphate may depress bicarbonate reabsorption in the dog which is alkaluric as the result of potassium loading (ROBERTS et al. 1956), while bicarbonate loading may depress phosphate reabsorption (MALVIN and LOTSPEICH). Phosphate reabsorption is also depressed during the alkaluria resulting from acetazolamide administration (MALVIN and LOTSPEICH). On the other hand, phosphate excretion (reabsorption was not measured) was decreased during alkaluria of hyperventilation in dog and man (BRASSFIELD and BEHRMANN; STANBURY and THOMSON 1952; BARKER et al. 1957) and increased in respiratory acidosis (BARKER et al. 1957). The mechanisms involved are unknown but a weak competition for reabsorption between bicarbonate and phosphate has been proposed (MALVIN and LOTSPEICH).

c) Acid
α) General description

Technically, acid is excreted when urine is more acid than the blood. Available evidence indicates that the difference between excretion of acid and excretion of alkali (bicarbonate) is largely one of degree, and that the same tubular transport systems are operative in both circumstances. These are two hydrogen-sodium exchange systems, one in the proximal and one in the distal convoluted segment, which transport hydrions into the lumen of the tubule in exchange for sodium ions which are reabsorbed. The secreted hydrions react with buffer salts present in the lumen to yield the corresponding buffer acids. When bicarbonate is present the reaction yields carbonic acid which, being tissue-permeable, diffuses along its concentration gradient into the blood. A similar process probably operates with respect to other tissue-permeable weak acids such as salicylic acid. With dissipation of bicarbonate, only tissue-impermeable weak acids remain in the tubular fluid. Secretion of hydrion into the lumen can continue whether or not buffer salts are present which can react with it, the concentration of unbound hydrion being measured as the pH of the urine. The total of all hydrion, free as well as bound to anions, which is introduced into the urine in excess of that sufficient to cause the urine to have the same pH as the blood is the *titratable acidity*. It is measured as the amount of strong alkali which must be added to urine to bring its pH to that of blood. Although the titratable acidity is an arbitrary measure of hydrogen secretory function, it is an important measure of the function of the kidney in maintaining the acid-base equilibrium of the body. In addition to salts of weak acids, which enter the tubule partly by filtration and partly by secretion, weak bases can also bind secreted hydrion and thus serve as buffers. The most important of these by far is ammonia. The sum of ammonia plus titratable acidity measures the total rate of acid excretion by the kidney.

The overall (proximal plus distal) process of hydrogen secretion varies with the carbon dioxide tension and potassium concentration of plasma and is subject to partial inhibition by carbonic anhydrase inhibitors. Although no evidence is available to indicate that the same mechanism is not operative in both proximal and distal processes, considerable importance attaches to possible quantitative differences between them. Acetazolamide (PITTS et al. 1958a) and sodium bicarbonate infusion (MALVIN, WILDE and SULLIVAN 1958b) produce a marked depression in distal hydrogen secretion. Since total bicarbonate reabsorption is only partially depressed by the first and not measurably by the second, a marked sensitivity of the distal process to inhibitors and, of particular importance, to blood pH can be inferred[1]. The increase in potassium excretion evoked by bicarbonate loading, with the potassium probably coming from the distal segment, also supports the view that the distal transport system is pH-sensitive. No information is available in mammals on the relative contributions of the proximal and distal processes to the titratable acidity, although in *Necturus* all of the titratable acidity is contributed by the distal system (MONTGOMERY and PIERCE).

Under a given set of conditions, most importantly blood pH, K and pCO_2 which, collectively, may be termed the acid-secretory drive, the rate of titratable acid excretion depends upon three major variables: 1. the quantity of exchangeable sodium ions delivered distally (i.e., available to both ion-exchange processes); 2. the quantity of buffer salts available for excretion either by filtration or tubular secretion; 3. pK of the respective buffers[2].

The importance of sodium is illustrated by the marked rise in titratable acidity and decrease in urinary pH when sodium excretion is abruptly increased in acidotic or sodium-retaining subjects by diuretics or loading with neutral or even somewhat alkaline sodium salts (RYBERG 1948c; METCOFF, GORDILLO and ANTONOWICZ; SCHWARTZ, JENSON and RELMAN; EPSTEIN et al. 1956; WILLIAMS). It is of interest that under these circumstances potassium as well as hydrogen excretion may increase, indicating that both transport systems were 'starved' for sodium. The higher urinary pH observed at very low urine flows

---

[1] Alkalinization of the blood (pH not reported) did not suppress acid secretion by the semiisolated, perfused distal tubule of *Necturus* (MONTGOMERY and PIERCE).

[2] pK measures the strength, or degree of dissociation, of any incompletely dissociated acid as follows. A weak acid is in equilibrium with hydrogen ion and its salt according to the equation, $HA \rightleftharpoons H^+ + A^-$. The proportions of the three components of the equilibrium which are present in any solution are given by the mass law equation,

$$\frac{[H^+] [A^-]}{[HA]} = K \tag{1}$$

where brackets signify molar concentration and K is an equilibrium constant which is characteristic of each acid. Rearranging equation (1) yields

$$\frac{1}{[H^+]} = \frac{1}{K} \frac{[A^-]}{[HA]} . \tag{2}$$

Taking the logarithm of both sides of equation (2) yields

$$\log \left(\frac{1}{[H^+]} \right) = \log \left(\frac{1}{K} \right) + \log \left(\frac{[A^-]}{[HA]} \right) . \tag{3}$$

$\log \left(\frac{1}{[H^+]} \right)$ and $\log \left(\frac{1}{K} \right)$ are, by definition, termed pH and pK, hence

$$pH = pK + \log \left(\frac{[A^-]}{[HA]} \right) . \tag{4}$$

When the acid is half dissociated (that is, when $[A^-] = [HA]$) the logarithm of the ratio vanishes so that $pH = pK$.

may result from diffusional loss of hydrogen ion through the lower urinary tract (LEVINSKY and BERLINER 1959a).

β) Buffers

The importance of buffer and its pK arises principally from the circumstance that the kidney, unlike the stomach, is unable to produce an intensely acid fluid. The most acid urine which can be produced by the human kidney has a p_H of about 4.5 (SCHIESS et al.) while values of 4.8 are more usually observed (HENDERSON and PALMER 1913). A liter of urine at p_H 4.5 and free of buffers could contain no more than 0.03 mM. of acid, which is insignificant in relation to usual excretory needs of the body. If buffer salts are present, they can react with the

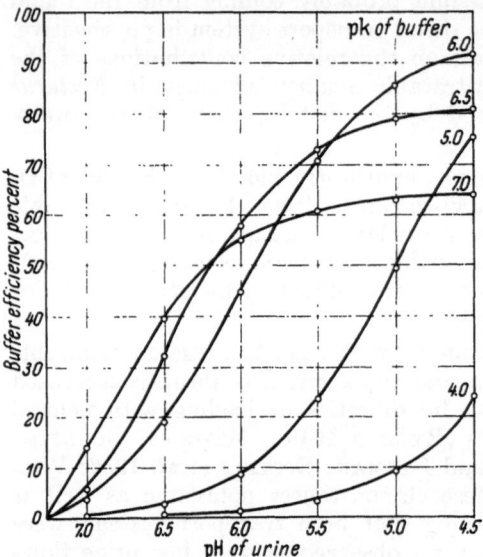

hydrions as rapidly as the latter are secreted, thus permitting considerable secretion before the concentration of free hydrion rises to the level at which further transport is suppressed. The total quantity of hydrogen which can be secreted into a urine of specified p_H and a single buffer species is an almost linear function of the total quantity of buffer present. The effect of buffer pK is illustrated in Fig. 53. The percentage of the buffer which can be utilized to excrete acid (efficiency) is measured by the difference between the quantity of buffer in the acid form at the p_H of plasma and the quantity in the acid form at the p_H of urine. As can be seen in Fig. 53, buffers with pK above 7.0 and below 5.0 are inefficient, the former because they are already largely in the acid form at blood p_H and the latter because the fraction convertible to the acid form in the urine is small.

Fig. 53. Efficiency of utilization of excreted buffer acids of different pK for the excretion of acid as related to p_H of urine. Efficiency is measured as the difference between the percentage of the buffer present as the acid form in the blood and the percentage present as the acid in the urine

If the quantity of a buffer in the urine and the urinary p_H are known, multiplying the quantity by the efficiency at that p_H yields the titratable acidity contributed by that buffer. Apart from excreted quantity and pK, no other properties of buffers are important for acid excretion (PITTS and ALEXANDER 1945; SCHIESS et al.).

Transport of hydrogen ion from plasma at a lower to urine at a higher concentration is necessarily an energy-consuming process with theoretical limitations imposed by the slowest reaction in the transport process. Although a maximal transport rate, or secretory Tm, probably exists, it has not been discovered. Titratable acid has been excreted at rates equivalent to 0.6 M/day in acidotic man during phosphate loading with no indication that excretion rate was approaching a limiting value (SCHIESS et al.).

Adrenocortical function is essential for normal operation of the Na-H exchange system as it is for Na-K exchange and NaCl reabsorption. Urinary p_H and titratable acidity are depressed in adrenal insufficiency. The defect is corrected rapidly and by relatively small quantities of steroids (SARTORIUS,

CALHOON and PITTS 1952, 1953). Unlike K secretion, however, steroid administration to normal animals does not noticeably increase secretory capacity or rate.

γ) Metabolic and other influences on acid excretion

Apart from the variables noted above, titratable acidity and urinary p_H are significantly affected by few metabolic and pharmacologic factors. Acidity is unaffected by mercurial or xanthine diuretics (BLUMGART et al. 1932, 1934; WESTON, GROSSMAN and LEITER 1951). It is depressed by carbonic anhydrase inhibitors, intravenous maleic acid (0.35 mg./kg.) in acidotic dogs (BERLINER, KENNEDY and HILTON 1950a) and by several hours of ureteral occlusion the dog (HASHIMOTO). Epinephrine and norepinephrine given intravenously is followed in about 10 minutes by an abrupt rise in urine p_H in acidotic rabbits. A similar response is reported in dog and man (SCHLEGEL). Cooling to 20^0 C in the dog abolishes acid secretory activity, causing urine p_H to equal that of plasma (SEGAR, RILEY and BARILA).

Experimental potassium depletion in man and animals as well as potassium depletion in various clinical states (D V 2 h) is associated with a low titratable acidity and a p_H which is usually between 6.7 and 7.1. Plasma pCO_2 is normal and plasma p_H and bicarbonate concentration tend to be slightly increased. Body acid-base balance is maintained by an increase in urinary ammoniation equal to the defect in titratable acidity. Low titratable acid excretion is contrary to what might be predicted from acute experiments in which alkalinization of the urine is associated with K excess rather than with K depletion. When K-depleted men or rats are subjected to severe metabolic acidosis, urine p_H seldom decreases below 5.5 (CLARKE et al.; HALL and RELMAN). If, however, additional buffer as phosphate is supplied to the kidney, titratable acidity increases normally but without change in p_H (CLARKE et al.). In the potassium-depleted rat, such acidification as occurs is principally in the collecting ducts with little change in p_H, in contrast to the normal animal, occurring in the proximal and distal segments (WINDHAGER and GIEBISCH 1960). Chronic potassium depletion apparently causes a metabolic lesion of the H-transport system such that the limiting concentration gradient of hydrogen ion between blood and urine has decreased from a factor of 500—800 to a factor of 10—100. Further evidence in support of the existence of such a lesion is the increase in renal carbonic anhydrase as well as glutaminase, which occurs in the potassium-deficient rat and dog (IACOBELLIS, MUNTWYLER and GRIFFIN 1954, 1955), and the rapid increase in titratable acidity observed during K-repletion in depleted patients (KLEEMAN et al. 1955b; EALES and LINDER).

δ) Acid excretion in man

Average rate of total acid excretion (titratable acidity plus ammonia) by an individual can be accurately predicted by analysis of the diet. Metabolism of fats, proteins and minerals yields both acids and bases as end products. The difference between the two measures the quantity of acid or alkali which must be excreted in order that body acid-base balance be maintained. In the average European and North American diet with its large protein component, acids exceed bases by about 40 to 80 mM. per day. Although excretion rate as averaged over several days is predictable, the rate of excretion at any one time, and the partition of total acid excretion between ammonia and titratable acidity is not subject to quantitative description because of numerous independent variables, such as rate of phosphate buffer excretion, upon which acid excretion depends.

The diurnal cycle, activity and feeding are physiological activities associated with marked changes in urine p_H and acid excretion.

a) **Diurnal cycle.** In inactive, healthy individuals, urinary p_H is lowest toward the end of the sleep period, generally 3 to 5 A.M., rising rapidly toward a weakly acid or neutral reaction during the first few hours after awakening. The maximum p_H is generally attained in midmorning, about 10 A.M., and sustained, with considerable fluctuation, until evening (CAMPBELL 1920; CAMPBELL and WEBSTER 1921; SIMPSON 1924, 1925; JORES; RYBERG 1943; STANBURY and THOMSON 1951; BRUNTON, review). Titratable acidity and ammonia excretion generally are correlated also with buffer excretion (mostly phosphate) and parallel p_H, but titratable acidity may depart from correlation with p_H during the daytime rise in phosphate excretion. The nocturnal aciduria followed by alkalinization after awakening has generally been attributed to the known rise in blood pCO_2 during sleep with subsequent compensatory hyperventilation, but this is not proven. Urine p_H may decrease slightly during daytime sleep (SIMPSON 1925) but in subjects who adopted a 12 hour cycle for 48 hours, urine p_H retained a 24 hour cycle (MILLS and STANBURY). Nocturnal aciduria ceased in sodium-depleted subjects (CLARKE et al.).

b) **Food.** Immediately following ingestion of food, the urine frequently becomes more acid for a few, perhaps 30, minutes. The reaction then rapidly becomes more alkaline than before eating and the alkaline phase lasts for several hours. This postprandial decrease in urine acidity has been termed the *alkaline tide.* It is particularly conspicuous following the first meal of the day when the matutinal and postprandial rises in p_H tend to be additive. Following other meals, however, and in patients with achlorhydria the postprandial alkaline phase may frequently be abortive or absent (CAMPBELL 1920; BRUNTON; BARNETT and BLUME; RYBERG 1943). Correlation with secretion of gastroenteric fluids, particularly acid gastric juice, remains the most plausible hypothesis of the cause of the postprandial p_H changes. Strict correlation with gastric secretion alone should not be expected, however, since the composition of the blood should respond to all gastroenteric secretions both during their secretion and during their reabsorption.

c) **Activity.** During and for several hours following both light and heavy exercise, urine p_H is markedly decreased and titratable acidity and ammonia excretion are increased (MACKEITH et al.; WILSON et al. 1925; EGGLETON 1942; BARCLAY and NUTT 1944b; GOVAERTS and DELANNE). Light to moderate exercise may abort the postprandial rise in urine p_H (CAMPBELL 1920) even when the exercise occurred during the preceding day (BARNETT and BLUME).

Orthostasis (quiet standing) may cause a decrease in p_H and increase in titratable acidity similar to exercise (WHITE et al.; EPSTEIN et al. 1956).

d) **Water diuresis.** Water diuresis following water ingestion in man is associated with an increase in urine p_H. The rise is generally 0.5 to 1.0 units (CARR; BARCLAY and NUTT 1944a). The mechanism is unknown. A similar rise in p_H was not observed during alcohol (water-type) diuresis (EGGLETON 1946).

e) **Acidosis.** Metabolic acidosis results from ingestion or production of non-volatile acids in the body at a rate greater than they can be excreted. Plasma bicarbonate is reduced. Pulmonary ventilation, stimulated by decrease in blood p_H, is moderately increased causing plasma pCO_2 to decrease. In this respect the respiratory system acts as a negative feed-back system in the regulation of blood p_H. Although bicarbonate reabsorptive capacity presumably is decreased by decrease in pCO_2, adequacy to reabsorb the more greatly decreased filtered load is not threatened, and parallel decreases in CO_2 tension and plasma bicarbonate (pH constant) are associated with an increase in acid excretion (SIM-MONS, ASSALI and AVEDON). Maximum titratable acidity in metabolic acidosis in healthy man and under constant conditions of urinary buffer is attained at a plasma bicarbonate of about 20 mM./L. (SCHIESS et al.). Unlike ammonia (D V 3 e δ), no adaptation or increase in acid excretory capacity occurs in chronic metabolic acidosis as measured within attainable limits of buffer excretion (PITTS and LOTSPEICH 1956b; SARTORIUS, ROEMMELT and PITTS).

Respiratory acidosis results from breathing a gas mixture containing 5 to 10 percent CO_2 or from impaired elimination of CO_2 from the blood. Plasma pCO_2 and bicarbonate are elevated and pH is decreased. Although concentration of bicarbonate in glomerular filtrate is increased, reabsorptive capacity as a result of increased pCO_2, and perhaps also as a result of decreased pH acting on the distal system, is also increased. Titratable acidity is increased and pH is decreased within a few minutes of the onset of respiratory acidosis (BRASS-FIELD and BEHRMANN; FULLER and MACLEOD; BARKER et al. 1957; KAIM et al.).

Acid excretion is well sustained in chronic BRIGHT'S disease until renal failure is far advanced. Ammonia secretory capacity deteriorates rapidly so that acid excretion in uremia is mostly as titratable acidity (HENDERSON and PALMER 1915; VAN SLYKE et al. 1926). So large is the apparent hydrogen secreting capacity in the normal man, however, that 5 percent of the total should be sufficient to excrete the usual daily production of fixed acids provided that buffers are available. The nephritic patient differs from the normal, however, in that acid production does not become efficient until plasma bicarbonate decreases to values which are relatively low and significantly less than 20 mM./L. (SCHWARTZ et al. 1959). The reasons for this are unknown but may be attributable in part to the relatively high rates of glomerular filtration and high filtered loads of bicarbonate and chloride per nephron.

d) Carbon dioxide and carbonic acid

Carbonic acid exists almost entirely in the form of its anhydride, dissolved carbon dioxide. The ratio, $H_2CO_3:CO_2$ is about 1:800 (ROUGHTON). The solubility and diffusibility of carbonic acid in tissues are therefore mostly the properties of CO_2. At any specified temperature, dissolved CO_2 attains an equilibrium with CO_2 in the gas phase or CO_2 tension (pCO_2) in a constant ratio expressed by a solubility constant. Since the solubility constants for blood and various urines are nearly equal, pCO_2 and carbonic acid concentration can be used interchangeably, as an approximation, in comparing various fluids. Theoretically, however, blood and urine are at equilibrium when the pCO_2 rather than the carbonic acid concentrations are equal. Since interest has centered in theoretical aspects of equilibria rather than in carbonic acid excretion, pCO_2 has been the preferred measure.

The carbonic acid concentration of urine is very close to that of arterial blood (GAMBLE 1922), rarely differing from the latter by a factor greater than two over the entire range of urine flow and urine pH. Because of the high renal blood flow as related to renal CO_2 production, the pCO_2 of renal venous blood is only slightly greater than that of arterial blood. Therefore, carbonic acid excretion varies roughly in proportion to urine flow (DORMAN, SULLIVAN and PITTS 1954b) which is compatible with the view that CO_2 can diffuse freely either into or out of the tubule during bicarbonate reabsorption and acid production. In spite of the near equality of pCO_2 (or carbonic acid concentration) between blood and urine, considerable interest centers on possible mechanisms which can account for observed differences. When pH of the urine is acid, the pCO_2 of urine is very nearly equal to that of blood with a significant tendency to be slightly lower in the more acid urines. As the urine becomes progressively more alkaline, and particularly in the range pH 7.0 to 8.0, urinary pCO_2 increases progressively, attaining values 2 to 2.5 times that of blood (Ryberg 1948b; Pitts, Ayer and Schiess; Kennedy, Orloff and Berliner; Dorman, Sullivan and Pitts 1954b; Hong and Rahn). Two principal hypotheses have been proposed to account for the high pCO_2 in alkaline urine (Ryberg 1948b). These are 1. delayed dehydration of carbonic acid combined with continuing hydrogen secretion during alkalosis; 2. mixing within the collecting ducts of urines of varying pH from different nephrons. Of these two hypotheses the delayed dehydration hypothesis, appropriately modified, is in best agreement with information. Hydrogen secretion is evidently continuing in alkalosis as measured by bicarbonate reabsorption. Because of saturation of the transport system, it is probable that more intratubular carbonic acid is generated during alkaluria from bicarbonate loading than during aciduria. High urinary pCO_2 is observed in alkaline urine following acetazolamide, which presumably depresses hydrogen secretion (Fig. 54) (Kennedy, Orloff Berliner; Dorman, Sullivan and Pitts 1954b; Capeci et al.; Portwood et al.), but bicarbonate reabsorption may be depressed no more than about 30 percent when carbonic anhydrase is totally inhibited. Urinary pCO_2 in both alkaline and acid urine can be elevated somewhat above values observed at the same pH in urine of low buffer content by increasing the urinary content of nonvolatile buffers (Kennedy, Orloff and Berliner; Portwood et al.; Kaim and Brodsky 1960), observations which are compatible with a function

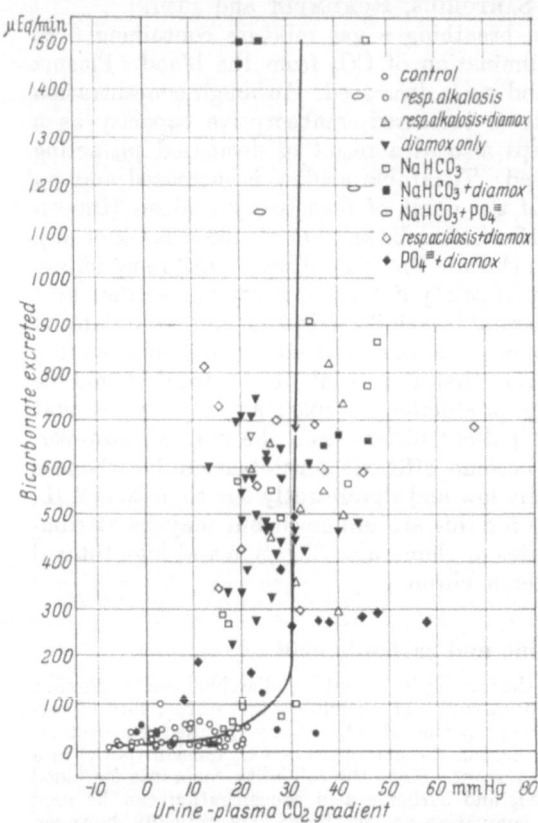

Fig. 54. Difference in carbon dioxide tension between plasma and urine as related to bicarbonate excretion in man. The tension difference is not evidently related to the mechanism causing alkaluria, particularly at high rates of bicarbonate excretion. After Portwood, Seldin, Rector and Cade. Reproduced by permission of the authors and the Journal of Clinical Investigation

which buffers theoretically could perform by storing hydrogen in the form of nondiffusible buffer acids. As CO_2 is lost by diffusion, buffer acids can release the stored hydrion into bicarbonate-containing urine for the generation of additional CO_2 (Kennedy, Eden and Berliner). Finally, injection of carbonic anhydrase during alkaluria abolishes the urine-blood pCO_2 difference (Ochwadt and Pitts 1956b; Kaim and Brodsky 1959). Alternatively, the "mixing" hypothesis is virtually eliminated by observation that high urinary pCO_2 may be generated under circumstances of low excretion of buffers such that, if all the nonbicarbonate buffer were being excreted from tubules forming strongly acid urine, the effect would be inadequate to generate observed CO_2 tensions (Rector et al. 1959; BRODSKY et al. 1958). Some of the conceptual and quantitative objections to the "delayed dehydration" hypothesis can be eliminated if due provision is made for the trapping property of the medulla. In alkaluria, extensive hydrogen secretion continues in the proximal segment. Because of the distribution of bicarbonate in the lumen, extensive carbonic acid formation may be presumed to occur up to, or even across, the corticomedullary junction so that little of the carbonic acid generated in the penultimate portion of the proximal segment need be lost before the tubular fluid enters the medulla. Alkalinity of tubular fluid in the range pH 7—8 can also favor delayed dehydration (FAURHOLT). Filtered carbonic anhydrase by virtually abolishing delay, will allow nearly all excess carbonic acid to return to the cortical blood. In the medulla, CO_2 released by dehydration may enter the medullary interstitium where it can be trapped by the countercurrent arrangement of the vasa recta. Irrespective of the pCO_2 of the fluid entering the collecting ducts from the distal segment, the duct fluid will attain diffusion equilibrium with the medulla before entering the renal pelvis. The general role of the medulla in determining the final CO_2 tension is exhibited also by the 30—60 minute delay, again attributable to the countercurrent system, between change in blood and change in urine CO_2 tensions (KAIM et al.).

An even less firm theoretical basis is available to explain low urine pCO_2 in acid urine. The mechanism may well be quite different from that operating in alkaline urine. Bicarbonate reabsorption is probably complete high in the proximal segment with little excess carbonic acid entering the medulla. Unlike alkaline urine, the acid urine-blood pCO_2 gradient is not abolished by carbonic anhydrase (KAIM and BRODSKY 1960). The low CO_2 tensions may be assumed to represent the effects of medullary metabolic or secretory activities on medullary interstitial pCO_2 (BRODSKY et al. 1958).

e) Ammonia
α) General description

Urinary ammonia (NH_3) is synthesized *de novo* within the kidney rather than extracted from blood. This is demonstrated by the observations that not only does urinary NH_3 exceed that entering the kidney in arterial blood but also that more NH_3 leaves the kidney through the renal vein in cat, dog and man than enters through the artery (NASH and BENEDICT; AMBARD and SCHMID; FONTÈS and YOVANOVITCH; FØLLING; POLONOVSKI, BIZARD and BOULANGER; POLONOVSKI, BOULANGER and BIZARD; VAN SLYKE et al. 1943; BERRY et al.). The primary source or substrate utilized by the kidney for ammonia synthesis may be glutamine. Glutamine is extracted from renal blood in amounts sufficient to account for 60 percent of ammonia excretion in acidotic dogs while extraction of amino acid is small, and glutamine extraction decreases to low values in alkalotic dogs excreting little ammonia (VAN SLYKE et al. 1943). Renal tissue contains large quantities of at least two enzymes (glutaminase I and glutaminase II) which can split glutamine to glutamate and ammonia[1]. Certain amino acids, including alanine, histidine, asparagine, tyramine, leucine, glycine, cysteine and methionine, may also serve as direct and indirect sources or precursors of urine ammonia as demonstrated by their causing increased production of NH_3 by acidotic animals or increased synthesis by kidney slices *in vitro* (BLISS; JIMENEZ-DIAZ; STEIGER and

---

[1] Glutaminase I is optimally active *in vitro* at about pH 7.4 while glutaminase II, which is somewhat more abundant in whole kidney, is optimally active about pH 8.8 (GOLDSTEIN, RICHTERICH-VAN BAERLE and DEARBORN).

Strehler; Lotspeich and Pitts; Davies and Yudkin; Kamin and Handler 1951 b; Orloff and Berliner; Madison and Seldin). Dextro-isomers of amino acids are particularly potent sources of ammonia (Bliss). Aspartate probably can supply urinary NH$_3$ while lysine, arginine (Lotspeich and Pitts) and proline (Madison and Seldin) are ineffective sources. Urea, also, is not a significant source of urinary NH$_3$ (van Slyke et al. 1943). Presence of both l- and d-amino-acid oxidases and glycine oxidase in the kidney indicates that NH$_3$ can be obtained directly from the amino acids utilized (Bénard and Gajdos, review). In addition, the kidney contains an enzyme system capable of synthesizing glutamine from glutamic acid and amino donors (Goldstein, Richterich-van Baerle and Dearborn). Unlike glutaminase I, however, amino acid oxidases, glycine oxidase, and the glutamine synthesizing system are absent from the inner medulla (collecting duct area) (Richterich-van Baerle and Goldstein 1958).

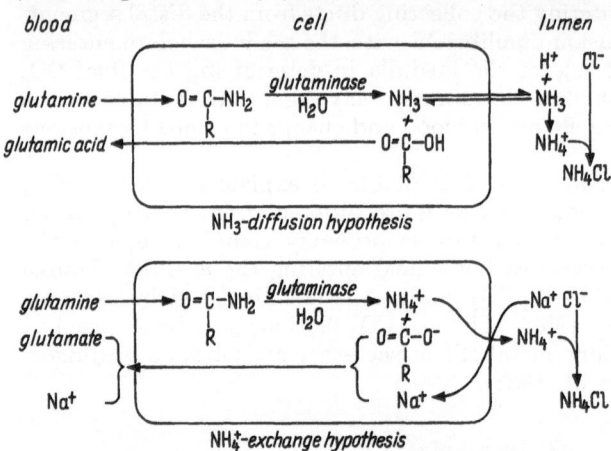

Fig. 55. Hypothetical mechanisms of ammonia secretion

Introduction of ammonia (NH$_3$) into the urine occurs near the end of the nephron and is one of the last events in urine formation. In the frog, NH$_3$ enters the urine from a narrow area a little below the middle of the distal convoluted tubule (Walker 1940). This region is the same which, in *Necturus*, secretes acid. In mammals, NH$_3$ enters the urine in some portion either of the distal tubule or the collecting duct. Two hypotheses have been proposed to describe the mechanism of entry of ammonia into the tubular fluid (Fig. 55). According to the *exchange* hypothesis, NH$_4$ ions are introduced into the tubular lumen by an exchange of intracellular NH$_4^+$ for Na$^+$ in the tubular fluid (Ryberg 1948c). According to the *diffusion* hypothesis (Sartorius, Roemmelt and Pitts), NH$_3$ which is formed as such within the cell diffuses through the permeable cell membrane into the lumen where, by reacting with free hydrogen ions to form ammonium ions (NH$_4^+$), acid is neutralized. A third mechanism, secretion of whole salt, is virtually excluded by studies which also exclude this mechanism for secretion of acid. It is evident, however, that the NH$_3$-diffusion hypothesis is also, indirectly, a cation exchange process since a sodium ion had to be reabsorbed by exchange to provide each hydrion for reaction with NH$_3$.

No final choice can be made as yet between these two concepts and it is possible that both systems exist. The diffusion hypothesis requires that NH$_3$ secretion occur in the same region of the nephron as acid secretion in order that NH$_3$ may facilitate the latter by providing buffer base. Coincidence of the two processes is almost certainly true in amphibia. High glutaminase content of cortex, NH$_3$ production by cortex *in vitro* and apparent simultaneous appearance of NH$_3$ and of K secretion in stopped-flow patterns in the dog (Pitts et al. 1958a; Sullivan, Wilde and Malvin) indicate that concurrent appearance of acid and ammonia in the distal convoluted tubule is probable in many mammals. Both acid and ammonia (but not potassium) appear in increased amounts in the collecting ducts of rodents concomitantly with sodium reabsorption (ULLRICH, HILGER and KLÜMPER; KLÜMPER, ULLRICH and HILGER; ULLRICH et al.). This and other evidence suggest that the acid- and ammonia-secretory function of the collecting ducts in rodents is rudimentary in other mammals. Other observations which are in good agreement with or best explained by the diffusion hypothesis are: the studies of ORLOFF and BERLINER indicating that total acid excretion (titratable acidity plus NH_3) may remain constant during increase in NH_3 production resulting from amino acid infusion in the dog; the high correlation between urine acidity and ammonia excretion; and the relatively high permeability to ammonia of most tissues. A theoretical weakness of the diffusion hypothesis is the extraordinarily high NH_3 and NH_4^+ concentrations which must exist in urine which are at the same time alkaline and abundant in ammonia. The concentration of intracellular NH_4^+ must be particularly high if it be assumed that intracellular p_H of the ammonia-secreting cells has approximately the same value, 6.8, as mammalian cells generally (YOSHIMURA et al.). The cation exchange hypothesis allows NH_4 secretion to be independent of both location and rate of hydrion secretion.

As indicated by the general description above, ammonia excretion depends upon the following variables: quantity of available substrates (glutamine and appropriate amino acids) from which NH_3 can be synthesized; quantity of sodium available to the cation exchange areas either for direct Na-NH_4 exchange or indirect Na-H exchange; p_H of the urine acting in some fashion to modify the rate of entry of NH_3 or NH_4 into the tubular lumen; and the mass of the NH_3-synthesizing system as measured in part by glutaminase and dependent, in turn, upon the acid-base balance of the body.

β) Urine acidity and ammonia excretion

During any reasonably short period, the rate of ammonia production by the kidney is roughly constant (POPPELL et al.; OWEN, FLANAGAN and TYOR). The fraction of this production which enters the urine as excretion is, however, closely correlated with urine p_H irrespective of the circumstances under which p_H has changed. Thus, in man and dog ammonia excretion decreases when p_H increases as the result of sodium bicarbonate administration (ÖSTBERG; PITTS et al. 1958a), hyperventilation (BRASSFIELD and BEHRMANN; BARKER et al. 1957; FULLER and MACLEOD), acetazolamide administration (LAAKE 1956), and potassium-loading (LOEB et al.; BRIGGS) and increases when urine p_H is acutely decreased by acid loading (ÖSTBERG) or respiratory acidosis (CO_2 inhalation) (BARKER et al. 1957; FULLER and MACLEOD). Excretion decreases with the rise in p_H following meals (CAMPBELL 1920) and increases with the fall in p_H during and following exercise (WILSON et al.; EGGLETON 1942) or during sodium sulfate infusion (BRIGGS; EGGLETON 1947). In the diurnal excretory cycle, NH_3 excretion is maximal during nocturnal aciduria and decreases during the morning rise in p_H (CAMPBELL 1920; CAMPBELL and WEBSTER 1921; SIMPSON 1924). In the dog, the logarithm of ammonia excretion appears linearly correlated with urine p_H (Fig. 56) (ORLOFF and BERLINER) so that a decrease of 1.0 units in urine p_H is correlated with an approximate doubling in NH_4 excretion. A similar factor of approximately 2.0 per unit change in p_H is observed in man (EGGLETON 1947; WOLF 1947; CLARKE et al.; BARKER et al. 1957).

γ) Ammonia excretion in diuresis

Variations in urine flow have no significant effect on NH_3 excretion in acid urine at constant p_H in the dog. At urine p_H above 6.0, however, excretion increases slowly with increasing urine flow as in the case of weak acids and bases (D III 5) (Orloff and Berliner). Mercurial and xanthine diuretics have no evident effect on NH_3 excretion (Blumgart et al. 1932, 1934; Hilton 1951; Weston, Grossman and Leiter 1951).

δ) Ammonia excretion in acidosis and alkalosis

Ammonia excretion under usual circumstances in man is about 20 to 40 mM./day and represents half or somewhat more of the total quantity of acid excreted daily. In infants with very low rate of excretion of phosphate buffer, nearly all of the acid is excreted as NH_3 (McCance and v. Finck). When metabolic acidosis is produced in healthy subjects by ingestion of acidifying salts such as ammonium chloride or calcium chloride, NH_3 excretion increases over several days without corresponding changes in urine p_H. Ammonia excretion is not proportional to the degree of acidosis, since acidosis is most severe during the first 2 to 4 days following adoption of an acidifying regime and becomes less severe as increasing NH_4 excretion eliminates some of the accumulated acid load (Gamble, Blackfan and Hamilton; Ryberg 1948a; Hilton 1951; Sartorius, Roemmelt and Pitts). A new constant rate of NH_3 excretion is attained after 5 to 10 days of acidosis (Fig. 57). The rate of NH_3 excretion attained is approximately equal to the increased daily acid ingestion if the acid is strong. This is because buffer excretion and titratable acidity increases only slightly and temporarily. Ammonia excretion of 200—400 mM./day is readily attained when this quantity of strong acid is ingested (300 mM. is equivalent to 15 g. of ammonium chloride) (Ryberg 1948a; Sartorius, Roemmelt and Pitts; Hilton 1951), but administration of supplementary amino acid substrates during acidosis can permit excretion to rise to a rate equivalent to 600 mM./day (Madison and Seldin). The maximum rate of NH_3 excretion attainable by the normal human kidney is unknown.

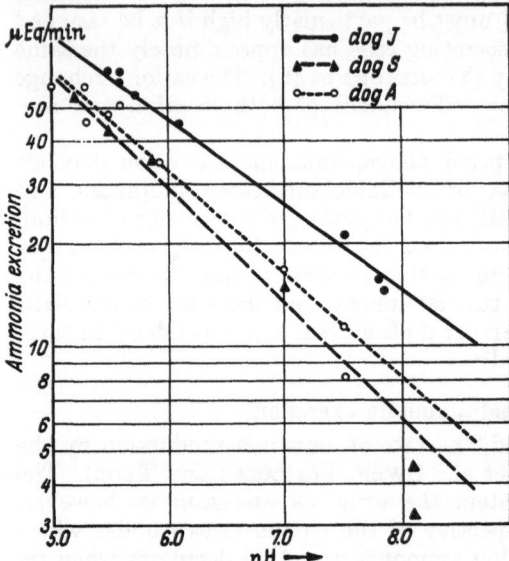

Fig. 56. Ammonia excretion as related to urinary p_H in the dog. After Orloff and Berliner. Reproduced by permission of the authors and the Journal of Clinical Investigation

The nature of the compensatory changes in the NH_3-synthesizing system in acidosis is unknown. Increased excretion reflects an increase in synthesis of ammonia rather than an increased fraction of a constant rate of synthesis (Poppell et al.). In the acidotic dog, presumably also in man but in contrast to the rat, few changes occur in the activity of either glutaminase I or II or in rate of NH_3 synthesis from glutamine *in vitro* (Rector and Orloff). Some increase in glutaminase may be observed in the dog during profound potassium depletion (Iacobellis, Muntwyler and Griffin 1955).

Because of extensive studies on ammonia excretion in the rat, and the temptation to generalize from rat to man, it is important to note the differences of rodents (rat, guinea pig and hamster) and perhaps also rabbits from dog or man. In rat, NH_4 excretion correlates poorly with urine pH and correlates best with acid-base state of the animal (LEONARD and ORLOFF; RECTOR et al.; RICHTERICH-VAN BAERLE, GOLDSTEIN and DEARBORN 1956a, 1958); in dog and man, NH_3 excretion correlates with pH under all circumstances. In rat, glutaminase I occurs in relatively high concentration in the inner stripe of the outer medulla and the inner medulla; in dog, both glutaminases are relatively more abundant in cortex (WEISS and LONGLEY; GOLDSTEIN, RICHTERICH-VAN BAERLE and DEARBORN; RICHTERICH-VAN BAERLE and GOLDSTEIN 1958). The high medullary glutaminase I content of the rat correlates well with demonstrated secretion of NH_3 in the collecting duct of the rodent (hamster) (ULLRICH, HILGER and KLÜMPER). In rat and guinea pig renal glutaminase activity, particularly glutaminase I, increases markedly during chronic metabolic acidosis (RECTOR, SELDIN and COPENHAVER; GOLDSTEIN, RICHTERICH-VAN BAERLE and DEARBORN;

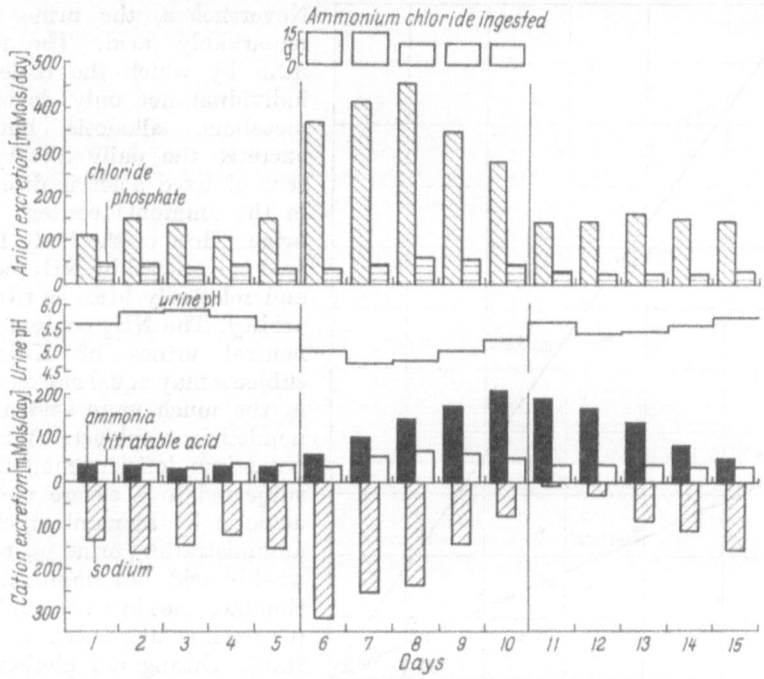

Fig. 57. Ammonia, chloride and sodium excretion during chronic ammonium chloride acidosis in a normal man. After PITTS (1948). Reproduced by permission of the author and Federation Proceedings

RICHTERICH-VAN BAERLE and GOLDSTEIN 1957, 1958) but the increased activity is principally in the cortex (WEISS and LONGLEY); in the dog, glutaminase changes during chronic acidosis are not evident. Interestingly, glutaminase activity in the guinea pig increases also during metabolic alkalosis due to alkali-loading or in the rat due to potassium depletion (GOLDSTEIN, RICHTERICH-VAN BAERLE and DEARBORN; IACOBELLIS, MUNTWYLER and GRIFFIN 1954; MUNTWYLER, IACOBELLIS and GRIFFIN; WILLIAMS et al.). The paradox could be resolved if NH_4 excretion in these rodents is viewed as responding to an intracellular acidosis which can result from potassium depletion from any cause including alkali loading. Failure of glutaminase activity to increase in the rat during chronic respiratory acidosis casts doubt on this hypothesis, however (CARTER, SELDIN and TENG). Although glutaminase activity is normal in the adrenoprival rat and activity increases normally during acidosis, such animals have a marked impairment in NH_3 excretion with relatively little increase in NH_3 excretion during acid-loading. The excretion defect is rapidly corrected by small quantities of steroids such as desoxycorticosterone (SARTORIUS, CALHOON and PITTS 1952, 1953; WHITE and ROLF 1953; WILSON and SELDIN; WILLIAMS et al.).

Correlation between NH_3 excretion and urine pH exists in the acidotic as well as the normal man or dog (Fig. 58). The acidotic differs from the normal animal in that NH_3 excretion in acidosis is greater than in the normal when the two are compared at any selected urine p_H. Therefore, neutral or even alkaline urine from acidotic animals may contain large quantities of NH_3.

Alkaline urine is commonly observed in human chronic potassium depletion (D V 2 h). Such individuals also have a slight to moderate extracellular metabolic alkalosis as measured by increase in plasma p_H and bicarbonate. The metabolic alkalosis is interpretable in terms of the general theory of intracellular cation equilibria, according to which K deficiency should induce an intracellular acidosis. The renal tubular cells, responding to the intracellular acidosis, excrete excessive quantities of acid from the body, thus contributing to bicarbonate accumulation in the plasma. Nevertheless, the urine is not remarkably acid. The mechanism by which the K-deficient individual not only develops a metabolic alkalosis but also excretes the daily dietary content of fixed acids is discovered in the ammonia content of the urine. Most of the body load of acid is excreted by NH_3 secretion and relatively little as titratable acidity. The NH_3 content of the neutral urines of K-deficient subjects may equal or exceed that in the much more acid urine of nondeficient subjects. When the potassium deficient man or rat is subjected to a severe metabolic acidosis by ammonium chloride administration, urine p_H remains weakly acid, but ammonia excretion increases in a normal fashion (CLARKE et al.; HALL and REL- MAN). During K-repletion, NH_3 excretion decreases at a time when urine is becoming more acid and titratable acidity is increasing (EALES and LINDER).

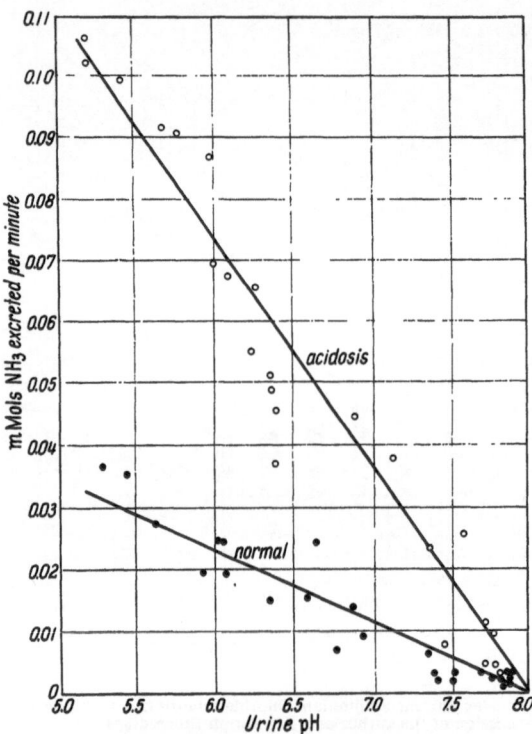

Fig. 58. Ammonia excretion during chronic acidosis in the dog. After PITTS (1948). Reproduced by permission of the author and Federation Proceedings

ε) Hypoadrenalism

Ammonia excretion is relatively low in man and dog with adrenal insufficiency (LOEB, ATCHLEY and STAHL; JIMENEZ-DIAZ; LEVY, POWER and KEPLER; HARRIS et al.). The deficiency in excretion is evident both in relation to urine p_H, in relation to the acidosis usually present in hypoadrenal patients and animals, and in the defective response to acid loading. Man and dog resemble the rodents in these respects. The defect in NH_3 excretion is repaired by very small quantities of adrenal steroids.

ζ) Chronic nephritis

Ammonia excretion is decreased in patients with severe, parenchymatous renal disease of whatever cause (HENDERSON and PALMER 1915; LINDER). The decrease in excretion is roughly proportional to loss in other tubular functions, such as p-aminohippurate transport and glucose transport. In the normal adult half to two thirds of the daily acid load may be excreted as NH_3, but in the patient with chronic nephritis, NH_3 represents less than half (VAN SLYKE et al. 1926). Ammonia excretion by the nephritic fails to increase or increases only very slowly during acidosis (GAMBLE, BLACKFAN and HAMILTON; DAVIES and WRONG; SCHWARTZ et al. 1959).

5. Calcium

Excreted Ca is that quantity of filtered Ca which escapes active reabsorption from the glomerular filtrate. Although Ca is secreted by the tubule of the aglomerular fish (EDWARDS and CONDORELLI; MARSHALL and GRAFFLIN 1928; BERGLUND and FORSTER), no evidence of a tubular secretory system has been observed in mammals or amphibia (LIANG).

The region of the nephron where Ca is reabsorbed is uncertain. "Stopped-flow" studies indicate that a major reabsorptive site is distal to the proximal convoluted tubule (p-aminohippurate secretory area) and proximal to the second quarter of the distal tubule (sodium reabsorptive area) WESSON and LAULER; HOWARD, WILDE and MALVIN; GLOBUS, KESSLER and THOMPSON; SAMIY et al.), suggesting the terminal segment or pars recta of the proximal tubule as a possible anatomical site. Some exchange between intratubular and peritubular Ca, as measured by radioisotopic Ca, apparently occurs proximal to the reabsorptive area (GLOBUS, KESSLER and THOMPSON; SAMIY et al.) but without evidence of active transport. Calcium and magnesium share the same reabsorptive area (WESSON and LAULER; SAMIY et al.) but, unlike the secretory system in the aglomerular fish (BERGLUND and FORSTER), existence of significant competition between these two cations in mammals is uncertain. A small increase in magnesium excretion is observed during calcium-loading in the dog (WOLF and BALL), while magnesium loading may evoke a large increase in calcium excretion (SAMIY et al.).

An accurate description of the tubular transport of Ca under various conditions is not yet available. This is because the concentration of calcium in glomerular filtrate (plasma ultrafiltrate) is difficult to measure accurately and cannot be estimated from serum or plasma concentrations with an accuracy acceptable for precision studies.

Approximately 35 percent of the calcium in normal human plasma is nonfilterable because of binding or adsorption to plasma proteins and electrostatic restriction in the DONNAN distribution. The filterable fraction of plasma Ca varies significantly with temperature, pH, quantity of each kind of plasma protein, and concentrations of Ca, PO_4, oxalate, citrate, sulfate, etc. (PINCUS, PETERSON and KRAMER; LOEB and NICHOLS; GREENBERG and LARSON 1939; HOPKINS, HOWARD and EISENBERG; TORIBARA, TEREPKA and DEWEY; PETERSON and CRISMON). The filterable fraction is not measurably altered in hyper- or hypoparathyroidism (HOPKINS, CONNOR and HOWARD).

The filterable calcium is divisible into ionized and nonionized moities, the latter representing compounds of calcium with substances such as oxalate and citrate. Analogy with other transport systems suggests that Ca ions rather than complexes are absorbed, but this is not proven. Moreover, each complex is in equilibrium with Ca ion so that complexed Ca^{++} can redissociate to yield ions until the tubular concentration of Ca decreases to some unknown value at which transport ceases. During loading with substances such as citrate (GOMORI and GULYAS), ethylenediamine tetracetate (SPENCER et al.) or sulfate (WALSER and BROWDER) which form poorly or incompletely ionized complexes with Ca, Ca excretion increases partly because of increase in the filterable fraction of plasma Ca but probably also because of decrease in Ca reabsorption. Calcium

excretion is extremely low at plasma concentrations below about 8 mg. percent
(Albright and Ellsworth) and most of such excretion that occurs is probably
obligated by complexing anions (Chen and Neumann 1955a). Above about
8 mg. percent (threshold) Ca excretion begins to rise significantly. At normal
plasma Ca concentration, excretion is about 1 percent of filtered load (assuming
65 percent filtrability of plasma Ca) and at 12—15 mg. percent during acute
loading excretion may be 10 percent of estimated load (Levitt et al. 1958). An
apparent Tm of 0.12 and 0.27 mM./min. was observed in 2 dogs weighing 15
and 22 kg. at plasma concentrations above 20 mg. percent (Poulos). Because
of the uniformly marked depression in filtration rate at these concentrations,
the constancy of the Tm values is not established. Available data suggests that
calcium probably has a Tm in man between 0.13 and 0.25 mM./min. (Bernstein et al. 1959).

Calcium excretion increases slightly to moderately during mercurial diuresis
in man (Keith and Whelan; Blumgart et al. 1932, 1934) and following injection of phlorhizin, dinitrophenol or azide to dogs, but increased excretion seldom
exceeded a few percent of filtered load. Following acetazolamide administration,
Ca excretion is reported to be increased in man (Barker, Elkinton and Clark)
and unchanged in the dog (Chen and Neuman 1955b). Strontium, chemically
closely related to Ca, exhibits a small to moderate depressant effect on Ca
reabsorption presumably by competition for reabsorptive transport (Chen and
Neumann 1955b). Calcium excretion is regularly increased (as is also phosphate)
in experimental acidosis in man (Albright and Reifenstein). The mechanism
is unknown. Filtration rate changes are irregular (Sartorius, Roemmelt and
Pitts). Plasma calcium concentration is unchanged or slightly decreased in acidotic
normal subjects (Sartorius, Roemmelt and Pitts; Schulthess-Sallmann) but
may increase in hypoparathyroid patients (Albright et al. 1931). On the other
hand, the filterable fraction of plasma calcium is increased (Hopkins, Howard
and Eisenberg; Toribara, Terepka and Dewey; Schulthess-Sallmann).
Calcium excretion, plasma calcium and filterable fraction are not clearly altered
in experimental alkalosis (Schulthess-Sallmann).

The parathyroid glands profoundly affect body balance and plasma concentrations of calcium and phosphate. In some studies in man or dog no clear
evidence that the parathyroids affected tubular calcium reabsorption has been
found (Albright et al. 1929; Albright and Ellsworth; Albright and Reifenstein; Jahan and Pitts; Ellsworth and Howard). In other studies on man
(Bernstein et al. 1959) or rat (Talmage and Kraintz 1954b; Talmage,
Kraintz and Buchanan 1955, 1959) Ca excretion has been depressed in hyperparathyroidism and in individuals on a low calcium diet as compared with hypoparathyroid patients and individuals on a high calcium diet provided excretion is
measured at the same plasma or filtrate Ca concentration. Calcium Tm is not
affected by the degree of parathyroid activity so that reported changes in excretion must represent changes in efficiency of reabsorption of filtered loads which
are less than Tm. Irrespective of changes in reabsorption of Ca, the principal
factor determining Ca excretion rates at various levels of parathyroid activity is
plasma concentration.

Factors determining the diurnal cycle of Ca excretion are unknown but are
probably related to ingestion and absorption. In some studies, Ca excretion
is maximal during the night (Norn), while in others it is maximal during the day
(Campbell and Webster 1921) or in late afternoon or evening (Wesson and
Lauler, unpublished). Ca excretion usually correlates better with Mg than
with Na, K, p_H or PO_4, but sometimes may differ from Mg (Campbell and

WEBSTER 1921). When the diurnal activity cycle was reversed, the cycle of calcium excretion also reversed (CAMPBELL and WEBSTER 1922).

Calcium excretion is increased in hyperthyroidism and decreased in hypothyroidism although plasma calcium and phosphate concentrations are usually unchanged (ALBRIGHT, BAUER and AUB).

6. Magnesium

Excreted Mg is that quantity of filtered Mg which escapes active reabsorption from glomerular filtrate. Although Mg is secreted by the tubule of the aglomerular fish in which it frequently is the principal urinary cation (MARSHALL and GRAFFLIN 1928; EDWARDS and CONDORELLI; MARSHALL and GRAFFLIN 1932; PITTS 1934; BRULL and CUYPERS; BERGLUND and FORSTER), no evidence of a tubular secretory system has been observed in mammals.

The region of the nephron where Mg is reabsorbed is uncertain. 'Stopped flow' studies indicate that a major reabsorptive site is distal to the proximal convoluted tubule (p-aminohippurate secretory area) and proximal to the first portions of the distal tubule (sodium reabsorptive area) (WESSON and LAULER; SAMIY, BROWN and GLOBUS) suggesting that the reabsorptive site may lie in the terminal segment (pars recta) of the proximal tubule. Extensive exchange between intratubular and peritubular Mg, as measured by radioisotopic Mg, occurs in the area of reabsorption (MURDAUGH and ROBINSON; GINN et al.). Magnesium and calcium appear to share the same reabsorptive area (WESSON and LAULER; SAMIY et al.; MURDAUGH and ROBINSON). They are competitive for the secretory system in the aglomerular fish (BERGLUND and FORSTER) and some competition may exist in mammals. Magnesium-loading in the dog enhances calcium excretion (SAMIY et al.) but calcium-loading increases magnesium excretion to a relatively small extent (WOLF and BALL; SAMIY et al.).

Because of difficulty in accurately measuring the concentration of Mg in glomerular filtrate, a satisfactory description of tubular transport of Mg under various conditions is not yet available.

Between 15 and 30 percent of the magnesium in normal human plasma is nonfilterable because of binding or adsorption to plasma proteins (WILLIS and SUNDERMAN; HOPKINS, HOWARD and EISENBERG). The fraction which is filterable is presumably subject to many of the variables which affect filterability of plasma calcium.

Daily urinary magnesium excretion in individuals on usual mixed diets is 5 to 15 mM./day (TIBBETTS and AUB 1937a). This represents 4 to 12 percent of the estimated filtered load. When subjects are transferred to an essentially magnesium-free diet (less than 0.1 mEq./day) urinary excretion decreases rapidly to about 1.0 mM./day (BARNES, COPE and HARRISON). Studies on magnesium excretion, like studies on calcium, are complicated by the fact that only a small and variable fraction, roughly 25 percent, of ingested magnesium is excreted in the urine.

The diurnal cycle of Mg excretion and factors that affect it are unclear. In some studies, Mg excretion has been greater during the night than during the day (NORN; DOE, VENNES and FLINK), while in others day and night excretion have been essentially equal (CAMPBELL and WEBSTER 1921) or it has been greater in late afternoon or evening (WESSON and LAULER, unpublished). In both circumstances, however, the cycle of Mg excretion correlates better with Ca than with Na, K or pH (NORN; WESSON and LAULER, unpublished) and is probably determined extensively by intestinal absorption. When Mg salts are infused intravenously in man, excretion rises rapidly. After a small increase in plasma Mg concentration, each additional increment in filtered Mg is excreted quantitatively with no evidence of tubular secretion. This suggests that the titration splay of the Mg transport system is quite small and that excretion occurs only when filtered load is close to Tm (HELLER, HAMMARSTEN and STUTZMAN; WOMERSLEY; HAMMARSTEN, ALLGOOD and SMITH; BARKER, CLARK and ELKINTON; CHESLEY and TEPPER).

Magnesium excretion in man is increased moderately by infusion of sodium salts of lactate, acetate, bicarbonate and p-aminohippurate. Excretion is increased slightly by probenecid and moderately by mercurial diuretics (KEITH and WHELAN 1926) and by calcium salts. The effect of Ca salts is not significantly greater than that of Na salts, however (BARKER, ELKINTON and CLARK). Unlike Ca, however, Mg excretion is decreased by acetazolamide possibly as the result of an average 15 percent decrease in filtration rate with this compound (JABIR, ROBERTS and WOMERSLEY; BARKER, ELKINTON and CLARK). Mg excretion is increased by ammonium chloride acidosis but is unaffected by KCl-loading (JABIR, ROBERTS and WOMERSLEY).

Mg excretion is affected temporarily by changes in parathyroid activity. Excretion decreases following removal of a parathyroid tumor and increases temporarily upon administration of parathyroid extract. In both circumstances, the changes in excretion appear to be greater than can be accounted for by changes in bone Mg (TIBBETTS and AUB 1937 b). The mechanisms are unknown.

7. Phosphate

a) General description

Phosphorus is present in the blood plasma in both organic and inorganic forms. Organic phosphorus is composed almost entirely of phospholipids which are bound to proteins and are filterable in significant amounts only under conditions such as nephrosis where glomerular permeability is increased. Inorganic phosphorus exists almost if not entirely in the form of orthophosphate (PO_4^{---}) and all references to "phosphorus" or "phosphate" unless otherwise noted may be assumed to refer to this substance. Phosphate is freely filterable through the glomeruli (WALKER 1933). Only during marked hyperphosphatemia or hypercalcemia does a portion of the phosphate become nonfilterable (GROLLMAN 1927; HARRISON and HARRISON 1941; LAMBERT, VAN KESSEL and LEPLAT; HOPKINS, HOWARD and EISENBERG). There is no chemical evidence that any significant fraction of organic phosphorus or phosphate esters is included in the usual chemical determinations of inorganic phosphate (LOWRY and LOPEZ; HANDLER and COHN 1951).

The question of the nature of plasma "inorganic" phosphate has remained open because of disparity between specific activity or urine and plasma phosphate observed by GOVAERTS and others during intravenous infusion of radioisotopic phosphate phosphorus. Following single injections or during intravenous infusion of radioactive phosphorus in man, dog and guinea pig the specific activity (quantity of radioactivity per unit of chemical phosphorus) is higher in the urine than in the blood at the same time. After one or two hours, the specific activities become equal (GOVAERTS 1947, 1947/48; STRÖM; ÖSTLING and TÖTTERMAN 1953, 1954; ÖSTLING and GÅSSTRÖM; FUCHS and FUCHS; GOVAERTS and MACHIROUX). During infusion of radioisotopic calcium, on the other hand, specific activity of urine and plasma calcium were essentially equal (GOVAERTS 1949). These observations suggested that some of the chemically determined plasma phosphate was derived from phosphate compounds which equilibrated slowly with inorganic isotope and which either were less freely filterable or, if filtered, were more completely reabsorbed than inorganic phosphate. This interpretation of the disparity between urine and plasma specific activity has received considerable criticism. In some studies, particularly those on man, venous blood samples have been employed without proof that the specific activity of venous and arterial blood is equal during infusion of radioisotope. Although the observations of Govaerts were confirmed by Handler and Cohn (1951), the latter found that the phosphate specific activities of plasma and its ultrafiltrate were equal thus eliminating incomplete filtration as an explanation of the differences. In addition, they observed that the same urine-plasma disparity of specific activity was observed in a dog which had received plasma from a donor animal in whom radioactive phosphate had time to equilibrate with various possible plasma phosphate fractions. They emphasized that the urine-plasma specific activity differences are compatible with the known rather long times required for equilibration between urine and plasma. Direct support for the concept that the disparity is due to equilibration delay is supplied by the experiments of Liljestrand and Swedin who injected a mass of inulin simultaneously with radioisotope in the dog. When the phosphate specific activity curves were adjusted to the experimentally observed equilibration delay in the inulin excretion, the urine-plasma disparity in specific activity vanished. Another possible explanation of Govaerts's results lies in the heterogeneity of the metabolic pool of intracellular phosphorus compounds, some of which exchange with radioactive tracer phosphate with extraordinary rapidity (Dratz and Handler). If the rapidly equilibrating moities can be assumed to exchange rapidly with intratubular phosphate as well, a mechanism is available by which activity from the plasma can bypass the glomerulus and enter the urinary phosphate ahead of that derived from glomerular filtration.

The mechanism of renal excretion of phosphate differs among various vertebrates just as do those of Ca, Mg, urea and many other substances. Phosphate apparently is secreted by the kidney of aglomerular fish (Marshall 1930; Marshall and Grafflin 1928; Edwards and Condorelli; Pitts 1934) and also by the glomerular kidneys of elasmobranchs (Clarke and Smith) and bird (chicken) (Davidson and Levinsky). In amphibian (Walker and Hudson 1937c) and mammal, phosphate is actively reabsorbed from glomerular filtrate, excretion representing the difference between filtration and reabsorption. In amphibia in particular, where the tubules can be perfused separately from the glomeruli by phosphate-containing fluids, no evidence of a secretory process has been found (Liang; Hogben and Bollman 1951a).

Evidence that phosphate can be secreted by the dog kidney has been reported occasionally. Phosphate/inulin clearance ratios above 1.0, indisputable evidence of secretion, have been reported during phosphate loading (Barclay, Cooke and Kenney 1947a, 1949) but such ratios have not been generally confirmed. When a mass of phosphate was injected into the renal artery of the dog, the fraction of phosphate excreted was greater than the fraction of a simultaneously injected mass of creatinine after deducting excretion from the contralateral kidney (Carrasquer and Brodsky). The data could be explained as well by transient depression of phosphate reabsorption as by activation of a phosphate secretory system. A phosphate secretory system responding to parathormone has been proposed since phosphaturesis following parathormone injection occurred in kidneys with tartrate nephrosis but not in kidneys with nephrosis from ureterally injected mercuric chloride (Nicholson 1959). Interpretation of this data is precarious because of the large number of assumptions which must be introduced.

When phosphate is infused intravenously, causing plasma phosphate concentration to rise, phosphate excretion rises rapidly. Ultimately, each additional increment of filtered load is excreted quantitatively indicating that an upper limit to phosphate reabsorption has been attained. Existence of such transport maxima has been demonstrated in man (Ollayos and Winkler; Barclay, Bray and Cooke; Anderson; Longson et al.; Thompson and Hiatt 1957a; Morgan and Williams), dog (Smith, Ollayos and Winkler; Pitts and Alexander 1944) probably in rabbit (Addis, Meyers and Bayer) but not in the cat (Eggleton and Shuster 1954a). Reabsorption occurs in those portions of the proximal convoluted tubule which are responsible for p-aminohippurate secretion and glucose reabsorption (Pitts et al. 1958a; Malvin, Wilde and Sullivan 1958a; Wilde and Malvin 1958; Rees et al.). When phosphate reabsorption is plotted against filtered load, a titration curve (D I 2) is generated which has a splay in man which is slightly greater than that for glucose (Morgan and Williams). Also, like glucose, phosphate Tm appears to be independent of reasonable variation in glomerular filtration rate in the dog (HARRISON and HARRISON 1941 a; AYER, SCHIESS and PITTS). The same degree of independence has not been observed in man (BARCLAY and COOKE) but the validity of presumed changes in filtration rate are unknown (LONGSON et al.). Most studies of the tubular phosphate reabsorption have been measurements of excretion under random, or uncontrolled conditions of filtered load. In a few studies, changes in Tm in physiological or pathological conditions have been measured by infusing phosphate to assure full saturation of the transport system. Titration curves, which are essential to determine the extent to which changes in reabsorption are due to changes in Tm or to efficiency of reabsorption at filtered loads less than Tm (titration splay), have rarely been made. Available studies indicate that the phosphate transport system is quite labile. Transport is depressed by glucose and by various anions in a fashion suggesting competitive interactions. Central to lability of phosphate transport in man, however, are the parathyroid glands whose secretion presumably can depress transport. Many changes in phosphate excretion or reabsorption observed during experimental procedures such as phosphate loading to measure Tm may be attributable to alterations in parathyroid function resulting from the procedures themselves.

b) Phosphate transport in normal man

Phosphate Tm in healthy subjects averages about 0.145 mM. (4.5 mg.) per minute with a standard deviation of 15 to 20 percent (BARCLAY, BRAY and COOKE; PITTS et al. 1948; LAMBERT, VAN KESSEL and LEPLAT; ANDERSON 1955; THOMPSON and HIATT 1957a). Sex and age differences are unclear. In 5 women between 40 and 50 years old, phosphate Tm (using creatinine to estimate filtration rate) averaged 0.131 mM. (NASSIM, SAVILLE and MULLIGAN). In 15 children aged 6 to 15 years, Tm averaged 0.20 mM./min.1.73 M^2 with a sigma of 0.04 (STALDER, SCHMID and GERSTNER). In infants, Tm averaged 0.12 mM./min./ 1.73 M^2 (McCRORY et al. 1952). Tm is attained at load/Tm ratios of 1.3 to 1.5 both in adults and children (STALDER, SCHMID and GERSTNER; MORGAN and WILLIAMS).

In persons following customary living patterns, phosphate excretion is lowest about the end of the sleep period and greatest in late afternoon or evening (BROADHURST; CAMPBELL and WEBSTER 1921, 1922; DEAN and McCANCE 1948). Unlike sodium and potassium which exhibit "intrinsic" diurnal excretory cycles, phosphate is closely dependent on the living pattern. In fasting subjects, both the morning minimum and the evening maximum occur earlier than in nonfasting subjects (SIMPSON 1929). The cycle was not altered by sleeplessness (KLEITMAN) but reversal or alteration of the diurnal cycle of activity and sleep is accompanied by corresponding changes in phosphate excretion so that the minimum and maximum occur in the same relative positions in the activity cycle (CAMPBELL and WEBSTER 1922; KLEITMAN; MILLS and STANBURY). The mechanisms controlling the phosphate excretory cycle are unknown but correlation between excretion and plasma phosphate, at least in normal subjects (HAVARD and REAY 1925; STANBURY 1958b), suggests that changes in filtered load resulting from intestinal absorption and intermediary metabolism of phosphorus is a major factor.

Phosphate excretion decreases during quiet standing (SIMPSON 1929; WHITE et al.) possibly as the result of decrease in filtration rate and increases during and immediately following moderate to severe exercise (WILSON et al.; HAVARD and REAY 1926; EGGLETON 1942, 1943), possibly as the result of increase in plasma phosphate (HAVARD and REAY 1926).

c) Metabolic and other influences on phosphate transport

Some situations in which phosphate transport is increased, decreased or unchanged are listed in Table 18. Many of these observations require confirmation before they can be accepted unreservedly.

Table 18. *Changes in phosphate transport in various conditions*

Reabsorption decreased

Acidosis (dog, man)[1, 28]
Alkaluria (dog)[2]
Cinchophen (dog)[3]
Cortisone and hydrocortisone (dog, rat)[4, 5, 32]
Cyanide (dog)[6]
Dehydroacetate (dog)[3]
Glucose loading (dog, man)[7–10, 27, 30]
Glucagon (man)[29]

Hyperparathyroidism (dog, man)[11]
Hypopituitarism (man)[12]
Hypothermia (dog)[13]
Malonate (dog)[3]
Phosphate loading (dog, man)[14, 15]
Potassium depletion, chronic (man)[16]
Urea diuresis (dog)[26]
Stilbestrol (women)[17]
Vitamin D sterols (man, rat)[18, 19]

Reabsorption increased

Calcium loading (man)[20]
Diabetes mellitus (man)[21]
Hypoparathyroidism (dog, man)[11]
Insulin (man, cat)[22, 29]

Mannitol diuresis (man)[10]
Phlorhizin (dog)[7, 8, 9]
Vitamin D sterols in Ca depletion (man, dog)[1, 18]

Reabsorption or excretion unchanged

Alkalosis, acute (dog)[7]
Azide (dog)[23]
Dinitrophenol (dog)[23]

Desoxycorticosterone (dog)[5]
Mercurial diuretics (man)[24, 25]
Xanthine diuretics (man)[12, 25]

[1] HARRISON and HARRISON 1941a; [2] MALVIN and LOTSPEICH; [3] SHIDEMAN and RENE; [4] ROBERTS 1952; [5] ROBERTS and RANDALL; [6] BAYLISS and LUNDSGAARD; [7] PITTS and ALEXANDER 1944; [8] COHEN, BERGLUND and LOTSPEICH 1955; [9] COHEN, BERGLUND and LOTSPEICH 1957; [10] SELDIN and TARAIL; [11] See text for references; [12] STALDER, SCHMID and GERSTNER; [13] SEGAR; [14] HOGBEN and BOLLMAN 1951b; [15] THOMPSON and HIAT 1957b; [16] MAHLER and STANBURY; [17] NASSIM, SAVILLE and MULLIGAN; [18] ALBRIGHT and REIFENSTEIN; [19] CRAWFORD, GRIBETZ and TALBOT; [20] HIATT and THOMPSON 1957b; [21] STALDER, SCHMID and GERSTNER; [22] EGGLETON and SHUSTER 1954b; [23] CHEN and NEUMAN 1955b; [24] KEITH and WHELAN; [25] BLUMGART et al. 1934; [26] MUDGE, FOULKS and GILMAN 1949; [27] HUFFMAN et al. 1958; [28] SARTORIUS, ROEMMELT and PITTS; [29] BUTTURINI and BONOMINI; [30] LEVITAN; [31] ROBERTS and PITTS 1953; [32] ARISON and STOERK.

Phosphate transport is reciprocally related to glucose transport, suggesting that some portion of the phosphate transport system is shared with glucose. In some representative studies in the dog phosphate Tm decreased 40 percent during glucose loading. Conversely, administration of phlorhizin which suppresses glucose reabsorption may increase phosphate transport 20 percent or more (PITTS and ALEXANDER 1944; COHEN, BERGLUND and LOTSPEICH 1956). A reciprocal relationship with glucose transport is also exhibited by acetoacetate and, in particular, by sulfate (COHEN, BERGLUND and LOTSPEICH 1956). A reciprocal, partial inhibition of transport exists also between phosphate and sulfate and phosphate and acetoacetate (COHEN, BERGLUND and LOTSPEICH 1957).

Phosphate reabsorption is depressed by other anions including bicarbonate (MALVIN and LOTSPEICH) and nitrate (COHEN, BERGLUND and LOTSPEICH 1957); and phosphate excretion in infants and adult patients is increased by p-aminohippurate or sodium thiosulfate loading (MCNAMARA and BARNETT; SCHNEIDER and CORCORAN; DESPOPOULOS 1958). Depression of phosphate reabsorption during alkaluria associated with respiratory alkalosis in the dog appears in disagreement with the decrease in phosphate excretion regularly observed in man during acute respiratory alkalosis (hyperventilation) (BRASSFIELD and BEHRMANN;

BROADHURST; STANBURY and THOMSON 1952; BARKER et al. 1957) and the increase during acute respiratory acidosis (BRASSFIELD et al.; HAVARD and REAY 1926; BARKER et al. 1957). In the human studies, however, filtered load of phosphate has not been explicitly measured or controlled, but plasma phosphate may increase during respiratory acidosis (HAVARD and REAY 1926). Increased phosphate excretion in man following acetazolamide (NADELL) is in agreement with the dog studies. The decrease in phosphate excretion in man acutely subjected to simulated high altitude may be due to hyperventilation (D'ANGELO). Reabsorption may be depressed during urea diuresis in the dog, although the depression may be secondary to hypernatremia (MUDGE, FOULKES and GILMAN 1949; HOGBEN and BOLLMAN 1951b), but not during mannitol diuresis in man (SELDIN and TARAIL).

An increased excretion of phosphate following mercurial injection in man has been reported (FARNSWORTH; BARKER, ELKINTON and CLARK) but an unequivocal mercurigenic phosphaturia was not observed in other studies in man (BLUMGART et al. 1934; DALE and SANDERSON) or dog (MUDGE, FOULKS and GILMAN 1949).

Probenecid has no acute effect upon phosphate transport in the dog (BEYER et al. 1951) nor does probenecid produce more than a very small negative phosphate balance in patients with disorders unrelated to phosphate metabolism (SPURR, FORD and MOYER; BRONSKY, KUSHNER and DUBIN). On the other hand, a decrease in plasma phosphate has frequently been reported in patients with high plasma phosphate concentrations associated with hypoparathyroidism, pseudohypoparathyroidism and related disorders when probenecid has been administered chronically (SCHNEIDER and CORCORAN; HOFFMAN, PASCALE and DUBIN; PASCALE, DUBIN and HOFFMAN; JACKSON et al.; BAER et al. 1957; BEIDELMAN). The mechanism is unknown, and a clear renal effect has been difficult to demonstrate (DESPOPOULOS 1958).

Phosphate transport is affected by several endocrine systems. It is depressed by cortisone, an effect which has been attributed to stimulation of the parathyroids since phosphaturia does not occur following hydrocortisone administration (5—50 mg./kg.) in the parathyroidectomized rat (ARISON and STOERK). It is almost certainly elevated by anterior pituitary growth hormone as indicated by the high plasma phosphate and known high filtration rate in acromegaly (REIFENSTEIN, KINSELL and ALBRIGHT). In hyperparathyroidism, reabsorption is usually depressed as measured by relatively high rates of phosphate excretion at relatively low filtered phosphate loads. In hypoparathyroidism, a normal rate of phosphate excretion can be attained only at high filtered loads, indicating an increase in reabsorption (ALBRIGHT and REIFENSTEIN).

Research on the nature of parathyroid-induced changes in phosphate transport has been complicated by lack of information on the chemistry of parathyroid secretion and by the probable existence of species differences in renal response to extracts of the glands. Extracts of the gland can mimic the effects of hyperparathyroidism in man by causing serum calcium to rise and phosphate excretion to increase, and can relieve the effects of parathyroidectomy in experimental animals (THOMPSON and COLLIP). The extracts are of a generally protein nature (THOMPSON and COLLIP; WOOD and ROSS; ROSS and WOOD) but under certain conditions the active principles appear to be partially separable from the protein fraction, suggesting that the activity may reside in polypeptides which are strongly bound to proteins of relatively low molecular weight (ROSS and WOOD; L'HEUREUX, TEPPERMAN and WILHELMI). Parathyroid activity travels electrophoretically with the beta and gamma globulin fractions in human serum and with the alpha globulins in the rat (L'HEUREUX and REICHERT). In addition, the calcium activity appears to be partially separable from the phosphate activity (DAVIES and GORDON; KENNY, VINE and MUNSON; HANDLER and COHN 1952; STEWART and BOWEN 1952; BERNSTEIN et al. 1960). Whether this indicates that the gland secretes two hormones, or whether extraction methods have split apart a single molecule containing two active centers is unknown. Since commercial extracts of the glands are assayed for calcium but not for phosphate effects (THOMSON and COLLIP), it is evident that preparations with equal calcemic potency may differ in phosphaturic potency. Variability in ratio of calcium to phosphate activity in various extracts could account for the great variation in phosphaturia reported in different studies (MILNE; DENT 1953; MUNSON).

Although the effects of the parathyroids on plasma calcium are quite uniform among various vertebrates (THOMSON and COLLIP) the same cannot be said for effects on phosphate excretion. In the chicken, extract causes phosphate excretion to increase either by a decrease in reabsorption or increase in secretion (DAVIDSON and LEVINSKY). No renal phosphaturic response to massive quantities of extract is evident in the normal sheep (LOTZ, TALMAGE and COMAR) and plasma phosphate is similarly refractory in the rabbit (COLLIP). In the dog, phosphate Tm has been found by some authors to be elevated (HOGBEN and BOLLMAN 1951 b) and by others to be unchanged (FOULKS and PERRY 1959 a) following parathyroidectomy. Administration of parathyroid extract to either normal or parathyroidectomized dogs is not associated with rapid changes in phosphate reabsorption, particularly in phosphate Tm (FAY, BEHRMANN and BUCK; JAHAN and PITTS; HANDLER, COHN and DE MARIA; HOGBEN and BOLLMAN 1951 b; FOULKS; FOULKS and PERRY 1959 b, c) but Tm decreases slowly over several hours in parathyroidectomized dogs (HOGBEN and BOLLMAN 1951 b). The evidence from some studies (FOULKS and PERRY 1959 c) suggests that an equally slow widening in the titration splay (lowering of the 'threshold') may occur in the normal dog without change in Tm, although others have failed to discover any changes in the phosphate titration curve within 6 hours (JAHAN and PITTS). Tm is decreased 24 hours after subcutaneous injection of extract, however (HARRISON and HARRISON 1941 a). Evaluation is rendered difficult by an apparent lability of phosphate Tm both in normal and parathyroidectomized dogs during prolonged phosphate infusion (HOGBEN and BOLLMAN 1951 b). In rat and mouse, parathyroidectomy is associated with an immediate decrease in phosphate excretion and a somewhat slower rise in plasma phosphate concentration. Parathyroid extract causes a prompt increase in phosphate excretion in the parathyroidectomized rat but little change in excretion in the normal rat except when it is given in large quantities (TWEEDY and CAMPBELL; TALMAGE and KRAINTZ 1954 a, b; TALMAGE, KRAINTZ and BUCHANAN 1955, 1959; STOERK and SILBER). The mechanism of the changes in renal phosphate reabsorption in these animals is unknown. In the above studies on dog and rat, and the same consideration applies to man, changes in reabsorption must be carefully distinguished from changes in excretion. When parathyroid extracts are administered, particularly by rapid intravenous injection, filtration rate generally increases acutely (HANDLER, COHN and DE MARIA; HOGBEN and BOLLMAN 1951 b). Also, in the dog as in the sheep (LOTZ, TALMAGE and COMAR), plasma phosphate may increase acutely (JAHAN and PITTS; HOGBEN and BOLLMAN 1951 b). Rearrangement ofe xperimental conditions could prevent the rise (HANDLER and COHN 1952) and an early (one hour) decrease in concentration associated with phosphaturia was observed in young, fasted dogs (LOGAN 1939). Increases in filtered load are quite sufficient to account for the increases in excretion.

The increase in filtered load, although transitory, may persist until alterations in transport have become detectable. A slow disappearance of parathyroid effect on tubular transport in the dog is affirmed by the studies of BRULL and CARBONESCO, who found that a normal kidney transplanted to a parathyroidectomized dog continued for several hours to excrete more phosphate than a kidney from a parathyroidectomized dog.

In man, phosphate Tm is not clearly increased above normal in hypoparathyroidism (THOMPSON and HIATT 1957a). Titration splay, however, is very small so that significant excretion does not appear until Tm is exceeded. Tm is somewhat decreased in hyperparathyroidism. In 2 hyperparathyroid patients Tm increased 9 and 26 percent following removal of parathyroid adenomas (SIROTA). The absolute values for transport in hyperparathyroidism are not easily comparable with normals because of variable degrees of renal deterioration. Injection of parathyroid extract regularly and rapidly increases phosphate excretion (ALBRIGHT et al. 1929; KLEEMAN and COOKE).

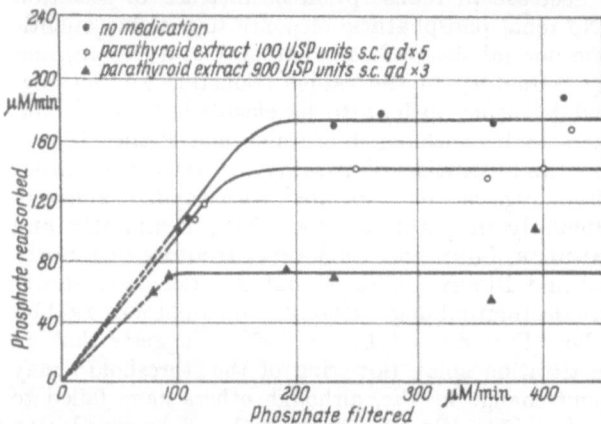

In normal adult subjects, much of the initial phosphaturia may be attributable to increases in filtration rate of 20 percent or more (KLEIN and GOW; HIATT and THOMPSON 1957a). Frequently, however, little or no increase in filtration rate follows injection of extract, in which case the decrease in reabsorption is unequivocal, begins rapidly, and is marked within an hour after injection (JACOBS and VERBANCK; BERTHOUD, COURVOISIER and

Fig. 59. Tubular phosphate reabsorption before and during chronic treatment with parathyroid extract in a patient with surgical hypoparathyroidism. After HIATT and THOMPSON (1957a). Reproduced by permission of the authors and the Journal of Clinical Investigation

ZAHND; GERSHBERG, SHIELDS and KOVE). Tm is decreased (JACOBS and VERBANCK), and titration splay is greatly widened as indicated by increased excretion at all loads. A more marked decrease in Tm (averaging 41%) is evident after repeated injection of extract (HIATT and THOMPSON 1957a). A marked phosphaturia follows extract injection in patients with hypoparathyroidism (ALBRIGHT and ELLSWORTH; ELLSWORTH and HOWARD). In these subjects, almost all of the increased excretion results from decrease in reabsorption both under phosphate loading (Tm) (HIATT and THOMPSON 1957a) and at less than Tm loads (CRAWFORD et al.) and relatively little from any increases in filtration rate (Fig. 59). A rapid decrease in reabsorption of about 20 percent also occurs in children and infants (KLEIN and GOW; McCRORY et al.) who probably can be considered functionally hypoparathyroid. Extract does not affect phosphate reabsorption or excretion in the various pseudohypoparathyroid states (ALBRIGHT et al. 1942; BERTHOUD, COURVOISIER and ZAHND; SMULYAN and RAISZ)[1].

---

[1] Pseudohypoparathyroidism: blood chemistry that of hypoparathyroidism, but resistant to parathyroid extract, in patients usually with characteristic skeletal changes (ALBRIGHT et al. 1942). Pseudo-pseudohypoparathyroidism: physical appearance and skeletal changes as in pseudohypoparathyroidism but blood chemistry normal (ALBRIGHT, FORBES and HENNEMAN).

Plasma phosphate concentration usually decreases rapidly following injection of extract in man (ELLSWORTH; ELLSWORTH and HOWARD; KLEIN and GOW) as it also decreases under certain conditions in the dog (HANDLER and COHN 1952). Early decreases lie in the range of 5 to 20 percent and in hypoparathyroid patients decreases seem greater than can be accounted for by increased excretion (MILNE).

8. Sulfate and Thiosulfate

a) Sulfate

In man, dog and probably mammals in general, sulfate is actively reabsorbed from the glomerular filtrate. In the dog, the titration splay is extremely small and excretion can be described very simply as that fraction of filtered load which is in excess of Tm (LOTSPEICH). In this respect, sulfate is probably the most nearly ideal of all known 'threshold' substances. In man, sulfate Tm lies between 0.04 and 0.10 mM./min./1.73 M^2 (GERSHBERG, HEINEMANN and STUMPF) but details of the titration curve are unknown.

Most information concerning tubular transport characteristics of sulfate come from studies on the dog. Radiosulfate enters tubular fluid in advance of filtered substances in dog and chicken, indicating that sulfate reabsorption involves bidirectional ion movements (BECKER and THOMPSON; GLOBUS, BECKER and THOMPSON). Sulfate excretion is increased by thiosulfate loading (BERGLUND and FORSTER; BERGLUND, HELANDER and HOWE) suggesting that these two divalent anions can compete for a common transport system. Collateral support for this view comes from the aglomerular fish, *Lophius*. In this animal, sulfate is actively secreted by the tubules (MARSHALL and GRAFFLIN 1928) and secretion is depressed by thiosulfate (BERGLUND and FORSTER). Competitive interactions are very extensive, however, and have been observed between sulfate and chloride (LOTSPEICH; BERGLUND and LOTSPEICH 1956a), nitrate (COHEN, BERGLUND and LOTSPEICH 1957), phosphate (COHEN, BERGLUND and LOTSPEICH 1957), acetoacetate (COHEN, BERGLUND and LOTSPEICH 1957), glucose (COHEN, BERGLUND and LOTSPEICH 1956, 1957) and amino acids (BERGLUND and LOTSPEICH 1956b). Osmotic diuretics such as urea, xylose and mannitol do not affect sulfate reabsorption, while the effect of aminophylline is unclear (BERGLUND and LOTSPEICH 1956a). The depressant effect of NaCl loading on sulfate Tm follows relatively small salt loads but nearly an hour is required for the maximal effect to appear (BERGLUND and LOTSPEICH 1956a). The depressant effect of glucose can be prevented by phlorhizin, while the depressant effect of amino acids on sulfate transport is proportional to the transport rate of the acid; that is, amino acids with high Tm depress sulfate reabsorption more than acids with low Tm.

Sulfate Tm is not affected by a single meat meal (LOTSPEICH) or by a high as compared with a moderate protein diet. In dogs on a low protein diet, Tm increased 75 percent above values on a moderate protein diet (GERSHBERG, HODLER and GASCH). The increase in Tm caused plasma sulfate concentration to rise although dietary sulfur was decreased. Sulfate Tm also increases during administration of cortisone (GERSHBERG, HODLER and GASCH) and growth hormone (GERSHBERG and GASCH) but not during desoxycorticosterone administration (GERSHBERG, HODLER and GASCH). In two patients with active acromegaly, sulfate transport maxima were 0.29 and 0.21 mM./min./1.73 M^2 compared with normal values of less than 0.1 (GERSHBERG, HEINEMAN and STUMPF).

14

b) Thiosulfate

Initial studies on man (NEWMAN, GILMAN and PHILLIPS; GALAN and FAEZ; BRUN; LANGERON et al.) and dog (GILMAN, PHILLIPS and KOELLE; PITTS and LOTSPEICH 1947) failed to reveal any evidence of tubular reabsorption or secretion of thiosulfate. That is, thiosulfate clearance was equal, within limits of measurement, to clearance of substances which measure filtration rate. Subsequent studies strongly suggest, however, that slow processes of both reabsorption and, more surprisingly, secretion occur. Lack of evidence of net transport in many studies must arise, therefore, from near equality between secretion and reabsorption. In female dogs given cortisone or testosterone for 5 to 10 days, thiosulfate/creatinine clearance ratio may attain values of 1.5 at plasma thiosulfate concentrations of 15 to 20 mg. percent (FOULKS et al.). Similar high clearance ratios are reported in untreated male dogs (LUETSCHER, pers. comm. to FOULKS et al.). In the cat (BING and EFFERSØE; EGGLETON and HABIB), rabbit (BING and EFFERSØE) and also in some studies on man (BLEGEN, ØRNING and AAS; BUCHT 1949; LAMBIOTTE, BLANCHARD and GRAFF), thiosulfate clearance was distinctly greater than that of inulin, consistent with a net secretion. Administration of caronamide abolished the secretory component of thiosulfate in man and dog and revealed a small but significant net reabsorption of the ion (BUCHT; LEBRUN; LAMBIOTTE, BLANCHARD and GRAFF; FOULKS et al.; BERGLUND, HELANDER and HOWE). Similarly, sodium benzoate in the rabbit depressed thiosulfate excretion and revealed a net reabsorption (EFFERSØE 1949). In some studies p-aminohippurate, diodrast and probenecid, did not depress thiosulfate clearance in the dog (FOULKS et al.) but in other studies, p-aminohippurate at sufficiently great plasma concentrations (25—50 mg. percent) depressed thiosulfate clearance in both man and dog (LAMBIOTTE, BLANCHARD and GRAFF). In the female dog, in which no secretion is evident under usual conditions, thiosulfate may slowly accumulate in the tubules in excess of the quantity filtered during brief arrest of urine flow (SULLIVAN et al.).

Since thiosulfate and sulfate depress the reabsorption of each other, it seems probable that both anions are reabsorbed by the same system (BERGLUND and FORSTER) with thiosulfate reabsorbed at about 0.65 times the rate of sulfate reabsorption (BERGLUND, HELANDER and HOWE).

9. Monovalent small anions:
Fluoride, Bromide, Iodide, Nitrate

The excretion of these three anions is correlated in a complex way with that of chloride but the exact reabsorptive mechanisms are unknown. Presumably, all three can share, to a certain extent, one or more of the chloride transport systems.

The radiofluoride/creatinine clearance ratio in the dog exceeds that of chloride but remains less than 1.0, averaging 0.3 (range, 0.06—0.77). The clearance of fluoride as well as chloride increases following chlorothiazide administration but the clearances of the two halides converge as the result of the relatively greater increase in chloride clearance (CARLSON et al.).

At low rates of bromide excretion in the dog, bromide is reabsorbed more efficiently than chloride, the clearance of bromide being half or less than the clearance of total halogen (McINTYRE and VAN DYKE; BODANSKY and MODELL 1941). The difference between bromide and chloride excretion tends to disappear as chloride excretion increases during mercurial or aminophylline diuresis

(BODANSKY and MODELL 1941) or as the bromide fraction of plasma total halide increases (BODANSKY and MODELL 1942; WOLF and EADIE).

The excretion of *iodide* as related to its plasma concentration (clearance) is greater than that of chloride in man, dog and rat. Reports that iodide clearance increases with increasing plasma concentration in dog and rat (RIGGS; HALMI et al.) have not been confirmed in man and dog (BRICKER and HLAD; GIEBISCH, MACLEOD and KAVALER). Irrespective of plasma concentration, iodide clearance in all three species rises rapidly with increasing rate of chloride excretion whether this results from mercurial diuretics (GIEBISCH, MACLEOD and KAVALER) or loading with mannitol or NaCl, $NaNO_3$ or $NaClO_4$ (RIGGS; GIEBISCH, MCLEOD and KAVALER; HALMI et al.). Iodide clearance also increases during bromide excretion (GIEBISCH, MACLEOD and KAVALER; HALMI et al.) but the effect of the latter ion is not clearly distinct from that of an equivalent quantity of chloride. Clearance is increased by mercurial and osmotic chloruretic agents (BRICKER and HLAD; GIEBISCH, MACLEOD and KAVALER). Saline diuretics which are not markedly chloruretic, such as ferrocyanide or thiosulfate, do not enhance iodide clearance nor does increase in urine flow by water loading enhance clearance (GIEBISCH, MACLEOD and KAVALER; HALMI et al.).

In man, under usual conditions, the ratio of iodide clearance to filtration rate is about 0.3 to 0.4 (CHILDS et al. 1950; MCCONAHEY, KEATING and POWER; BRICKER and HLAD) and is essentially independent of plasma iodide concentration within attainable limits (CHILDS et al. 1950; BRICKER and HLAD). When urine flow exceeds 10 percent of filtration rate, as during osmotic diuresis or following relief of ureteral obstruction (BRICKER and HLAD; BRICKER et al. 1957) the ratio rises rapidly to 0.6 or higher but never exceeds 1.0. Although iodide clearance varies with thyroid status, being lower in hypothyroid than in euthyroid or hyperthyroid man or rat (MCCONAHEY, KEATING and POWER; GILBERT and LANGE) the ratio of iodide clearance to filtration rate (C V 11) remains constant (HLAD and BRICKER; BRICKER and HLAD). Iodide clearance in the rat is depressed following adrenalectomy and hypophysectomy to extents compatible with filtration rate change and is not significantly affected by corticosteroids (PARIS et al.).

Nitrate which, like bromide, can replace chloride to a considerable extent in plasma in the dog, is also a potent chloruretic and obligates chloride excretion even when plasma chloride is quite low (HIATT 1940; GREENE and HIATT 1954). At low plasma nitrate concentrations and low chloride excretion rates, nitrate is almost completely reabsorbed. Higher plasma nitrate (10—30 mM./L.) regularly evokes marked excretion of both nitrate and chloride. Excretion of nitrate is greater than of chloride as related to their respective plasma concentrations, and at these greater excretion rates the nitrate-chloride clearance ratio in the dog is 4 to 6 (GREENE and HIATT 1955; RICE, FRIEDEN and SMITH). Mercurial diuresis during nitrate loading in the dog evokes a relatively greater increase in chloride than in nitrate excretion (RICE, FRIEDEN and SMITH). Although this is cited as evidence that mercury affects chloride specifically as between these two anions, the data is also compatible with an equiproportional depression in the total reabsorption of each ion.

VI. Passive reabsorption

Certain substances which can pass freely across cell membranes are present in plasma water. When such substances have passed into the lumen of the tubule with the glomerular filtrate they become subject to progressive concentration by tubular reabsorption of salts and water. Since these substances are capable of passing through cells, the molecules diffuse from the tubular lumen into the blood at a rate which is a product of their concentration difference and the ┊permeability of the epithelium. Among such substances are the rather simply described ethanol and acetone, the gases, oxygen and carbon dioxide, and the exceedingly complex urea and water. The role of passive reabsorption in the excretion of weak acids and bases has been discussed in section D III 5 a. Because diffusion between tubular fluid and medulla is the final stage of urine formation, the properties of the medulla and the chemistry of its interstitial fluid are important factors in the excretion of any tissue-permeable substance. The more permeable the substance, the more completely will its excretory pattern be determined by the medulla alone.

1. Some properties of the medulla

The potential for accumulation formed by the bunching of parallel loops of HENLE and vasa recta is described in section B VIII 4. If a metabolite is formed in the medulla (by synthesis or transport) its concentration will rise or (in the negative case of consumption fall) to values which depart greatly from those of plasma. In essence, the corticomedullary junction behaves as a barrier to diffusion out of or into the medulla. The magnitude of the difference between medullary and plasma concentrations is determined by the permeabilities of the tube systems, the lengths of the loops, the rates of flow (blood or urine) through the loops and the rates of flow through the two tube systems, the lymphatics and collecting ducts, which flow unidirectionally through the medulla. These elements represent so many potential variables, most of which have not been measured, that it is possible to do no more than describe some of the respects in which medullary fluid differs from plasma.

a) Medullary flows

The medullary blood flow is probably fairly abundant, but not nearly as abundant as cortical flow (DANIEL, PEABODY and PRICHARD 1950). From rates of accumulation of radioiodinated or of T-1824-labelled albumin, flow in the papilla is estimated at about 20 ml. of plasma per minute per 100 g. tissue (LILIENFIELD, MAGANZINI and BAUER 1960 b; THURAU et al.), a perfusion rate which is roughly 10 percent that of the cortex. Since the erythrocyte space of papilla is roughly half that of cortex (LILIENFIELD, ROSE and LASSEN), the high ratio of space to flow both explains and measures the slow transit of radiopaque particles through the medulla as compared with cortex (DANIEL, PEABODY and PRICHARD 1950). The medulla is heterogeneous, however, and both vascular volumes and flows are probably greater in the outer medulla than in the inner medulla and papilla (LILIENFIELD, ROSE and LASSEN). The importance of flow through the vasa recta lies in the high dependence of medullary concentrations on this flow. As conceived by BERLINER et al. 1958) the concentration gradient between medulla and extramedullary blood may vary inversely with perhaps the square of the flow, so that a small change in flow can cause a proportionally large change in gradient. Under some circumstances, cortical and medullary flow may vary more or less proportionally but under other circumstances, flow through the two areas may diverge: Autoregulation is absent from the medulla under circumstances in which it is present in the cortex (THURAU et al.); and papillary perfusion may decrease markedly during osmotic (mannitol) diuresis although total renal blood flow is usually little altered (LILIENFIELD, MAGANZINI and BAUER 1960a). The possibility is therefore great that the medullary flow is susceptible to control independent from that of the cortex and that medullary composition is controlled through the vascular system. The role of flow through the vasa recta is relatively simple to evaluate qualitatively since the assumption of high permeability of the vessel walls to all except erythrocytes seems admissible. The role of flow through the loops of HENLE and the collecting ducts is difficult to evaluate since no general assumptions concerning permeability can be made. Lymphatic flow is quite unknown.

b) Medullary concentrations

Cortico-medullary concentration gradients have been reported for plasma proteins, urea, sodium, chloride, total osmotic pressure, calcium, creatinine, amino acids and phosphates[1]. The list will probably be greatly extended as other substances are examined. Gradients are small and of questionable significance with respect to potassium and magnesium (ULLRICH and JARAUSCH; MALVIN and WILDE). Probably the most significant gradients, because of their probable importance in water reabsorption, are those of total osmotic pressure, urea, and Na and Cl, the solutes which contribute most of the osmotic activity of the medullary water.

Osmotic pressure was the first corticomedullary gradient to be described in a long-neglected paper by HIROKAWA (1908). Osmotic pressure of cortex was constant and slightly greater than that of blood (a difference now recognized as due to rapid autolytic changes (MAFFLY and LEAF). Osmotic pressure of medulla was much greater and varied in direct proportion to urine osmotic pressure. The findings of HIROKAWA were rediscovered by WIRZ, HARGITAY and KUHN and widely confirmed and extended (ULLRICH, DRENCKHAHN and JARAUSCH; APPEL-BOOM and BRODSKY; SCHMIDT-NIELSEN and O'DELL 1959). In nondiuretic conditions osmotic pressure rises progressively, although not necessarily linearly from cortex to apex of papilla. The degree of the concentration rise is closely correlated with the osmotic pressure of the urine but it does not necessarily equal that of urine. When urine is hypertonic, papillary osmotic pressure is usually somewhat less than that of urine (ULLRICH, DRENCKHAHN and JARAUSCH; APPELBOOM and BRODSKY) but occasionally, as in the sheep, may be slightly greater (SCHMIDT-NIELSEN and O'DELL 1959). At the apex of the papilla, the osmotic pressures of urine and medullary blood are essentially identical (WIRZ 1953). During water diuresis, osmotic pressure of inner medulla and papilla decreases to that of cortex or blood although urine osmotic pressure may be much lower. Osmotic pressure of outer medulla, however, tends to remain somewhat elevated with a pressure about twice that of blood (ULLRICH, DRENCK-HAHN and JARAUSCH; BRAY). During urea or sulfate diuresis, urine may be hypertonic to medulla while the corticomedullary gradient itself resembles that during water diuresis (ULLRICH, DRENCKHAHN and JARAUSCH).

The concentration of urea in the medulla may attain values up to 20 times that of the cortex (MARSHALL and CRANE; ULLRICH, JARAUSCH and OVERBECK; ULLRICH and JARAUSCH). Both the absolute medullary concentration and the gradient decrease during water or osmotic (mannitol) diuresis, in animals on low protein diets and following reduction in filtration rate (MARSHALL and CRANE;

---

[1] Most studies have been made by analysing serial slices of medulla cut parallel to the cortico-medullary junction. Such analyses yield the composition of whole tissue and generally do not permit more than rough conclusions with regard to the compositions of the intra-tubular, intracellular, interstitial and intravascular subdivisions of the tissue slice. Similar slices of cortex may be taken for reference.

ULLRICH and JARAUSCH; LEVINSKY, DAVIDSON and BERLINER; LEVINSKY and
BERLINER 1959b; SCHMIDT-NIELSEN and O'DELL 1959). The concentration of
urea in the medulla as a whole is almost always less than that of urine, and in
the papilla of the desert rat may be 1,000 mM. less than in the urine (SCHMIDT-
NIELSEN and O'DELL 1960). In view of a probably slow rate of movement of
urea from the papilla into the blood, these observations indicate a relatively
low permeability of the collecting duct epithelium to urea. Most of the increase
in tissue urea concentration occurs between cortex and outer zone, with less
of a further increase between outer and inner zones. This tendency is exhibited
in exaggerated form in the sheep on low protein diet, in which inner zone and
urine may have a lower urea concentration than that of the outer zone (SCHMIDT-
NIELSEN and O'DELL 1959).

Medullary concentrations of chloride and sodium increase at a nearly uniform
rate from the corticomedullary junction to the apex of the pyramid in dehydrated
animals, attaining concentrations at the apex of 250 to 400 mM./L. in rabbit,
dog and cat and higher values in the desert rat (SCHMIDT-NIELSEN and O'DELL
1960; LJUNGBERG 1947, 1949; ULLRICH, JARAUSCH and OVERBECK; ULLRICH
and JARAUSCH; MALVIN and WILDE; BARCLAY, CRAMPTON and MATTHEWS).
Lower maximal values are observed in pig and sheep (BARCLAY, CRAMPTON and
MATTHEWS; SCHMIDT-NIELSEN and O'DELL 1959). During either water or
osmotic diuresis, medullary concentrations decrease and become nearly uniform
throughout the medulla at levels only moderately exceeding those of the cortex
(ULLRICH and JARAUSCH; MALVIN and WILDE). To a large extent, the decrease
in medullary sodium concentration with diuresis represents displacement of
salt from the tissue rather than addition of water, since sodium content is also
decreased when expressed on a dry weight basis (MALVIN and WILDE). Comparing the NaCl and the urea gradients as functions of urine flow and composition, the NaCl gradient varies less than the urea gradient with variation in urine
flow, and is independent of dietary protein. Neither the NaCl nor the urea
gradient correlates well with the corresponding urine concentrations. However,
the sum of these two in the medulla correlates fairly well with the osmotic pressure
of the urine. The mechanisms of medullary urea and NaCl accumulation will be
considered in discussion of urea and water excretion.

Creatinine is concentrated in the medulla 4 to 12 times above the cortical
concentration in the dehydrated dog. Like urea, the concentration gradient
disappears during water diuresis (ULLRICH and JARAUSCH). Presumably, the
collecting ducts are not wholly impermeable to creatinine so that small amounts
can diffuse into the medullary interstitium.

Calcium and phosphate gradients, unlike those of urea or NaCl, do not necessarily vary with diuresis. Calcium increases from 3—5 mM. in cortex to 8—29
in papilla and may represent accumulated calcium phosphate deposits. It does
not vary with diuresis. Phosphates are a heterogeneous group, each member
of which must be considered separately. Phospholipids and adenosine mono-
and diphosphate decrease from cortex to papilla, while inorganic phosphate
increases. Both groups are independent of urine flow. Organic acid-soluble
phosphate, however, increases in concentration from cortex to medulla and also
varies with urine flow as does urea (ULLRICH, JARAUSCH and OVERBECK; ULL-
RICH and JARAUSCH; ULLRICH). Amino acids decrease in concentration in the
outer zone and increase again in the papilla to the cortical concentration. The
gradient is unaffected by diuresis (ULLRICH and JARAUSCH).

Medullary content of plasma proteins is high. The albumin space of the
papilla (the apparent volume containing albumin at the concentration of blood)

is about 35 to 38 percent of the total tissue (LASSEN, LONGLEY and LILIENFIELD; LONGLEY and BURSTONE; LILIENFIELD, ROSE and LASSEN). Since the corresponding red cell space is not nearly as large, the apparent hematocrit of the papilla is much below that of large-vessel blood or of other regions of the kidney (C I 3 d). Because radioiodinated globulin equilibrates in the papilla much more slowly than iodinated albumin, a large fraction of the proteins is probably extravascular (LASSEN, LONGLEY and LILIENFIELD). It seems unlikely, however, that the anatomical space occupied by plasma proteins together with red cells is actually about 40 percent of the volume of the papilla. More likely, the plasma proteins are restricted to a smaller space but at a concentration considerably exceeding plasma. A feasible explanation of such a concentration is the countercurrent multiplier system as described by KUHN and RYFFEL and by HARGITAY and KUHN. Plasma water, extruded in small amounts by hydrostatic pressure from the descending limbs of the vasa recta at any level, can enter the ascending limb at the same level. The extrusion results in a slight concentration of plasma proteins. The process of extrusion and concentration integrated along the full length of the loops of vasa recta can result in substantial concentration of proteins at the tip of the loops. Since the concentrated proteins, but not cells, can diffuse slowly into interstitial fluid space, the possibility of substantial protein accumulation is present.

2. Reabsorption of highly permeable substances

a) Ethanol and acetone

The urine-plasma concentration ratio of these two substances is very close to 1.0 in man and experimental animals at all plasma concentrations and urine flows which have been studied and is probably due to their diffusion through the epithelium as rapidly as the tubular fluid is concentrated. Since urine concentration is independent of urine flow, the excretion rate of these substances is directly dependent on the rate of flow. When plasma concentration is changing rapidly, as following ingestion of an alcoholic beverage, urine concentration is slightly lower during rising and slightly higher than that of plasma during falling plasma concentration. This difference is attributable to delay in equilibration of the substance between blood and renal tissue water and in passage of urine into the bladder. The rather long time difference between the occurrence in urine and plasma of the same ethanol concentration, which may be as long as 30 minutes (WIDMARK; HAGGARD, GREENBERG and CARROLL; BLOTNER; EGGLETON 1942a), is probably attributable to slow exchange between medulla and extramedullary circulation. Other ketone bodies, acetoacetate and beta-hydroxybutyrate, do not exhibit the same excretory pattern as acetone but are actively reabsorbed from the glomerular filtrate (STARK and SOMOGYI).

b) Oxygen and carbon dioxide

The tissue-soluble gases, oxygen and carbon dioxide, are also apparently excreted by diffusion since the urine/plasma concentration ratios of these substances never depart greatly from 1.0. Variations in the ratio are presumably related to renal metabolism. In dogs breathing room air, the urine/plasma oxygen concentration ratio is 0.5 to 0.6 (RENNIE, REEVES and PAPPENHEIMER). The urinary oxygen tension increases in animals breathing pure oxygen, but remains significantly less than that of renal venous blood and is not affected by temporary arrest of urine flow (RENNIE). The data are consistent with equilibration of urine with a low oxygen tension in the medulla.

The urine/plasma carbon dioxide ratio is very close to or slightly below 1.0 in acid urine in man and dog, but may exceed 1.0 and attain values as high as 2.5 in alkaline urine. The mechanisms causing deviation of the U/P values from 1.0 are unknown but are probably attributable in part to aspects of delayed dehydration of carbonic acid. Excretion of carbonic acid is discussed more extensively in section D V 4 d.

3. Urea

Few substances have a more diverse set of excretory patterns in vertebrates than urea. Urea is not actively secreted by the aglomerular fish tubule (EDWARDS and CONDORELLI; MARSHALL and GRAFFLIN 1928). It is actively reabsorbed from the glomerular filtrate in elasmobranchs by a process which is unaffected by phlorhizin or probenecid (SMITH 1931, 1936; CLARKE and SMITH; FORSTER and BERGLUND; KEMPTON 1953). In the frog, urea has long been known to be actively secreted by a transport system which is located in the proximal segment and can be inhibited by cyanide, p-aminohippurate, probenecid and dinitrophenol (NUSSBAUM; CULLIS; MARSHALL and CRANE; CRANE; HÖBER 1930b; MARSHALL 1932/33; CONWAY and KANE; WALKER and HUDSON 1937b; FORSTER 1954). In all other vertebrates including the amphibians *Necturus* (WALKER and HUDSON 1937b) and the Japanese toad (TERUI), birds (PITTS and KORR) and mammals, no clear evidence of active transport of urea has been found.

a) Descriptions of urea excretion

The first widely employed description of urea excretion is that of AMBARD and WEILL. They defined a "ureosecretory constant", K, which correlates plasma concentration, excretion rate and urine concentration and which roughly resembles in its dimensions the 'clearance' expression evolved later.

AMBARD and WEILL concluded that excretion of urea was directly proportional to the square of plasma urea concentration and inversely proportional to the square root of the urine urea concentration. Combining these 2 expressions in the arrangement used in later studies yields $\dfrac{U^{\frac{1}{2}} \cdot V^{\frac{1}{2}}}{P} = \dfrac{1}{K^{\frac{1}{2}}}$, where U, P, V and K are urine and plasma urea concentrations, urine flow and ureosecretory constant, respectively. The correlation of excretion with the square of plasma concentration in their studies instead of with the first power is probably the consequence of the great rise in filtration rate which follows feeding of meat to dogs as in their experiments.

VAN SLYKE and coworkers (AUSTIN, STILLMAN and VAN SLYKE; MÖLLER, MCINTOSH and VAN SLYKE; VAN SLYKE) found that urea excretion in man could be described simply as the ratio of excretion rate to plasma urea concentration. This ratio they termed 'clearance'. The relationship yielded a constant, however, only at urine flows above about 2 ml./min. (augmentation limit). At lower rates of urine flow, constancy of clearance, independent of urine flow, could be obtained only by dividing the urea clearance by the square root of the urine flow. The result of this operation, which measured the extent to which urea excretion was dependent upon urine flow and which, in essence, corrects the simple clearance to the value expected at a urine flow of 1.0 ml./min., was termed the 'standard clearance'. At very low urine flows (below 0.35 ml./min.), the standard clearance fails to yield constant values (CHESLEY). DOMINGUEZ and POMERENE (DOMINGUEZ 1935) eliminated some of the clumsiness inherent in using two equations (one for high and one for low flows) by expressing the effect of urine flow as an exponential term. Their equation, the last of the empirical formulations, did not offer sufficient advantages in relation to its complexity, however, to be adopted for clinical measurements.

These equations can be expressed as follows:

Urea clearance (simple): $Cu = \dfrac{UV}{P}$.

Standard urea clearance (MÖLLER et al.): $C_s = \dfrac{UV\frac{1}{2}}{P}$.

Equation of DOMINGUEZ and POMERENE: $C = A\,(1-e^{-kv}) + bv$. In the above expressions, U, P and V are urine and plasma urea concentrations and urine flow; A, k and b are constants.

REHBERG suggested that urea excretion in man could be described in terms of filtration from which variable amounts of urea are reabsorbed passively. This concept, that urea excretion should be expressed as a function of filtration rate, has formed the basis for subsequent descriptions. SHANNON (1936, 1938b) in the dog and CHASIS and SMITH in man showed that urea clearance could be described with considerable accuracy provided that filtration rate and

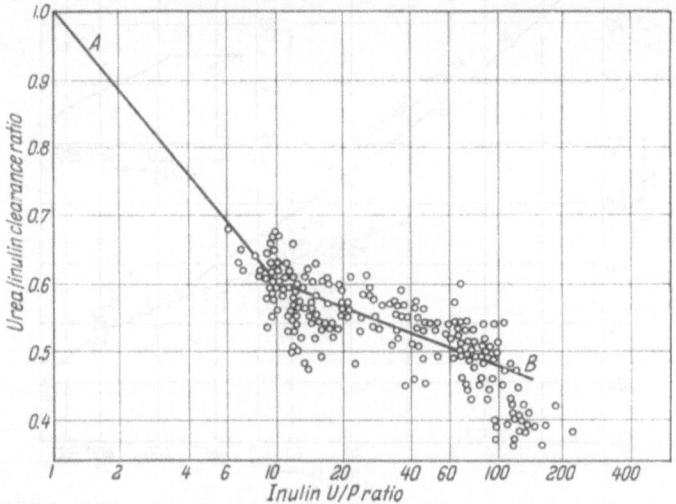

Fig. 60. The urea/inulin clearance ratio in man as related to concentration of the glomerular filtrate. Clearance ratio is plotted arithmetically and concentration, measured by the inulin urine/plasma ratio, is plotted logarithmically. Variations in U/P ratio were produced by water-loading. After CHASIS and SMITH. Reproduced by permission of the authors and the Journal of Clinical Investigaton

urine flow were known. Urea clearance as a fraction of filtration rate (urea/inulin or urea/creatinine clearance ratio) approaches 1.0 as urine flow approaches equality with filtration rate (that is, as the degree of concentration of glomerular filtrate, or inulin U/P ratio, approaches 1.0). This is the general pattern to be expected in a passive reabsorption system: the less concentrated the urine, the lower the urea diffusion gradient between tubular fluid and blood and the less filtered urea is lost from the tubules by diffusion. When no urea is lost, the clearance ratio is 1.0. If filtration rate and urine flow remain constant, then urea excretion must be a strictly linear function of plasma urea concentration. The diffusion process is quite evidently complex. To achieve approximate linearity between urea/inulin clearance ratio and inulin U/P ratio, the latter must be arranged logarithmically as in Fig. 60 and 61. Even so, two distinct limbs are generated. One limb, lying at low urine flows as measured by U/P ratios of 10 or greater is relatively flat and is usually generated by varying degrees of water diuresis. If extrapolated to maximum flow (U/P ratio of 1.0) the urea/inulin clearance ratio would be about 0.7 in dog and man. The second limb, lying at U/P ratios between 10 and 1.0, rises steeply toward a clearance ratio of 1.0 and is generated by osmotic loading. Because water diuresis is believed to be due to changes restricted to distal tubule and collecting ducts, while osmotic diuresis reflects alterations in reabsorption in the proximal tubule, the observations suggest that the lower limb measures the effects on urea reabsorption resulting from changes in urea concentration in distal portions of the nephron while the upper limb, at low U/P ratios, measures the corresponding effects caused by changes in concentration in the proximal segment.

A theoretical treatment by JUNG, in which urea is viewed as diffusing in accord with concentration gradient through the walls of a tube of uniform characteristics, successfully fitted limited data. A similar treatment by DOLE successfully fitted the data lying in the lower (water-diuresis) limb. Whereas JUNG assumed that

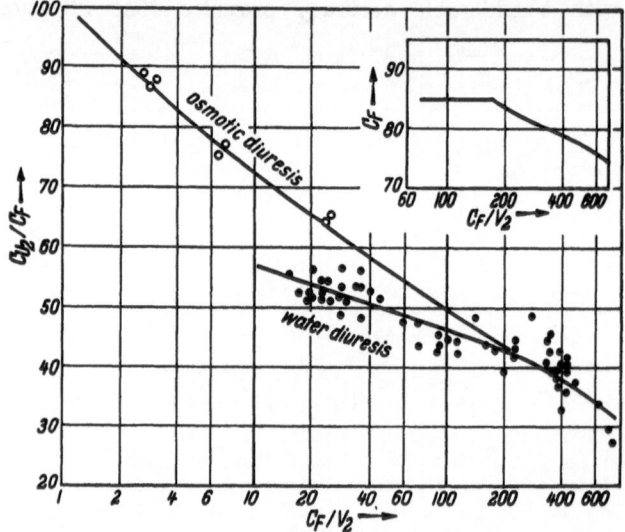

Fig. 61. Urea/creatinine clearance ratio, Cu_2/C_F, in the dog (dog G, SHANNON 1936, 1938b) plotted against C_F/V_2. Solid dots are data obtained during water loading; circles are data obtained during osmotic loading. Insert shows changes in filtration rate observed at low urine flows (high values of C_F/V_2) which accounts for the curvature in the 'water diuresis' curve. C_F and V_2 are filtration rate and urine flow. The lines are calculated from the theoretical equation (2). Reproduced by permission American Journal of Physiology

water was reabsorbed linearly, DOLE assumed that water reabsorption occurred as a single step at the beginning of the distal segment. The concept of JUNG was extended by WESSON (1954) to permit description of the effects of changes in water reabsorption in a two-component system, "proximal" and "distal", representing both the upper and lower limbs of the urea curves, and in filtration rate. The fit of this equation to data from SHANNON is illustrated in Fig. 61.

1) Equation of DOLE:
$$\frac{Cu}{C_F} = \Phi e^{-k_1/V_2}.$$

2) Equation of WESSON:
$$\frac{Cu_2}{C_F} = \frac{1}{k_1 + V_1 - C_F} \left[\frac{k_1 V_1}{C_F} - (C_F - V_1) \left(\frac{V_1}{C_F} \right) \frac{k_1}{C_F - V_1} \right] \left(\frac{V_2}{V_1} \right) \frac{k_2}{V_1 - V_2}.$$

In these equations, Cu and C_F are urea clearance and filtration rate, k_1 and k_2 are the permeability constants of the 'proximal' and the 'distal' areas of the nephron, V_1 and V_2 are the volumes of fluid issuing from the proximal segments and the collecting ducts (urine) respectively, Φ is the fraction of filtered urea absorbed in the proximal area.

The theoretical formulations of urea excretion described above assume that urea diffuses from a tube divisible, for practical purposes, into two regions which differ, one from another, in urea concentrations and in permeability. The fluid into which urea diffuses is assumed to have the concentration of blood. These assumptions seem entirely adequate for urea reabsorption from the proximal segment. Urea penetrates freely throughout the total tissue water of cortex without evidence of accumulation (CONWAY and FITZGERALD). During stopped flow, urea progressively disappears from proximal tubular fluid in the dog (ROBINSON et al. 1959). Isotopically labelled urea moves freely in both directions across the epithelium of the frog kidney (LOVE and LIFSON) and of both proximal and distal segments of the dog kidney (PENA and MALVIN). These assumptions are patently inapplicable to the medulla, where 'distal' portions of the nephron represented by the loops of HENLE and the collecting ducts flow through areas in which the interstitial fluid and blood contain urea at concentrations which not only are nonuniform but which greatly exceed that in the general circulation. Nevertheless, the medulla can, in operational terms, be described as a 'tubular' compartment from which urea is passively reabsorbed across the corticomedullary junction. This simplifying description of the medulla explains, perhaps, how the simple, 2-compartment system of earlier descriptions was able to provide a reasonable fit of the data, since the number and operation of the variables will be little changed in another system in which the 'distal' area is replaced by a medullary compartment from which urea can escape only by diffusion or by excretion. Questions for future research are measurement of the quantitative contribution of medullary blood flow and of the medullary urea concentration to urea transport across the cortico-medullary junction, and the extent of urea transport from the cortical distal convoluted tubule. Should the epithelium of this segment be significantly permeable to urea, then theoretical descriptions must be enlarged to provide a third area of urea transport.

The mechanism by which urea attains high concentrations in the medulla unquestionably rests upon the accumulating properties of that tissue, but in other respects is not wholly clear. Urea passes into the medulla from the collecting ducts of the hamster presumably by diffusion (KLÜMPER, ULLRICH and HILGER). In the dog, medullary urea concentration is rarely if ever greater than that of urine, suggesting that a major source of medullary urea in this species is derived from passive diffusion from the collecting ducts whose urea concentration is elevated by reabsorption of water. In protein-depleted ruminants (see below) and possibly also in the protein-depleted rat (BRAY and PRESTON) urinary urea may be lower than that of the medulla. The contribution to medullary urea from urea entering the medulla from the proximal tubules is unknown. However, from the circumstances that radioisotopic urea injected into the renal artery of the dog is excreted almost as rapidly as creatinine (CHINARD and ENNS), that such delay as is evident can be accounted for in the collecting ducts, and that the urea concentration in the loop, of HENLE is much lower than the concentration within the collecting ducts at the corresponding level of the medulla (LASSITER, GOTTSCHALK and MYLLE), it seems probable that little urea crosses the epithelium of the loop of HENLE and that the epithelium of the thin segment is, in fact, highly impermeable to urea. In this view, medullary urea concentration represents an intermediate point in the diffusion gradient of urea between collecting duct and corticomedullary junction.

b) Exaltation and abatement of urea clearance

When urine flow rises rapidly, urea/inulin (or creatinine) clearance ratios are observed which, for a few minutes, are substantially greater than the ratios observed at a later time when urine flow is constant. The changes represent an absolute increase in urea clearance rather than a decrease in filtration rate. The transitory high values of the clearance ratio have been referred to as 'exaltation' of the urea clearance, and values 50 percent or greater than those expected at the same urine flow under stable conditions may be observed (Shannon 1936). Alternatively, rapid decrease in urine flow is associated with lower than expected values of the clearance ratio and has been termed 'abatement' of the urea clearance (Schmidt-Nielsen 1958). The excess of urea appearing during exaltation and the deficit during abatement are compatible in the sheep with changes in the urea content of the medulla and probably also in the dog (Schmidt-Nielsen et al. 1958). During increasing urine flow, the diffusion gradient between collecting ducts and medulla presumably is reversed so that medullary urea is mobilized in the urine. During decreasing flow, the gradient is increased with the result that diffusion from the collecting ducts is accelerated. Reports of secretion of urea in mammals such as the kangaroo rat (Schmidt-Nielsen 1952) probably represent examples of 'exaltation' such that the clearance ratio exceeds 1.0. The possibility of such an event is favored in the rat by its large medulla with high urea concentration.

A phenomenon which is analogous to exaltation and abatement of clearance is anomalous urea extraction ratios. Normally, the kidney exhibits little evidence of synthesis or utilization of urea. The concentration of urea in renal venous blood is lower than that in arterial blood by an amount which corresponds to urinary excretion of urea. Occasionally, however, the urea concentration of renal venous blood may be momentarily higher than expected from excretion rate and may exceed the arterial concentration. Anomalously low concentrations may be observed at other times (van Slyke et al. 1934; Gordon et al. 1937). A possible explanation of the anomalous arterio-venous differences in urea concentration may lie in variation in renal medullary blood flow which could alternately mobilize or accumulate medullary stores of urea.

c) Metabolic and other influences on urea clearance

Because of its close dependence on filtration rate and urine flow, little value is derived from describing urea clearance separately from these two terms. The probable magnitude of urea clearance in various physiological and pathological states may be estimated to a reasonable approximation from known values of filtration rate in those states. Detailed reviews are available (Herrin). States of particular interest are those in which the urea/inulin clearance ratio departs from the expected values as represented in Figs. 60 and 61.

Urea/inulin clearance ratio is not significantly inhibited by certain inhibitors of active transport processes such as phlorhizin (Chasis, Jolliffe and Smith; Shannon and Smith), caronamide (Beyer et al. 1947b), or hypothermia (Andersen and Nielsen). The clearance ratio is significantly depressed by cyanide (Nicholson 1949) although filtration rate is not significantly altered. The clearance ratio is also depressed in mercurial or bismuth nephritis (Govaerts 1948), in tartrate nephritis (Nicholson, Urquhart and Selby), during excitement in the rat (Schmidt-Nielsen 1955), following acute decrease in filtration rate in man caused by blood sequestration or hypotension (Levitt, Levy and Polimeros), in adrenal insufficiency (Hills et al.) and in acute glomerulonephritis (Earle et al. 1951 b). The clearance ratio is increased in chronic glomerular nephritis (Chasis and Smith) and following relief of urinary tract obstruction (Bricker et al. 1957). The mechanism involved in these changes in urea clearance must necessarily remain unknown as long as the entire urea reabsorptive system is not understood. In some instances, such as those related to excitement, blood sequestration and adrenal insufficiency, decreases in filtration rate in an otherwise stable system (WESSON 1954) appear sufficient to account for much if not all of the change in clearance ratio, but the possibility of significant changes in fractions of water reabsorbed in different permeability areas as well as changes in permeability (or medullary blood flow in the case of the medullary compartment) cannot be determined.

The effect of diet, particularly of dietary protein content, on urea/inulin clearance ratio is ambiguous. In man, the clearance ratio is significantly greater during normal or high than during low protein diets. The differences are most clearly marked as between low and normal protein diets and at low urine flows (GOLDRING et al. 1934; NIELSEN and BANG; MURDAUGH et al.). At low urine flow, for example at inulin U/P ratios of 200, the urea/inulin clearance ratio in subjects on a low protein diet may be $1/3$ of corresponding values on a normal protein diet. At high urine flows (inulin U/P ratio of 10), differences between the two diets are not evident (MURDAUGH et al.). The effect of dietary protein in dog (SHANNON, JOLLIFFE and SMITH 1932a; SHANNON 1936) and rat (SCHMIDT-NIELSEN 1955) is of the same order of magnitude as in man. The effect of dietary protein change in ruminants, however, is of such a different order of magnitude compared with that in other mammals as to suggest the possibility that a different mechanism controlling urea excretion may be operative in these animals.

SCHMIDT-NIELSEN and her coworkers have written this interesting chapter in comparative physiology. When dietary nitrogen is abundant in the diet of camel and sheep, urea/creatinine clearance ratios are of the magnitudes observed in other mammals. During protein deprivation, however, as during growth, lactation or on a low protein diet, urine urea concentration approaches that of plasma, which is the lowest excretion rate possible in a passive reabsorption system (SCHMIDT-NIELSEN et al. 1957, 1958; SCHMIDT-NIELSEN and OSAKI). No changes of comparable magnitude occur in filtration rate, urine flow or plasma urea concentration. Acquisition of the capacity to conserve urea appears correlated with the ability of ruminants to utilize urea through the action of intestinal bacteria by protein synthesis (SCHMIDT-NIELSEN et al. 1957). The mechanism by which the changes in urea excretion are effected is unknown. The data suggest that the permeability to urea of some distal region of the nephron such as the distal convoluted tubule is subject to extrarenal control. Correspondingly, urea content of the inner medulla is low in the sheep on a low protein diet, indicating that urea reabsorption is completed before the fluid enters the collecting ducts (SCHMIDT-NIELSEN and O'DELL 1959).

Unlike ruminants, other mammals appear unable to utilize urea, even when on a low protein diet and for them urea is always a metabolite requiring excretion. Although objections have been raised against the view that permeability of the tubular epithelium may be considered as a more or less constant term in man and dog (BJERING 1949; SCHMIDT-NIELSEN 1958), there is no support for the concept that a facultative control of urea excretion exists to a measurable extent in these species. Available data concerning dietary influences on urea/inulin clearance ratio in man are interpretable in terms of non specific changes in factors such as filtration rate (Section C IV 5), intrarenal redistribution of water reabsorption and medullary blood flow, which variables are difficult to measure.

In infants, the urea/inulin clearance ratio is an approximately linear function of log (inulin U/P), with no clear division of the curve into two limbs as in adults. This probably reflects the great lability of inulin clearance in infants as related to hydration. At an inulin U/P of 100, the clearance ratio is 0.3 while at U/P of 6 it is about 0.9 (BARNETT et al. 1948a).

d) Thiourea and derivatives

Excretion of thiourea closely resembles that of urea in man and dog (NICHOLES and HERRIN; BERGMANN et al.) as related to filtration rate and urine flow. Like urea, thiourea exhibits exaltation when urine flow is rising rapidly (NICHOLES and HERRIN). Reabsorption of derivatives of thiourea is more complete than that of the parent compound at low urine flows, to a degree which is roughly proportional to their ether/water partition ratios (NICHOLES and HERRIN).

4. Water
a) General description

Normally, 85 to 99 percent of more of the water filtered at the glomeruli is returned to the blood stream. Although reabsorption occurs throughout most

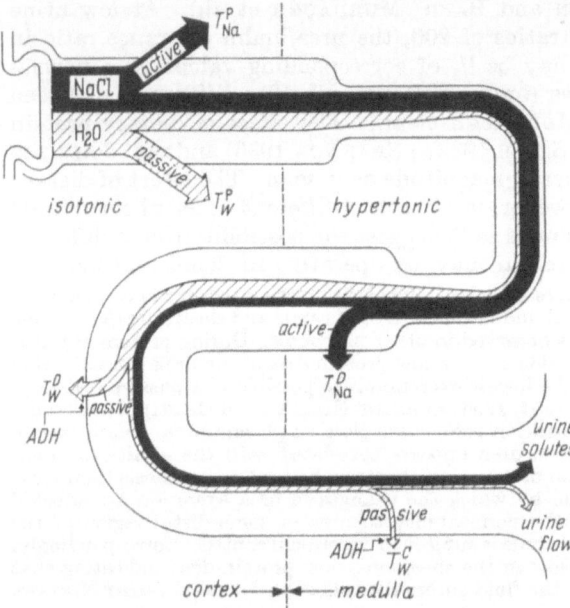

of the nephron, reabsorption is a far from uniform process. Our concepts of the excretion of water may be said to originate in CUSHNY's "Modern Theory". Earlier views had attributed water excretion to variable secretion on the part of glomerulus or tubules. CUSHNY proposed that urine was no more than the water and solids remaining after the tubules had reabsorbed an ultrafiltrate as nearly 'ideal' as possible. Water diuresis represented the water remaining after an 'ideal' plasma ultrafiltrate had been reabsorbed from a hypotonic glomerular filtrate. This view, although emphasizing the role of reabsorption, could not, however, provide an acceptable explanation of the antidiuretic action of posterior pituitary

Fig. 62. Diagram of water transport in the nephron. Water movements from the proximal, distal and collecting divisions are indicated by T_w^p, T_w^d and T_w^c, respectively. Principal solute movements are those of sodium salts, indicated by T_{Na}^p and T_{Na}^d

principles, and the volume of water released during water diuresis was greater than the excess water of dilution carried in the glomerular filtrate or even in the renal blood. REHBERG (1926) suggested that water (and chloride) reabsorption occurred principally in the proximal segment. BURGESS, HARVEY and MARSHALL, noting that hypertonic urine is formed only by those orders, mammals and birds, which possess a loop of HENLE, attributed to the thin segment the function of adjusting the final concentration. Reabsorption in the proximal segment was viewed as producing a normally hypotonic urine. Antidiuretic hormone, in proportion to its blood concentration, caused fluid issuing from the proximal segment to become variably concentrated and even to become hypertonic. SHANNON (1942a) followed BURGESS, HARVEY and MARSHALL in viewing the thin segment of the loop of HENLE as the site of facultative osmotic equilibration but attributed to the distal segment the property of concentrating the urine. SMITH (1937, 1947) and WESSON, ANSLOW and SMITH rejected this role of the thin segment but offered no satisfactory alternative. Adhering closely to the implications of the micropuncture studies of individual nephrons by

WALKER and his coworkers in the laboratory of Prof. A. N. RICHARDS, they viewed proximal water reabsorption as rigidly isosmotic throughout, and hence 'obligatory'. A hypotonic tubular fluid did not appear until the distal segment, where it was generated by selective reabsorption of solutes. The hypotonicity could be variably abolished or a hypertonic urine formed in relation to the blood concentration of antidiuretic hormone. Because of logical difficulties presented by assigning both concentration and dilution to a single process, WESSON and ANSLOW (1952) and SMITH (1951) combined the three-component system of SHANNON with the isosmotic proximal-hypotonic distal system of SMITH. They assigned the concentrating process to the collecting ducts where water was presumably removed from tubular fluid by an active transport process. Active transport of water was shown to be thermodynamically feasible by FRANCK and MAYER and by GRIM et al. Finally, WIRZ and others demonstrated that solute and water were reabsorbed in separate regions of the distal segment and that medullary hypertonicity rendered active transport of water in the collecting ducts unnecessary.

Three distinct transport systems are recognized (Fig. 62): a transport system located in the proximal convoluted tubule, T_w^p; a transport system located in the distal convoluted tubule, T_w^d; and a transport system located in the collecting ducts, T_w^c. All three transport processes have in common the feature that water movement is passive in the sense that water does not move against its concentration gradient or from a higher osmotic pressure within the tubular lumen to a lower osmotic pressure in the peritubular fluid.

The proximal and distal systems of water transport have been discussed in part in the chapter on sodium chloride transport. The proximal system is obligatory, functioning automatically at all times. The distal and collecting duct systems are facultative, the permeability of the epithelium being subject to variation under the influence of the antidiuretic hormone. The collecting duct system depends in addition upon the capacity of the medulla to accumulate solutes. Changes in any one of these systems will affect the flow and osmotic concentration of the urine.

b) Proximal tubular reabsorption of water

Throughout the length of the proximal segment in amphibia, tubular fluid is isotonic with or very slightly hypotonic to plasma (Fig. 33) (WALKER et al., 1937b; WIRZ 1956). At the same time, considerable quantities of water are reabsorbed as indicated by increase in phlorhizinized-glucose or inulin concentration of the tubular fluid to values 40 to 80 percent above those in the original filtrate (WALKER and HUDSON 1937a; GIEBISCH 1956; BOTT 1957; SOLOMON et al. 1957). When solute movement is arrested by introducing into the lumen of the proximal tubule a saline solution appropriately diluted with mannitol, net water movement ceases. These relationships permit proximal water transport to be defined very exactly since the fraction of filtered water reabsorbed in the proximal segment equals the fraction of filtered solute (expressed in osmotic pressure units) reabsorbed in the proximal segment (Fig. 36)[1] (WINDHAGER et al.; WHITTEMBURY et al. 1959a). Plasma albumin at a concentration of about 3 percent did not significantly affect water transport from the proximal tubule of *Necturus* (WHITTEMBURY et al. 1959a). However, colloidal solutions perfused

---

[1] When expressed symbolically, this takes the form:

$$\frac{T_w^p}{\text{GFR}} = \frac{T_{osm}^p}{P_{osm}} \cdot \text{GFR} \qquad \text{or,} \qquad T_w^p = T_{osm}^p / P_{osm}$$

through the portal circulation of the frog are reported to decrease urine flow (HEYM).

The bidirectional permeability of the proximal segment to water is extremely high, which accounts for the circumstance that the tubular fluid is seldom if ever significantly hypotonic to plasma (HOSHIKO, SWANSON and VISSCHER; SWANSON and VISSCHER; WHITTEMBURY et al. 1959a; TOSTESON and WHITE). Chick mesonephric proximal tubules *in vitro* are, however, reported to generate a hypotonicity of 4 to 15 percent below ambient TYRODE's medium (KEOSIAN). Correspondingly, in the mammal (rat, guinea pig) large quantities of fluid are

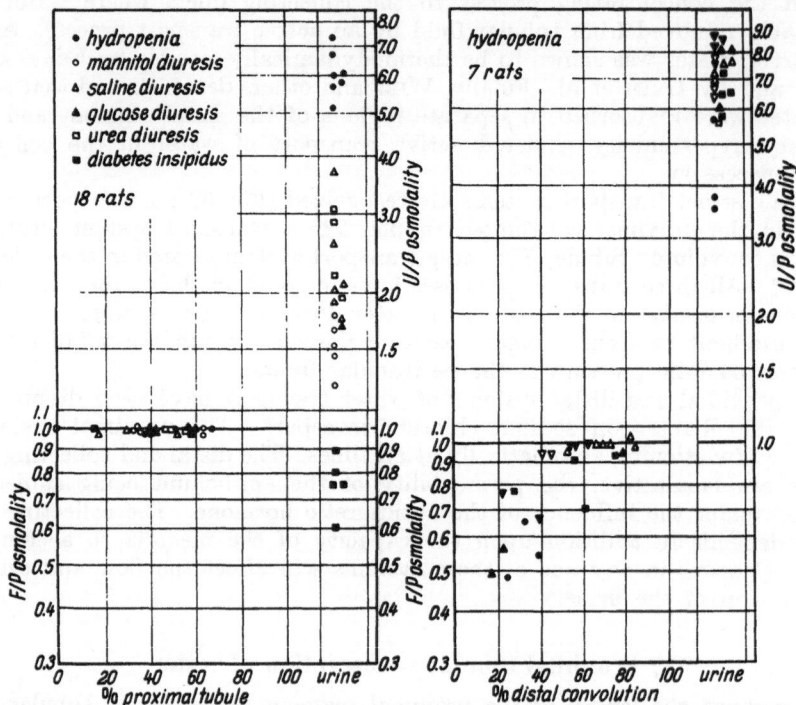

Fig. 63. Osmotic concentration ratio of tubular fluid to plasma (F/P) obtained by micropuncture in the rat. Left: the F/P ratio in the proximal tubule is isosmotic (close to 1.0) throughout irrespective of the simultaneous concentration ratio in the urine (U/P). Right: Distal tubular fluid is invariably hypotonic (F/P less than 1.0) at the beginning of the segment during hydropenia but becomes isosmotic near the distal end of the segment. Urine hypertonicity appears distal to the distal convoluted tubule in the collecting ducts. After GOTTSCHALK and MYLLE (1959). Reproduced by permission of the authors and the American Journal of Physiology

reabsorbed in the proximal segment as measured by a 2.5 to 3 fold concentration of filtered substances at the midpoint of the segment (Fig. 35). Nevertheless, proximal tubular fluid is at all times isotonic with plasma (Fig. 34 and 63) (WALKER et al. 1941; GOTTSCHALK and MYLLE 1959) and is unaffected by induction of water diuresis or administration of antidiuretic hormone, vasopressin (WIRZ 1955a, 1956).

c) Distal tubular reabsorption of water (dilution system)

Operations upon tubular fluid as it traverses the loop of HENLE were, until recently, largely speculative. It is now reasonably clear from micropuncture studies (GOTTSCHALK and MYLLE 1958), which confirm earlier experiments with ferrocyanide indicator (GERSH and STIEGLITZ; GERSH; HOWELL and GERSH), that tubular fluid becomes progressively more concentrated as it passes deeper into the medulla along the descending limb. At any level of the medulla, the tubular fluid has approximately the osmotic pressure common to that level of the medulla (WIRZ, HARGITAY and KUHN; BRAY) and to the collecting duct urine at that level (GOTTSCHALK and MYLLE 1958; LASSITER, GOTTSCHALK and MYLLE). As the fluid returns to the cortex along the ascending limb, it becomes progressively more dilute and presumably is not far from isosmotic when it reaches the broad segment of the ascending limb in the outer zone of the medulla. From this point the tubular fluid presumably becomes rapidly hypotonic. The only direct evidence that this hypotonicity results from reabsorption of sodium chloride (the only solute available in sufficient amounts) rather than secretion

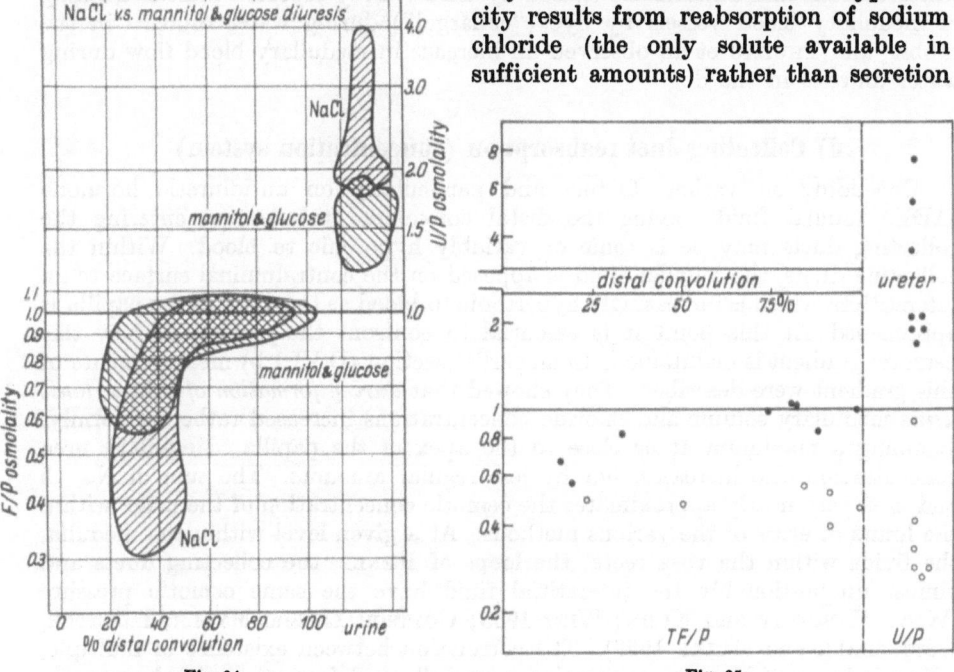

Fig. 64.

Fig. 65

Fig. 64. Osmotic concentration ratios of distal tubular fluid to plasma (F/P) in the rat during saline or mannitol diuresis. Mannitol, which as a nonreabsorbable solute obligates water excretion, causes early distal fluid to be less hypotonic and urine to be less hypertonic than does saline. After GOTTSCHALK and MYLLE (1959). Reproduced by permission of the authors and the American Journal of Physiology

Fig. 65. Osmotic concentration ratio of distal tubular fluid to plasma (TF/P) during hydropenia (dots) and watertype (ethanol) diuresis in the rat (circles). During water diuresis, early distal tubular fluid remains hypotonic and the urine (ureter) is hypotonic. After WIRZ (1956). Reproduced by permission of the author and Helvetica Physiologica Pharmacologica Acta

of water is that concentration of solutes destined for excretion does not decrease during formation of hypotonic tubular fluid in amphibia (BOTT 1957). Indirectly, it seems unlikely that water would be continually secreted only to be reabsorbed again more distally. Hypotonicity of the tubular fluid persists as far as the pars convoluta of the distal tubule within the cortex (Figs. 63—65) (WALKER et al. 1941; WIRZ 1956; GOTTSCHALK and MYLLE 1959). The hypotonicity is greater during saline loading than during mannitol loading (Fig. 64), probably because mannitol, unlike NaCl, cannot be abstracted from tubular fluid. From the beginning of the pars convoluta, water transport and composition of the tubular fluid depend on antidiuretic hormone of the posterior pituitary. When antidiuretic hormone (ADH) secretion is suppressed, as during ethanol narcosis in the rat (Fig. 65), the epithelium remains essentially impermeable to water. The tubular fluid remains hypotonic and is discharged into the bladder as hypotonic urine. In the presence of sufficient quantities of ADH, tubular fluid rapidly becomes isotonic with plasma (Figs. 63—65) and unquestionably because ADH has rendered the epithelium more permeable to water (Wirz 1956). Even in the presence of unknown but considerable quantities of circulating ADH, the distal tubule of the dog is substantially less permeable to water than the proximal segment (Tosteson and White).

Preliminary studies suggest that medullary blood flow varies as between water diuresis and antidiuresis caused by ADH. Frey reported increased filling of medullary blood vessels by dye ("collargol") during water diuresis in the rabbit; and Thurau et al. observed an increase in medullary blood flow during water diuresis in the dog.

d) Collecting duct reabsorption (concentration system)

Depending on various factors and particularly on antidiuretic hormone (ADH) tubular fluid leaving the distal convoluted tubule and entering the collecting ducts may be isotonic or variably hypotonic to blood. Within the collecting ducts, the tubular fluid is apposed on the contraluminal surface to an interstitium which is increasingly hypertonic to blood as the apex of the papilla is approached. At this point it is essential to confront the problem of how this osmotic gradient is maintained. In an earlier section (D VI 1 b) measurements of this gradient were described. They showed that *during formation of a hypertonic urine* medullary sodium and chloride concentrations increased rather uniformly, attaining a maximum at or close to the apex of the papilla. Medullary urea concentration also increases, but by less regular amounts. The sum of Na, Cl and urea very nearly approximates the osmotic concentration of the urine within the limits of error of the various methods. At a given level within the medulla, the fluids within the vasa recta, the loops of Henle, the collecting ducts and almost unquestionably the interstitial fluid have the same osmotic pressure (Wirz, Hargitay and Kuhn; Wirz 1953; Gottschalk and Mylle; Lassiter, Gottschalk and Mylle 1959). The correlation between existence of multiple, adjacent loops of Henle constituting a medulla and formation of a hypertonic urine is so overwhelming, as noted by Burgess, Harvey and Marshall, as to be considered a demonstrated fact. Of particular importance is the observation that it is the medullary structure itself, and not the thin segment, which is essential for urine concentration. In birds, and in mammals such as pig, and certain rodents (beaver and *Aplodontia*) an inner medulla is absent and the thin segment is short and frequently absent, particularly in birds (v. Möllendorf; Sperber 1944; O'Dell and Schmidt-Nielsen; Nungesser et al.). In these species, osmotic concentration of the urine to values 2 to 3 times the plasma is usual. Elongation of the thin segment to form an inner medulla apparently represents an elaboration of the intrinsic medullary concentrating system. A clear correlation exists between maximal urinary concentration and percentage of nephrons with loops entering the inner medulla (long loops) and the length of those loops (Howell and Gersh; Sperber 1944; Vimtrup 1949; Barclay, Crampton and Matthews). In carnivores (dog and cat) most or all of the loops of Henle enter the inner medulla, and this group forms more concentrated urine than man, in whom only a fraction of the nephrons form long loops. In the rodents, short loop nephrons are present but the long loops may be extremely long. Development of medulla and particularly the papilla in association with extremely long loops of HENLE is maximal in desert rodents, which excrete extremely concentrated urine (KOEFOED; SCHMIDT-NIELSEN, SCHMIDT-NIELSEN and SCHNEIDERMAN).

Solutions to the problem of medullary accumulation which could explain many observations have been proposed by HARGITAY and KUHN, and WIRZ (1956) and by BERLINER et al. (1958). HARGITAY and KUHN demonstrated that hydrostatic pressure within the loops of HENLE and transferring water from the descending to the ascending limbs cannot, alone, account for the known urine volumes and concentrations and they and WIRZ suggested as an alternative source of energy that sodium and chloride could be transported from the ascending to the descending limb of the loop of HENLE throughout its length, thus carrying an increasingly concentrated tubular fluid to the apex of the loop. At no point need the sodium concentration gradient between the two limbs be large yet a high concentration could be delivered to the apex of the loop (counter-current multiplier). In the system of WIRZ, it is also essential to postulate that the ascending limb be impervious to water while the descending limb is pervious. Thus, water is able to move into the descending limb from the collecting ducts in relation to absorbed sodium. BERLINER, however, proposed that sodium and chloride are transported into the medullary interstitium at the apex of the loops. The hypotonic fluid thus formed continues into the distal convoluted tubule to be reabsorbed or not according to ADH concentration. The experimental evidence, noted above, indicates that, if either of these two processes is operative, it is not sufficient to produce a measurable change in the osmotic pressure of fluid within the loops. Nevertheless, this evidence is not a sufficient reason for rejecting either of these hypotheses. In the steady state, the fluid in the ascending limb need be hypotonic to the descending limb only to the extent of the quantity of water entering the medulla from the collecting ducts. This quantity may be so small as a fraction of the total flow through the loops of HENLE that the degree of dilution is not readily detectable by current methods. An alternative view represents a rearrangement and combination within the loop of HENLE of the water transport and the salt transport concepts of HARGITAY and KUHN. In this view, the initial step in medullary accumulation is reabsorption of salt without water within the broad ascending segment of the loop of HENLE in the outer zone of the medulla. Large quantities of sodium chloride are removed from the tubular fluid creating a rapid decrease in its osmotic pressure. The hypotonicity does not become marked within the confines of the medulla itself (BRAY), however, indicating that only a fraction of distal sodium transport is available for medullary accumulation. The solute which is accumulated within the medulla is sufficient in amount to account for observed urinary concentrations. This salt effects an initial concentration of fluid in the adjacent first portions of the thin segment and therefore is the partial equivalent of salt exchange across the loops. Considerable concentration might be attained by the countercurrent multiplier principle within the limited thickness of the inner stripe. Although solute transport in the outer medulla should be associated with a marked increase in osmotic concentration in this area, an abrupt increase in concentration in the outer medulla as compared with cortex is not evident during formation of a concentrated urine. A system must be postulated by which accumulated solute can be transported from the outer to the inner medulla, but no experimental basis for such a system is yet clearly evident although the function is assignable hypothetically to the thin segments. The loops of the thin segment, by transporting water from the descending to the ascending limb, again according to the countercurrent multiplier principle, may accumulate solute in a high concentration at the apex of the loop. The energy for the water transport could be the hydrostatic pressure gradient across the loop which, in the rat, may be 15 to 20 millimeters of mercury (C I 1 d). Since the primary function of the thin segment has in this view become the lending of efficiency to the concentrating process and is not required to perform the major work of concentration, a very small hydrostatic pressure may suffice for establishment of a medullary concentration gradient increasing to the papilla.

Radioisotopic sodium injected intravenously in the rat is rapidly accumulated in high concentration in the medulla, beginning with the papilla (KRAKUSIN and JENNINGS), but these studies cannot distinguish clearly between entry by the *vasa recta* and entry by the loops of HENLE. During stopped-flow, radioisotopic sodium enters the medulla of the dog nearly twice as rapidly as tritiated water which attains only about 20 percent of equality between medulla and blood in five minutes (WHITE, TOSTESON and ROLF). Radioisotopic sodium is excreted more rapidly than creatinine following a single injection into the renal artery of the dog, indicating that medullary sodium probably does not interchange freely with intratubular sodium (CHINARD and ENNS) as would seem to be implicit in the concept of WIRZ.

No provision for urea exists in these concepts of medullary solute accumulation. Most of the available data is interpretable in terms of a slow, passive diffusion of urea from the collecting ducts into the medullary interstitium. Nevertheless, observations such as those of SCHMIDT-NIELSEN and O'DELL (1959) on the sheep, in which urea is accumulated in the outer medulla, and of the effects of urea on water excretion require that the possibility of active medullary accumulation of urea be retained for the present.

Reabsorption of water in the collecting ducts is demonstrated both indirectly as the difference in concentration between urine and fluid in the distal convoluted tubule, and directly by analyses of collecting duct fluid (HILGER, KLÜMPER and ULLRICH). The water transport must be considered as a process of passive diffusion from tubule into medulla since energy is not necessary to effect transport (HIROKAWA). Permeability of the collecting ducts may be under the control of ADH but this is not proven. The inference is supported by the intramedullary osmotic concentrations attained during water diuresis (which, although depressed, do not approach that of the urine) and by localization of radioisotopically labelled (I^{131}) vasopressin in the collecting ducts as well as the distal convoluted tubule (DARMADY and STRANACK).

During diuresis, large quantities of isotonic fluid enter the collecting ducts and appear in the urine at concentrations considerably below those observed at low urine flows. During solute diuresis (urea, sulfate, mannitol) in the presence of vasopressin, the urine is slightly to moderately hypertonic indicating that water has been abstracted from the tubular fluid within the medulla. Medullary osmotic pressure decreases, particularly in the papilla. Osmotic pressure and sodium concentration attain maximum values in the outer half of the inner zone (that is, close to the outer zone), where the osmotic concentration may be roughly twice that of blood. These concentrations may then be essentially uniform throughout the inner zone (ULLRICH, DRENCKHAHN and JARAUSCH; ULLRICH and JARAUSCH; MALVIN and WILDE). During water diuresis, however, urine is hypotonic to blood. Medullary concentration may be somewhat lower toward the papilla from the maximum closer to the cortex (ULLRICH, DRENCKHAHN and JARAUSCH) but the concentration does not become hypotonic. Thus, water diuresis is the only circumstance in which disparity exists between the osmotic pressures of collecting duct fluid and medullary fluid. Presumably, this is attributable to decreased permeability of the collecting ducts in the absence of vasopressin. Decrease in medullary osmotic pressure must be attributed to increased rate of water transport during solute diuresis and to residual permeability of the duct epithelium to water during water diuresis. Existence of such a residual permeability is implied by the observations that inulin may be somewhat concentrated in the collecting ducts during water diuresis in the hamster (HILGER, KLÜMPER and ULLRICH) and that both osmotic pressure and inulin concentration of urine arrested in the collecting ducts during water diuresis may increase, the former attaining an osmotic pressure 26 percent greater than blood (MUR-DAUGH, GALLOWAY and HAYES; JAENIKE and BERLINER).

The maximum rate of water removal from the collecting duct urine, Tm_w^c (see below), during osmotic diuretic conditions and after a steady state has been attained, necessarily equals the rate at which solute-free water leaves the medulla. Whether solute-free water leaves the medulla by being transported into vessels, or is generated by removal of salt from the loop of HENLE, is not completely resolved. If the latter mechanism, which seems more likely, is true, then Tm_w^c constitutes an approximate measure of the rate of transport of water-free solute into the medulla.

e) Osmolar and free-water clearances

Urine is considered to be concentrated or dilute according to whether it has an osmotic pressure (OP) which is greater or less than that of the concurrent plasma. Conventional values of OP as measured in millimeters of mercury or of weight per unit area are temperature-dependent and of less use than the relative differences between the OPs of various fluids. A convenient relative measure is obtained by expressing the quantity of osmotically active solutes in a fluid in molar units as estimated from depression of the freezing point. A 1.0 molal (1.0 gram mole per kilogram of water) solution of an 'ideal' solute (no dissociation, no binding of water, no interactions between particles) has a freezing point depression of 1.86° C. Any other solution containing nonideal solutes irrespective of their concentrations but with a freezing point depression of 1.86° C is defined as a 1.0 osmolal (or 1000 milliosmolal) solution and the units of solute per kilogram of water are termed osmols or milliosmols. The number of milliosmols per kilogram of water is, by definition, a linear function of the depression of the freezing point. The terms 'osmolarity' and 'osmolality' have been employed interchangeably to designate the concentration of solutions in osmolal units and both terms refer to the same standard of reference. Although the relative osmotic strengths of two solutions at 37° C may differ slightly from their relative strengths at 0° C, the error is small.

If urine has the same osmotic concentration as plasma, then no separation of water from solute has occurred in the overall operation of urine formation. If, on the other hand, the concentration of urine is different from plasma, then separation has occurred. The quantity of water which has been thus separated is termed the 'free-water clearance', C_w. In a concentrated urine, C_w is measured as the amount of water which must be restored to the urine to render it isotonic. Correspondingly, C_w in a dilute urine is the quantity which must be removed from urine to render it isotonic. The isotonic urine which would be formed in either case, representing the urine flow in the absence of concentration or dilution, is termed the 'osmolar clearance', C_{osm} (WESSON and ANSLOW 1952; WESSON 1952)[1]. C_{osm} is usually calculated directly from freezing point measurements

---

[1] This method of analysis was proposed independently by WEST and RAPOPORT who suggested the terms 'solute clearance' and 'water economy' to designate the functions, 'osmolar clearance' and 'free-water clearance'.

on urine and plasma as $C_{osm} = \dfrac{V \cdot U_{osm}}{P_{osm}}$, where V is rate of urine flow in ml./min. and U_{osm} and P_{osm} are concentrations of plasma and urine expressed in osmolar units. Urine flow and osmolar and freewater clearances are related by $C_w = V - C_{osm}$. Thus, C_w is negative in a concentrated urine, since water appears to have been abstracted during urine formation, and is positive in a dilute urine since, as a virtual operation, water appears to have been added to an antecedent isotonic fluid. C_{osm} measures the minimum volume of fluid issuing from the distal convoluted tubule and entering the collecting ducts. During antidiuresis, when the distal tubular fluid presumably becomes isotonic, C_{osm} may closely approximate the true volume leaving the segment. C_w, when positive, affords an estimate of the minimum quantity of solute which has been reabsorbed without water in the distal segment. This quantity, which may be termed the 'osmotic equivalent', T_{osm}, of the free-water clearance, is given by $T_{osm} = C_w \cdot P_{osm}$. C_w, when negative, represents the least volume of water (T_w^c) transported from the collecting ducts into the medulla. Under conditions such that fluid issuing from the distal tubule may be considered isotonic with blood. C_w $(= T_w^c)$ may closely approximate the true rate of water transport within the collecting ducts. T_{osm} now represent the least quantity of solute transported without water into the medulla.

f) Summary of variables determining urine flow and concentration

From the foregoing description of the water transport system it is evident that urine flow and concentrations are determined by a large number of variables. These are so numerous that in relatively few physiological or pathological states has it proven possible to recognize the exact cause of a change in urine flow or concentration. These variables in summary and considered broadly are:

Filtration rate and plasma composition. These factors determine the quantity and composition of solutes presented to the proximal segment for reabsorption.

Proximal tubular reabsorption. This factor determines the quantity of isotonic fluid delivered to the loop of HENLE and the quantity of reabsorbable NaCl in that fluid. Mercurial diuresis is an example of disturbance in proximal tubular reabsorption.

Distal (or loop of HENLE) NaCl reabsorption. This factor determines the quantity of water available for water diuresis. It is dependent upon the quantity of NaCl discharged from the proximal segment and probably, also, upon adrenal steroids.

Distal tubular and collecting duct permeability to water. This factor determines the rate of water transport from the tubule at any specified osmotic concentration gradient. The *relative* effect of water transport on the composition of the urine is, of course, related to the concentration gradient and the volume of water available for transport. If the volume of the tubular fluid is very large and its tonicity is close to that of blood, significant quantities of water may fail to be transported even when permeability is high as in the presence of ADH. Conversely, if the volume flow of tubular fluid is very small even a low rate of water transport as related to residual tubular permeability in the absence of ADH may be sufficient to largely dissipate hypotonicity within the distal segment and permit significant concentration within the collecting ducts.

Efficiency of medullary solute accumulation. This represents the rate of salt (and perhaps urea) transport into the medulla, the activity of the intramedullary solute distributive system (countercurrent multiplier) and the volume and distribution of the medullary blood flow.

g) Antidiuretic hormone, vasopressin and antidiuretic substance

α) Antidiuretic hormone

The hypothalamus and the posterior pituitary are the sources of a humoral factor which causes the urine to become concentrated (E II 2) and which is termed antidiuretic hormone (ADH). The antidiuretic activity of extracts of these tissues can be accounted for almost entirely by their content of the octapeptide, vasopressin. The octapeptide, oxytocin, which is the other active extract of the posterior pituitary in mammals, possesses a residual antidiuretic activity which is too small to contribute significantly to the antidiuretic activity of the gland (STEHLE 1934; FRASER 1937; BOYD and GARAND; VAN DYKE, ADAMSONS and ENGEL). The antidiuretic activity of commercial oxytocic pituitary extracts (e.g., Pitocin) is attributable partly to contamination by traces of vasopressin and partly to this intrinsic antidiuretic activity within the oxytocin molecule.

In the absence of vasopressin, as in the dog heart-lung-kidney preparation, the urine is hypotonic. The urine becomes hypertonic if pituitary extract is injected, but not if the kidney is perfused with hypertonic saline (STARLING and VERNEY; BAYLISS and FEE). When vasopressin is injected into one renal artery of the water-diuresing dog, antidiuresis is largely restricted to the injected side (BARGER, BERLIN and TULENKO). The renal nerves are not essential to formation of hyper- or hypotonic urine (BAYLISS and BROWN) although they may affect urine tonicity through a separate, hemodynamic mechanism (E II 2 e). In a 70 kg. man, vasopressin must be infused intravenously at about 16 milliunits per hour to attain maximal antidiuresis (LAUSON 1951). The corresponding rate for a dog (about 12 kg.) is 5 mU. per hour (SHANNON 1942b). At submaximal rates of vasopressin infusion, the decrease in urine flow below the maximum attainable under water loading is a curvilinear, asymptotic function of the infusion rate (HOLLANDER et al. 1957a). No distinction can be made between the effects of exogenous vasopressin and of endogenously liberated ADH since vasopressin does not cause further urine concentration in dehydrated subjects (JONES and DE WARDENER; SODEMAN and ENGELHARDT; SCHNEEBERG; BJERRE-CHRISTENSEN; RAISZ, McNEELY and SAXON), water administration to subjects who have received vasopressin causes no decrease in concentration (WEST, TRAEGER and KAPLAN), and neither acute dehydration nor vasopressin (Pitressin) following chronic hyperhydration can cause the urine to achieve concentrations observed prior to hyperhydration (DE WARDENER and HERXHEIMER).

Available evidence indicates, therefore, that ADH is, in fact, vasopressin possibly associated with a protein carrier molecule. In extracts of the posterior pituitary which are prepared with minimal chemical treatment, the antidiuretic, and also oxytocic, activity is bound to a small protein molecule (mol. wt. about 30,000) (VAN DYKE et al.; HAM and LANDIS; HAM and ROSENFELD). Treatment with dilute acid separates the polypeptides from the protein fraction. Antidiuretic activity (equivalent to 100 to 400 microunits of Pitressin per ml.) in the jugular venous blood of the hemorrhaged dog was similar to vasopressin in thioglycollate reduction and susceptibility to proteolytic enzymes (BOCANEGRA and LAUSON, pers. comm.) and was ultrafilterable to the extent of 70 to 80 percent as compared with 100 percent for Pitressin (LAUSON and BOCANEGRA 1960). In the rat, however, very little of either endogenous ADH or exogenous Pitressin is ultrafilterable (THORN and SILVER).

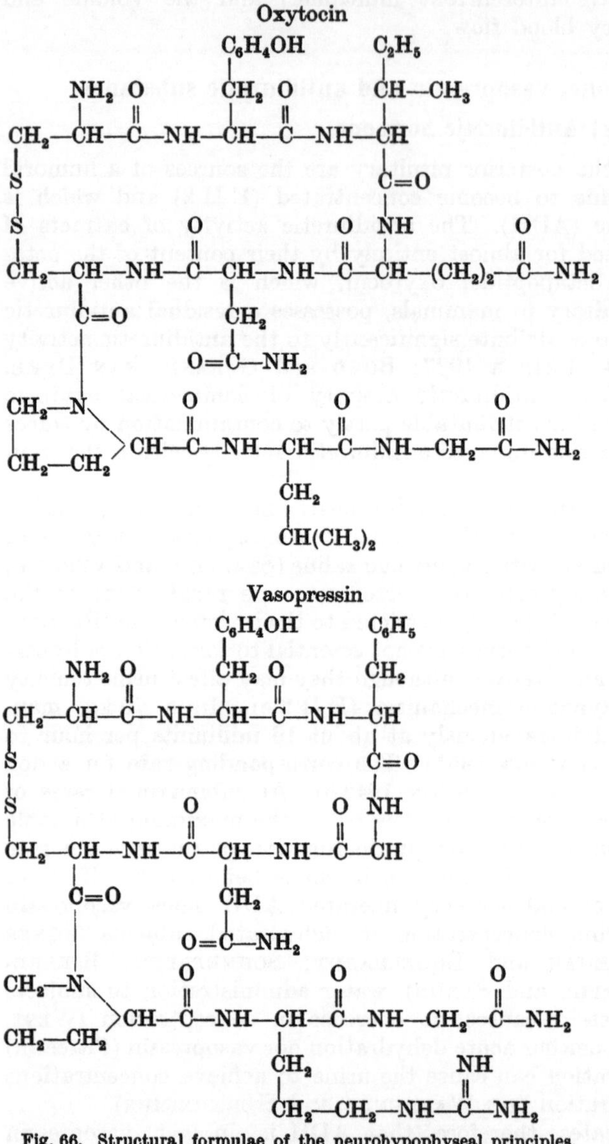

Oxytocin

C_6H_4OH C_2H_5

NH_2 O CH_2 O $CH—CH_3$

$CH_2—CH—C—NH—CH—C—NH—CH$

|

S $C=O$

|

S   O   O NH   O

$CH_2—CH—NH—C—CH—NH—C—CH—(CH_2)_2—C—NH_2$

| |

$C=O$ CH_2

| |

$O=C—NH_2$

$CH_2—N$

$CH_2—CH_2$ $\rangle$ $CH—C—NH—CH—C—NH—CH_2—C—NH_2$

|

O   O   O

CH_2

|

$CH(CH_3)_2$

Vasopressin

C_6H_4OH C_6H_5

NH_2 O CH_2 O CH_2

$CH_2—CH—C—NH—CH—C—NH—CH$

|

S $C=O$

|

S   O   O NH

$CH_2—CH—NH—C—CH—NH—C—CH$

| |

$C=O$ CH_2

|

$O=C—NH_2$

$CH_2—N$

$CH_2—CH_2$ $\rangle$ $CH—C—NH—CH—C—NH—CH_2—C—NH_2$

O   O   O

| |

CH_2 NH

| |

$CH_2—CH_2—NH—C—NH_2$

Fig. 66. Structural formulae of the neurohypophyseal principles, oxytocin and arginine vasopressin

β) Vasopressin

Vasopressin is a polypeptide extracted from the anterior hypothalamus and the posterior pituitary glands of mammals. It has been highly purified by STEHLE (1934) and POTTS and GALLAGHER (1942, 1944) and its structure defined and confirmed by synthesis by DU VIGNEAUD and his coworkers (DU VIGNEAUD, LAWLER and POPENOE; POPENOE, LAWLER and DU VIGNEAUD; DU VIGNEAUD, GISH and KATSOYANNIS; DU VIGNEAUD et al.). These and other studies have shown that vasopressin is an octapeptide with the structural formula shown in Fig. 66. The similarity between vasopressin and oxytocin is evident. Among mammals, vasopressin occurs in two forms distinguished by the penultimate aminoacid residue of the side chain. Arginine vasopressin (Fig. 66) is the form probably existing in most mammals including rat, ox, sheep, camel, dog, monkey and man (VAN DYKE, ADAMSONS and ENGEL; LIGHT and DU VIGNEAUD). Lysine vasopressin, with lysine instead of arginine in the penultimate position on the side chain, is found in the pig.

In representative species of cyclostomes (Petromyzon), teleosts, (Pollachius), reptiles (Chelonia), amphibians (Rana) and birds, but not elasmobranchs (Squalus), the role of vasopressin in control of water balance is filled by vasotocin (SAWYER, MUNSICK and VAN DYKE). This octapeptide, which, interestingly, was synthesized by KATSOYANNIS and DU VIGNEAUD (1958b, 1959) prior to its identification in natural extracts, is constructed of the ring of oxytocin and the side chain of arginine vasopressin.

The vasopressins exhibit two major biological activities: in small quantities they are antidiuretic, preventing or aborting a water diuresis and, in appropriate quantities, causing the urine to attain concentrations observed during water deprivation; in large quantities they are intensely vasoconstrictor and cause the blood pressure to rise. Injections of larger quantities in experimental animals are frequently associated with an increase in urine flow as compared with flows observed during maximal antidiuresis. This pituitrin diuresis is essentially a solute diuresis since sodium chloride excretion is also increased (C V 1 e) and urine remains hypertonic. Both the relative antidiuretic and the pressor activities of neurohypophyseal polypeptides (arginine-, lysine-, histidine- and leucine-vasopressin, arginine-vasotocin and oxytocin) depend extensively upon the basicity of the penultimate amino acid residue and in part upon other as yet unidentified components of the molecule. Antidiuretic activity may be somewhat more species-specific (KATSOYANNIS and DU VIGNEAUD 1958a; VAN DYKE, ADAMSONS and ENGEL; SAWYER; MUNSICK, SAWYER and VAN DYKE 1958, 1960). Reports that pressor activity is separable from antidiuretic activity by various procedures such as heating, dialysis, reduction, or adsorption (HELLER 1940; DONALDSON; CROXATTO, ALMEYDA and TUDELA; DUMM, LESLIE and LAKEN) require confirmation in terms of molecular alteration.

Injected vasopressin disappears rapidly from the circulation. Removal is accomplished almost entirely by liver and kidney (BIRNIE; EVERSOLE, BIRNIE and GAUNT; GINSBURG; DICKER 1954; DICKER and GREENBAUM; DICKER and NUNN 1957a; HELLER and ZAIDI; LAUSON and BOCANEGRA). The removal rate in the intact dog is such that the half-life of the plasma concentration is approximately 5 minutes (LAUSON and BOCANEGRA, pers. comm.). Inactivating factors are present in liver homogenates (LARSON) and in placenta and pregnancy serum (CROXATTO, BARNAFI and FERRER; HAWKER). With respect to the hepatic removal, no difference in rate of inactivation could be observed between normal and cirrhotic human liver homogenates (MILLER and TOWNSEND), but inactivation by liver of adrenalectomized rats is depressed (BIRNIE). The suggestion that neither liver nor kidney is capable of complete inactivation of vasopressin, but that an active residue remains from one organ which can be inactivated by the other organ, requires confirmation (DICKER and GREEN-BAUM).

γ) Antidiuretic substance

Demonstration of humoral transmission of antidiuretic influences has prompted intensive search for antidiuretic activity in plasma and urine of patients with impaired ability to excrete water. Evidences of antidiuretic activity are detected and quantitated by various bioassays which usually consist of injecting various quantities of serum, urine or urine extracts subcutaneously, intraperitoneally or intravenously into water-loaded animals, usually rats. Impairment in rate of excretion of the water load is compared with rates of excretion following corresponding injection of graded quantities of posterior pituitary pressor activity (vasopressin). In a variation, increase in chloride excretion rather than decrease in water excretion has been employed as the measure of activity (HAM 1943) since vasopressin is chloruretic in the rat. Other assay animals and the usual route of administration are: rabbit, subcutaneously (WALKER 1939); toad, subcutaneously (BUCHBORN 1955); normal or diabetes-insipidus dog, intravenously (HARE, HICKEY and HARE 1941b; HARE et al. 1945); and man, intravenously (LAUSON et al. 1952). Serum or blood is usually injected unaltered or treated in various ways as by acidification, concentration, dialysis, or adsorption of antidiuretic activity on substances such as collodion or alumina. Although the assays in some studies may truly reflect changes in circulating ADH, identity of antidiuretic substance or a major fraction thereof with vasopressin or its metabolites remains to be demonstrated and the results, generally, are uninterpretable (VAN DYKE, ADAMSONS and ENGEL). Because the same technique does not appear to have been employed in any two laboratories no attempt will be made in the following summary to report the technical details of the assay.

Urinary antidiuretic substance (per unit time) has been reported to be increased during dehydration in man (LLOYD and LOBOTSKY), dog (HARE, HICKEY and HARE 1941b), cat (INGRAM, LADD and BENBOW; MARTIN, HERRLICH and FAZEKAS), rat (GILMAN and GOODMAN 1937; DICKER and NUNN 1957b; MARTIN, HERRLICH and FAZEKAS; AMES and VAN DYKE) and rabbit (WALKER 1939), and in patients with congestive heart failure (DOCHIOS and DREIFUS; BERÇU, ROKAW and MASSIE), cirrhosis (DOCHIOS and DREIFUS; RALLI et al.; ORTI, LAKEN and RALLI; HALL, FRAME and DRILL; FAULKNER, HAMMERSCHMIDT and NEWMAYR), pregnancy (HAM 1941; CROXATTO, BARNAFI and FERRER), toxemia of pregnancy (HAM and LANDIS) and hypoadrenalism or panhypopituitarism (SLESSOR). Urinary antidiuretic activity is increased in the adrenalectomized dog (LLOYD and LOBOTSKY), rat (BIRNIE et al. 1949), and cat (MARTIN, HERRLICH and FAZEKAS), in the dog following hypertonic saline injection (AMES, MOORE and VAN DYKE), posttransfusional oliguria (ZUIDEMA et al.), injection of epinephrine or norepinephrine (ERANKO et al.), in the rat following morphine (WINTER, GAFFNEY and FLATAKER; GIARMAN and CONDOURIS; GIARMAN, MATTIE and STEVENSON; LIPSCHITZ and STOKEY), anesthesia (DICKER and GREENBAUM), trauma (BACHRACH et al. 1956) or hypertonic saline administration (GILMAN and GOODMAN). The effect of morphine in the rat is blocked by the morphine antagonist, N-allylmorphine (WINTER, GAFFNEY and FLATAKER; GIARMAN and CONDOURIS). Urinary antidiuretic substance is decreased following hydration and in diabetes insipidus in man (BELLENS) and following hypophysectomy in rat (GILMAN and GOODMAN), cat (INGRAM, LADD and BENBOW) and dog (HARE, HICKEY and HARE 1941b).

Reports on antidiuretic activity of plasma or serum generally parallel roughly those of urine. Serum antidiuretic activity has been reported to be increased in cirrhosis, congestive heart failure, hypertension (STEIN, SCHWARTZ and MIRSKY), nephrosis (LAUSON et al. 1952), exercise (VERA and CROXATTO), following paracentesis (WOLFF, KOCZOREK and BUCHBORN 1958) or 18-hour dehydration (LEWIS 1953) in man; following dehydration (LEAF and MAMBY 1952a), hypertonic saline injections (BARATZ and INGRAHAM; AMES, MOORE and VAN DYKE) or hemorrhage (BARATZ and INGRAHAM; LAUSON and BOCANEGRA) in the dog; following excitement or pain (MIRSKY, STEIN and PAULISCH), hypertonic saline, anesthesia (THORN and SILVER), adrenalectomy (BIRNIE et al. 1949, 1950; MIRSKY, PAULISCH and STEIN) or hemorrhage (GINSBURG) in the rat. Decreases in serum antidiuretic activity are reported following hydration in man (VERA and CROXATTO) and hypophysectomy in the rat (MIRSKY, PAULISCH and STEIN; BIRNIE et al. 1949). Antidiuretic activity of human serum (toad test) is reported to vary in proportion to serum osmotic activity (BUCHBORN 1957).

Although these studies appear consistent in suggesting that plasma and urine may reflect the quantity of circulating antidiuretic hormone, further information indicates that they are largely uninterpretable and that vasopressin itself constitutes relatively little of the urinary activity and an undetermined fraction of the plasma activity. Numerous substances such as sympathomimetic amines, serotonin (ERSPAMER and CORREALE) and ferritin (BAEZ, MAZUR and SHORR) are present in plasma and urine and are known to be antidiuretic. In addition, urine in dog and man may contain specifically diuretic substances (LLOYD and LOBOTSKY; LITTLE). Some authors have been unable to detect significant increases in antidiuretic activity of urine or serum from cirrhotic or cardiac patients, or activity may be increased during the normal daytime diuresis (GOLDMAN and LUCHSINGER; PERRY and FYLES; WOLFF et al.). ADS may remain at high levels during water diuresis in the dog (LIPSCHITZ and STOKEY). Serum antidiuretic activity may increase following adrenalectomy in hypophysectomized rats (MIRSKY, PAULISCH and STEIN); and no correlation between changes in serum ADS and urine flow following ACTH administration in patients with panhypopituitarism is evident (CHALMERS and LEWIS 1951b). Three distinct antidiuretic fractions are separable from the urine of cirrhotic patients, of which only two occur to a significant extent in normal urine. Of these latter, one is antidiuretic to the rat but not to the dog (ORTI, LAKEN and RALLI). Urine from normal and eclamptic subjects contains numerous substances, particularly heavy metals, which have the effect of enhancing the apparent antidiuretic potency of added vasopressin when it is injected subcutaneously in the rat (SCHAFFER, CADDEN and STANDER; NOBLE, RINDERKNECHT and WILLIAMS). WALKER (1939) found that the relative antidiuretic activity or urine from dehydrated as compared with hydrated animals depends extensively upon the details of treatment of the urine, although the activity remains always greater in the dehydrated urine. When large quantities of posterior pituitary extract are injected intravenously in cat, dog, rat and rabbit, some increase in antidiuretic activity can be detected in the urine (INGRAM, LADD and BENBOW; WALKER 1939; HARE, HICKEY and HARE 1941b). In the rat, about 4.5 percent of the activity of injected Pitressin was excreted (DICKER and NUNN 1957a). Smaller or subcutaneous doses of Pitressin are not detectably excreted (HELLER 1943). A major component representing most of the urinary antidiuretic substance differs significantly from vasopressin: it is nondialysable from neutral urine and is ultracentrifugable (BERÇU, ROKAW and MASSIE; HAM 1941; HAM and LANDIS; AMES, MOORE and VAN DYKE); is more stable at neutral to alkaline p_H (WALKER 1939; SCHAFFER, CADDEN and STANDER); is more resistant to reducing agents such as sulfite (GIARMAN, MATTIE and STEVENSON); is not chloruretic in the rat (HAM 1941; HAM and LANDIS) and migrates at a different velocity electrophoretically (WILSON and MUIRHEAD). Nevertheless, the circumstances that this component qualitatively resembles vasopressin in many chemical properties has kept open the question that it may be related to, or perhaps be a metabolite of, vasopressin (GILMAN and GOODMAN 1937). With respect to the latter possibility, DICKER and GREENBAUM reported that urinary ADS in the rat can be inactivated by liver but not by kidney. Since exposure of Pitressin to kidney tissue also leaves a residue of antidiuretic activity which can be inactivated by liver but not kidney, they suggest that some excreted ADS may represent such an active residue of renal metabolism. Similarly, much of the activity in rat plasma resembles vasopressin in that it is inactivated by reducing agents and can be dialysed into an acid solution (BIRNIE et al. 1950). In nephrotic patients, plasma antidiuretic activity is similar to, but differs slightly from vasopressin (WILSON and MUIRHEAD). Further difficulties arise from lack of agreement among the assay procedures themselves. Different assay results are obtained when different injection routes are used in the same animal, or the same injection route is employed in different species. Thus, in the rat, subcutaneous or intraperitoneal injection of the test solutions generally yield higher values than intravenous injection; and a positive assay by intravenous injection in the rat may yield negative results when the same technique is employed in the dog (VAN DYKE, ADAMSONS and ENGEL). Normal human serum, for example, is antidiuretic when injected intraperitoneally in the rat (PERRY and FYLES) but has no detectable activity when injected intravenously in water-loaded man or dog. In studies on dehydrated subjects, the serum antidiuretic titers, as assayed by transfusion in a water-diuresing recipient, yielded values $1/_{10}$ of that obtained by rat assay, the first method indicating a total blood content of about 26 milliunits (LEWIS 1953). Hence, provisional identification of ADS with some substance having the general properties of vasopressin can be made only if the same activity is obtained by more than one method of assay (VAN DYKE, ADAMSONS and ENGEL). Although few studies have met these rigid assay criteria, certain studies in which test blood is infused into a water-diuresing recipient of the same species will probably be found to yield valid assays of circulating antidiuretic hormone. Among such studies are those of AMES, MOORE and VAN DYKE; and BOCANEGRA and LAUSON who observed increases in ADH in jugular venous blood of the dog following hemorrhage or hypertonic saline injection; and those of GINSBURG and of THORN and SILVER who observed increases in plasma ADH titer in the rat following hemorrhage, hypertonic saline injection or ether anesthesia.

Improved methods for the separation of vasopressin from other biological materials (ARIMURA and DINGMAN; WEINSTEIN, BERNE und SACHS) may resolve much of the confusion concerning the nature and significance of antidiuretic substance.

h) Normal values of concentration and dilution in man

Maximal concentration and dilution of urine and maximal (absolute values) of positive and negative free-water clearances depend on dietary salt and protein contents, degree of hydration and rates of solute excretion (see below).

On unrestricted diets and 12 to 24 hours dehydration, maximum osmotic urine/plasma ratio (U/P_{max}) is about 4.0, ranging from about 3.5 to 4.8 (ADOLPH; McCANCE and YOUNG 1943; McCANCE 1945; GAMBLE 1946; BRODSKY et al. 1952; MILES, PATON and DE WARDENER; JONES and DE WARDENER; RAISZ, McNEELY and SAXON; RAISZ and SCHEER). Highest values are observed at urine flows of 0.5 ml./min. or somewhat less. At flows of 1.0 ml./min., the maximum U/P ratio is about 3.0 to 3.5 in young men (RAISZ and SCHEER) and 2.2 to 3.3 in older subjects (BOYARSKY and SMITH; MERONEY, RUBINI and

BLYTHE). A similar decrease in maximal concentration with age is observed in the rat (DICKER and NUNN 1958). The maximum value decreases progressively with increasing urine flows resulting from increased solute excretion (Fig. 67). Highest values reported are 4.8 in fasting, thirsting young men receiving 100 g. glucose daily as nourishment (GAMBLE and BUTLER; GAMBLE 1946), and 5.0 in chronically dehydrated young men on a high protein diet (JOHNSON et al.).

Urine of infants is usually hypotonic but this is probably related to large fluid volumes ingested (McCANCE and YOUNG 1941). During fluid restriction or following injection of posterior pituitary extract, urine of infants becomes hypertonic but seldom exceeds about one half the adult values (HELLER 1944; McCANCE and WIDDOWSON 1954; EDELMANN, TROUPKOU and BARNETT). The depressed maximal concentration of infancy may well be a physiological equivalent of the depressed concentration observed in adults following chronic hyperhydration.

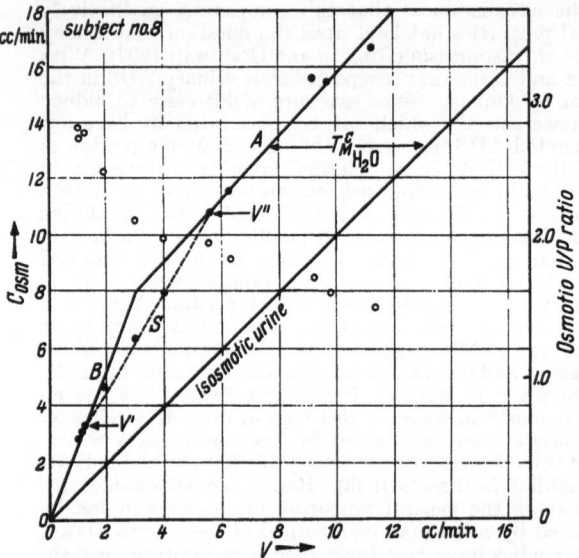

Fig. 67. Osmotic U/P ratio and free-water reabsorption, $T_w^c H_2O$ as related to urine flow and osmolar clearance, C_{osm}, during mannitol diuresis in a normal subject. After BOYARSKY and SMITH. Reproduced by permission of the authors and Journal of Urology

Free water reabsorption, T_w^c, increases when urine flow (osmolar clearance) is increased by solute loading under conditions of dehydration and with supplementary vasopressin administered to prevent possible dilution as a result of decreased endogenous antidiuretic hormone production during fluid infusion. T_w^c attains a maximum, Tm_w^c, of 7.5 to 10 ml./min. in young men (BRODSKY et al. 1952; RAISZ, AU and SCHEER 1959b) and 4 to 6 in older subjects (ZAK, BRUN and SMITH; BOYARSKY and SMITH) at urine flows of 6 ml./min. or greater (Fig. 67). Tm_w^c as related to surface area is low in infants but may attain near-adult values when adjusted to 100 ml. of filtration rate (EDELMANN, TROUPKOU and BARNETT).

Minimum osmotic concentration of the urine during water diuresis is 40 to 80 mOsm./liter and is observed at the lowest osmolar clearances, about 2 ml./min. (KLEEMAN, EPSTEIN and WHITE 1956; SCHOEN). Infants dilute urine to the same extent as adults (BARNETT et al. 1952). Maximum free-water clearance, Cm_w, is 10 to 15 ml./min. (LADD 1952; KLEEMAN, EPSTEIN and WHITE) varying somewhat with osmolar clearance. Cm_w averages about 10 ml./min. at C_{osm} of 2, and 15 at C_{osm} of 4 ml./min. Cm_w as high as 28.8 ml./min. has been reported during saline loading (LADD 1952).

Concentration and dilution values in man may be compared with those in some other mammals. In the cat, U/P$_{max}$ averaged about 7.2 (DRESER). In dog and seal, *Phoca*, U/P$_{max}$ averaged 4 to 8 and 5.6, respectively, with Tm_w^c in the dog averaging about 7 ml./min./100 ml. GFR (WEST and RAPOPORT; PAGE and RHEEM; PAGE et al. 1954b; ANSLOW and WESSON 1955a). A maximum value for Tm_w^c in the seal was not discovered. In the kangaroo rat, U/P$_{max}$ may attain about 20 (SCHMIDT-NIELSEN; SCHMIDT-NIELSEN and SCHNEIDERMAN). Minimum osmotic U/P ratio in the dog has the same range as in man (BERLINER and DAVIDSON) and Cm_w is 15 to 20 ml./min./100 ml. of GFR.

Multiplying osmotic U/P ratio by plasma osmotic concentration (about 280 mOsm./L. in man and 310 in the dog) yields the osmotic concentration of the urine.

j) Concentration of the urine as affected by metabolic and other factors

The most important factor, by far, which affects the concentration of the urine is the quantity of circulating antidiuretic hormone (ADH). Mechanisms governing the secretion of ADH will be considered in a later section. The principal pathological states in which concentration is impaired are listed in Table 19. Concentration (U/P_{max}), as considered here, refers to the osmotic U/P ratio attained in the presence of presumably maximal quantities of ADH. This is attained either by deprivation of fluids for 12 to 24 hours or by injection of vasopressin preparations such as Pitressin.

Table 19. *Physiological and pathological states associated with diminished concentration or dilution*

Concentration diminished

hypoadrenalism[1,2]   mercurial diuresis[21-25]
hypercalcemia[3-8]   nephritis[26-29]
filtration decrease[9-11]   protein restriction[30-35]
hyperhydration[12-15]   sicklemia[36-38]
hypokalemia[16-20]   hyperthyroidism[39,40]

Dilution diminished

hypoadrenalism[41-45]   hypopituitarism[42,50]
filtration decrease[46-49]   sodium-retaining states[51-56]

[1] KOTTKE, CODE and WOOD; [2] REFORZO-MEMBRIVES, POWER and KEPLER; [3] CARONE et al.; [4] EPSTEIN, RIVERA and CARONE; [5] EPSTEIN et al. 1959; [6] GROSSMAN, GOLDMAN and MINES; [7] BECK, LEVITIN and EPSTEIN; [8] HAUSER, POLIMEROS and LEVITT; [9] LEVINSKY, DAVIDSON and BERLINER 1959b; [10] LEVITT, LEVY and POLIMEROS; [11] RAISZ, AU and SCHEER 1959a; [12] HOLLAND and STEAD 1951; [13] DAVIS, HOWELL and HYATT 1954; [14] EPSTEIN, KLEEMAN and HENDRIKX; [15] LEVINSKY, DAVIDSON and BERLINER 1959a; [16] DUSTAN, CORCORAN and PAGE; [17] HOLLANDER et al. 1957b; [18] MULINOS, SPINGARN and LOJKIN; [19] GIEBISCH and LOZANO; [20] RUBINI; [21] GROSSMAN et al. 1955; [22] WELT et al. 1953; [23] AU and RAISZ; [24] SPRITZ et al.; [25] HAUSER, POLIMEROS and LEVITT; [26] WHITE and RUBIN; [27] KLEEMAN and EPSTEIN; [28] FRANKLIN, NIALL and MERRILL; [29] BRICKER et al. 1959; [30] McCANCE 1945; [31] CRAWFORD, DOYLE and PROBST; [32] MILES, PATON and DE WARDENER; [33] EPSTEIN et al. 1957; [34] LEVINSKY and BERLINER 1959b; [35] MERONEY, RUBINI and BLYTHE; [36] ZARAFONETIS et al; [37] KUNZ et al.; [38] KEITEL, THOMPSON and ITANO; [39] WESTON et al. 1956; [40] EPSTEIN and RIVERA; [41] REFORZO-MEMBRIVES, POWER and KEPLER; [42] SLESSOR; [43] LEWIS 1953; [44] RENZI et al.; [45] GROSS and DETTBARN; [46] KLEEMAN, MAXWELL and ROCKNEY 1957; [47] BRADLEY et al. 1955; [48] DEL GRECO and DE WARDENER; [49] BERLINER and DAVIDSON; [50] LAMDIN et al.; [51] JAMES, GORDILLO and METCOFF; [52] HANENSON et al. 1956; [53] LAMDIN et al.; [54] WHITE, RUBIN and LEITER 1951; [55] GABUDZA, TRAEGER and DAVIDSON; [56] BIRCHARD et al.

α) Osmolar clearance

As indicated in the preceding section, urine osmotic concentration is a smooth curvilinear function of the rate of solute excretion, the latter measurable as the osmolar clearance. U/P_{max} is highest at osmolar clearances of about 2 ml./min. (urine flows of 0.5 ml./min.) and declines from this value both with increasing and decreasing C_{osm}. With increasing C_{osm}, U/P_{max} approaches a value of 1.0 as an asymptote and can be described reasonably satisfactorily by any of a variety of empirical asymptotic equations (RAPOPORT et al. 1948; RAISZ, AU and SCHEER 1959b). The curve of U/P_{max} as related to C_{osm} is generally independent of the chemical nature of the solutes which comprise C_{osm} (HERVEY, MCCANCE and TAYLOR; BRODSKY, RAPOPORT and WEST; BRODSKY). At high osmolar clearances, above 6 ml./min., the curve is best described in terms of Tm_w^c which is usually constant and independent of C_{osm}. U/P_{max} declines at urine flows less than 0.5 ml./min. (ROSCOE), probably as the result of decrease in filtration or filtered solute load (see below). U/P_{max} (at low flows) and Tm_w^c (at high flows) are usually, but not invariably, affected in a parallel fashion in various physiological and pathological states.

In occasional human subjects, Tm_w^c may increase or decrease with increasing C_{osm} (ZAK, BRUN and SMITH). The number of such individuals is approximately equal so that, on the average, Tm_w^c is constant (BOYARSKY and SMITH). A tendency for Tm_w^c to decrease at high osmolar clearances is observed regularly in the dog (ANSLOW and WESSON 1955a; ORLOFF, WAGNER and DAVIDSON; BRESLER, MONROE and GILMARTIN). The decrease is not reversible by vasopressin injections or hypertonic saline but is temporary, the original values of Tm_w^c returning after several hours at elevated C_{osm} (ANSLOW and WESSON 1955a).

β) Filtration rate

Small decreases in filtration rate produced in the dog by renal artery compression (LEAF et al. 1954; LEVINSKY, DAVIDSON and BERLINER 1959b) and in man by hypotension (LEVITT, LEVY and POLIMEROS) are associated with little change; but decreases greater than 30 percent are associated with a small to moderate decrease in U/P_{max}. How much of the effect is due to decrease in filtration or renal blood flow and how much is due to attendant decrease in C_{osm} is not clear. At low urine flows, urine hypertonicity can be significantly diminished by passive equilibration in the lower urinary tract (LEVINSKY and BERLINER 1959a). Severe exercise, which is associated with decrease in filtration rate and renal blood flow was also accompanied by decrease in U/P_{max} but Tm_w^c, measured during mannitol infusion, remained unchanged (RAISZ, AU and SCHEER 1959a).

γ) Hypercalcemia and hypokalemia

Both hypercalcemia and hypokalemia are associated with decrease in U/P_{max} and Tm_w^c. Severe hypercalcemia induced by parathyroid extract or vitamin D administration in dog or rat is associated with severe histological lesions, particularly in the collecting ducts, and with decrease in filtration rate. U/P_{max} decreases to 1.5 from about 5 and Tm_w^c approaches zero in the dog. In man, Tm_w^c may decrease to less than 1.0 ml./min. (WALKER and CARPENTER). How much of the effect is secondary to cellular damage is unknown (CARONE et al.; EPSTEIN, RIVERA and CARONE; EPSTEIN et al. 1959). In both man and dog, however, U/P_{max} and T_w^c decrease during acute hypercalcemia caused by calcium gluconate infusion (GROSSMAN, GOLDMAN and MINES; GROSSMAN et al. 1958; HAUSER, POLIMEROS and LEVITT; BECK, LEVITIN and EPSTEIN; YOFFEE and DINGMAN). The absolute magnitude rather than the change in calcium appears to be important since impaired concentration is not observed when calcium increases from low toward normal concentrations in hypoparathyroid patients. The reverse process (increase in U/P_{max}) following lowering of plasma calcium in hyperparathyroid patients occurs more slowly (YOFFEE and DINGMAN).

In hypokalemic states, depression in U/P_{max} is proportional to the degree of potassium deficit (HOLLANDER et al. 1957b) but may not become significant until the deficit, in man, exceeds 200 mM. (RUBINI). In both man and dog,

Tm_w^c is depressed more rapidly and to a greater extent than U/P_{max} (RUBINI; GIEBISCH and LOZANO). In hyperaldosteronism, U/P_{max} may be depressed to 1.0 or less (DINGMAN, GAITAN and STAUB) but Tm_w^c may be well sustained in other patients although some potassium depletion is present (DUSTAN, CORCORAN and PAGE). Chronic hypokalemia may be associated with histological changes in the nephron (RELMAN and SCHWARTZ 1958) which, in experimental animals, is particular conspicuous in the collecting duct cells as periodic acid-Schiff-positive droplets (STRAUS and SPARGO). Hypokalemia is, however, seldom associated with significant depression in filtration rate. The mechanism involved in depression of water transport by changes in plasma concentrations of these two ions is unknown, but the antagonism between calcium and potassium in many cell membrane phenomena suggests that the mechanism may be the same for both. The defect apparently lies in the medullary-collecting duct system since water equilibration in the distal convoluted tubule of the potassium-deficient rat proceeds normally (GOTTSCHALK et al.). Medullary solute concentration is decreased both in hypokalemia and in hypercalcemia in dog and rat, but remains greater than plasma both with respect to sodium concentration and to total solute concentration (MANITIUS et al. 1960a and b; HOLLIDAY, EGAN and WIRTH). Urine solute concentration is significantly less than that of the medulla in spite of the presence of presumably adequate quantities of circulating ADH. For example, papillary solute concentration was decreased 30 percent in hypercalcemic rats at a time when urine solute concentration was decreased 50 percent. Whether or not the solute concentration of the medullary interstitium is decreased at all remains to be determined. The principal element in the concentration defect therefore appears to be decreased permeability of the collecting ducts to water.

Recovery is rapid. A significant increase in concentration occurs immediately following acute potassium administration to hypokalemic patients, and essentially normal concentration is recovered within 3 days in hypokalemic man and rat (HOLLANDER et al. 1958; WALKER and CARPENTER). Recovery of concentration also is rapid in hypercalcemic patients who respond to treatment (WALKER and CARPENTER).

δ) Sicklemia

Sicklemia is associated with marked impairment in urine concentration (KUNZ et al.; ZARAFONETIS et al.). U/P_{max} generally ranges between 1.5 and 2.5 (KEITEL, THOMPSON and ITANO). Tm_w^c, however, was normal in a child although depressed about 50 percent in adults (HEINEMANN and CHEUNG). The concentration defect is not related to anemia since it is present in nonanemic individuals. It appears to be directly related to the defective erythrocytes, since urine concentration temporarily approaches normal following extensive transfusion (KEITEL, THOMPSON and ITANO) and dilution is normal as also is response to Pitressin during water diuresis (LEVITT et al. 1959).

Tm_w^c is essentially normal in nonsicklemic anemia although U/P_{max} may be somewhat decreased to 2.3—3.1 (HEINEMANN and CHEUNG).

ε) Dehydration and hyperhydration

Chronic dehydration of 48 hours or longer is associated with an increase in U/P_{max}. The amount of the increase is related to the duration of the dehydration and the previous state of the individuals, but the increases are generally of the order of 10 to 20 percent (GAMBLE 1946; JONES and DE WARDENER; JOHNSON et al.; EPSTEIN, KLEEMAN and HENDRIKX).

Hyperhydration resulting from prolonged ingestion of large fluid volumes is associated with a decrease in U/P_{max}. In these studies, U/P_{max} is defined as the concentration ratio attained during Pitressin administration. Following three days of consumption of 5 to 6 liters of water daily, U/P_{max} averaged 2.6 compared with 3.2 on unrestricted diet and 4.0 in the same subjects following three days of fluid restriction (EPSTEIN, KLEEMAN and HENDRIKX). Following 11 days of drinking 10 liters of water daily, U/P_{max} decreased from 3.2 to 1.7 (DE WARDENER and HERXHEIMER). Markedly impaired concentration attributable to chronic hyperhydration has been reported clinically in psychogenic polydipsia (KLEEMAN, MAXWELL and WITLIN). Tm_w^c also varies with hydration, averaging 6.7 following fluid restriction and 4.1 following fluid supplementation. The hydration effect is not dependent upon the antecedent urine flow since a progressive decrease in U/P_{max} is observed in hydrated individuals in whom diuresis is prevented by administration of Pitressin tannate (HOLLAND and STEAD 1951; EPSTEIN, KLEEMAN and HENDRIKX; JAENIKE and WATERHOUSE) nor is it evidently correlated with changes in filtration rate or solute excretion. The phenomenon is prominent in the dog, in which U/P_{max} may decrease from 6.0 to 1.5 during 15 days of sustained hyperhydration (DAVIS, HOWELL and HYATT 1954; LEVINSKY, DAVIDSON and BERLINER 1959a).

ζ) Diet

The protein content and to a lesser extent the salt content of the diet exert a marked effect on urine concentration. In various studies in man, U/P_{max} averages 10 to 25 percent greater on a high than on a low protein diet (McCANCE 1945; MILES, PATON and DE WARDENER 1954; EPSTEIN et al. 1957; MERONEY, RUBINI and BLYTHE). The dietary protein effect is preserved qualitatively in potassium deficiency (RUBINI) and in dehydration (HENDRIKX and EPSTEIN). Decrease in U/P_{max} on a low protein diet is also observed in the dog (LEVINSKY and BERLINER 1959b) and rat (HENDRIKX and EPSTEIN) but not clearly in the sheep (SCHMIDT-NIELSEN and O'DELL 1959). Tm_w^c is decreased 15 to 50 percent on low protein diet in man (EPSTEIN et al. 1957) and may decrease to zero or below (hypotonic urine) during mannitol diuresis in the dog (LEVINSKY and BERLINER 1959b). The dietary effect is attributable only in part to the urea formed from protein metabolism. Urea administered to the rat or dog on a normal or low protein diet results in increase in both U/P_{max} and in Tm_w^c but values observed on a high protein diet are not attained (CRAWFORD, DOYLE and PROBST; KELLOGG and KOIKE; LEVINSKY and BERLINER 1959b). In man, supplemental urea is associated acutely with an increase in U/P_{max} in subjects on a low protein diet (LEVINSKY and BERLINER 1959b) but no clear effect is observed either in U/P_{max} or Tm_w^c in subjects on an unrestricted diet (RAISZ and SCHEER; RAISZ, AU and SCHEER 1959b). Sodium restriction results in a slightly lower U/P_{max} in subjects on a low protein diet but no effect from sodium restriction is evident in subjects on unrestricted or high protein diets (MERONEY, RUBINI and BLYTHE).

η) Hypoadrenalism

Impairment of renal concentrating capacity, as measured by a low urinary-specific gravity, has long been recognized in patients with hypoadrenalism (REFORZO-MEMBRIVES, POWER and KEPLER). A similar impairment occurs in the adrenalectomized dog (KOTTKE, CODE and WOOD). Because of the marked depression in filtration rate and renal blood flow in hypoadrenalism (C V 12),

it is not yet clear whether the impairment is a nonspecific consequence of hemodynamic changes or represents withdrawal of a specific effect of adrenal steroids
on tubular functions. Water content of both cortex and medulla is increased
in the adrenalectomized rat (CRABBÉ and NICHOLS). In the normal man or dog,
hydrocortisone has no significant effect on U/P_{max} or Tm_w^c (KLEEMAN et al.
1959; GIEBISCH and LOZANO).

ϑ) Mercury

Tm_w^c is decreased in man by amounts which vary from slight to as much as
48 percent by mercurial diuretics such as mercaptomerin and meralluride (WELT
et al. 1953; GROSSMAN et al. 1955; SPRITZ et al.; AU and RAISZ; HAUSER, POLI-
MEROS and LEVITT). In the dog, however, little apparent change in Tm_w^c is
observed under the influence of mercury (BRODSKY and GRAUBARTH 1953b).

ι) Chronic nephritis

Concentration is regularly impaired in chronic renal disease. To a considerable extent, depression in U/P_{max} is attributable to increased concentration
of urea, sulfate, phosphate and other solutes present in excess in the glomerular
filtrate and capable of establishing a solute diuresis in each of a diminished
number of viable nephrons. Nevertheless, depression in U/P_{max} to a degree
related to the severity of the disease persists when filtered solute load is diminished by hypotension (FRANKLIN, NIALL and MERRILL; LEVITT, LEVY and POLI-
MEROS) or hemodialysis to remove urea (FRANKLIN, NIALL and MERRILL). In
uremic patients, therefore, urine flow and C_{osm} are roughly equal (WHITE and
RUBIN). In many patients with chronic nephritis, the urine may be persistently
hypotonic to plasma by as much as 100 milliosmols per liter. Both the
frequency and degree of dilution of such persistently hypotonic urines are related
more closely to the degree of renal failure (being frequent at filtration rates
less than 10 ml./min.) than to the nature of the pathological process (glomerulo-
nephritis, pyelonephritis, nephrosclerosis, diabetes) (SCHÜCK, SMAHELOVA and
STRIBRNA; KLEEMAN and EPSTEIN). Impaired concentration is also observed
in dogs with unilateral experimental nephritis in which the contralateral normal
kidney prevents the glomerular filtrate from becoming abnormal (BRICKER
et al. 1959). Tm_w^c is depressed both absolutely and relative to glomerular filtration rate in nephritic patients with filtration rate below 50 percent of normal,
but at higher filtration rates Tm_w^c per 100 ml. of filtrate is essentially normal.
In experimental nephritis in the dog, Tm_w^c is well sustained down to filtration rates
as low as 25 percent of control levels (BRICKER et al. 1959). An exception must
be noted in patients recovering from acute renal failure. Tm_w^c remains very low,
with values of 0.8 to 2.8 per 100 ml. of filtrate. at filtration rates of 60 ml./min.
(BALDWIN et al. 1955).

Other states which are probably associated with depressed maximal concentration are hyperthyroidism in man: U/P_{max} decreased 20 to 50 percent (EP-
STEIN and RIVERA; WESTON et al. 1956); severe, chronic alcoholism in man:
specific gravity depressed in 30 percent of patients (SCHULTZ and COWEN);
hypothermia in the dog: Tm_w^c decreased to 30 percent of control values at 25° C
(HONG and BOYLAN); pyrogens (PIROMEN) in the dog: Tm_w^c frequently decreased
to zero (BRANDT et al. 1955, 1956).

k) Dilution of the urine as affected by metabolic and other factors

Dilution refers to the decrease in urine osmotic concentration which follows
water ingestion or infusion. Conventionally, the volume of water should be

sufficiently large that secretion of antidiuretic hormone (ADH) is suppressed. Suppression of ADH secretion in normal subjects is inferred when C_w does not increase with increasing water load and is of the order of magnitude observed in hydrated patients with diabetes insipidus. A volume of not less than one and probably two liters of water is essential to assure suppression of ADH secretion in the majority of healthy subjects. Unfortunately, in many pathological states in which dilution is poor, it is impossible to determine whether ADH secretion has been suppressed by the same water load which suppresses secretion in the normal. A larger water load, particularly in patients with hyponatremia, may induce symptoms of water intoxication. The problem will be solved ultimately by development of a sensitive and specific assay for ADH. Until then, impaired dilution represents failure to attain with a 1 to 2 liter water load the C_w expected from the same individual in the normal state, and it is accepted that persistent secretion of ADH may be part or all of the cause of the impaired dilution. The positive free-water clearance attained under such loading conditions will be termed the maximal free-water clearance, Cm_w, and the urine/plasma osmotic concentration ratio will be termed U/P_{min}. Some of the pathological states in which dilution is impaired are listed in Table 19.

α) Osmolar clearance

Both U/P_{min} and Cm_w are dependent on solute excretion, which can be measured by the osmolar clearance, C_{osm}. U/P_{min} usually decreases with decreasing C_{osm} provided filtration rate is not depressed. The data suggest a limiting value in man of about 0.12 at C_{osm} of zero (KLEEMAN, EPSTEIN and WHITE). Under certain conditions, however, as in somewhat dehydrated patients with diabetes insipidus, an increase in solute excretion may be associated with a decrease in U/P_{min} (DE WARDENER and DEL GRECO) similar to the changes observed with increased solute excretion in cirrhosis and other states. Both Cm_w and U/P_{min} increase with increasing C_{osm} (DE WARDENER and DEL GRECO). Cm_w attains a limiting maximal value at C_{osm} of about 10 ml./min. (STRAUSS and ROSENBAUM; WELT et al. 1954; KLEEMAN, EPSTEIN and WHITE) and is constant at all greater values of C_{osm} (BRODSKY and RAPOPORT; WEST et al.; WESSON and ANSLOW 1952). The increase in Cm_w as between low and high rates of solute excretion is about 30 percent (KLEEMAN, EPSTEIN and WHITE). Cm_w is not significantly correlated with the composition of the loading solute as measured by C_{osm}. Thus, Cm_w attains approximately the same values as related to control rates when the solute is mannitol, urea or sodium chloride, during mercurial diuresis (WESSON and ANSLOW 1952; BLACKMORE 1959; LARAGH; HEINEMANN and BECKER) or chlorothiazide diuresis (LARAGH, HEINEMANN and DEMARTINI; JANUSZEWICZ et al.; BLACKMORE 1959), although Cm_w has been depressed following mercury in some studies (CAPPS et al.; LADD 1952; DALE and SANDERSON). The effect of solute excretion on Cm_w has been attributed to the sodium chloride component which is regularly increased in urea and mannitol as well as in mercurial diuresis (STRAUSS and ROSENBAUM), although this has been denied as it relates to urea (KLEEMAN, EPSTEIN and WHITE). When Cm_w is constant, U/P_{min} becomes a simple function of Cm_w and urine flow, V, as described by the equation, $U/P_{min} = 1 - \dfrac{Cm_w}{V}$.

A similar correlation between solute excretion, as related to dietary content of protein and salt, and urine flow is reported in the diabetes insipidus dog and cat (WINTER, INGRAM and EATON).

β) Filtration rate

Decrease in filtration rate regularly results in a rise in U/P_{min} although C_{osm} is diminished. Cm_w is profoundly decreased. The effect is not attributable to ADH secretion since an increase in U/P_{min} to values which may be greater than 1.0 may be observed in patients with diabetes insipidus in whom filtration rate is depressed by abdominal compression (BRADLEY et al. 1955) or hypotension (KLEEMAN, MAXWELL and ROCKNEY 1957) and in water-loaded dogs in which filtration rate in one or both kidneys is depressed by constriction of a renal artery or the abdominal aorta (BERLINER and DAVIDSON; DEL GRECO and DE WARDENER). In the animals with one renal artery constricted, continuing low urine concentration and high flow in the contralateral kidney indicated that ADH was absent. The small or absent C_w in these studies presumably results from inadequate delivery of reabsorbable solutes (NaCl) to the loop of HENLE or the distal tubule where free water is generated, while hypertonicity of the urine is compatible with the view that residual permeability of collecting duct epithelium permits partial equilibration of urine with hypertonic medulla. Dogs with experimental diabetes insipidus frequently form hypertonic urine during dehydration (SHANNON 1942a; LEVKOFF et al. 1952). Alternatively, Cm_w increases with increasing filtration rate. An increase in filtration rate, effected in both normal subjects and subjects with diabetes insipidus by aminophylline, resulted in an increase in Cm_w as compared with control values at the same C_{osm} (KLEEMAN et al. 1960). In dogs maximal urine flow (uncorrected for C_{osm}) per 100 ml. of filtration rate was greater in animals with high filtration rate on a meat diet than when filtration rate was lower as the result of a low protein diet (LUDEMANN, RAISZ and WIRZ).

γ) Hypoadrenalism

Low urine flow and impaired dilution following water-loading has long been recognized in patients with adrenocortical deficiency (REFORZO-MEMBRIVES, POWER and KEPLER; THOMSON, BROWNELL and CUMMING). As noted above with respect to impairment in concentration, filtration rate and renal blood flow are depressed in such patients. In addition, a tendency toward hypotension constitutes a potentially significant nonosmotic stimulus to ADH secretion and persistent secretion of ADH has been suggested as the cause of the impaired diuretic response to water (LEAF and MAMBY 1952b). No significant depletion of the neurohypophyseal content of the posterior pituitary could be detected in the adrenalectomized rat (as compared with the depletion observed following dehydration) (SAWYER and ROTH) and the possibility remains that a significant increase in the plasma ADH concentration may arise because of impaired inactivation by the liver of the adrenoprival animal (BIRNIE; GINSBURG). Loss of the adrenal medulla, alone, does not affect water excretion in the rat (GAUNT, LILING and CORDSEN).

Following water loading, urine flow and concentration may not change for as much as 12 hours, but a small diuresis up to about 2 ml./min., with some associated decrease in concentration, appears eventually in most patients who are not severely ill. Whether the appearance of this small diuresis is the result of a delayed suppression of ADH secretion or to renal hemodynamic or other changes in unknown. Urinary antidiuretic activity which persists following water-loading and which decreases with onset of diuresis has been reported (SLESSOR) but the validity of the assay (BURN rat test) as a measure of ADH remains to be established. Dilution was also impaired in a hypoadrenal patient

16*

with diabetes insipidus, but the circumstance that the impairment was much less than in non diabetic patients suggests that ADH is continually secreted in the latter group (SKILLERN, CORCORAN and DUSTAN; SKILLERN, CORCORAN and SCHERBEL). Aminophylline, which may cause both filtration rate and solute excretion to increase, is associated with an increase in Cm_w in hypoadrenal patients (KLEEMAN and MAXWELL 1957), as also is mercurial diuresis which increases solute excretion but does not affect filtration rate (KLEEMAN, MAXWELL and ROCKNEY 1958). Cm_w does not attain normal values, however. Loading hypoadrenal patients with saline or albumin also causes Cm_w to increase to a much greater extent than does mannitol infusion (GILL et al.), but whether the fluid-loading acts by increase in filtration rate or suppression of ADH secretion, in addition to increasing solute excretion, is unknown.

Normal dilution is restored rapidly by cortisone, and by adrenocortical steroids generally, in hypoadrenal man and adrenalectomized rat (GARROD and BURSTON; SKILLERN, CORCORAN and DUSTAN; RENZI et al.; GROSS and LICHTLEN; THOMSON, BROWNELL and CUMMING; OLEESKY; KLEEMAN, MAXWELL and ROCKNEY 1958; LAMDIN et al.), although the adrenalectomized dog frequently exhibits impaired diuretic response in the presence of steroid administration (GROSS and DETTBARN; GROSS and LICHTLEN). In addition, cortisone administration frequently is associated with an increase in Cm_w in subjects with normal adrenal function (RAISZ et al. 1957; KLEEMAN et al. 1959a). The effect of steroids has frequently been attributed to a specific diuretic or anti-ADH effect on the renal tubules (SILVETTE and BRITTON; COREY and BRITTON; GAUNT, BIRNIE and EVERSOLE; GARROD and BURSTON; KLEEMAN et al. 1959a) but little direct evidence is available to support this view. Cortisone or hydrocortisone fails to correct delayed water excretion in hypoadrenal patients until fluid depletion has been corrected (GROSS and LICHTLEN), while little increase in Cm_w is observed in normal subjects on a low salt diet during cortisone administration (RAISZ et al. 1957). The adrenalectomized dog, carefully maintained on a high sodium-low potassium diet and without adrenal steroids may exhibit an essentially normal response to water-loading (KOTTKE, CODE and WOOD). Desoxycorticosterone does not inhibit the antidiuretic effect of Pitressin (SARTORIUS and ROBERTS). Therefore, the diuretic effect of adrenal steroids appears more likely to be exerted through a complex group of nonspecific factors such as increase in filtration rate, increase in solute excretion, and decrease in ADH secretion as the result of rise in blood pressure, fluid retention and improved cardiovascular tone (RAMEY and GOLDSTEIN).

δ) Hypopituitarism

The dilutional defect in patients with hypopituitarism is similar in many respects to that observed in hypoadrenal patients. A load of water is excreted slowly, onset of diuresis is delayed, and maximum urine flow is small (SLESSOR; IKKOS, LUFT and OLIVECRONA; CHALMERS and LEWIS 1951b; SOFFER and GABRILOVE). Interpretation is complicated in many patients by uncertainty as to the degree of involvement of the neurohypophysis in the pathological process. In a patient in whom posterior pituitary function is clearly vestigial, the urine may remain slightly hypotonic during dehydration. C_{osm} is usually low because of hypometabolism (LEAF et al. 1952a, b). When C_{osm} is increased by infusion of iso- or hypertonic sodium chloride or urea solutions in patients with panhypopituitarism, Cm_w may increase markedly and the increase can be prevented by Pitressin (FORBES and CLAFFEY; LEAF et al. 1952a, b). In the absence of a change in C_{osm}, replacement hormones such as thyroxine, cortisone, adrenocorticotropin and pituitary somatotropin may have little effect on Cm_w (LEAF et al. 1952a, b). Other patients with hypopituitarism have exhibited small although significant increases in Cm_w in association with aminophylline or mercurial diuresis (KLEEMAN and MAXWELL 1957; KLEEMAN, MAXWELL and ROCKNEY 1958). In other studies, increases in Cm_w following cortisone, prednisolone or adrenocorticotropin have been relatively large (LEWIS 1953; GARROD and BURSTON; HOEL; KLEEMAN, KOPLOWITZ and MAXWELL; IKKOS, LUFT and OLIVECRONA; CHALMERS and LEWIS 1951b; THOMSON, BROWNELL and CUMMING; OLEESKY). Removal of the anterior hypophysis in animals with experimental diabetes insipidus regularly results in rapid or slow subsidence of the polyuria which can be restored by administration of anterior pituitary extract. As a result of these and related studies, secretion of a 'diuretic' hormone by the anterior pituitary has been postulated (BOURQUIN; WHITE and HEIN-BECKER 1937). In the broader sense that anterior pituitary principles are essential to excretion of a water load at the normal rate, one or more of these principles may be considered as diuretic. In the narrower sense of a specific effect on renal tubular water transport, no diuretic effect has been demonstrated, and the data are compatible with a general dependence of renal hemodynamics and tubular solute transport on anterior pituitary function (SMITH 1951).

Panhypophysectomy in experimental animals is usually followed by a transitory polyuria which soon subsides (PENCHARZ, HOPPER and RYNEARSON; FISHER, INGRAM and RANSON). In the hypophysectomized rat, polyuria can usually be restored by administration of anterior pituitary extract, with adrenocortico-tropin or desoxycorticosterone being less effective restoratives (RICHTER; SCHWEITZER et al.), although opposite results have been reported by others (JOSEPH et al.). In the hypophysectomized dog, anterior pituitary extract as well as adrenocorticotropin and various steroids usually fail to restore polyuria but thyroid extract is usually effective (BARNES, REGAN and BUENO; HEIN-BECKER, WHITE and ROLF; EARLE et al. 1953). Absence of permanent polyuria in the hypophysectomized dog appears to depend upon the presence of residual functioning neurohypophyseal tissue (HEINBECKER and WHITE 1941).

ε) Sodium-retaining states

Water diuresis is frequently impaired in nephrosis, cirrhosis and congestive heart failure. The mechanism is probably complex and represents variable combinations of persistence of ADH secretion, depression in filtration rate, and depression in either C_{osm} or rate of sodium excretion. Water diuresis is closely correlated with the severity of the disease. In the less severely ill, diuresis is nearly normal, while frequently in the severely ill no diuresis may be observed.

In a nephrotic child, blood ADH concentration (as measured by transfusion of nephrotic blood into a water-diuresing recipient) was high during edema formation and the concentration decreased during diuresis of the edema fluid, but the concentration was not measured during water loading (LAUSON et al. 1952). Intravenous dextran in nephrotic children was associated with an increase in Cm_w. Renal blood flow and possibly filtration rate also increased, but the blood volume expansion could well have caused suppression of ADH secretion (JAMES, GORDILLO and METCOFF).

Impaired diuresis in cirrhosis has frequently been attributed to impaired inactivation by the liver of circulating ADH or to accumulation of nonspecific antidiuretic substances. However, cirrhotic human liver inactivates vasopressin *in vitro* at essentially the same rate as normal liver (MILLER and TOWNSEND) and the delay in onset of water diuresis, duration of antidiuresis after injection of Pitressin and response to nicotine during diuresis are not prolonged in cirrhotic patients as compared with normal subjects (WHITE, RUBIN and LEITER 1951; NELSON and WELT; BERNSTEIN et al. 1953; HARRIS, LLOYD and LOBOTSKY; EARLEY and SANDERS; BIRCHARD et al.). The diuretic response to ethanol, which presumably suppresses ADH secretion temporarily, has been variously reported as good (STRAUSS, BIRCHARD and SAXON 1956) or poor (LAMDIN et al.). Although time factors are usually normal in cirrhotics as noted above, Cm_w is regularly depressed. The magnitude of Cm_w is correlated directly with either C_{osm} or sodium excretion but the data do not permit a clear choice to be made between these two terms (BIRCHARD et al.). In some cirrhotics, in whom the urine may remain hypertonic or very slightly hypotonic following water-loading, dilution may occur and Cm_w may approach normal values during increase in C_{osm} by mannitol infusion (SCHEDL and BARTTER). Further impairment in dilution may occur following paracentesis (GABUDZA, TRAEGER and DAVIDSON) at which time an increase in concentration of blood antidiuretic substance (toad test) has been reported (WOLFF, KOCZOREK and BUCHBORN).

Dilution is essentially normal in congestive heart failure of mild to moderate severity. In severe congestive heart failure, dilution may fail irrespective of the size of a water load and the dilutional failure is reflected in an increasingly severe hyponatremia (HANENSON et al. 1956). Such patients also respond poorly to ethanol (LAMDIN et al.) but the assumption that ethanol has suppressed vasopressin secretion seems unwarranted. The importance of other factors in the dilution failure of severely ill cardiacs has not been examined.

The diuretic response to water-loading of salt-depleted normal man and dog is impaired although the urine, at the time of water loading, need not be maximally concentrated (BLACK, PLATT and STANBURY; DARROW and YANNETT; CIZEK et al.).

ζ) Nephrogenic diabetes insipidus

Diabetes insipidus is a syndrome characterized by continuous excretion of large quantities of very hypotonic urine. Renal function in other aspects is essentially normal. Among the various causes of diabetes insipidus is failure of the kidney to concentrate to more than a very small extent when antidiuretic hormone (Pituitrin, Pitressin) is injected. Since a defect lies in the kidney irrespective of whether or not endogenous ADH is circulating, the disease is termed 'nephrogenic' or 'Pituitrin refractory' diabetes insipidus.

According to FORSSMAN, the disease is hereditary. It occurs almost entirely in males and, where family histories are available, is transmitted by females (FORSSMAN; WARING, KAJDI and TAPPAN; WILLIAMS and HENRY; DANCIS, BIRMINGHAM and LESLIE; MACDONALD 1955; FLAX and GERSH; ELLBORG and FORSSMAN; LINNEWEH, BUCHBORN and DELBRÜCK; WEST and KRAMER). The incidence is 5 to 15 percent of all patients with hereditary diabetes (FORSSMAN). The diabetes has been mild in the few reported female patients. The mechanism is unknown. Water deprivation fails to stimulate release of any alternative, endogenous antidiuretic substance. Plasma of patients contains no substances which block the action of vasopressin in the rat (WILLIAMS and HENRY), and the loop of HENLE of their kidneys is anatomically normal (MACDONALD).

η) Miscellaneous factors

Dilution has been reported as essentially normal in sicklemia (as compared with impaired concentration) (LEVITT et al. 1959), but impaired, statistically, in patients with hypochromic anemia (TAYLOR). Dilution is normal in potassium depletion in the dog (MULINOS, SPINGARN and LOJKIN) and rat (LEVITIN, MANITIUS and EPSTEIN) and Cm_w may be greater than normal during acute calcium loading in man (HAUSER, POLIMEROS and LEVITT). Cm_w per 100 ml. of glomerular filtrate is normal or greater than normal in patients with chronic nephritis (KLEEMAN, ADAMS and MAXWELL) and is normal in experimental chronic nephritis in the dog (BRICKER et al. 1959). Water excretion is impaired in the rat by glutamine inhibitors (GIRERD et al.) and in the diabetes insipidus dog by serotonin (infused at 10 gamma/kg./min.) (BLACKMORE 1958): renal hemodynamics were not examined in the former, and in the latter decreased filtration rate can account for at least some of the impaired excretion. A small diuresis follows water loading during hypothermia in rat and ground squirrel at 16° and 5° C, respectively, but the magnitude cannot be evaluated because of profound depression in renal blood flow (HONG). Aminopterin (antimetabolite to folic acid) administered chronically to rats at 50 mg./kg./day causes the urine to become abundant and dilute (RABASA and BERGMANN). Persistence of serum and pituitary antidiuretic activity and of posterior pituitary neurosecretory material (SCHOR and FERRER) suggests that the defect may be a primary failure of the distal tubule to respond to ADH, in which event a close similarity to nephrogenic diabetes insipidus is afforded. Caffeine (30 mg./kg.) resulted in excretion of a hypotonic urine (U/P of 0.65) in the rabbit under chloral anesthesia (DRESER).

The effects of thyroid on urinary dilution are not clear. Thyroid administration to normal dog may result in a small increase in urine flow, perhaps in relation to decreased concentration. Thyroid administration to the dog or cat with diabetes insipidus, however, results in an augmentation which may more than double the urine flow (FISHER, INGRAM and RANSON; BIGGART and ALEXANDER; MAHONEY and SHEEHAN 1935). In the hypophysectomized dog, thyroidectomy is followed by cessation of polyuria which returns with the feeding of thyroid extract but not with the administration of anterior pituitary extract (BARNES, REGAN and BUENO; HEINBECKER, WHITE and ROLF). The effect of thyroidectomy is present but small, however, if neurohypophysectomy is complete (HEINBECKER, WHITE and ROLF). The augmenting effect of thyroid may decrease as the duration of the polyuria lengthens (HEINBECKER and WHITE 1939). The effect of thyroid may be attributable at least in part to change in filtration rate, since GFR decreases following initiation of diabetes insipidus in the dog, returns slowly to the control levels (HEINBECKER and WHITE 1939) and is augmented by thyroid (HARE et al. 1944). Polyuria decreased following thyroidectomy in a patient with diabetes insipidus (HEINBECKER and WHITE 1939).

Cm_w is reportedly depressed about 50 percent in patients with essential hypertension (BRODSKY and GRAUBARTH 1953a).

VII. Protein excretion

1. General description

Numerous macromolecular substances, or colloids, are present in normal urine. The origins of many of these, such as mucopolysaccharides, various peptides and others as yet unidentified, are unknown. Most of the urinary colloids comprise proteins which are indistinguishable from plasma albumin and globulins and which are excreted in the aggregate at 20 to 75 mg. per day (RIGAS and HELLER; GUKELBERGER and ABPLANALP; MCGARRY, SEHON and ROSE). Under circumstances too numerous to record in detail but including states such as lordotic posture (KING and BALDWIN), exercise (GOVAERTS and

DELANNE; WHITE and ROLF 1948), elevated venous pressure (WEGRIA et al.), transitory or sustained hypertension, congestive heart failure and innumerable fevers the urinary content of plasma proteins is increased. The mechanisms by which proteins enter the urine in the 'normal' state as well as during the proteinurias not clearly associated with disease of the kidneys are unknown. A generally sufficient explanation lies in the filtration-reabsorption hypothesis. Physiological and anatomical evidence are in good agreement that filtration occurs for the most part through pores about 80 Angstrom units in diameter (C II 3). The rate of filtration of any protein through such pores can be calculated if its molecular size and concentration in plasma are known and glomerular filtration rate is known. No plasma protein occurs in urine in amounts greater than the amount theoretically filtered. The concept of tubular secretion of protein, particularly of foreign proteins, has been generally abandoned (RATHER). Nevertheless, passive diffusion of proteins through the epithelium of the urinary tract (BARETZ, HARTEN and WALSER) and retrograde passage of protein-containing lymph (LÖWGREN), remain alternative sources of 'normal' and certain of the 'benign' proteinurias. At present, the significance of the nonfiltration sources of urinary protein remains speculative with the possible exception of the chylurias.

When identifiable or labelled proteins are injected into the blood, these may be detected in the cells of the proximal convoluted tubule, designating this segment as the site of the reabsorptive process (SMETANA and JOHNSON; SMETANA; RATHER; SELLERS et al.; STRAUS and OLIVER; GOODMAN and BAXTER). Because these cells are capable of absorbing particles of highly variable size and composition, it has been suggested that all macromolecules including proteins are reabsorbed by a single process to which the term 'athrocytosis' has been applied and which is considered to be allied to phagocytosis (GÉRARD). It is not known, however, whether all such particles are transported. Many, including some employed for experimental studies, may be stored in cells until the latter are desquamated and voided in the urine. Storage of recognizable materials occurs with greatest intensity in the distal half of the proximal segment (GÉRARD; OLIVER 1944, 1948). The considerable quantities of plasma proteins which are filtered daily are normally reabsorbed without a trace. When excessive filtration occurs, as following a glomerular injury or when a foreign protein is injected into the blood, the protein accumulates in the cell and aggregates into microscopically visible particles. Simultaneously with or perhaps contributing to aggregate formation, mitochondria dissolve and their content of ribonucleic acid becomes incorporated in the protein aggregates and affects their staining reactions. Accumulated lipids from filtered and reabsorbed lipoproteins produce fat droplets. If the protein loading is interrupted, the aggregates slowly dissolve and the mitochondria are reconstituted (OLIVER 1948; STRAUS and OLIVER; OLIVER et al. 1955; OLIVER and MacDOWELL 1958). Presumably, proteins can be absorbed from the tubular fluid more rapidly than they can be liberated into the blood. When the slower rate is exceeded, accumulation, with the characteristic picture of proximal tubular cells in the nephrotic syndrome, results.

2. Hemoglobin and myoglobin

When hemoglobin is injected intravenously, it does not appear in the urine until the plasma concentration exceeds 125 mg. percent in man (GILLIGAN, ALTSCHULE and KATERSKY; LATHEM and WORLEY) or 100 mg. in the dog (MONKE and YUILE). Excretion of hemoglobin, once it has commenced, is linearly related to plasma hemoglobin concentration. The change in hemoglobin excretion per unit change in plasma concentration has the dimensions of a clearance and is usually expressed as a fraction of the filtration rate. This fraction has been variously termed the 'filterability', 'permeability coefficient' or 'glomerular clearance ratio' of hemoglobin. This may be abbreviated for convenience to GCR. Values of GCR in man have been reported as 0.05 (LATHEM 1959) to 0.10 (McDONALD, MILLER and ROACH) and in the dog as 0.03 to 0.05 (MONKE and YUILE; YUILE et al.; LATHEM 1957b; LAMBERT et al. 1957). The plasma hemoglobin threshold results from two factors. Most importantly, much of the plasma hemoglobin is bound to certain of the plasma proteins (haptoglobin) which have a molecular weight of about 85,000 and which move electrophoretically in the alpha-2 globulin fraction (JAYLE and BOUSSIER). Not until the hemoglobin binding capacity of the plasma, equivalent to about 128 mg. percent, is exceeded and free hemoglobin is present can significant filtration of hemoglobin commence (LAMBERT et al. 1957; LATHEM and WORLEY). In addition, hemoglobin is reabsorbed, and filtered hemoglobin, corrected for plasma binding, must exceed reabsorptive capacity, or Tm, before significant excretion commences. Tm in man is about 1.3 mg./min. (LATHEM 1959) and in the dog 3 to 4 mg./min. (LAMBERT et al. 1957). Decrease in filtration rate is associated with an increase in GCR as predicted by filtration theory (LAMBERT et al. 1957). Epinephrine administration in the dog is associated with an increase in hemoglobin GCR which is greater than that attributable to decrease in filtration rate (LAMBERT et al. 1957; LATHEM 1957a, b), suggesting that this amine has increased the diameter of the filtration pores either directly or indirectly through hypertension. Renin, however, does not increase excretion of hemoglobin although excretion of other proteins is increased in rabbit and rat (BRANDT and GRUHN; ADDIS et al. 1949). Steroids, particularly glucocorticoids, increase hemoglobin threshold in the dog (LAMBERT and GRÉGOIRE) by increasing plasma binding capacity (LAMBERT et al. 1957). Following single or repeated injections of hemoglobin in the dog the plasma threshold decreases (YUILE et al.). This is attributable for the most part to rapid disappearance from the circulation of the hemoglobin-haptoglobin complex, and in patients with hemolytic anemia very little haptoglobin is present (LAURELL and NYMAN). In addition, hemoglobin Tm may be depressed (LAMBERT et al. 1957). Hemoglobin loading is occasionally associated with a small increase in excretion of nonhemoglobin protein, suggesting possible competition for reabsorption.

Myoglobin, a small protein with a molecular weight of about 17,000 compared with 60,000 for hemoglobin, has a glomerular clearance ratio of about 0.75 or nearly 20 times that of hemoglobin (YUILE and CLARK). Like hemoglobin, myoglobin is partially bound to certain plasma proteins which may be haptoglobins, but the binding is neither as firm nor as extensive (about 20 mg. percent in man) as with hemoglobin (WILLOUGHBY).

3. Plasma proteins

The mechanism of albumin excretion can be examined by methods similar to those for hemoglobin. When plasma proteins are injected in the dog, proteinuria appears at a threshold concentration of 8 to 10 g. percent (TERRY et al.). The albumin glomerular clearance ratio (GCR) is about 0.006 which is about $1/5$ that of hemoglobin and in agreement with the value expected from the larger size of the albumin molecule. Albumin Tm, likewise in the dog, is 10 to 12 mg./min. (MALMENDIER and LAMBERT; LAMBERT et al. 1957).

Albumin GCR in 4 healthy men averaged 0.003 which, at a filtration rate of 120 ml./min. and an albumin threshold of 7.3 g. percent indicates that albumin Tm is about 26 mg./min. or 37 g./24 hours (LAMBERT et al. 1957). Rapid increase in urinary excretion of proteins following increase in plasma protein concentration has long been recognized in patients with renal disease (KEUTMAN and BASSETT; LUETSCHER 1944). The glomerular clearance of albumin is greatly increased in such patients. In patients with nephrosis, glomerular clearance ratios of 0.02 to 0.06, values roughly 10 times normal, have been reported (HARDWICK and SQUIRE; CHINARD et al. 1954; LAMBERT et al. 1957). The marked tendency in some nephrotic patients for the clearance ratio to increase with increasing plasma albumin concentration (CHINARD et al. 1954; LAMBERT et al. 1957) has been attributed to existence of two or more discrete nephron populations which differ in their glomerular permeability and albumin Tm (MALMENDIER, GREGOIRE and LAMBERT).

Albumin Tm in nephrosis is somewhat decreased, with values of 9 to 30 mg./min. reported (LAMBERT et al. 1957; HARDWICK and SQUIRE; MALMENDIER, GREGOIRE and LAMBERT). The GCR are of the same magnitude (0.01 to 0.03) in azotemic albuminurics as in nephrotics (LAMBERT et al. 1957). In patients with amyloid nephrosis, GCR of 0.006 to 0.01 and very low albumin Tm, 2 to 8 mg./min., have been reported (LAMBERT et al. 1957). Steroid administration (adrenocorticotropin or prednisone) in patients with 'lipoid' nephrosis is associated with a decrease in albumin GCR of 50 to 90 percent (LAUSON et al. 1952, 1954) with little or irregular changes in albumin Tm (LAMBERT et al. 1957; MALMENDIER, GREGOIRE and LAMBERT).

Other plasma proteins in man have glomerular clearance ratios compatible with their molecular weights. The GCR of alpha-1 globulin is very close to that of albumin while that of the beta and gamma globulins vary from 20 to 80 percent of the albumin GCR and, in proteinuric patients, averaging 42 and 38 percent, respectively. GCR of alpha-2 globulin ranges from 5 to 46 percent of the albumin value. Variation in globulin/albumin clearance ratios presumably represents variation in pore size in the diseased glomerulus (HARDWICK and SQUIRE).

E. Extrarenal control of renal function

I. General considerations

CLAUDE BERNARD first recognized the importance to the body of stabilizing the composition of the extracellular fluid. This stability of composition, expressed in terms of variations about normal values of various constituents, has long been a cardinal principle of physiology, to which the term 'homeostasis' was applied by CANNON (1932). It is now clear, however, that constancy of body fluid composition (later broadened to include volume as well) is only a particular instance of stabilization of all aspects of body function, such as blood pressure, metabolic rate, total body composition and, ultimately, growth and form itself. Moreover, a relative stability of a particular quantity is not a property peculiar to living things. Rather it is a property of most natural processes describable as steady states. A relative stability in a steady state system results from the circumstance that a change in one variable is followed by changes in one or more other variables such that the effects of the first change are minimized. An example from the nonliving world which offers an analogy to some kidney functions is the depth of a lake. Large changes in the inflow to a lake are followed by corresponding large changes in outflow with the result that the depth of the lake may change very little. Such a degree of stability would, if observed in the body, be termed homeostasis. Because of the difficulty of assigning any precise definition to homeostasis as a property of living systems, it is more useful to classify body quantities according to the type of system within which they are stabilized. Two principal types of control systems can be recognized:

A. Simple steady state systems. The elements of these systems are the controlled quantity and the tissue or organ which controls it, the effector organ.

B. Negative feed-back systems. The elements of these systems are the controlled quantity, the effector organ, and a third element, the feed-back element, whose output responds to changes in the controlled quantity in such a way that a counter change is made in the effector organ.

Simple steady state systems are represented by the example of the lake level described above. They are usually quite easily described. Usually, but far from always, variables in these systems are less closely controlled than are systems containing feed-back elements. In addition, oscillation in these simple systems cannot be sustained. Blood urea, uric acid, creatinine and sulfate concentrations in man appear to be largely or entirely controlled within simple steady-state systems, the renal glomeruli constituting the effector organ.

In negative feed-back systems, a change in the controlled quantity causes a second system to operate in such a way as to tend to drive the controlled quantity in the direction opposite to the change. The system of the lake level control, described above, can be converted to a negative feed-back system by introducing a device by which a rise in lake level, the controlled quantity, could enlarge the outlet to the lake. Other familiar negative feed-back systems are the speed-controls of motors and temperature controls of houses and other units. In speed controls an increase or decrease in the controlled quantity, engine speed, actuates a mechanism which decreases or increases the supply of energy to the motor. In temperature control, an increase or decrease in temperature actuates a thermostat which causes the fuel supply to a heater to decrease or increase. Negative feed-back systems are frequently complex and are difficult to describe mathematically[1]. They usually permit a much higher degree of control of the subject quantity than is possible without them. Of great theoretical importance is the fact that sustained oscillation is possible in negative feed-back systems because a delay always exists between a change in the subject quantity and attainment of full response on the part of the feed-back element.

If a feed-back system is present, it may be either remote from the effector organ (external feed-back) or within the effector organ itself (internal feed-back). The internal feed-back system, unfortunately, has thus far proven difficult to analyse and its existence in specific cases must be inferred. The renal excretion of potassium and of acid may be controlled by internal feed-back systems. Although potassium excretion is greatly modified by many extrarenal influences, no clear evidence is available that any of these vary reciprocally (external negative feed-back) with plasma potassium concentration. Similarly, no extrarenal variable affecting the renal mechanisms for the excretion of acid (hydrogen ion and ammonia production) and responding to changes in blood pH have been detected. The renal acid excreting mechanisms must, in fact, operate in the presence of opposition from the respiratory system since a decrease in blood

---

[1] For some mathematical treatments of biological feed-back systems see, for example, DANZIGER and ELMERGREEN, and ROSTON.

carbon dioxide tension resulting from increased pulmonary ventilation in acidosis tends to limit the capacity of the kidney to excrete acid.

External feed-back systems are represented by the extrarenal controls of renal function. Two such systems are clearly recognized. These are the systems regulating the excretion of water and of sodium chloride. A third system may regulate excretion of calcium and phosphate, and other systems may exist whose existence as yet can be no more than suspected.

II. Extrarenal control of water and salt excretion
1. General description

The negative feed-back systems controlling water and salt excretion are diagrammed in Fig. 68. For simplicity, the interactions between the water and the salt systems are not indicated. The 'negative' aspect of the feed-back is illustrated by the circumstance that the effects on the kidney of the nervous system control mechanism are opposite in sign to the direction of change of the kidney function.

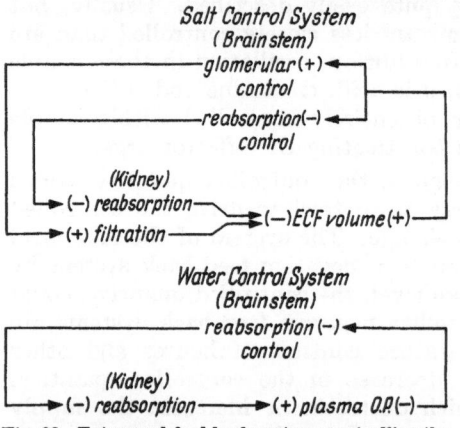

Fig. 68. Extrarenal feed-back systems controlling the excretion of water and salt. The systems illustrate the changes attendant upon an increase (+) in extracellular fluid volume or a decrease (−) in plasma osmotic pressure. Reversal of these signs should be attended by a reversal of all other signs in the circuit

Interdependence of the salt and water systems is illustrated in Fig. 69. Important interrelationships occur in 2 areas: in the kidney, the osmotic pressure, reflected in plasma sodium concentration, directly affects the excretion of NaCl. In the hypothalamus, extracellular fluid volume which, in this simplified system is assumed to represent the state of the circulation, directly affects the response of the osmoreceptor system to a given plasma osmotic pressure. This last relationship has the effect of causing plasma sodium concentration to reflect the overall state of the circulation (Fig. 71).

The complete body system governing salt and water balance and of which the renal system, illustrated in Fig. 69, is no more than a component is illustrated in Fig. 70. In this view, the kidney is one of several effector organs regulating the cardiovascular system. The primary cardiovascular variable which is regulated is 'adequacy of perfusion of body tissues', or simply, 'cardiovascular adequacy'. This term, which is not susceptible to further definition, is designed to allow for variations in body need for circulating blood as well as for variation in volume and distribution of cardiac output[1]. The afferent pathways which signal the degree of cardiovascular adequacy are largely unknown. They include the "volume receptors", the search for which has involved immense research effort, although it appears increasingly probable that 'volume receptors' in the sense of a specialized organ responding sensitively to a change in some fraction or quality of the extracellular fluid volume probably do not exist. Some afferent nerve pathways such as from stretch receptors in the right atrium and from endings in the walls of the large arteries (Henry, Gauer and

---

[1] This concept represents no important difference from the views of Borst.

REEVES; HENRY and PEARCE; BARTTER, MILLS and GANN) have been identified. These may well represent particularly conspicuous examples of afferents arising from the entire cardiovascular system. The possibility of humoral as well as neurogenically mediated afferent signals must also be considered. For example, renin, liberated by the kidney in response to alteration in the character of its blood flow, can be viewed as a special example of a humoral agent of peripheral origin.

The search for the 'volume receptor' has consisted in the testing of one after another of conceivable functions of the extracellular and vascular volumes. Of particular interest are the generally negative results associated with intracerebral (LEWIS et al. 1950; CATHCART and WILLIAMS; LOMBARDO and HARRISON; NETRAVISESH; NICKEL, LEVINE and GAGNON; FISHMAN) and intrathoracic venous pressure and volume changes (SURTSHIN, HOELTZENBEIN and WHITE; LOVE et al.) and the vascular and extracellular fluid volumes themselves. With each succeeding set of negative observations the dimensions of the 'volume receptor' have been broadened. EPSTEIN, POST and MCDOWELL have identified the 'volume receptor' as coextensive with the arterial system, while ROBINSON (1954a) has taken the final step in the evolution of this thought and identified the 'volume receptor' with the entire vascular system. In ROBINSON'S view, with which the present author agrees, volume as a controlled quantity is represented by "all the afferent information from the vascular system [which] is co-ordinated somewhere, perhaps in the hypothalamus". Some

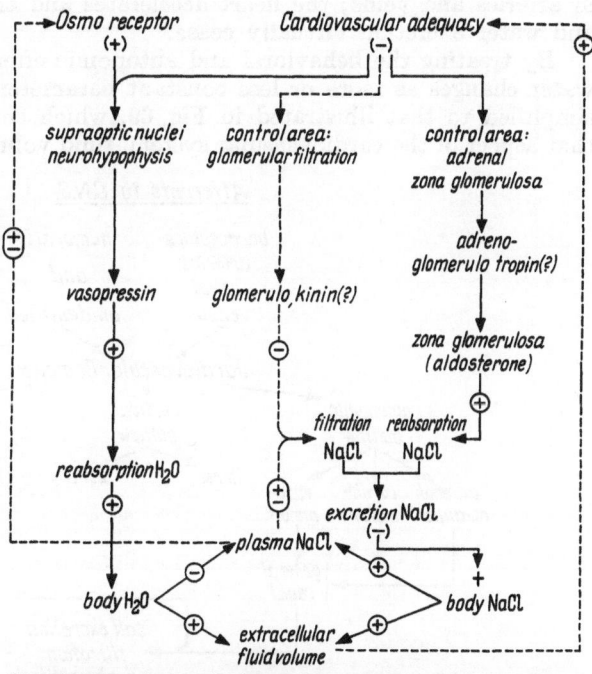

Fig. 69. Interrelationships between the salt and the water control systems. The diagram illustrates the events following a primary cardiovascular stress (decrease in cardiovascular adequacy) combined with plasma hypertonicity (increase in osmoreceptor activity). Solid lines represent increases in quantity or functional activity. Broken lines indicate either decreasing quantity, decreasing activity, or inhibitory or releasing influences. Ambiguity of effect arising from variation in the proportions of the NaCl and H_2O changes is indicated by ($\pm$)

review articles which consider volume control are: PETERS (1948, 1952), LEITER (1948), STEAD (1952), WELT (1952, 1955, 1960), BULL (1955), BARGER (1956), COLEBATCH (1956), GROSSMAN (1957), SMITH (1957).

Afferent signals from the vascular system to the central nervous system probably have a double distribution. Part of the distribution (either by separate fibers or by collaterals) may be to local functional areas. The other part of the distribution may be combined in the brain stem into a single signal, the intensity of which directly measures 'cardiovascular adequacy'. Three major effector systems, behavioral, motor and humoral appear responsive to this signal: The *Behavioral* system comprises efferents to the cerebral cortex and governs energy expenditure and salt and water consumption. A hypothalamic center originating thirst activity is demonstrable. The *Motor* system comprises vasomotor and cardiomotor fibers which alter cardiac output, the size of blood reservoirs (FREIS and ROSE), the distribution of the cardiac output, and total and regional arterial resistances. The *Humoral* system comprises hormones whose liberation is controlled by the hypothalamus and which determine the blood volume or, more generally, the circulating volume of extracellular fluid by their effects on renal salt and water excretion. In addition, the humoral system probably controls the efficiency of salt conservation by intestine and sweat glands. The role of these three systems in maintaining cardiovascular adequacy is seen following simple hemorrhage: the organism avoids exertion and is thirsty; blood is drained from venules and veins; vasoconstriction occurs in arteries and veins; the heart accelerates and empties more completely; salt and water excretion virtually cease.

By treating the behavioral and autonomic efferents and extrarenal salt and water changes as more or less constant parameters, the general system can be simplified to that illustrated in Fig. 69, which comprises only the kidney and that aspect of the cardiovascular system, fluid volume, which it governs directly.

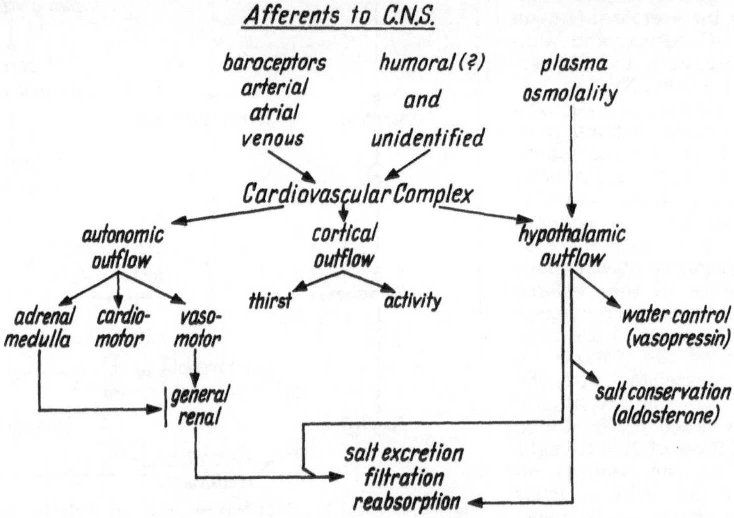

Fig. 70. Body mechanisms governing cardiovascular adequacy. Salt and water balance is one of several elements determining 'adequacy'. Balance can be controlled by either renal or extrarenal systems

2. Control of water reabsorption (hypothalamico-neurohypophyseal system)

a) General description

Reabsorption and excretion of water are determined by numerous variables described in section D VI 4 g. Of these variables, three appear to be subject to some degree of direct extrarenal control. These are: rate of filtration of water, described in section E II 4; rate of liberation of antidiuretic hormone; and a mechanism whose nature is as yet unknown which responds to the state of hydration of the body and determines the responsiveness of the kidney to antidiuretic hormone (D VI 4). The most important of these is liberation of antidiuretic hormone which, for practical purposes, constitutes extrarenal control of water excretion.

Experimental studies which elucidate the structure of this system have led to a voluminous literature. These have been the subject of numerous reviews such as those of WHITE and HEINBECKER (1937); FISHER, INGRAM and RANSON; FISHER; VERNEY (1946, 1947, 1954, 1957); PICKFORD (1945); O'CONNOR (1947); SMITH (1947); MAHONEY and SHEEHAN (1936); HARRIS (1948, 1955); WELT

(1952); LEAF and MAMBY (1952a); LEAF (1960); DINGMAN; and THORN (1958) and the reader is referred to these for details. In the prevailing view, antidiuretic hormone (ADH) appears to arise from neurons of the supraoptic nuclei, the rostroventral portions of the paraventricular hypothalamic nuclei (HEINBECKER and WHITE) and possibly from the ventromedial, anterior hypothalamic and dorsal paraventricular nuclei (FISHER, INGRAM and RANSON). Within the neurons, ADH is tentatively identified with granular 'neurosecretory material' which is presumed to represent the polypeptides vasopressin or, in other neurons, oxytocin bound to a protein carrier. The axons of the supraoptic and paraventricular nuclei pass downward and posteriorly as the supraoptico-hypophyseal tracts to terminate around the pituicytes of the pars nervosa of the pituitary body (RENNELS and DRAGER). Many of the axons do not pass as far as the pars nervosa, however, but terminate in relation to similar cells in the pituitary stalk and the median eminence of the hypothalamus. Neurosecretory material is transmitted along the axons to the vicinity of the pituicytes which are presumed to function in a storage and release capacity. The functional unit is, therefore, the neuron with its terminal pituicytes. Section of the axon at any point in the supraoptico-hypophyseal tract or destruction of the cell bodies of the supraoptic nuclei is followed by disappearance of neurosecretory material from the neurons and pituicytes and nearly complete disappearance of antidiuretic material from the entire neurohypophysis (median eminence, pituitary stalk and pars nervosa) (FISHER, INGRAM and RANSON; MELVILLE and HARE; HARE, HICKEY and HARE 1941a, b; PHILLIPS and HARE; BAILEY and BREMER). Some species variation exists with respect to the distribution of terminations of supraopticohypophyseal fibers. In cat and rat, these fibers appear to terminate almost entirely in the pars nervosa (FISHER, INGRAM and RANSON). In dog and monkey, median eminence and stalk represent 15 to 30 percent of neurohypophyseal tissue or the terminus of this fraction of the neurons (HEINBECKER and WHITE 1941; MAGOUN, FISHER and RANSON). Permanent polyuria does not occur if 5 or at most 15 percent of the neurons remain intact (HEINBECKER and WHITE 1941; O'CONNOR and VERNEY 1941). When renal function also is depressed as following removal of the anterior pituitary, persistence of very small quantities of functional tissue is sufficient to prevent the appearance of an overt polyuria (KELLER). Failure to obtain permanent polyuria following surgical hypophysectomy suggests that in man as in dog and monkey significant quantities of neurohypophyseal tissue lie outside the pars nervosa (LIPSETT et al.). The alternative view, that pressor-antidiuretic material is synthesized within the neurohypophysis, has neither received experimental support nor been clearly disproven.

Not only formation but also release of ADH requires integrity of the neurohypophyseal neurons, release occurring in response to impulses passing over the axons (HATERIUS; ANDERSSON and MCCANN). Whether ADH can be released directly from cell bodies of supraoptic neurons is unknown. Neural connections to the supraoptic nuclei, by which the latter can be stimulated to release ADH, arise from an immense variety of sensory areas. For the most part, but with significant exceptions, these connections arise from two principal areas. These are the 'osmoreceptors' and the cardiovascular system. The nature of the osmoreceptors is unknown. The term is employed to designate hypothetical sensory endings which respond to changes in the osmotic pressure of the blood and synapse with the supraoptic neurons. The osmoreceptors are located in the anterior hypothalamus (VERNEY 1957) and may, in fact, be the supraoptic neurons themselves or certain ones of them. Large vesicles or vesiculated neurons, 60 micra in diameter, have been described in the supraoptic nuclei and which could function mechanically as organs sensitive to volume changes arising from changes in osmotic pressure of the blood (VERNEY 1957). Only solutes incapable of passing freely through cell membranes should be capable of effecting a change in cell volume.

Stimuli to the neurohypophysis from the cardiovascular system are clearly recognized but their origin is uncertain. Such stimuli are typified by the anti-diuretic effects of blood sequestration. No evidence of direct communication between the neurohypophysis and peripheral cardiovascular stimulatory afferents is available although it would seem reasonable to suppose that such may exist. Rather, the neurohypophysis appears to respond to stimuli of cardiovascular origin concomitantly with the diencephalic-adrenal system and the glomerular filtration control system, suggesting the probable existence of an integrative area through which a large number of cardiovascular afferents are transmitted to the neurohypophysis as a single signal.

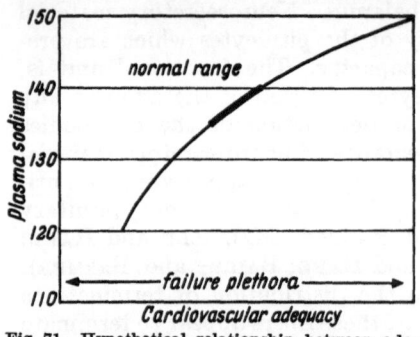

Fig. 71. Hypothetical relationship between adequacy of the circulation and the plasma sodium concentration at which water diuresis appears

In addition to afferent stimuli, certain afferent connections exert an inhibitory influence on neurohypophyseal function. Among these are stretch receptors of the atria, and exposure to cold, although the latter influence may be an indirect one and related to redistribution of blood.

The relationship of cardiovascular to osmotic influences is not clear. It is evident that a change in either osmotic pressure or the cardiovascular system is capable of effecting a change in ADH secretion. Under appropriate circumstances, influences from the two areas may either cancel or reinforce each other, suggesting an algebraic addition. Alternatively, however, highly indirect evidence suggests that the osmotic stimulus is prepotent. A working hypothesis which is in agreement with most of the data is that the primary signal to the supraoptic neurons arises from the osmoreceptors and that the intensity of this signal is a continuous although not necessarily linear function of plasma osmotic pressure. This signal may then be subject to amplication (and possibly to inhibition) by impulses arising from the cardiovascular system or a cardiovascular integrative center. Rate of ADH release should then be a function of the intensity of the modified signal. Conversely, the plasma osmotic pressure (determined for the most part by salts of sodium) at which significant release of ADH occurs should be a function of the state of the cardiovascular system (Fig. 71).

Vasopressin appears in the neurohypophysis during fetal life at about 70 days, earlier than oxytocin, and for some time after oxytocin has appeared is present in relatively greater amounts (DICKER and TYLER; VAN DYKE, ADAMSONS and ENGEL). By birth, however, both polypeptides are present in approximately equal amounts and a ratio of 1.0 continues to maturity although the hormone content of the gland is increasing. The ratio of vasopressin to oxytocin is regularly greater in the hypothalamus than in the pars nervosa (VAN DYKE, ADAMSONS and ENGEL).

The pars nervosa at birth contains about 166 milliunits of pressor-antidiuretic substance per milligram dry weight and at maturity about 741 mU. (HELLER and ZAIMIS). The entire gland in man contains about 15 and occasionally as much as 30 units, an immense store in view of the fact that infusion of 10—15 milliunits per hour is sufficient to maintain maximal antidiuresis (LAUSON 1951a; HOLLANDER et al. 1957a).

b) Osmotic control of vasopressin release

The presence of antidiuresis during water deprivation or infusion of hypertonic solutions, and diuresis following water ingestion, is well known. In either circumstance, a change in osmotic or solute concentration of the plasma is demonstrable (SMITH 1951, review). The osmotic response is independent of the renal nerves (BAYLISS and BROWN; BAYLISS and FEE; KLISIECKI et al. 1933a, b; BRICKER et al. 1956), and of local peripheral osmotic pressure changes (ZUIDEMA and CLARKE). A prompt antidiuretic response without significant change in filtration rate is, however, elicited by intracarotid injection of small amounts of hypertonic solutions of sodium chloride, sodium sulfate or sucrose but not of urea (VERNEY 1946, 1947, 1948; ZUIDEMA and CLARKE; ZUIDEMA, CLARKE and MINTON, SQUIRES, HAN and ZEMACH). Antidiuretic activity of jugular venous blood is increased (AMES, MOORE and VAN DYKE). Since a response is elicited by substances which are largely restricted to the extracellular fluid compartment, but not by urea which readily enters cell water, the term 'effective osmotic pressure' is employed to designate that fraction of plasma solute which affects the activity of the osmoreceptors. Infusion of hypertonic urea in normal man is followed by a water diuresis (EARLEY). The antidiuretic effect of blood hypertonicity is abolished by section of the supraoptico-hypophyseal tracts (VERNEY 1946, 1947, 1948) and the effect is limited to that fraction of the cerebral blood which perfuses the anterior hypothalamus (VERNEY 1957). Slow potentials can be recorded from the hypothalamus of the cat during intracarotid infusion of hypertonic NaCl, and potentials of opposite polarity can be recorded during infusion of water, but these are not clearly correlated with osmoreceptor activity (v. EULER). Prolonged osmotic stimulation, as occurs during water deprivation or salt loading, is associated with progressive depletion of the ADH content of the pars nervosa of the rat (HARE, HICKEY and HARE 1941a; DICKER and NUNN 1957b) and an increase in mitoses among the pituicytes (CHAMBERS).

The osmotically-stimulated release of ADH is undiminished by aging in the rat, and decreasing urine concentration with aging cannot be attributed to neurohypophyseal failure (DICKER and NUNN 1958).

c) Nonosmotic factors stimulating antidiuretic hormone release

A large number of factors of a nonosmotic character stimulate the release of ADH. Release of ADH is detected by suppression or abolition of a water diuresis without significant changes in filtration rate or solute excretion. In neurohypophysectomized animals, or patients with diabetes insipidus, the stimulus should be ineffective. ADH is released in response to pain, excitement or exercise in dog (THEOBALD and VERNEY; RYDIN and VERNEY; O'CONNOR and VERNEY 1941; O'CONNOR 1946; DEMPSTER and JOEKES), and rabbit (HATERIUS). In man, antidiuresis occurs during and following syncope (BRUN, KNUDSEN and RAASCHOU 1945, 1945b, c), pain (CHALMERS and LEWIS 1951a), exercise in normal or cardiac subjects (BARCLAY and NUTT 1944b; BARCLAY et al. 1947; DUNCAN), quiet standing (SURTSHIN and WHITE), breathing against a positive pressure (DRURY, HENRY and GOODMAN) or application of limb tourniquets (JUDSON et al. 1950, 1952). With the possible exceptions of pain and excitement, the factor common to all of these situations is some form of circulatory stress.

The stimulus to ADH release is probably mediated by largely unknown afferents from the cardiovascular system and is not mediated by peripherally released epinephrine.

ADH release is stimulated by numerous drugs and related substances. Ether, cyclopropane or nitrous oxide anesthesia is antidiuretic to man (APRAHAMIAN et al.). Barbiturates (amytal, pheno- and pentobarbital) are weakly antidiuretic in the dog (DE BODO and PRESCOTT) but thiopental has little antidiuretic effect in man or rat (APRAHAMIAN et al.; SILVETTE 1942). Morphine is a potent stimulant of ADH release in the dog (DE BODO; HANDLEY and KELLER 1950b). In man, however, the ADH-releasing effect of morphine is weak or absent (PAPPER et al. 1957; BOYD and SCHERF; WALKER 1949) and some evidence suggests that the principal effect of morphine is reinforcement of the antidiuretic effect of other stimuli such as pain or hypotension (LEWIS 1953; LE QUESNE and LEWIS). Acetylcholine, particularly by intracarotid injection, elicits antidiuresis in the dog. The effect is enhanced by eserine (DUKE and PICKFORD; PICKFORD and WATT 1952), can be blocked by intracarotid injection of 1—3 micrograms of epinephrine 20 seconds prior to the acetylcholine, but cannot be blocked by atropine. No effect is observed in the diabetes insipidus dog (PICKFORD 1939). A similar antidiuretic response to acetylcholine is observed in man (CHALMERS and LEWIS 1951a). Of particular interest is the effect of nicotine. This base, probably acting through the same mechanism as that of acetylcholine, is profoundly antidiuretic to normal man and rat but not to subjects with diabetes insipidus (BURN, TRUELOVE and BURN; CATES and GARROD; CHALMERS and LEWIS 1951a; BISSET and WALKER 1951; WALKER 1949; HANENSON et al. 1956). Nicotine antidiuresis cannot be blocked by either ethanol or hexamethonium in the rat (BISSET and WALKER 1951). The effects of nicotine can be duplicated by 1—3 cigarettes (BURN, TRUELOVE and BURN; CHALMERS and LEWIS 1951a) with nonsmokers being the more sensitive (WALKER 1949). Among other agents which are antidiuretic, probably by stimulating release of ADH, are dimercaptopropanol in the dog (EARLE and BERLINER 1947), novocaine in the dog (PRONINA), derivatives of cinchoninic acid (MARSHALL and BLANCHARD), serotonin in the rat (KIVALO, MARJANEN and RINNE), and histamine in the dog (BLACKMORE and CHERRY). Renin appears to stimulate ADH release in the dog in addition to depressing filtration rate (WHITNEY et al.). Epinephrine and norepinephrine exert in the dog an irregular but generally antidiuretic effect which is independent of changes in renal blood flow and glomerular filtration and which can be abolished by hypothalamic injury (PICKFORD and WATT 1950; ABRAHAMS and PICKFORD 1956; DEARBORN and LASAGNA). In man, epinephrine in tolerable quantities is not significantly antidiuretic (CHALMERS and LEWIS 1951a).

d) Nonosmotic factors inhibiting antidiuretic hormone release

Release of ADH can be inhibited by certain drugs or chemicals and by influences which are probably or certainly mediated by afferent nervous pathways. Inhibition is detected by the appearance of a water-type diuresis: a decrease in urine osmotic concentration and corresponding increase in urine flow which can be inhibited by exogenous vasopressin.

Diuresis may be evoked in man by infusion of isotonic or slightly hypertonic saline solutions (LADD 1951a, 1952; MURPHY and STEAD; BIRCHARD; BIRCHARD and STRAUSS; BLOMHERT et al.). The diuretic response is enhanced if the subject is prehydrated by water or saline 12 to 24 hours previous to the infusion (LADD 1951a, 1952; BIRCHARD and STRAUSS), and is inhibited if the subject is not recumbent during the infusion (STRAUSS et al. 1951). Diuresis may be elicited by rapid saline infusion in subjects with cirrhosis (STRAUSS, BIRCHARD and SAXON), hypoadrenalism (GILL et al.) or panhypopituitarism (FORBES and CLAFFEY); by Dextran infusion in nephrotics (JAMES, GORDILLO and METCOFF); by breathing 5 to 7 percent carbon dioxide (BARBOUR et al.); by breathing against a negative pressure (SIEKER, GAUER and HENRY; SURTSHIN, HOELTZEN-BEIN and WHITE; LOVE et al.; BOYLAN and ANTKOWIAK; HULET and SMITH); by exposure to cold (BADER, ELIOT and BASS) and under certain conditions of emotional stress and anxiety (HINKLE, EDWARDS and WOLF; MILES, DE WAR-DENER and McSWINEY). Diuresis, presumably water-type, has been reported as elicited by hypnotic suggestion (MARX 1926). In the dog, water-type diuresis may be elicited by infusion of 25 percent albumin (ORLOFF and BLAKE) and by negative pressure breathing. The diuretic response to negative pressure breathing can be duplicated by distention or filling of the right atrium and abolished by block of certain afferent fibers which travel in the vagi and which discharge during atrial distention (GAUER et al.; HENRY and PEARCE; HENRY, GAUER and REEVES; SURTSHIN, HOELTZENBEIN and WHITE). Filtration rate and sodium excretion do not change in either dog or man during negative pressure breathing, but the brevity of the experiments may have precluded detection of slower changes in filtration or adrenal control. Diuresis is reported in the dog as a conditioned reflex response to presentation of water or dilute milk (GROSSMAN 1929; MARX 1931; BYKOW and ALEXEJEW-BERKMANN), and during exposure to low barometric pressure in the rat (SILVETTE). Diuresis is not elicited in man by increased cerebral venous pressure produced by head-down position (WILKINS, BRADLEY and FRIEDLAND; CATHCART and WILLIAMS).

Drugs which inhibit ADH secretion are promazine in man (SMITH, PAPPER and ROSENBAUM) and ethanol in man, dog and rat (HAGGARD, GREENBERG and CARROLL; EGGLETON 1942a; RUBINI, KLEEMAN and LAMDIN; STRAUSS, ROSEN-BAUM and NELSON; VAN DYKE and AMES; WIRZ 1956). The diuretic effect of ethanol is principally a direct one upon the central nervous system (VAN DYKE and AMES) and in man and dog is significant only during rising blood ethanol concentration (HAGGARD, GREENBERG and CARROLL; EGGLETON 1942a; VAN DYKE and AMES). Ethanol can block the antidiuretic effect of moderate degrees of blood sequestration or hypertonic saline infusion provided it has become effective prior to the antidiuretic stimulus. It is ineffective following the antidiuretic stimulus or if the hypertonicity is marked (KLEEMAN et al. 1955a; STRAUSS, ROSENBAUM and NELSON). In some but not in all subjects who are exhibiting a declining urine flow under a sustained water load, ethanol may restore the diuresis (ROSENBAUM et al. 1957). Ethanol diuresis is minimal or absent in patients with congestive heart failure, nephrosis, cirrhosis, panhypopituitarism or hypoadrenalism (LAMDIN et al.).

· e) Thirst center

Located in the anterolateral hypothalamus is a region which, when stimulated, elicits drinking behavior in rat and goat; and lesions in the area may abolish the normal drinking response to water deprivation or hypertonic saline (GREER; ANDERSSON and McCANN; for reviews: WELT et al. 1952; ROSENBAUM 1956). It is close to, but distinguishable from, the supraoptic and paraventricular nuclei. The importance of the 'thirst center' in maintaining water balance is equal to or greater than that of the neurohypophysis. Both the thirst and the ADH-releasing areas appear to be stimulated by the same afferents. As in the case of ADH-release, the thirst center responds to hypertonic saline but not

to hypertonic urea (GILMAN), suggesting that thirst osmoreceptors are similar
to or the same as those supplying the neurohypophysis. It is significant, however,
that atrophy of the supraoptic and paraventricular neurons following destruction of the neurohypophysis does not notably impair thirst response to hyperosmolarity of the blood.

f) Renal nerves and water diuresis

Nerve impulses mediated by the renal nerves are capable of inhibiting water
diuresis. Thus, antidiuresis attending ether anesthesia in the diabetes insipidus
dog is abolished by renal denervation (BAYLISS and BROWN) and urine hypotonicity is abolished by stimulation of the splanchnic nerves in the dog heart-
lung-kidney preparation (BAYLISS and FEE). In the intact dog, emotional antidiuresis is a combination of neurogenic and ADH inhibition of urine flow, the
former being rapid in onset and abolished by renal denervation, the latter being
slower and abolished by neurohypophysectomy (O'CONNOR and VERNEY 1941,
1945; O'CONNOR 1946). The mechanism of renal nervous inhibition of diuresis
is undoubtedly the consequence of reduction in glomerular filtration rate and
in rate of solute excretion (D VI 4 k). This mechanism probably accounts for many
occurrences of oliguria, such as that following syncope (BRUN, KNUDSEN and RAA-
SCHOU 1945c), in patients with diabetes insipidus.

g) Diurnal variation in urine flow

As with several other excretory functions, urine flow and concentration
exhibit a characteristic diurnal cycle. Flow is lowest and concentration is maximal
by night, with rapidly rising flow and decreasing concentration during the first
hours after awakening. The cycle appears to be determined in part by the
corresponding cycle of nocturnal minimum and diurnal maximum in solute
(Na, K, Cl, urea, phosphate) excretion, and in part by cyclical increase in ADH
activity by night and decrease by day. In normal man, exogenous vasopressin
fails to cause a further increase in urine concentration at night, although concentration is usually submaximal during the day (LABBÉ, VIOLLE and AZERAD)
and response to water-loading is delayed and impaired at night (BLOMHERT
et al.; PAPPER and ROSENBAUM). Subjects ingesting water at a fixed rate during
the 24 hours exhibit a positive water balance by night and a negative balance
by day (SIMPSON 1924). The cycle is unaffected by fasting (SIMPSON 1929). It
tends to persist as a 24-hour cycle in subjects who have adopted a 12, 22 or 27
hour "day" (MILLS 1951; LEWIS, LOBBAN and SHAW; LEWIS and LOBBAN 1957a, b),
but is less rigid than the potassium cycle and about as rigid as the NaCl cycle
(LEWIS and LOBBAN 1957a, b). In patients with panhypopituitarism, the cycle
in urine flow is abolished or reversed, although the normal NaCl cycle persists
(LEWIS 1953).

h) Diabetes insipidus

Clinical diabetes insipidus is a syndrome characterized by the more or less
continuous production of abundant (2.5 liters or more per day), hypotonic urine
in patients with grossly normal renal function. Diabetes insipidus is to be
distinguished from clinical situations characterized by isotonic or weakly hypotonic urine formation such as occurs in chronic BRIGHT's disease, sicklemia,
potassium depletion and other states (D VI 4 j). Several forms of diabetes insipidus are recognized (BLOTNER; JONES; CANNON 1955; LEAF 1960). These
are: psychogenic polydipsia (excluded from diabetes insipidus by some authors),
posttraumatic diabetes insipidus, idiopathic diabetes insipidus, and nephrogenic

diabetes insipidus. Psychogenic polydipsia is recognized by demonstration of a normal antidiuretic response to neurohypophyseal stimuli such as infusion of hypertonic (2.5 percent) saline (HICKEY and HARE; CARTER and ROBBINS), subcutaneous injection of 1—3 mg. of nicotine (CATES and GARROD), or smoking sufficient cigarettes to produce symptoms (LEWIS and CHALMERS). Nephrogenic diabetes insipidus (D VI 4 k) is recognized by failure to obtain a significant antidiuretic response to vasopressin (CARTER and ROBBINS). It is familial, the trait appearing in males and transmitted by females.

Posttraumatic diabetes insipidus occurs concurrent with or following infections of the central nervous system or tumors, injuries or vascular accidents in the infundibular region and is probably identifiable in most cases with the diabetes insipidus which follows neurohypophysectomy in experimental animals. As with the experimental form, the diabetes insipidus may subside if the lesion (as carcinoma) extends to involve the anterior hypophysis but may reappear if cortisone is administered (HOEL). However, since surgical hypophysectomy with cortisone replacement frequently fails to produce a permanent polyuria, lesions probably must involve the median eminence or interrupt the supraopticohypophyseal tracts if diabetes insipidus is to be produced (LIPSETT et al.). Also as in experimental animals, 'neurosecretory material' disappears from the supraoptic nuclei (RUSSELL and DRAGER). Diagnosis is established by rapid subsidence of the polyuria following injection of vasopressin, together with failure of the polyuria to respond to osmotic or nicotine stimuli. Water deprivation is not a satisfactory test for diabetes insipidus since dehydration in the thirsting patient is associated with a marked decrease in urine flow and creatinine clearance (GREINER and PODHRADSZKY).

Idiopathic diabetes insipidus is recognized partly by exclusion of recognizable infundibular disease and partly by its marked familial tendency (FORSSMAN; LEVINGER and ESCAMILLA). This form of diabetes is apparently transmitted as a simple dominant and accounts for 85 percent or more of patients with familial diabetes insipidus as compared with 5 to 15 percent with the nephrogenic form (FORSSMAN). The neurohypophysis is normal pathologically and the nature of the neurohypophyseal defect is unknown.

Some authors have argued that patients with diabetes insipidus may have a primary polydipsia (KOURILSKY et al.) which may be wholly or partially relieved by administration of Pitressin without replacement of water loss (PASQUALINI and CODEVILLA). Others, however, have argued that the polydipsia is wholly secondary to water loss and in their cases have shown that the polydipsia can be relieved by rehydration alone (HOLMES and GREGERSEN). In view of the juxtaposition of the thirst center to the neurohypophysis and the apparent production of primary polydipsia experimentally both by hypothalamic stimulation and as an immediate, transitory response to neurohypophyseal trauma (LEVKOFF, DEMUNBRUN and KELLER; LIPSETT et al.), an element of primary polydipsia may well exist in certain cases of human diabetes insipidus. Most studies have, however, employed inadequate methods and criteria for its recognition. Renal function is grossly normal both in this and the posttraumatic form (WINER). Reports have been published both of exaggeration and of remission of diabetes insipidus during pregnancy (FORSSMAN). Pregnancy causes little change in polyuria in the diabetes insipidus cat, however, and changes in polyuria in pregnant diabetic patients may be secondary to changes in renal function and salt balance.

Diabetes insipidus produced in experimental animals by neurohypophyseal lesions or in man by surgical hypophysectomy evolves in three stages, the first two of which are incompletely understood (Fisher, Ingram and Ranson; Magoun, Fisher and Ranson). Immediately following production of the lesion occurs a phase of polyuria lasting about 3 days. The degree of this polyuria is not closely correlated with either the exact location or the extent of the lesion and has been attributed to inhibition of the normal mechanism of ADH release. It may appear while the animals are still under anesthesia (Magoun, Fisher and Ranson), but some authors have observed an apparently normal response to osmotic stimuli during this phase (Levkoff, Demunbrun and Keller; Lipsett et al.). Following the initial polyuria, the urine again becomes scanty and hypertonic for 3 to 6 days, the 'normal interphase'. During this period, the diuretic response to water-loading is poor or absent and the antidiuresis is attributed to pathological release of stored vasopressin (Mudd et al.). If neuro-hypophysectomy has been sufficiently complete, polyuria resumes and endures for months or years, the 'permanent phase'. This phase is attributed to atrophy of the supraoptic and paraventricular neurons and their subtended neurohypophyseal tissue.

j) Hyponatremia

Hyponatremia may be defined somewhat arbitrarily as a plasma sodium concentration less than 130 mM./L. in man. Since sodium salts constitute the bulk of osmotically active solutes in the extracellular fluid, hyponatremia signifies a lowering of the 'effective' osmotic pressure. Hyponatremia has been observed in a wide variety of clinical and experimental situations (Cheek). Two principal types may be recognized: hyponatremia occurring in association with sodium-retaining states (secondary hyponatremia); and hyponatremia occurring in the absence of a tendency to sodium retention (primary hyponatremia).

Examples of secondary hyponatremia are the well-known hyponatremia observed in patients with congestive heart failure or advanced cirrhosis, hyponatremia observed following surgery (Le Quesne and Lewis; Goodyer and Glenn) and in salt depletion in normal man (Aitken; McCance 1936; Nadal, Pedersen and Maddock; Black, Platt and Stanbury; Watkin et al.) and dog (Darrow and Yannett; Cizek et al.; Holmes). Diuresis following administration of a water load tends to be delayed or impaired (p. 245) although a good diuresis may frequently be obtained by sufficiently intense water-loading in subjects who are not severely ill (Harris, Lloyd and Lobotsky; Earley and Sanders; Hanenson et al. 1956; White, Rubin and Leiter 1951, 1953). Interpretation of the mechanisms involved is complicated by the tendency for renal function and solute excretion to be depressed in most sodium-retaining states, and by lack of a sufficiently sensitive and reliable method for assaying plasma vasopressin concentration. In some subjects, such as nephrotics, an increased titer of circulating ADH may be detected during periods of edema formation (Lauson et al. 1952), or presumed by failure of exogenous vasopressin to elicit an increase in urine concentration as during mercurial diuresis in patients with congestive heart failure (Spritz et al.). Alternatively, submaximal secretion of ADH may be presumed in salt-deficient normal subjects who respond to osmotic stimuli with a decrease in urine flow (Black, Platt and Stanbury) and in edematous but not hyponatremic cardiacs whose plasma antidiuretic activity lies within normal limits (Wolff et al.). The most probable explanation of hyponatremia in sodium-retaining states is that increased inflow of stimuli to the hypothalamus from the cardiovascular system results in an increase in thirst and in ADH secretion. A positive balance of water is achieved and maintained until increasing plasma hypotonicity results in withdrawal of that component of stimuli to the hypothalamus which is contributed by the osmo-receptors (Fig. 71). With decreasing osmotic stimulus, ADH-release and thirst subside to the point where water balance is regained. Much the same hypothetical mechanism, related both to salt depletion and to absence of the vasotonic effects of cortisol, may be assumed to operate in generation of the hyponatremia of hypoadrenal or adrenoprival subjects. Although a functional neurohypophysis is probably essential to the formation of hyponatremia, it is apparently not essential to fluid accumulation since edema and ascites may form in the diabetes insipidus dog with inferior vena caval constriction (LARAGH et al. 1956) and in a patient with diabetes insipidus and edema of unknown cause (WHITE 1954).

Primary hyponatremia has been described in patients with tuberculous meningitis (HARRISON, FINBERG and FLEISHMAN; RAPOPORT, WEST and BRODSKY), cerebral tumor (CORT), cerebral trauma (CARTER, RECTOR and SELDIN) and bronchogenic carcinoma with and without cerebral metastases (SCHWARTZ et al. 1957; ROBERTS 1959). The syndrome has also been described in a subject with no discernible organic disease (EPSTEIN and LEVITIN). These patients usually resemble normal subjects in most respects but with the differences that plasma sodium, and to some extent chloride, are decreased and body sodium and water balance is more labile. Concentration and dilution of the urine in response to water deprivation or loading is normal; additionally administered sodium chloride is rapidly excreted; chronic water deprivation or loading leads to further gains or losses of sodium, respectively (CARTER, RECTOR and SELDIN); and isotonic saline infusion may lead acutely to a water-type diuresis (SCHWARTZ et al. 1957). The sodium balance changes closely resemble those observed in experimental hyponatremia caused by sustained antidiuresis with Pitressin tannate. The hypothesis has been proposed that primary hyponatremia arises from excessive secretion of ADH at normal levels of plasma osmotic pressure but the nature of the sensitization of the neurohypophysis is as yet unexplained.

k) Hypernatremia

Hypernatremia (plasma sodium concentration in excess of 150 mM./L.) is observed in a variety of clinical situations (KNOWLES). The common denominator is excessive loss of water caused by impairment of the normal mechanisms for acquisition or retention of water. Hypernatremia has been observed in comatose patients with diabetes insipidus (ULLMAN) or with excessive water loss resulting from a high protein diet (KNOWLES), and in noncomatose subjects with probable diabetes insipidus secondary to meningitis or tumor (ENGSTROM and LIEBMAN; LEVITT, BALSKY and POLIMEROS). In the latter group, thirst has not been a prominent symptom and failure to maintain adequate water intake is probably the consequence of damage to the thirst center. Transitory hypernatremia has been described in a patient with panhypopituitarism, secondary to a craniopharyngeoma, in whom sodium retention was obligated by desoxycorticosterone administration (McGAVACK et al.).

l) Oxytocin release and effects

The function, if any, of oxytocin in the control of renal function is unknown. Oxytocin is stored in large quantities in the pars nervosa of both male and female (HELLER and ZAIMIS) and is present at birth in quantities, on a unitage basis, equal to vasopressin. Oxytocin may be formed predominantly by the paraventricular nuclei, since lesions in this region cause a relatively greater depletion of oxytocic than of antidiuretic activity in the neurohypophysis (OLIVECRONA).

Oxytocin is reported to cause a marked increase in RPF and a lesser increase in GFR in the water-diuresing dog, but to be ineffective in the presence of small quantities of vasopressin (ALI). Oxytocin (Pitocin) and also Pituitrin but not vasopressin (Pitressin) cause GFR and RPF to increase in the neurohypophysectomized dog with depressed renal function (DEMUNBRUN et al.) but failure of GFR to decrease regularly in the stalk-sectioned dog (PICKFORD and RITCHIE) renders a sustaining function of oxytocin on the renal circulation questionable.

Oxytocin is released from the neurohypophysis in significant quantities concomitantly with vasopressin in response to ether anesthesia or nicotine in the rat (BISSET and WALKER 1954, 1957), emotional antidiuresis in the dog (ABRAHAMS and PICKFORD 1954), hypertonic saline infusion in the rabbit (HOLLAND, CROSS and SAWYER) or stimulation in the region of the paraventricular nuclei of the goat (ANDERSSON and McCANN). Conversely, variable degrees of antidiuresis, suggesting release of ADH, are observed during the oxytocin release associated with lactation in man (KALLIALA and KARVONEN), dog (KALLIALA, KARVONEN and LAPPÄNEN) and rabbit (CROSS). The vasopressin/oxytocin ratios in the blood, as estimated from the physiological responses of the target organs, are quite different as between osmotic and reproductive stimuli and in neither circumstance are the ratios equal to that of the hormones stored in the neurohypophysis (LAUSON 1960, review). During parturition, the neurohypophysis is preferentially depleted of oxytocin (DICKER and TYLER). Such observations suggest a certain degree of separate control of the release of the two polypeptides.

m) Vasopressin effects on anterior pituitary and adrenocortical function

In addition to its function in the control of renal tubular reabsorption of water, vasopressin is capable, under certain conditions, of affecting renal function indirectly by stimulation of the adrenal cortex and the anterior pituitary. Injection of relatively large quantities of Pitressin into rat or guinea pig causes depletion of adrenocortical ascorbate, evidence of cortical stimulation (McCANN; McCANN and BROBECK; ROYCE and SAYERS; ITOH; MARTINI and MORPURGO; MARTINI and DE POLI; CASENTINI et al.; SOBEL et al.), and repeated injections of Pitressin or Pitocin induce enlargement of the cortex (MARTINI, DE POLI and CURRI). These effects upon the adrenal cortex evidently could arise either by direct stimulation of the cortex or indirectly by stimulating secretion of adrenocorticotropin by the anterior pituitary. Stimulation of corticotropin secretion is suggested but not proven by the observation that the ascorbate depletion of cortical hypertrophy is diminished or indetectable in the hypophysectomized animal (McCANN; MARTINI, DE POLI and CURRI; CASENTINI et al.; SOBEL et al.), and that ascorbate depletion can be elicited by Pitressin or lysine vasopressin (but not by Pitocin or other agents) in the presence of intraocularly transplanted anterior pituitary tissue (CASENTINI et al.). A significant increase in 17-hydroxycorticoid excretion follows intracarotid injection of lysine vasopressin in the dog, but the quantity required is more than 2,000 times that required to produce maximal antidiuresis (NICHOLS, GUILLEMIN and SIEBERT) and should be sufficient to stimulate adrenal cortical secretion directly. Alternatively, however, small quantities (2 milliunits) of arginine vasopressin which, unlike lysine vasopressin, occurs normally in the dog, elicits a significant increase in corticoid excretion when injected intraventricularly (KWAAN and BARTELSTONE). In the same studies, oxytocin and vasotocin were ineffective. Interpretation of the evidence suggesting an anterior pituitary-stimulating effect of vasopressin is further complicated by the observations that release of corticotropin by anterior pituitary tissue *in vitro* is stimulated when the tissue is incubated with posterior pituitary or hypothalamic tissue or extracts of these (SAFFRAN and SHALLY; SAFFRAN, SHALLY and BENFEY; GUILLEMIN et al.; GUILLEMIN and ROSENBERG). The extracts contain an active principle, termed 'corticotropin-releasing factor', which is a polypeptide distinguishable from vasopressin or oxytocin and which may be present in hypothalamic tissue devoid of the two latter substances.

A direct effect of vasopressin on the adrenal cortex is suggested by the observation that, under appropriate conditions, adrenal ascorbate depletion may follow injection of Pitressin in the hypophysectomized rat (ROYCE and SAYERS). Other studies have shown that lysine and arginine vasopressin perfused through the isolated adrenal gland of the dog increases the rate of secretion of cortisol but not of aldosterone (HILTON et al. 1959a, b; HILTON 1960; SCIAN et al.). The effect is additive to and the mechanism is probably different from that of adrenocorticotropin. The quantities required, although relatively small, are considerably in excess of those sufficient to produce maximal antidiuresis and are sufficient to produce vasoconstriction in the adrenal circulation.

Although vasopressin in sufficient quantities has some stimulating effect on the anterior pituitary and adrenal cortex, other studies indicate that these actions are not significant under physiological conditions: No correlation has been observed in dog or man between diuresis and antidiuresis (reflecting absence or presence of ADH liberation) and the rate of 17-hydroxycorticoid secretion (NICHOLS and GUILLEMIN; MCDONALD, WAGNER and WEISE); and the usual response of corticotropin liberation to stress persists in an apparently normal fashion in animals with diabetes insipidus (NICHOLS et al.).

3. Control of sodium reabsorption (adrenal system)

Renal tubular reabsorption of sodium and chloride is subject to innumerable factors such as compensatory hypertrophy, dietary elements, potassium balance, metabolic (thyroid) activity, adenohypophyseal growth hormone and (probably) body temperature (WESSON 1957, review). Primary variations in such factors appear to be largely independent of the state of the circulation or of body fluid volume. Variations in tubular reabsorption occurring as the effect of these factors are continually balanced by counter variations in glomerular filtration rate so that glomerulo-tubular balance is preserved. A clear correlation between the state of the cardiovascular system and the rate of secretion of a humoral agent which unequivocally affects renal tubular sodium transport is evident only with respect to the aldosterone component of the secretions of the adrenal cortex. The principal but not exclusive stimulus to the secretion of aldosterone is *cardiovascular* stress, while the principal stimulus to the secretion of cortisol is stress in the more general sense, such as injury, pain and emotion although severe, acute cardiovascular stress, such as hemorrhage, can elicit an increase in cortisol secretion.

a) Adrenocortical hormones

In experimental mammals, and presumably also in man, the adrenal cortex has two principal secretions, cortisol and aldosterone. Cortisol (17-hydroxycorticosterone) arises from the zonae fasciculata and reticularis of the adrenal cortex. It influences virtually all body metabolic processes such as glucose, fat and protein metabolism, leucocyte production and tissue inflammatory responses. Its rate of synthesis is sensitively controlled by the adrenocorticotropic hormone of the adenohypophysis. Secretion of adrenocorticotropin is, in turn, controlled

by the hypothalamus probably by an as yet unidentified hormone which enters
the adenohypophysis in relatively high concentration through the hypothalamico-
hypophyseal portal system. Thus, the role of the adenohypophysis is that of an
amplifier. Aldosterone is secreted by the zona glomerulosa and primarily influences electrolyte metabolism. Its secretion is not sensitively controlled by
adrenocorticotropin although influenced by it. Other steroids such as corticosterone (compound B) and desoxycorticosterone (cortexone) are secreted in
relatively small quantities as measured in terms of functional activity, and no
specific physiological role has been discovered for them. Since the adrenocortico-
tropin-cortisol system appears to play little more than a supportive role in body
electrolyte control, it will not be described in more detail. Sprague et al.;
INGLE (1950), NOBLE (1950) and SAYERS (1950, 1951) may be consulted for reviews.

The fascinating history of the discovery of aldosterone and its relation to
body salt metabolism has been detailed in numerous review articles (JOHNSON
and LUETSCHER; LUETSCHER and CURTIS 1955a, b; GAUNT, RENZI and CHART;
NEHER and WETTSTEIN; LUETSCHER 1956a, b; BARTTER 1955, 1956, 1957, 1958;
DAVIS 1957; AUGUST, NELSON and THORN). Extracts of urine were observed
to contain material in trace quantities which, injected into adrenalectomized
rats, resulted in marked decrease in sodium and increase in potassium content
in the urine. Urine obtained from patients with edema-forming states contained
larger quantities of the salt-retaining factor. Isolation procedures first in nephrosis
(LUETSCHER, NEHER and WETTSTEIN) and later in other states demonstrated
that virtually all of the increased urinary salt-retaining activity was represented
by aldosterone (SIMPSON et al. 1954a), a steroid which had been earlier isolated
from the amorphous fraction of adrenocortical extracts and adrenal venous
blood (MATTOX et al.; SIMPSON et al. 1953, 1954a, b, c; FARRELL and RICHARDS).

Aldosterone is produced almost, if not entirely, by the glomerulose zone of
the adrenal cortex. This is suggested indirectly by the observation that hypertrophy occurs only in this zone in rats on a salt-restricted diet (DEANE, SHAW
and GREEP; GOLDMAN, RONZONI and SCHROEDER; KOVACS and DAVID) or
in dogs with experimental heart failure (DEANE and BARGER). The zona glomerulosa, unlike the zona fasciculata, fails to atrophy in dogs given large quantities
of cortisone or cortisol (FARRELL, BANKS and KOLETSKY) or following hypophysectomy, but atrophy occurs both in normal and hypophysectomized rats if large
quantities of desoxycorticosterone are given (GREEP and DEANE). Aldosterone
is synthesized *in vitro* in significant quantities from slices of the zona glomerulosa
but not from other regions of the cortex (GIROUD et al.; GIROUD, STACHENKO
and VENNING).

In healthy subjects on a diet unrestricted in salt, the average 24 hour excretion rate of aldosterone is about 10 gamma (micrograms) per 24 hours[1]. This
quantity is about 5 percent of the average rate of secretion of aldosterone by the
adrenal (AYRES et al. 1957a, b, 1958; WOLFF, KOCZOREK and BUCHBORN; ULICK,
LARAGH and LIEBERMAN). No difference in excretion is evident between men
and women (VENNING, DYRENFURTH and GIROUD 1956; HERNANDO et al.) and
excretion is not clearly affected by urine flow (HERNANDO et al.).

b) Aldosterone excretion in physiological and pathological conditions

When a normal subject is placed on a nearly salt-free diet (LUETSCHER and
JOHNSON 1954a; LUETSCHER and AXELRAD 1954b; LIDDLE, DUNCAN and BART-
TER; DUNCAN, LIDDLE and BARTTER; AYRES et al. 1957) or is subjected to water

---

[1] Lower published values are based on methods known to give incomplete recovery.

or blood loss (FALBRIARD et al. 1955b; FINE, MEISELAS and AUERBACH; BARTTER 1957) aldosterone excretion increases markedly. Excretion decreases below normal levels in subjects on a high salt diet, following hypertonic saline or albumin infusion, or with forced water retention (DUNCAN, LIDDLE and BARTTER; MULLER, RIONDEL and MACH; MULLER, RIONDEL and MANNING 1956; BECK et al. 1955a; BARTTER 1957). Aldosterone excretion is moderately increased in congestive heart failure (GORDON, CHART and MEYERS; LUETSCHER and JOHNSON 1954b; WOLFF, KOCZOREK and BUCHBORN; DUNCAN, LIDDLE and BARTTER; HERNANDO et al.; WOLFF et al.; BUCHBORN, KOCZOREK and WOLFF), and markedly increased in nephrosis (GORDON, CHART and MAYER; LUETSCHER and JOHNSON 1954a, b; LUETSCHER and CURTIS 1955a, b; LUETSCHER et al. 1955) and cirrhosis (GORDON, CHART and MEYER; CHART and SHIPLEY; LUETSCHER and JOHNSON 1954b; DUNCAN, LIDDLE and BARTTER; LIDDLE, DUNCAN and BARTTER; WOLFF, KOCZOREK and BUCHBORN; BUCHBORN, KOCZOREK and WOLFF; DYRENFURTH et al.). The changes in urinary excretion both in normals on high and low salt diets and in pathological states represent a genuine and roughly proportional change in the secretion rate of the gland (WOLFF, KOCZOREK and BUCHBORN; ULICK, LARAGH and LIEBERMAN; WOLFF et al.) although the excreted fraction tends to increase at higher secretion rates (WOLFF, KOCZOREK and BUCHBORN; BECK et al. 1955; VENNING et al. 1955). Improvement in the clinical status of patients with heart failure, nephrosis or cirrhosis (in the latter following successful construction of a portocaval shunt) is associated with a significant decrease in excretion rate, frequently to normal (HERNANDO et al.; DYRENFURTH et al.; MITTLEMAN, GORE and BARKER; WOLFF et al.; VEYRAT et al.). Excretion rate is slightly to moderately increased in hypertension (HERNANDO et al.; GENEST et al.; GARST et al.) and moderately increased in pregnancy (GORDON et al. 1954; WOLFF, KOCZOREK and BUCHBORN; VENNING and DYRENFURTH; VENNING et al. 1957; RINSLER and RIGBY; GENEST et al. 1957; LAIDLAW, COHEN and GORNALL). In preeclamptic toxemia of pregnancy, excretion has been variously reported as increased (GORDON et al. 1954) or decreased (RINSLER and RIGBY) as compared with normal pregnancy. Excretion is increased in salt-losing nephritis (LUETSCHER and CURTIS 1955a, b; AYRES et al. 1957a; HERNANDO et al.), an important observation since these people have impaired renal function as well a sodium-rich urine. On high or low salt diets and in edema-forming states excretion of other steroids does not differ significantly from normal (DAUGHADAY and MACBRYDE; HERNANDO et al.; LIDDLE, DUNCAN and BARTTER; JOHNSON, LIEBERMAN and MULROW). In experimental animals changes in aldosterone secretion as related to functional states are qualitatively similar to that observed in man. In experimental animals, however, the rate of aldosterone secretion can be measured directly in adrenal vein blood. Secretion is increased in the nephrotic rat (SINGER 1957) and in dogs on a low salt diet (ROSNAGLE and FARRELL; GOODKIND, BALL and DAVIS), with congestive heart failure[1] (DAVIS et al. 1956, 1957; BALL, DAVIS and GOODKIND), forming ascites as the result of intrathoracic inferior vena caval constriction (DAVIS et al. 1956, 1957; BALL, DAVIS and GOODKIND; BALL et al.), or subjected to acute or chronic hemorrhage (MULROW and GANONG; GOODKIND, BALL and DAVIS). The renal sodium retention and the formation of ascites by dogs is independent of the location of the kidney

---

[1] No increase in secretion was observed by DRISCOL et al. (1957) in dogs with experimental heart failure although their animals formed ascites. The cardiac lesion in their animals appears to have been less severe than in those of DAVIS et al., which agrees with the observation that humans in mild congestive failure may not exhibit a significant increase in aldosterone excretion.

(*in situ* or transplanted to the neck), a further demonstration of the independence
of the renal response from renal nerves or renal venous pressure (CARPENTER
et al. 1960).

c) Control of aldosterone secretion

The single denominator common to the changes in aldosterone excretion
described above is a change in the volume, distribution or circulation of the
extracellular fluid. In nephrotics and cirrhotics, excessive quantities of fluid
are diverted into poorly circulating areas; in pregnancy, a significant fraction
of the cardiac output is diverted through the placental circulation, the latter
constituting, in essence, an arteriovenous fistula; patients with salt-losing
nephritis are subject to continual depletion of body salt and water content.
The aldosterone secretory response to cardiovascular stresses is rapid. A marked
increase in secretion appears within a few minutes following acute hemorrhage
(MULROW and GANONG; FARRELL, ROSNAGLE and RAUSCHKOLB) or vena caval
constriction (YANKOPOULOS et al. 1958; BARTTER, MILLS and GANN) in the dog
or following certain postural changes in man (GOWENLOCK, MILLS and THOMAS).
The immediate stimulus to aldosterone secretion in the fluid-depleted sheep
and caval-constricted dog is a humoral factor which is absent from the blood
of unstressed animals (DENTON, GODING and WRIGHT; YANKOPOULOS et al. 1959).

Injection of adrenocorticotropin (ACTH) causes a moderate increase in
aldosterone secretion acutely in normal or hypophysectomized man (LUETSCHER
and CURTIS 1955; GIROUD et al.; LIEBERMAN et al.; VENNING, DYRENFURTH
and BECK; LIDDLE, DUNCAN and BARTTER; MULLER, RIONDEL and MANNING;
TRONCHETTI, MUCIO and ROMANELLI; SCIAN et al.; CRABBÉ) dog (FARRELL,
RAUSCHKOLB and ROYCE) and rat (SINGER and STACK-DUNNE) and stimulates
an increase in aldosterone production in the isolated adrenal (ROSENFELD et al.),
while hypophysectomy in both the normal and the caval-constricted dog is
followed acutely by a moderate decrease in secretion (RAUSCHKOLB, FARRELL
and KOLETSKY 1956; DAVIS et al. 1959, 1960). That adrenocorticotropin is not
the significant humoral factor which determines aldosterone response to cardiovascular stress is indicated by the observations that aldosterone excretion is
generally within normal limits in patients with panhypopituitarism (LUETSCHER
and CURTIS 1955c; LUETSCHER and AXELRAD 1954a; VENNING, DYRENFURTH
and BECK; LLAURADO; HERNANDO et al.; HÖKFELT et al.), although secretion
of other adrenal steroids is depressed. Aldosterone excretion generally increases
in patients with panhypopituitarism who have been placed on a low sodium diet
(LUETSCHER 1956) and in the hypophysectomized dog following caval constriction or hemorrhage (BALL et al.; MULROW and GANONG), and no increase in ACTH
activity, as measured by excretion of cortisol and corticosterone and their metabolites, is present in association with the increased aldosterone excretion. An
occasional patient with panhypopituitarism fails to respond to sodium deprivation with increased aldosterone secretion (LUETSCHER 1956; HERNANDO et al.).
Whether or not this failure signifies hypothalamic involvement is unknown.

Cortisone has no evident effect on aldosterone secretion although it may
inhibit secretion of corticotropin (LIDDLE, DUNCAN and BARTTER; VENNING,
DYRENFURTH and BECK). Other pituitary principles such as growth hormone
(somatotropin) (VENNING et al. 1955, 1956; GIROUD et al. 1956; ROSENFELD
et al.; BECK et al. 1957), thyrotropin (TRONCHETTI, MUCIO and ROMANELLI),
interstitial cell-stimulating hormone (TRONCHETTI, MUCIO and ROMANELLI),
vasopressin and oxytocin (SCIAN et al.; GIROUD, STACHENKO and PILETTA)
have little effect on aldosterone excretion in man and the small increases observed

occasionally with somatotropin and thyrotropin are probably secondary to effects on total body metabolism. Evidence that the humoral factor stimulating aldosterone secretion arises from the brain is suggested by decreases in secretion to about 30 percent of control values following exclusion of the head in the dog. Equally significant decreases in secretion were observed following decerebration (diencephalic section) or removal of the pineal body and adjacent structures in the roof of the diencephanol or the production of lesions in the dorsal or central diencephalon (NEWMAN et al. 1958; NEWMAN, REDGATE and FARRELL; DAVIS et al. 1959). Decortication, spinal cord section and hypothalamic lesions, however, caused no change in secretion (RAUSCHKOLB and FARRELL; FARRELL, KOLETSKY and LAPHAM; DAVIS et al. 1959). In the sheep, brain stem section rostral of the corpora quandrigemina did not affect sodium depletion and repletion responses but section rostral of the pons was followed by partial abolition of the depletion response (DENTON, GODING and WRIGHT). Neutral, cold saline extracts of diencephalon and particularly of the pineal gland or immediately adjacent areas are reported to stimulate secretion of aldosterone in the dog without stimulating cortisol secretion (FARRELL 1959a, b) or to prevent sodium-repletion from restoring to normal the low salivary Na/K ratio in the sodium-depleted sheep (DENTON, GODING and WRIGHT). The diencephalic active principle is relatively soluble in acetone and hexane (FARRELL 1959b).

The origins and pathways of the signals to the brain which stimulate release of the aldosterone secretory factor is unclear. The signals probably include many, but not all, of the signals controlling filtration rate and anti-diuretic hormone secretion. Section of the vagi at the level of the thyroid in the dog fails to prevent the rise in aldosterone secretion which results from inferior vena caval constriction. On the other hand, aldosterone secretion fails to return to control values following release of constriction in vagal-sectioned animals (MILLS, CASPER and BARTTER), but this may indicate no more than that recovery of circulatory equilibrium in the vagal-sectioned animal is impaired. Infusion of blood or Dextran solution in the caval-constricted dog failed to prevent rise in aldosterone secretion, but proof of adequacy of the replacement is difficult to obtain (YANKOPOULOS 1958). Bilateral common carotid artery constriction in the dog increased aldosterone secretion and both the effects of carotid constriction as well as the effects of inferior vena caval constriction could be prevented by denervation of the region at the origin of the thyroid arteries, but section of the carotid sinus nerves had no effect on aldosterone secretion (BARTTER, MILLS and GANN). Although these studies suggest an arterial pressor-sensitive control of aldosterone secretion, others have been unable to detect a change in blood pressure during the sodium-retaining response of the caval-constricted dog (CARPENTER et al. 1960).

The postulated humoral factor which arises from the brain stem in response to cardio- vascular stress and which stimulates the adrenal cortex to secrete aldosterone has been termed 'aldosteronotropic factor' by SAYERS et al. (1958) and 'adrenoglomerulotropin' by FARRELL. For detailed reviews of the literature relating to diencephalic control of aldosterone and other hormones see SAYERS, REDGATE and ROYCE; DINGMAN; and FARRELL (1958).

Direct humoral control by the brain of adrenal aldosterone secretion may be due to the possibility that the minute quantities of aldosterone secreted require correspondingly minute quantities of trophic hormone. Hence, introduction of an adenohypophyseal 'amplifier' would be unnecessary.

d) Aldosterone and potassium balance

The mechanisms by which aldosterone secretion or excretion is correlated with body potassium balance are not clear. The problem is complicated by the circumstance that sodium balance tends to change in a direction opposite to that of potassium. Potassium-loading in man or dog is regularly associated with loss of body sodium (BUNGE) and generally some increase in plasma potassium concentration, while sodium is retained, often to the point of edema formation, in human potassium deficiency (BLACK and MILNE; BLAHD and BASSETT; REIMER, SCHOCH and NEWBURGH; WOMERSLEY and DARRAGH; VERMET, DUCKERT and MULLER; JOHNSON, LIEBERMAN and MULROW). Correspondingly, aldosterone excretion is increased during potassium-loading although sodium is lost, and is decreased in potassium depletion although sodium is retained (FALBRIARD et al. 1955b; VERMET, DUCKERT and MULLER; MULLER, MANNING and RIONDEL 1958a; SINGER and STACK-DUNNE). The effect of potassium-loading is small or insignificant in subjects on high sodium diets (BARTTER et al. 1956; LIEBERMAN et al.; ROSNAGLE and FARRELL; LARAGH and STOERK; MILLER, FALOON and LLOYD) and is exaggerated on low sodium diets (LARAGH and STOERK). The effect of potassium deficiency is small in man and dog on a sodium restricted diet (JOHNSON, LIEBERMAN and MULROW; LARAGH and STOERK). The degree of hypertrophy of the zona glomerulosa of the rat on diets deficient in both Na and K is less than in those deficient in Na alone (DEANE, SHAW and GREEP; KOVACS and DAVID). The possibility of direct response of the adrenal to plasma potassium concentration is demonstrated by augmentation of rate of secretion of aldosterone by the isolated calf adrenal when the Na/K ratio of the medium is changed from 149/3.5 to 125/25 (ROSENFELD et al.). More moderate decreases in the Na/K ratio, such as are compatible with life, do not stimulate secretion in the sheep although they may delay return of secretory rate to the resting values following a period of fluid depletion (DENTON, GODING and WRIGHT). Studies of MULLER, MANNING and RIONDEL (1958a) suggest that the effects of potassium balance on aldosterone excretion in man are to some extent, at least, secondary to changes in extracellular fluid or plasma volume. In potassium excess, fluid volume tends to decrease with attendant stimulation of aldosterone secretion unless adequacy of dietary sodium prevents a significant fluid deficit from appearing. In potassium deficiency, fluid volume tends to expand, with the possibility of attendant suppression of aldosterone secretion. That change in extracellular fluid volume, as estimated from sodium balance, is not the only factor involved is shown by the fact that prevention of sodium losses or gains diminishes but does not prevent the changes in aldosterone following potassium excess or deficiency (BARTTER 1957; BARTTER et al. 1959). The mechanisms responsible for the potassium-induced changes in sodium balance are unknown but could depend in part, at least, upon changes in renal tubular reabsorption of sodium chloride.

Potassium-depleted man responds to sodium loss normally with augmented aldosterone excretion (LUETSCHER and CURTIS 1955b; BARTTER et al. 1956; LIEBERMAN et al.); and potassium depletion in an ascites-forming patient with cirrhosis was not associated with a detectable decrease in rate of excretion of sodium-retaining steroids (WESSON, SUNSHINE and EPSTEIN).

e) Noncorrelations between aldosterone and sodium balance

The close correlation between aldosterone production and sodium balance or cardiovascular stress has been noted. In other circumstances, particularly when sodium and aldosterone excretion are followed closely, the correlation is less close. In normal man, changes in aldosterone excretion do not correlate closely with changes in sodium excretion during the diurnal cycle (VENNING,

DYRENFURTH and GIROUD 1955; MULLER, RIONDEL and MANNING 1957; LUET-
SCHER 1956; MULLER, MANNING and RIONDEL 1958b; BARTTER et al. 1958),
during acute changes in posture (GOWENLOCK, MILLS and THOMAS), during the
first one or two days after changing the dietary salt intake (CRABBÉ, ROSS and
THORNE; RENWICK, ROBSON and STEWART 1955a, b), following moderate alterations in blood volume in normal and cirrhotic subjects (BARTTER et al. 1958)
or during postoperative salt retention (CASEY, BICKEL and ZIMMERMANN; VEN-
NING et al. 1958). Natriuresis during compensation in a patient with congestive
heart failure was not accompanied by reciprocal changes in aldosterone excretion (WOLFF et al.) nor is the magnitude of diuresis in cardiac or cirrhotic
patients correlated with the degree of change in aldosterone excretion (MULLER,
MANNING and RIONDEL 1956). When a subject is deprived of sodium, the sweat
sodium concentration, presumably responding to aldosterone secretion, decreases
more slowly than does urine sodium (ROBINSON et al. 1955). No clear correlation
exists between sodium and aldosterone excretion when various states in man
(cirrhosis, salt deprivation in normal subjects, and congestive heart failure,
in order of decreasing aldosterone excretion) are compared (WOLFF, KOCZOREK
and BUCHBORN). Alternatively, the pattern of sodium balance in the adrenoprival human closely resembles the normal following surgery (ROBSON et al.;
MASON; WILKINSON; RANDALL and PAPPER), application of venous tourniquets
(ROSENBAUM, PAPPER and ASHLEY; EPSTEIN 1956), or dietary salt restriction
(RANDALL and PAPPER).

4. Glomerular filtration control

Evaluation of the role of tubular reabsorption in regulation of renal salt
excretion is not possible unless filtered load of salt is considered simultaneously.
Unfortunately, virtually nothing is known of the mechanisms which regulate
filtration rate, and explanations of the fragmentary evidence must be viewed
as highly speculative. The available data can best be interpreted by postulating
the existence of two controlling mechanisms: one, mediated by the renal nerves
and circulating sympathomimetic amines, can decrease filtration rate in response
to stress; the other, whose existence is inferred and presumably is humorally
mediated, can increase filtration rate in response to the need to excrete more salt.

a) Depression of filtration rate:
renal nerves and sympathomimetic amines

In resting, unanesthetized man (CORCORAN and PAGE; FOA et al. 1943;
BRICKER et al. 1956) or dog (MALUF; SURTSHIN, MUELLER and WHITE; BERNE
and LEVY; BERNE et al.; SURTSHIN and SCHMANDT; PAGE et al. 1954b; BRICKER
et al. 1958; BALINT et al. 1959) no significant difference can be observed between
an innervated and a denervated kidney. In stress states, however, a clear
difference appears between the two kidneys. When a dog, one kidney of which
has been denervated, is subjected to stresses such as excitement, positive pressure respiration, anesthesia or hemorrhage filtration rate in the innervated
kidney decreases relatively more than that of the denervated kidney (SURTSHIN,
MUELLER and WHITE; SURTSHIN and SCHMANDT; KNOEFEL, HANDLEY and
HUGGINS; BERNE; HELLER 1958; BALINT et al. 1959). In the same studies,
sodium excretion is regularly less from the innervated kidney. The effect of
the renal nerves on filtration rate during stress is also reflected in the rise in
filtration rate following acute denervation under anesthesia (KRISS, FUTCHER
and GOLDMAN; KAPLAN, FOMON and RAPOPORT 1951) and these filtration rate

changes are correlated with the long-known effects of renal nerve section or stimulation on increasing or decreasing renal blood flow and NaCl excretion under anesthesia (Smith 1939 for review). Nevertheless, filtration rate is also frequently decreased in the denervated kidney during the same stress states and a decrease in filtration rate has been reported in the denervated human kidney following blood sequestration by leg tourniquets (Wilkins et al.; Epstein) or orthostasis (Bricker et al. 1956). A partial and perhaps sufficient explanation of this response on the part of a denervated kidney is liberation from the autonomic nervous system of the animal, stressed by hemorrhage or excitement, of epinephrine and norepinephrine (Watts; Walker et al. 1959a, b) which mimic the effect of renal nervous activity. Whether the increase in epinephrine and norepinephrine secretion associated with orthostasis is sufficient to account for all of the depression in function is not clear. During orthostasis in man norepinephrine excretion may increase 0.01 to 0.02 gamma/min. (v. Euler, Luft and Sundin; Sundin) and plasma concentration of vasoconstrictor activity increases (Camp). Assuming that excretion represents two percent of secretion (v. Euler, Luft and Sundin; Goldenberg et al.), this is equivalent to intravenous infusion of 0.5—1.0 gamma per minute. Although this quantity is not of itself sufficient to cause a significant decrease in filtration rate in unstressed subjects (C V 2 a), other significant factors such as absence of acute blood pressure elevation may also be present. It is probable, therefore, that filtration rate and sodium excretion are under the control of the autonomic nervous system to the extent that during acute cardiovascular stress they can be caused to decrease below resting values. In addition, reabsorption may be accelerated by the rise in intrarenal temperature which results from epinephrine-induced renal ischemia (Grupp 1957).

The experimental evidence is less clear as to whether a significant degree of renal nervous activity is present in chronic stress states. In the dog, moderate congestive heart failure is not associated with a significant decrease either in postabsorptive filtration rate or renal blood flow (Fishman et al. 1951; Davis and Howell 1953a; Davis, Hyatt and Howell; Barger, Rudolph and Yates), suggesting that no significant degree of renal vasomotor activity is present[1]. In advanced failure, postabsorptive filtration rate and blood flow are decreased but the effects of denervation have not been studied. In patients with congestive heart failure high spinal anesthesia was not associated with a significant increase in filtration rate (Mokotoff and Ross), but ephedrine, administered to maintain blood pressure, could have prevented a rise from occurring. On the other hand, an increase in filtration rate and renal blood flow was observed in about 8 of 15 patients with heart failure following dibenamine infusion (Brod, Fejfar and Fejfarova). Until evidence is obtained to the contrary, it seems reasonable to postulate that man differs from dog in that vasoconstrictor tone, with or without an increase in blood concentration of sympathomimetic amines, may be present at rest in many patients with congestive heart failure.

b) Augmentation of filtration rate

The relation of intact renal nerves to filtration rate in acute stress states is in contrast with an absence of correlation between integrity of the renal nerves

---

[1] Dibenzyline, an adrenergic blocking agent, is reported to cause natriuresis from the kidney into whose renal artery it is injected in dogs with heart failure. Filtration rate and renal blood flow measurements are not reported in these studies, however (Barger, Liebowitz and Muldowney).

and hemodynamic and excretory responses in the presence of body fluid excess. When saline is infused into a dog with one kidney denervated, filtration rate increases at least as much in the denervated as in the innervated kidney (SELLWOOD and VERNEY; BRICKER et al. 1958) and salt excretion is equal from the two kidneys (SURTSHIN, MUELLER and WHITE; O'CONNOR 1955; BRICKER et al. 1958). In a human subject with denervated (homotransplanted) kidney no significant changes in creatinine clearance were observed during or immediately following infusion of 3 liters of isotonic saline, while a tendency to a small increase in creatinine clearance was observed in his donor twin with innervated kidney. The responses of both kidneys are within normal limits, however, since the human kidney usually does not exhibit large changes in filtration rate acutely in response to the rates of saline infusion employed (C V 3 b). In chronic fluid loading, whether resulting from retention of water or salt as forced by pitressin tannate or steroid administration or from increased salt intake, filtration rate may attain values twice those observed on a low salt diet. No more than 2 or 3 days are necessary for the changes to occur (LEVITT and BADER; PECHET, BOWERS and BARTTER; BURNETT; INGBAR et al. 1950; ALEXANDER et al.; WESSON and LAULER, unpublished). The mechanism responsible for the rise in filtration rate above the resting value is unknown. That this is not the result of decreased colloid osmotic pressure is indicated by the fact that the greatest increases in filtration rate are observed chronically, when plasma protein concentrations are essentially normal (STEWART and ROURKE), rather than immediately following loading when protein concentrations may be measurably depressed. Blood pressure may not change significantly in normal subjects ingesting 20—30 g. daily supplements of salt (GRANT and REISCHMAN). Filtration rate is not controlled, at least directly, by glucocorticoid secretion since intravenous infusion of steroids such as hydrocortisone at 10 or more mg./hr. for 24 hours affected neither the magnitude nor the character of the diurnal cycle of filtration in normal subjects (DINGMAN et al.). Moreover, the diurnal cycle of 17-hydroxysteroid excretion and plasma concentration is nearly opposite in phase to that of filtration rate and sodium excretion (PINCUS; PINCUS et al.; LAIDLAW et al. 1954; TYLER et al.; MIGEON et al.; DOE, FLINK and GOODSELL)[1], and the diurnal cycle of 17-hydroxysteroid excretion, unlike that of sodium excretion (LEWIS and LOBBAN 1956, 1957a, b, c), is not readily reversed by reversing sleep (TYLER et al.; MIGEON et al.). These observations, together with persistence of a normal diurnal cycle of filtration rate and sodium excretion in adrenoprival man (GARROD and BURSTON; ROSENBAUM, PAPPER and ASHLEY; DINGMAN et al.), constancy of glucocorticoid excretion during dietary NaCl variation (DAUGHADAY and MACBRYDE) and the ability of the adrenalectomized man or dog to excrete massive quantities of NaCl in a normal fashion (CHASE and HALL; ROEMMELT, SARTORIUS and PITTS; BURNETT, SELDIN and WALSER; MADSEN; RANDALL and PAPPER) indicate that neither the adrenal cortex nor its trophic hormones are part of a mechanism which directly controls *variation* in filtration rate. No clearly evident alternative remains except to postulate the existence of an as yet unidentified humoral agent which has the capacity of dilating the afferent glomerular arterioles. Provisionally, this agent may be termed, *glomerulokinin*. Analogy with the aldosterone-control system suggests that' glomerulokinin' may, like 'adrenoglomerulotropin', be a neurohumor elaborated in the brain stem where it is secreted in proportion to the intensity of signals from cardiovascular afferents measuring circulatory plethora. This

[1] Contrary results are reported by GOLDMAN and BASSETT who observed a coincidence of sodium and steroid excretory peaks.

concept leads to the conclusion that filtration rate levels attained after a few days on a low salt diet represent the effects of virtual absence of 'glomerulokinin' but without, necessarily, supervention of neurogenic depression of function. The normal diurnal cycle, and its inversion in various disease states, should represent a corresponding cyclical release of 'glomerulokinin' analogous to the diurnal cyclical release of adrenocorticotropin and adrenoglomerulotropin.

The mechanisms responsible for the filtration rate responses following acute saline loading in the dog are undoubtedly complex. O'CONNOR (1955, 1958a) has emphasized that rise in blood pressure and decrease in colloid osmotic pressure can account for much and perhaps all of the filtration rate rise observed acutely in the dog during saline loading and that the filtration rate responses occur more rapidly than is usually observed in endocrine systems. That the mechanism is more complex than this is suggested by several observations. Mannitol loading in the dog, although associated with a marked decrease in colloid osmotic pressure usually does not cause filtration rate to increase (WESSON and ANSLOW 1948). Filtration rate during saline loading, although elevated, may exhibit marked fluctuations without corresponding changes in plasma protein concentration (WESSON et al. 1950). Filtration rate in the dog and seal exhibits large, immediate increases in response to eating a meat meal and without significant fluid ingestion (SHANNON, JOLLIFFE and SMITH 1932a; PITTS 1944; TANK and HERRIN; PAGE et al. 1954; MITCHELL et al.). Chloruresis and natriuresis (associated with an increase in filtration rate where this was measured) occur in the dog following infusion of colloidal solutions such as Dextran, oxypolygelatin, albumin and plasma (RAISZ; STAMLER et al.; PEARCE and ROBERTS; PEARCE; ATKINS and PEARCE), in the rabbit following infusion of acacia or blood (KOIWA), and in man following infusion of plasma (WILSON and HARRISON). In the studies on the dog (PEARCE and ROBERTS; PEARCE; ATKINS and PEARCE), chloruresis occurred following section of both vagi and the carotid sinus nerves. Although the immediate effects of food and salt on filtration rate in the dog and of *massive* fluid infusions in man may well represent responses of the kidney to nonhormonal changes in blood composition, the later, secondary rise in filtration rate in the dog (WESSON et al. 1950) and the late rise in man must, in the absence of evidence to the contrary, be viewed as of humoral origin.

c) Relative roles of filtration control and tubular reabsorption control in body salt balance

Few studies are available in which filtered load and tubular reabsorption have been studied simultaneously in relation to alterations of NaCl excretion. Inferences must be derived from a large number of incomplete observations such as have been described in the preceding and also in the following section. These lead to the view that the primary control of NaCl balance in man is a hemodynamic one acting through variations in glomerular filtration. Within wide limits, changes in renal tubular reabsorptive capacity do not appear to be important. The functions of the adrenal cortex may be viewed as supplementing the hemodynamic system and constituting an auxiliary control mechanism which permits a primary filtration control of body fluid volume to function more efficiently. These supplementary functions are: 1. a constant, small quantity of adrenal steroids are necessary to prevent NaCl depletion at low filtration rate. In the absence of adrenal steroids, the hemodynamic mechanisms are incapable of conserving NaCl efficiently. 2. Adrenal steroids, particularly the glucocorticoids, evoke significant increases in filtration rate in the hypoadrenal (but not sodium-deficient) man (DINGMAN et al.; GARROD and BURSTON; SKILLERN, CORCORAN and SCHERBEL; SALA and LUETSCHER; RENZI et al.; GARROD, DAVIES and CAHILL). The mechanism of this effect is completely unknown but provisionally may be interpreted as indicating that steroids have enhanced the responsiveness of the glomerular arterioles to 'glomerulokinin' or other humoral agents. Indirect support for this view, which is in accord with the 'permissive' theory of glucocorticoid action (INGLE 1956), comes from the observation that desoxycorticosterone, although a potent sodium-retaining steroid is a poor potentiator of the actions of sympathomimetic amines and of the autonomic nervous system compared with the glucocorticoids (RAMEY and GOLDSTEIN) and that adrenoprival patients treated with desoxycorticosterone or 9-alpha-fluorohydrocortisone alone frequently become edematous (LOEB; FERREBEE et al.; MuCULLAGH and RYAN; WILSON, RYNEARSON and DRY; CURRENS and WHITE; THORN, ENGEL and LEWIS; THORN, DORRANCE and DAY; THORN et al.; SANDERSON; OWEN, ENGEL and WESTER). 3. Release of aldosterone in cardiovascular stress states augments the efficiency of hemodynamic NaCl conservation. Possibly more important to salt conservation than the renal effects of aldosterone are the extrarenal effects on sweat, salivary glands and intestinal salt reabsorption which minimizes extrarenal salt losses. Aldosterone and salt-retaining steroids generally are relatively unimportant as controlling factors in hour to hour or even day to day changes in sodium excretion and are not essential to edema formation. Administration of a renal tubular aldosterone antagonist (SC 8109) to rats is followed by a large increase in aldosterone excretion if the animals are on a low salt diet, but no change in excretion is observed if the animals are on a normal salt diet (SINGER 1959). 4. Increasing aldosterone secretion during states of low sodium excretion may act as an important mechanism anticipating a need to facilitate potassium and hydrogen secretion in the presence of a diminished supply of sodium to exchange areas in the nephron (BARTTER 1956).

5. Sodium chloride balance in various conditions
a) Diurnal variation

Sodium chloride excretion is lower at night than during the day in normal man, thus correlating with other diurnal rhythms. Average excretion rate during the day is greater than the average rate during the night by ratios of 1.5 to 2.0 (VÖLKER; CAMPBELL and WEBSTER 1921, 1922; KLEITMAN; SIMPSON 1924, 1925, 1929; NORN; MANCHESTER 1933; BARBOUR et al.; BORST and DE VRIES; GOLDMAN 1951; NOBLE; DOE, VENNES and FLINK). Ratio of maximum daytime to minimum nighttime rate, however, may be much greater and range from 3.0 to 6.0 (STANBURY and THOMSON 1951; GERRITZEN 1937, 1940; AZERAD et al.; LEWIS and LOBBAN 1956, 1957a, b). The maximum and minimum are generally attained about 5 hours after arising and retiring, respectively, in subjects on a regular daily routine. The diurnal cycle is not dependent on meals, activity, or salt content of the diet since it persists during fasting, evenly spaced feeding, complete rest, and sodium restriction or supplementation (CAMPBELL and WEBSTER 1921; SIMPSON 1929; STANBURY and THOMPSON 1951; GARROD and BURSTON; ROSENBAUM, PAPPER and ASHLEY; WRONG 1957; WESSON 1957; NORN). Although the cycle is disturbed by sleeplessness and is reversed in night workers (SIMPSON 1925; NORN), it is not immediately dependent on sleep since it can be partially dissociated from the sleep rhythm in subjects whose daily routine is organized around a 22 or 27 hour day or following acute reversal of the sleep rhythm (LEWIS and LOBBAN 1957a, b; NORN). Degree of dissociation between the excretion rhythm and the sleep-activity rhythm in the former studies did not exceed 2 hours, however, and the relationship of the two rhythms must be close. The 24-hour cycle persisted in subjects who adopted a 12-hour day for 4 cycles (48 hours) (MILLS and STANBURY).

Since GFR has a diurnal cycle (see Section C-IV-4) in which filtration is larger in the daytime than in the nighttime it is evident that a positive correlation between filtration and excretion must exist. This is shown in the few studies in which both have been measured simultaneously. Correlation between the maximal values of GFR and chloride or sodium excretion (whether the maxima

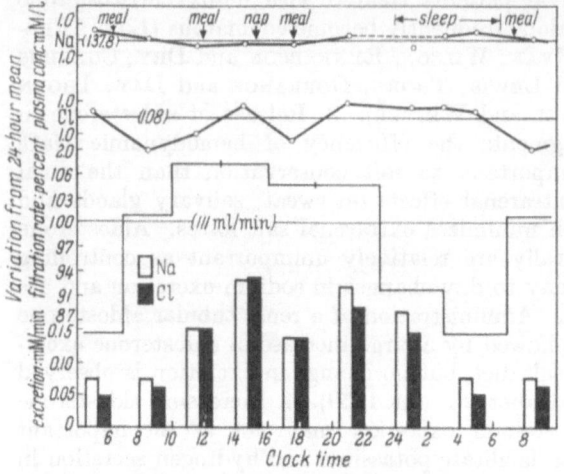

Fig. 72. Diurnal cycle of sodium and chloride excretion as correlated with plasma sodium and chloride concentrations and with glomerular filtration rate in a healthy 22 year old man. The values are the means of 5 nonconsecutive 24 hour cycles under a fixed regimen. (Wesson and Lauler, unpublished)

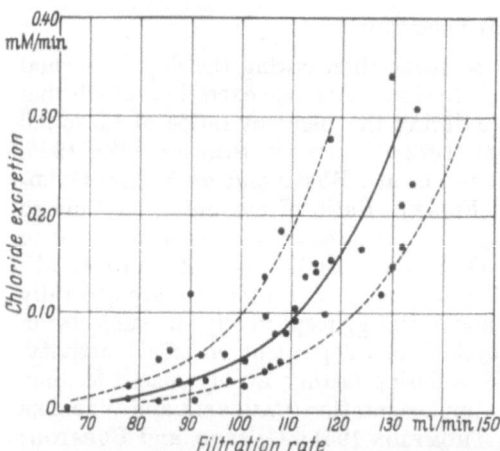

Fig. 73. Correlation between chloride excretion and filtration rate during the diurnal cycle in the subject illustrated in Fig. 72. The solid curve is the hypothetical relationship between excretion and filtration rate illustrated in Fig. 40. Filtration rate values in Fig. 40 have been multiplied by 0.82 to adjust the hypothetical curve to the average filtration rate observed in this subject. The effect on excretion of diurnal variation in plasma chloride concentration has been approximately compensated by increasing or decreasing observed filtration rate values at the rate of 4 ml./min. per mM./L. that plasma chloride concentration is above or below the mean of 108 mM./L.

occurred in the day as usual, or in the night as occasionally) was positive in all 3 subjects studied by Stanbury and Thomson (1951), in 7 of 8 experiments on 6 subjects studied by Fejfar and Brod and in 3 of 5 subjects studied by Baldwin et al. (Wesson 1957). In all of 8 cycles on one subject studied by Wesson and Lauler (unpubl.) the maxima and minima of the two cycles coincide (Fig. 72 and 73) but whether a change in one cycle is regularly accompanied by a change in the other remains to be determined. In cirrhosis and in congestive heart failure the diurnal excretion cycle is frequently reversed. Sodium excretion was greater in the night than in the day in 12 of 13 cirrhotic patients and in 6 of 8 patients with congestive heart failure (Goldman). Correspondingly, the filtration rate cycle is frequently reversed, particularly in ascitic cirrhotics (Jones, McDonald and Last). Of 7 patients with congestive heart failure, sodium excretion was greater during the night in 4 with persistent edema and in one of 3 who were edema-free or diuresing. GFR was correspondingly greater during the night in all 4 subjects with reversed excretion cycles (Baldwin, Sirota and Villarreal). In 22 studies of 16 patients with heart failure, chloride excretion was greater in the night in 13 and in the day in 9. In almost all instances, the GFR cycle corresponded with that of chloride (Fig. 74) (Fejfar and Brod).

Subjects on a high salt diet may exhibit fluctuations in daily NaCl excretion. The fluctuations occur in a regular pattern and are consistent with existence of a rhythm in the amplitude of the diurnal cycle which has a 2 to 3 day period. The period could represent the natural frequency of sustained oscillation in the salt-control system (Baldwin, Alexander and Warner).

The diurnal cycle of NaCl excretion is not dependent on a functioning adrenal cortex since the cycle is present in both treated and untreated adrenoprival patients (LEVY, POWER and KEPLER; GARROD and BURSTON; ROSENBAUM, PAPPER and ASHLEY; DOE, VENNES and FLINK). In persons with normally functioning adrenal glands, cortisol excretion is generally high and aldosterone excretion low toward the end of the sleep period and at the beginning of daily activity while filtration rate and NaCl excretion are at their minima shortly before or after the end of sleep. Cortisol excretion begins to decline and, if the individual becomes active, aldosterone excretion increases during the hours after arising, concurrent with rising filtration rate and NaCl excretion (VENNING, DYRENFURTH and GIROUD 1955, 1956; MULLER, RIONDEL and MANNING 1957;

LUETSCHER and CURTIS 1955; MULLER, MANNING and RIONDEL 1958b; BARTTER et al. 1958). If the individual is not active, little variation in aldosterone excretion may be observed, or excretion may be greater at night although the diurnal cycle of sodium excretion is unaffected. Relatively large quantities of cortisone (200 to 500 mg. daily) were capable of suppressing or reversing the diurnal cycle of excretion in normal subjects (ROSENBAUM et al. 1952) and a reversed cycle may occur in patients with hyperadrenocorticalism (DOE, VENNES and FLINK). Provisionally, there-

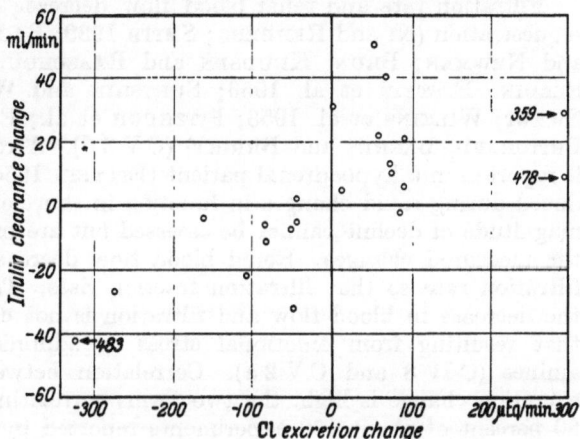

Fig. 74. Correlation between changes in filtration rate (inulin clearance) and changes in chloride excretion in diurnal cycles of cardiac patients (FEJFAR and BROD). Reproduced by permission of the Williams and Wilkins Co., Baltimore

fore, the normal diurnal cycle of NaCl excretion (Fig. 72), must be viewed as hemodynamically controlled perhaps by cyclic variations in secretion of a hypothetical 'glomerulokinin', with the adrenal cortex contributing relatively minor and irregular effects.

b) Acute blood sequestration

Acute blood sequestration refers to any of a group of procedures which prevent a portion of the blood volume from circulating freely. Among such procedures are application of venous tourniquets, partial occlusion of superior or inferior vena cava by catheters, orthostasis, phlebotomy, and supine position in pregnancy (BRUN, KNUDSEN and RAASCHOU 1945a, 1946; LEWIS et al. 1950; VIAR et al.; LOMBARDO et al.; CARGILL 1952; LEVITT, TURNER and SWEET; NETRAVISESH; GOODYER and SELDIN; FITZHUGH et al.; WILKINS et al. 1953; FARBER, BECKER and EICHNA; BACKMAN and YOUMANS; HOLLAND and STEAD 1954; PEARCE and NEWMAN; PRITCHARD, BARNES and BRIGHT; SURTSHIN and WHITE; EPSTEIN et al. 1956; DOYLE and MERRILL; GOMBOS et al.).

Without exception, such maneuvers in normal subjects are followed by a rapid decrease in NaCl excretion. The decrease in excretion following application of venous tourniquets can be prevented by simultaneously infusing blood into the general circulation (JUDSON et al. 1952). A decrease in excretion may fail to occur (or excretion may increase) in patients in congestive heart failure, particularly if cardiac output has increased as a result of removing some blood from the general circulation (Judson et al. 1952, 1955c; Lombardo).

In normal subjects, aldosterone excretion increases significantly within a short time and perhaps within 30 minutes of blood sequestration (Fine, Meiselas and Auerbach; Gowenlock, Mills and Thomas). NaCl excretion during tourniquet application decreases rapidly, however, in patients with Addison's disease (Decourt et al. 1945; Rosenbaum, Papper and Ashley) and also in normal subjects given large quantities of salt-retaining steroid (1.5—6 mg. daily of 9 alpha-flurohydrocortisone) (Strauss and Earley). It is evident, therefore, that secretions of the adrenal cortex may modify but do not govern the principal response to blood sequestration.

Filtration rate and renal blood flow decrease regularly during acute blood sequestration (Ni and Rehberg; Smith 1939; Bachman and Youmans; Pearce and Newman; Brun, Knudsen and Raaschou 1945a, 1946; Goodyer and Seldin; Epstein et al. 1956; Surtshin and White; Levitt, Turner and Sweet; Wilkins et al. 1953; Fitzhugh et al.; Farber, Becker and Eichna; Pritchard, Barnes and Bright) (C V 3 d). A response similar to the normal is reported in a hypoadrenal patient (Epstein 1956). Because of artefacts introduced during rapid changes in function in short experiments, the true rate and magnitude of decline cannot be assessed but are probably significantly less than the measured changes. Renal blood flow decreases relatively more than does filtration rate so that filtration fraction rises. The mechanism responsible for the decrease in blood flow and filtration is not clear, but resembles somewhat that resulting from emotional stress or administration of sympathomimetic amines (C IV 8 and C V 2 a). Correlation between filtration rate and NaCl excretion change is high, the two terms correlating positively in approximately 80 percent of about 100 experiments reported by various authors, both during and on recovery from blood sequestration. Inherent errors in measurement, particularly of filtration rate, can account for most or all of the noncorrelations. Correlation is particularly high if provision is made for the observation that change in NaCl excretion occurs 15 to 30 minutes (one clearance period) later than the apparent change in filtration rate (Wesson 1957). This observation is unexplained but may represent differences between inulin and sodium in equilibration time.

c) Acute fluid loading

Immediate changes in NaCl excretion in response to oral or intravenous fluid loading in man depend upon composition of the infusate, rapidity of infusion and the physiological or pathological state of the individual.

Fluids infused at rates in excess of 25 ml./min. usually result in significant increases in filtration rate. Hypertonic saline solutions increase plasma NaCl concentrations and, in addition, are associated with significant increases in filtration rate when infused at rates less than 25 ml./min. (C V 3 b). Two liters of isotonic (0.15 M.) saline is sufficient to elevate plasma NaCl concentrations 2 to 4 mM./L. (Papper et al.). Varying combinations of filtration rate and plasma composition change in different experimental studies are sufficient to explain natriuresis resulting from fluid loading (Wesson 1957). Natriuresis following isotonic or hypotonic solutions given relatively slowly may be small or absent and variably related to body position (Blomhert et al.; Welt and Orloff; Crawford and Ludemann). The same quantity of salt, probably for the reasons outlined above, is associated with a more profuse natriuresis when given concentrated in a small volume than in a large volume of water (Darragh

et al.). A large volume of water orally, with or without administration of vasopressin, is seldom associated with a significant immediate increase in NaCl excretion although filtration rate may increase (LADD 1951 b).

Concentrated, salt-poor albumin in normal subjects is not regularly associated
with a significant natriuresis and frequently is associated with a decrease in
excretion, although plasma volume is expanded (GOODYER, PETERSON and
RELMAN; EPSTEIN et al. 1951; WELT and ORLOFF; PETERSDORF and WELT).
Change in plasma albumin concentration is not reported. Presumably, the
expanded plasma volume occupied the depleted interstitial fluid space following
shifts of fluid into the vascular compartment so that a true intravascular plethora
did not occur. In cirrhosis and nephrosis, however, concentrated albumin or
Dextran is regularly associated with a rise in filtration rate and usually, also,
sodium excretion (PATEK et al.; ORLOFF, WELT and STOWE; LUETSCHER, HALL
and KREMER; JAMES, GORDILLO and METCOFF).

The physiological or pathological state of the subject markedly affects the
response to fluid loading. The difference between normal subjects and patients
with cirrhosis and nephrosis in response to injection of concentrated albumin
was noted above, and differences in response are noted in other circumstances.
Ingestion of a large volume (1—2 L.) of water with ensuing water diuresis (prehydration) 12 hours before a saline infusion results in a more massive natriuretic
response to saline infusion than when prehydration is omitted (LADD 1951 a, b,
1952). Plasma sodium concentrations and postinfusion filtration rates were
the same in both groups. Prehydrated subjects, however, had a higher rate of
filtration and of sodium excretion at the start of the infusion, and in view of
the effects of a water load on aldosterone excretion (MULLER, RIONDEL and
MANNING) it seems reasonable to suppose that the mechanism of the prehydration effect otherwise may be related to lower aldosterone secretion in the prehydrated group.

Patients with hypertension frequently exhibit a more pronounced natriuretic response to infusion of hypertonic saline than do normal subjects (GREEN
et al. 1952; THOMPSON et al. 1954; BIRCHALL et al.; HOLLANDER and JUDSON
1957, 1958; COTTIER, WELLER and HOOBLER 1958a, b; WELLER and HOOBLER;
ULLMAN et al. 1959). Hypertensive pregnant women, however, did not exhibit
increased excretion rate as compared with pregnant and nonpregnant normotensive women (CHESLEY, VALENTI and REIN). The mechanisms involved are
not clear, and in no study have all the major variables been examined. The
importance of the control rate of sodium excretion is illustrated from a theoretical
view point in Fig. 41, in which the increment in sodium excretion per unit change
in filtration rate when control excretion is 0.40 mM./min. is nearly twice the
increment predicted at a control excretion of 0.15 mM./min. In the studies on
hypertensive pregnant women, control rate of sodium excretion was lower than
in the other groups (CHESLEY, VALENTI and REIN), while in other studies, in
which the hypertensive group excreted sodium more rapidly, control sodium
excretion in the hypertensives has been higher than in normotensive subjects
(COTTIER, WELLER and HOOBLER 1958a; BIRCHALL et al.; HOLLANDER and
JUDSON). When attention is limited to normotensive and hypertensive groups
having subequal control rates of sodium excretion, some, but not all, of the
difference between the two groups vanishes (HOLLANDER and JUDSON 1957;
COTTIER, WELLER and HOOBLER 1958a, b). Insufficient studies are available
in the restricted groups (equal control excretion rate) to determine whether significant differences exist in other variables such as plasma composition or filtration rate. Plasma sodium concentration in hypertensives may average slightly

higher than in normotensives (WELLER and HOOBLER), while changes in filtration rate, considered alone, do not correlate with the difference between normotensives and hypertensives. The enhanced excretory response in hypertensives is decreased following splanchnicectomy (THOMPSON et al. 1954) or treatment with antihypertensive drugs, reserpine or hydralazine (HOLLANDER and JUDSON 1958) but only if blood pressure is lowered (HOLLANDER and JUDSON 1957). The exaggerated natriuretic response is abolished in hypertensives on a low sodium diet (HANENSON et al. 1959; BALDWIN et al. 1959). In such patients, however, control excretion rate, plasma sodium concentration and filtration rate are depressed. The effects of hypertonic saline infusion on aldosterone excretion, reported to be increased in many hypertensive patients (HERNANDO et al.; GENEST et al. 1958; GARST et al.), remains to be examined, while the effects of high arterial blood pressure on tubular sodium reabsorption are unknown.

Both normal and hypertensive subjects given an injection of hypertonic saline following acute administration of a salt-retaining steroid, desoxycorticosterone (DOC), excrete the salt more slowly than when the DOC is not given (SOFFER et al.; SOFFER, GABRILOVE and JACOBS; LONDON and TERRY). However, if normal subjects have been maintained on DOC, 9-alpha-fluorohydrocortisone or large quantities of cortisone for several days until normal excretion of salt has resumed (escape), the response to hypertonic saline is equal to or greater than normal (BIRCHALL et al.; STRAUSS and EARLEY). Patients with CUSHING's disease (hyperadrenalism) and primary aldosteronism resemble the normal subject in steroid escape. They exhibit no change or an enhanced chloruretic response when given additional, exogenous salt-retaining steroids (SOFFER et al.; SOFFER, GABRILOVE and JACOBS) and their response to a challenge saline load is greater than normal (KRISS and FUTCHER; BIRCHALL et al.; BIGLIERI, WATLINGTON and FORSHAM; HANENSON et al. 1959). Both the subjects in steroid escape (STRAUSS and EARLEY) and the patients with aldosteronism (BIGLIERI, WATLINGTON and FORSHAM) exhibited further increase in GFR during loading.

d) Chronic salt restriction or depletion

When a person transfers from a diet which is normal or unrestricted in salt (4—6 grams NaCl daily) to a diet which is low in salt, daily excretion decreases rapidly. Within 3 to 5 days following adoption of the low-salt diet, excretion and consumption are approximately equal. Body salt content, however, is lower than on the unrestricted diet by the cumulative difference between consumption and excretion during the several days before equality of the two terms is attained. The 'deficit' is permanent: there is no evidence that excretion decreases below consumption so that the prior body content is regained. The body is, in fact, in a new 'steady state', emphasizing that 'normal' body salt content is a term which has no meaning without reference to the concurrent state of the circulation, daily salt intake and numerous other less significant variables. If negative NaCl balance is produced abruptly following adoption of a low-salt diet, as by a mercurial diuresis, salt excretion decreases at once, remains low, and the progressive daily decline in excretion rate is not seen (STRAUSS et al. 1958).

Concurrently with decreasing NaCl excretion, plasma sodium and chloride concentrations decrease probably as the result of increasing nonosmotic stimulation of the neurohypophysis (AITKEN; McCANCE 1936; NADAL, PEDERSON and MADDOCK; BLACK, PLATT and STANBURY; WESTON et al. 1950; WATKIN et al.; WIGGINS et al.). In subjects on a rigidly sodium-restricted diet (15 mM./day or less), plasma NaCl decreases 3 to 8 mM./L. Filtration rate also decreases in most studies of the effects of low salt diets (BLACK, McCANCE and YOUNG; BLACK, PLATT and STANBURY; CHASIS et al. 1950; WESTON et al. 1950; WIGGINS et al.) with relatively less change in RPF (C V 3 e). The decline in filtration rate is significant in the first day following adoption of the low-salt regime (WESSON and LAULER, unpubl.). Hypoadrenal patients maintained on cortisone exhibited decreases in creatinine clearance (LIPSETT and PEARSON). Patients with uremia due to chronic nephritis exhibited decreases in filtration rate averaging 45 percent (NICKEL, LOWRANCE and LEIFER).

Aldosterone excretion rises markedly one or two days after adoption of a low-sodium diet and while sodium excretion is still decreasing. The maximum aldosterone excretion rate is generally not sustained but declines to lower although still elevated values (CRABBÉ, ROSE and THORN). Other evidences of increased steroid activity, such as increased potassium excretion and decreased sweat Na concentration, also appear toward the end of the period of rapid decrease in sodium excretion (RENWICK, ROBSON and STEWART; ROBINSON et al. 1955; WESSON and LAULER, unpubl.). Immediately following resumption of un-restricted salt diet, aldosterone excretion decreases to normal values although sodium excretion remains low (CRABBÉ, ROSE and THORN). Excretion of other steroids is unchanged on low-salt diets (DAUGHADAY and MACBRYDE). These observations, together with the circumstance that the adrenalectomized patient maintained on cortisol responds normally to adoption of a low salt diet (RANDALL and PAPPER), measure the relatively subsidiary function contributed by the adrenal cortex in adjustment to changes in salt intake. The significance of adrenocortical function is indicated by the facts that renal conservation of salt is less complete and extrarenal salt losses are greater than normal in cortisol-maintained adrenoprival patients (LIPSETT and PEARSON).

e) Chronic salt- or fluid-loading

The responses to acquisition of excess body fluid differ somewhat according to the state of the body and the nature and manner of acquisition of the fluid excess. The importance of body state is illustrated by patients with heart failure, nephrosis or cirrhosis (see below). Hypertonic saline or salt administration is associated with an acute increase in NaCl excretion. The increase in plasma NaCl concentration is a stimulus to increased water retention and water consumption (thirst activation) which convert into an isotonic expansion of extracellular fluid any excess salt which is not excreted acutely. Isotonic or slightly hypotonic saline loading in normal subjects may or may not be associated with a small, acute increase in excretion. Irrespective of the immediate response, however, excretion increases rapidly, generally within 24 hours, so that within one or two days the excess salt is excreted or, if the individual has adopted a high salt diet, excretion approximately equals intake. Although few studies are available on renal function during chronic or sustained saline loading, these are in agreement in showing elevation of glomerular filtration rate, a slight elevation in plasma NaCl concentrations (MARKLEY et al.; WESSON and LAULER, unpubl.) and decrease in aldosterone excretion (DUNCAN, LIDDLE and BARTTER; MULLER, RIONDEL and MANNING 1956b).

A slightly different pattern is exhibited in individuals whose body fluids are expanded by water-loading combined with vasopressin (Pitressin tannate) injections. NaCl excretion does not increase or may decrease somewhat for 2 to 4 days, following which a marked natriuresis usually occurs (LEAF et al.

1953; WESTON et al. 1960; WRONG 1956). When the natriuresis occurs, filtration
rate is elevated (WESSON and LAULER, unpubl.) and aldosterone excretion is
depressed (DUNCAN, LIDDLE and BARTTER; MULLER, RIONDEL and MANNING).
The natriuresis can be blunted but not suppressed by administration of adrenocorticotropin or desoxycorticosterone (WESTON et al. 1960).

Potassium depletion is associated with NaCl retention, often to the point
of edema formation, together with a decrease in aldosterone excretion. The
mechanisms involved are unknown and probably complex.

f) Sodium-retaining states

The critical element in edema formation is a persistently positive NaCl
balance. Although body salt and water content increase indefinitely, excretion
fails to rise to the point that balance is attained. According to the concepts
outlined in this section, excretion will fail to respond to increase in body fluid
under either of two circumstances: the integrated signal to the nervous system
registering degree of cardiovascular adequacy may fail to change with fluid
retention; or the nervous system may be incapable of responding to the signal.
The latter circumstance, although suggested (MACH; KLOTZ and KAHN), is not
yet clearly recognized in human clinical states.

Failure of the cardiovascular signal to change significantly with fluid expansion
carries no necessary implication with respect to the absolute magnitude of cardiovascular adequacy. In theory, therefore, a person with apparently normal
cardiovascular status and who is not forming edema on a diet with average salt
content can become edematous on a high salt diet if his cardiovascular system
fails to register a change of status. A more frequently encountered situation,
however, is that in which a patient with a mild degree of cardiovascular inadequacy and with a somewhat depressed NaCl excretion rate forms edema on an
unrestricted salt diet but becomes edema-free on a low-salt diet. Congestive
heart failure, nephrosis and cirrhosis represent conditions of mild to severe
cardiovascular inadequacy in which the cardiovascular state fails to improve,
or even deteriorates further in association with indefinite expansion of body
fluid volume.

The term "compensated", as applied to patients with edema-forming states, generally
refers to sustained freedom from gross fluid accumulations. The term does not clearly
distinguish between patients who retain or have reacquired a significant degree of intrinsic
control of their extracellular fluid volume (physiologically compensated) from those patients
(physiologically decompensated) who have lost this capacity and can remain edema-free
only by salt-restriction and diuretics.

Heart failure. Congestive heart failure is characterized by a low NaCl excretion rate as manifested by the need of sodium-restricted diets or of diuretics
in order to control excessive salt retention. The failure can arise from depression
of cardiac output below body needs for 'adequate' perfusion at rest or from
inability of the cardiac output to meet increase in physiological need, as during
slight to moderate exercise or 'pathological' need as in hyperthyroidism, fever,
pregnancy, liver disease, beriberi, and arteriovenous aneurysm (high output
failure). The mechanisms responsible for failure to attain salt balance in high-
output failure are frequently difficult to analyse because of extensive metabolic
or endocrine disturbances. Heart failure in the presence of hypertension is
complicated by deterioration of both renal hemodynamic and tubular functions.
In the least complicated group of patients, those with failure secondary to
cardiac valvular or vascular disease, filtration rate is moderately, and renal
blood flow is markedly lower than in normal populations of the same age and

sex (C V 4). If, however, the cardiacs are compared with normals who, because of dietary salt restriction or salt depletion are also excreting little salt, then much of the difference in filtration rate between cardiac and noncardiac populations disappears (C V 3 e). In addition to an apparent failure of the normal mechanisms augmenting filtration rate, an additional depression in glomerular filtration probably occurs in the more severely ill patients secondary to neurogenic or humoral depression in renal blood flow.

An increase in aldosterone secretion probably contributes to NaCl retention in both the moderately and severely ill patients but definitive studies are not available. In the less severely ill, it is possible that aldosterone secretion may increase significantly only during mild exertion, but in the more severely ill patients secretion is markedly increased at all times. That aldosterone secretion is not essential for the formation of cardiac edema is indicated by edema formation in a patient with ADDISON's disease (BLACKET). Hypochloremia and hyponatremia probably contribute significantly to impaired NaCl excretion in the very ill patients (WESTON et al. 1952), but plasma concentrations are essentially normal in less ill, ambulatory cardiac patients even though they are edematous (BRICKER and WESSON). Whether other variables such as renal venous pressure (BRADLEY and BLAKE) or unrecognized metabolic or humoral agents play a significant contributory role in cardiac edema remains to be determined. Improvement of the patient is accompanied by increase in renal blood flow and glomerular filtration rate (DAVIES; EICHNA et al. 1953) and decrease in aldosterone excretion (LUETSCHER and CURTIS 1955b; HERNANDO et al.).

Exercise has many physiological properties in common with high-output heart failure. Unfortunately, reliable renal function measurements during moderately severe exercise in normal subjects are not available (C IV 6). Chloride excretion regularly decreases, frequently to very low levels and recovers slowly during the postexercise period (MACKEITH et al.; WILSON et al.; HAVARD; EGGLETON 1943; BARCLAY et al. 1947; KATTUS et al.; BUCHT et al. 1953; DUNCAN). More extensive studies are available of the effects of exercise on patients with heart disease. Relatively mild exercise in cardiac patients is generally associated with decreased chloride excretion, and where normals and cardiacs are subjected to the same exercise, the decrease is significantly greater in the latter. Filtration rate and renal plasma flow decrease roughly in proportion to the degree to which the exercise is exhausting, the latter more than the former, so that filtration fraction increases further (C V 4). A good correlation exists between NaCl excretion and filtration rate change (WERKO et al. 1954a; FREEMAN et al.; JUDSON et al. 1955b; WESSON 1957).

Nephrosis. The cardiovascular lesion in nephrosis is probably a deficient blood volume caused by a deficient quantity of intravascular albumin, the latter deficiency arising, for the most part, from excessive urinary excretion. Salt and water retained by the kidneys pass into the interstitial spaces instead of restoring the blood volume. There seems little doubt that the extraordinarily efficient salt retention in nephrosis is attributable in large part to the high rate of aldosterone secretion which may reach 20 to 30 times normal (ULICK, LARAGH and LIEBERMAN). The role of hemodynamic changes is not clear. Filtration rate may be low, normal or elevated and renal blood flow is not significantly depressed (C V 10). Interpretation of the low values is complicated by the high incidence of nephritic changes in patients with the nephrotic syndrome. A partial explanation for failure of salt excretion in patients with supranormal filtration rate is offered by the observation that those tubular functions which have been measured, p-aminohippurate secretion and glucose reabsorption

(D III 1 d and D IV 1 a), are also elevated in these patients. Of more significance is the increase in filtration rate observed during natriuresis whether spontaneous or as the result of albumin administration or steroid therapy (LUETSCHER, HALL and KREMER; METCOFF, KELSEY and JANEWAY; METCOFF, NAKASONE and RANCE; BARNETT et al. 1951; LAUSON et al.; EDER et al.) but the relative contributions to natriuresis of rising filtration rate and of decreasing aldosterone secretion are unknown. A small, variable degree of hyponatremia and hypochloremia related to dietary salt restriction may also contribute to decreased salt excretion rate in nephrosis (McQUARRIE and ZIEGLER).

Cirrhosis. Renal function has been relatively little studied in patients with cirrhosis. The general pattern appears to resemble that in nephrosis rather more than that in congestive heart failure. Aldosterone excretion is generally and often markedly elevated and plasma Na concentration tends to be low (AMATUZIO et al.). Filtration rate, renal plasma flow and p-aminohippurate secretory capacity are frequently elevated suggesting that the renal hemodynamic contribution to salt retention is a persistent glomerulo-tubular imbalance. This view is supported by the observation that ascites may continue to form in adrenalectomized cirrhotic patients (MARSON; GIUSEFFI et al.) who are receiving no more than the normal daily maintenance dose of cortisone (McLEAN et al. 1955; HILLS, ZINTEL and PARSONS). Similarly, adrenalectomized dogs with intrathoracic inferior vena caval constriction form ascites during administration of relatively small quantities of steroids. Release of the constriction during steroid administration is followed by prompt diuresis and rise in filtration rate (DAVIS, HOWELL and SOUTHWORTH).

g) Anesthesia and surgery

During anesthesia and surgery, GFR, RPF and NaCl excretion are greatly depressed (C V 1). After anesthesia or surgery and in the absence of hypotension or dehydration, GFR and RPF return to or close to preoperative values within 24 hours (CRAWFORD and GAUDINO; HABIF et al.) but occasionally significant depression, particularly of GFR, may be more prolonged (ARIEL and MILLER). NaCl excretion remains low for 4 to 8 days with perhaps a small, temporary increase in excretion of 1 to 2 days duration in the middle of this period (FEYEL and VARANGOT; LE QUESNE and LEWIS). An intense antidiuresis, beginning with anesthesia, continues for 1 to 3 days postoperatively. The antidiuresis is enhanced by various drugs such as morphine and results in retention of excess water and production of hyponatremia which is terminated, ultimately, by a spontaneous diuresis (LE QUESNE and LEWIS). Sodium retention continues, or reappears following remission of the antidiuretic phase, and retention cannot be averted by preventing postoperative hyponatremia (JØRGENSEN and SCHLEGEL). Aldosterone excretion is significantly elevated only during the first 1 to 2 days postoperatively (CASEY, BICKEL and ZIMMERMANN; VENNING et al. 1958) and is coincident with but not proven to be the cause of a brief period of increased renal potassium excretion (LE QUESNE and LEWIS). Evidence of increased secretion of glucocorticoids (ACTH dependent) persists much longer (VENNING et al. 1958). On the other hand, a phase of postoperative sodium retention closely resembling that observed in normals is observed following surgery in adrenalectomized patients (ROBSON et al.; MASON; WILKINSON; RANDALL and PAPPER) and following injury in the adrenalectomized rat (INGLE et al.; SHARE and STADLER) so that it is evident that the mechanism of postoperative NaCl retention is unsettled. Hyponatremia and increased adrenocortical activity probably play contributory roles in the immediate postoperative period. The degree of later NaCl retention could be lessened by increased dietary potassium, suggesting that a small degree of potassium depletion might be present and contributing to excessive NaCl retention. That no intrinsic abnormality of renal function exists is shown by the circumstance that the patient excretes a salt load as efficiently postoperatively as preoperatively provided that, as a result of prior salt administration, the control rate of NaCl excretion is equal in the 2 states (RANDALL and PAPPER). These observations are consistent with but do not prove that a critical element in postoperative retention is delayed recovery of the normal control of glomerular filtration.

h) Steroid escape and hyperaldosteronism

Administration of excessive quantities of steroids such as adrenocorticotropin, hydrocortisone, desoxycorticosterone, 9-α-fluorohydrocortisone and aldosterone is unable to effect more than a transitory positive sodium balance in healthy man or dog. Following a period of NaCl retention, whose duration is related to the antecedent body salt content and to the dietary salt intake during the period of steroid administration, further salt retention ceases and much of the previously retained salt may be lost, constituting the phenomenon of 'steroid escape' (ZIERLER and LILIENTHAL; ALEXANDER et al.; LUFT and SJÖGREN 1951; RELMAN and SCHWARTZ 1952; SPRAGUE et al.; HETZEL et al.; AUGUST, NELSON and THORN; OWEN, ENGEL and WESTER; PECHET, BOWERS and BARTTER; STAHL et al.; STRAUSS and EARLEY; RELMAN, STEWART and SCHWARTZ; AUGUST and NELSON 1959b). The time required for escape to appear is related directly to degree of hydration at commencement of steroid loading and to salt intake. If individuals are well hydrated and on a high salt diet, 'escape' is essentially immediate (STRAUSS and EARLEY; AUGUST and NELSON). 'Escape' does not require a functioning adrenal cortex (AUGUST and NELSON 1959b). A more or less chronic form of naturally occurring 'steroid escape' is seen in primary aldosteronism. Tumors of the adrenal may secrete variably increased and sometimes large amounts of aldosterone without overt edema formation unless heart disease supervenes (FOYE and FEICHTMEIR; MACH et al.; MADER and ISERI; EALES and LINDER; DUSTAN, CORCORAN and PAGE; CONN and LOUIS; HEWLETT et al.; MILNE, MUEHRCKE and AIRD; GOLDSMITH et al.; BARTTER and BIGLIEREI; AYRES et al. 1958; ULICK, LARACH and LIEBERMAN (1958). Filtration rate increases during 'steroid escape' (ZIERLER and LILIENTHAL; LUFT and SJÖGREN 1949b, c; ALEXANDER et al.; PECHET, BOWERS and BARTTER; WESSON and LAULER, unpubl.). In the studies of LUFT and SJÖGREN, average filtration rate of 12 subjects on a regime of 20 mg. desoxycorticosterone (cortexone) with 5 to 10 grams of supplemental dietary NaCl daily was 20 ml./min. greater than on a moderately salt-restricted (less than 3 g. daily) regime. Omitting from the averages one subject with advanced renal disease and a second who failed to adjust (i.e. became markedly edematous) average GFR increased 26 ml./min. or about 30 percent above the low-salt values. Renal blood flow, as also in chronic fluid loading, did not change significantly. Filtration rate in primary aldosteronism is generally in the high normal range (after making appropriate corrections for age and mannitol clearance measurements) (DUSTAN, CORCORAN and PAGE; EALES and LINDER; HEWLETT et al.) although the frequent occurrence of pyelonephritis (MUEHRCKE and MILNE; STANBURY 1958) and potassium depletion in patients with the diagnosis of primary aldosteronism, with their deleterious effects on tubular functions, render interpretation of absolute magnitudes difficult. Filtration rate decreases postoperatively, however (DUSTAN, CORCORAN and PAGE).

III. Control of calcium and phosphate excretion

Experimental studies have generally failed to indicate that an extrarenal feedback system must be postulated to explain calcium and phosphate balance in normal man. Nearly all of the data relating to excretion of these substances are compatible with a simple steady state system in which plasma concentrations measure the balance between extrarenal metabolism (utilization and net intestinal absorption) and renal excretion. Variations in excretion compatible with a simple filtered load-dependence are readily observed when filtration rate or plasma concentrations of either calcium or phosphate are altered acutely, but technical difficulties have delayed accumulation of precise information on the mechanism of calcium excretion under such conditions. Information on phosphate is somewhat more abundant. Although precise measurements of filtration rate are frequently lacking, the phosphate data in short term studies show a generally good correlation between phosphate excretion and plasma phosphate concentration (Milne; Talpers and Stein; Goldman and Basset 1958). In advanced renal disease, although some control of phosphate excretion is possible by variation in tubular transport (Gershberg, Shields and Kove) such control is of little significance (Goadby) and excretion for practical purposes is determined by filtered load (Kleeman and Cooke; Goldman and Bassett 1954). Nevertheless, two circumstances combine to render a simple steady state system unlikely. These are an apparent need for a precise control of calcium and phosphate concentrations, together with existence in the parathyroid glands of a system which is quite adequate to stabilize these concentrations. (For reviews, see Dragstedt; Thomson and Collip; Greep 1948; Bartter 1954.) This system is illustrated hypothetically in Fig. 75. It is based upon the effects of excess or deficient parathyroid activity and the effects of changes in calcium and phosphate balance. Nevertheless, the system must remain hypothetical until development of suitable assay methods can determine whether the glands do in fact respond in the way they are presumed to respond. The reality of the problem of whether the parathyroids respond reciprocally to changes in calcium or phosphate concentration can be illustrated by the analogous problem of the relation of glucocorticoids to sodium excretion. Although sodium balance is disturbed in the presence of either excess or deficiency of these steroids there is, however, no evidence that they play more than a conditioning role in sodium balance.

The apparent need for control of plasma calcium and phosphate concentrations arises from the narrowness of the range of tolerable concentrations. Sufficient concentrations of both ions are necessary not only for bone formation but also for numerous other metabolic functions. An upper limit to concentrations is rigidly established by the low solubility of various calcium phosphate salts. The solubility of $CaHPO_4$, which is both the simplest and the most soluble of these salts, appears to be the most important, and serum is normally not too far from saturation with this salt (Albright and Reifenstein; Neuman).

The solubility product of $CaHPO_4$ is the product of the concentrations of Ca and HPO_4, expressed in molar or activity units, when both ions are in equilibrium with the solid phase. The molar solubility product in serum is about 2.5×10^{-6} (Logan). When the product of the ionic concentrations of Ca^{++} and $HPO_4^=$ is less than this value, the serum is undersaturated. The product in normal serum is about 2.1×10^{-6}, indicating a significant degree of undersaturation with respect to this salt (Logan; Albright and Reifenstein; Neuman). Plasma is supersaturated with respect to $Ca_3(PO_4)_2$ and other more complex salts, but at plasma pH these salts apparently cannot form directly but require formation of $CaHPO_4$ as a first step (Logan). Factors which may prevent indefinite precipitation of Ca and PO_4 at bone surface have been considered by Logan and by Neuman.

If concentrations are allowed to rise above the solubility levels of calcium phosphates, precipitation can occur. Since the concentrations of Ca and PO_4 cannot be independently varied, it follows that control of the concentration of one ion automatically establishes the maximum concentration attainable by the other ion. However, to prevent random precipitation of calcium phosphates in blood or tissues, the ionic concentration product of Ca and PO_4 must be kept below the solubility limit, yet, within the limitations of this restriction, each ion should be kept as close as possible to its optimum concentration.

When the parathyroid glands are removed, serum calcium and calcium excretion decline, bone turnover decreases and plasma phosphate increases. Urine phosphate excretion comes into equilibrium with intake. In hyperparathyroidism resulting from an active parathyroid adenoma or injections of extract, the converse findings are observed: plasma calcium and calcium excretion increase, bone turnover increases and plasma phosphate decreases (ALBRIGHT and REIFENSTEIN). Views that all of the effects of parathyroid excess or deficit could be attributed to a primary action on bone with excretion changes secondary (THOMSON and CLLIP) or to a primary action on excretion with bone secondary (ALBRIGHT et al. 1931; ALBRIGHT and REIFENSTEIN) are now recognized to be oversimplified. Parathyroid excess or deficit directly affects tubular reabsorption of both calcium and phosphate. In man, extracts increase calcium reabsorption slightly (D V 5) and decrease phosphate reabsorption slightly to moderately as compared with the normal and markedly as compared with hypoparathyroid states (D V 7). Alternatively, studies

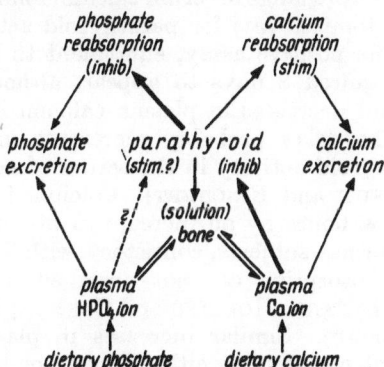

Fig. 75. Mechanisms controlling the plasma concentrations of calcium and phosphate, lhypothetical

on nephrectomized rat and dog indicate that bone histology and plasma calcium concentration remain sensitive to presence of parathyroid or to administration of extract (SELYE; STOERK; INGALLS, DONALDSON and ALBRIGHT; ELLSWORTH and FUTCHER; MONAHAN and FREEMAN; STEWART and BOWEN 1951, 1952; TALMAGE et al. 1953; GROLLMAN 1954; TOFT and TALMAGE)[1]. A direct action on bone is further shown when bone which is juxtaposed to parathyroid tissue dissolves (BARNICOT; CHANG). Plasma phosphate shows little response to parathyroid extract in the nephrectomized animal, suggesting that, in the absence of the kidneys, the glands have little influence over extraosseous distribution of that ion (MONAHAN and FREEMAN; TALMAGE et al. 1953).

The phosphaturic action of hydrocortisone in the rat requires the presence of functioning parathyroid glands, and no specific phosphaturic effect from hydrocortisone is observed in parathyroidectomized rats to which parathyroid extract has been given (ARISON and STOERK). Moreover, tumors frequently occur simultaneously in both anterior pituitary and parathyroid glands (TÖRNBLOM). Nevertheless, regulation of parathyroid secretion through the pituitary or adrenal glands remains to be demonstrated. Although nerves enter the parathyroids, the glands function well following denervation (TÖRNBLOM, review). Evidence that the parathyroid glands respond directly to plasma concentrations

---

[1] NEUFELD and COLLIP observed no effect of parathyroid extract on plasma calcium in animals with suppressed renal function, but their animals were not parathyroidectomized and their controls were inadequate.

of calcium and perhaps phosphate are indirect but rather convincing. Hypertrophy and hyperplasia of the parathyroids are observed in human and animal rickets and osteomalacia, in uremia associated with low plasma calcium concentrations (Thomson and Collip; Albright and Reifenstein) and in animals on calcium-deficient diets (Ham et al.; Stoerk and Carnes). Osteoclastic activity in nephrectomized rats fails to appear if calcium supplements are fed or if the animals are parathyroidectomized (Toft and Talmage). Repeated injections of phosphate are associated with hypertrophy of the parathyroids in rats while calcium injections are associated with decrease in gland size (Albright and Reifenstein). Parathyroidectomized rabbits, which required about 40 units of parathyroid extract/kg./24 hours to sustain blood chemistry and phosphate excretion equal to unoperated controls, required about 60 units to duplicate the pattern of the control group during phosphate loading (Törnblom). A positive assay (change in serum calcium following injection of test serum into a parathyroidectomized rat) for parathyroid activity is obtained in the calcium-depleted rat. The positive assay, equivalent to 20 to 40 units of parathyroid extract per ml. required 8 days to appear, although histological changes in the parathyroids and decreases in plasma calcium had appeared by the fourth day of depletion. The delay probably represents insensitivity of the assay method since parathyroid activity in the serum of normal man is about 0.4 units per ml. (L'Heureux and Reichert). Calcium infusions are associated with or followed in a few hours by an increase in plasma phosphate or in phosphate reabsorption in normal subjects, consistent with inhibition of the parathyroid, but changes in reabsorption are not observed in either hypo- or hyperparathyroid subjects (Howard, Hopkins and Connor; Hiatt and Thompson 1957b; Kleeman et al. 1959b). Similar increases in plasma phosphate from calcium infusions were not observed in either hyper- or hypoparathyroid patients (Howard, Hopkins and Connor). An increase in phosphate reabsorption was observed in an adult subject (Thompson and Hiatt 1957a) and in infants (McCrory et al.) on a low phosphate diet while a decrease in reabsorption followed phosphate loading. In 4 normal subjects, phosphate Tm decreased 28, 36 and 57 percent and decreased to zero in the fourth after 3 days of loading. In 3 hypoparathyroid patients, Tm decreased 10, 24 and 61 percent. Plasma calcium, however, did not increase, suggesting that if the decrease in phosphate transport is due to secretion of a parathyroid principle, this principle has little calcium-mobilizing potency (Thompson and Hiatt 1957b). Injection of 250 mg. calcium in man was not associated with an acute change in phosphate excretion, however (Milne). In these studies change in phosphate reabsorption constitutes a presumptive indication of change in activity of the glands, which presumably can respond in the normal but not in dysfunctional states. Unknown is whether phosphate-loading inhibits parathyroid function directly, or indirectly through effects on calcium ionization.

Many changes in calcium and phosphate excretion are perhaps too easily explained by postulating changes in parathyroid function: The rise in phosphate reabsorption following vitamin D administration to rachitic puppies may be attributed to decrease in parathyroid secretion (Harrison and Harrison 1941a). Decrease in phosphate reabsorption resulting from cortisone may result from parathyroid stimulation (Arison and Stoerk). Increase in phosphate excretion in acidosis may result from parathyroid stimulation secondary to excessive urinary calcium loss (Albright and Reifenstein). For the final answer to these and many other questions, the parathyroid hormone or hormones must be characterized and a sensitive assay developed.

F. Renal function tests

I. General considerations

The capacity of the kidney as an excretory organ is measured by the three general functions of plasma or blood flow, filtration rate, and tubular transport. Tubular transport is a general term including a large number of semi-independent transport systems each of which must be measured separately. With the exception of blood flow, which may be measured directly in surgically-prepared experimental animals, all function measurements are based on clearances. The choice of methods of measurement is related to the use to which the information will be put. For research purposes, the separate functions should be measured explicitly and accurately. For clinical purposes, simplicity and rapidity are usually more important than accurate measurement of discrete functions.

Clearances and clearance ratios

Except under rare circumstances in which an excreted substance is transported in significant quantities by erythrocytes as well as by plasma, clearance measurements are preferably limited to plasma. The clearance of a substance is the least amount of plasma, measured as volume per unit of time and usually as milliliters per minute, required to supply the amount of the substance appearing in the urine. Consider, for example, formation of urine with a volume flow, V, containing a substance, S, at a concentration, U_s. The rate of excretion of S is $V \cdot U_s$. Consider further that S exists in plasma at a concentration, P_s. Let C_s be the volume of plasma in which the quantity, $V \cdot U_s$, must be dissolved to attain the concentration, P_s. Then by definition, $C_s \cdot P_s = V \cdot U_s$, or: $C_s = \dfrac{V \cdot U_s}{P_s}$. C_s is the 'clearance' of S. Clearance measurements have little significance except in relation to the properties of the substance cleared. Consider the excretion of a substance, F, with the following properties: it is not bound to plasma proteins, it is freely filterable through the glomerular membranes, it is not transported in either direction by the tubular epithelium and it is not metabolized by the tubular cells. In these circumstances, the rate of excretion of F is identically equal to the rate of filtration of F: $\mathrm{GFR} \cdot P_F = V \cdot U_F$, or: $\mathrm{GFR} = \dfrac{V \cdot U_F}{P_F} = C_F$.

It therefore follows that the clearance of any substance which has the properties attributed to F is equal to the glomerular filtration rate. Inulin is the only substance which has been clearly demonstrated to fulfill these conditions, although creatinine appears to fulfill them in many mammals under most circumstances (D III 3). When a high degree of accuracy is not required, clearances of creatinine, urea, mannitol or thiosulfate may afford an acceptable approximation to filtration rate. It can be demonstrated in a similar fashion that the clearance of any substance which is entirely removed or extracted from the renal arterial plasma, and which is not metabolized, is identically equal to the renal plasma flow. No substance fulfills these conditions entirely although numerous substances, of which the best known are various aromatic acids, are extracted to the extent of 90 to 95 percent and constitute a good approximation to the total renal plasma flow. This approximation, represented by the clearance of acids such as diodrast and p-aminohippuric acid, measures the least amount of renal plasma which has perfused secretory elements of the kidney and is termed for this reason the 'effective' renal plasma flow. Clearances of substances which do not approximately fulfill the above limiting conditions convey relatively little information, and expressing excretion of such substances in terms of clearances more frequently obscures than clarifies significant relationships between excretion and plasma concentration.

The excretion pattern of one substance may be compared with that of a second in terms of the ratio of the two clearances. For practical purposes, such 'clearance ratios' usually are useful only when the second clearance, preferably measured simultaneously, is that of a substance such as inulin or creatinine which measures filtration rate. In this circumstance, deviation of the clearance ratio from unity indicates the presence of tubular transport. A clearance ratio greater than 1.0 indicates the presence of tubular secretion while a clearance ratio less than 1.0 (provided binding to plasma proteins is absent, or clearance of the filterable fraction is measured if binding is present) indicates the presence of tubular reabsorption. A clearance ratio of 1.0 indicates that the data contain no evidence of tubular transport. The absolute magnitudes of clearance ratios are of little significance.

The relationship of inulin clearance ratios to tubular transport can be illustrated as follows: Let the clearance ratio to inulin of a substance, S, be C_s/C_{in} and the excretion rate of S, $(VU)_s$, be the sum of two components, $(VU)_{Fs}$ and $(VU)_{Ts}$, derived from filtration and tubular transport, respectively. $(VU)_{Ts}$ can take either positive or negative values according to whether transport is secretory or reabsorptive. By definition, $C_s \equiv \dfrac{(VU)_s}{P_s}$ and $C_{in} \equiv \mathrm{GFR}$.

Then, $C_s/C_{in} = \dfrac{(VU)_s}{P_s \cdot \mathrm{GFR}} = \dfrac{(VU)_{Fs} \pm (VU)_{Ts}}{P_s \cdot \mathrm{GFR}} = \dfrac{(VU)_{Fs}}{P_s \cdot \mathrm{GFR}} \pm \dfrac{(VU)_{Ts}}{P_s \cdot \mathrm{GFR}}$. By definition, the term, $\dfrac{(VU)_{Fs}}{P_s}$, is identical with GFR so that the clearance ratio reduces to $C_s/C_{in} = 1 \pm \dfrac{(VU)_{Ts}}{P_s \cdot \mathrm{GFR}}$.

II. Clinical measurement of renal function
1. Criteria and general concepts

Clinical measurements of renal function can, for practical purposes, only supply information concerning the extent to which a pathological process has interfered with the excretory capacity of the kidney. As such, they are useful in detecting the existence of a pathological process and in evaluating the ability of the kidney to supply the excretory needs of the patient. Function measurements as a group are generally of little value in discovering the cause of a functional impairment. The cause must be discovered from other sources such as from the history, radiography, and study of the urinary sediment. It is evident from these objectives of clinical function measurement that neither great accuracy in the measurement of specific renal function nor absolute standards of reference have much clinical value. Of greater value are simplicity, reproducibility, and accuracy of analytical procedures. Since the individual is his own standard of reference, tests generally should measure the balance between excretory needs and renal excretory capacity. To a considerable extent, this is equivalent to measurement of the degree of uremia or of the effects of uremia. Many of the manifestations of uremia, however, such as anemia and acidosis are susceptible to so many day-to-day fluctuations or are modified by so many extrarenal factors that they cannot supply the important quality of reproducibility. Other manifestations of uremia which can be employed as renal function tests are measured by the degree of accumulation in the blood of renally excreted metabolites such as sulfate and urate. Most of these measurements have little to recommend them and are of academic interest only. Those and other tests are described in numerous text books on nephritis, such as that of Fishberg, and will not be considered here. The most useful tests are related to creatinine, urea, phenolsulfonphthalein and specific gravity.

2. Plasma concentrations

a) Plasma creatinine concentration

In normal subjects, the plasma creatinine concentration is quite constant. The normal values are about 1.0 mg./100 ml. in men and 0.80 in women. It is largely independent of diet, body size and age. The standard deviation in the normal population is about 0.2 mg. (ADDIS 1951; BARRETT and ADDIS; SULLIVAN and IRREVERE; EDWARDS and WHYTE). The normal values tend to be somewhat higher in children (MATTAR et al. 1952). Constancy of plasma creatinine arises from the circumstances, first, that the rate of creatinine production by the body is highly constant. Creatinine arises as a by-product of muscle metabolism. Synthesis of creatine, the precursor of creatinine, by liver and kidney apparently is controlled by an incompletely understood feedback system related to muscle needs of creatine. In moderately advanced to advanced uremia, however, renal excretion of creatinine may decrease by as much as 30 percent either because of decreased formation or because of extrarenal elimination (GOLDMAN 1954; EFFERSØE 1957; MONGE et al.). Creatinine production, therefore, constitutes a useful measure of the metabolism of muscle. Since muscle is the largest tissue mass of the body, metabolism of this tissue and of body structures subservient to muscle needs represents the major source of the load of renally excreted metabolites. The second circumstance critical to the constancy of plasma creatinine is that creatinine is excreted for the most part by glomerular filtration. Hence, plasma creatinine approximately measures the ratio of body metabolism to filtration rate, and a normal plasma creatinine concentration indicates that filtration rate is normal in relation to needs for the excretion of muscle-dependent metabolites in a given individual (GOLDMAN 1956; HAUGEN and BLEGEN 1955; EFFERSØE 1957; STEINITZ and TURKAND; MONGE et al.). For these reasons and because of simplicity of measurement, plasma creatinine concentration is probably the most useful of all renal function tests.

The relationship of plasma creatinine concentration to filtration rate can be illustrated as follows: Let the rate of formation of creatinine be a constant, K. When the individual is close to equilibrium, that is, when neither renal function nor metabolism are changing rapidly, excretion = formation = K. But excretion, by definition, equals the creatinine clearance, C_c, multiplied by the plasma creatinine concentration, P_c, whence: $C_c \cdot P_c = K$. Let the subscripts n and d refer to function in the normal state and in renal disease. Then, $Cc_n \cdot Pc_n = K = Cc_d \cdot Pc_d$. Rearranging, and substituting GFR as an approximation to C_c, $\dfrac{\text{GFR}_d}{\text{GFR}_n} \approx \dfrac{Pc_n}{Pc_d}$. Since GFR$_n$ can be written as 100 percent of normal function for each individual, GFR$_d$, as a fraction of this normal value, can be approximated as,

$$\text{GFR}_d \approx 100 \cdot \frac{Pc_n}{Pc_d}.$$

b) Plasma urea concentration

Like creatinine, plasma urea concentration measures the balance between urea formation and excretion. Unlike creatinine, however, urea formation is highly variable and intimately dependent on protein content of the diet and on rate of body protein anabolism or catabolism (AMBARD and WEILL; ADDIS 1947). In the studies of ADDIS, for example, blood urea nitrogen concentration averaged 19 mg./100 ml. in subjects on a diet containing 0.5 g. protein/kg./day and 45 mg. on a diet of 2.5 g. In addition, although urea is excreted by filtration and constitutes a measure of this, reabsorption is highly variable, ranging from 15 to 70 percent of the quantity filtered (D VI 3), and is correlated only in part with intrinsic alterations in renal function. The excreted fraction tends to increase in renal failure. As a consequence, variation in plasma urea concentration in the normal population is greater than that of creatinine, and azotemia is not regularly present until loss of function exceeds 50 percent and filtration rate is less than 40 ml./min. (MacKay and MacKay; Edvall 1957a).

3. Clearances
a) Creatinine clearance

The clearance of creatinine can be measured as the clearance of exogenously administered creatinine, of endogenous true creatinine or of endogenous total creatinine-like chromogen. None of these clearances constitutes a precise measurement of glomerular filtration rate in primates (D III 3), yet the creatinine clearance irrespective of method of measurement usually lies within 30 percent of the inulin clearance (Smith, Finkelstein and Smith; Steinitz and Turkand; Dodge and Daeschner; van Pilsum and Seljesky; Barclay and Kenney; Blegen, Haugen and Aas; Brod and Sirota; Dean and McCance 1947; Galan et al.; Miller and Winkler, Brun et al. 1953). The creatinine/inulin clearance ratio tends to increase in uremia, but rarely exceeds 2.0 (Miller and Winkler; Platt; Brod and Sirota; Steinitz and Turkand). The clearance ratio may also vary either in an apparently random fashion or in response to influences on renal function to such an extent that changes in creatinine clearance cannot safely be employed as an index to changes in inulin clearance up to 30 percent (Talbott 1951; Patalano and Vivone; Burnett; Ingbar et al. 1950; Barnett et al. 1951; Dodge and Daeschner).

The creatinine clearance, unlike plasma concentration, yields an absolute measure of renal function, and size age, sex and metabolic state of the individual must be considered in its interpretation. Creatinine clearance is most usefully employed during rapidly changing renal function when lack of equality between creatinine formation and excretion renders plasma creatinine concentration unreliable. Creatinine clearance is also useful in comparing the separate functions of the two kidneys (Nesbitt). Since the exogenous and the endogenous true creatinine clearances have no evident advantage over the creatinine total chromogen clearance, the latter, as the simpler, is preferable for clinical purposes.

b) Creatinine concentration and clearance measurements

One or more methods for the quantitative measurement of creatinine concentration of blood and urine may be found in most standard text books of clinical chemistry and will not be described in detail here. Alkaline picrate (trinitrophenol) is the chromogenic reagent employed most frequently, but dinitrobenzoate (Gukelberger and Wyss) and napthoquinone sulfonate (Sullivan and Irreverre) are among other reagents described.

Color development by alkaline picrate methods does not follow the Lambert-Beers law and is subject to numerous variables including concentrations of alkali and picric acid and the temperature of the solution. Color development of creatinine is complete in 10 to 15 minutes at room temperature, but further color development from noncreatinine chromogens in plasma filtrates may continue much longer. Twenty minutes is probably the most frequently used development time. Occasionally, endogenous or exogenous chromogens such as ketone bodies, salicylates or reducing substances may occur in relatively large amounts (Steinitz and Turkand). The effects of these and other variables are described by Bonsnes and Taussky, Lauson (1951), Owen et al. (1954), and Edwards and Whyte (1958). Most plasma filtrates are suitable for clinical plasma creatinine analyses. Trichloroacetic acid filtrates yield 100 percent recovery of added creatinine.

A 5 to 10 percent failure of recovery may occur with tungstic acid and cadmium sulfate filtrates (MANDEL and JONES) but the recovery failure with tungstate can be minimized if the reagents are adjusted so that the pH of the filtrate is greater than 5.0 (OWEN et al. 1954). Cadmium filtrates are undesirable because of the precipitation of residual cadmium following addition of alkaline picrate. Zinc sulfate (SOMOGYI) filtrates yield excessively high recovery failure.

Creatinine and urea clearances consist of collecting a urine specimen over an accurately timed interval (clearance period) together with a plasma specimen. One clearance period is generally sufficient for clinical purposes but two are desirable to detect the presence of errors. The precise timing of the procedure is not important but should be adapted to the clinic or hospital schedule. Fasting is unnecessary for a creatinine clearance but is desirable for a urea clearance. Fluids may be given an hour prior to the test to promote an increase in urine flow but, since clearances are frequently performed on patients with renal disease or who are unable to diurese, fluid administration is generally of little value. Beverages, including coffee and tea, do not affect the clearances significantly. The length of the clearance period is determined by the time required to obtain a reasonably accurate estimate of urine flow. Generally, the longer the period, the more accurate is the estimate of average rate of flow because errors in bladder emptying become relatively less significant. Twenty-four hour periods may be employed with creatinine but these are unsuitable for urea; and possible contamination or inadvertent loss of urine together with the circumstance that clearances have their greatest clinical use under acute conditions makes one 3 to 4 hour or two $1^1/_2$ to 2 hour periods more desirable. If bladder emptying and rinsing are good, accurate clearances can be performed with 10 minute periods. Generally, the bladder should be catheterized using acceptable sterile precautions. When rapid drainage of urine from the catheter has ceased, the bladder should be rinsed at least three times in rapid succession with 50 ml. of sterile water. Saline may be substituted for water if electrolytes are not being measured or if inflammatory conditions of the bladder exist. The bladder may be gently massaged to promote evacuation of the rinse, and 25 cc. of air may be injected immediately following the last rinse. Return of the air, or cessation of flow of the last rinse if air is not injected, marks the beginning of the clearance period and this time, t_0, should be noted accurately. The rinse fluids should be discarded save for the last which may be analysed for creatinine or urea to confirm adequacy of the washing procedure. Two facts should be noted with respect to bladder washing: return of injected air does not necessarily indicate that the bladder is empty; and failure to recover all injected rinsing fluid does not seriously impair the accuracy of the clearance if the rinsing has been adequate. At the termination of the clearance period, the bladder washing procedure is repeated and the time of return of air or of termination of free flow of the last rinse, t_1, is noted. All returns of bladder washing fluid at this time are carefully saved and added to the urine collected during the period. The combined urine and wash fluid is mixed and the volume is measured. All except a sample sufficient for analyses may now be discarded. The gross rate of 'urine' flow, V', is the measured volume divided by $t_1 - t_0$. Voluntary voiding of urine specimens may be permitted if the patient is ambulatory and is believed capable of adequate evacuation. With voluntary voiding the procedure is somewhat different. The patient is instructed to avoid urination until he feels capable of voiding freely. The termination of the first voiding, t_0, performed standing, is noted and the urine discarded. The patient then waits until he again is capable of voiding freely. The time of the second volume, t_1, is noted, the urine sample retained, its volume measured, and an aliquot taken for analysis. A venous blood sample is obtained approximately in the middle of each clearance period. If the specimens cannot be analysed quickly, attention should be paid to their preservation. In addition to losses from bacterial contamination, creatinine is extensively converted to creatine at neutral or alkaline pH. The conversion can be prevented, however, by acidifying to pH 3.0 (Cannan and Shore).

In measuring the concentrations of creatinine or urea, analyses of plasma and urine should be made concurrently. In addition, the urine should be diluted to yield approximately the same concentration as the plasma filtrate. The appropriate dilution for the urine, D_u, can be approximated as follows:

$$D_u = \frac{C' \cdot D_P}{V'},$$

where C' is the clearance predicted from clinical or other laboratory data, D_P is the dilution of the plasma in preparing a suitable filtrate, and V' is the gross rate of urine flow. When the colorimetric readings for urine and plasma are subequel, the effects of random variation attributable to analytical methods are minimized. The true clearance then is calculated as, $C = \dfrac{u \cdot D_u \cdot V'}{p \cdot D_p}$ where u and p are the concentrations as measured

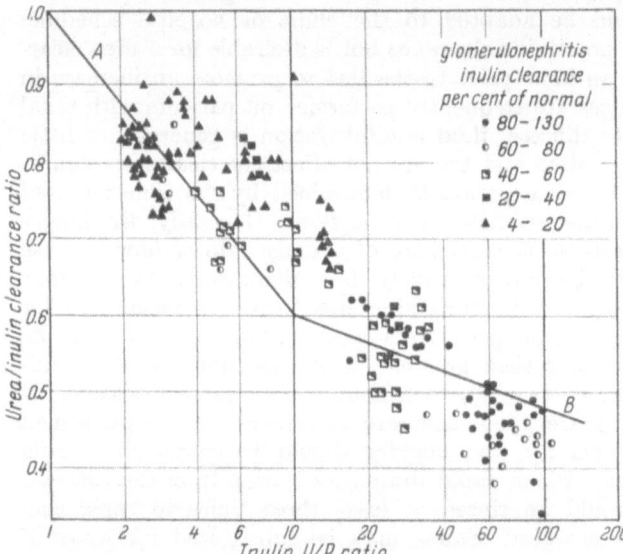

Fig. 76. Urea-inulin clearance ratio as related to concentration of the glomerular filtrate (inulin U/P ratio) in chronic glomerulonephritis (Chasis and Smith). Reproduced by permission of the authors and the Journal of Clinical Investigation

in the diluted urine and plasma. The true, or net, rate of urine flow, V, may be calculated by subtracting the volume of the wash fluid from the gross urine volume prior to dividing by the duration of the clearance period. This term is essential for the calculation of the standard urea clearance, or may be important for reasons unrelated to clearance measurements.

c) Urea clearance

The urea clearance offers a clinical measure of renal function which is largely independent of protein metabolism or plasma urea concentration and is related to intrinsic renal functional capacity (Addis 1917, 1922; Goldring et al. 1934). Urea clearance in chronic renal disease, as in normal kidneys, is related to glomerular filtration rate and to the degree of concentration of the filtrate as measured by the inulin U/P ratio (Fig. 76). Dividing the urea clearance by $V^{\frac{1}{2}}$ to yield the standard clearance (D VI 3) partially eliminates the effects of variation in V. Whether measured as the simple clearance or as the standard clearance, urea clearances have few advantages over creatinine clearance as a measure of renal function. The urea and creatinine clearances together generally set lower and upper limits to the probable level of filtration rate in renal disease.

4. Phenolsulfonphthalein test

Phenolsulfonphthalein (PSP) was selected by ROWNTREE and GERAGHTY from among a variety of renally excreted substances on largely pharmacological considerations. PSP is an aromatic acid which enters the urine almost entirely by tubular secretion. Although the clearance of PSP is distinctly less than that of PAH and diodrast (D III 1 e), the PSP clearance generally varies in proportion to renal plasma flow, and the PSP test constitutes a semiempirical crude index of RPF (MITCHELL, OWENS and VOLK). Blood concentrations attained following injection of the usual six milligram quantity are far below the concentrations required to approach saturation of tubular transport capacity.

The test, as customarily performed, is as follows. The patient consumes 600 to 800 ml. of water about 40 minutes before injection of the dye. This effectively increases urine flow in normals but is often of little value in patients with renal disease. Six milligrams of the dye are then injected. The quantity is arbitrary, and the excretion curve is similar with quantities between 3 and 25 mg. (SHAW). If different quantities are injected, appropriate adjustment must be made in either the color standards or the calculations. The intravenous injection route is preferred. If intramuscular or subcutaneous routes are employed, comparison must be made with normal excretion curves obtained under the same conditions. The bladder generally should be catheterized at the time of or immediately prior to injection of the dye, since many if not most patients will be unable to void accurately at short intervals unless they are diuresing profusely. The urine present in the bladder at the time of injection may be discarded, but this is not necessary and does not affect the accuracy of the test. If voluntary voiding is employed, it is advisable for the patient to accumulate an easily voidable volume of bladder urine prior to injection of the dye. This volume is then retained until the time for the collection of the first specimen and permits an accurate collection of dye secreted during this period. Urine specimens are collected at 15, 30 and 60 minutes following injection of the dye, preferably with a bladder wash in the case of catheterized subjects. The wash is added to the urine collected during the period. One to two ml. of concentrated alkali (10 percent $NaOH$) is added to the urine, which is then diluted to one liter. The red color is compared with a series of standards prepared by diluting various fractions of the quantity of injected dye to one liter after alkalinizing. For example, a 10 percent standard represents 0.6 mg. of PSP diluted to one liter If the urine contains little dye, it should be diluted to 250 or 500 ml. instead of to 1000 ml., in which circumstance the apparent percent of excreted dye should be divided by 4 or 2. Normally, 30 to 50 percent of the dye is excreted during the first 15 minute period, 13 to 22 percent during the second 15 minutes and 9 to 16 percent during the following 30 minute period About 20 percent of the injected dye does not appear in the urine of normal subjects and greater fractions may fail to appear in the urine of patients with renal disease (SHAW; CHAPMAN and HALSTEAD). The most important period is the first, because this period is the most sensitive to depression in renal function. Depressed excretion of the dye observed in the first period is caused, first, by decrease in renal blood flow and, second, by a delay in onset of excretion which is present in chronic nephritis but which is particularly evident in obstructive uropathy. In normals, dye begins to appear in the bladder about 5 minutes after injection, and the excretion rate attains a maximum about 10 minutes after injection. In renal disease, dye may not appear in significant quantities until 10 or 15 minutes after injection, and the maximal rate of excretion may not be attained until 30 or 45 minutes after injection. A similar delay in onset of excretion from the diseased kidney is observed with p-aminohippurate and inulin (BRADLEY, LEIFER and NICKEL).

The PSP test furnishes a useful means of detecting clinically significant impairment of renal function under conditions where quantitative blood or urine analyses are not feasible. Where routine clearances and plasma concentrations of urea or creatinine can be measured, the PSP test seldom contributes significant additional information, although occasionally a marked delay in excretion may suggest the existence of obstruction.

5. Concentration and dilution tests
a) Concentration tests

A concentration test consists of measurement of the urinary concentration of solids attained following procedures designed to stimulate water conservation. Urinary concentration is dependent on a great variety of factors including proximal and distal tubular reabsorption of solutes, permeability of collecting duct epithelium, integrity of the medullary countercurrent concentration system, and volume and composition of the glomerular filtrate. As such, concentration is affected by a great variety of functional disturbances and impairment of concentration is nonspecific.

Theoretically, concentration should be measured in osmotic units. In practice, however, the circumstance that most urines have roughly similar proportions of urea and salts permits specific gravity of the urine to be employed as an empirical index of osmotic concentration. The simplicity and rapidity of hydrometric measurements of specific gravity are obtained in exchange for the precision of freezing point measurements.

Several concentration tests have been described, all of which are satisfactory. That one should be chosen which is most adaptable to the particular hospital or clinic routine. The test of ADDIS and SHEVSKY consists of witholding all fluids from the patient for one day. The urine formed during the ensuing night is then collected and its specific gravity measured. The FISHBERG test consists of witholding all fluids from midday of the day before the test and of giving the patient a dry diet. The nighttime urine is collected, together with four, subsequent, one-hourly urine specimens on the following day. The highest specific gravity among these specimens is recorded. Vasopressin may also be employed as a concentration test. Ten units of vasopressin (e.g., Pituitrin or Pitressin) are injected subcutaneously in the morning. Urine specimens are collected half hourly or hourly for 3 hours, and the highest specific gravity among these is recorded (SODEMAN and ENGELHARDT; BJERRE-CHRISTENSEN; SCHNEEBERG). Finally, Pituitrin injection may be combined with the dehydration type of test as a precaution against the deficiencies of each. If concentration exceeds 1.025 in young adult and 1.018 in older subjects, significant impairment of renal function is probably absent (ELLIS and WEISS; EDVALL 1957a).

A number of precautions should be taken both in measurement and interpretation of specific gravity. The hydrometer should be checked for accuracy with water and with a solution of known specific gravity, both at the proper temperature. Urine should be allowed to cool to room temperature, since the specific gravity is lower by about 0.003 units at body temperature than at 20° C. Presence of large quantities of solutes with high molecular weight may produce a disproportionately high specific gravity. Glucose adds about 0.002 specific gravity units for each gram percent concentration and albumin adds about

0.0026 units. These and similar contingencies are not present if concentration is measured cryoscopically (D VI 4 e).

Concentration tests are of value as a screening procedure and for supplementing information obtained from PSP tests or plasma creatinine or urea concentrations. They are of little or no value as an index of the degree of general functional impairment. Impairment of concentration, considered alone, does not indicate that renal disease is present.

b) Dilution tests

A dilution test consists of measuring the specific gravity of the urine specimens collected at 15 to 30 minute intervals for 2 hours following ingestion of 1.0 to 1.5 liters of water. The lowest value is recorded. In normal subjects, this should be 1.003 or less. The commonest cause of impaired dilution is persistent secretion of antidiuretic hormone associated with excitement, edema-forming states, dehydration, smoking and various drugs, so that impairment is an unreliable sign that renal disease is present. Dilution tests find their greatest usefulness in confirming the cause of certain types of impairment of concentration such as hypercalcemia, hypokalemia, and sicklemia since dilution in these conditions is normal. With the discovery of cortisone and the development of accurate methods for measuring urinary excretion of corticosteroids, dilution tests such as that of ROBINSON, POWER and KEPLER are employed with decreasing frequency for the diagnosis of ADDISON'S disease. A significant improvement in dilution (usually measured as increase in urine flow) following administration of cortisone or ACTH usually indicates hypoadrenalism (OLEESKY; SOFFER and GABRILOVE; THOMSON, BROWNELL and CUMMING).

III. Measurement of discrete renal functions
1. Glomerular filtration rate
a) Physiological and chemical properties of inulin

Inulin is the only substance whose clearance is generally accepted to represent glomerular filtration rate in man. The evidence supporting this belief may be summarized, briefly, as follows: It is present in the glomerular filtrate of amphibia in the same concentration as in plasma water (HENDRIX, WESTFALL and RICHARDS). A nearly complete diffusion equilibrium of inulin across the glomerular membranes is predicted from theoretical considerations (Fig. 17). Inulin is not bound to plasma proteins (SHANNON and SMITH; COTLOVE 1955). In normal man and dog as well as in renal disease excretion rate of inulin is directly proportional to plasma concentration over a wide concentration range, which is equivalent to stating that the clearance is independent of plasma concentration (RICHARDS, WESTFALL and BOTT; SHANNON and SMITH; SHANNON 1935a, b; MILLER, ALVING and RUBIN; MATTAR et al.; KENNEDY and KLEH)[1]. Under conditions such that the relative contributions of tubular transport to the total excretory pattern progressively diminish, the clearance of substances other than inulin converge on the inulin clearance as a limiting value: the clearances of glucose, diodrast and other substances as their plasma concentrations are indefinitely increased (SMITH 1951); the clearance of glucose following phlorhizin and of diodrast or p-aminohippurate following probenecid; the clearance of urea as urine flow is indefinitely increased. Inulin is absent from the urine of aglomerular

---

[1] Only one group, employing a single injection technique, has failed to observe this relationship (BARNARD, BASSIR and HOUGH).

fish (Shannon 1934) and is nearly absent from the urine of the frog when perfused through the renal portal venous system (Hogben and Bollman 1951a). In one or more respects, other substances proposed as alternatives to inulin for the measurement of filtration rate have proven unsatisfactory. Synthetic polymers such as Dextran or polyvinyl are difficult to measure or exhibit excessive heterogeneity of molecular weight. Clearances of ferrocyanide (Miller and Winkler 1936), allantoin (Friedman, Byers and Abrahm 1948; Miller et al. 1952b) and creatinine fail to agree with that of inulin or with one another in man. Creatinine, even in the dog in which it agrees closely with that of inulin under most circumstances, may fail to agree when inulin clearance is greatly depressed (D III 3). Initial reports suggested that the clearances of inulin and mannitol were equal (Smith, Finkelstein and Smith) but subsequent studies have shown that, for unknown reasons, the clearance of mannitol in both man and dog is regularly about 10 percent less than that of inulin (Berger, Farber and Earle; Corcoran and Page 1947a; Schwartz, Breed and Maxwell). The observation that the clearance of sucrose may coincide with that of inulin requires further study (Steinitz 1940b).

Inulin is a polyfructoside with a molecular weight of approximately 5,000 (Westfall and Landis; Haworth and Learner; Drew and Haworth). It is difficultly soluble in cold water but the solubility increases rapidly above 80° C. Solutions can remain supersaturated for several days. It hydrolyses slowly with prolonged boiling and at acid pH (Drew and Haworth). Commercial inulin preparations are moderately heterogeneous, containing fractions of differing molecular weight (including fructose itself) and chemical properties. Differences in alkali-lability, fermentability, ethanol solubility and electrophoretic migration have been described (Cotlove 1954; Bassir). The clearances of all fractions, with the exception of fructose and possibly of some fermentable oligofructosides, are identical (Walser, Davidson and Orloff). Crude inulin preparations, particularly those from dahlia roots, may be pyrogenic. The pyrogen cannot be separated by repeated precipitation or destroyed by boiling (Smith, Chasis and Ranges; Bunim, Smith and Smith), although it may be partially removed by adsorption with Norit. The pyrogen may be completely removed, however, by filtering inulin solutions through a number 3 Seitz filter (Co Tui et al.). Chemical methods for the analysis of inulin depend upon acid-hydrolysis of inulin to fructose and measurement of the fructose so formed by any of several methods such as diphenylamine (Corcoran and Page 1939a; Alving et al. 1941; Harrison; Rojel), anthrone (Young and Raisz), vanillin (Levine and Becker), skatol (Ranney and McCune 1943) and resorcinol (Steinitz 1938; Roe, Epstein and Goldstein). Resorcinol is the most widely employed agent, and numerous variations of this method have been described (Fritz and Nüssgens; Kruhoffer 1946; Higashi and Peters; Schreiner). Either cadmium sulfate or zinc sulfate (Somogyi) plasma filtrates may be employed.

b) Inulin determination

The following procedure incorporating fermentation and the modification by Schreiner of the resorcinol method is employed in our laboratory and will be described as representative of most methods.

1. To 1 ml. each of plasma and urine specimens (assuming a plasma inulin concentration of 20 to 40 mg./100 ml.) in 25 ml. Erlenmeyer flasks add 8 ml. of a 1 percent washed, fresh suspension of yeast. Stopper and let stand overnight at room temperature. A 1 ml. sample of inulin-free plasma should be treated similarly as a blank. A urine blank is usually unnecessary because the blank value is insignificant.

2. After overnight fermentation, add to all flasks 1 ml. of acid zinc sulfate (10 g $ZnSO_4$ · 7 H_2O plus 4 ml. of 6 N H_2SO_4 to 100 ml. with H_2O), then 1 ml. of 0.75 N NaOH. Shake well, centrifuge, and decant or filter the supernatant.

3. Dilute the urine filtrates by the amount calculated to yield the approximate inulin concentration of the plasma filtrates. This dilution equals the estimated filtration rate divided by the gross rate of urine flow (urine volume plus wash, divided by the duration of the clearance period).

4. Place 2 ml. aliquots, in triplicate, of plasma filtrate or diluted urine filtrate in screw-capped vials and add 7 ml. of resorcinol reagent. This is prepared by adding 2 volumes of alcoholic resorcinol (100 mg. of resorcinol in 100 ml. of 95 percent ethanol) to 5 volumes of 30 percent HCl. Stopper tightly, heat in a water bath at 80° C for 25 minutes, and cool rapidly to room temperature. The vial caps should contain acid-resistant seals such as polyethylene. The resorcinol reagent should be freshly prepared from a refrigerated 1 percent stock solution in 95 percent ethanol. The water bath should be well-stirred to assure uniformity of temperature. Appropriate standard inulin solutions may be included with the group of plasma and urine samples. Routine employment of standard solutions is unnecessary for the calculation of inulin clearance when urine and plasma specimens are measured concurrently but is useful to assure reliability of the methods.

5. When the specimens are cool, they are read in a photoelectric colorimeter at a wave length of 490—500, against a blank prepared by adding 7 ml. of resorcinol reagent to 2 ml. of distilled water.

6. Inulin clearance, $C_{in} = \dfrac{u \cdot Du \cdot V'}{p - po}$ where p, po and u are concentrations of inulin (either absolute or arbitrary units) in plasma filtrate, plasma blank and diluted urine filtrate. Du is the dilution of the urine filtrate, and V' is the gross rate of urine flow.

In experiments of short duration in which the inulinoid blank of unfermented plasma and urine may be assumed to be reasonably constant, fermentation is unnecessary. In longer studies, to which the above method is adapted, this assumption is not valid. The fermented inulinoid blank of plasma is quite constant, is derived largely from the yeast, and is equivalent to roughly 1 mg. inulin/100 ml. The fermented inulinoid blank of urine is insignificant as a fraction of total urine inulin concentration.

c) Clearance techniques

Every effort must be made to establish and maintain a reasonably steady state, since only under this condition can clearances be measured accurately and reliably. Steady state refers to constancy of urine flow, plasma concentrations and renal function. Corrections can be introduced under certain circumstances for distortions arising from changing plasma concentration, but no method is available by which the effects of rapidly changing renal function on the apparent clearances can be corrected. The usual method of measuring inulin clearance requires establishment of a suitable plasma concentration by a priming injection, maintenance of this concentration by a continuous intravenous infusion, accurately timed collection of urine specimens, and plasma sampling. Details have been described by SMITH, GOLDRING and CHASIS; GOLDRING and CHASIS; and SMITH (1956).

a) Priming injection. The quantity of inulin to be injected is calculated from body weight, estimated volume of distribution (extracellular fluid volume) and desired plasma concentration. Assuming a volume of 200 ml./kg. body weight in normal subjects and a desired plasma inulin concentration of 300 mg./L., the prime is 60 mg./kg. Appropriate adjustments in this quantity may be made for infants or edematous subjects (increased) or obese or dehydrated subjects (decreased). During intravenous injection of the prime, consideration should be given to the circumstances that excretion commences within a few minutes of the start of the injection, and that distribution of the prime through the extracellular fluid volume proceeds rather slowly and exponentially. If the prime is injected rapidly, very high plasma concentrations are attained and, in normal subjects, much of the prime is excreted. Ideally, about one third of the prime may be injected rapidly and the remainder injected at a decreasing rate over about 20 minutes. The sustaining infusion is started within a few minutes of starting the prime injection to insure continuous replacement of the excreted portion. If, for technical reasons, it is desirable to inject the entire prime rapidly in subjects with essentially normal renal function, the quantity should be increased by 25 to 35 percent.

b) **Sustaining infusion.** A continuous intravenous infusion of an inulin solution is essential to maintain a constant plasma concentration. The rate of injection of inulin is calculated by multiplying the desired plasma inulin concentration (about 0.3 mg./ml.) by the probable value of the inulin clearance. In resting normal subjects this can be estimated from information such as that illustrated in Fig. 19. In subjects with renal disease, GFR can be estimated from the plasma creatinine concentration or other data. The volume of infusate is based on technical requirements such as the capacity of the infusion apparatus and the fluid requirements of the subject. Inulin may be infused as a supersaturated solution provided no particles of undissolved inulin are present to initiate precipitation. Meticulous attention should be devoted to constancy of the rate of infusion. An infusion pump should be employed and its delivery rate checked at frequent intervals. Free flow through the infusion tubing and the intravenous needle or catheter should be assured at all times. The infused limb should be maintained close to heart level to avoid large fluctuations in venous drainage and it should remain as quiet as possible.

c) **Equilibration.** All preliminary estimates of inulin space and clearance in a particular individual are subject to a probable 15 percent error. In addition, at least 20 minutes are required following establishment of a constant plasma concentration before a constant rate of urinary excretion of inulin is attained. This is attributed to variation in time of passage of filtrate through different nephrons (BRADLEY, LEIFER and NICKEL; CHILDS et al. 1955). For these reasons, at least 40 minutes should elapse between commencement of the prime and the beginning of the first clearance period.

d) **Urine collection.** Voluntary voiding may be employed with young subjects provided they are known to be capable of voiding freely and completely. Considerable variation in bladder residual volumes on successive urinations by the same subject may be expected, however (MILLS, THOMAS and YATES). If the experiment includes relatively short (20 minute) clearance periods, a diuresis should be initiated by drinking 800 to 1,000 ml. water prior to the experiment in order to facilitate bladder emptying and to minimize the relative error arising from bladder residual volumes. Diuresis should be sustained, if necessary, by drinking supplentary volumes of about 200 ml. at half-hourly intervals. With longer clearance periods (one hour or more) water-loading may often be omitted.

Bladder catheterization is usually desirable for accurate studies. This is particularly the case in studies on elderly, immobilized or enfeebled subjects, in studies on subjects who do not diurese well following water-loading, in studies in which the effects of water-loading on renal function should be avoided, in studies in which short (10 to 15 minute) clearance periods are desired, and in studies in which antidiuretic stimuli (pain, excitement, hypotension, dehydration, exercise, drugs, hypertonic solutions, smoking) may be present. A soft-rubber, multi-eyed, single-lumen catheter is satisfactory. Sterile technique should be employed with its insertion and with subsequent irrigations. A diuresis is unnecessary with bladder catheterization since washing can remove excreted inulin from the bladder as thoroughly as the experimenter desires. An increase in urine flow by diuresis does not increase the rate of washout of the renal dead space represented by kidney and renal pelvis since this space varies in size in direct proportion to rate of urine flow (BOJESEN 1949, 1954; McSWINEY and DE WARDENER). Moreover, rapid changes in urine flow associated with anti-diuretic stimuli during water diuresis may distort the clearance measurements.

Rinsing the bladder three times in rapid succession with 50 ml. of distilled water following suprapubic manual expression of urine at the termination of the clearance period has, in our experience, provided an adequate washing. Air (25 to 30 ml.) may be injected following cessation of return of the final wash to improve recovery of the wash. Subjects excreting very concentrated urine or who have dilated or diverticulous bladders may require more extensive washing. During diuresis, washing may be decreased, and at urine flows consistently above 8 ml./min. may be omitted entirely (SMITH 1956). Cessation of free drainage of the last wash, or return of air following air injection, marks the beginning or end of the period. Washing the bladder at the termination of the equilibration and commencement of the first clearance period should be as thorough as all subsequent washings. Wash fluids, apart from a small, measured volume of the final wash which may be set aside to be analysed for inulin content, are added to and mixed with the urine collected during the period. The total volume (urine plus wash) divided by the duration of the period is the gross rate of urine flow, V', which is employed in all subsequent clearance calculations.

In order to estimate the probable error of measurement in a given experiment and to evaluate stability of clearance, several shorter clearance periods are superior to a single long period.

e) **Plasma concentrations.** Accurate knowledge of the mean inulin concentration of the plasma from which urine collected during the period was formed is equal in importance to accurate urine collection. When plasma concentration is nearly constant, the mean concentration is known quite exactly. When plasma concentrations are changing at an approximately uniform rate during the period, the value of the mean concentration corresponding to a period generally lies about 7 minutes before the midpoint of the period for arterial blood samples (BRUN, HILDEN and RAASCHOU 1949; BRADLEY, NICKEL and LEIFER). Because venous plasma concentrations are regularly lower than arterial during rising and greater than arterial during falling plasma concentrations as the result of movements of inulin into and out of peripheral tissues, the mean venous concentration occurs later than the arterial and, on the average, about $1/2$ minute before the midpoint of the period (SMITH, GOLDRING and CHASIS). Generally, an effort is made to obtain the samples at the appropriate time before the expected midpoint of the period since the measured values can then be employed directed in the clearance equation. If this cannot be accomplished, a graph of the plasma concentration must be prepared and the probable values obtained by interpolation. To be assured of the plasma concentrations throughout the study, supplementary plasma specimens should be obtained near the end of the equilibration period, at the termination of the final clearance period, and at intervals during any periods of several hours duration or in which renal function is changing rapidly.

f) **Subject factors.** Numerous factors associated with the experimental procedures, such as pain of venepuncture, excitement, bladder catheterization, and filling of the urinary bladder may affect renal function (MILES and DE WARDENER; PRÁT; SHUCK and STRIBRNA). Bladder catheterization, trial urine collections and other procedures should therefore be performed well in advance of the first clearance period in order that the subject may become accustomed to the experimental conditions. Smoking (nicotine) may increase urinary concentration but does not appear to affect other renal functions in habitual smokers. Large meals may be followed by a transitory decrease in inulin clearance, and absorbed fructose may markedly increase the nonfermented inulinoid blank. Mild sedation may be employed in apprehensive subjects without affecting clearances.

d) Other techniques of inulin clearance

Inulin may be injected subcutaneously, in association with a suitable intravenous prime, to maintain a satisfactorily constant plasma concentration for several hours (FINDLEY and WHITE 1940; DUPRÉ and COXON).

A technique which avoids urine collection depends upon attainment of infusion equilibrium (EARLE and BERLINER 1946; DEANE). Following injection of a suitable prime, a sustaining solution is infused at a very constant and accurately measured rate. After an hour, a nearly constant plasma inulin concentration is attained, indicating that excretion approximately equals rate of intravenous infusion. Since infusion rate is known, this term may be substituted for excretion and, divided by plasma concentration when this has become constant, yields inulin clearance. Much longer equilibration periods are required in subjects with poor circulation, edema or fluid accumulations. Values obtained by this method average about 3 percent greater than those obtained by urine collection, probably because complete uniformity of distribution of inulin in the extracellular fluid compartment has not been attained. This method may be employed on subjects, such as patients with ureterocolic anastomoses, in whom urine collection is not feasible, but the method is not reliable if renal function is significantly reduced.

Numerous methods have been devised which employ a single large injection of inulin or mannitol without a sustaining infusion. Diodrast or PAH may be included to measure renal plasma flow or, if sufficiently large quantities are employed, the Tm of these substances may be measured (LANDOWNE and ALVING 1947; BARNETT; NEWMAN, BORDLEY and WINTERNITZ; NEWMAN et al. 1949; ROBSON et al. 1949; ALVING and MILLER; FOA and FOA). In some single injection methods, clearances are calculated in the usual way from urine collections and estimated mean plasma concentration during each period. Other methods omit bladder collections entirely, and clearance is measured from the slope of the plasma concentration. The latter methods, in particular, require numerous simplifying assumptions and detailed calculations (DOMINGUEZ, CORCORAN and PAGE; DOMINGUEZ 1952; ROBSON; SMITH 1956). The results are irregular and agreement with the results obtained by the constant infusion technique are not very good, particularly with respect to plasma flow and Tm measurements. The results are also unreliable if renal function is changing. Single injection techniques have been recommended for situations in which the usual methods are not feasible, as in infants (BARNETT), or as clinical function tests. A single injection together with urine collections may also be employed reliably when renal function is very poor, since plasma concentration declines slowly in such subjects.

2. Effective renal plasma flow
a) Clearance techniques

The clearance of substances which are extracted almost completely from plasma during its passage through the kidneys constitutes a measure of ERPF.

The necessary additional assumption is that the substance is not metabolized and that the quantity extracted is excreted intact. Diodrast (diodone) and p-aminohippurate have been employed almost exclusively for this purpose. Both substances yield essentially identical clearance values and little if any of the excreted quantities are derived from the red cell water in man (SMITH 1951). PAH is the agent of choice because of the simplicity and accuracy of its analytical method.

Clearance techniques are similar to those described for inulin. Constancy of rate of intravenous infusion is even more important, however, and single injection techniques yield grossly aberrant results.

The priming injection of PAH is calculated from a volume of distribution of PAH of about 400 ml./kg. body weight and a desired plasma concentration of 0.02 mg./ml., yielding a value of 8 mg./kg.

The rate of injection of PAH in the sustaining solution is the product of plasma PAH concentration and estimated ERPF. For healthy subjects, probable ERPF may be estimated from data in section C IV. In renal disease, ERPF may be estimated from the ratio, expected GFR/FF, recognizing that FF tends to increase somewhat in chronic BRIGHT's disease from its usual value of 0.20, and may be decreased in acute glomerulonephritis, pyrogenic toxemia and other situations. The PAH may be combined with inulin in both priming and sustaining infusions. Glucose, however, must be omitted from all solutions containing PAH since aberrantly low PAH clearances occur in the presence of glucose due to slow formation of a poorly excreted addition compound between the two substances (KLOPP, YOUNG and TAYLOR 1944; GRIMELLI et al.; BALDWIN et al. 1950). In addition, exogenous substances such as sulfonamides or procaine which contain diazotizable amino groups cannot be given to the subject. PAH cannot be taken orally since it is absorbed poorly from the interstinal tract and satisfactory blood concentrations cannot be attained (HAGENSEN, KEIDING and SCHMIDT). Small amounts of contaminating p-aminobenzoate are absorbed preferentially from the intestinal tract and result in significantly lower clearance values (SCHREINER, WESSON and ANSLOW). A plasma specimen is taken immediately prior to the experiment as a blank, the value of which is subtracted from subsequent plasma PAH analyses in calculating the clearances. A urine blank is unnecessary.

b) Analytical methods

Analytical methods for diodrast based upon iodine content have been described by SMITH, GOLDRING and CHASIS, by ALPERT and by many others and will not be described here. PAH is usually analysed by the method of SMITH et al. (1945).

1. Prepare cadmium or zinc sulfate plasma filtrates (SMITH 1956). Quantities of water added during the precipitation should yield a final concentration in the filtrate appropriate to the sensitivities of the instrument employed. A 25-fold dilution yielding a filtrate concentration of 1 to 2 micrograms/ml. is usually sufficient. Urine specimens should be diluted with water to yield concentrations approximately the same as those of the plasma filtrates.

2. To 5 ml. of plasma filtrate, diluted urine and appropriate standard solutions, each in duplicate, add 1.0 ml. of 1.2 N HCl and 0.5 ml. of $NaNO_2$ solution (100 mg. $NaNO_2$ to 100 ml. with distilled water; freshly prepared before each analysis). Mix well and wait not less than 3 nor more than 5 minutes.

3. Add 0.5 ml. of ammonium sulfamate (500 mg. $NH_4SO_3NH_2$ to 100 ml. of dist. water; refrigerated and reasonably fresh), mix, wait 3 minutes for the sulfamate to react with residual nitrous acid.

4. Add 0.5 ml. of diamine reagent [100 mg. N-(1-naphthyl) ethylenediamine hydrochloride to 100 ml. of distilled water; refrigerated], mix, wait 15 minutes for the purple diazonium compound to form.

5. Read in a photoelectric colorimeter at a wave length of 540 against a reagent blank prepared with 5 ml. of water. The color follows the LAMBERT-BEERS law closely and is quite stable.

3. Extraction ratios

The renal extraction ratio of a substance is the arterio-venous concentration difference divided by the arterial concentration or, $(a—v)/a$. The term is applied to substances removed from the renal arterial plasma or blood by metabolism or excretion and measures the fraction of the plasma so cleared. Measurement requires simultaneous collection of arterial (from any artery) and renal venous blood samples. The latter technique has been described in detail by WARREN, BRANNAN and MERRILL and by NICKEL and BRADLEY and is essentially the same as that employed in cardiac catheterization studies. The catheter, instead of remaining in the cardiac chambers, is passed into the inferior vena cava and thence into a renal vein. The right renal vein is preferred because of relative freedom from collaterals, particularly ovarian or spermatic veins, but satisfactory placement of the catheter distally in the left vein yields values similar to the right. The plasma should be separated as soon as possible to prevent possible outward diffusion of PAH or diodrast from the red cells.

Extraction ratios of excreted substances are performed for the most part to measure total renal plasma or blood flow, and of metabolized substances to study renal metabolism. The extraction ratio of PAH (E_{pah}) averages about 0.91 in healthy subjects (SMITH 1951) but may be decreased both acutely and chronically. In chronic BRIGHT'S disease, E_{pah} decreases roughly proportionally to the logarithm of the clearance of p-aminohippurate and averages about 0.2 at a clearance of 40 ml./min. (EDVALL 1957b). The extraction of radioiodinated diodrast may also be employed as a useful alternative to PAH (BERGSTROM, BUCHT and JOSEPHSON).

The 8 to 10 percent of PAH or diodrast entering the renal artery which fails to be extracted has been attributed to blood which has perfused non-excretory tissue such as stroma, capsule and major vessels, to arteriovenous anastomoses, to inability of the transport system to remove all PAH molecules from the peritubular fluid, and to medullary perfusion since the medullary portions of the *partes rectae* of the proximal segments are probably incapable of aromatic acid transport (LONGLEY, BURG and BURTNER).

4. Total renal plasma and blood flow

Total renal plasma flow is measured by $VU/(a—v)$ where VU is the excretion rate of any substance not metabolized by the kidney, and $a—v$ is its simultaneous renal arteriovenous difference. It is evident that this expression is also equal to the clearance, VU/P, divided by the extraction ratio, $(a—v)/a$, where a and P are interchangeable terms.

The expression is derived rigorously as follows: Let TRPF, a, v and VU equal total renal plasma flow, arterial and renal venous concentrations and excretion rate of a substance. Since metabolism does not occur, all of the substance entering in the renal arterial blood, TRPF $\cdot$ a must appear either in the urine, VU, the renal vein, TRPF $\cdot$ v, or in both. Hence, TRPF $\cdot$ a = TRPF $\cdot$ v + VU which, on rearrangement, yields the previous expression: TRPF = $VU/(a—v)$. This expression does not provide for the fact that renal venous blood flow is smaller than the arterial by the volume of fluid escaping from the kidney as urine and lymph. The error is very small, however, the correct value in normal subjects employing PAH extraction being lower than the measured value by less than 0.5 percent.

Although all nonmetabolized, excreted substances should yield the same TRPF, accuracy increases when the terms in the equation, particularly the *a—v* difference, are as large as possible. Since this is the circumstance with diodrast and PAH, these substances are employed almost exclusively to measure TRPF. Total renal blood flow, TRBF, can be measured directly provided that the *a—v* difference of whole blood instead of plasma is measured. In practice, however, TRBF is usually calculated indirectly as TRPF/(1-hematocrit).

Variations of the extraction technique may be employed to measure TRPF during oliguria or anuria, when excretion of PAH is too small for accurate measurements. A substance which is soluble in renal tissue, such as radioactive krypton (BRUN et al. 1955) or nitrous oxide (CROSLEY et al.), is introduced into the blood stream. Simultaneous arterial and renal venous blood samples are obtained in rapid succession from immediately before introduction of the substance until a time several minutes later. Renal venous concentrations are at first lower than arterial, the difference representing solution of the substance in renal tissue. The two concentrations approach equality as saturation of the tissue at the concurrent arterial concentration is attained. Total uptake, measured as the product of renal mass × solubility × arterial concentration, divided by the average *a—v* difference over the time interval until saturation is complete yields TRBF. In a group of anuric subjects, TRBF, measured by this method, averaged 20 percent of normal (BRUN et al. 1955).

5. Tubular transport maxima
a) General principles

Maximal rate of tubular transport of a substance is measured by presenting the tubules with progressively increasing quantities, or load, for transport. Ultimately, with increasing load (L) transport attains a constant value (Tm) and does not change with further increases in L. The technique employing progressively increasing load is not generally used, but is restricted to measurement of titration curves and studies of less well known substances. In routine studies of the Tm of substances such as PAH and glucose whose transport characteristics are well known, a load calculated to assure Tm is established rapidly by appropriate prime and sustaining solutions.

Inulin clearance must generally be measured during Tm determinations since filtration rate must be known in order to calculate the load presented for transport in reabsorptive Tm measurements or to calculate the excreted quantity contributed by filtration in secretory Tm measurements. As with clearance measurements in general, stable plasma concentrations are desirable.

Direct measurement of inulin clearance is omitted in an alternate method. The equation, $UV = P \cdot \text{GFR} \pm Tm$, is linear at all values of plasma concentration, P, above that required to attain Tm, if GFR is constant. When excretion rate as the ordinate is plotted against 2 or more values of P as the abscissa, the slope of the line generated measures GFR and the extrapolated intercept on the UV axis measures Tm. If GFR is decreasing or increasing, falsely low or high values for Tm will be obtained.

b) Transport maximum of PAH

The following method is that of SMITH (1956). The PAH prime should be calculated to yield a plasma concentration of not less than 20 and preferably closer to 40 mg. percent. Assuming a PAH volume of distribution of 400 ml./kg., the prime is 160 mg./kg. The prime should be injected slowly to avoid vasomotor and autonomic nervous disturbances: the method described for injecting the inulin prime is satisfactory. The sustaining infusion rate is set equal to the probable magnitude of Tm plus the probable rate of excretion of PAH by filtration. Because some of the plasma PAH is bound to plasma proteins and is unable to pass into the glomerular filtrate, filtrate concentration is less than plasma by a factor, k. Hence, the quantity of PAH excreted by filtration is $\text{GFR} \cdot P_{pah} \cdot k$. In an average, healthy young subject, assuming a Tm of 75 mg./min., GFR of 130 ml./min., P_{pah} of 0.4 mg./ml. and k of 0.8, the infusion rate should be approximately 117 mg./min. The PAH can be combined with inulin in the prime and sustaining solutions, but glucose should be omitted. Measurements of ERPF are frequently desired in conjunction with Tm_{pah}. In this case, a second PAH prime sufficient to elevate plasma PAH to values above 30 mg./100 ml. is injected, slowly, upon the termination of the last clearance period measuring ERPF; and the sustaining solution is exchanged for another containing an appropriately increased quantity of PAH. A second equilibration period should elapse, however, in order to attain stability of excretion.

Tm is calculated from the equation, $Tm_{pah} = V \cdot U_{pah} - \text{GFR} \cdot P_{pah} \cdot k$. The factor, k, is of considerable importance in the calculation and is the ratio of unbound to total PAH in the plasma. Since the ratio is fairly constant over a wide concentration range, the most important variable is the concentration of plasma proteins. The diffusible fraction at any plasma protein concentration can be calculated from the adsorption equation, $\dfrac{x}{m} = Kc^{1/n}$, where x and c are the concentrations of bound and unbound PAH in mg./100 ml. of plasma water, m is plasma protein concentration in g./100 ml., and K and n are constants. For whole plasma in man, K is 0.076 and $1/n$ is 0.88. For the albumin fractions alone, K is 0.112 and $1/n$ is 0.84 (Taggart 1951). For simplicity in calculating k, c can be taken arbitrarily as 80 percent of the measured total plasma PAH concentration. x is readily calculated from the adsorption equation and k then equals $x/(c + x)$. At a plasma protein concentration of 6 g./100 ml., this equation yields a value of k of 0.77, which is slightly less than the value of 0.83 obtained indirectly from clearance data in normal subjects by Chasis et al. (1945).

Expected values of Tm_{pah} are recorded in D III 1 c, d. They may also be estimated roughly from GFR. In chronic Bright's disease, the ratio, GFR/Tm_{pah}, is essentially normal until renal function is less than 50 percent of normal. The ratio then rises progressively with decreasing function (Earle 1950).

c) Transport maximum of glucose

For several reasons, glucose Tm is more difficult to measure satisfactorily than that of PAH: the large volumes of fluid required to produce and sustain satisfactory plasma concentrations of glucose as well as dehydration which may result from massive glucosuria may cause considerable fluctuations in filtration rate; the sustaining infusion must provide not only for glucose excretion but also for an unpredictable and frequently very high rate of extrarenal removal by oxidation and storage; the range of plasma concentrations within which Tm can be measured satisfactorily utilizing inulin clearances is narrower than for PAH and the L/Tm ratio should lie between 1.5 and 3.0. A ratio of 2.0 is desirable. Frequently, a study must be repeated one or more times before satisfactory measurements are obtained. The following method is based upon the studies of Smith et al. (1943) and of Bradley (pers. comm.).

The glucose prime should be calculated to produce a plasma glucose concentration of about 600 mg./100 ml. Assuming a resting plasma glucose concentration of 100 mg./100 ml. in nondiabetic subjects and a glucose volume of distribution of 200 ml./kg., the prime is 1 g./kg. Initially, glucose may be infused in a sustaining solution at 500 mg./min. This may be modified either during the first study or in a subsequent study but the sustaining infusion should not be less than the desired rate of glucose excretion, while excretion should approximately equal the probable glucose Tm. The glucose sustaining solution should, if possible, be infused separately from the inulin sustaining solution since it is often necessary to modify the rate of glucose infusion. In our laboratory, much of the uncertainty inherent in attempting to establish and maintain a prescribed plasma glucose concentration is avoided by infusing glucose at about 20 mg./kg./min. After about one hour, plasma glucose concentration is high and still rising. When glucosuria, as determined by testing, is adequate the blood and urine samples for Tm measurements may be obtained. The disadvantages of this method are that a relatively long equilibration period is necessary, and a constant plasma glucose concentration is seldom attained within a practicable length of time. PAH may be infused during measurement of glucose Tm but should not be present in a glucose-containing solution. Clearance periods may be as short as 10 minutes but should be about 15 minutes. Rapid, semiquantitative measurements of urine glucose should be made during the study in order to be assured that a satisfactory degree of glucosuria is being maintained. Arterial plasma samples should be taken because of the unpredictability of the arteriovenous difference of glucose in peripheral blood. The interpolated plasma glucose value 5—8 minutes before the midpoint of the period is employed in the calculations.

Any suitably accurate method may be employed for the analysis of glucose in urine and plasma. Nonglucose reducing substances are relatively insignificant at the high blood and urine concentrations attained and may be ignored. In the inulin analyses, plasma and urine samples should be yeast-fermented to remove glucose.

d) Titration curves

Titration curves provide one method for analysis of the kinetics of tubular transport (D I 2). The method has been applied to relatively few substances (glucose, PAH, sulfate, phosphate, urate) but is available for the study of all active transport systems. The region of interest is the titration splay, from that load at which excretion begins to increase perceptibly to that load at which Tm is attained. Although a continuous series of L and T measurements in this region is desirable, the necessity of maintaining stable plasma concentrations prevents more than a few points being measured during a single study. The method, in essence, consists of a sequence of sets of three clearance periods at successively higher plasma concentrations, each set with appropriate prime, sustaining solution and equilibration period. The sustaining solutions must be calculated from the anticipated rates of excretion at the plasma concentrations attained.

With both PAH and glucose it is often desirable to measure Tm in a separate preliminary study. The first prime should establish the tubular load at a point just below the titration splay. In normal subjects this will be at a plasma PAH concentration of about 8 mg./100 ml. Three successive primes with their sustaining solutions are calculated to provide equal increments in tubular load to a L/Tm ratio of approximately 1.2.

Glucose titration curve is more difficult to measure than PAH because highly variable extrarenal disposal of glucose renders predictable, stepwise increments in plasma concentration almost impossible to attain. The procedure is therefore empirical. A moderately concentrated (10 to 20 percent) glucose solution is infused separately from inulin. The glucose infusion rate is increased stepwise at one to two hourly intervals until the infusion rate is at least 500 mg./min.

In an initial study, the first step may be at $^1/_3$ and the second at $^2/_3$ of the probable final infusion rate which is calculated to attain Tm levels. Clearance periods in which urine flow has increased abruptly, as with the onset of glucosuria, frequently yield anomalous values and should be discarded. Similarly, periods during which plasma glucose changes rapidly, as, for example, exceeding a change rate of 5 mg/100 ml/min, are unreliable. The region of the titration splay is difficult to attain, and several studies are generally necessary before a satisfactory number of measurements have been made in this region (Bradley, pers. comm.).

Bibliography

Aas, K., and E. Blegen: The renal blood flow and the glomerular filtration rate in congestive heart failure and some other clinical conditions. Scand. J. clin. Lab. Invest. 1, 22 (1949). — Abrahams, V. C., and Mary Pickford: Simultaneous observations on the rate of urine flow and spontaneous uterine movements in the dog, and their relationship to posterior lobe activity. J. Physiol. (Lond.) 126, 329 (1954). — Observations on a central antagonism between adrenaline and acetylcholine. J. Physiol. (Lond.) 131, 712 (1956). — Adams, W., A. S. Alving, I. Sandiford, K. S. Grimson and C. Scott: The effect of bilateral paravertebral sympathectomy on the cardio-renal system in essential hypertension. Amer. J. Physiol. 133, P 190 (1941) (abstract). — Addis, T.: The ratio between the urea content of the urine and of the blood after the administration of large quantities of urea. An approximate index of the quantity of actively functioning kidney tissue. J. Urol. (Baltimore) 1, 263 (1917). — Renal function and the amount of functioning tissue. Arch. intern. Med. 30, 378 (1922). — Addis, T., Evalyn Barrett, R. I. Boyd and Helen J. Ureen: Renin proteinuria in the rat. I. The relation between the proteinuria and the pressor effect of renin. J. exp. Med. 89, 131 (1949). — Addis, T., Evalyn Barrett, L. J. Poo, Helen J. Ureen and R. W. Lippman: The relation between protein consumption and diurnal variations of endogenous creatinine clearance in normal individuals. J. clin. Invest. 30, 206 (1951). — Addis, T., Evalyn Barrett, L. J. Poo and D. W. Yuen: The relation between the serum urea concentration and the protein consumption of normal individuals. J. clin. Invest. 26, 869 (1947). — Addis, T., B. A. Meyers and Leona Bayer: The regulation of renal activity. XI. The rate of phosphate excretion by the kidney. The effect of variation in the concentration of phosphate in the plasma on the rate of phosphate excretion. Amer. J. Physiol. 12, 125 (1925). — Addis, T., and Marian C. Shevky: A test of the capacity of the kidney to produce a urine of high specific gravity. Arch. intern. Med. 30, 559 (1922). — Adolph, E. F.: The excretion of water by the kidneys. Amer. J. Physiol. 65, 419 (1923). — Ahlborg, Nils G.: Ascorbic acid excretion by human kidney. A study on the renal reabsorption mechanism. Acta physiol. scand. 12, Suppl. 36 (1946). — Aikawa, J. K., and R. H. Fitz: The distribution of Hg^{203}-labeled mercaptomerin in human tissues. J. clin. Invest. 35, 775 (1956). — Aitken, R. S.: On the renal threshold for chloride in man. J. Physiol. (Lond.) 67, 199 (1929). — Albright, F., W. Bauer and J. C. Aub: Studies of calcium and phosphorus metabolism. VIII. The influence of the thyroid gland and the parathyroid hormone upon the total acid-base metabolism. J. clin. Invest. 10, 187 (1931). — Albright, F., W. Bauer, Jessie R. Cockrill and R. Ellsworth: Studies on the physiology of the parathyroid glands. II. The relation of the serum calcium to the serum phosphorus at different levels of parathyroid activity. J. clin. Invest. 9, 659 (1931). — Albright, F., W. Bauer, Marion Ropes and J. C. Aub: Studies of calcium and phosphorus metabolism. IV. The effect of the parathyroid hormone. J. clin. Invest. 7, 139 (1929). — Albright, F., C. H. Burnett, Patricia H. Smith and W. Parson: Pseudo-hypoparathyroidism — an example of 'Seabright-Bantam syndrome'. Endocrinology 30, 922 (1942). — Albright, F., and R. Ellsworth: Studies on the physiology of the parathyroid glands. I. Calcium and phosphorus studies on a case of idiopathic hypoparathyroidism. J. clin. Invest. 7, 183 (1929). — Albright, F., Anne P. Forbes and P. H. Henneman: Pseudopseudohypoparathyroidism. Trans. Ass. Amer. Phycns 65, 337 (1952). — Albright, F., and E. C. Reifenstein jr.: The parathyroid glands and metabolic bone disease. Selected studies. Baltimore: Williams & Wilkins Company 1948. — Alexander, C. S.: Response of rats with experimental diabetes insipidus to water and salt loading. Amer. J. Physiol. 197, 173 (1959). — Alexander, J. D., E. D. Pellegrino, S. J. Farber and D. P. Earle: Observations on the relation of renal function changes to the electrolyte and glycosuric effects of ACTH in man. Endocrinology 49, 136 (1951). — Ali, M. N.: Some activities of arginine vasopressin and lysine vasopressin on kidney function in conscious dogs. Brit. J. Pharmacol. 13, 131 (1958). — Allen, T. H., and E. B. REEVES: Distribution of 'extra plasma' in the blood of some tissues in the dog as measured with P^{32} and T-1824. Amer. J. Physiol. 175, 218 (1953). — ALPERT, L. K.: A rapid method for the determination of diodrast-iodine in blood and urine. Bull. Johns Hopk. Hosp. 68, 522 (1941). — ALVING, A. S., J. FLOX, I. PITESKY and B. F. MILLER: Further notes on colorimetric determination of inulin in blood and urine. J. Lab. clin. Med. 27, 115 (1941). — ALVING, A. S., and B. F. MILLER: Practical method for measurement of glomerular filtration rate (inulin clearance), with evaluation of clinical significance of this determination. Arch. intern. Med. 66, 306 (1940). — ALVING, A. S., J. RUBIN and B. F. MILLER: A direct colorimetric method for the determination of inulin in blood and urine. J. biol. Chem. 127, 609 (1939). — AMATUZIO, D. S., F. STUTZMAN, N. SHRIFTER and S. NESBITT: A study of serum electrolytes (Na, K, Ca, P) in patients with severely decompensated portal cirrhosis of the liver. J. Lab. clin. Med. 39, 26 (1952). — AMBARD, L., et F. SCHMID: De la formation de l'ammoniaque urinaire au niveau du rein. Arch. Mal. Reins 1, 196 (1922). — AMBARD, L., et A. WEILL: Les lois numeriques de la sécrétion rénale de l'urée et du chlorure de sodium. J. Physiol. Path. gén. 14, 753 (1912). — AMES, R. G., and H. B. VAN DYKE: Antidiuretic hormone in the urine and pituitary of the kangaroo rat. Proc. Soc. exp. Biol. (N.Y.) 75, 417 (1950). — AMES, R. G., D. H. MOORE and H. B. VAN DYKE: The excretion of posterior pituitary antidiuretic hormone in the urine and its detection in the blood. Endocrinology 46, 215 (1950). — AMINI, F., N. L. PETRAKIS, W. MANDEL and MARIE DOHERTY: The effect of intravenous administration of pyrazinamide on tubular reabsorption of uric acid. Clin. Res. Proc. 7, 76 (1959) (abstract). — ANDERSEN, A. H.: On fixation of sulfathiazole, sulfapyridine, sulfanilamide and para-aminobenzoic acid by plasma. Acta pharmacol. (Kbh.) 1, 141 (1945). — ANDERSEN, A. H., K. O. MELLER u. MARGRETHE H. SIMESEN: Über die Zustandsform von Sulfathiazol im Blut, Urin und in der Cerebrospinalflüssigkeit. Naunyn-Schmiedeberg's Arch. exp. Path. Pharmak. 199, 528 (1942). — ANDERSEN, M., and K. C. NIELSEN: Studies on the renal function under experimental hypothermy in rabbits. Acta med. scand. 151, 191 (1955). — ANDERSON, E., and H. W. BEAMS: Light and electron microscope studies on the cells of the labyrinth in the "green gland" of Cambarus sp. Proc. Iowa Acad. Sci. 63, 681 (1956). — ANDERSON, HELEN M. and J. H. LARAGH: Renal excretion of potassium in normal and sodium depleted dogs. J. clin. Invest. 37, 323 (1958). — ANDERSON, I. A., A. MILLER and A. P. KENNY: Osteomalacia and renal glycosuria in adults. Metabolic investigation of a case with particular reference to its relation to the Fanconi syndrome and to treatment. Quart. J. Med. 21, 33 (1952). — ANDERSON, J.: A method for estimating Tm for phosphate in man. J. Physiol. (Lond.) 130, 268 (1955). — ANDERSON, J. A., and W. R. MURLIN: Antagonism of pitressin and adrenal cortical extract in human diabetes insipidus. J. Pediat. 21, 326 (1942). — ANDERSSON, B., and S. M. McCANN: Drinking, antidiuresis and milk ejection from electrical stimulation within the hypothalamus of the goat. Acta physiol. scand. 35, 191 (1955). — ANDREWS, J. C., and W. E. CORNATZER: The effect of acid and alkali on the absorption and metabolism of quinine. J. Pharmacol. exp. Ther. 82, 261 (1944). — ANSLOW jr., W. P., and L. G. WESSON jr.: Effect of sustained, graded urea diuresis on water and electrolyte excretion. Amer. J. Physiol. 180, 605 (1955a). — Some effects of pressor-antidiuretic and oxytocic fractions of posterior pituitary extract on sodium, chloride, potassium and ammonium excretion in the dog. Amer. J. Physiol. 182, 561 (1955b). — APPELBOOM, J. W. T., and W. A. BRODSKY: Osmotic activity of renal papillae of dogs during formation of hypertonic urine. Fed. Proc. 17, 5 (1958) (abstract). — APRAHAMIAN, H. A., J. L. VANDERVEEN, J. P. BUNKER, ANNA J. MURPHY and J. D. CRAWFORD: The influence of general anesthetics on water and solute excretion in man. Ann. Surg. 150, 122 (1959). — ARIEL, I. M., and F. MILLER: The effects of hypochloremia upon renal function in surgical patients. Surgery 28, 553 (1950a). — The effects of abdominal surgery upon renal clearance. Surgery 28, 716 (1950b). — ARIMURA, A., and J. F. DINGMAN: Specific and sensitive assay method for vasopressin and oxytocin using glasspaper chromatography. Nature (Lond.) 184, 1874 (1959). — ARISON, R., and H. C. STOERK: Mediation of phosphaturia in hydrocortisone-injected rats by parathormone. Fed. Proc. 19, 159 (1960) (abstract). — ARMSTRONG, P. B.: The embryonic origin of function in the pronephros through differentiation and parenchyma-vascular association. Amer. J. Anat. 51, 157 (1932). — ARROW, V. K., and R. G. WESTALL: Amino acid clearances in cystinuria. J. Physiol. (Lond.) 142, 141 (1958). — ASSALI, N. S., S. A. KAPLAN, S. J. FOMON and R. A. DOUGLASS jr.: Renal function studies in toxemia of pregnancy: excretion of solutes and renal hemodynamics during osmotic diuresis in hydropenia. J. clin. Invest. 32, 44 (1953). — ASSALI, N. S., S. A. KAPLAN, S. J. FOMON, R. A. DOUGLASS and Y. TADA: The effect of high spinal anesthesia on the renal hemodynamics and the excretion of electrolytes during osmotic diuresis in the hydropenic normal pregnant woman. J. clin. Invest. 30, 916 (1951). — ATKINS, E. L., and J. W. PEARCE: Mechanisms of the renal response to plasma volume expansion. Canad. J. Biochem. 37, 91 (1959). — ATKINSON, MILDRED, G. A. CLARK and J. A. MENZIES: The function of the urinary tubules in the frog. J. Physiol. (Lond.) 55, 253 (1921). — AU, W.

Y. W., and L. G. Raisz: The impairment of renal concentrating ability during mercurial diuresis. Clin. Res. Proc. 7, 280 (1959) (abstract). — August, J. T., S. S. Franklin, S. B. Rees, E. D. Robin and D. H. Nelson: Potassium excretion in the canine stop-flow preparation. Clin. Res. Proc. 8, 114 (1960) (abstract). — August, J. T., and D. H. Nelson: The dual action of aldosterone on renal sodium reabsorption in normal subjects. Clin. Res. Proc. 7, 274 (1959a) (abstract). — Adjustment to aldosterone or desoxycorticosterone acetate-induced sodium retention in patients with Addison's disease. J. clin. Invest. 38, 1964 (1959b). — August, J. T., D. H. Nelson and G. W. Thorn: Response of normal subjects to large amounts of aldosterone. J. clin. Invest. 37, 1549 (1958a). — Aldosterone. New Engl. J. Med. 259, 917 (1958b). — Austin, J. H., E. Stillman and D. D. van Slyke: Factors governing the excretion rate of urea. J. biol. Chem. 46, 91 (1921). — Averbeck, G., H. J. Meitner u. M. Schneider: Über die nervöse Beeinflussung der Nierendurchblutung und der Harnausscheidung. Z. ges. exp. Med. 111, 436 (1942). — Axelrod, D. R., and R. F. Pitts: The relationship of plasma pH and anion pattern to mercurial diuresis. J. clin. Invest. 31, 171 (1952a). — Effects of hypoxia on renal tubular function. J. appl. Physiol. 4, 593 (1952b). — Ayer, J. L., W. A. Schiess and R. F. Pitts: Independence of phosphate reabsorption and glomerular filtration in dog. Amer. J. Physiol. 151, 168 (1947). — Ayres, P. J., J. Barlow, O. Garrod, A. E. Kellie, Sylvia A. S. Tait, J. F. Tait and G. Walker: Aldosterone, p. 73. Boston: Little, Brown & Co. 1958. — Ayres, P. J., O. Garrod, S. A. Simpson and J. F. Tait: A method for the determination of aldosterone, cortisol and corticosterone in biological extracts, particularly applied to human urine. Biochem. J. 65, 639 (1957). — Ayres, P. J., O. Garrod, Sylvia A. S. Tait and J. F. Tait: Primary aldosteronism (Conn's syndrome). Aldosterone, p. 143. Boston: Little, Brown & Co. 1958. — Ayres, P. J., O. Garrod, Sylvia A. S. Tait, J. F. Tait and G. Walker: The use of (16-^{3}H) aldosterone in studies on human peripheral blood. Ciba foundation colloquia on endocrinology. II. Hormones in blood, p. 309. 1957. — Azerad, E., H. Lestradet, A. Reinberg et J. Gatha: Variations nycthémerales de l'élimination urinaire du potassium, du sodium et du chlore chez l'homme normal. Ann. Méd. 54, 431 (1953).

Babics, A., u. F. Renyi-Vamos: Das Lymphgefäßsystem der Niere und seine Bedeutung in der Nierenpathologie und Chirurgie. Budapest: Ungarische Akademie der Wissenschaften 1957. — Bachman, D. M., and W. B. Youmans: Effects of posture on renal excretion of sodium and chloride in orthostatic hypotension. Circulation 7, 413 (1953). — Bachrach, D., S. Scultety, J. Jaki u. B. Korpassy: Antidiuretischer Wirkstoff im Urin bei experimenteller traumatischer Oligurie. Z. ges. exp. Med. 127, 250 (1956). — Bader, R. A., J. W. Eliot and D. E. Bass: Renal and hormonal mechanisms of cold diuresis. Fed. Proc. 8, 7 (1949) (abstract). — Baer, J. E., K. H. Beyer, H. F. Russo and D. C. Titus: Renal tubular secretion of chlorothiazide (6-chloro-7-sulfamyl-1,2,4-benzothiadiazine-1,1-dioxide). Fed. Proc. 17, 346 (1958) (abstract). — Baer, J. E., H. Loraine Leidy, Antonia V. Brooks and K. H. Beyer: The physiological disposition of chlorothiazide (Diuril) in the dog. J. Pharmacol. exp. Ther. 125/126, 295 (1959). — Baer, J. E., Sue F. Paulson, H. F. Russo and K. H. Beyer: Renal elimination of 3-methylaminoisocamphane hydrochloride (mecamylamine). Amer. J. Physiol. 186, 180 (1956). — Baer, R. B., T. Benedek, I. M. Rosenthal and H. J. Zimmerman: Renal excretion of phosphorus in pseudohypoparathyroidism. Arch. intern. Med. 99, 14 (1957). — Baez, S., A. Mazur and E. Shorr: Mechanism of antidiuretic action of crystalline ferritin in dogs. Fed. Proc. 10, 8 (1951) (abstract). — Bahn, R. C., and J. B. Longley: Quantitative effects of a mercurial diuretic on the distribution of renal succinic dehydrogenase in the rat. J. Pharmacol. exp. Ther. 118, 365 (1956). — Bailey, P., and F. Bremer: Experimental diabetes insipidus. Arch. intern. Med. 28, 773 (1921). — Bainbridge, F. A., S. H. Collins and J. A. Menzies: Experiments on the kidneys of the frog. (Preliminary communication.) Proc. roy. Soc. B 86, 355 (1912/13). — Baldwin, D., R. W. Alexander and E. G. Warner jr.: Chronic sodium chloride challenge studies in man. Clin. Res. Proc. 7, 283 (1959) (abstract). — Baldwin, D. S., H. J. Berman, H. O. Heinemann and H. W. Smith: The elaboration of osmotically concentrated urine in renal disease. J. clin. Invest. 34, 800 (1955). — Baldwin, D. S., A. W. Biggs, W. Goldring, W. H. Hulet and H. Chasis: Exaggerated natriuresis in essential hypertension. Amer. J. Med. 24, 893 (1958). — Baldwin, D. S., E. M. Kahana and R. W. Clarke: Renal excretion of sodium and potassium in the dog. Amer. J. Physiol. 162, 655 (1950). — Baldwin, D. S., and P. G. McLean: Effect of acetate on Tm-pah in man. J. appl. Physiol. 4, 797 (1952). — Baldwin, D. S., G. E. Schreiner, E. S. Breed, L. G. Wesson jr. and M. H. Maxwell: Depression of apparent p-aminohippurate extraction ratio by glucose. J. clin. Invest. 29, 614 (1950). — Baldwin, D. S., J. H. Sirota and H. Villarreal: Diurnal variations of renal function in congestive heart failure. Proc. Soc. exp. Biol. (N.Y.) 74, 578 (1950). — Balint, P.: Experimentelle Daten über die Innervation der Nierentubuli. Klin. Wschr. 35, 597 (1957) (abstract). — Balint, P., A. Fekete, A. Hajdu and E. Kiss: An interoceptive reflex in the regulation of renal function. Acta med. scand. 154, 407 (1956). — Balint, P., A.

FEKETE and S. SZALAY: Tubular factors in the renal response to arterial hypotension. Experientia (Basel) 12, 228 (1956). — BALINT, P., A. HAJDU, E. KISS and J. STURZ: On the function of the denervated kidney. Acta physiol. Acad. Sci. hung. 15, 1 (1959). — BALL jr., W. C., R. C. BAHN, M. J. GOODKIND and J. O. DAVIS: Aldosterone excretion from hypophysectomized dogs with thoracic inferior vena cava constriction. Fed. Proc. 16, 5 (1957) (abstract). — BALL jr., W. C., J. O. DAVIS and M. J. GOODKIND: Ascites formation without sodium intake in dogs with thoracic inferior vena cava constriction and in dogs with right-sided congestive heart failure. Amer. J. Physiol. 188, 578 (1957). — BANG, H. O., and A. L. NIELSEN: Influence of proteins in diet on renal function measured by inulin and diodrast clearance. Nord. méd. 37, 518 (1948). — BARATZ, R. A., and R. C. INGRAHAM: Sensitive bioassay method for measuring antidiuretic hormone in mammalian plasma. Proc. Soc. exp. Biol. (N.Y.) 100, 296 (1959). — BARBOUR, A., G. M. BULL, B. M. EVANS, N. C. HUGHES-JONES and J. LOGOTHETOPOULOS: The effect of breathing 5 to 7 percent carbon dioxide on urine flow and mineral excretion. Clin. Sci. 12, 1 (1953). — BARCLAY, J. A., H. G. BRAY and W. T. COOKE: The renal tubular reabsorption of phosphate in man. J. Physiol. (Lond.) 103, 7P (1944) (abstract). BARCLAY, J. A., and W. T. COOKE: Reabsorption of electrolytes in renal tubules. Nature (Lond.) 154, 85 (1944). — BARCLAY, J. A., W. T. COOKE and R. A. KENNEY: Evidence for 3-component system of renal excretion. Acta med. scand. 128, 500 (1947a). — Observations on effects of adrenalin on renal function and circulation in man. Amer. J. Physiol. 151, 621 (1947). — The renal excretion of inorganic phosphate in man and dog. Acta med. scand. 134, 107 (1949). — BARCLAY, J. A., W. T. COOKE, R. A. KENNEY and MARJORIE E. NUTT: Effects of water diuresis and exercise on volume and composition of urine. Amer. J. Physiol. 148, 327 (1947). — BARCLAY, J. A., R. F. CRAMPTON and D. M. MATTHEWS: Henle's loops and the sodium content of the medullae of mammalian kidneys. J. Physiol. (Lond.) 147, 48P (1959) (abstract). — BARCLAY, J. A., and R. A. KENNEY: Method for estimation of creatinine. Biochem. J. 41, 586 (1947). — BARCLAY, J. A., and MARJORIE E. NUTT: Urinary changes during water diuresis. J. Physiol. (Lond.) 103 20P (1944a) (abstract). — The effect of exercise on the composition of the urine. J. Physiol. (Lond.) 103, 21P (1944b) (abstract). — BARETZ, L. H., M. HARTEN and M. WALZER: The absorption of protein from the urinary bladder. J. Urol. (Baltimore) 50, 71 (1943). — BARGER, A. C.: The pathogenesis of sodium retention in congestive heart failure. Metabolism 5, 480 (1956). — BARGER, A. C., R. D. BERLIN and J. F. TULENKO: Infusion of aldosterone, 9-α-fluorohydrocortisone and antidiuretic hormone into the renal artery of normal and adrenalectomized, unanesthetized dogs: effect on electrolyte and water excretion. Endocrinology 62, 804 (1958). — BARGER, A. C., M. R. LIEBOWITZ and F. P. MULDOWNEY: Role of sympathetic nervous system in sodium and water retention of experimental congestive heart failure. Fed. Proc. 18, 7 (1959) (abstract). — BARGER, A. C., R. S. ROSS and H. L. PRICE: Reduced sodium excretion in dogs with mild valvular lesions of the heart and in dogs with congestive failure. Amer. J. Physiol. 180, 249 (1955). — BARGER, A. C., A. M. RUDOLPH and E. F. YATES: Sodium excretion and renal hemodynamics in normal dogs, dogs with mild valvular lesions of the heart and dogs in frank congestive heart failure. Amer. J. Physiol. 183, 595 (1955) (abstract). — BARGMANN, W., A. KNOOP u. T. H. SCHIEBLER: Histologische, cytochemische und electron-mikroskopische Untersuchungen am Nephron (mit Berücksichtigung der Mitochondrien). Z. Zellforsch. 42, 386 (1955). — BARKER, E. S., J. K. CLARK, A. P. CROSLEY jr. and A. J. CUMMINS: The effect of salt poor human albumin on renal oxygen consumption in man. Amer. J. med. Sci. 218, 715 (1949) (abstract). — BARKER, E. S., J. K. CLARK and J. R. ELKINTON: Renal response to magnesium loading in the dog. Fed. Proc. 16, 6 (1957) (abstract). — BARKER, E. S., J. R. ELKINTON and J. K. CLARK: Studies of the renal excretion of magnesium in man. J. clin. Invest. 38, 1733 (1959). — BARKER, E. S., R. B. SINGER, J. R. ELKINTON and J. K. CLARK: The renal response in man to acute experimental respiratory alkalosis and acidosis. J. clin. Invest. 36, 515 (1957). — BARNAFI, L., R. ROSAS, M. DE LA LASTRA and H. CROXATTO: Influence of oxytocin and vasopressin on sodium-retaining activity of aldosterone in the rat. Amer. J. Physiol. 198, 255 (1960). — BARNARD, H. F., O. BASSIR and J. M. HOUGH: Fall in the inulin clearance following a single injection. Quart. J. exp. Physiol. 40, 217 (1955). — BARNES, B. A., O. COPE and T. HARRISON: Magnesium conservation in the human being on a low magnesium diet. J. clin. Invest. 37, 430 (1958). — BARNES, B. O., J. F. REGAN and J. G. BUENO: Is there a specific diuretic hormone in the anterior pituitary? Amer. J. Physiol. 105, 559 (1933). — BARNETT, A. J., R. B. BLACKET, A. E. DEPOORTER, P. H. SANDERSON and G. M. WILSON: The action of noradrenalin in man and its relation to phaeochromocytoma and hypertension. Clin. Sci. 9, 151 (1950). — BARNETT, G. D., and F. E. BLUME: Alkaline tides. J. clin. Invest. 17, 159 (1938). — BARNETT, H. L.: Renal physiology in infants and children: method for estimation of glomerular filtration rate. Proc. Soc. exp. Biol. (N.Y.) 44, 654 (1940). — BARNETT, H. L., C. W. FORMAN, HELEN MCNAMARA, W. W. MCCRORY, M. RAPOPORT, A. J. MITCHIE and G. BARBERO: The effect of adrenocorticotrophic hormone on children with the nephrotic syndrome.

II. Physiologic observations on discrete kidney functions and plasma volume. J. clin. Invest. 30, 227 (1951). — BARNETT, H. L., K. HARE, HELEN MCNAMARA and RUTH HARE: Measurement of glomerular filtration rate in premature infants. J. clin. Invest. 27, 691 (1948a). — BARNETT, H. L., HELEN MCNAMARA, R. S. HARE and K. HARE: Inulin, urea, mannitol and PAH clearance ratios in premature infants. Fed. Proc. 7, 5 (1948b) (abstract). — BARNETT, H. L., HELEN MCNAMARA, SELMA SHULTZ and R. TOMPSETT: Renal clearances of sodium penicillin G, procaine penicillin G, and inulin in infants and children. Pediatrics 3, 418 (1949). — BARNETT, H. L., A. M. PERLEY and H. G. MCGINNIS: Renal physiology in infants and children; inulin clearances in newborn infant with extrophy of bladder. Proc. Soc. exp. Biol. (N.Y.) 49, 90 (1942). — BARNETT, H. L., J. VESTERDAL, HELEN MCNAMARA and H. D. LAUSON: Renal water excretion in premature infants. J. clin. Invest. 31, 1069 (1952). — BARNICOT, N. A.: The local action of the parathyroid and other tissues on bone in intracerebral grafts. J. Anat. (Lond.) 82, 233 (1948). — BARRETT, EVALYN, and T. ADDIS: The serum creatinine concentration of normal individuals. J. clin. Invest. 26, 875 (1947). — BARRON, E. S. G., and T. P. SINGER: Studies on biological oxidations. XIX. Sulfhydryl enzymes in carbohydrate metabolism. J. biol. Chem. 157, 221 (1945). — BARTRAM, E. A.: Experimental observations on the effect of various diuretics when injected directly into one renal artery of the dog. J. clin. Invest. 11, 1197 (1932). — BARTTER, F. C.: The parathyroids. Ann. Rev. Physiol. 16, 429 (1954). — New adrenal cortical steroid. Science 121, 581 (1955). — The role of aldosterone in normal homeostasis and in certain disease states. Metabolism 5, 369 (1956). — The role of aldosterone in the regulation of body fluid volume and composition. Scand. J. clin. Lab. Invest. Suppl. 28—32, 50 (1957). — The physiological control of aldosterone secretion. Proc. roy. Soc. Med. 51, 201 (1958). — BARTTER, F. C., and E. G. BIGLIERI: Primary aldosteronism: Clinical staff conference at the National Institutes of Health. Ann. intern. Med. 48, 647 (1958). — BARTTER, F. C., E. G. BIGLIERI, P. PRONOVE and C. S. DELEA: Effect of changes in intravascular volume on aldosterone secretion in man. Aldosterone, p. 100. Boston: Little, Brown & Co. 1958. — BARTTER, F. C., G. W. LIDDLE, L. E. DUNCAN jr., JOAN K. BARBER and CATHERINE DELEA: The regulation of aldosterone secretion in man: the role of fluid volume. J. clin. Invest. 35, 1306 (1956). — BARTTER, F. C., I. H. MILLS, E. G. BIGLIERI and CATHERINE DELEA: Studies on the control and physiologic action of aldosterone. Recent Progr. Hormone Res. 15, 311 (1959). — BARTTER, F. C., I. H. MILLS and D. S. GANN: Increase of aldosterone secretion by carotid artery constriction and its prevention by thyro-carotid arterial junction denervation. J. clin. Invest. 38, 986 (1959) (abstract). — BASSIR, O.: Molecular inhomogeneity as a source of error in inulin clearance studies. J. Physiol. (Lond.) 131, 586 (1956). — BAYLISS, L. E., and A. BROWN: Part played by renal nerves in production of water diuresis in hypophysectomized and decerebrate dog. J. Physiol. (Lond.) 99, 190 (1940). — BAYLISS, L. E., and A. R. FEE: Studies on water diuresis. III. A comparison of the excretion of urine by innervated and denervated kidneys perfused with the heart lung preparation. J. Physiol. (Lond.) 69, 135 (1930). — BAYLISS, L. E., and E. LUNDSGAARD: The action of cyanide on the isolated mammalian kidney. J. Physiol. (Lond.) 74, 279 (1932). — BAYLISS, L. E., and A. M. WALKER: The electrical conductivity of glomerular urine from the frog and from Necturus. J. biol. Chem. 87, 523 (1930). — BAYLISS, R. I. S., D. MARRACK, JEANETTE PIRKIS, J. R. REES and JOAN F. ZILVA: The use of chlorothiazide in the treatment of edema: a comparison with other diuretic agents. Ann. N.Y. Acad. Sci. 71, 442 (1958). — BECK, D., H. LEVITIN and F. H. EPSTEIN: Effect of intravenous infusions of calcium on renal concentrating ability. Amer. J. Physiol. 197, 1118 (1959). — BECK, J. C., INGE DYRENFURTH, C. GIROUD and ELEANOR H. VENNING: Observations on the regulatory mechanisms of aldosterone secretion in man. Arch. intern. Med. 96, 463 (1955). — BECK, J. C., C. P. GIROUD, INGE DYRENFURTH and ELEANOR H. VENNING: The metabolic effects of intravenously administered aldosterone in a totally adrenalectomized human. Canad. J. Biochem. 33, 884 (1955). — BECK, J. C., E. E. MCGARRY, INGE DYRENFURTH and ELEANOR H. VENNING: Metabolic effects of human and monkey growth hormone in man. Science 125, 884 (1957). — BECK, L. V.: Action of phlorizin on acid phosphatase activity and on glucose phosphorylation of kidney cortex extracts. Proc. Soc. exp. Biol. (N.Y.) 49, 435 (1942). — BECK, L. V., and R. CHAMBERS: Secretion in tissue cultures. II. Effect of Na iodoacetate on the chick kidney. J. cell. comp. Physiol. 6, 441 (1935). — BECKER, E. L.: Renal function in polycythemic dogs. J. appl. Physiol. 10, 75 (1957). — BECKER, E. L., J. A. SCHILLING and R. B. HARVEY: Renal function in man acclimatized to high altitude. J. appl. Physiol. 10, 79 (1957). — BECKER, E. L., and D. D. THOMPSON: Radiosulfate excretion by the normal dog kidney. Fed. Proc. 18, 9 (1959) (abstract). — BECKER-CHRISTENSEN, P., and P. SCHOU: Experimental studies on the excretion of sulfathiazole by the kidneys with normal and greatly increased diuresis (sulphate diuresis). Acta pharmacol. (Kbh.) 1, 357 (1945). — BEER, E.: Über das Vorkommen von zweigeteilten Malpighischen Körperchen in der menschlichen Niere. Z. Heilk. 24, 334 (1903). — BEIDELMAN, B.: Treatment of chronic hypoparathyroidism with probenecid. Metabolism 7, 690 (1958). — BELLENS, R.: Différenciation de certaines polyuries par le dosage de l'activité antidiurétique urinaire. Arch. int. Pharmacodyn. 116, 113 (1958). — BÉNARD, H., et A. GAJDOS: Activité métabolique du rein et son rôle dans l'éxcretion urinaire. Paris: Masson et Cie. 1954. — BENSLEY, R. R., and W. B. STEEN: The functions of the differentiated segments of the uriniferous tubule. Amer. J. Anat. 41, 75 (1928). — BERCU, B. A., S. N. ROKAW and E. MASSIE: Antidiuretic action of the urine of patients in cardiac failure. Circulation 2, 409 (1950). — BERGER, E. Y., S. J. FARBER and D. P. EARLE jr.: Renal excretion of mannitol. Proc. Soc. exp. Biol. (N.Y.) 66, 62 (1947). — BERGER, E. Y., M. GALDSTON and S. HOROWITZ: The effect of anoxic anoxia on the human kidney. J. clin. Invest. 28, 648 (1949). — BERGER, L., TSAI F. YÜ and A. B. GUTMAN: Effect of drugs that alter uric acid excretion in man on uric acid clearance in the chicken. Amer. J. Physiol. 198, 575 (1960). — BERGLUND, F., and R. P. FORSTER: Renal tubular transport of inorganic divalent ions by the aglomerular marine teleost, Lophius americanus. J. gen. Physiol. 41, 429 (1958). — BERGLUND, F., C.-G. HELANDER and R. B. HOWE: Inorganic sulfate and thiosulfate: Transport and competition in renal tubules of the dog. Amer. J. Physiol. 198, 586 (1960). — BERGLUND, F., and W. D. LOTSPEICH: Renal tubular reabsorption of inorganic sulfate in the dog, as affected by glomerular filtration rate and sodium chloride. Amer. J. Physiol. 185, 533 (1956a). — Effect of various amino acids on the renal tubular reabsorption of inorganic sulfate in the dog. Amer. J. Physiol. 185, 539 (1956b). — BERGMANN, F., S. DIKSTEIN, J. MENCZEL and T. D. ULLMANN: Renal clearance of uncharged particles, as exemplified by thioureas. J. Physiol. (Lond.) 145, 22 (1959). — BERGSTRÖM, J., H. BUCHT and J. EK: The influence of chlorothiazide on the renal functions. Scand. J. clin. Lab. Invest. 10, 402 (1958). — BERGSTRÖM, J., H. BUCHT and B. JOSEPHSON: Determination of the renal blood flow in man by means of radioactive Diodrast and renal vein catheterization. Scand. J. clin. Lab. Invest. 11, 71 (1959). — BERLINER, R. W.: Renal secretion of potassium and hydrogen ions. Fed. Proc. 11, 695 (1952). — Some aspects of ion exchange in electrolyte transport by the renal tubules. Metabolic aspects of transport across cell membranes, p. 203. Madison: University of Wisconsin Press 1957. — Ion exchange mechanisms in the nephron. Circulation 21, 892 (1960). — BERLINER, R. W., and D. G. DAVIDSON: Production of hypertonic urine in the absence of pituitary antidiuretic hormone. J. clin. Invest. 36, 1416 (1957). — BERLINER, R. W., J. G. HILTON, T. F. YÜ and T. J. KENNEDY: The renal mechanism for urate excretion in man. J. clin. Invest. 29, 396 (1950). — BERLINER, R. W., and T. J. KENNEDY jr.: Renal tubular secretion of potassium in the normal dog. Proc. Soc. exp. Biol. (N.Y.) 67, 542 (1948). — BERLINER, R. W., T. J. KENNEDY jr. and J. G. HILTON: Salyrgan and renal tubular secretion of para-aminohippurate in the dog and man. Amer. J. Physiol. 154, 537 (1948). — Effect of maleic acid on renal function. Proc. Soc. exp. Biol. (N.Y.) 75, 791 (1950a). — Renal mechanisms for excretion of potassium. Amer. J. Physiol. 162, 348 (1950b). — BERLINER, R. W., T. J. KENNEDY jr. and J. ORLOFF: Relationship between acidification of the urine and potassium metabolism. Amer. J. Med. 11, 274 (1951). — Factors affecting the transport of potassium and hydrogen ions by the renal tubules. Arch. int. Pharmacodyn. 97, 299 (1954). — BERLINER, R. W., N. G. LEVINSKY, D. G. DAVIDSON and M. EDEN: Dilution and concentration of the urine and the action of antidiuretic hormone. Amer. J. Med. 24, 730 (1958). — BERLINER, R. W., and J. ORLOFF: Carbonic anhydrase inhibitors. Pharmacol. Rev. 8, 137 (1956). — BERNE, R. M.: Hemodynamics and sodium excretion of denervated kidney in anesthetized and unanesthetized dog. Amer. J. Physiol. 171, 148 (1952). — BERNE, R. M., W. K. HOFFMAN jr., A. KAGAN and M. N. LEVY: Response of the normal and denervated kidney to l-epinephrine and l-nor-epinephrine. Amer. J. Physiol. 171, 564 (1952). — BERNE, R. M., and M. N. LEVY: Effect of acute reduction in cardiac output on the denervated kidney. Amer. J. Physiol. 171, 558 (1952). — BERNSTEIN, D., C. R. KLEEMAN, J. T. DOWLING and M. H. MAXWELL: The renal clearance of diffusable calcium associated with clinical and experimental alterations in parathyroid function. Clin. Res. 7, 246 (1959) (abstract). — Heterogeneity of partially purified human and animal parathyroid hormone. Clin. Res. Proc. 8, 139 (1960) (abstract). — BERNSTEIN, S. H., R. E. WESTON, G. ROSS, J. GROSSMAN, I. B. HANENSON and L. LEITER: Studies on intravenous water diuresis and nicotine and pitressin antidiuresis in normal subjects and patients with liver disease. J. clin. Invest. 32, 422 (1953). — BERRY, J. N., J. F. FLANAGAN, E. E. OWEN and M. P. TYOR: The kidney as a source of blood ammonia in resting and hyperventilated cirrhotics. Clin. Res. Proc. 7, 154 (1959) (abstract). — BERTHOUD, E., B. COURVOISIER et G. ZAHND: Action de l'hormone parathyroïdienne sur la clearance rénale du phosphore dans l'hypoparathyroïdisme. Helv. med. Acta 24, 524 (1957). — BESKIND, H., and G. H. MUDGE: Effect of potassium deficiency on renal tubular reabsorption and assimilation of glucose. Bull. Johns Hopk. Hosp. 104, 252 (1959). — BEYER, K. H.: New concept of competitive inhibition of renal tubular excretion of penicillin. Science 105, 94 (1947). — Factors basic to the development of useful inhibitors of renal transport mechanisms. Arch. int. Pharmacodyn. **98**, 97 (1954). — Metabolic aspects of transport across cell membranes, p. 263. Madison: University Wisconsin Press 1957. — The mechanism of action of chlorothiazide. Ann. N.Y. Acad. Sci. **71**, 363 (1958). — BEYER, K. H., H. FLIPPIN, W. F. VERWEY and R. WOODWARD: The effect of para-aminohippuric acid on plasma concentration of penicillin in man. J. Amer. med. Ass. **126**, 1007 (1944a). — BEYER, K. H., P. A. MATTIS, ELIZABETH A. PATCH and H. F. RUSSO: Para-aminohippuric acid; its pharmacodynamic actions. J. Pharmacol. exp. Ther. **84**, 136 (1945a). — BEYER, K. H., A. K. MILLER, H. F. RUSSO, ELIZABETH A. PATCH and W. F. VERWEY: Inhibitory effect of caronamide on renal elimination of penicillin. Amer. J. Physiol. **149**, 355 (1947a). — BEYER, K. H., R. H. PAINTER and V. D. WIEBELHAUS: Enzymatic factors in renal tubular secretion of phenol red. Amer. J. Physiol. **161**, 259 (1950). — BEYER, K. H., L. PETERS, R. WOODWARD and W. F. VERWEY: The enhancement of the physiological economy of penicillin in dogs by the simultaneous administration of para-aminohippuric acid. II. J. Pharmacol. exp. Ther. **82**, 310 (1944b). — BEYER, K. H., H. F. RUSSO, S. R. GASS, KATHERINE M. WILHOYTE and ALICE A. PITT: Renal tubular elimination of N'-methylnicotinamide. Amer. J. Physiol. **160**, 311 (1950a). — BEYER, K. H., H. F. RUSSO, ELIZABETH A. PATCH, L. PETERS and K. L. SPRAGUE: The formation and excretion of acetylated sulfonamides. J. Lab. clin. Med. **31**, 65 (1946a). — BEYER, K. H., H. F. RUSSO, ELIZABETH A. PATCH, ELIZABETH K. TILLSON and GRACE SHANER: Certain pharmacologic properties of 4'-carboxyphenylmethanesulfonaniliide (caronamde), including its effect on renal clearance of compounds other than penicillin. J. Pharmacol. exp. Ther. **91**, 272 (1947b). — BEYER, K. H., H. F. RUSSO, ELIZABETH K. TILLSON, A. KATHERINE MILLER, W. F. VERWEY and S. R. GASS: 'Benemid', p-(di-n-propylsulfamyl)-benzoic acid: Its renal affinity and its elimination. Amer. J. Physiol. **166**, 625 (1951). — BEYER, K. H., ELIZABETH K. TILLSON, H. F. RUSSO, JACQUELINE K. FISHMAN and F. T. BRENNAN: Darstine: interrelationship of renal tubular secretion and tissue sequestration in the physiological economy of a quaternary anticholinergic agent, 1-(3-hydroxy-5-methyl-4-phenylhexyl)-1-methylpiperidinium bromide. Fed. Proc. **12**, 301 (1953) (abstract). — BEYER, K. H., ELIZABETH K. TILLSON, H. F. RUSSO, GRACE S. SCHUCHARDT and ALICE A. PITT: Elimination (metabolism and excretion) of p-aminobenzoic acid by the dog. Fed. Proc. **11**, 13 (1952) (abstract). — BEYER, K. H., W. F. VERWEY, R. WOODWARD, L. PETERS and P. A. MATTIS: The enhancement of the plasma concentration of penicillin in dogs by the simultaneous administration of para-aminohippuric acid. III. Amer. J. med. Sci. **200**, 608 (1945b). — BEYER, K. H., V. D. WIEBELHAUS, H. F. RUSSO, H. M. PECK and S. E. McKINNEY: Benemid, p-(di-n-propylsulfamyl)-benzoic acid. An anticatabolite: its pharmacological properties. Fed. Proc. **9**, 258 (1950b) (abstract). — BEYER, K. H., V. D. WIEBELHAUS, ELIZABETH K. TILLSON, H. F. RUSSO and KATHERINE M. WILHOYTE: Benemid, p-(di-n-propylsulfamyl)-benzoic acid: Inhibition of glycine conjugative reactions. Proc. Soc. exp. Biol. (N.Y.) **74**, 772 (1950c). — BEYER, K. H., R. WOODWARD, L. PETERS, W. F. VERWEY and P. A. MATTIS: The prolongation of penicillin retention in the body by means of para-aminohippuric acid. Science **100**, 107 (1944c). — BEYER, K. H., L. D. WRIGHT, H. F. RUSSO, HELEN R. SKEGGS and ELIZABETH A. PATCH: Renal clearance of essential amino acids: tryptophane, leucine, isoleucine and valine. Amer. J. Physiol. **146**, 330 (1946b). — BEYER, K. H., L. D. WRIGHT, HELEN R. SKEGGS, H. F. RUSSO and G. A. SHANER: Renal clearance of essential amino acids; their competition for reabsorption by renal tubules. Amer. J. Physiol. **151**, 202 (1947c). — BIALESTOCK, DORA: The extra-glomerular arterial circulation of the renal tubules. Anat. Rec. **129**, 53 (1957). — BICKERS, J. N., and E. H. BRESLER: Effect of an organomercurial on the rat kidney. Clin. Res. Proc. **8**, 62 (1960) (abstract). — BICKFORD, R. G., and F. R. WINTON: Influence of temperature on the isolated kidney of the dog. J. Physiol. (Lond.) **89**, 198 (1937). — BIETER, R. N.: The effect of the splanchnics upon glomerular blood flow in the frog's kidney. Amer. J. Physiol. **91**, 436 (1929). — The action of some diuretics upon the aglomerular kidney. J. Pharmacol. exp. Ther. **43**, 399 (1931). — BIETER, R. N., and A. D. HIRSCHFELDER: The excretion of dyes and other substances in the frog's kidney and its bearing upon the theories of renal secretion. Amer. J. Physiol. **68**, 326 (1924). — BIGGART, J. H., and G. L. ALEXANDER: Experimental diabetes insipidus. J. Path. Bact. **48**, 405 (1939). — BIGLIEREI, E. G., C. WATLINGTON and P. H. FORSHAM: The rigidity of the expanded extracellular fluid compartments in primary aldosteronism. Clin. Rec. Proc. **8**, 106 (1960) (abstract). — BING, J., and P. EFFERSØE: Comparative tests of the thiosulphate and creatinine clearance in rabbits and cats. Acta physiol. scand. **15**, 231 (1948). — BING, R. J.: Effect of vitamin A on some renal functions of dog. Amer. J. Physiol. **140**, 240 (1944). — BIRCHALL, R., S. W. TUTHILL, W. S. JACOBS, W. J. TRAUTMAN jr. and T. FINDLEY: Renal excretion of water, sodium and chloride. Comparison of the responses of hypertensive patients with those of normal subjects, patients with specific adrenal or pituitary defects and a normal subject primed with various hormones. Circulation **7**, 258 (1953). — BIRCHARD, W. H.: The effect of expansion of extracellular fluid volume in conditioning the diuretic response to ingested isotonic saline. J. clin. Invest. **31**, 617 (1952) (abstract). —

BIRCHARD, W. H., T. E. PROUT, T. F. WILLIAMS and J. D. ROSENBAUM: Diuretic responses to oral and intravenous water loads in patients with hepatic cirrhosis. J. Lab. clin. Med. 48, 26 (1956). — BIRCHARD, W. H., and M. B. STRAUSS: Factors influencing the diuretic response of seated subjects to the ingestion of isotonic saline solution. J. clin. Invest. 32, 807 (1953). — BIRNIE, J. H.: The inactivation of posterior pituitary antidiuretic hormone by liver extracts. Endocrinology 52, 33 (1953). — BIRNIE, J. H., W. J. EVERSOLE, W. R. BOSS, C. M. OSBORN and R. GAUNT: An antidiuretic substance in the blood of normal and adrenalectomized rats. Endocrinology 47, 1 (1950). — BIRNIE, J. H., ROSEMARY JENKINS, W. J. EVERSOLE and R. GAUNT: An antidiuretic substance in the blood of normal and adrenalectomized rats. Proc. Soc. exp. Biol. (N.Y.) 70, 595 (1949). — BISNO, A., I. KASSER, D. ROLF, D. C. TOSTESON and H. L. WHITE: Effect of a mercurial diuretic on sodium flux across proximal tubular epithelium. Fed. Proc. 19, 365 (1960) (abstract). — BISSET, G. W., and J. M. WALKER: Assay of oxytocin in blood. J. Physiol. (Lond.) 126, 588 (1954). — Nicotine, hexamethonium and ethanol on the secretion of the antidiuretic and oxytocin hormones of the rat. Brit. J. Pharmacol. 12, 461 (1957). — BJERING, T.: The influence of histamine on renal function. Acta med. scand. 91, 267 (1937). — Renal excretion of urea. Acta med. scand. Suppl. 234, 33 (1949). — BJERRE-CHRISTENSEN, K.: The pitressin test of renal concentrating capacity. A comparative evaluation of the Addis-Shevky and pitressin tests. Acta med. scand. 142, 215 (1952). — BJØRNEBOE, M., S. DALGAARD-MIKKELSEN and F. RAASCHOU: On the excretion of salicylic acid in man. A preliminary report. Scand. J. clin. Lab. Invest. 1, 287 (1949). — BLACK, A. B., and J. A. LITCHFIELD: Uraemia complicating low salt treatment of heart failure. Quart. J. Med. 20, 149 (1951). — BLACK, D. A. K., H. E. F. DAVIES, E. W. EMERY and E. G. WADE: Renal handling of radioactive potassium in man. Clin. Sci. 15, 277 (1956). — BLACK, D. A. K., R. A. McCANCE and W. F. YOUNG: Function of the kidney in dehydration. Nature (Lond.) 150, 461 (1942). — BLACK, D. A. K., and M. D. MILNE: Experimental potassium depletion in man. Clin. Sci. 11, 397 (1952). — BLACK, D. A. K., R. PLATT and S. W. STANBURY: Regulation of sodium excretion in normal and salt-depleted subjects. Clin. Sci. 9, 205 (1950). — BLACK, D. A. K., J. F. POWELL and A. F. SMITH: Inulin and perabrodil clearance after alimentary haemorrhage in man. J. Physiol. (Lond.) 99, 344 (1941). — BLACKET, R. B.: Oedema in heart failure: Lessons from the beri-beri heart. Aust. Ann. Med. 4, 261 (1955). — BLACKMORE, W. P.: Effect of serotonin on renal hemodynamics and sodium excretion in the dog. Amer. J. Physiol. 193, 639 (1958). — Comparative effects of chlorothiazide and mersalyl (mersalyl sodium and theophylline) on the kidney. J. Pharmacol. exp. Ther. 125, 303 (1959). — BLACKMORE, W. P., and G. R. CHERRY: Antidiuretic action of histamine in the dog. Amer. J. Physiol. 180, 596 (1955). — BLACKMORE, W. P., V. E. WILSON and T. R. SHERROD: The effect of histamine on renal hemodynamics. J. Pharmacol. exp. Ther. 109, 206 (1953). — BLAHD, W. H., and S. H. BASSETT: Potassium deficiency in man. Metabolism 2, 218 (1953). — BLAKE, W. D.: Some effects of dihydrogenated ergot alkaloids on renal hemodynamics, water and electrolyte excretion in the dog. Amer. J. Physiol. 173, 337 (1953). — Pathways of adrenaline action on renal function with observations on a blood pressure reflex regulating water and electrolyte excretion. Amer. J. Physiol. 181, 399 (1955a). — Some effects of single, subcutaneous injections of adrenal medullary hormones on renal excretion of water and electrolytes in the dog. Amer. J. Physiol. 181, 417 (1955b). — BLAKE, W. D., and D. G. DAVIDSON: Some effects of repeated injections of epinephrine and of an adrenergic blocking agent on the daily excretion of water and electrolytes in the dog. Amer. J. Physiol. 181, 423 (1955). — BLATTEIS, C. M., and S. M. HORVATH: Renal, cardiovascular and respiratory responses and their interrelations during hypothermia. Amer. J. Physiol. 192, 357 (1958). — BLEGEN, E.: Kidney function in heart failure. Scand. J. clin. Lab. Invest. 1, 298 (1949). — BLEGEN, E., H. N. HAUGEN and K. AAS: Endogenous "creatinine" clearance. Scand. J. clin. Lab. Invest. 1, 191 (1949). — BLEGEN, E., K. ØRNING and K. AAS: The renal clearance of thiosulphate in man. Scand. J. clin. Lab. Invest. 1, 102 (1949). — BLISS, S.: Increased excretion of urinary ammonia in the dog following the intravenous injection of both natural and unnatural forms of certain amino acids. J. biol. Chem. 137, 217 (1941). — BLOMHERT, G., J. A. MOLHUYSEN, J. GERBRANDY, L. A. DE VRIES and J. G. G. BORST: Diuretic effect of isotonic saline solution compared with that of water. Influence of diurnal rhythm. Lancet 1951 II, 1011. — BLOTNER, H.: Diabetes insipidus. Oxford Medicine, vol. 4, chap. 6. New York: Oxford University Press 1949. — BLUMGART, H. L., D. R. GILLIGAN, R. C. LEVY and M. G. BROWN: The effect of diuretics on water and salt metabolism. Trans. Ass. Amer. Phycns 47, 304 (1932). — BLUMGART, H. L., D. R. GILLIGAN, R. C. LEVY, M. G. BROWN and M. C. VOLK: Action of diuretic drugs: Action of diuretics in normal persons. Arch. intern. Med. 54, 40 (1934). — BODANSKY, O., and W. MODELL: Differential excretion of bromide and chloride ions and its role in bromide retention. J. Pharmacol. exp. Ther. 73, 51 (1941). — The fecal and urinary excretion, the tissue distribution, and the serum concentration of bromide and chloride during prolonged bromide administration. Fed. Proc. 1,

101 (1942) (abstract). — BODO, R. C. DE: Antidiuretic action of morphine and its mechanism. J. Pharmacol. exp. Ther. **82**, 74 (1944). — BODO, R. C. DE, and K. F. PRESCOTT: Antidiuretic action of barbiturates (phenobarbital, amytal, pentobarbital) and mechanism involved in this action. J. Pharmacol. exp. Ther. **85**, 222 (1945). — BOGER, W. P., J. O. BEATTY, F. W. PITTS and H. F. FLIPPIN: The influence of a new benzoic acid derivative on the metabolism of para-aminosalicylic acid (PAS) and penicillin. Ann. intern. Med. **33**, 18 (1950). — BOGER, W. P., and H. F. FLIPPIN: Penicillin plasma concentrations. J. Amer. med. Ass. **139**, 1131 (1949). — BOGER, W. P., M. E. GALLAGHER and F. W. PITTS: The effect of a new benzoic acid derivative on penicillin and para-amino-salicylic acid (PAS). J. Philad. gen. Hosp. **1**, 51 (1950). — BOGER, W. P., F. W. PITTS and M. E. GALLAGHER: Benemid and carinamide: Comparison of effect on para-aminosalicylic acid (PAS) plasma concentrations. J. Lab. clin. Med. **36**, 276 (1950). — BOJESEN, E.: The function of the urinary tract as "dead space" in clearance experiments. A preliminary report. Scand. J. clin. Lab. Invest. **1**, 290 (1949). — The transport of urine in the upper urinary tract. Acta physiol. scand. **32**, 39 (1954). — BONGIOVANNI, A. M., and W. R. EBERLEIN: The renal clearance of neutral 17-ketosteroids in man. J. clin. Endocr. **17**, 238 (1957). — BONSNES, R. W., and E. S. DANA: Increased uric acid clearance following intravenous infusion of hypertonic glucose solutions. J. clin. Invest. **25**, 386 (1946). — BONSNES, R. W., L. V. DILL and E. S. DANA: The effect of diodrast on the normal uric acid clearance. J. clin. Invest. **23**, 776 (1944). — BONSNES, R. W., and W. A. LANGE: Inulin clearance during pregnancy. Fed. Proc. **9**, 154 (1950) (abstract). — BONSNES, R. W., and HELEN H. TAUSSKY: On the colorimetric determination of creatinine by Jaffe reaction. J. biol. Chem. **158**, 581 (1945). — BOOK, M. H.: The secreting area of the glomerulus. J. Anat. (Lond.) **71**, 91 (1936). — BORDLEY, J. 3rd, J. P. HENDRIX and A. N. RICHARDS: Quantitative studies of the composition of glomerular urine. XI. The concentration of creatinine in glomerular urine from frogs determined by an ultramicro-adaptation of the Folin method. J. biol. Chem. **101**, 255 (1933). — BORDLEY, J. 3rd, and A. N. RICHARDS: Quantitative studies of the composition of glomerular urine. VIII. The concentration of uric acid in glomerular urine of snakes and frogs, determined by an ultra-microadaptation of Folin's method. J. biol. Chem. **101**, 193 (1933). — BORGHGRAEF, R. R. M., R. H. KESSLER and R. F. PITTS: Plasma regression, distribution and excretion of radiomercury in relation to diuresis following the intravenous administration of Hg^{203} labelled chlormerodrin to the dog. J. clin. Invest. **35**, 1055 (1956). — BORGHGRAEF, R. R. M., and R. F. PITTS: The distribution of chlormerodrin (Neohydrin) in tissues of the rat and dog. J. clin. Invest. **35**, 31 (1956). — BORGSTÖM, B.: Detoxification of benzoic acid by glycuronic acid under normal conditions and in liver disease. Acta med. scand. **133**, 7 (1949). — BORSOOK, H., and J. W. DUBNOFF: The biological synthesis of hippuric acid in vitro. J. biol. Chem. **132**, 307 (1940). — BORST, J. G. G.: The maintenance of an adequate cardiac output by the regulation of the urinary excretion of water and sodium chloride; an essential factor in the genesis of oedema. Acta med. scand. **130**, Suppl. 207 (1948). — BORST, J. G. G., and L. A. DE VRIES: The three types of "natural" diuresis. Lancet **1950 II**, 1. — BOTT, PHYLLIS A.: Quantitative studies of composition of glomerular urine; concentration of sodium in glomerular urine of Necturi. J. biol. Chem. **147**, 653 (1943). — Josiah Macy Conf. on Renal Function 5, 42 (1953). — The concentration of potassium in glomerular urine of Necturi. J. biol. Chem. **215**, 287 (1955). — Transport of micromolecules in mammalian and *Necturus* nephrons. A. Evidences from the concentrations of electrolytes in tubule fluid, serum and urine, especially in amphibia. Proc. 8th Ann. Conf. on the Nephrotic Syndrome, p. 39, 1957. — Region of tubule fluid sodium concentration drop in *Necturus* kidney. Fed. Proc. **17**, 18 (1958) (abstract). — BOTT, PHYLLIS A., and A. N. RICHARDS: Passage of protein molecules through glomerular membranes. J. biol. Chem. **141**, 291 (1941). — BOURQUIN, HELEN: Studies on diabetes insipidus. IV. Amer. J. Physiol. **96**, 66 (1931). — BOUYOUCOS, B. G.: La chlorurie, l'hydrurie, la chloremie et l'hydremie au cours de la diurese par les sels mercuriels organiques. C. R. Soc. Biol. (Paris) **115**, 1170 (1934). — BOWMAN, W.: On the structure and use of the Malpighian Bodies of the kidney, with observations on the circulation through that gland. Phil. Trans. B **132**, 57 (1842). — BOYARSKY, S., and H. W. SMITH: Renal concentrating operation at low urine flows. J. Urol. (Baltimore) **78**, 511 (1957). — BOYD, E. M., and N. D. GARAND: Effect of pressor and oxytocic fractions of posterior pituitary extract on loss of water administered to albino rats. Endocrinology **30**, 433 (1942). — BOYD, L. J., and D. SCHERF: The effect of sedatives on diuresis. Med. Clin. N. Amer. **24**, 869 (1940). — BOYER, C. C.: The vascular pattern of the renal glomerulus as revealed by plastic reconstruction from serial sections. Anat. Rec. **125**, 433 (1956). — BOYLAN, J. W., and DOROTHY E. ANTKOWIAK: Mechanism of diuresis during negative pressure breathing. J. appl. Physiol. **14**, 116 (1959). — BOYLAN, J. W., and S. K. HONG: Sodium chloride excretion in hypothermic dogs. Fed. Proc. **18**, 15 (1959) (abstract). — BRADLEY, S. E.: The validity of the clearance technique in the measurement of renal blood flow in normal man and in patients with essential hypertension. Trans. Conf. on Factors Regulating

Blood Pressure 1, 118 (1947). — The thyroid, p. 546, edit. by S. C. Werner. New York: Hoeber-Harper 1955. — Kidney. Ann. Rev. Physiol. 19, 513 (1957). — BRADLEY, S. E., and W. D. BLAKE: Pathogenesis of renal dysfunction during congestive heart failure. Amer. J. Med. 6, 470 (1949). — BRADLEY, S. E., and G. P. BRADLEY: Renal function during chronic anemia in man. Blood 2, 192 (1947a). — Effect of increased intra-abdominal pressure on renal function in man. J. clin. Invest. 26, 1010 (1947b). — BRADLEY, S. E., G. P. BRADLEY, C. J. TYSON, J. J. CURRY and W. D. BLAKE: Renal function in renal diseases. Amer. J. Med. 9, 766 (1950). — BRADLEY, S. E., E. LEIFER and J. F. NICKEL: Distribution of functional activity among the nephron population. The kidney. Ciba foundation symposium. Boston: Little, Brown & Co. 1954. — BRADLEY, S. E., G. H. MUDGE, W. D. BLAKE and P. ALPHONSE: The effect of increased intra-abdominal pressure on the renal excretion of water and electrolytes in normal human subjects and in patients with diabetes insipidus. Acta clin. belg. 10, 209 (1955). — BRADLEY, S. E., J. F. NICKEL and E. LEIFER: The distribution of nephron function in man. Trans. Ass. Amer. Phycns 65, 147 (1952). — BRADLEY, S. E., and H. O. WHEELER: On the diversities of structure, perfusion and function of the nephron population. Amer. J. Med. 24, 692, 1958. — BRANDT, J. L., and J. G. GRUHN: Effect of renin on proteinuria and PAH clearance at low plasma levels. Amer. J. Physiol. 153, 458 (1948). — BRANDT, J. L., H. D. RUSKIN, B. ZUMOFF, L. CASTLEMAN and S. ZUCKERMAN: Inhibition of renal tubular responsiveness to antidiuretic hormone by pyrogens. Proc. Soc. exp. Biol. (N.Y.) 88, 451 (1955). — BRANDT, J. L., B. ZUMOFF, L. CASTLEMAN, H. D. RUSKIN, AUDREY JONES and S. ZUCKERMAN: Studies of the effects of large doses of bacterial pyrogen in the dog. I. The renal handling of salt and water. J. clin. Invest. 35, 1080 (1956). — BRASSFIELD, C. R., and V. G. BEHRMANN: A correlation of p_H of arterial blood and urine as affected by changes in pulmonary ventilation. Amer. J. Physiol. 132, 272 (1941). — BRAUN, W., V. P. WHITTAKER and W. D. LOTSPEICH: Renal excretion of phlorizin and phlorizin glucuronide. Amer. J. Physiol. 190, 563 (1957). — BRAY, G. A.: The determination of osmolality in frozen kidney slices. Fed. Proc. 19, 366 (1960) (abstract). — BRAY, G. A., and A. S. PRESTON: Urinary concentration and the urea concentration of the papilla and urine in the rat. Fed. Proc. 20, 406 (1961) (abstract). — BRAZEAU, P., and A. GILMAN: Effect of plasma CO_2 tension on renal tubular reabsorption of bicarbonate. Amer. J. Physiol. 175, 33 (1953). — BRESLER, E., J. MONROE and J. GILMARTIN: Hyposmolar urine formation during plasma hyperosmolality. Fed. Proc. 19, 360 (1960) (abstract). — BRICKER, N. S., R. R. DEWEY, H. LUBOWITZ, J. STOKES and T. KIRKENSGAARD: Observations on the concentrating and diluting mechanisms of the diseased kidney. J. clin. Invest. 38, 516 (1959). — BRICKER, N. S., W. R. GUILD, J. B. REARDAN and J. P. MERRILL: Studies on the functional capacity of a denervated homotransplanted kidney in an identical twin with parallel observations in the donor. J. clin. Invest. 35, 1364 (1956). — BRICKER, N. S., and C. J. HLAD jr.: Observations on the mechanism of the renal clearance of I^{131}. J. clin. Invest. 34, 1057 (1955). — BRICKER, N. S., E. I. SHWAYRI, J. B. REARDAN, D. KELLOG, J. P. MERRILL and J. H. HOLMES: An abnormality in renal function resulting from urinary tract obstruction. Amer. J. Med. 23, 554 (1957). — BRICKER, N. S., R. A. STRAFFON, E. P. MAHONEY and J. P. MERRILL: The functional capacity of the kidney denervated by autotransplantation in the dog. J. clin. Invest. 37, 185 (1958). — BRICKER, N. S., and L. G. WESSON jr.: Plasma electrolyte concentrations in ambulatory cardiac patients. Circulation 7, 687 (1953). — BRIGGS, A. P.: Excretion of ammonia and neutrality regulation. J. biol. Chem. 104, 231 (1934). — BROADHURST, H. C.: The excretion of phosphoric acid in the urine. J. Physiol. (Lond.) 54, P28 (1920) (abstract). — BROD, J., and Z. FEJFAR: The origin of oedema in heart failure. Quart. J. Med. 19, 187 (1950). — BROD, J., Z. FEJFAR and M. H. FEJFAROVA: The role of neurohumoral factors in the genesis of renal hemodynamic changes in heart failure. Acta med. scand. 148, 273 (1954). — BROD, J., and V. FENCL: Diurnal variations of systemic and renal haemodynamics in normal subjects and in hypertensive disease. Cardiologia (Basel) 31, 494 (1957). — BROD, J., and J. H. SIROTA: The renal clearance of endogenous "creatinine" in man. J. clin. Invest. 27, 645 (1948). — BRODIE, T. G.: A new conception of glomerular function. Proc. roy. Soc. B 87, 571 (1913). — BRODIE, T. G., and J. J. MACKENZIE: On changes in the glomeruli and tubules of the kidney accompanying activity. Proc. roy. Soc. B 87, 593 (1914). — BRODSKY, W. A.: Regulation of urine flow and solute excretion during acute acidosis induced by loading with strong mineral acids in hydropenic dogs. Amer. J. Physiol. 181, 616 (1955). — BRODSKY, W. A., and H. N. GRAUBARTH: Excretion of water and electrolytes in patients with essential hypertension. J. Lab. clin. Med. 41, 43 (1953a). — Mechanism of mercurial diuresis in hydropenic dogs. Amer. J. Physiol. 172, 67 (1953b). — BRODSKY, W. A., J. T. KAIM and G. CARRASQUER: The nature of urinary acidification process during transient obstruction of renal artery and ureter. J. clin. Invest. 38, 991 (1959) (abstract). — BRODSKY, W. A., J. F. MILEY, J. T. KAIM and N. P. SHAH: Characteristics of acidic urine after loading with weak organic acids in dogs. Current concepts on renal mechanisms of acidification in relation to data on CO_2 tension. Amer. J. Physiol.

193, 108 (1958). — BRODSKY, W. A., and S. RAPOPORT: The mechanism of polyuria of diabetes insipidus in man. The effect of osmotic loading. J. clin. Invest. **30**, 282 (1951). — BRODSKY, W. A., S. RAPOPORT, H. N. GRAUBARTH and A. H. LEVKOFF: Osmotic diuresis as a measurement of renal function in man. J. appl. Physiol. **5**, 62 (1952). — BRODSKY, W. A., S. RAPOPORT and C. D. WEST: The mechanism of glycosuric diuresis in diabetic man. J. clin. Invest. **29**, 1021 (1950). — BRODSKY, W. A., and R. SATRAN: Comparison of effects of acidosis and alkalosis on the renal action of diamox. Amer. J. Physiol. **197**, 585 (1959). — BRODY, T. M., and J. A. BAIN: Effect of barbiturates on oxidative phosphorylation. Proc. Soc. exp. Biol. (N.Y.) **77**, 50 (1951). — BRONSKY, D., A. DUBIN and D. S. KUSHNER: Diuretic action of benemid. Its effect upon the urinary excretion of sodium, chloride, potassium and water in edematous subjects. Amer. J. Med. **18**, 259 (1955). — BRONSKY, D., D. KUSHNER and A. DUBIN: Effect of phosphaturic agents on renal excretion of urate and electrolytes in hyperuricemic subjects. Clin. Res. Proc. **3**, 135 (1955) (abstract). — BROOKS, F. P., and MARY PICKFORD: The effect of posterior dituitary hormones on the excretion of electrolytes in dogs. J. Physiol. (Lond.) **142**, 468 (1958). — BRUCK, ERIKA: Renal function in anemia. J. Dis. Child. **86**, 511 (1953). — BRUCK, ERIKA, M. RAPOPORT and M. I. RUBIN: Renal functions in the course of the nephrotic syndrome in children. J. clin. Invest. **33**, 699 (1954). — BRULL, L., et G. CARBONESCO: L'action de la parathyroide sur le rein. C. R. Soc. Biol. (Paris) **131**, 800 (1939). — BRULL, L., and Y. CUYPERS: Blood perfusion of the kidney of *Lophius piscatorius* L. IV. Magnesium excretion. J. Mar. biol. Assoc. U. Kingd. **34**, 637 (1955). — BRULL, L., et D. LOUIS-BAR: Énervation anatomique et énervation pharmacologique du rein. Arch. int. Physiol. **62**, 140 (1954). — BRULL, L., D. LOUIS-BAR and H. LYBECK: The action of chronic denervation and of the use of a gangliopleqic or a sympatholytic agent on the baresthetic device of the renal arteries. Acta physiol. scand. **34**, 175 (1955). — BRUN, C.: Thiosulfate as a measure of the glomerular filtration rate in normal and diseased human kidneys. Acta med. scand. Suppl. **234**, 63 (1949). — BRUN, C., C. CRONE, H. G. DAVIDSEN, J. FABRICIUS, A. T. HANSEN, N. A. LASSEN and O. MUNCK: Renal blood flow in anuric human subject determined by use of radioactive krypton 85. Proc. Soc. exp. Biol. (N.Y.) **89**, 687 (1955). — Renal interstitital pressure in normal and in anuric man: Based on wedged renal vein pressure. Proc. Soc. exp. Biol. (N.Y.) **91**, 199 (1956). — BRUN, C., H. GORMSEN, T. HILDEN, P. IVERSEN and F. RAASCHOU: Diabetic nephropathy. Kidney biopsy and renal function tests. Amer. J. Med. **15**, 187 (1953). — BRUN, C., T. HILDEN and F. RAASCHOU: On the effects of mersalyl on the renal function. Acta pharmacol. (Kbh.) **3**, 1 (1947a). — Maximum tubular excretion of diodrast in normal human kidney. Acta med. scand. **127**, 464 (1947b). — On excretion of p-aminohippuric acid through kidneys. Acta med. scand. **127**, 471 (1947c). — Para-aminohippursyre. Et middel til bestemmelse af nyrernes plasmagennemstrømning og af den maximale, tubulaere secretion. Nord. méd. **34**, 803 (1947d). — The significance of the difference in systemic arterial and venous plasma concentrations in renal clearance methods. J. clin. Invest. **28**, 144 (1949). — BRUN, C., E. O. E. KNUDSEN and F. RAASCHOU: Influence of posture on kidney function; fall of diuresis in erect posture. Acta med. scand. **122**, 315 (1945). — Influence of posture on kidney function; glomerular dynamics in passive erect posture. Acta med. scand. **122**, 332 (1945a). — Post-syncopal oliguria. Kidney function and circulatory collapse. Acta med. scand. **122**, 381 (1945b). — On cause of post-syncopal oliguria. Acta med. scand. **122**, 486 (1945c). — Kidney function and circulatory collapse; post-syncopal oliguria. J. clin. Invest. **25**, 568 (1946). — BRUNNER, H., G. KUSCHINSKY, O. MÜNCHOW u. G. PETERS: Der Einfluß von natürlichem und synthetischem Oxytocin auf endogene Kreatinin-Clearance, Salzausscheidung und Säureausscheidungsfähigkeit der Ratte und auf die Diurese des Menschen. Naunyn-Schmiedeberg's Arch. exp. Path. Pharmak. **230**, 80 (1957). — BRUNNER, H., G. KUSCHINSKY u. G. PETERS: Die Wirkung von Vasopressin auf die renale Wasser- und Salzausscheidung der Ratte bei Veränderungen der Salzkonzentration des Trinkwassers und nach Nierenparenchymresektionen. Naunyn-Schmiedeberg's Arch. exp. Path. Pharmak. **228**, 434 (1956a). — Der Einfluß von Oxytocin auf renale Wasser- und Salzausscheidung der Ratte. Naunyn-Schmiedeberg's Arch. exp. Path. Pharmak. **228**, 457 (1956b). — BRUNTON, C. E.: The acid output of the kidney and the socalled alkaline tide. Physiol. Rev. **13**, 372 (1933). — BRYNER, S., W. H. CLARK, ELIZABETH RANDALL and L. A. RANTZ: Renal tubular excretory capacity for penicillin in health and in subacute bacterial endocarditis. Amer. J. Med. **5**, 202 (1948). — BRYNER, S., ELIZABETH RANDALL and L. A. RANTZ: Penicillin clearance as a test of renal function, using potassium penicillin in beeswax and peanut oil. Stanford med. Bull. **6**, 411 (1948). — BUCHBORN, E.: Ein quantitativer biologischer Adiuretin-(Vasopressin-)Nachweis an der Kröte. Z. ges. exp. Med. **125**, 614 (1955). — Plasma level of antidiuretic hormone and serum osmolarity in normal human adults. Endocrinology **61**, 375 (1957). — BUCHBORN, E., K. R. KOCZOREK u. H. P. WOLFF: Aldosteron, Glomerulusfiltrat und Natriumretention. Klin. Wschr. **37**, 71 (1959). — BUCHT, H.: On the tubular excretion of thiosulphate and creatinine under the influence of caronamide. Scand. J. clin. Lab. Invest. **1**, 270 (1949). — Studies on renal function in man with special reference to glomerular filtration and renal plasma flow in pregnancy. Scand. J. clin. Lab. Invest. **3**, Suppl. 3 (1951). — BUCHT, H., J. EK, H. ELIASCH, A. HOLMGREN, B. JOSEPHSON and L. WERKO: The effect of exercise in the recumbent position on the renal circulation and sodium excretion in normal individuals. Acta physiol. scand. **28**, 95 (1953). — BUCHT, H., J. EK, B. JOSEPHSON, B. THOMASSON, E. VARNAUSKAS and L. WERKO: Rapid infusion and renal function. Clin. Sci. **15**, 617 (1956). — BUCHT, H., L. WERKO and B. JOSEPHSON: The oxygen consumption of the human kidney during heavy tubular excretory work. Scand. J. clin. Lab. Invest. **1**, 277 (1949). — BUCKLEY, NANCY M., D. G. VIDT and L. A. SAPIRSTEIN: Renal clearance of para-amino salicylic acid in the dog. Proc. Soc. exp. Biol. (N.Y.) **90**, 10 (1955). — BUCKNER, B., and J. E. NELLOR: Parathormone-like activity in the sera of rats with induced hyperparathyroidism. Fed. Proc. **19**, 150 (1960) (abstract). — BÜHLMANN, A., A. LABHART, H. J. HOLTMEIER u. O. SPÜHLER: Verschiebungen im Elektrolyt- und Säure-Basen-Gleichgewicht beim Menschen unter Carboanhydrase-Hemmung. Helv. med. Acta **20**, 323 (1953). — BULL, G. M.: Body water control. Lectures on the Scientific Basis of Medicine **3**, 219 (1953). — BUNGE, G.: Lehrbuch der physiologischen und pathologischen Chemie. Leipzig: F. C. W. Vogel 1894. — Text-book of physiological and pathological chemistry. Philadelphia: P. Blakistons Son & Co. 1902. — BUNGE, G., u. O. SCHMIEDEBERG: Über die Bildung der Hippursäure. Naunyn-Schmiedeberg's Arch. exp. Path. Pharmak. **6**, 233 (1877). — BUNIM, J. J., W. W. SMITH and H. W. SMITH: The diffusion coefficient of inulin and other substances of interest in renal physiology. J. biol. Chem. **118**, 667 (1937). — BURG, M., and J. ORLOFF: The effect of strophanthidin on electrolyte transport in slices of rabbit renal cortex. Fed. Proc. **18**, 20 (1959) (abstract). — BURGEN, A. S. V.: A theoretical treatment of glucose reabsorption in the kidney. Canad. J. Biochem. **34**, 466 (1956). — BURGESS, W. W., A. M. HARVEY and E. K. MARSHALL: The site of the antidiuretic action of pituitary extract. J. Pharmacol. exp. Ther. **49**, 237 (1933). — BURN, J. H., L. H. TRUELOVE and I. BURN: Antidiuretic action of nicotine and of smoking. Brit. med. J. **1945 I**, 403. — BURNETT, C. H.: Actions of ACTH and cortisone on renal function in man. Trans. Conf. on Renal Function Josiah Macy, Jr. Found., N.Y., p. 106, 1950. — BURNETT, C. H., ESTHER L. BLOOMBERG, G. SHORTZ, D. W. COMPTON and H. K. BEECHER: A comparison of the effects of ether and cyclopropane anesthesia on the renal function of man. J. Pharmacol. exp. Ther. **96**, 380 (1949). — BURNETT, C. H., B. A. BURROWS and R. R. COMMONS: The lack of correlation between glomerular filtration rate, and serum electrolyte concentration changes, urinary electrolyte excretion or edema formation following sodium loads in subjects with normal kidneys, glomerulonephritis, and the nephrotic syndrome. J. clin. Invest. **28**, 773 (1949) (abstract). — BURNETT, C. H., D. W. SELDIN and M. WALSER: Observations on the electrolyte and water metabolism in Addison's disease during oral salt loading. Trans. Ass. Amer. Phycns **66**, 65 (1953). — BURNS, J. J., T. F. YÜ, A. RITTERBAND, J. M. PEREL, A. B. GUTMAN and B. B. BRODIE: A potent new uricosuric agent, the sulfoxide metabolite of the phenylbutazone analogue, G-25671. J. Pharmacol. exp. Ther. **119**, 418 (1957). — BURRILL, M. W., S. FREEMAN and A. C. IVY: Sodium, potassium, and chloride excretion of human subjects exposed to simulated altitude of 18,000 feet. J. biol. Chem. **157**, 297 (1945). — BURSTON, R. A., and O. GARROD: The variability of the lowered glomerular filtration rate in Addison's disease and panhypopituitarism, and the effect of cortisone thereon. Clin. Sci. **2**, 129 (1952). — BUTTURINI, U., u. V. BONOMINI: Über die Wirkung von Glukagon und Insulin auf Nierenfunktion, Harnausscheidung der Phosphat-, Bicarbonat- und Ammoniakionen und titrierbarer Acidität beim Menschen. Helv. med. Acta **25**, 617 (1958). — BYKOW, K. M., u. I. A. ALEXEJEW-BERKMANN: Die Ausbildung bedingter Reflexe auf die Harnausscheidung. II. Bedingte Reflexe bei denervierte Niere. Pflügers Arch. ges. Physiol. **227**, 301 (1931).

CADE, J. R., R. J. SHALHOUB and M. L. CANESSA: Effect of strophanthidin on transport mechanisms of the renal tubule. Fed. Proc. **19**, 370 (1960) (abstract). — CAFRUNY, E. J., and A. FARAH: Effects of the mercurial diuretic, mersalyl, on the concentration of protein-bound sulfhydryl in the cytoplasm of dog kidney cells. J. Pharmacol. exp. Ther. **117**, 101 (1956). — CAFRUNY, E. J., and C. ROSS: Effects of 2,4-dinitrophenol on renal binding and excretion of mercurial compounds. Fed. Proc. **19**, 361 (1960) (abstract). — CALDWELL, F. T., DORIS ROLF and H. L. WHITE: Effects of acute hypoxia on renal circulation in man. J. appl. Physiol. **1**, 597 (1948). — CALDWELL, P. C.: Intracellular pH. Int. Rev. Cytol. **5**, 229 (1956). — CAMERON, GLADYS, and R. CHAMBERS: Direct evidence of function in kidney of an early human fetus. Amer. J. Physiol. **123**, 482 (1938). — CAMP, J. L.: Effect of posture on salt and water retention. II. Appearance of a circulating vasoconstrictor substance in the blood on assuming the erect position. J. Lab. clin. Med. **52**, 202 (1958). — CAMPBELL, D.: Excretion and diuretic action of mercurial diuretics. Experientia (Basel) **13**, 327 (1957). — CAMPBELL, D. E. S.: The excretion of mercaptomerin and its diuretic effect modified by bromcresol green and probenecid. Acta pharmacol. (Kbh.) **16**, 151 (1959). — CAMPBELL, J. A.: Ammonia excretion, amino acid excretion and the alkaline tide in Singapore. Biochem.

J. **14**, 603 (1920). — CAMPBELL, J. A., and T. A. WEBSTER: Day and night urine during complete rest, laboratory routine, light muscular work and oxygen administration. Biochem. J. **15**, 660 (1921). — Note on urinary tides and excretory rhythm. Biochem. J. **16**, 507 (1922). — CANNAN, R. K., and AGNES SHORE: The creatine-creatinine equilibrium. The apparent dissociation constants of creatine and creatinine. Biochem. J. **22**, 920 (1928). — CANNON, J. F.: Diabetes insipidus. Clinical and experimental studies with consideration of genetic relationships. Arch. intern. Med. **96**, 215 (1955). — CANNON, W. B.: The wisdom of the body. New York: W. W. Norton & Co. 1932. — CAPECI, N. E., O. R. KRUESI, D. C. WEAVER and J. G. HILTON: Effect of diamox (acetazoleamide) on the carbon dioxide tension of the urine. Amer. J. Physiol. **191**, 55 (1957). — CAPPS, J. N., W. S. WIGGINS, D. R. AXELROD and R. F. PITTS: The effect of mercurial diuretics on the excretion of water. Circulation **6**, 82 (1952). — CARGILL, W. H.: Effect of the intravenous administration of human serum albumin on renal function. Proc. Soc. exp. Biol. (N.Y.) **68**, 189 (1948). — The measurement of glomerular and tubular plasma flow in the normal and diseased human kidney. J. clin. Invest. **28**, 533 (1949). — Factors influencing excretion of chloride. Fed. Proc. **11**, 22 (1952) (abstract). — CARLSON, C. H., W. D. ARMSTRONG, L. SINGER and L. B. HINSHAW: Renal excretion of radiofluoride in the dog. Amer. J. Physiol. **198**, 829 (1960). — CARONE, F. A., F. H. EPSTEIN, D. BECK and H. LEVITIN: The effects upon the kidney of transient hypercalcemia induced by parathyroid extract. Amer. J. Path. **36**, 77 (1960). — CARPENTER, C. C. J., J. HOLMAN, C. R. AYERS and J. O. DAVIS: Experimental ascites with marked sodium retention after transplant of the left kidney to the neck and right nephrectomy. Fed. Proc. **19**, 365 (1960) (abstract). — CARR, A. D.: The effect of water diuresis on the elimination of certain urinary constituents. J. Pharmacol. exp. Ther. **18**, 221 (1921). — CARRASQUER, G., and W. A. BRODSKY: Transient secretion of phosphate in the mammalian kidney. Proc. Soc. exp. Biol. (N.Y.) **101**, 477 (1959). — CARTER, ANNE C., and J. ROBBINS: Use of hypertonic saline infusions in differential diagnosis of diabetes insipidus and psychogenic polydipsia. J. clin. Endocr. **7**, 753 (1947). — CARTER, N. W., F. C. RECTOR jr. and D. W. SELDIN: Pathogenesis of persistent hyponatremia with water retention in cerebral disease. Clin. Res. **7**, 273 (1959) (abstract). — CARTER, N. W., D. W. SELDIN and H. C. TENG: Tissue and renal response to chronic respiratory acidosis. J. clin. Invest. **38**, 949 (1959). — CARVALHO, A. A. M. S. DE: Estudo comparativo dos glomerulos corticais e justamedulares no rim do coelho. Folia anat. (Coimbra) **32**, 1 (1957). — CASENTINI, S., A. DE POLI, S. HUKOVIC and L. MARTINI: Studies on the control of corticotrophin release. Endocrinology **64**, 483 (1959). — CASEY, J. H., E. Y. BICKEL and B. ZIMMERMANN: The pattern and significance of aldosterone excretion by the postoperative surgical patient. Surg. Gynec. Obstet. **105**, 179 (1957). — CASTEX, M. R., A. BIASOTTI and A. PATALANO: La reabsorcion tubular de glucosa en la diabetes renal. Rev. Soc. argent. Biol. **18**, 351 (1942). — CATES, J. E., and O. GARROD: The effect of nicotine on urinary flow in diabetes insipidus. Clin. Sci. **10**, 145 (1951). — CATHCART, E. S., and I. T. D. WILLIAMS: The effect of the headdown position on the excretion of certain urinary constituents. Clin. Sci. **14**, 121 (1955). — CHAIT, A., and P. B. CAMPONOVO: Glomerular filtration during the application of torniquetes of limbs. Effects chemical denervation of the renal artery. Rev. Soc. argent. Biol. **29**, 66 (1953). — CHALMERS, J. H., R. W. CRANSTON, H. L. TAYLOR and A. KEYS: Effect of a psychiatric interview on renal plasma flow and finger skin temperature. Fed. Proc. **8**, 23 (1949) (abstract). — CHALMERS, T. M., and A. A. G. LEWIS: Stimulation of the supraoptico-hypophysial system in man. Clin. Sci. **10**, 127 (1951a). — The effect of adrenocorticotropic hormone on the diuretic response to water in panhypopituitarism. Lancet **1951**IIb, 1158. — CHALMERS, T. M., A. A. G. LEWIS and G. L. S. PAWAN: The effect of posterior pituitary extracts on the renal excretion of sodium and chloride in man. J. Physiol. (Lond.) **112**, 238 (1951). — CHAMBERS, G. H.: Changes in the rat's posterior pituitary following sodium chloride administration. Anat. Rec. **92**, 391 (1945). — CHAMBERS, R., L. V. BECK and M. BELKIN: Secretion in tissue cultures. I. Inhibition of phenol red accumulation in the chick kidney. J. cell. comp. Physiol. **6**, 425 (1935). — CHAMBERS, R., and GLADYS CAMERON: Intracellular hydrion concentration studies. VII. The secreting cells of the mesonephros in the chick. J. cell. comp. Physiol. **2**, 99 (1932). — CHAMBERS, R., and R. T. KEMPTON: Indications of function of the chick mesonephros in tissue culture with phenol red. J. cell. comp. Physiol. **3**, 131 (1933). — The elimination of neutral red by the frog's kidney. J. cell. comp. Physiol. **10**, 199 (1937). — CHANG, H.-Y.: Grafts of parathyroid and other tissues to bone. Anat. Rec. **111**, 23 (1951). — CHAPMAN, C. B., A. HENSCHEL and A. FORSGREN: Renal plasma flow during moderate exercise of several hours' duration in normal male subjects. Proc. Soc. exp. Biol. (N.Y.) **69**, 170 (1948). — CHAPMAN, C. B., A. HENSCHEL, J. MINCKLER, A. FORSGREN and A. KEYS: The effect of exercise on renal plasma flow in normal male subjects. J. clin. Invest. **27**, 643 (1948). — CHAPMAN, D. W., and S. A. PEOPLES: Sulfathiazole as a substitute for inulin in determining the glomerular filtration rate. J. clin. Invest. **26**, 1177 (1947) (abstract). — CHAPMAN, E. M., and J. A. HALSTEAD: The fractional phenolsulfonephthalein test in Bright's diesease. Amer. J. med. Sci. 186, 223 (1933). — CHART, J. J., and E. S. SHIPLEY: The mechanism of sodium retention in cirrhosis of the liver. J. clin. Invest. 32, 560 (1953) (abstract). — CHASIS, H., W. GOLDRING, E. S. BREED, G. E. SCHREINER and A. A. BOLOMEY: Salt and protein restriction: Effects on blood pressure and renal hemodynamics in hypertensive patients. J. Amer. med. Ass. 142, 711 (1950). — CHASIS, H., N. JOLLIFFE and H. W. SMITH: The action of phlorizin on the excretion of glucose, xylose, sucrose, creatinine and urea by man. J. clin. Invest. 12, 1083 (1933). — CHASIS, H., H. A. RANGES, W. GOLDRING and H. W. SMITH: The control of renal blood flow and glomerular filtration in normal man. J. clin. Invest. 17, 683 (1938). — CHASIS, H., and J. REDISH: Effective renal blood flow in separate kidneys of subjects with essential hypertension. J. clin. Invest. 20, 655 (1941). — CHASIS, H., J. REDISH, W. GOLDRING, H. A. RANGES and H. W. SMITH: Use of sodium p-aminohippurate for functional evaluation of human kidney. J. clin. Invest. 24, 583 (1945). — CHASIS, H., and H. W. SMITH: The excretion of urea in normal man and in subjects with glomerulonephritis. J. clin. Invest. 17, 347 (1938). — CHEEK, D. B.: Hyponatremia and central nervous system disease. Med. J. Aust. 44, 649 (1957). — CHEEK, D. B., and D. C. WEST: Effect of desoxycorticosterone on distribution of water and on electrolyte excretion during enforced hydration in the dog and rat. Amer. J. Physiol. 184, 69 (1956). — CHEN jr., P. S., and W. F. NEUMAN: Renal excretion of calcium by the dog. Amer. J. Physiol. 180, 623 (1955a). — Renal reabsorption of calcium through its inhibition by various chemical agents. Amer. J. Physiol. 180, 632 (1955b). — CHESLEY, L. C.: The validity of the calculation of standard urea clearances from low urine flows. J. clin. Invest. 16, 653 (1937). — CHESLEY, L. C., and E. R. CHESLEY: Diodrast clearance and renal blood flow in normal pregnant and non-pregnant women. Amer. J. Physiol. 127, 731 (1939). — CHESLEY, L. C., E. J. CONNELL, E. R. CHESLEY, J. D. KATZ and C. S. GLISSEN: Diodrast clearance and renal blood flow in toxemias of pregnancy. J. clin. Invest. 19, 219 (1940). — CHESLEY, L. C., and I. TEPPER: Some effects of magnesium loading upon renal excretion of magnesium and certain other electrolytes. J. clin. Invest. 37, 1362 (1958). — CHESLEY, L. C., C. VALENTI and H. REIN: Excretion of sodium loads by nonpregnant and pregnant normal, hypertensive and pre-eclamptic women. Metabolism 7, 575 (1958). — CHESLEY, L. C., and L. O. WILLIAMS: Renal glomerular and tubular function in relation to the hyperuricemia of pre-eclampsia and eclampsia. Amer. J. Obstet. Gynec. 50, 367 (1945). — CHIARINI, P.: Meccanismi di compenso renale in corso di policitemia, in riferimento all'osservazione personale di un caso. Minerva nefrol. (Torino) 4, 23 (1957). — CHILDS, A. W., H. O. WHEELER, B. COMINSKY, E. LEIFER, O. L. WADE and S. E. BRADLEY: The distribution of "nephron delay time" in normal man. J. clin. Invest. 34, 926 (1955) (abstract). — CHILDS jr., D. S., F. R. KEATING jr., J. E. RALL, M. M. D. WILLIAMS and MARSCHELLE H. POWER: The effect of varying quantities of inorganic iodide (carrier) on the urinary excretion and thyroidal accumulation of radioiodine in exophthalmic goiter. J. clin. Invest. 29, 726 (1950). — CHINARD, F. P.: Derivation of an expression for the rate of formation of glomerular fluid (GFR). Applicability of certain physical and physicochemical concepts. Amer. J. Physiol. 171, 578 (1952). — CHINARD, F. P., and T. ENNS: Relative renal excretion patterns of sodium ion, chloride ion, urea, water and glomerular substances. Amer. J. Physiol. 182, 247 (1955). — CHINARD, F. P., H. D. LAUSON, H. A. EDER, R. L. GREIF and ALMA HILLER: A study of the mechanism of proteinuria in patients with the nephrotic syndrome. J. clin. Invest. 33, 621 (1954). — CHINARD, F. P., W. R. TAYLOR, MARY F. NOLAN and T. ENNS: Transport of glucose by the renal tubule cells of anesthetized dogs. Science 125, 736 (1957). — Renal handling of glucose in dogs. Amer. J. Physiol. 196, 535 (1959). — CHINARD, F. P., G. J. VOSBURGH and T. ENNS: Transcapillary exchange of water and of other substances in certain organs of the dog. Amer. J. Physiol. 183, 221 (1955). — CHRISTENSEN, P. J.: Tubular reabsorption of glucose during pregnancy. Scand. J. clin. Lab. Invest. 10, 364 (1958). — CHRISTENSEN, P. J., and O. R. STEENSTRUP: Uric acid excretion with increasing plasma glucose concentration (pregnant and non-pregnant cases). Scand. J. clin. Lab. Invest. 10, 182 (1958). — CHRISTIAN, H. A., and E. A. BARTRAM: Experimental observations on the action of diuretics. Trans. Ass. Amer. Phycns 47, 292 (1932). — CHROMETZKA, F., u. K. UNGER: Untersuchungen über die Größe des Glomerulusfiltrats unter dem Einfluß von Diureticis und Hormonen. Z. ges. exp. Med. 80, 261 (1931). — CHURCHILL-DAVIDSON, H. C., and W. D. WYLIE: The effects of adrenaline, noradrenaline and methedrine on the renal circulation during anesthesia. Lancet 1951 II, 803. — CIZEK, L. J., R. E. SEMPLE, K. C. HUANG and M. I. GREGERSEN: Effect of extracellular electrolyte depletion on water intake in dogs. Amer. J. Physiol. 164, 415 (1951). — CLARK, G. A.: Glucose absorption in the renal tubules of the frog. J. Physiol. (Lond.) 56, 201 (1922). — CLARK, J. K., and H. G. BARKER: Studies in renal oxygen consumption in man. I. The effect of tubular loading (PAH), water diuresis and osmotic (mannitol) diuresis. J. clin. Invest. 30, 745 (1951). — CLARKE, E., BARBARA M. EVANS, I. MACINTYRE and M. D. MILNE: Acidosis in experimental electrolyte depletion. Clin. Sci. 14, 421 (1955). — CLARKE, R. W., and H. W. SMITH: Absorption and excretion of water and salts by the Elasmobranch fishes. III. The use of xylose as a measure of the glomerular filtrate in *Squalus acanthias*. J. cell. comp. Physiol. **1**, 131 (1932). — COHEN, J. J., F. BERGLUND and W. D. LOTSPEICH: Renal tubular reabsorption of acetoacetate, inorganic sulfate, and inorganic phosphate in the dog as affected by glucose and phlorizin. Amer. J. Physiol. **184**, 91 (1956). — Interrelations during renal tubular reabsorption in the dog among several anions showing a sensitivity to glucose and phlorizin. Amer. J. Physiol. **189**, 331 (1957). — COLE, D. F.: Effect of aldosterone on renal excretion of intravenously administered saline. Endocrinology **60**, 562 (1957). — COLEBATCH, H. J. H.: The mechanism of fluid retention in heart failure. Med. J. Aust. **43**, 1087 (1956). — COLLER, F. A., V. L. REES, K. N. CAMPBELL, VIVIAN L. IOB and C. A. MOYER: Effects of ether and cyclopropane anesthesia upon renal function in man. Ann. Surg. **118**, 717 (1943). — COLLINGS, W. D., and H. G. SWANN: Blood and interstitial spaces of the functional kidney. Fed. Proc. **17**, 28 (1958) (abstract). — COLLIP, J. B.: A study of parathyroidectomized rabbits. Amer. J. Physiol. **76**, 219 (1926) (abstract). — CONN, J. W., and L. H. LOUIS: Primary aldosteronism, a new clinical entity. Ann. intern. Med. **44**, 1 (1956). — CONWAY, E. J., and O. FITZGERALD: Diffusion relations of urea, inulin and chloride in some mammalian tissues. J. Physiol. (Lond.) **101**, 86 (1942). — CONWAY, E. J., and F. KANE: Diffusion equilibria for the isolated frog's kidney. II. Urea. Biochem. J. **29**, 1446 (1935). — COOMBS, F. S., L. J. PECORA, ELIZABETH THOROGOOD, W. V. CONSOLAZIO and J. H. TALBOTT: Renal function in patients with gout. J. clin. Invest. **19**, 525 (1940). — COOPER, A. M., R. D. ECKHARDT, W. W. FALOON and C. S. DAVIDSON: Investigation of the aminoaciduria in Wilson's disease (hepatolenticular degeneration). Demonstration of a defect in renal function. J. clin. Invest. **29**, 265 (1950). — COPE, C. L.: The excretion of non-metabolized sugars by the mammalian kidney. J. Physiol. (Lond.) **80**, 238 (1934). — COPENHAVER jr., J. H., and R. P. FORSTER: Displacement characteristics of intracellularly accumulated p-aminohippurate in a mammalian renal transport system *in vitro*. Amer. J. Physiol. **195**, 327 (1958). — CORA, D., F. ABRIGNANI e S. DEBIASI: Influenza della 5-idrossitriptamina sulla diuresi. Studio clinico-sperimentale mediante le clearances renale. Minerva nefrol. (Torino) **4**, 21 (1957). — CORCORAN, A. C., J. S. BROWNING and I. H. PAGE: Renal hemodynamics in orthostatic hypotension; effects of angiotonin and head-up bed. J. Amer. med. Ass. **119**, 793 (1942). — CORCORAN, A. C., K. G. KOHLSTAEDT and I. H. PAGE: Changes of arterial blood pressure and renal hemodynamics by injection of angiotonin in human beings. Proc. Soc. exp. Biol. (N.Y.) **46**, 244 (1941). — CORCORAN, A. C., G. MASSON, RUTH REUTING and I. H. PAGE: Measurement of renal functions in rats. Amer. J. Physiol. **154**, 170 (1948). — CORCORAN, A. C., and I. H. PAGE: Effects of renin, pitressin, and pitressin and atropine on renal blood flow and clearance. Amer. J. Physiol. **126**, 354 (1939). — Applications of diphenylamine in the determination of levulose in biological media. I. The determination of inulin. II. The determination of levulose in small amounts of blood. J. biol. Chem. **127**, 601 (1939a). — Effects of angiotonin on renal blood flow and glomerular filtration. Amer. J. Physiol. **130**, 335 (1940). — Renal function in late toxemia of pregnancy. Amer. J. med. Sci. **201**, 385 (1941a). — Renal blood flow and sympathectomy in hypertension. Arch. Surg. (Chicago) **42**, 1072 (1941b). — Renal aspects of experimental and clinical hypertension. J. Lab. clin. Med. **26**, 1713 (1941c). — Renal blood flow in experimental renal hypertension. Amer. J. Physiol. **135**, 361 (1942). — Effects of anesthetic dosage of pentobarbital sodium on renal function and blood pressure in dogs. Amer. J. Physiol. **140**, 234 (1943a). — Effects of hypotension due to hemorrhage and of blood transfusion on renal function in dogs. J. exp. Med. **78**, 205 (1943b). — Specific renal functions in hyperthyroidism and myxedema. Effects of treatment. J. clin. Endocr. **7**, 801 (1947). — A method for the determination of mannitol in plasma and urine. J. biol. Chem. **170**, 165 (1947a). — CORCORAN, A. C., H. W. SMITH and I. H. PAGE: Removal of diodrast from blood by dog's explanted kidney. Amer. J. Physiol. **134**, 333 (1941). — CORCORAN, A. C., R. D. TAYLOR and I. H. PAGE: Immediate effects on renal function of the onset of shock due to partially occluding limb tourniquets. Ann. Surg. **118**, 871 (1943). — Circulatory responses to spinal and caudal anesthesia in hypertension; relation to effect of sympathectomy. II. Effect on renal function. J. Lab. clin. Med. **32**, 1421 (1947). — Functional patterns in renal disease. Ann. intern. Med. **28**, 560 (1948). — COREY, E. L., and S. W. BRITTON: Antagonistic action of desoxycorticosterone and post-pituitary extract on chloride and water balance. Amer. J. Physiol. **133**, 511 (1941). — CORT, J. H.: Cerebral salt wasting. Lancet **1954 I**, 752. — COTLOVE, E.: Heterogeneity of inulin: chemical, physical and physiologic aspects. Fed. Proc. **13**, 30 (1954) (abstract). — C^{14} carboxyl-labeled inulin as a tracer for inulin. Fed. Proc. **14**, 32 (1955) (abstract). — COTTIER, P. T., J. M. WELLER and S. W. HOOBLER: Effect of an intravenous sodium chloride load on renal hemodynamics and electrolyte excretion in essential hypertension. Circulation **17**, 750 (1958a). — Sodium chloride excretion following salt loading in hypertensive subjects. Circulation **18**, 196 (1958b). — Co TUI, M., H. SCHRIFT, K. L. MCCLOSKEY and A. L. YATES: Filtration studies on pyrogenic inulin. Proc. Soc. exp.

Biol. (N.Y.) **36**, 227 (1937). — COULSON, R. A., and T. HERNANDEZ: Renal excretion of CO_2 and ammonia by the alligator. Proc. Soc. exp. Biol. (N.Y.) **88**, 682 (1955). — Role of carbonic anhydrase in anion excretion in the alligator. Amer. J. Physiol. **188**, 121 (1957). — COUNIHAN, T. B., B. M. EVANS and M. D. MILNE: Observations on the pharmacology of the carbonic anhydrase inhibitor "Diamox". Clin. Sci. **13**, 583 (1954). — CRABBÉ, J., and G. NICHOLS jr.: Effects of adrenalectomy and aldosterone on sodium concentration in renal medulla of hydropenic rats. Proc. Soc. exp. Biol. (N.Y.) **101**, 168 (1959). — CRABBÉ, J., W. T. REDDY, E. J. ROSS and G. W. THORN: The stimulation of aldosterone secretion by adrenocorticotropic hormone (ACTH). J. clin. Endocr. **19**, 1185 (1959). — CRABBÉ, J., E. J. ROSS and G. W. THORN: The significance of the secretion of aldosterone during dietary sodium deprivation in normal subjects. J. clin. Endocr. **18**, 1159 (1958). — CRAIG, F. N.: Renal tubular reabsorption, metabolic utilization, and isomeric fractionation of lactic acid in the dog. Amer. J. Physiol. **146**, 146 (1946). — CRAIG, F. N., F. E. VISSCHER and C. R. HOUCK: Renal function in dogs under ether or cyclopropane anesthesia. Amer. J. Physiol. **143**, 108 (1945). — CRAIG, J. W., M. MILLER, J. E. OWENS and H. WOODWARD jr.: Renal malic acid metabolism *in vivo*. Fed. Proc. **12**, 29 (1953) (abstract). — CRANE, M. M.: Observations on the function of the frog's kidney. Amer. J. Physiol. **81**, 232 (1927). — CRANE, R. K., R. A. FIELD and C. F. CORI: Studies of tissue permeability. I. The penetration of sugars into the Ehrlich ascites tumor cells. J. biol. Chem. **224**, 649 (1957). — CRAWFORD, ELIZABETH: Depression of exogenous creatinine/inulin or thiosulfate clearance ratios in man by diodrast and p-aminohippuric acid. J. clin. Invest. **27**, 171 (1948). — CRAWFORD, ELIZABETH. J., and M. GAUDINO: Changes in extracellular fluid volume, renal function, and electrolyte excretion induced by intravenous saline solution and by short periods of anesthesia. Anesthesiology **13**, 374 (1952). — CRAWFORD, ELIZABETH, and H. LUDEMANN: The renal response to intravenous injection of sodium chloride solutions in man. J. clin. Invest. **30**, 1456 (1951). — CRAWFORD, J. D., ANTOINETTE P. DOYLE and J. H. PROBST: Service of urea in renal water conservation. Amer. J. Physiol. **196**, 545 (1959). — CRAWFORD, J. D., D. GRIBETZ and N. B. TALBOT: Mechanism of renal tubular phosphate reabsorption and the influence thereon of vitamin D in completely parathyroid-ectomized rats. Amer. J. Physiol. **180**, 156 (1955). — CRAWFORD, J. D., M. M. OSBORNE jr., N. B. TALBOT, MARY L. TERRY and MARY F. MORRILL: The parathyroid glands and phosphorus homeostasis. J. clin. Invest. **29**, 1448 (1950). — CRONE, C., and U. V. LASSEN: The action of probenecid (p-[di-n-propylsulphamyl]-benzoic acid) on uric acid excretion and plasma uric acid level in normal human subjects. Acta pharmacol. (Kbh.) **11**, 295 (1955a). — The effect of salicylic acid and acetylsalicylic acid on uric acid excretion and plasma uric acid concentration in the normal human subject. Acta pharmacol. (Kbh.) **11**, 355 (1955b). — Mechanism of increased renal urate excretion during administration of salicylic acid. Acta pharmacol. (Kbh.) **11**, 362 (1955c). — CROSLEY jr., A. P., J. F. BROWN, J. H. HUSTON, D. A. EMANUEL, H. TUCHMAN, C. COSTILLO and G. G. ROWE: The adaptation of the nitrous oxide method to the determination of renal blood flow and *in vivo* renal weight in man. J. clin. Invest. **35**, 1340 (1956). — CROSLEY jr., A. P., G. G. ROWE and C. W. CRUMPTON: The hemodynamic and metabolic response of the human hypertensive kidney to a standard dose of 1-hydrazinophthalazine (hydralazine). J. Lab. clin. Med. **44**, 104 (1954). — CROSS, B. A.: Suckling antidiuresis in rabbits. J. Physiol. (Lond.) **114**, 447 (1951). — CROSS, R. J., and J. V. TAGGART: Renal tubular transport: Accumulation of p-aminohippurate by rabbit kidney slices. Amer. J. Physiol. **161**, 181 (1950). — CROXATTO, H., M. ALMEYDA and L. TUDELA: Action of thiosorbitol on vasopressin. Acta physiol. lat.-amer. **4**, 68 (1954). — CROXATTO, H., L. BARNAFI and R. FERRER: The antidiuretic potency of pregnant women serum. Acta physiol. lat.-amer. **4**, 166 (1954). — CROXATTO, H., R. ROSAS and L. BARNAFI: Effect of vasopressin and oxytocin on the excretion of water and electrolytes (Na, Cl and K) in the albino rat. Acta physiol. lat.-amer. **6**, 147 (1956). — CROXATTO, H., and B. ZAMORANO: Effect of purified vasopressin and oxytocin on water and sodium excretion in hypophysectomized rats. Acta physiol. lat.-amer. **7**, 33 (1957). — CRUTCHFIELD jr., A. J., and J. E. WOOD jr.: Urine volume and total renal sodium excretion during water diuresis. Ann. int. Med. **28**, 28 (1948). — CULLIS, WINIFRED C.: On secretion in the frog's kidney. J. Physiol. (Lond.) **34**, 250 (1906). — CURRENS, J. H., and P. D. WHITE: Congestive heart failure and electrocardiographic abnormalities resulting from excessive desoxycorticosterone acetate therapy in the treatment of Addison's disease. Amer. Heart J. **28**, 611 (1944). — CUSHNY, A. R.: The secretion of urine. London: Longmans, Green & Co. 1917. London and New York: Longmans, Green & Co. 1926.

DALE, R. A., and P. H. SANDERSON: The mode of action of a mercurial diuretic in man. J. clin. Invest. **33**, 1008 (1954). — DALGAARD-MIKKELSEN, S.: On the renal excretion of salicylate. Acta pharmacol. (Kbh.) **7**, 243 (1951). — DALTON, A. J.: Structural details of some of the epithelial cell types in the kidney of the mouse as revealed by the electron microscope. J. nat. Cancer Inst. **11**, 1163 (1951). — DANCIS, J., J. R. BIRMINGHAM and S. H.

324   LAURENCE G. WESSON:

LESLIE: Congenital diabetes insipidus resistant to treatment with pitressin. Amer. J. Dis.
Child. 75, 316 (1948). — D'ANGELO, S. A.: Urinary output and phosphorus excretion in
human subjects during prolonged exposures at low simulated altitudes. Proc. Soc. exp.
Biol. (N.Y.) 62, 13 (1946). — DANIEL, P. M., C. N. PEABODY and MARJORIE M. L. PRICHARD:
Observations on the circulation through the cortex and the medulla of the kidney. Quart.
J. exp. Physiol. 36, 199 (1950). — Cortical ischaemia of the kidney with maintained blood
flow through the medulla. Quart. J. exp. Physiol. 37, 11 (1952). — DANN, W. J., and J. H.
QUASTEL: The effects of phloridzin and other substances on fermentations by yeast. Biochem. J. 22, 245 (1928). — DANZIGER, L., and G. L. ELMERGREEN: Mathematical models
of endocrine systems. Bull. math. Biophysics 19, 9 (1957). — DARMADY, E. M., and FAY
STRANACK: Autoradiography of the isolated nephron. Proc. Soc. exp. Biol. (N.Y.) 100,
658 (1959). — DARRAGH, J. H., L. G. WELT, A. V. N. GOODYER and W. A. ABELE: Influence
of the tonicity of body fluids on rate of excretion of electrolytes. J. appl. Physiol. 5, 658
(1953). — DARROW, D. C., and H. YANNETT: Metabolic studies on the changes in body
electrolyte and distribution of body water induced experimentally by deficit of extracellular
electrolyte. J. clin. Invest. 15, 419 (1936). — DATE, J. W.: Quantitative determination
of some carbohydrates in normal urine. Scand. J. clin. Lab. Invest. 10, 155 (1958). —
DAUGHADAY, W. H., and C. M. MACBRYDE: Renal and adrenal mechanisms of salt conservation: The excretion of urinary formaldehydogenic steroids and 17-ketosteroids during
salt deprivation and desoxycorticosterone administration. J. clin. Invest. 29, 591 (1950). —
DAVENPORT, H. W.: Carbonic anhydrase in tissues other than blood. Physiol. Rev. 26, 560
(1946). — DAVENPORT, H. W., and A. E. WILHELMI: Renal carbonic anhydrase. Proc. Soc.
exp. Biol. (N.Y.) 48, 53 (1941). — DAVENPORT, L. F., M. N. FULTON, H. A. VAN AUKEN,
and R. J. PARSONS: The creatinine clearance as a measure of glomerular filtration in dogs
with particular reference to the effect of diuretic drugs. Amer. J. Physiol. 108, 99 (1934). —
DAVID, E.: Über die Harnbildung in der Froschniere. Über den Einfluß der Temperatur
auf die Funktion der überlebenden Froschniere. Pflügers Arch. ges. Physiol. 208, 529 (1925). —
DAVIDSON, D. G., and N. LEVINSKY: Effect of parathyroid extract on renal excretion of
phosphate in the chicken. Fed. Proc. 16, 28 (1957) (abstract). — DAVIDSON, D. G., N. G.
LEVINSKY and R. W. BERLINER: Maintenance of potassium excretion despite reduction
of glomerular filtration during sodium diuresis. J. clin. Invest. 37, 548 (1958). — DAVIES,
BERYL M. A., and A. H. GORDON: Hormonal nature of extracts of parathyroid gland
stimulating phosphate excretion. Nature (Lond.) 171, 1122 (1953). — DAVIES, BERYL M. A.,
and J. YUDKIN: Studies in biochemical adaptation. The origin of urinary ammonia as
indicated by the effect of chronic acidosis and alkalosis on some renal enzymes in the rat.
Biochem. J. 52, 407 (1952). — DAVIES, C. E.: The effect of treatment on renal circulation
in heart failure. Lancet 1951 II, 1052. — DAVIES, C. E., and J. A. KILPATRICK: Renal circulation in "low output" and "high output" heart failure. Clin. Sci. 10, 53 (1951). — DAVIES,
C. E., J. MACKINNON and M. M. PLATTS: Renal circulation and cardiac output in "low-
output" heart failure and in myxoedema. Brit. med. J. 1952 II, 595. — DAVIES, D. F., and
N. W. SHOCK: Age changes in glomerular filtration rate, effective renal plasma flow and
tubular excretory capacity in adult males. J. clin. Invest. 29, 496 (1950). — DAVIES, H. E. F.,
and O. WRONG: Acidity of urine and excretion of ammonium in renal disease. Lancet
1957 II, 625. — DAVIES, H. W., J. B. S. HALDANE and E. L. KENNAWAY: Experiments on
the regulation of the blood's alkalinity. J. Physiol. (Lond.) 54, 32 (1920). — DAVIES, R. E.:
Hydrochloric acid production by isolated gastric mucosa. Biochem. J. 42, 609 (1948). —
DAVIES, R. E., and NORAH M. LONGMUIR: Production of ulcers in isolated frog gastric mucosa.
Biochem. J. 42, 621 (1948). — DAVIS, J. O.: Some aspects of the physiology of aldosterone.
J. nat. med. Ass. (N.Y.) 49, 42 (1957). — DAVIS, J. O., R. C. BAHN, N. A. YANKOPOULOS,
B. KLIMAN and R. E. PETERSON: Acute effects of hypophysectomy and diencephalic lesions
on aldosterone secretion. Amer. J. Physiol. 197, 380 (1959). — DAVIS, J. O., C. C. J. CAR-
PENTER, C. R. AYERS and R. C. BAHN: Relation of anterior pituitary function to aldosterone
and corticosterone secretion in conscious dogs. Fed. Proc. 19, 166 (1960) (abstract). —
DAVIS, J. O., M. J. GOODKIND, M. M. PECHET and W. C. BALL jr.: Increased excretion of
aldosterone in urine from dogs with right-sided congestive heart failure and from dogs with
thoracic inferior vena cava constriction. Amer. J. Physiol. 187, 45 (1956). — DAVIS, J. O.,
and D. S. HOWELL: Mechanisms of fluid and electrolyte retention in experimental preparations in dogs. Circulat. Res. 1, 171 (1953a). — Comparative effect of ACTH, cortisone and
DCA on renal function, electrolyte excretion and water exchange in normal dogs. Endocrinology 52, 245 (1953b). — DAVIS, J. O., D. S. HOWELL and R. E. HYATT: Effect of
chronic pitressin administration on electrolyte excretion in normal dogs and in dogs with
experimental ascites. Endocrinology 55, 409 (1954). — Effects of acute and chronic digoxin
administration in dogs with right-sided congestive heart failure produced by pulmonary
artery constriction. Circulat. Res. 3, 259 (1955). — DAVIS, J. O., D. S. HOWELL and J. L.
SOUTHWORTH: Mechanisms of fluid and electrolyte retention in experimental preparations

in dogs. III. Effect of adrenalectomy and subsequent desoxycorticosterone acetate administration on ascites formation. Circulat. Res. 1, 260 (1953). — DAVIS, J. O., R. E. HYATT and D. S. HOWELL: Right-sided congestive heart failure in dogs produced by controlled progressive constriction of the pulmonary artery. Circulat. Res. 3, 252 (1955). — DAVIS, J. O., M. M. PECHET, W. C. BALL jr. and M. J. GOODKIND: Increased aldosterone secretion in dogs with right-sided congestive heart failure and in dogs with thoracic inferior vena cava constriction. J. clin. Invest. 36, 689 (1957). — DAVIS, J. O., and N. W. SHOCK: The effect of theophylline ethylenediamine on renal function in control subjects and in patients with congestive heart failure. J. clin. Invest. 28, 1459 (1949). — DAVIS, P. L., and P. K. SMITH: Relation of rate of excretion of salicylate to urinary acidity. Arch. int. Pharmacodyn. 86, 303 (1951). — DEAN, A. L., J. C. ABELS and H. C. TAYLOR: The effects of certain hormones on the renal function of man. J. Urol. (Baltimore) 53, 647 (1945). — DEAN, R. F. A., and R. A. McCANCE: Inulin, diodone, creatinine and urea clearances in newborn infants. J. Physiol. (Lond.) 106, 431 (1947). — Phosphate clearances in infants and adults. J. Physiol. (Lond.) 107, 182 (1948). — The renal responses of infants and adults to the administration of hypertonic solutions of sodium chloride and urea. J. Physiol. (Lond.) 109, 81 (1949). — DEANE, HELEN W., and A. C. BARGER: Histophysiology of the adrenal cortex in dogs with mild and severe cardiac damage. Endocrinology 61, 758 (1957). — DEANE, HELEN W., J. H. SHAW and R. O. GREEP: The effect of altered sodium or potassium intake on the width and cytochemistry of the zona glomerulosa of the rat's adrenal cortex. Endocrinology 43, 133 (1948). — DEANE, N.: Infusion technique for measurement of renal function. Meth. med. Res. 5, 156 (1952). — DEARBORN, E. H., and L. LASAGNA: The antidiuretic action of epinephrine and norepinephrine. J. Pharmacol. exp. Ther. 106, 122 (1952). — DECOURT, J., L. FISCHER et L. GUILLEMIN: A propos de l'action des diurétiques mercuriels. Bull. Soc. méd. Hôp. Paris 52, 1540 (1936). — DECOURT, J., R. GORIN, R. CHATEAU et R. LOUCHART: Insuffisance surrénale et diurése provoquée action des hormones surrenales. Ann. Endocr. (Paris) 6, 172 (1945). — DE FELICE, E. A.: Effect of reserpine (Serpasil) on renal hemodynamics and sodium and chloride excretion in the anesthetized dog. Arch. int. Pharmacodyn. 114, 1 (1958). — DEL GRECO, F., and H. E. DE WARDENER: The effect on urine osmolarity of a transient reduction in glomerular filtration rate and solute output during a "water" diuresis. J. Physiol. (Lond.) 131, 307 (1956). — DEMETRY, J. P., and J. K. AIKAWA: Effect of Hg^{203}-labeled mercaptomerin on renal sulfhydryl concentration in normal rabbits. Proc. Soc. exp. Biol. (N.Y.) 90, 413 (1955). — DEMPSTER, W. J., M. GRACE EGGLETON and S. SHUSTER: The effect of hypertonic infusions on glomerular filtration rate (GFR) and glucose reabsorption in the kidney of the dog. J. Physiol. (Lond.) 132, 213 (1956). — DEMPSTER, W. J., and A. M. JOEKES: Functional studies of the kidney autotransplanted to the neck of dogs. Acta med. scand. 147, 99 (1953). — Emotional antidiuresis in the autotransplanted kidney. J. Physiol. (Lond.) 128, 122 (1955). — DEMUNBRUN, T. W., A. D. KELLER, A. H. LEVKOFF and R. M. PURSER jr.: Pitocin restoration of renal hemodynamics to pre-neuro-hypophysectomy levels; effect of administering neurohypophysial extraction products upon the reduced renal functions associated with neurohypophysectomy. Amer. J. Physiol. 179, 429 (1954). — DE MUYLDER, C. G.: The "Neurility" of the kidney. A monograph on nerve supply to the kidney. Oxford: Blackwell Sci. Publ. 1952. — DENT, C. E.: Discussion on the physiology and clinical disorders of the parathyroid glands. Physiology of the parathyroid glands. Proc. roy. Soc. Med. 46, 291 (1953). — The renal amino-acidurias. Exp. Med. Surg. 12, 229 (1954). — DENT, C. E., B. SENIOR and J. M. WALSHE: The pathogenesis of cystinuria. II. Polarographic studies of the metabolism of sulfur-containing amino acids. J. clin. Invest. 33, 1216 (1954). — DENTON, D. A., J. R. GODING and R. D. WRIGHT: Control of adrenal secretion of electrolyte-active steroids. Brit. med. J. 1959 II a, 447. — Control of adrenal secretion of electrolyte-active steroids. Adrenal stimulation by cross-circulation experiments in conscious sheep. Brit. med. J. 1959 II b, 522. — DESPOPOULOS, A.: Probenecid in hypoparathyroidism: Absence of phosphaturic response. J. clin. Endocr. 18, 769 (1958). — Renal excretory transport of organic acids: Inhibition by oxypurines. Amer. J. Physiol. 197, 1107 (1959). — DESPOPOULOS, A., D. ARCHER, K. C. HUANG and P. K. KNOEFEL: Renal tubular transport of amino and acetamido benzoic and hippuric acids. Fed. Proc. 17, 363 (1958) (abstract). — DESPOPOULOS, A., and E. H. KAUFMAN: Effect of desoxycorticosterone glucoside on renal tubular reabsorption of glucose in dogs. Amer. J. Physiol. 170, 11 (1952). — DICKENS, F., and G. E. GLOCK: Direct oxidation of glucose-6-phosphate, 6-phosphogluconate and pentose-5-phosphates by enzymes of animal origin. Biochem. J. 50, 81 (1951). — DICKER, S. E.: Action of mersalyl, calomel and theophylline sodium acetate on kidney of rat. Brit. J. Pharmacol. 1, 194 (1946). — The fate of the antidiuretic activity of Pitressin in rats. J. Physiol. (Lond.) 124, 464 (1954). — DICKER, S. E., and A. L. GREENBAUM: The degree of inactivation of the antidiuretic activity of vasopressin by the kidneys and the liver of rats. J. Physiol. (Lond.) 126, 116 (1954). — DICKER, S. E., and H. HELLER: Renal action of posterior pituitary extract and its fractions as analysed by clearance experiments on rats. J. Physiol. (Lond.) **104**, 353 (1946). — Dicker, S. E., and Joan Nunn: Fate and excretion of the pressor activity of vasopressin in rats. J. Physiol. (Lond.) **138**, 11 (1957a). — The role of the antidiuretic hormone during water deprivation in rats. J. Physiol. (Lond.) **136**, 235 (1957b). — Antidiuresis in adult and old rats. J. Physiol. (Lond.) **141**, 332 (1958). — Dicker, S. E., and Christine Tyler: Vasopressor and oxytocic activities of the pituitary glands of rats, guinea-pigs and cats and of human foetuses. J. Physiol. (Lond.) **121**, 206 (1953). — Diczfalusy, E.: Turnover of acid-soluble phosphorus in kidneys of phlorhizinized rats. Acta endocr. (Kbh.) **7**, 60 (1951). — Dignam, W. J., N. S. Assali and K. Dasgupta: Homeostatic responses to blood volume sequestration in normal pregnancy. Clin. Res. **7**, 78 (1959) (abstract). — Dignam, W. J., P. Titus and N. S. Assali: Renal function in human pregnancy. I. Changes in glomerular filtration rate and renal plasma flow. Proc. Soc. exp. Biol. (N.Y.) **97**, 512 (1958). — Dignam, W. S., J. Voskian and N. S. Assali: Effects of estrogens on renal hemodynamics and excretion of electrolytes in human subjects. J. clin. Endocr. **16**, 1032 (1956). — Dill, L. V., C. E. Isenhour, J. F. Cadden and N. K. Schaffer: Glomerular filtration and renal blood flow in toxemias of pregnancy. Amer. J. Obstet. Gynec. **43**, 32 (1942a). — Dill, L. V., C. E. Isenhour, J. F. Cadden and C. E. Robinson: Glomerular filtration and renal blood flow in "normal" patients following toxemias of pregnancy. Amer. J. Obstet. Gynec. **44**, 66 (1942b). — Dingman, J. F.: Hypothalamus and the endocrine control of sodium and water metabolism in man. Amer. J. med. Sci. **235**, 79 (1958). — Dingman, J. F., J. T. Finkenstaedt, J. C. Laidlaw, A. E. Renold, D. Jenkins, J. P. Merrill and G. W. Thorn: Influence of intravenously administered adrenal steroids on sodium and water excretion in normal and Addisonian subjects. Metabolism **7**, 608 (1958). — Dingman, J. F., E. Gaitan and M. C. Staub: Effects of vasopressin on electrolyte and water metabolism in primary aldosteronism. J. clin. Invest **38**, 999 1959. — Dochios, Mary, and L. S. Dreifus: Antidiuretic hormone studies in patients presenting edema. Amer. J. med. Sci. **222**, 538 (1951). — Dodge, W. F., and C. W. Daeschner: Factors influencing the short-term measurement of glomerular filtration rate by endogenous creatinine clearance. Clin. Res. **8**, 62 (1960) (abstract). — Doe, R. P., E. B. Flink and Marilyn G. Goodsell: Relation of diurnal variation in 17-hydroxycorticosteroid levels in blood and urine to eosinophils and electrolyte excretion. J. clin. Endocr. **16**, 196 (1956). — Doe, R. P., J. A. Vennes and E. B. Flink: Diurnal variation of 17-hydroxycorticosteroids, sodium, potassium, magnesium and creatinine in normal subjects and in cases of treated adrenal insufficiency and Cushing's syndrome. J. clin. Endocr. **20**, 253 (1960). — Dole, V. P.: Back-diffusion of urea in mammalian kidney. Amer. J. Physiol. **139**, 504 (1943). — Domer, F. R.: Cationic excretion by the dog kidney. Amer. J. Physiol. **198**, 1053 (1960). — Dominguez, R.: On the renal excretion of urea. Amer. J. Physiol. **112**, 529 (1935). — Kinetics of renal excretion of injected substances. Meth. med. Res. **5**, 135 (1952). — Dominguez, R., A. C. Corcoran and I. H. Page: Mannitol: kinetics of distribution, excretion and utilization in human beings. J. Lab. clin. Med. **32**, 1192 (1947). [Correction in J. Lab. clin. Med. **33**, 396 (1948).] — Dominguez, R., and E. Pomerene: Urea clearance and diuresis in man. J. clin. Invest. **22**, 1 (1943). — Donaldson, W.: Dialyzability of pressor and antidiuretic activities of pitressin. J. clin. Invest. **26**, 1023 (1947). — Doolan, P. D., H. A. Harper, M. E. Hutchim and W. W. Shreeve: Renal clearance of eighteen individual amino acids in human subjects. J. clin. Invest. **34**, 1247 (1955). — Dorman, P. J., W. J. Sullivan and R. F. Pitts: The renal response to acute respiratory acidosis. J. clin. Invest. **33**, 82 (1954a). — CO_2 tension in urine. Amer. J. Physiol. **179**, 181 (1954b). — Doty, J. R.: Reabsorption of certain amino acids and derivatives by kidney tubules. Proc. Soc. exp. Biol. (N.Y.) **46**, 129 (1941). — Doyle, A. E., and J. M. Merrill: The influence of posture on renal function in heart failure. Clin. Sci. **16**, 155 (1957). — Dragstedt, L. R.: The physiology of the parathyroid glands. Physiol. Rev. **7**, 499 (1927). — Dratz, A. F., and P. Handler: Renal phosphate and carbohydrate metabolism studied with the aid of radiophosphorus. J. biol. Chem. **197**, 419 (1952). — Dreser, H.: Über Diurese und ihre Beeinflussung durch pharmakologische Mittel. Naunyn-Schmiedeberg's Arch. exp. Path. Pharmak. **29**, 303 (1892). — Drew, H. D. K., and W. N. Haworth: Polysaccharides. III. The molecular complexity of inulin. J. chem. Soc. **2**, 2690 (1928). — Drinker, C. K., and J. M. Yoffey: Lymphatics, lymph and lymphoid tissue. Cambridge, Mass: Harvard University Press 1941. — Driscol, T. E., M. M. Maultsby, G. L. Farrell and R. M. Berne: Aldosterone secretion in experimental congestive heart failure. Amer. J. Physiol. **191**, 140 (1957). — Drovanti, S., C. Cei e C. Strada: Azione diuretica della Rauwolfia Serpentina. Minerva med. (Torino) **45**, 1403 (1954). — Drury, D. R., J. P. Henry and J. Goodman: The effects of continuous pressure breathing on kidney function. J. clin. Invest. **26**, 945 (1947). — Duggan, J. J., and R. F. Pitts: Studies on diuretics. I. The site of action of mercurial diuretics. J. clin. Invest. **29**, 365 (1950). — Duke, Helen N., and Mary Pickford: Observations on the action of acetylcholine and adrenaline on the hypothalamus. J. Physiol. (Lond.) **114**, 325 (1951). — Dumm, Mary E.,

S. H. LESLIE and B. LAKEN: Methods of fractionating Pitressin. Fed. Proc. 11, 38 (1952) (abstract). — DUNCAN jr., L. E.: The effect of exercise on the excretion of water by patients with congestive failure. Circulation 12, 90 (1955). — DUNCAN jr., L. E., G. W. LIDDLE and F. C. BARTTER: The effect of changes in body sodium on extracellular fluid volume and aldosterone and sodium excretion by normal and edematous men. J. clin. Invest. 35, 1299 (1956). — DUNCAN jr., L. E., D. H. SOLOMON, M. P. NICHOLES and E. ROSENBERG: The effect of the chronic administration of adrenal medullary hormones to man on excretion of electrolytes. J. clin. Invest. 30, 908 (1951). — DUNIHUE, F. W., and W. VAN B. ROBERTSON: The effect of desoxycorticosterone acetate (DCA) and of sodium on the juxtaglomerular apparatus. Endocrinology 61, 293 (1957). — DUNN jr., J. R., S. DEAVERS, R. A. HUGGINS and E. L. SMITH: Effect of hemorrhage on red cell and plasma volume of various organs of the dog. Amer. J. Physiol. 195, 69 (1958). — DUPRÉ, J., and R. V. COXON: Use of subcutaneous depots of test substances in the measurement of renal clearances. Quart. J. exp. Physiol. 43, 74 (1958). — DUSTAN, HARRIET P., A. C. CORCORAN and I. H. PAGE: Renal function in primary aldosteronism. J. clin. Invest. 35, 1357 (1956). — DUSTAN, HARRIET P., A. C. CORCORAN, R. D. TAYLOR and I. H. PAGE: Renal vasodilator effects of 1-hydrazinophthalazine in hypertensive patients. Amer. J. Med. 14, 502 (1953) (abstract). — DUSTIN, J. P.: De l'élimination des acides aminés dans les urines de nourrisson. Exp. Med. Surg. 12, 233 (1954). — DYRENFURTH, INGE, C. H. STACEY, J. C. BECK and ELEANOR H. VENNING: Aldosterone excretion in patients with cirrhosis of the liver. Metabolism 6, 544 (1957). — DYKE, H. B. VAN, K. ADAMSONS jr. and S. L. ENGEL: Aspects of the biochemistry and physiology of the neurohypophyseal hormones. Recent Progr. Hormone Res. 11, 1 (1955). — DYKE, H. B. VAN, and ROSE G. AMES: Alcohol diuresis. Acta endocr. (Kbh.) 7, 110 (1951). — DYKE, H. B. VAN, B. F. CHOW, R. O. GREEP and A. ROTHEN: The isolation of a protein from the pars neuralis of the ox pituitary with constant oxytocic, pressor and diuresis-inhibiting activities. J. Pharmacol. exp. Ther. 74, 190 (1942). — DYKE, H. B. VAN, S. L. ENGEL and K. ADAMSONS: Comparison of pharmacological effects of lysine and arginine vasopressins. Proc. Soc. exp. Biol. (N.Y.) 91, 484 (1956).

EAGLE, H., and E. NEWMAN: The renal clearance of penicillins F, G, K and X in rabbits and man. J. clin. Invest. 26, 903 (1947). — EALES, L., and G. C. LINDER: Primary aldosteronism. Some observations on a case in a cape colored woman. Quart. J. Med. 25, 539 (1956). — EARLE jr., D. P.: Renal excretion of sulfamerazine. J. clin. Invest. 23, 914 (1944). — Renal function tests in the diagnosis of glomerular and tubular disease. Bull. N.Y. Acad. Med. 26, 47 (1950). — EARLE jr., D. P., J. D. ALEXANDER, S. J. FARBER and E. D. PELEGRINO: Observations on the relation of renal function changes to the electrolyte and glycosuric effects of ACTH. Proc. 2nd ACTH Conf., p. 139, 1951a. — EARLE jr., D. P., and R. W. BERLINER: Simplified clinical procedure for measurement of glomerular filtration rate and renal plasma flow. Proc. Soc. exp. Biol. (N.Y.) 62, 262 (1946). — Effect of 2,3-dimercaptopropanol on diuresis. Amer. J. Physiol. 151, 215 (1947). — EARLE jr., D. P., and B. B. BRODIE: Renal excretion of 4'-carboxyphenylmethane sulfonanilide (caronamide). J. Pharmacol. exp. Ther. 91, 250 (1947). — EARLE jr., D. P., S. J. FARBER, J. D. ALEXANDER and L. W. EICHNA: Effect of treatment on renal function and electrolyte excretion in congestive heart failure. J. clin. Invest. 28, 778 (1949) (abstract). — EARLE jr., D. P., S. J. FARBER, J. D. ALEXANDER and E. D. PELEGRINO: Renal function and electrolyte metabolism in acute glomerulonephritis. J. clin. Invest. 30, 421 (1951b). — EARLE jr., D. P., S. J. FARBER, R. C. DE BODO, M. KURTZ and M. W. SINKOFF: Effects of ACTH, cortisone and hydrocortisone on renal functions in hypophysectomized dogs. Amer. J. Physiol. 173, 189 (1953). — Personal communication 1957. — EARLE jr., D. P., S. SHERRY, L. W. EICHNA and N. J. CONAN: Low potassium syndrome due to defective renal tubular mechanisms for handling potassium. Amer. J. Med. 11, 283 (1951c). — EARLE jr., D. P., J. V. TAGGART and J. A. SHANNON: Glomerulonephritis. A survey of the functional organization of the kidney in various stages of diffuse glomerulonephritis. J. clin. Invest. 23, 119 (1944). — EARLEY, L. E.: Water diuresis following ingestion of large volumes of slightly hypertonic urea solution by hydropenic subjects. J. clin. Invest. 38, 1000 (1959) (abstract). — EARLEY, L. E., and C. A. SANDERS: The effect of changing serum osmolality on the release of antidiuretic hormone in certain patients with decompensated cirrhosis of the liver and low serum osmolality. J. clin. Invest. 38, 545 (1959). — EATON, A. G., F. P. FERGUSON and F. T. BYER: Renal reabsorption of amino acids in dogs: valine, leucine and isoleucine. Amer. J. Physiol. 145, 491 (1946). — EDELMAN, I. S., B. W. ZWEIFACH, DORIS J. W. ESHER, J. GROSSMAN, R. MOKOTOFF, R. E. WESTON, L. LEITER and E. SCHORR: Studies on VEM and VDM in blood in relation to renal hemodynamics and renal oxygen extraction in chronic congestive heart failure. J. clin. Invest. 29, 925 (1950). — EDELMANN jr., C. M., V. TROUPKOU and H. L. BARNETT: Renal concentrating ability in newborn infants. Fed. Proc. 18, 40 (1959) (abstract). — EDER, H. A., H. D. LAUSON, F. P. CHINARD, R. L. GREIF, G. C. COTZIAS and D. D. VAN SLYKE: A study of the mechanisms of edema formation in patients with the

328   LAURENCE G. WESSON:

nephrotic syndrome. J. clin. Invest. **33**, 636 (1955). — EDVALL, C. A.: Renal function tests: a comparison between routine clinical tests and selective clearances. Acta chir. scand. **114**, 293 (1957a). — Determination of unilateral renal function in urology. Unilateral selective clearances and the extraction ratio of PAH (E-pah) determined by renal vein catheterization. Acta chir. scand. **114**, 303 (1957b). — EDWARDS, J. G.: The vascular pole of the glomerulus in the kidney of vertebrates. Anat. Rec. **76**, 381 (1940). — The renal tubule (nephron) as affected by mercury. Amer. J. Path. **18**, 1011 (1942). — Efferent arterioles of glomeruli in the juxtamedullary zone of the human kidney. Anat. Rec. **125**, 521 (1956). — EDWARDS, J. G., and L. CONDORELLI: Studies on aglomerular and glomerular kidneys. II. Physiological. Amer. J. Physiol. **86**, 383 (1928). — EDWARDS, J. G., and E. K. MARSHALL jr.: Microscopic observations of the living kidney after injection of phenolsulphonephthalein. Amer. J. Physiol. **70**, 489 (1924). — EDWARDS, K. D. G., and H. M. WHYTE: The measurement of creatinine in plasma and urine. Aust. J. exp. Biol. med. Sci. **36**, 383 (1958). — Plasma creatinine level and creatinine clearance as test of renal function. Aust. Ann. Med. **8**, 218 (1959). — EFFERSØE, P.: Comparative investigations into the inulin, creatinine and thiosulfate clearances of rabbits after ingesting sodium benzoate. Scand. J. clin. Lab. Invest. **1**, 343 (1949) (abstract). — Relationship between endogenous 24-hour creatinine clearance and serum creatinine concentration in patients with chronic renal disease. Acta med. scand. **156**, 429 (1957). — EGGLETON, M. GRACE: Diuretic action of alcohol in man. J. Physiol. (Lond.) **101**, 172 (1942a). — A class experiment on urinary changes after exercise. J. Physiol. (Lond.) **101**, 1 P (1942) (abstract). — Effect of exercise on chloride excretion in man during water diuresis and during tea diuresis. J. Physiol. (Lond.) **102**, 140 (1943). — Urine acidity in alcohol diuresis in man. J. Physiol. (Lond.) **104**, 312 (1946). — Some factors affecting the acidity of urine in man. J. Physiol. (Lond.) **106**, 456 (1947). — EGGLETON, M. GRACE, and Y. A. HABIB: Action of thiosulfate on the kidney of the cat. Nature (Lond.) **163**, 1000 (1949). — EGGLETON, M. GRACE, J. R. PAPPENHEIMER and F. R. WINTON: Mechanisms of dilution diuresis in isolated kidney and anesthetized dog. J. Physiol. (Lond.) **98**, 336 (1940a). — Relation between ureter, venous, and arterial pressures in isolated kidney of dog. J. Physiol. (Lond.) **99**, 135 (1940b). — EGGLETON, M. GRACE, and S. SHUSTER: Glucose and phosphate excretion in the cat. J. Physiol. (Lond.) **124**, 613 (1954a). — The effect of insulin on the excretion of glucose and phosphate by the kidney of the cat. J. Physiol. (Lond.) **124**, 623 (1954b). — EICHNA, L. W., S. J. FARBER, A. R. BERGER, D. P. EARLE, BERTHA RADER, E. PELLEGRINO, R. E. ALBERT, J. D. ALEXANDER, H. TAUBE and S. YOUNGWIRTH: The interrelationships of the cardiovascular, renal and electrolyte effects of intravenous digoxin in congestive heart failure. J. clin. Invest. **30**, 1250 (1951). — Cardiovascular dynamics, blood volumes, renal functions and electrolyte excretion in the same patients during congestive heart failure and after recovery of cardiac compensation. Circulation **7**, 674 (1953). — EILER, J. J., T. L. ALTHAUSEN, and M. STOCKHOLM: Effect of thyroxin on maximum rate of transfer of glucose and diodrast by renal tubules. Amer. J. Physiol. **140**, 699 (1944a). — Absorption of galactose by renal tubules of dog. Proc. Soc. exp. Biol. (N.Y.) **56**, 67 (1944b). — EK, J.: The influence of heavy hydration on the renal function in normal and hypertensive man. Scand. J. clin. Lab. Invest. **7**, Suppl., 19 (1955). — EK, J., and B. JOSEPHSON: On the influence of beer and a purine derivitive on the renal clearance of creatinine, inulin and paraaminohippuric acid (PAH). Acta physiol. scand. **28**, 347 (1953a). — The influence of beer on the renal excretion of water, sodium and potassium. Acta physiol. scand. **28**, 355 (1953b). — EKEHORN, G.: On the principles of renal function. Acta med. scand. Suppl. **36** (1931). — ELIAS, A. H.: De structura glomeruli renalis. Anat. Anz. **104**, 26 (1957). — ELKINTON, J. R., R. TARAIL, and J. P. PETERS: Transfers of potassium in renal insufficiency. J. clin. Invest. **28**, 378 (1949). — ELLBORG, A., and H. FORSSMAN: Nephrogenic diabetes insipidus in children. Acta paediat. (Uppsala) **44**, 209 (1955). — ELLINGER, P.: The formation of urine in the amphibian and the mammalian kidney. J. Physiol. (Lond.) **97**, 433 (1940a). — Site of acidification of urine in frog's and rat's kidney. Quart. J. exp. Physiol. **30**, 205 (1940b). — ELLIOT jr., H. C., and H. V. MURDAUGH jr.: Renal excretion of endogenous metabolites in man. The glycine effect. Fed. Proc. **19**, 359 (1960) (abstract). — ELLIS, L. B., and S. WEISS: Normal variations in renal function tests with discussion of their physiological significance. Amer. J. med. Sci. **186**, 233 (1933). — ELLSWORTH, R.: Studies on the physiology of the parathyroid glands. V. Action of parathyroid extract on the renal threshold for phosphorus. J. clin. Invest. **11**, 1011 (1932). — ELLSWORTH, R., and P. H. FUTCHER: The effect of parathyroid extract upon the serum calcium of nephrectomized dogs. Bull. Johns Hopk. Hosp. **57**, 91 (1935). — ELLSWORTH, R., and J. E. HOWARD: Studies on the physiology of the parathyroid glands. VII. Some responses of normal human kidneys and blood to intravenous parathyroid extract. Bull. Johns Hopk. Hosp. **55**, 296 (1934). — ELSOM, K. A., PHYLLIS A. BOTT and E. H. SHIELS: On the excretion of skiodan, diodrast and hippuran by the dog. Amer. J. Physiol. **115**, 548 (1936). — EMANUEL, D. A., J. SCOTT, R. COLLINS and F. J. HADDY: Local effect of serotonin on renal vascular resistance and urine flow rate. Amer. J. Physiol. **196**, 1122 (1959). — EMERSON, K., and V. P. DOLE: Diodrast and inulin clearances in nephrotic children with supernormal urea clearances. J. clin. Invest. **22**, 447 (1943). — EMERSON jr., K., P. H. FUTCHER and L. E. FARR: Relation of high and low urea clearances to inulin and creatinine clearances in children with nephrotic syndrome. J. clin. Invest. **20**, 361 (1941). — ENGSTRÖM, A., and B. JOSEPHSON: Historadiographic demonstration of diodrast in the rabbit kidney. Amer. J. Physiol. **174**, 61 (1953). — ENGSTROM, W. W., and A. LIEBMAN: Chronic hyperosmolarity of the body fluids with a cerebral lesion causing diabetes insipidus and anterior pituitary insufficiency. Amer. J. Med. **15**, 180 (1953). — EPSTEIN, F. H.: Renal excretion of sodium and the concept of a volume receptor. Yale J. Biol. Med. **29**, 282 (1956). — EPSTEIN, F. H., D. BECK, F. A. CARONE, H. LEVITIN and A. MANITIUS: Changes in renal concentrating ability produced by parathyroid extract. J. clin. Invest. **38**, 1214 (1959). — EPSTEIN, F. H., A. V. N. GOODYER, F. D. LAWRASON and A. S. RELMAN: Studies of the antidiuresis of quiet standing: the importance of changes in plasma volume and G.F.R. J. clin. Invest. **30**, 63 (1951). — EPSTEIN, F. H., R. C. KLEEMAN and A. HENDRIKX: The influence of bodily hydration on the renal concentrating process. J. clin. Invest. **36**, 629 (1957). — EPSTEIN, F. H., C. R. KLEEMAN, E. LAMDIN and M. E. RUBINI: Studies of the antidiuresis of quiet standing: observations upon electrolyte and acid-base excretion during sulfate diuresis. J. clin. Invest. **35**, 308 (1956). — EPSTEIN, F. H., C. R. KLEEMAN, S. PURSEL and A. HENDRIKX: The effect of feeding protein and urea on the renal concentrating process. J. clin. Invest. **36**, 635 (1957). — EPSTEIN, F. H., and H. LEVITIN: "Cerebral salt-wasting": an example of sustained inappropriate release of antidiuretic hormone. J. clin. Invest. **38**, 1001 (1959) (abstract). — EPSTEIN, F. H., R. S. POST and M. McDOWELL: The effect of an arteriovenous fistula on renal hemodynamics and electrolyte excretion. J. clin. Invest. **32**, 233 (1953). — EPSTEIN, F. H., and M. J. RIVERA: Renal concentrating ability in thyrotoxicosis. J. clin. Endocr. **18**, 1135 (1958). — EPSTEIN, F. H., M. J. RIVERA and F. A. CARONE: The effect of hypercalcemia induced by calciferol upon renal concentrating ability. J. clin. Invest. **37**, 1702 (1958). — ERANKO, O., M. J. KARVONEN, A. LAAMANEN and M. E. PITKANEN: The antidiuretic action of adrenaline and noradrenaline in the water-loaded dog. Acta pharmacol. (Kbh.) **9**, 345 (1953). — ERSPAMER, V., and P. CORREALE: Further observations on the action of 5-hydroxytryptamine (5-HT) on the urine flow and chloride excretion in the rat. Arch. int. Pharmacodyn. **101**, 99 (1955). — ERSPAMER, V., and A. OTTOLENGHI: Pharmacological studies on enteramine. VIII. Action of enteramine on the diuresis and the renal circulation of the rat. Arch. int. Pharmacodyn. **93**, 177 (1953). — ETHRIDGE, C. B., D. W. MEYERS and M. N. FULTON: Modifying effect of various inorganic salts on the diuretic action of salyrgan. Arch. intern. Med. **57**, 719 (1936). — ETTLEDORF, J. N., J. D. SMITH, A. H. TUTTLE and L. W. DIGGS: Renal hemodynamic studies in adults with sickle cell anemia. Amer. J. Med. **18**, 243 (1955). — ETTLEDORF, J. N., A. H. TUTTLE and G. W. CLAYTON: Renal function studies in pediatrics. I. Renal hemodynamics in children with sickle cell anemia. Amer. J. Dis. Child. **83**, 185 (1952). — EULER, C. v.: A preliminary note on slow hypothalamic "osmo-potentials". Acta physiol. scand. **29**, 133 (1953). — EULER, U. S. v., R. LUFT and T. SUNDIN: Excretion of urinary adrenaline in normals following intravenous infusion. Acta physiol. scand. **30**, 249 (1953/54). — The urinary excretion of noradrenaline and adrenaline in healthy subjects during recumbency and standing. Acta physiol. scand. **34**, 169 (1955). — EVANS, BARBARA M., N. C. HUGHES-JONES, M. D. MILNE and S. STEINER: Electrolyte excretion during experimental potassium depletion in man. Clin. Sci. **13**, 305 (1954). — EVANS, BARBARA M., I. MACINTYRE, C. R. MACPHERSON and M. D. MILNE: Alkalosis in sodium and potassium depletion (with special reference to organic acid excretion). Clin. Sci. **16**, 53 (1957). — EVERED, D. F.: The excretion of amino acids by the human. Biochem. J. **62**, 416 (1956). — EVERSOLE, W. J., J. H. BIRNIE and R. GAUNT: Inactivation of posterior pituitary antidiuretic hormone by the liver. J. clin. Endocr. **8**, 616 (1948) (abstract). — EVERSOLE, W. J., F. A. GIERE and M. H. ROCK: Effects of adrenal medullary hormones on renal excretion of water and electrolytes. Amer. J. Physiol. **170**, 24 (1952).

FALBRIARD, A.: Action rénale des sulfamides inhibiteurs de la carboanhydrase. Praxis **43**, 265, 293 (1954). — FALBRIARD, A., A. F. MULLER, J. CRABBÉ et A. DUCKERT-MAULBETSCH: Actions comparées du Diamox, du potassium et leur association sur l'élimination urinaire des electrolytes. Reaction surrenalienne (aldosterone). Helv. med. Acta **22**, 495 (1955a). — FALBRIARD, A., A. F. MULLER, R. NEHER et R. S. MACH: Étude des variations de l'aldostéronurie sous l'effet de surcharges en potassium et déperditions rénales et extrarénales de sel et d'eau. Schweiz. med. Wschr. **85**, 1218 (1955b). — FARAH, A.: Metabolic aspects of transport across cell membranes, p. 257. Madison: University of Wisconsin Press 1957. — FARAH, A., C. H. BENDER, R. KRUSE and E. CAFRUNY: The influence of acidosis and alkalosis on mercurial-induced diuresis and sulfhydryl changes in the kidney. J. Pharmacol. exp. Ther. **125**, 309 (1959). — FARAH, A., E. J. CAFRUNY and H. S. DISTE-

330   Laurence G. Wesson:

Fano: Histochemical studies on the site of action of mercurial diuretics. J. Histochem. Cytochem. **3**, 271 (1955). — Farah, A., T. C. Cobbey and W. Mook: Renal action of mercurial diuretics as affected by sodium load. J. Pharmacol. exp. Ther. **104**, 31 (1952). — Farah, A., M. Frazer and E. Porter: Studies on the uptake of N-methylnicotinamide by renal slices of the dog. J. Pharmacol. exp. Ther. **126**, 202 (1959). — Farah, A., and G. Maresh: Influence of sulfhydryl compounds on diuresis and renal and cardiac circulatory changes caused by mersalyl. J. Pharmacol. exp. Ther. **92**, 73 (1948). — Farah, A., and B. Rennick: Studies on the renal tubular transport of tetraethylammonium ion in renal slices of the dog. J. Pharmacol. exp. Ther. **117**, 478 (1956). — Farah, A., B. Rennick and M. Frazer: The influence of some basic substances on the transport of tetraethylammonium ion. J. Pharmacol. and exp. Ther. **119**, 122 (1957). — Farber, S. J., J. D. Alexander, E. D. Pellegrino and D. P. Earle: The effect of intravenously administered digoxin on water and electrolyte excretion and on renal functions. Circulation **4**, 378 (1951). — Farber, S. J., W. H. Becker and L. W. Eichna: Electrolyte and water excretions and renal hemodynamics during induced congestion of the superior and inferior vena cava of man. J. clin. Invest. **32**, 1145 (1953). — Farber, S. J., E. Y. Berger and D. P. Earle: Effect of diabetes and insulin on the maximum capacity of the renal tubules to reabsorb glucose. J. clin. Invest. **30**, 125 (1951). — Farber, S. J., N. J. Conan jr. and D. P. Earle jr.: Effect of diabetes and insulin on glucose Tm and other renal functions. Amer. J. Physiol. **155**, 436 (1948) (abstract). — Farnsworth, Edith B.: Clearance of inulin, diodrast, chloride and phosphate under mercurial diuresis; intensive study of patient in severe cardiac failure. Amer. J. Med. **1**, 246 (1946). — Farquhar, Marilyn G., R. L. Vernier and R. A. Good: Studies on familial nephrosis. II. Glomerular changes observed with the electron microscope. Amer. J. Path. **33**, 791 (1957). — Farr, L. E.: The effect of dietary protein on the urea clearance of children with nephrosis. J. clin. Invest. **15**, 703 (1936). — Farrell, G. L.: Steroids in adrenal venous blood of the dog: Venous-arterial differences across the adrenal. Proc. Soc. exp. Biol. (N.Y.) **86**, 338 (1954). — Regulation of aldosterone secretion. Physiol. Rev. **38**, 709 (1958). — Steroidogenic properties of extracts of beef diencephalon. Endocrinology **65**, 29 (1959a). — Glomerulotropic activity of an acetone extract of pineal tissue. Endocrinology **65**, 239 (1959b). — Farrell, G. L., R. C. Banks and S. Koletsky: The effect of corticosteroid injection on aldosterone secretion. Endocrinology **58**, 104 (1956). — Farrell, G. L., S. Koletsky and L. W. Lapham: Decreased aldosterone secretion following pinealectomy. Fed. Proc. **18**, 44 (1959) (abstract). — Farrell, G. L., Elizabeth W. Rauschkolb and P. C. Royce: Secretion of aldosterone by the adrenal of the dog. Effects of hypophysectomy and ACTH. Amer. J. Physiol. **182**, 269 (1955). — Farrell, G. L., Elizabeth W. Rauschkolb, P. C. Royce and H. Hirschmann: Isolation of desoxycorticosterone from adrenal venous blood of the dog; effect of hypophysectomy and ACTH. Proc. Soc. exp. Biol. (N.Y.) **87**, 587 (1954). — Farrell, G. L., and J. B. Richards: Isolation of a potent sodium-retaining substance from adrenal venous blood of the dog. Proc. Soc. exp. Biol. (N.Y.) **83**, 628 (1953). — Farrell, G. L., R. S. Rosnagle and Elizabeth W. Rauschkolb: Increased aldosterone secretion in response to blood loss. Circulat. Res. **4**, 606 (1956). — Farrell, G. L., P. C. Royce, Elizabeth W. Rauschkolb and H. Hirschmann: Isolation and identification of aldosterone from adrenal venous blood. Proc. Soc. exp. Biol. (N.Y.) **87**, 141 (1954). — Faulkner, M., R. Hammerschmidt and A. Newmayr: The urinary output of antidiuretic substances in man during therapy of liver cirrhosis with a total-liver-extract. Acta med. scand. **151**, 473 (1955). — Faurholt, C.: Relationship between carbon dioxide, carbonic acid, carbamates, and carbonates. Kgl. Veterin.-Landsbohøjsk. Aarskr. **3**, 122 (1924). — Fawaz, G., and E. N. Fawaz: Mechanism of action of mercurial diuretics. Proc. Soc. exp. Biol. (N.Y.) **77**, 239 (1951). — Fay, M., Vivian G. Behrmann and Dorothy M. Buck: The parathyroids and the clearance of inorganic phosphate. Amer. J. Physiol. **136**, 716 (1942). — Fejfar, E., and J. Brod: The excretion of chlorides in patients with heart failure. Quart. J. Med. **19**, 221 (1950). — Ferguson, F. P., A. G. Eaton and J. S. Ashman: Renal reabsorption of methionine in normal dogs. Proc. Soc. exp. Biol. (N.Y.) **66**, 582 (1947). — Ferrannini, A., e S. Castorina: Diuretici mercuriali e ricambio dell'acido urico. Omnia med. (Pisa) **20**, 39 (1942). — Ferrannini, A., e G. Fontana: L'azione dei diuretici mercuriali sulla eliminazione dell'acido urico nei soggetti normali ed in quelli con fegato leso. Boll. Soc. ital. Biol. sper. **14**, 557 (1939). — Ferrebee, J. W., C. Ragan, D. W. Atchley and R. F. Loeb: Desoxycorticosterone esters. Certain effects in the treatment of Addison's disease. J. Amer. med. Ass. **113**, 1725 (1939). — Feyel, P., et J. Varangot: Sur l'élimination rénale des électrolytes apres les interventions chirurgicales non choquantes. C. R. Soc. Biol. (Paris) **135**, 1356 (1941). — Filomeni, M.: Ostacolo ed inibizione della diuresi da Mersalyl per azione del CaEDTANa₂ e dell'EDTANa₂ nel ratto. Ric. sci. **29**, 779 (1959). — Filomeni, M., e I. Palumbi: Influenza del complesso mercurico bisodico dell'acido etilendiamminotetracetico sulla diuresi da Mersalyl nell ratto. Ric. sci. **29**, 1018 (1959). — Findley, T., J. C. Edwards, Etta Clinton and H. L. White: Clearance of diodrast, phenolsulfonphthalein and inulin in hypertension and in nephritis. Arch. intern. Med. 70, 935 (1942). — Simplified technique for measuring renal blood flow and tubular excretory mass. J. Lab. clin. Med. 28, 916 (1943). — FINDLEY, T., and H. L. WHITE: Measurement of diodrast and inulin clearances in man after subcutaneous administration. Proc. Soc. exp. Biol. (N.Y.) 45, 623 (1940). — FINE, D., L. E. MEISELAS and THERESA AUERBACH: The effect of acute hypovolemia on the release of "aldosterone" and on the renal excretion of sodium. J. clin. Invest. 37, 232 (1958). — FISCHER, A., L. TAKACS u. S. VARGA: Glomerulusfiltrat und Natriumausscheidung der denervierten Niere. Z. ges. exp. Med. 129, 33 (1957). — FISHBERG, A. M.: Hypertension and nephritis, 5th edit. Philadelphia: Lea and Febiger 1954. — FISHER, C.: Diabetes insipidus and neurohormonal control of water balance. Proc. Inst. Med. Chicago 13, 117 (1940). — FISHER, C., W. R. INGRAM and S. W. RANSON: Diabetes insipidus and the neuro-hormonal control of water balance: a contribution to the structure and function of the hypothalamico-hypophyseal system. Ann. Arbor: Edwards Brothers 1938. — FISHER, S. H., L. TROAST, ALICE WATERHOUSE and J. A. SHANNON: The relation between chemical structure and physiological disposition of a series of substances allied to sulfanilamide. J. Pharmacol. exp. Ther. 79, 373 (1943). — FISHMAN, A. P., M. H. MAXWELL, C. H. CROWDER and P. MORALES: Kidney function in cor pulmonale. Particular consideration of changes in renal hemodynamics and sodium excretion during variation in level of oxygenation. Circulation 3, 703 (1951). — FISHMAN, A. P., J. STAMLER, L. N. KATZ, A. J. MILLER, E. N. SILBER and L. RUBENSTEIN: Mechanisms of edema formation in chronic experimental pericarditis with effusion. J. clin. Invest. 29, 521 (1950). — FISHMAN, R. A.: The failure of intracranial pressure-volume change to influence renal function. J. clin. Invest. 32, 847 (1953). — FITZGERALD, M. G., and P. FOURMAN: The renal factor in the alkalosis of potassium deficiency. Lancet 1955 II, 848. — FITZHUGH jr., F. W., R. L. McWHORTER jr., E. H. ESTES jr., J. V. WARREN and A. J. MERRILL: The effect of application of tourniquets to the legs on cardiac output and renal function in normal human subjects. J. clin. Invest. 32, 1163 (1953). — FLAX, L. J., and I. GERSH: Congenital renal tubular dysfunction (nephrogenic diabetes insipidus). Amer. J. Dis. Child. 89, 602 (1955). — FOA, P. P., and N. L. FOA: Simple method for determining effective renal blood flow and tubular excretory mass in man. Proc. Soc. exp. Biol. (N.Y.) 51, 375 (1942). — FOA, P. P., W. W. WOODS, M. M. PEET and N. L. FOA: Effective renal blood flow, glomerular filtration rate and tubular excretory mass in arterial hypertension. Arch. intern. Med. 69, 822 (1942). — Effective renal blood flow, glomerular filtration rate and tubular excretory mass in arterial hypertension; effect of supradiaphragmatic splanchnicectomy with lower dorsal sympathetic ganglionectomy. Arch. intern. Med. 71, 357 (1943). — FOLLI, G., V. E. POLLAK, R. T. W. REID, C. L. PIRANI and R. M. KARK: Electronmicroscopic studies of reversible glomerular lesions in the adult nephrotic syndrome. Ann. intern. Med. 49, 775 (1958). — FØLLING, A.: On the mechanism of ammonium chloride acidosis. Acta med. scand. 71, 221 (1929). — FONTES, M. M. G., et A. YOVANOVITCH: Exist-ils des sels ammoniacaux dans le sang? Bull. Soc. Chim. biol. Paris 7, 1044 (1925). — FORBES, ANNE P., and JANE CLAFFEY: The response of patients with panhypopituitarism to the infusion of 3 percent saline solution. Clin. Res. Proc. 7, 240 (1959) (abstract). — FORD, R. V., J. C. MADISON and J. H. MOYER: Pharmacology of mecamylamine. Amer. J. med. Sci. 232, 129 (1956). — FORD, R. V., J. H. MOYER and C. L. SPURR: Hexamethonium in the chronic treatment of hypertension — its effect on renal hemodynamics and on the excretion of water and electrolytes. J. clin. Invest. 32, 1133 (1953). — FORSSMAN, H.: On hereditary diabetes insipidus. Acta med. scand. Suppl. 159 (1945). — FORSTER, R. P.: The use of inulin and creatinine as glomerular filtrate measuring substances in the frog. J. cell. comp. Physiol. 12, 213 (1938a). — Xylose, inulin and creatinine clearance in the normal frog. Proc. Soc. exp. Biol. (N.Y.) 38, 258 (1938b). — Nature of glucose reabsorptive process in frog renal tubule. Evidence for intermittency of glomerular function in intact animal. J. cell. comp. Physiol. 20, 55 (1942). — An examination of some factors which alter glomerular activity in the rabbit kidney. Amer. J. Physiol. 150, 523 (1947). — Use of thin kidney slices and isolated renal tubules for direct study of cellular transport kinetics. Science 108, 65 (1948). — A comparative study of renal function in marine teleosts. J. cell. comp. Physiol. 42, 487 (1953). — Active cellular transport of urea by frog renal tubules. Amer. J. Physiol. 179, 372 (1954). — FORSTER, R. P., and F. BERGLUND: Contrasting inhibitory effects of probenecid on the renal tubular excretion of p-aminohippurate and on the active reabsorption of urea in the dogfish, Squalus acanthias. J. cell. comp. Physiol. 49, 281 (1957). — FORSTER, R. P., F. BERGLUND and BARBARA RENNICK: Tubular secretion of creatine, trimethylamine oxide and other organic bases by the aglomerular kidney of Lophius americanus. J. gen. Physiol. 42, 319 (1958). — FORSTER, R. P., and J. H. COPENHAVER jr.: Intracellular accumulation as an active process in a mammalian renal transport system in vitro. Energy dependence and competetive phenomena. Amer. J. Physiol. 186, 167 (1956). — FORSTER, R. P., and S. K. HONG: In vitro transport of dyes by isolated renal tubules of the flounder as disclosed by direct visualization. Intracellular accumulation and transcellular movement. J. cell. comp. Physiol. 51, 259 (1958). — Forster, R. P., and J. P. Maes: Effect of experimental neurogenic hypertension on renal blood flow and glomerular filtration rates in intact denervated kidneys of unanesthetized rabbits with adrenal glands demedullated. Amer. J. Physiol. 150, 534 (1947). — Forster, R. P., I. Sperber and J. V. Taggart: Transport of phenolsulfonphthalein dyes in isolated tubules of the flounder and in kidney slices of the dogfish. Competetive phenomena. J. cell. comp. Physiol. 44, 315 (1954). — Forster, R. P., and J. V. Taggart: Use of isolated renal tubules for the examination of metabolic processes associated with active cellular transport. J. cell. comp. Physiol. 36, 251 (1950). — Foulkes, E. C., and B. F. Miller: Transport of p-amino-hippurate from cell to lumen in kidney tubule. Amer. J. Physiol. 196, 83 (1959). — Steps in p-aminohippurate transport by kidney slices. Amer. J. Physiol. 196, 86 (1959). — Foulks, J., P. Brazeau, E. S. Koelle and A. Gilman: Renal secretion of thiosulfate in the dog. Amer. J. Physiol. 168, 77 (1952). — Foulks, J., G. H. Mudge and A. Gilman: Renal excretion of cation in the dog during infusion of isotonic solutions of lithium chloride. Amer. J. Physiol. 168, 642 (1952). — Foulks, J. G.: Homeostatic adjustment in the renal tubular transport of inorganic phosphate in the dog. Canad. J. Biochem. 33, 638 (1955). — Foulks, J. G., and Florence A. Perry: Renal excretion of phosphate following para-thyroidectomy in the dog. Amer. J. Physiol. 196, 554 (1959a). — Mechanism of the phosphat-uric action of parathyroid extract in the dog. Amer. J. Physiol. 196, 561 (1959b). — Altera-tions in renal tubular phosphate transport during intravenous infusion of parathyroid extract in the dog. Amer. J. Physiol. 196, 567 (1959c). — Fourman, P.: The ability of the normal kidney to conserve potassium. Lancet 1952 I, 1042. — Fourman, P., R. A. McCance and R. A. Parker: Chronic renal disease in rats following a temporary deficiency of potas-sium. Brit. J. exp. Path. 37, 40 (1956). — Fourman, P., and J. R. Robinson: Diminished urinary excretion of citrate during deficiencies of potassium in man. Lancet 1953 II, 656. — Foye jr., L. V., and T. V. Feichtmeir: Adrenal cortical carcinoma producing solely min-eralocorticoid effect. Amer. J. Med. 29, 966 (1955). — Franck, J., and J. E. Mayer: An osmotic diffusion pump. Arch. Biochem. 14, 297 (1947). — Frankl, W., and M. S. Dunn: Apparent concentration of free tryptophan, histidine and cystine in normal human urine measured microbiologically. Arch. Biochem. 13, 93 (1947). — Franklin, S. S., J. T. Au-gust, S. B. Rees, E. D. Robin and J. P. Merrill: The effect of salicylate on renal tubular transport of p-aminohippuric acid (PAH), phosphate and potassium. Clin. Res. Proc. 7, 276 (1959) (abstract). — Franklin, S. S., J. F. Niall and J. P. Merrill: The influence of solute load on the isosthenuria of renal disease. J. clin. Invest. 38, 1005 (1959) (abstract). — Fraser, A. M.: The diuretic action of the oxytocic hormone of the pituitary gland and its effect on the assay of pituitary extracts. J. Pharmacol. exp. Ther. 60, 89 (1937). — Action of oxytocic hormone of pituitary gland on urine secretion. J. Physiol. (Lond.) 101, 236 (1942). — Freeman, O. W., G. W. Mitchell, J. S. Wilson, F. W. Fitzhugh and A. J. Merrill: Renal hemodynamics, sodium and water excretion in supine exercising normal and cardiac patients. J. clin. Invest. 34, 1109 (1955). — Freis, E. D., and J. C. Rose: The sympathetic nervous system, the vascular volume and the venous return in relation to cardiovascular integration. Amer. J. Med. 22, 175 (1957). — Freis, E. D., J. C. Rose, E. A. Partenope, T. F. Higgins, R. T. Kelley, H. W. Schnaper and R. L. Johnson: The hemodynamic effects of hypotensive drugs in man. III. Hexamethonium. J. clin. Invest. 32, 1285 (1953). — Freis, E. D., H. W. Schnaper, J. C. Rose and L. S. Lilienfield: Renal transcapillary net exchange in the dog. Circulat. Res. 6, 432 (1958). — French, D. M., P. A. Molano and W. M. Booker: Renal function related to acutely and chronically raised intraabdominal pressure in anesthetized and unanesthetized dogs. Amer. J. Physiol. 167, 241 (1951). — Frey, E.: Schaltstelle des Blutstromes in der Niere und Hypophysenhinter-lappenhormon. Naunyn-Schmiedeberg's Arch. exp. Path. Pharmak. 182, 633 (1936). — Friedberg, C. K., M. Halpern and R. Taymor: The effect of intravenously administered 6063, the carbonic anhydrase inhibitor, 2-acetylamino-1,3,4-thiadiazole-5-sulfonamide, on fluid and electrolytes in normal subjects and patients with congestive heart failure. J. clin. Invest. 31, 1074 (1952). — Friederiszick, F. K.: Nieren-Clearance-Untersuchungen im Kindesalter. Bibl. paediat. (Basel) (suppl. Ann. Paed.) fasc. 57 (1954). — Friedlich, A., C. B. Holman and R. P. Forster: Renal clearance studies in the fresh-water turtle, Pseudemys elegans. Bull. Mt. Desert I. Biol. Lab. 25 (1940). — Friedman, G. J., S. Sherry and E. P. Ralli: Mechanism of excretion of vitamin C by human kidney at low and normal plasma levels of ascorbic acid. J. clin. Invest. 19, 685 (1940). — Friedman, H. L.: Relation-ship between chemical structure and biological activity in mercurial compounds. Ann. N.Y. Acad. Sci. 65, 461 (1957). — Friedman, M.: Creatinine, inulin and hippurate clearance in rat. Amer. J. Physiol. 148, 387 (1947a). — The effect of glycine on the production and excretion of uric acid. J. clin. Invest. 26, 815 (1947b). — Observations concerning the effects of (1) sodium salicylate and (2) sodium salicylate and glycine upon the production and excre-tion of uric acid and allantoin in the rat. Amer. J. Physiol. 152, 302 (1948). — Friedman, M., and S. O. BYERS: Effect of sodium salicylate upon the uric acid clearance of the Dalmatian dog. Amer. J. Physiol. **154**, 167 (1948). — Increased renal excretion of urate in young patients with gout. Amer. J. Med. **9**, 31 (1950). — FRIEDMAN, M., S. O. BYERS and P. M. ABRAHM: Allantoin clearance as measure of glomerular filtration rate in man. Proc. Soc. exp. Biol. (N.Y.) **66**, 522 (1947). — Renal clearance of allantoin as a measure of glomerular filtration rate. Amer. J. Physiol. **155**, 278 (1948). — FRIEDMAN, M., A. SELZER and H. ROSENBLUM: The renal blood flow in coarctation of the aorta. J. clin. Invest. **20**, 197 (1941 a). — Renal blood flow in hypertension as determined in patients with variable, with early and with long-standing hypertension. J. Amer. med. Ass. **117**, 92 (1941 b). — FRIEDMAN, M., A. SELZER, J. SUGARMAN and M. SOKOLOW: The renal blood flow, glomerular filtration rate and degree of tubular reabsorption of glucose in renal glycosuria. Amer. J. med. Sci. **204**, 22 (1942). — FRISK, A. R.: Sulfanilamide derivitives. Chemotherapeutic evaluation of N'-substituted sulfanilamides. Acta med. scand. Suppl. **142** (1943). — FRITZ, K. W., u. H. NÜSSGENS: Methodische Fehlermöglichkeiten der Inulinclearance. Z. ges. exp. Med. **128**, 393 (1957). — FROESCH, E. R., A. I. WINEGRAD u. A. E. RENOLD: Die tubuläre Nierenfunktion bei verschiedenen Formen des renalen Diabetes mellitus. Helv. med. Acta **24**, 548 (1957). — FROESCH, E. R., A. I. WINEGRAD, A. E. RENOLD and G. W. THORN: Mechanism of the glycosuria produced by the administration of steroids with glucocorticoid activity. J. clin. Invest. **37**, 524 (1958). — FROMHERZ, K.: Über die Wirkung der Hypophysenextrakte auf die Nierenfunktion. Naunyn-Schmiedeberg's Arch. exp. Path. u. Pharmak. **100**, 1 (1923). — FUCHS, ANNA-RITA, and F. FUCHS: Investigations on the plasma phosphate. I. The renal excretion of phosphate in the guinea pig. Acta physiol. scand. **30**, 191 (1954). — FULLER, G. R., and MARTHA B. MACLEOD: Excretion of titratable acid during acute respiratory disturbances of acid-base balance. Amer. J. Physiol. **186**, 505 (1956). — FULLER, G. R., MARTHA B. MACLEOD and R. F. PITTS: Influence of administration of potassium salts on the renal tubular reabsorption of bicarbonate. Amer. J. Physiol. **182**, 111 (1955). — FULTON, M. N., H. A. AUKEN, R. J. PARSONS and L. F. DAVENPORT: The comparative effect of various diuretics in dogs with special reference to the excretion of urine, chloride and urea. J. Pharmacol. exp. Ther. **50**, 223 (1934). — FURMAN, R. H., R. G. GALE, E. M. ORY and A. WEINSTEIN: Renal function studies in acute syphilitic nephrosis before and after treatment with penicillin. Ann. intern. Med. **35**, 444 (1951).

GABUDZA jr., G. J., H. S. TRAEGER and C. S. DAVIDSON: Hepatic cirrhosis: Effects of sodium chloride administration and restriction and of abdominal paracentesis on electrolyte and water balance. J. clin. Invest. **33**, 780 (1954). — GAGNON, J. A., and R. W. CLARKE: Renal functions in the chimpanzee. Amer. J. Physiol. **190**, 117 (1957). — GALAN, E.: Nephrosis in children. I. Observations on 84 patients. II. Clearance and saturation tests. Amer. J. Dis. Child. **77**, 328 (1949). — GALAN, E., y O. G. FAEZ: Aclaramientos simultaneos de thiosulfato e inulina en el nino normal. Rev. cubana Pediat. **20**, 32 (1948). — GALAN, E., M. PEREZ-STABLE, J. MAS MARTIN y O. GARCIA FAEZ: Las Pruebas renales de aclaramiento y saturacion en el nino normal. Arch. Med. infant. **16**, 102 (1947). — GALIMARD, J. E.: Métabolism du salicylate de sodium. I. Salicylurie et gluconurie. Bull. Soc. Chem. biol. **26**, 185 (1944). — GAMBLE, J. L.: Carbonic acid and bicarbonate in urine. J. biol. Chem. **51**, 295 (1922). — Physiological information gained from studies on the life raft ration. Harvey Lect. **42**, 247 (1946/47). — GAMBLE, J. L., K. D. BLACKFAN and B. HAMILTON: A study of the diuretic action of acid producing salts. J. clin. Invest. **1**, 359 (1924/25). — GAMBLE, J. L., and A. M. BUTLER: Measurement of renal water requirement. Trans. Ass. Amer. Phycns **58**, 157 (1944). — GAMBLE, J. L., G. S. ROSS and F. F. TISDALL: Studies of tetany. I. The effect of calcium chloride ingestion on acid-base metabolism of infants. Amer. J. Dis. Child. **25**, 455 (1923). — GAMMELTOFT, A., and K. KJERULF-JENSEN: The mechanisms of renal excretion of fructose and galactose in rabbit, cat, dog and man (with special reference to the phosphorylation theory). Acta physiol. scand. **6**, 369 (1943). — GANONG, W. F., and P. J. MULROW: Rate of change in sodium and potassium excretion after injection of aldosterone into the aorta and renal artery of the dog. Amer. J. Physiol. **195**, 337 (1958). — GARBY, L.: On the mechanism of formation of the glomerular fluid. Acta physiol. scand. **35**, 88 (1955). — GARDNER, L. I., E. A. MACLACHLAN and H. BERMAN: Effect of potassium deficiency on carbon dioxide, cation, and phosphate content of muscle. J. gen. Physiol. **36**, 153 (1952). — GARROD, O., and R. A. BURSTON: The diuretic response to ingested water in Addison's disease and panhypopituitarism and the effect of cortisone thereon. Clin. Sci. **11**, 113 (1952). — GARROD, O., S. A. DAVIES and G. CAHILL jr.: The action of cortisone and desoxycorticosterone acetate on glomerular filtration rate and sodium and water exchange in the adrenalectomized dog. J. clin. Invest. **34**, 761 (1955). — GARST, JOSEPHINE B., N. P. SHUMWAY, H. SCHWARTZ and G. L. FARRELL: Aldosterone excretion in hypertension. Fed. Proc. **19**, 166 (1960) (abstract). — GAUDINO, M., and M. F. LEVITT: Influence of the adrenal cortex on body water distribution and renal function. J. clin. Invest. **28**, 1487 (1949). — GAUER, O. H., J. P. HENRY, H. O. SIEKER and W. E. WENDT: The effect of negative pressure breathing on urine flow. J. clin. Invest. **33**, 287 (1954). — GAUNT, R., J. H. BIRNIE and W. J. EVERSOLE: Adrenal cortex and water metabolism. Physiol. Rev. **29**, 281 (1949). — GAUNT, R., MILDRED LILING and MARGARET CORDSEN: Adrenal medulla in water diuresis and water intoxication. Endocrinology **37**, 136 (1945). — GAUNT, R., A. A. RENZI and J. J. CHART: Aldosterone. A review. J. clin. Endocr. **15**, 621 (1955). — GAVAZZENI, M.: Filtrato glomerulare e diuretici. Policlinica, Sez. med. **39**, 236 (1932). — GENEST, J., E. KOIW, W. NOWACZYNSKI and G. LEBOEUF: Further studies on urinary aldosterone in human arterial hypertension. Proc. Soc. exp. Biol. (N.Y.) **97**, 676 (1958). — GENEST, J., E. V. NEWMAN, A. A. KATTUS, B. SINCLAIR-SMITH and A. GENECIN: Renal function before and after surgical resection of coarctation of the aorta. Bull. Johns Hopk. Hosp. **83**, 429 (1948). — GENEST, J., W. NOWACZYNSKI, E. KOIW, J.-M. PEPIN, B. THERIEN and B. VITYE: Aldosterone excretion in late normal pregnancy. Clin. Res. Proc. **5**, 190 (1957) (abstract). — GÉRARD, P.: Comparative histophysiology of the vertebrate nephron. J. Anat. (Lond.) **70**, 354 (1936). — GERRITZEN, F.: Der 24-Stunden-Rhythmus der Chlorausscheidung. Pflügers Arch. ges. Physiol. **238**, 483 (1937). — The rhythmic function of the human liver. Acta med. scand. Suppl. **108**, 121 (1940). — GERSH, I.: Reabsorption of water during pituitary antidiuresis. J. Pharmacol. exp. Ther. **52**, 231 (1934). — GERSH, I., and E. J. STIEGLITZ: Histochemical studies on the mammalian kidney. I. The glomerular elimination of ferrocyanide in the rabbit and some related problems. Anat. Rec. **58**, 349 (1933/34). — GERSHBERG, H., and J. GASCH: Effect of growth hormone on sulfate Tm, urea clearance and fasting blood glucose. Proc. Soc. exp. Biol. (N.Y.) **91**, 46 (1956). — GERSHBERG, H., H. O. HEINEMANN and H. H. STUMPF: Renal function studies and autopsy report in a patient with gigantism and acromegaly. J. clin. Endocr. **17**, 377 (1957). — GERSHBERG, H., J. HODLER and J. GASCH: Diet and hormones on plasma sulfate and Tm$_{SO_4}$. Fed. Proc. **13**, 53 (1954) (abstract). — GERSHBERG, H., D. R. SHIELDS and SALLY S. KOVE: The acute effects of parathyroid extract in states of edema, diminished renal function and parathyroid disease. J. clin. Endocr. **19**, 681 (1959). — GIARMAN, N. J., and G. A. CONDOURIS: The antidiuretic action of morphine and some of its analogs. Arch. int. Pharmacodyn. **97**, 28 (1954). — GIARMAN, N. J., L. R. MATTIE and W. F. STEPHENSON: Studies on the antidiuretic action of morphine. Science **117**, 225 (1953). — GIBSON 2nd, J. G., A. M. SELIGMAN, W. C. PEACOCK, J. C. AUB, J. FINE and R. D. EVANS: The distribution of red cells and plasma in large and minute vessels of the normal dog, determined by radioactive isotopes of iron and iodine. J. clin. Invest. **25**, 848 (1946). — GIEBISCH, G.: Measurements of p$_H$, chloride and inulin concentrations in proximal tubule fluid of *Necturus*. Amer. J. Physiol. **185**, 171 (1956). — Electrical potential measurements on single nephrons of *Necturus*. J. cell. comp. Physiol. **51**, 221 (1958). — GIEBISCH, G., and P. J. DORMAN: Comparative study of uptake and distribution of Hg^{203} given as labelled chlormerodrin (Neohydrin). Proc. Soc. exp. Biol. (N.Y.) **98**, 50 (1958). — GIEBISCH, G., H. D. LAUSON and R. F. PITTS: Renal excretion and volume of distribution of various dextrans. Amer. J. Physiol. **178**, 168 (1954). — GIEBISCH, G., and R. LOZANO: The effects of adrenal steroids and potassium depletion on the elaboration of an osmotically concentrated urine. J. clin. Invest. **38**, 843 (1959). — GIEBISCH, G., MARTHA B. MACLEOD and F. KAVALER: Renal excretion of radioiodide in the dog. Amer. J. Physiol. **187**, 529 (1956). — GIEBISCH, G., MARTHA B. MACLEOD and R. F. PITTS: Effect of adrenal steroids on renal tubular reabsorption of bicarbonate. Amer. J. Physiol. **183**, 377 (1955). — GIEBISCH, G., and E. E. WINDHAGER: Chloride fluxes across single proximal tubules of *Necturus* kidney. Fed. Proc. **18**, 52 (1959) (abstract). — GIERE, F. A.: Further studies on the effects of adrenal medullary hormones on renal excretion of water and electrolytes in the intact rat. Endocrinology **55**, 448 (1954). — GILBERT, J. L., and GERTRUDE LANGE: Renal clearance of I^{131} in hypothyroid and euthyroid rats. Endocrinology **59**, 181 (1955). — GILL jr., J. R., D. S. GANN, CATHERINE S. DELEA and F. C. BARTTER: Correction of the defect in water excretion in untreated Addisonian patients by volume expansion alone. Clin. Res. Proc. **7**, 254 (1959) (abstract). — GILLIGAN, D. R., M. D. ALTSCHULE and EVELYN M. KATERSKY: Studies of hemoglobinemia and hemoglobinuria produced in man by intravenous injection of hemoglobin solutions. J. clin. Invest. **20**, 177 (1941). — GILMAN, A.: The relation between blood osmotic pressure, fluid distribution and voluntary water intake. Amer. J. Physiol. **120**, 323 (1937). — GILMAN, A., and L. GOODMAN: The secretory response of the posterior pituitary to the need for water conservation. J. Physiol. (Lond.) **90**, 133 (1937). — GILMAN, A., F. S. PHILIPS and ETHOL S. KOELLE: The renal clearance of thiosulfate with observations on its volume distribution. Amer. J. Physiol. **146**, 348 (1946). — GINN, H. E., W. O. SMITH, J. F. HAMMARSTEN and D. SNYDER: Renal tubular secretion of magnesium in dogs. Proc. Soc. exp. Biol. (N.Y.) **101**, 691 (1959). — GINSBURG, M.: The secretion of antidiuretic hormone in response to haemorrhage and the fate of vasopressin in adrenalectomized rats. J. Endocr. **11**, 165 (1954). — GIRERD, R. J., L. E. TENEBAUM, J. BERKOWITZ, C. L. RASSAERT et D. M. GREEN: Diurèse et inhibition de la glutaminase rénale. Rev. canad. Biol. **16**, 411 (1957). — GIROUD, C. J. P., M. SAFFRAN, A. V. SCHALLY, J. STACHENKO and ELEANOR H. VENNING: Production of aldosterone by rat adrenal glands *in vitro*. Proc. Soc. exp. Biol. (N.Y.) **92**, 855 (1956). — GIROUD, C. J. P., J. STACHENKO and P. PILETTA: *In vitro* studies of the functional zonation of the adrenal cortex and of the production of aldosterone. Aldosterone, p. 56. Boston: Little, Brown & Co. 1958. — GIROUD, C. J. P., J. STACHENKO and ELEANOR H. VENNING: Secretion of aldosterone by the zona glomerulosa of rat adrenal glands incubated *in vitro*. Proc. Soc. exp. Biol. (N.Y.) **92**, 154 (1956). — GIUSEFFI, J., E. E. WERK jr., P. U. LARSON, L. SCHIFF and D. W. ELLIOTT: Effect of bilateral adrenalectomy in a patient with massive ascites and postnecrotic cirrhosis. New Engl. J. Med. **257**, 796 (1957). — GJORUP, S., and T. HILDEN: The effect of hydralazine (apresolin) on kidney function and sodium excretion. Scand. J. clin. Lab. Invest. 8, 273 (1956). — GLAUSER, K. F., and E. E. SELKURT: Effect of barbiturates on renal function in the dog. Amer. J. Physiol. **168**, 469 (1952). — GLOBUS, D. L., E. L. BECKER and D. D. THOMPSON: Renal excretion of inorganic sulfate in the chicken. Fed. Proc. **19**, 369 (1960) (abstract). — GLOBUS, D. L., R. H. KESSLER and D. D. THOMPSON: Localization of calcium transport in the nephron of the dog. Fed. Proc. **18**, 53 (1959) (abstract). — GOADBY, H. K.: On the action of parathormone. III. Biochem. J. **31**, 1530 (1937). — GOLDBAUM, L. R., and T. F. HUBBARD: Effect of carinamide (4′ carboxyphenylmethane sulfonanilide) on the metabolism of thiopental in mice. J. Pharmacol. exp. Ther. **99**, 366 (1950). — GOLDENBERG, M., I. SERLIN, THEODORA EDWARDS and M. M. RAPPORT: Chemical screening methods for the diagnosis of Pheochromocytoma. Amer. J. Med. **16**, 310 (1954). — GOLDMAN, H., and L. A. SAPIRSTEIN: Determination of blood flow to the rat pituitary gland. Amer. J. Physiol. **194**, 433 (1958). — GOLDMAN, M. L., ETHEL RONZONI and H. A. SCHROEDER: The response of the adrenal cortex of the rat to dietary salt restriction and replacement. Endocrinology **58**, 57 (1956). — GOLDMAN, R.: Studies in diurnal variation of water and electrolyte excretion: Nocturnal diuresis of water and sodium in congestive cardiac failure and cirrhosis of the liver. J. clin. Invest. **30**, 1191 (1951). — Creatinine excretion in renal failure. Proc. Soc. exp. Biol. (N.Y.) **85**, 446 (1954). — The clinical evaluation of renal function. Calif. Med. **85**, 376 (1956). — GOLDMAN, R., and S. H. BASSETT: Diurnal variation in steroid excretion of neutral, lipid soluble reducing steroids in congestive cardiac failure and cirrhosis of the liver with ascites. J. clin. Invest. **31**, 253 (1952). — Phosphorus excretion in renal failure. J. clin. Invest. **33**, 1623 (1954). — Renal regulation of phosphorus excretion. J. Clin. Endocr. **18**, 981 (1958). — GOLDMAN, R., and ELIZABETH B. LUCHSINGER: Relationship between diurnal variations in urinary volume and the excretion of antidiuretic substance. J. clin. Endocr. **16**, 28 (1956). — GOLDRING, W.: The effects on renal activity of the oral administration of phlorizin in man. J. clin. Invest. **13**, 749 (1934). — GOLDRING, W., and H. CHASIS: Hypertension and hypertensive disease. New York: Commonwealth Fund 1944. — GOLDRING, W., H. CHASIS, H. A. RANGES and H. W. SMITH: Relations of effective renal blood flow and glomerular filtration to tubular excretory mass in normal man. J. clin. Invest. **19**, 739 (1940). — Effective renal blood flow in subjects with essential hypertension. J. clin. Invest. **20**, 637 (1941). — GOLDRING, W., R. W. CLARKE and H. W. SMITH: The phenol red clearance in normal man. J. clin. Invest. **15**, 221 (1936). — GOLDRING, W., L. RAZINSKY, M. GREENBLATT and S. COHEN: The influence of protein intake on the urea clearance in normal man. J. clin. Invest. **13**, 743 (1934). — GOLDSMITH, R. S., F. C. BARTTER, P. J. ROSCH, W. H. MERONEY and E. G. HERNDON jr.: "Primary aldosteronism" with edema. Clin. Res. Proc. **6**, 27 (1958) (abstract). — GOLDSTEIN, L., R. RICHTERICH-VAN BAERLE and E. H. DEARBORN: Increased activity of renal glutaminases in guinea pig following prolonged administration of acid or alkali. Proc. Soc. exp. Biol. (N.Y.) **93**, 284 (1956). — GOMBOS, E. A., P. BOPP, D. S. BALDWIN and H. CHASIS: Effect of induced congestion of the limbs on the function of the separate kidneys in normal man. Fed. Proc. **18**, 55 (1959) (abstract). — GOMEZ, D. M.: Evaluation of renal resistances with special reference to changes in essential hypertension. J. clin. Invest. **30**, 1143 (1951). — GOMORI, G., and E. GULYAS: Effect of parenterally administered citrate on renal excretion of calcium. Proc. Soc. exp. Biol. (N.Y.) **56**, 226 (1944). — GOODKIND, M. J., W. C. BALL jr. and J. O. DAVIS: Effect of chronic hemorrhage on urinary aldosterone-like activity and sodium excretion in dogs. Amer. J. Physiol. **189**, 181 (1957). — GOODKIND, M. J., R. E. HYATT and J. O. DAVIS: Failure of large doses of desoxycorticosterone acetate to block mercurial natriuresis in adrenalectomized dogs with thoracic inferior vena cava constriction and ascites. Amer. J. Physiol. **187**, 361 (1956). — GOODMAN, H. C., and J. H. BAXTER: Tubular reabsorption of protein in experimentally produced proteinuria in rats. Proc. Soc. exp. Biol. (N.Y.) **93**, 136 (1956). — GOODMAN, J. I., J. F. CORSARO and R. STACY: Mercurial and xanthine diuretics in chronic congestive heart failure. Arch. intern. Med. **70**, 975 (1942). — GOODWIN, W. E., and J. J. KAUFMAN: The renal lymphatics. I. Review of some of the pertinent literature. Urol. Surv. **6**, 305 (1956a). — Renal lymphatics. II. Preliminary experiments. J. Urol. (Baltimore) **76**, 702 (1956b). — GOODWIN, W. E., R. D. SLOAN and W. W. SCOTT: The "Trueta" renal vascular "shunt". J. Urol. (Baltimore) **61**, 1010 (1949). — GOODYER, A. V. N., and W. W.

336   LAURENCE G. WESSON:

L. GLENN: Relation of arterial pulse pressure to renal function. Amer. J. Physiol. 167, 689 (1951). — Observations on the hyponatremia following mitral valvulotomy. Circulation 11, 584 (1955). — GOODYER, A. V. N., and C. A. JAEGER: Renal response to nonshocking hemorrhage: Role of the autonomic nervous system and of the renal circulation. Amer. J. Physiol. 180, 69 (1955). — GOODYER, A. V. N., L. R. MATTIE and A. CHETRICK: Renal response to nonshocking hemorrhage: The role of intrarenal shunts. Amer. J. Physiol. 193, 360 (1958). — GOODYER, A. V. N., E. R. PETERSON and A. S. RELMAN: Some effects of albumin infusions on renal function and electrolyte excretion in normal man. J. appl. Physiol. 1, 671 (1949). — GOODYER, A. V. N., and D. W. SELDIN: The effects of quiet standing on solute diuresis. J. clin. Invest. 32, 242 (1953). — GOORMAGHTIGH, N.: L'appareil neuro-myo-artériel juxtaglomerulaire du rein; ses réactions en pathologie et ses rapports avec le tube urinifère. C. R. Soc. Biol. (Paris) 124, 293 (1937). — Existence of an endocrine gland in the media of the renal arterioles. Proc. Soc. exp. Biol. (N.Y.) 42, 688 (1939). — GOORMAGHTIGH, N., and K. S. GRIMSON: Vascular changes in renal ischemia cell mitosis in the media of arteries. Proc. Soc. exp. Biol. (N.Y.) 42, 227 (1939). — GORDILLO, G., R. A. SOTO, J. METCOFF, ELIZABETH LOPEZ and L. G. ANTILLON: Intracellular composition and homeostatic mechanisms in severe chronic infantile malnutrition. III. Renal adjustments. Pediatrics 20, 303 (1957). — GORDON, E. S., J. J. CHART, DOROTHY HAGEDORN and ELVA G. SHIPLEY: Mechanism of sodium retention in preeclamptic toxemia. Obstet. and Gynec. 4, 39 (1954). — GORDON, E. S., J. J. CHART and E. S. MEYER: The importance of a 'sodium retaining factor' in the urine in the mechanism of edema formation. J. clin. Invest. 31, 633 (1952) (abstract). — GORDON, G. B., A. EICHENHOLZ, F. MacDONALD and T. SEMBA: Studies on the mechanism of bicarbonate reabsorption in man. Clin. Res. Proc. 7, 76 (1959) (abstract). — GORDON, W., A. S. ALVING, N. R. KRETZSCHMAR and L. ALPERT: Variations in the extraction of urea by the kidney and their relation to the amount of urea reabsorbed. Amer. J. Physiol. 119, 483 (1937). — GOTTSCHALK, C. W.: An experimental and comparative study of renal interstitial pressure. Amer. J. Physiol. 163, 716 (1950) (abstract). — A comparative study of renal interstitial pressure. Amer. J. Physiol. 169, 180 (1952). — GOTTSCHALK, C. W., W. E. LASSITER and MARGARET MYLLE: Localization of urine acidification in the mammalian kidney. Amer. J. Physiol. 198, 581 (1960). — GOTTSCHALK, C. W., and MARGARET MYLLE: Micropuncture study of pressures in proximal tubules and peritubular capillaries of the rat kidney and their relation to ureteral and renal venous pressures. Amer. J. Physiol. 185, 430 (1956). — Micropuncture study of pressures in proximal and distal tubules and peritubular capillaries of the rat kidney during osmotic diuresis. Amer. J. Physiol. 189, 323 (1957). — Evidence that the mammalian nephron functions as a countercurrent multiplier system. Science 128, 594 (1958). — Micropuncture study of the mammalian urinary concentrating mechanism: Evidence for the countercurrent hypothesis. Amer. J. Physiol. 196, 927 (1959). — GOTTSCHALK, C. W., MARGARET MYLLE, R. W. WINTERS and L. G. WELT: Micropuncture study of the osmolality of renal tubular fluid in potassium-depleted rats. J. clin. Invest. 37, 898 (1958) (abstract). — GOVAERTS, A., and R. DELANNE: Influence of intensity of muscular exertion on diuresis, albumin and cylindruria. Brux.-méd. 20, 361 (1940). — GOVAERTS, J.: Urinary excretion of phosphate with $^{32}_{15}$P as indicator. Nature (Lond.) 160, 53 (1947). — Étude de l'état physico-chimique de l'ion phosphorique dans le plasma a l'aide du radiophosphore $^{32}_{15}$P en rapport avec le seuil d'élimination urinaire de l'ion phosphorique. Arch. int. Pharmacodyn. 75, 261 (1947/48). — Studies in calcium urinary excretion with the aid of radiocalcium. Amer. J. Physiol. 159, 542 (1949). — GOVAERTS, J., and R. MACHIROUS: L'éxistence de deux formes de phosphore dans le plasma. Proc. First (UNESCO) Internat. Conf. Sci. Res. 4, 52 (1958). — GOVAERTS, M. P., et M. P. CAMBIER: Élimination comparée du glucose, de la créatinine et de l'urée sous l'influence de la phlorizine. Bull. Acad. roy. Méd. Belg. 14, 226 (1934). — GOVAERTS, P.: Origin rénale ou tissulaire de la diurèse par un composé mercuriel organique. C. R. Soc. Biol. (Paris) 99, 647 (1928). — Ratio of creatinine clearance to urea clearance in toxic nephropathies. Stanf. med. Bull. 6, 71 (1948). — Physiopathology of glucose excretion by the human kidney. Brit. med. J. 1952 II, 4777. — GOVAERTS, P., and P.-P. LAMBERT: Pathogénie du diabète rénal. Acta clin. belg. 4, 341 (1949). — GOWENLOCK, A. H., J. N. MILLS and S. THOMAS: Acute postural changes in aldosterone and electrolyte excretion in man. J. Physiol. (Lond.) 146, 133 (1959). — GRABFIELD, G. P., and D. SWANSON: Uricosuric effects of certain polyhydric alcohols and saccharides. J. Pharmacol. exp. Ther. 74, 106 (1942). — GRAFFLIN, A. L.: The normal, the acromegalic and the hyperplastic nephritic human nephron. A further consideration of the plastic reconstructions of Louis A. Turley. Arch. Path. (Chicago) 27, 691 (1939). — Storage and distribution of iron-containing pigment and problem of segmental differentiation in proximal tubule of rat nephron. Amer. J. Anat. 70, 399 (1942). — GRAFFLIN, A. L., and E. H. BAGLEY: Glomerular activity in the frog's kidney. Bull. Johns Hopk. Hosp. 91, 306 (1952). — GRANT, H., and F. REISCHSMAN: The effects of the ingestion of large amounts of sodium chloride on the arterial and venous pressures of normal subjects. Amer. Heart J.

32, 704 (1946). — GREEN, D. M., and A. FARAH: Influence of sodium load on sodium excretion. Amer. J. Physiol. **158**, 444 (1949). — GREEN, D. M., A. D. JOHNSON, W. C. BRIDGES, J. H. LEHMANN, F. GRAY and A. FARAH: Effect of desoxycorticosterone glycoside on the tubular reabsorption of glucose. Endocrinology **46**, 338 (1950). — GREEN, D. M., H. G. WEDELL, M. H. WALD and B. LEARNED: The relation of water and sodium excretion to blood pressure in human subjects. Circulation **6**, 919 (1952). — GREEN, H. D., R. N. LEWIS, N. D. NICKERSON and A. L. HELLER: Blood flow, peripheral resistance and vascular tonus, with observations on the relationship between blood flow and cutaneous temperature. Amer. J. Physiol. **141**, 518 (1944). — GREEN, R. E., and L. PETERS: Inhibition of renal tubular excretion of N'-methylnicotinamide (NMN) by tetraalkylammonium derivatives in the chicken. Fed. Proc. **16**, 302 (1957) (abstract). — GREEN, R. E., W. E. RICKER, W. L. ATTWOOD, Y. S. KOH and L. PETERS: Studies of the renal tubular transport characteristics of N'-methylnicotinamide and tetraalkylammonium compounds in the avian kidney. J. Pharmacol. exp. Ther. **126**, 195 (1959). — GREENBERG, D. M., and C. E. LARSON: The relation of calcium proteinate and colloidal calcium phosphate in the partition of calcium in the blood stream. J. physic. Chem. **43**, 1139 (1939). — GREENE, INEZ, and E. P. HIATT: Behavior of the nitrate ion in the dog. Amer. J. Physiol. **176**, 463 (1954). — Renal excretion of nitrate and its effect on excretion of sodium and chloride. Amer. J. Physiol. **180**, 179 (1955). — GREEP, R. O.: The physiology and chemistry of the parathyroid hormone. Hormones **1**, 255 (1948). — GREEP, R. O., and HELEN W. DEANE: Cytochemical evidence for the cessation of hormone production in the zona glomerulosa of the rat's adrenal cortex after prolonged treatment with desoxycorticosterone acetate. Endocrinology **40**, 417 (1947). — GREER, M. A.: Suggestive evidence of a primary "drinking center" in the hypothalamus of the rat. Proc. Soc. exp. Biol. (N.Y.) **89**, 59 (1955). — GREGORY, R., W. C. LEVIN, G. T. Ross and A. BENNETT: Studies on hypertension; effect of lowering blood pressures of hypertensive patients by high spinal anesthesia on renal function as measured by inulin and diodrast clearances. Arch. intern. Med. **77**, 385 (1946). — GREIF, R. L., and GLORIA S. JACOBS: Effect of mercurial diuretics upon oxidative phosphorylation in rat kidney mitochondria. Amer. J. Physiol. **192**, 599 (1958). — GREIF, R. L., W. J. SULLIVAN, GLORIA S. JACOBS and R. F. PITTS: Distribution of radiomercury administered as labelled chlormerodrin (Neohydrin) in the kidneys of rats and dogs. J. clin. Invest. **35**, 38 (1956). — GREINER, A., and L. PODHRADSZKY: Kidney function in diabetes insipidus. Lancet **1947II**, 499. — GREVE, M. J., E. E. EDDLEMAN jr., K. WILLIS, S. EISENBERG and T. R. HARRISON: The effect of digitoxin on sodium excretion, creatinine clearance and apparent cardiac output. Circulation **3**, 405 (1951). — GRIBETZ, D., K. VAN LOON and J. D. CRAWFORD: Comparison of renal endogenous creatinine and inulin clearances in the rat. Amer. J. Physiol. **183**, 401 (1955). — GRIBOFF, S. I., ROSLYN WIENER, J. EISENBERG, A. IANNACCONE and L. J. SOFFER: Metabolic studies with aldosterone in a patient with Addison's disease and in a normal subject. Metabolism **4**, 289 (1955). — GRIGGS, D. E., and V. J. JOHNS: Influence of mercurial diuretics on the excretion of sodium, potassium and chlorides. Calif. Med. **69**, 133 (1948). — GRIM, E., W. H. BRODSKY, W. S. REHM and W. H. DENNIS: Osmotic gradients across cellular membranes. Science **124**, 221 (1956). — GRIMELLI, L. J., M. M. CHERTACK, H. L. RHETTA, A. B. KENDRICK and R. A. FORREST: Effect of hyperglycemia on the clearances of inulin and paraaminohippuric acid. J. Lab. clin. Med. **33**, 1617 (1948) (abstract). — GROLLMAN, A.: The combination of phenol red and proteins. J. biol. Chem. **64**, 141 (1925). — The condition of the inorganic phosphorus of the blood with special reference to the calcium concentration. J. biol. Chem. **72**, 565 (1927). — The role of the kidney in the parathyroid control of the blood calcium as determined by studies on the nephrectomized dog. Endocrinology **55**, 166 (1954). — GROSS, F., and W. D. DETTBARN: Water and salt loading in adrenalectomised dogs treated with cortexone, aldosterone, and 9-α-fluororcortisol. Acta endocr. (Kbh.) **22**, 335 (1956). — GROSS, F., and H. GYSEL: The action of electrocortin in the adrenalectomized dog. Acta endocr. (Kbh.) **15**, 199 (1954). — GROSS, F., and P. LICHTLEN: Further evidence for a qualitative difference between aldosterone and cortexone. Aldosterone, p. 39. Boston: Little, Brown & Co. 1958. — GROSSMAN, J.: Volume factors in body fluid regulation. Arch. intern. Med. **99**, 93 (1957). — GROSSMAN, J., A. G. GOLDMAN and M. F. MINES: Calcium diuresis: Effects on urinary composition and renal concentrating function in man. Fed. Proc. **17**, 62 (1958) (abstract). — GROSSMAN, J., M. F. MINES, A. G. GOLDMAN and M. WOLFMAN: Effects of calcium on urine concentrating ability. J. clin. Invest. **37**, 899 (1958) (abstract). — GROSSMAN, J., R. E. WESTON, E. R. BORUN and L. LEITER: Factors influencing the course of mercurial diuresis during pitressin infusion in normal subjects. J. clin. Invest. **34**, 1611 (1955). — GROSSMAN, J., R. E. WESTON, I. S. EDELMAN and L. LEITER: Studies on thiomerin — a subcutaneously administerable mercurial diuretic. Circulation **1**, 508 (1950a). — GROSSMAN, J., R. E. WESTON, J. P. HALPERIN and L. LEITER: The nature of the renal circulatory changes in chronic congestive failure as refleted by renal tubular maximal functions. J. clin. Invest. **29**, 1320 (1950b). — GROSSMAN,

J., R. E. WESTON, R. A. LEHMAN, J. P. HALPERIN, T. D. ULLMANN and L. LEITER: Urinary and fecal excretion of mercury in man following administration of mercurial diuretics. J. clin. Invest. **30**, 1208 (1951). — GROSSMAN, W.: Diurese als bedingter Reflex beim Hunde. Klin. Wschr. **8**, 1500 (1929). — GRUBER, C. M.: The autonomic innervation of genito-urinary system. Physiol. Rev. **13**, 497 (1933). — GRUPP, G.: Der Einfluß von Adrenalin und Nor-Adrenalin auf die Durchblutung und Wärmebildung der Niere. Naunyn-Schmiede-berg's Arch. exp. Path. Pharmak. **232**, 254 (1957). — Das Verhalten der Selbststeuerung des Nierenkreislaufs und der Wärmebildung der Niere auf die Erhöhung des Venendrucks. Z. ges. exp. Med. **131**, 174 (1959). — GUILLEMIN, R., W. E. DEAR, B. NICHOLS jr. and H. S. LIPSCOMB: ACTH releasing activity *in vivo* of a CRF preparation and of lysine vasopressin. Proc. Soc. exp. Biol. (N.Y.) **101**, 107 (1959). — GUILLEMIN, R., and B. ROSENBERG: Humoral hypothalamic control of anterior pituitary: A study with combined tissue cultures. Endocrinology **57**, 599 (1955). — GUKELBERGER, M.: Über das Wesen der natürlichen und künst-lichen Diurese. Helv. med. Acta **11**, 17 (1944). — GUKELBERGER, M., u. A. ABPLANALP: Der Nachweis geringer Eiweiß- und Polypeptidmengen im Urin und seine Bedeutung für die Beurteilung der Durchlässigkeit der Nierencapillaren. Dtsch. Arch. klin. Med. **187**, 392 (1940/41). — GUKELBERGER, M., u. F. WYSS: Zur stufenphotometrischen Bestimmung des Kreatinins in Plasma und Urin mit Hilfe der m-Dinitrobenzoesäure. Z. ges. exp. Med. **111**, 352 (1942). — GUTMAN, A. B.: Benemid (p-di-n-propylsulfamyl)-benzoic acid as uricosuric agent in chronic gouty arthritis. Trans. Ass. Amer. Phycns **64**, 279 (1951). — GUTMAN, A. B., and TSAI F. YÜ: Effects of adrenocorticotropic hormone (ACTH) in gout. Amer. J. Med. **9**, 24 (1950). — Effect of salicylate in varying dosage on urinary urate excretion in gouty subjects. Ann. rheum. Dis. **14**, 444 (1955) (abstract). — Renal function in gout. With a commentary on the renal regulation of urate excretion, and the role of the kidney in the pathogenesis of gout. Amer. J. Med. **23**, 600 (1957). — GUTMAN, A. B., TSAI F. YÜ and L. BERGER: Tubular secretion of urate in man. J. clin. Invest. **38**, 1778 (1959). — GUTMAN, A. B., TSAI F. YÜ and J. H. SIROTA: A study, by simultaneous clearance techniques, of sali-cylate excretion in man. Effect of alkalinization of the urine by bicarbonate administration; effect of probenecid. J. clin. Invest. **34**, 711 (1955).

HAAG, H. B., and P. S. LARSON: Studies on the fate of nicotine in the body. I. The effect of pH on the urinary excretion of nicotine by tobacco smokers. J. Pharmacol. exp. Ther. **76**, 235 (1942). — HAAG, H. B., P. S. LARSON and J. J. SCHWARTZ: The effect of urinary pH on the elimination of quinine in man. J. Pharmacol. exp. Ther. **79**, 136 (1943). — HABIF, D. V., E. M. PAPPER, H. F. FITZPATRICK, P. LOWRANCE, C. McC. SMYTHE and S. E. BRADLEY: The renal and hepatic blood flow, glomerular filtration rate, and urinary output of electrolytes during cyclopropane, ether and thiopental anesthesia, operation and immediate postoperative period. Surgery **30**, 241 (1951). — HADDY, F. J., J. SCOTT, M. FLEISHMAN and D. EMANUEL: Effect of change in renal venous pressure upon renal vascular resistance, urine and lymph flow rates. Amer. J. Physiol. **195**, 97 (1958a). — Effect of change in flow rate upon renal vascular resistance. Amer. J. Physiol. **195**, 111 (1958b). — HAGENSEN, N. R., R. KEIDING and V. SCHMIDT: Clearance determinations after oral administration of para-aminohippuric acid. Scand. J. clin. Lab. Invest. **2**, 12 (1950). — HAGGARD, H. W., L. A. GREENBERG and R. P. CARROLL: Studies in absorption, distribution and elimination of alcohol; diuresis from alcohol and its influence on elimination of alcohol in urine. J. Pharmacol. exp. Ther. **71**, 349 (1941). — HALL, B. V.: Further studies on the normal structure of the renal glomerulus. Proc. 6th Ann. Conf. on the Nephrotic Syndrome, 1955. — The protoplasmic basis of glomerular ultrafiltration. Amer. Heart. J. **54**, 1 (1957). — HALL, C. A., B. FRAME and V. A. DRILL: Renal excretion of water and antidiuretic substances in patients with hepatic cirrhosis and rats with dietary liver injury. Endocrinology **44**, 76 (1949). — HALL, P. W., and A. S. RELMAN: Acid excretion in rubidium- and cesium-substi-tuted rats. J. clin. Invest. **39**, 171 (1960). — HALMI, N. S., L. T. KING, R. R. WIDNER, A. C. HASS and R. G. STUELKE: Renal excretion of radioiodide in rats. Amer. J. Physiol. **193**, 379 (1958). — HAM, A. W., N. LITTNER, T. G. H. DRAKE, E. C. ROBERTSON and F. F. TISDALL: Physiological hypertrophy of the parathyroids, its cause and its relation to rickets. Amer. J. Path. **16**, 277 (1940). — HAM, G. C.: A comparison of pituitrin and the antidiuretic substance in human urine and placenta. J. clin. Invest. **20**, 439 (1941) (abstract). — Repro-ducible diuresis and chloruresis for bioassay of antidiuretic activity. Proc. Soc. exp. Biol. (N.Y.) **53**, 210 (1943). — HAM, G. C., and E. M. LANDIS: A comparison of pituitrin with the antidiuretic substance found in human urine and placenta. J. clin. Invest. **21**, 455 (1942). — HAM, G. C., and M. ROSENFELD: Ultracentrifugation of antidiuretic, chloruretic and pressor factors of posterior pituitary extracts. Bull. Johns Hopk. Hosp. **71**, 18 (1942). — HAMAR, N.: Sugar, water and creatinine excretion in normal and in B-avitaminotic dogs. Quart. J. exp. Physiol. **30**, 289 (1941). — HAMBURGER, J.: Physiologie de l'innervation renale. Paris theses, 1936. — HAMMARSTEN, J. F., M. ALLGOOD and W. O. SMITH: Effects of magnesium sulfate on renal function, electrolyte excretion and clearance of magnesium. J. appl. Physiol.

10, 476 (1957). — HAMMOND, J., and W. WHITAKER: Effects of intravenous digoxin in uncontrolled auricular fibrillation. Brit. Heart J. **19**, 23 (1957). — HANDLER, J. S.: The significance of lactic acid in the reduced uric acid excretion of toxemia of pregnancy. Clin. Res. Proc. **7**, 279 (1959) (abstract). — HANDLER, P., and D. V. COHN: Use of radiophosphorus in studies of glomerular permeability of plasma inorganic phosphate. Amer. J. Physiol. **164**, 646 (1951). — Effect of parathyroid extract on renal function. Amer. J. Physiol. **169**, 188 (1952). — HANDLER, P., D. V. COHN and W. J. A. DEMARIA: Effect of parathyroid extract on renal excretion of phosphate. Amer. J. Physiol. **165**, 434 (1951). — HANDLEY, C. A., D. CHAPMAN and J. H. MOYER: Some pharmacological properties of three new mercurial diuretics. Proc. Soc. exp. Biol. (N.Y.) **78**, 433 (1951). — HANDLEY, C. A., and A. D. KELLER: Changes in renal functions associated with diabetes insipidus precipitated by anterior hypothalamic lesions. Amer. J. Physiol. **160**, 321 (1950a). — Changes in renal function produced by morphine in normal dogs with diabetes insipidus. J. Pharmacol. exp. Ther. **99**, 33 (1950b). — HANDLEY, C. A., and M. LaFORGE: Effect of thiols on mercurial diuresis. Proc. Soc. exp. Biol. (N.Y.) **65**, 74 (1947). — HANDLEY, C. A., and P. S. LAVIK: Inhibition of the kidney succinic dehydrogenase system by mercurial diuretics. J. Pharmacol. exp. Ther. **100**, 115 (1950). — HANDLEY, C. A., and J. H. MOYER: Changes in sodium and water excretion produced by vasoactive and ganglionic and adrenergic blocking agents. Amer. J. Physiol. **178**, 309 (1954a). — Unilateral renal adrenergic blockade and the renal response to vasopressor agents and to hemorrhage. J. Pharmacol. exp. Ther. **112**, 1 (1954b). — HANDLEY, C. A., R. B. SIGAFOOS and M. LaFORGE: Proportional changes in renal tubular reabsorption of dextrose and excretion of p-aminohippurate with changes in glomerular filtration rate. Amer. J. Physiol. **159**, 175 (1949). — HANDLEY, C. A., JANE TELFORD and MARGUERITE LaFORGE: Xanthine and mercurial diuretics and renal tubular transport of glucose and p-aminohippurate in the dog. Proc. Soc. exp. Biol. (N.Y.) **71**, 187 (1949). — HANENSON, I. B., B. GOULUBOFF, J. GROSSMAN, R. E. WESTON and L. LEITER: Studies on water excretion following intravenous hydration and the administration of pitressin or nicotine in congestive heart failure. Circulation **13**, 242 (1956). — HANENSON, I. B., HERTHA TAUSSKY, N. POLASKY, W. RAHNSOHOFF and B. F. MILLER: Renal excretion of sodium in arterial hypertension. Circulation **20**, 498 (1959). — HANLEY, T., G. H. JOWETT, R. KILPATRICK and MARGARET M. PLATTS: The role of carbonic anhydrase in renal reabsorption of bicarbonate. J. Physiol. (Lond.) **145**, 277 (1959). — HANSEN, H. L., L. S. FOSDICK and C. A. DRAGSTEDT: A study of the effects of certain diuretics on the concentration of blood chlorides in dogs. J. Pharmacol. exp. Ther. **41**, 325 (1931). — HANSEN, P. G., E. A. JACOBSEN and M. F. PETERSEN: The renal excretion of fructose. Acta physiol. scand. **6**, 195 (1943). — HARDIN, R., J. SCOTT and F. HADDY: Relation of pressure to flow in the intact kidney. Fed. Proc. **19**, 95 (1960) (abstract). — HARDING, V. J., T. F. NICHOLSON and R. M. ARCHIBALD: Some properties of the reducing material in certain fractions of normal urines. I. The nature of the "free" fermentable sugars and the fermentable sugars produced on hydrolysis in "fasting" urines. Biochem. J. **30**, 326 (1936). — HARDWICK, J., and J. R. SQUIRE: The relationship between plasma albumin concentration and protein excretion in patients with proteinuria. Clin. Sci. **14**, 509 (1955). — HARE, RUTH S., and K. HARE: The renal excretion of chloride by the dog. Amer. J. Physiol. **133**, P316 (1941) (abstract). — HARE, K., R. C. HICKEY and RUTH S. HARE: The effect of withdrawal of drinking water upon the antidiuretic potency of the posterior lobe of the rat. Amer. J. Physiol. **133**, P316 (1941a) (abstract). — Renal excretion of antidiuretic substance by dog. Amer. J. Physiol. **134**, 240 (1941b). — HARE, K., E. V. MELVILLE, G. H. CHAMBERS and RUTH S. HARE: Assay of antidiuretic material in blood and urine. Endocrinology **36**, 323 (1945). — HARE, K., D. N. PHILLIPS, J. BRADSHAW, G. CHAMBERS and RUTH S. HARE: Diuretic action of thyroid in diabetes insipidus. Amer. J. Physiol. **141**, 187 (1944). — HARGITAY, B., u. W. KUHN: Das Multiplikationsprinzip als Grundlage der Harnkonzentrierung in der Niere. Z. Elektrochem. **55**, 539 (1951). — HARMAN, P. J., and HELEN DAVIES: Intrinsic nerves in the mammalian kidney. I. Anatomy in mouse, rat, cat and macque. J. comp. Neurol. **89**, 225 (1948). — HARRIS, E. J., and T. A. J. PRANKERD: Phloridzin and red cell phosphate turnover. Experientia (Basel) **14**, 249 (1958). — HARRIS, F. D., A. F. HARTMANN jr., DORIS ROLF and H. L. WHITE: Ammonia excretion in adrenal insufficiency. Amer. J. Physiol. **168**, 20 (1952). — HARRIS, G. W.: Neural control of the pituitary gland. Physiol. Rev. **28**, 139 (1948). — The function of the pituitary stalk. Bull. Johns Hopk. Hosp. **97**, 358 (1955). — HARRIS, H.: Genetic aspects of tubular function. Modern views on the secretion of urine. Cushny Memorial Lectures. Boston: Little, Brown & Co. 1956. — Renal aminoaciduria. Brit. med. Bull. **13**, 26 (1957). — HARRIS, I. E., L. RUBIN and J. S. LAWRENCE: Salyrgan and ammonium chloride as diuretics in cardiac oedema. Acta med. scand. **83**, 23 (1934). — HARRIS, J. F., C. W. LLOYD and J. LOBOTSKY: Some studies of posterior pituitary and adrenal cortical interrelationships in patients with and without cirrhosis of the liver. J. clin. Invest. **32**, 885 (1953). — HARRIS, J. S., W. C. SEALY and

W. DeMaria: Hypertension and renal dynamics in aortic coarctation. Amer. J. Med. 9, 734 (1950). — Harrison, H. E.: A modification of the diphenylamine method for determination of inulin. Proc. Soc. exp. Biol. (N.Y.) 49, 111 (1942). — Harrison, H. E. , L. Finberg and Evelyn Fleishman: Disturbances in ionic equilibrium of intracellular and extracellular electrolytes in patients with tuberculous meningitis. J. clin. Invest. 31, 300 (1952). — Harrison, H. E., and Helen C. Harrison: The renal excretion of inorganic phosphate in relation to the action of vitamin D and parathyroid hormone. J. clin. Invest. 20, 47 (1941a). — Effect of acidosis upon renal tubular reabsorptions of phosphate. Amer. J. Physiol. 134, 781 (1941b). — Inhibition of urine citrate excretion and the production of renal calcinosis in the rat by acetazoleamide (Diamox) administration. J. clin. Invest. 34, 1662 (1955). — Hartmann, H., S. L. Ørskov and H. Rein: Die Gefäßreaktionen der Niere im Verlaufe allgemeiner Kreislauf-Regulationsvorgänge. Pflügers Arch. ges. Physiol. 238, 239 (1937). — Hartroft, Phyllis M.: Studies on renal juxtaglomerular cells. III. The effects of experimental renal disease and hypertension in the rat. J. exp. Med. 105, 501 (1957). — Harvey, R. B.: Effect of temperature on function of isolated dog kidney. Amer. J. Physiol. 197, 181 (1959). — Hashimoto, K.: Studies of the renal function in experimental hydronephrosis. I. Urine volume and variation in the excretion of urine components after ligation of dog ureters for a short period, supplemented with excretion of dyes. Folia pharmacol. jap. 39, 554 (1943). — Haterius, H. O.: Evidence of pituitary involvement in experimental control of water diuresis. Amer. J. Physiol. 128, 506 (1940). — Hauck, Hazel M.: Plasma levels and urinary excretion of ascorbic acid in women during the menstrual cycle. J. Nutr. 33, 511 (1947). — Haugen, H. N., and E. M. Blegen: Plasma creatinine concentration and creatinine clearance in clinical work. Ann. intern. Med. 43, 731 (1955). — Hauser, A. D., D. Polimeros and M. F. Levitt: Effect of calcium loads on renal tubular function. Clin. Res. Proc. 8, 33 (1960) (abstract). — Havard, R. E.: Effect of exercise on the excretion of chloride in man. J. Physiol. (Lond.) 90, 90P (1937) (abstract). — Havard, R. E., and G. A. Reay: Normal variations of the inorganic phosphate of blood. Biochem. J. 19, 882 (1925). — The influence of exercise on the inorganic phosphates of the blood and urine. J. Physiol. (Lond.) 61, 35 (1926). — Hawker, R. W.: Inactivation of antidiuretic hormone and oxytocin during pregnancy. Quart. J. exp. Physiol. 41, 301 (1956). — Haworth, W. N., and A. Learner: Polysaccharides. I. The structure of inulin. J. chem. Soc. 1, 619 (1928). — Hayman jr., J. M.: Estimations of afferent arteriole and glomerular capillary pressures in the frog kidney. Amer. J. Physiol. 79, 389 (1926/27). — Hayman jr., J. M., and A. N. Richards: Deposition of dyes, iron and urea in the cells of a renal tubule after their injection into its lumen: glomerular elimination of the same substances. Amer. J. Physiol. 79, 149 (1926). — Hecht, G., u. W. Scholtan: Über die Ausscheidung von Polyvinylpyrrolidon durch die normale Niere. Z. ges. exp. Med. 130, 577 (1959). — Heidenhain, R.: Versuche über den Vorgang der Harnabsonderung. Pflügers Arch. ges. Physiol. 9, 1 (1874). — Physiologie der Absonderungsvorgänge. In Hermanns Handbuch der Physiologie, Bd. 5, S. 1. 1880. — Heijkenskjold, F., and L. Sandberg: Carbohydrate excretion in renal glycosuria; investigation of two cases. Acta med. scand. 157, 141 (1957). — Heinbecker, P., Doris Rolf and H. L. White: Effects of extracts of the hypophysis, the thyroid and the adrenal cortex on some renal functions. Amer. J. Physiol. 139, 543 (1943). — Heinbecker, P., and H. L. White: The role of the pituitary gland in water balance. Ann. Surg. 110, 1037 (1939). — Hypothalamico-hypophysial system and its relation to water balance in dog. Amer. J. Physiol. 133, 582 (1941). — Heinbecker, P., H. L. White and Doris Rolf: The essential lesion in experimental diabetes insipidus. Endocrinology 40, 104 (1946). — Heinemann, H. O., and E. L. Becker: Effect of a mercurial diuretic on the excretion of "free water" in diabetes insipidus. J. appl. Physiol. 12, 51 (1958). — Heinemann, H. O., and M. W. Cheung: Renal concentrating mechanism in sickle-cell anemia. J. Lab. clin. Med. 49, 923 (1957). — Heller, B. I., J. F. Hammarsten and F. L. Stutzman: Concerning the effects of magnesium sulfate on renal function, electrolyte excretion, and clearance of magnesium. J. clin. Invest. 32, 858 (1953). — Heller, B. I., and W. E. Jacobson: Renal hemodynamics in heart disease. Amer. Heart J. 39, 188 (1950). — Heller, B. I., R. E. Smith and R. I. Lubin: Renal functional status in patients with acromegaly. J. Lab. clin. Med. 44, 811 (1954) (abstract). — Heller, H.: Action of antidiuretic principle of posterior pituitary extracts on urine excretion of anaesthetized animals. J. Physiol. (Lond.) 98, 405 (1940). — Renal excretion of pituitary (posterior lobe) extracts. Nature (Lond.) 151, 502 (1943). — Renal function of newborn infants. J. Physiol. (Lond.) 102, 429 (1944). — Heller, H., and S. M. A. Zaidi: Metabolism of exogenous and endogenous antidiuretic hormone in the kidney and liver in vitro. Brit. J. Pharmacol. 12, 284 (1957). — Heller, H., and E. J. Zaimis: The antidiuretic and oxytocic hormones in the posterior pituitary glands of newborn infants and adults. J. Physiol. (Lond.) 109, 162 (1949). — Heller, J.: The influence of the nervous system on renal function. I. Effects of denervation. Physiol. Bohemosl. 7, 255 (1958). — Heller, J., and L. Krulich: The influence of the nervous system on renal function. III. Notes on the mechanism of conditioned water diuresis. Physiol. Bohemosl. **7**, 370 (1958). — HENDERSON, L. J., and W. W. PALMER: On the intensity of urinary acidity in normal and pathological conditions. J. biol. Chem. **13**, 393 (1913). — On the several factors of acid excretion in nephritis. J. biol. Chem. **21**, 37 (1915). — HENDRIKX, A., and F. H. EPSTEIN: Effect of feeding protein and urea on renal concentrating ability in the rat. Amer. J. Physiol. **195**, 539 (1958). — HENDRIX, J. P., B. B. WESTFALL and A. N. RICHARDS: Quantitative studies of the composition of glomerular urine. XIV. The glomerular excretion of inulin in frogs and *Necturi*. J. biol. Chem. **116**, 735 (1936). — HENRY, J. P., O. H. GAUER and J. L. REEVES: Evidence of the atrial location of receptors influencing urine flow. Circulat. Res. **4**, 85 (1956). — HENRY, J. P., and J. W. PEARCE: The possible role of cardiac atrial stretch receptors in the induction of changes in urine flow. J. Physiol. (Lond.) **131**, 572 (1956). — HERNANDO, L., J. CRABBÉ, E. J. ROSS, W. J. REDDY, A. E. RENOLD, D. H. NELSON and G. W. THORN: Clinical experience with a physicochemical method for estimation of aldosterone in urine. Metabolism **6**, 518 (1957). — HERRIN, R. C.: Factors affecting the tests of kidney function. Physiol. Rev. **21**, 529 (1941). — HERRIN, R. C., and C. C. LARDINOIS: Renal clearance of citric acids in the dog. Proc. Soc. exp. Biol. (N.Y.) **97**, 294 (1958). — HERRMANN, G., and G. M. DECHERD jr.: Further studies on the mechanism of diuresis with special reference to the action of some newer diuretics. J. Lab. clin. Med. **22**, 767 (1937). — HERRMANN, G., C. T. STONE and E. H. SCHWAB: Some studies in the mechanism of diuresis in patients with congestive heart failure. Trans. Ass. Amer. Phycns **47**, 279 (1932). — HERVEY, G. R., R. A. McCANCE and R. G. O. TAYLOR: Further observations on the causes of a diuresis during hydropenia. J. Physiol. (Lond.) **104**, 43P (1946). — HETZEL, B. S., R. R. McSWINEY, I. H. MILLS and F. T. G. PRUNTY: Observations on the effects of aldosterone in man. J. Endocr. **13**, 112 (1956). — HEWLETT, J. S., E. P. McCULLAGH, G. L. FARRELL, HARRIET P. DUSTAN, E. F. POUTASSE and W. L. PROUDFIT: Aldosterone-producing tumors of the adrenal gland. Report of three cases. J. Amer. med. Ass. **164**, 719 (1957). — HEYM, E.: Über die Bedeutung der Plasmakolloide für die Flüssigkeitsrückresorption in der Niere. Ber. ges. physiol. **179/180**, 131 (1956) (abstract). — HIATT, E. P.: Extreme hypochloremia in dogs induced by nitrate administration. Amer. J. Physiol. **129**, 597 (1940). — Effect of denervation on filtration rate and blood flow in dog kidneys rendered hyperemic by administration of pyrogen. Amer. J. Physiol. **136**, 38 (1942). — HIATT, H. H., and D. D. THOMPSON: The effects of parathyroid extract on renal function in man. J. clin. Invest. **36**, 557 (1957a). — Some effects of intravenously administered calcium on inorganic phosphate metabolism. J. clin. Invest. **36**, 573 (1957b). — HICKEY, R. C., and K. HARE: The renal excretion of chloride and water in diabetes insipidus. J. clin. Invest. **23**, 768 (1944). — HIERHOLZER, K., R. F. PITTS, R. S. GURD and R. H. KESSLER: Effects of acetazoleamide and chlorothiazide on distal tubular processes in nephron of the dog. Fed. Proc. **17**, 70 (1958) (abstract). — HIGASHI, A., and L. PETERS: A rapid colorimetric method for the determination of inulin in plasma and urine. J. Lab. clin. Med. **35**, 475 (1950). — HILDEN, T.: Glomerular filtration rate and maximal tubular excretory capacity in congestive heart failure. Scand. J. clin. Lab. Invest. **1**, 305 (1949). — HILGER, H. H., J. D. KLÜMPER u. K. J. ULLRICH: Wasserrückresorption und Ionentransport durch die Sammelrohrzellen der Säugetierniere. Pflügers Arch. ges. Physiol. **267**, 218 (1958). — HILLS, A. G., D. W. PARSONS, O. ROSENTHAL and IRIS KIEM: Excessive renal tubular reabsorption of filtered urea in human adrenal insufficiency, J. Clin. Invest. **38**, 1011, 1959 (abstract). — HILLS, A. G., H. A. ZINTEL and D. W. PARSONS: Observations of human adrenal cortical deficiency with special reference to replacement therapy with cortisone. Amer. J. Med. **21**, 358 (1956). — HILTON, J. G.: Potentiation of diuretic action of mercuhydrin by ammonium chloride. J. clin. Invest. **30**, 1105 (1951). — Effects of mercurial diuresis in patients with ascites due to cirrhosis. Amer. J. Med. **12**, 311 (1952). — Adrenocorticotropic action of antidiuretic hormone. Circulation **21**, 1038 (1960). — HILTON, J. G., N. E. CAPECI, G. T. KISS, O. R. KRUESI, V. V. GLAVIANO and R. WEGRIA: The effect of acute elevation of the plasma chloride concentration on the renal excretion of bicarbonate during acute respiratory acidosis. J. clin. Invest. **35**, 481 (1956). — HILTON, J. G., L. F. SCIAN, C. D. WESTERMANN and O. R. KRUESI: Direct stimulation of adrenocortical secretion by synthetic vasopressin in dogs. Proc. Soc. exp. Biol. (N.Y.) **100**, 523 (1959a). — Effect of synthetic lysine vasopressin on adrenocortical secretion. Science **129**, 971 (1959b). — HILTON, J. G., C. D. WESTERMANN, S. S. BERGEN and R. S. CRAMPTON: Syndrome of mineralocorticoid excess due to bilateral adrenocortical hyperplasia. New Engl. J. Med. **260**, 202 (1959c). — HINKLE jr., L., C. J. EDWARDS and S. WOLF: The occurrence of diuresis in humans in stressful situations and its possible relation to the diuresis of early starvation. J. clin. Invest. **30**, 809 (1951). — HINSHAW, L. B., H. M. BALLIN, S. B. DAY and C. H. CARLSON: Tissue pressure and autoregulation in the dextran-perfused kidney. Amer. J. Physiol. **197**, 853 (1959). — HINSHAW, L. B., S. B. DAY and C. H. CARLSON: Tissue pressure as a causal factor in the autoregulation of blood flow in the isolated perfused kidney. Amer. J. Physiol. **197**, 309 (1959). — HIROKAWA, W.: Über den osmotischen Druck des Nierenparenchyms. Beitr. chem. Physiol. Path. **11**, 458 (1908). — HIX, E. L.: Uretero-renal reflex facilitating renal vasoconstrictor responses to emotional stress. Amer. J. Physiol. **192**, 191 (1958). — HLAD, C. F., and N. S. BRICKER: Renal function and I^{131} clearance in hyperthyroidism and myxedema. J. clin. Endocr. **14**, 1539 (1954). — HODLER, J., H. O. HEINEMANN, A. P. FISHMAN and H. W. SMITH: Urine p_H and carbonic anhydrase activity in the marine dogfish. Amer. J. Physiol. **183**, 155 (1955). — HÖBER, R.: Beweis selektiver Sekretion durch die Tubulusepithelien der Niere. Pflügers Arch. ges. Physiol. **224**, 72 (1930a). — Über die Harnbildung in der Froschniere. XIX. Mitteilung. Über die Ausscheidung des Harnstoffs. Pflügers Arch. ges. Physiol. **224**, 422 (1930b). — Über die Ausscheidung von Zuckern durch die isolierte Froschniere. Pflügers Arch. ges. Physiol. **233**, 181 (1933). — The secretion of dyestuffs by the kidney. J. cell. comp. Physiol. **6**, 117 (1935). — Effect of some sulfonamides on renal secretion. Proc. Soc. exp. Biol. (N.Y.) **49**, 87 (1942). — HÖBER, R., and P. M. BRISCOE-WOOLLEY: Correlation between secretion of dyestuffs by kidney and molecular structure of these dyes. Proc. Soc. exp. Biol. (N.Y.) **41**, 624 (1939). — Conditions determining the selective secretion of dyestuffs by the isolated frog kidney. J. cell. comp. Physiol. **15**, 35 (1940a). — Further studies on conditions determining selective renal secretion of dyestuffs. J. cell. comp. Physiol. **16**, 63 (1940b). — HÖBER, R., P. M. BRISCOE-WOOLLEY, J. W. GREEN and M. ZIMMERMAN: Correlation between secretory power of frog kidney and molecular configuration of organic compounds; further studies. J. cell. comp. Physiol. **19**, 183 (1942). — HÖBER, R., and A. MEIROWSKY: Über die Ausscheidung lipoidunlöslicher Säurefarbstoffe durch die Froschniere. Pflügers Arch. ges. Physiol. **230**, 331 (1932). — HÖKFELT, B., R. LUFT, D. IKKOS, H. OLIVECRONA and J. SEKKENES: The immediate effect of hypophysectomy and section of the pituitary stalk on the urinary steroid excretion in man. Acta endocr. (Kbh.) **30**, 29 (1958). — HOEL, J.: Cortisone induced recurrence of diabetes insipidus by total destruction of the hypophysis. Acta endocr. (Kbh.) **21**, 15 (1956). — HOFF, F.: Untersuchungen über den Einfluß von Lactoflavin und Corticosteron auf den künstlichen renalen Diabetes. Klin. Wschr. **17**, 1535 (1938). — HOFFMAN, W. S., L. PASCALE and A. DUBIN: Effect of benemid on phosphate excretion in parathyroid tetany. Fed. Proc. **11**, 231 (1952) (abstract). — HOGBEN, C. A. M., and J. L. BOLLMAN: Excretion of phosphate by isolated frog kidney: an 'adsorption semipermeability' model for maximal tubular transport. Amer. J. Physiol. **164**, 662 (1951a). — Renal reabsorption of phosphate: Normal and thyroparathyroidectomized dog. Amer. J. Physiol. **164**, 670 (1951b). — HOLLAND, B. C., and E. A. STEAD jr.: Effect of vasopressin (Pitressin)-induced water retention on sodium excretion. Arch. intern. Med. **88**, 571 (1951). — Electrolyte excretion after single doses of ACTH, cortisone, desoxycorticosterone glucoside and motionless standing. J. clin. Invest. **33**, 132 (1954). — HOLLAND, R., B. A. CROSS and C. H. SAWYER: Milk ejection in the rabbit in response to intracarotid injections of hypertonic saline. Fed. Proc. **17**, 73 (1958) (abstract). — HOLLANDER, W., and W. E. JUDSON: The relationship of cardiovascular and renal hemodynamic function to sodium excretion in patients with severe heart disease but without edema. J. clin. Invest. **35**, 970 (1956). — Electrolyte and water excretion in arterial hypertension. I. Studies in non-medically treated subjects with essential hypertension. J. clin. Invest. **36**, 1460 (1957). — Electrolyte and water excretion in arterial hypertension. II. Studies in subjects with essential hypertension after antihypertensive drug treatment. Circulation **17**, 576 (1958). — HOLLANDER, W., A. L. MICHELSON and R. W. WILKINS: Serotonin and antiserotonins. I. Their circulatory, respiratory and renal effects in man. Circulation **16**, 246 (1957). — HOLLANDER jr., W., T. F. WILLIAMS, C. C. FORDHAM III and L. G. WELT: A study of the quantitative relationship between antidiuretic hormone (vasopressin) and the renal tubular reabsorption of water. J. clin. Invest. **36**, 1059 (1957a). — HOLLANDER jr., W., R. W. WINTERS, J. BRADLEY, T. F. WILLIAMS, W. E. LORING, J. OLIVER and L. G. WELT: The effect of potassium repletion on the renal-concentrating defect, the renal structural changes, and the cardiac and skeletal muscle lesions produced by potassium depletion in rats. Clin. Res. Proc. **6**, 287 (1958) (abstract). — HOLLANDER jr., W., R. W. WINTERS, T. F. WILLIAMS, J. BRADLEY, J. OLIVER and L. G. WELT: Defect in the renal tubular reabsorption of water associated with potassium depletion in rats. Amer. J. Physiol. **189**, 557 (1957b). — HOLLIDAY, M. A., T. J. EGAN and PATRICIA WIRTH: Changes in electrolyte composition of renal papillae in potassium-deficient rats having a urinary-concentrating defect. Clin. Res. **6**, 286 (1958) (abstract). — HOLMES, J. H.: Studies of water exchange in dogs with reduced serum electrolyte concentrations. Amer. J. Physiol. **129**, 384 (1940). — HOLMES, J. H., and M. I. GREGERSEN: Origin of thirst in diabetes insipidus. Amer. J. Med. **4**, 503 (1948). — HOLZEL, A., G. M. KOMROWER and V. SCHWARZ: Galactosemia. Amer. J. Med. **22**, 703 (1957). — HONG, S. K.: Renal function during hypothermia. Am. J. Physiol. **183**, 628 (1955) (abstract). — HONG, S. K., and J. W. BOYLAN: Renal concentrating operation in hypothermic dogs. Amer. J. Physiol. **196**, 1150 (1959). — HONG, S. K., and R. P. FORSTER: Run-out of chlorphenol red following luminal accumulation by isolated renal tubules of the flounder *in vitro*. J. cell. comp. Physiol. **51**, 241 (1958). — HONG, S. K., and H. RAHN: Total and partial gas tensions of human urine. Fed. Proc. **16**, 61 (1957) (abstract). — HOPKINS, THEDA R., T. B. CONNOR and J. E. HOWARD: Ultrafiltration studies on calcium and phosphorus in pathological human serum. Bull. Johns Hopk. Hosp. **93**, 249 (1953). — HOPKINS, THEDA R., J. E. HOWARD and H. EISENBERG: Ultrafiltration studies on calcium and phosphorus in human serum. Bull. Johns Hopk. Hosp. **91**, 1 (1952). — HORNE, N. W., and W. M. WILSON: Effect of caronamide on excretion of p-aminosalicylic acid. Lancet **1949 II**, 507. — HOSHIKO, T.: Effect of temperature on sodium reabsorption in the perfused bullfrog kidney. Amer. J. Physiol. **185**, 545 (1956). — HOSHIKO, T., R. E. SWANSON and M. B. VISSCHER: Excretion of Na^{22} and K^{42} by the perfused bullfrog kidney and the effect of some poisons. Amer. J. Physiol. **184**, 542 (1956). — HOUCK, C. R.: Mutual depression of reabsorption and excretory maxima in renal tubules. Proc. Soc. exp. Biol. (N.Y.) **63**, 398 (1946). — Alterations in renal hemodynamics and function in separate kidneys during stimulation of renal artery nerves in dogs. Amer. J. Physiol. **167**, 523 (1951). — HOWARD, J. E., THEDA R. HOPKINS and T. B. CONNOR: The use of intravenous calcium as a measure of activity of the parathyroid glands. Trans. Ass. Amer. Phycns **65**, 351 (1952). — HOWARD, P. J., W. S. WILDE and R. L. MALVIN: Localization of renal calcium transport; effect of calcium loads and of gluconate anion on water, sodium and potassium. Amer. J. Physiol. **197**, 337 (1959). — HOWELL, A. B., and I. GERSH: Conservation of water by the rodent *Dipodomys*. J. Mammalogy **16**, 1 (1935). — HOWELL, D. S., and J. O. DAVIS: Relationship of sodium retention to potassium excretion by the kidney during administration of desoxycorticosterone acetate to dogs. Amer. J. Physiol. **179**, 359 (1954). — HOWELL, D. S., J. O. DAVIS and G. L. LAQUER: Effect of hypophysectomy on electrolyte excretion in dogs with ascites produced by thoracic inferior vena cava constriction. Circulat. Res. **3**, 264 (1955). — HUANG, K. C.: Renal excretion of l-tyrosine derivatives. Fed. Proc. **19**, 368 (1960) (abstract). — HUANG, K. C., N. B. KING and E. GENAZZANI: Effects of xanthine diuretics on renal tubular transport of PAH and glycine conjugation of PABA. Amer. J. Physiol. **192**, 373 (1958). — HUANG, K. C., and P. K. KNOEFEL: Biochemorphology of renal tubular transport: Halogenated amino acids and derivatives. J. Pharmacol. exp. Ther. **121**, 443 (1957). — HUBER, G. C.: The arteriolae rectae of the mammalian kidney. Brit. med. J. **1906 II**, 1700. — Renal tubules. In: Special cytology, edit. by E. V. COWDRY. New York: P. B. Hoeber 1928. — The form and structure of the mammalian renal tubule. The kidney in health and disease 1. Philadelphia: Lea and Febiger 1935. — HUFFMAN, E. R., C. J. HLAD jr., N. E. WHIPPLE and H. ELRICK: The influence of blood glucose on the renal clearance of phosphate. J. clin. Invest. **37**, 369 (1958). — HUFFMAN, E. R., G. M. WILSON jr., G. M. CLARK and C. J. SMYTH: The acute renal effects of 9-alpha fluorohydrocortisone in human subjects with intact adrenals. J. Lab. clin. Med. **47**, 747 (1956). — HUGHES, W. L.: A physicochemical rationale for the biological activity of mercury and its compounds. Ann. N.Y. Acad. Sci. **65**, 454 (1957). — HUGHES, W. M., E. DENNIS and J. H. MOYER: Treatment of hypertension with oral reserpine alone and in combination with hydralazine or hexamethonium. Amer. J. med. Sci. **229**, 121 (1955). — HULET, W. H., and H. W. SMITH: Negative pressure respiration, water diuresis and natriuresis in normotensive, hypertensive, and prehydrated normotensive subjects. J. clin. Invest. **38**, 1972 (1959). — HUTH, E. J., R. D. SQUIRES and J. R. ELKINTON: Experimental potassium depletion in normal human subjects. II. Renal and hormonal factors in the development of extracellular alkalosis during depletion. J. clin. Invest. **38**, 1149 (1959). — HWANG, K., H. K. IWAMOTO, L. COEN and H. E. JOHNSON: Diuretic effect of some 2- and 3-substituted analogues of hydrochlorothiazide. Fed. Proc. **19**, 363 (1960) (abstract). — HYMAN, A. L., W. E. JAQUES and E. S. HYMAN: Observation on the direct effect of digoxin on renal excretion of sodium and water. Amer. Heart J. **52**, 592 (1956).

IACOBELLIS, M., E. MUNTWYLER and GRACE E. GRIFFIN: Enzyme concentration changes in the kidneys of protein and/or potassium-deficient rats. Amer. J. Physiol. **178**, 477 (1954). — Kidney glutaminase and carbonic anhydrase activity and tissue electrolyte composition in potassium-deficient dogs. Amer. J. Physiol. **183**, 395 (1955). — IKKOS, D., H. LJUNGGREN and R. LUFT: Glomerular filtration rate and renal plasma flow in acromegaly. Acta endocr. (Kbh.) **21**, 226 (1956). — IKKOS, D., R. LUFT and H. OLIVECRONA: Hypophysectomy in man: Effect of water excretion during the first two postoperative months. J. clin. Endocr. **15**, 553 (1955). — INGALLS, T. H., G. DONALDSON and F. ALBRIGHT: The locus of action of the parathyroid hormone: Experimental studies with parathyroid extract on normal and nephrectomized rats. J. clin. Invest. **22**, 603 (1943). — INGBAR, S. H., E. H. KASS, C. H. BURNETT, A. S. RELMAN, B. A. BURROWS and J. H. SISSON: The effects of ACTH and cortisone on the renal tubular transport of uric acid, phosphorus and electrolytes in patients with normal renal and adrenal function. Proc. 2nd Clin. ACTH Conf. **1**, 130 (1951). — INGBAR, S. H., A. S. RELMAN, B. A. BURROWS, E. H. KASS, J. H. SISSON and C. H. BURNETT:

344   LAURENCE G. WESSON:

Changes in normal renal function resulting from ACTH and cortisone. J. clin. Invest.
29, 824 (1950) (abstract). — INGLE, D. J.: The biologic properties of cortisone: A review.
J. clin. Endocr. **10**, 1312 (1950). — The functional interrelationship of the anterior pituitary and the adrenal cortex. Ann. intern. Med. **35**, 652 (1951). — The role of the adrenal
cortex in homeostasis. Pediatrics **17**, 407 (1956). — INGLE, D. J., R. C. MEEKS and KATHRYN
E. THOMAS: The effect of fractures upon urinary electrolytes in non-adrenalectomized rats
and in adrenalectomized rats treated with adrenal cortex extract. Endocrinology **49**, 703
(1951). — INGRAM, W. R., L. LADD and J. T. BENBOW: Excretion of antidiuretic substance
and its relation to hypothalamico-hypophyseal system in cats. Amer. J. Physiol. **127**, 544
(1939). — ITOH, S.: Role of vasopressin in the release of ACTH. Jap. J. Physiol. **7**, 213
(1957). — IYER, G. Y. N.: Estimation of free amino acids in normal human plasma by
paper-chromatography. Indian J. med. Res. **43**, 189 (1955).
    JABIR, F. K., S. D. ROBERTS and R. A. WOMERSLEY: Studies on the renal excretion
of magnesium. Clin. Sci. **16**, 119 (1957). — JACKSON, W. P. U., R. HOFFENBERG, G. C.
LINDER and LOUISE IRWIN: Syndrome of steatorrhea, pseudohypoparathyroidism and
amenorrhea. Observations on the calcium infusion test, and the effect of probenecid on
calcium and phosphorus metabolism. J. clin. Endocr. **16**, 1043 (1956). — JACOBS, E., and
M. VERBANCK: The renal action of parathyroid hormone in man. Acta med. scand. **145**,
143 (1953). — JACOBSON, H. N., and R. H. KELLOGG: Isotonic NaCl diuresis in rats. Antidiuresis and chloruresis produced by posterior pituitary extracts. Amer. J. Physiol. **184**,
376 (1956). — JACOBSON, W. E., J. F. HAMMARSTEN and B. I. HELLER: The effects of
adrenaline upon renal function and electrolyte excretion. J. clin. Invest. **30**, 1503 (1951). —
JAENIKE, J. R., and R. W. BERLINER: A study of distal renal tubular functions by a modified stop flow technique. J. clin. Invest. **39**, 481 (1960). — JAENIKE, J. R., and CHRISTINE
WATERHOUSE: The effects of sustained vasopressin administration in man. Clin. Res. Proc.
7, 272 (1959) (abstract). — JAFFEE, O. C.: Phenol red transport in the pronephros and
mesonephros of the developing frog *(Rana pipiens)*. J. cell. comp. Physiol. **44**, 347 (1954). —
JAHAN, I., and R. F. PITTS: Effect of parathyroid on renal tubular reabsorption of phosphate
and calcium. Amer. J. Physiol. **155**, 42 (1948). — JAILER, J. W., M. ROSENFELD and J. A.
SHANNON: The influence of orally administered alkali and acid on the renal excretion of
quinacrine, chloroquine and santoquine. J. clin. Invest. **26**, 1168 (1947). — JAMES, J.,
G. GORDILLO and J. METCOFF: Effects of infusion of hyperoncotic dextran in children with
the nephrotic syndrome. J. clin. Invest. **33**, 1346 (1954). — JANUSZEWICZ, W., H. O. HEINE-
MANN, F. E. DEMARTINI and J. H. LARAGH: A clinical study of the effects of hydrochlorothiazide on the renal excretion of electrolytes and free water. New Engl. J. Med. **261**, 264
(1959). — JARDETSKY, O.: On the distinction between the effects of agents on active and
passive transport of ions. Science **125**, 931 (1957). — JAYLE, M.-F., et GENEVIÈVE BOUS-
SIER: Les séromucoides du sang leurs rélations avec les mucoprotéines de la substance
fondamentale du tissu conjonctif. Expos. ann. Biochim. méd. **17**, 157 (1955). — JEAN-
NERET, P., A. F. ESSELLIER u. H. J. HOLTMEIER: Über den Einfluß des Natriumions auf den
Kalium-, Chlorid- und Wasserhaushalt unter Mineralcorticoidwirkung. Helv. med. Acta
23, 60 (1956). — JENSEN, K. A., K. O. MOLLER and K. OVERGAARD: Studies on the excre-
tion of penicillin through the kidney and the mechanism of this process. Acta pharmacol.
(Kbh.) **1**, 184 (1945). — JENSON, R. L., G. J. TOBIAS, J. F. GREANEY, A. S. RELMAN and
W. B. SCHWARTZ: Renal tubular function during severe metabolic acidosis. Amer. J. Physiol.
179, 188 (1954). — JIMENEZ-DIAZ, C.: Death in Addison's disease (functional renal failure).
Lancet **1936 II**, 1135. — JOHNSON, B. B., A. H. LIEBERMAN and P. J. MULROW: Aldosterone
excretion in normal subjects depleted of sodium and potassium. J. clin. Invest. **36**, 757
(1957). — JOHNSON, B. B., and J. A. LUETSCHER jr.: The possible role of aldosterone in
edema. Ann. N.Y. Acad. Sci. **61**, 605 (1955). — JOHNSON, R. E., F. SARGENT II, T. W.
NIELSEN and I. J. LICHTON: Osmotic concentrating ability: Measure of renal function in
man. Amer. J. Physiol. **183**, 632 (1955) (abstract). — JOHNSTON, W. B.: A reconstruction
of a glomerulus of the human kidney. Anat. Anz. **16**, 260 (1899). — JOLLIFFE, N., J. A.
SHANNON and H. W. SMITH: The excretion of urine in the dog. III. The use of non-metabolized sugars in the measurement of the glomerular filtrate. Amer. J. Physiol. **100**, 301
(1932). — JONES, G. M.: Diabetes insipidus: Clinical observations in 42 cases. Arch. intern.
Med. **74**, 81 (1944). — JONES, R. A., G. O. McDONALD and J. H. LAST: Reversal of diurnal
variation in renal function in cases of cirrhosis with ascites. J. clin. Invest. **31**, 326 (1952). —
JONES, R. T., and W. D. BLAKE: Renal excretion of *l*-epinephrine in the dog. Amer. J.
Physiol. **193**, 371 (1958). — JONES, R. V. H., and H. E. DE WARDENER: Urine concentration
after fluid deprivation or pitressin tannate in oil. Brit. med. J. **1956 I**, 271. — JORES, A.:
Die Urineinschränkung in der Nacht. Dtsch. Arch. klin. Med. **175**, 244 (1933). — JØRGENSEN,
H. E., and J. U. SCHLEGEL: Posttraumatic sodium retention. Fed. Proc. **17**, 82 (1958)
(abstract). — JOSEPH, S., M. SCHWEIZER, N. Z. ULMER and R. GAUNT: Anterior pituitary
and its relation to adrenal cortex in water diuresis. Endocrinology **35**, 338 (1944). — JOSEPH-

SON, B.: The mechanism of renal tubular excretion. Scand. J. clin. Lab. Invest. 1, 344 (1949) (abstract). — JOSEPHSON, B., A. GRIEG, G. KAKOSSAIOS and J. KALLAS: Renal tubular excretion from high plasma levels of para-aminohippurate (PAH) and Diodrast (D) in unanesthetized rabbits. Acta physiol. scand. 30, 11 (1953/54). — JOSEPHSON, B., and JULIA KALLAS: Inulin and creatinine clearance of unanesthetized rabbits. Acta physiol. scand. 30, 1 (1953/54a). — Iodine concentration in rabbit kidneys after diodrast injection. Mechanism of renal tubular excretion. Amer. J. Physiol. 174, 65 (1953b). — JUDSON, W. E., F. H. EPSTEIN, C. M. TINSLEY, B. H. BURROWS and R. W. WILKINS: The hemodynamic and renal functional effects of venous congestion of the limbs in patients with diabetes insipidus. J. clin. Invest. 29, 826 (1950) (abstract). — JUDSON, W. E., J. D. HATCHER, M. H. HALPERIN and R. W. WILKINS: Further studies on the antidiuresis and decrease in sodium excretion during venous congestion of the limbs: Its prevention in normal subjects by a large transfusion; its absence or presence in cardiac patients with or without congestive failure. J. clin. Invest. 31, 642 (1952) (abstract). — JUDSON, W. E., J. D. HATCHER, W. HOLLANDER and M. H. HALPERIN: The effects of mitral valvuloplasty on cardiovascular and renal function at rest and during exercise. J. clin. Invest. 34, 1297 (1955a). — JUDSON, W. E., J. D. HATCHER, W. HOLLANDER and M. H. HALPERIN and R. W. WILKINS: The effects of venous congestion of the limbs and phlebotomy upon renal clearances and the excretion of water and salt. II. Studies in patients with congestive failure. J. clin. Invest. 34, 1591 (1955c). — JUDSON, W. E., W. HOLLANDER, J. D. HATCHER and M. H. HALPERIN: The effects of exercise on cardiovascular and renal function in cardiac patients with and without heart failure. J. clin. Invest. 34, 1546 (1955b). — JUDSON, W. E., W. HOLLANDER and R. W. WILKINS: The effects of intravenous apresoline (hydralazine) on cardiovascular and renal function in patients with and without congestive heart failure. Circulation 13, 664 (1956). — JULIAN, L. M.: The static intravascular extracapillary blood volume of the kidney of the dog as estimated by the vinylite corrosion technique. Amer. J. vet. Res. 7, 276 (1956). — JUNG, C.: La sécrétion de l'urine envisagée au point de vue de la permeabilité des membranes. Schweiz. med. Wschr. 71, 282 (1941).

KAGAWA, C. M.: Blocking urinary electrolyte effects of desoxycorticosterone with progesterone in rats. Proc. Soc. exp. Biol. (N.Y.) 99, 705 (1958). — KAGAWA, C. M., and R. S. JACOBS jr.: Action of testosterone in blocking urinary electrolyte effects of desoxycorticosterone. Proc. Soc. exp. Biol. (N.Y.) 102, 521 (1959). — KAIM, J. T., and W. A. BRODSKY: Effect of carbonic anhydrase on CO_2 tension of urine and plasma during respiratory acidosis. Amer. J. Physiol. 197, 1097 (1959). — Factors affecting direction of urine-plasma gradients of pCO_2 during production of acidic urine. Fed. Proc. 19, 370 (1960) (abstract). — KAIM, J. T., G. CARRASQUER, R. SHAPIRO and W. A. BRODSKY: Diffusion of CO_2 across the renal tubule. Fed. Proc. 16, 69 (1957) (abstract). — KALCKAR, H.: Phosphorylation in kidney tissue. Enzymologia 2, 47 (1937). — The nature of phosphoric esters formed in kidney extracts. Biochem. J. 33, 631 (1939). — KALLIALA, H., and M. J. KARVONEN: Antidiuresis during suckling in lactating women. Ann. Med. exp. Fenn. 29, 233 (1951). — KALLIALA, H., M. J. KARVONEN and V. LAPPANEN: Release of antidiuretic hormone during nursing in the dog. Ann. Med. exp. Fenn. 30, 96 (1952). — KAMIN, H., and P. HANDLER: Effect of infusion of single amino acids upon excretion of other amino acids. Amer. J. Physiol. 164, 654 (1951a). The metabolism of parenterally administered amino acids. III. Ammonia formation. J. biol. Chem. 193, 873 (1951b). — KANDEL, A., and F. R. DOMER: Renal tubular secretion of potassium and basic organic compounds. Fed. Proc. 16, 310 (1957) (abstract). — KANDEL, A., R. E. GREEN, R. L. VOLLE and L. PETERS: Observations concerning the renal tubular transport of priscoline (tolazoline). J. Pharmacol. exp. Ther. 122, 327 (1958). — KANDEL, A., and L. PETERS: Observations concerning the renal tubular transport characteristics of three quaternary bases in dogs. J. Pharmacol. exp. Ther. 119, 550 (1957). — KANTER, G. S.: Renal clearance of glucose in hypothermic dogs. Amer. J. Physiol. 196, 866 (1959). — KAPLAN, A., M. FRIEDMAN and H. E. KRUGER: Observations concerning origin of renal lymph. Amer. J. Physiol. 138, 553 (1943). — KAPLAN, B. I., and H. W. SMITH: Excretion of inulin, creatinine, xylose and urea in the normal rabbit. Amer. J. Physiol. 113, 354 (1935). — KAPLAN, S. A., S. J. FOMON and S. RAPOPORT: Effect of splanchnic nerve division on urinary excretion of electrolytes during mannitol loading in the hydropenic dog. Amer. J. Physiol. 166, 641 (1951). — Effects of epinephrine and l-norepinephrine on renal excretion of solutes during mannitol diuresis in the hydropenic dog. Amer. J. Physiol. 169, 588 (1952). — KAPLAN, S. A., and S. RAPOPORT: Urinary excretion of sodium and chloride after splanchnicotomy; effect on the proximal tubule. Amer. J. Physiol. 164, 175 (1951). — KAPP, ELEANOR M., and A. F. COBURN: Urinary metabolites of sodium salicylate. J. biol. Chem. 145, 549 (1942). — KARIHER, D. H., and R. H. GEORGE: Toxemias of pregnancy and inulin-diodrast clearance tests. Proc. Soc. exp. Biol. (N.Y.) 52, 245 (1943). — KATSOYANNIS, P. G., and V. DU VIGNEAUD: The synthesis of the histidine analog of the vasopressins. Arch. Biochem. 78, 555 (1958a). — Arginine-vasotocin, a synthetic analogue of the posterior pituitary hormones containing the ring of oxytocin and the side chain of vasopressin. J. biol. Chem. **233**, 1352 (1958 b). — Arginine vasotocin. Nature (Lond.) **184**, 1463 (1959). — KATTUS, A. A., B. SINCLAIR-SMITH, J. GENEST and E. V. NEWMAN: The effect of exercise on the renal mechanism of electrolyte excretion in normal subjects. Bull. Johns Hopk. Hosp. **84**, 344 (1949). — KATZ, Y. J.: Some factors affecting renal lymphatic pressure. Circulat. Res. **6**, 452 (1958). — KATZ, Y. J., and A. T. K. COCKETT: Elevation of inferior vena cava pressure and thoracic lymph and urine flow. Circulat. Res. **7**, 118 (1959). — KEITEL, H. G., D. THOMPSON and H. A. ITANO: Hyposthenuria in sickle cell anemia: A reversible renal defect. J. clin. Invest. **35**, 998 (1956). — KEITH, N. M.: The human tolerance for potassium. Proc. Mayo Clin. **21**, 385 (1946). — KEITH, N. M., H. E. KING and A. E. OSTERBERG: Serum concentration and renal clearance of potassium in severe renal insufficiency in man. Arch. intern. Med. **71**, 675 (1943). — KEITH, N. M., A. E. OSTERBERG and M. W. BINGER: The effect of certain potassium salts on acid base excretion in the normal individual. Amer. J. Physiol. **119**, 347 (1937) (abstract). — KEITH, N. M., A. E. OSTERBERG and H. E. KING: Excretion of potassium by normal and diseased kidney. Trans. Ass. Amer. Phycns **55**, 219 (1940). — KEITH, N. M., and M. WHELAN: A study of the action of ammonium chloride and organic mercury compounds. J. clin. Invest. **3**, 149 (1926). — KELLER, A. D.: Elimination of pars nervosa without eliciting diabetes insipidus. Endocrinology **30**, 408 (1942). — KELLEY, V. C., and R. K. McDONALD: Observations of effects of altitude on renal function. Proc. Soc. exp. Biol. (N.Y.) **68**, 475 (1948). — KELLOGG, R. H., and T. I. KOIKE: Difference between mannitol and urea diuresis in the rat. Amer. J. Physiol. **183**, 633 (1955) (abstract). — KEMPTON, R. T.: Differences in the elimination of neutral red and phenol red by the frog kidney. J. cell. comp. Physiol. **14**, 73 (1939). — Studies on the elasmobranch kidney. I. The structure of the renal tubule of the spiny dogfish *(Squalus acanthias)*. J. Morph. **73**, 247 (1943). — Studies on the elasmobranch kidney. II. Reabsorption of urea by the smooth dogfish, *Mustelus canis*. Biol. Bull. **104**, 45 (1953). — KENNEDY jr., T. J., M. EDEN and R. W. BERLINER: Interpretation of urine CO_2 tension. Fed. Proc. **16**, 72 (1957) (abstract). — KENNEDY jr., T. J., and J. KLEH: The relationship between the clearance and the plasma concentration of inulin in normal man. J. clin. Invest. **32**, 90 (1953). — KENNEDY jr., T. J., J. ORLOFF and R. W. BERLINER: Significance of carbon dioxide tension in urine. Amer. J. Physiol. **169**, 596 (1952). — KENNY, A. D., B. H. VINE and P. L. MUNSON: Estimation of ratio of phosphaturic and calcium-mobilizing activities in parathyroid extracts. Fed. Proc. **13**, 240 (1954) (abstract). — KEOSIAN, J.: Secretion in tissue cultures. III. Tonicity of fluid in chick mesonephric cysts. J. cell. comp. Physiol. **12**, 23 (1938). — KERR jr., W. S.: Effect of complete ureteral obstruction for one week on kidney function. J. appl. Physiol. **6**, 762 (1954). — Effects of complete ureteral obstruction in dogs on kidney function. Amer. J. Physiol. **184**, 521 (1956). — KESSLER, R. H., O. P. A. HEIDENREICH and R. F. PITTS: Evaluation of the cell separation hypothesis of autoregulation of renal blood flow and filtration rate. Glucose titrations in normal and anemic dogs. Amer. J. Physiol. **191**, 501 (1957). — KESSLER, R. H., K. HIERHOLZER and RUTH S. GURD: Localization of urate transport in the nephron of the mongrel and Dalmation dog kidney. Amer. J. Physiol. **197**, 601 (1959). — KESSLER, R. H., K. HIERHOLZER and R. F. PITTS: Localization of diuretic action of chlormerodrin in the nephron of the dog. Amer. J. Physiol. **194**, 540 (1958). — KESSLER, R. H., R. LOZANO and R. F. PITTS: Studies on structure diuretic activity relationships of organic compounds of mercury. J. clin. Invest. **36**, 656 (1957a). — A comparison of the pharmacological behavior of chlormerodrin, meralluride, mersalyl and mercuric chloride in the dog. J. Pharmacol. exp. Ther. **121**, 432 (1957b). — KEUTMANN, E. H., and S. H. BASSETT: Studies on the mechanism of proteinuria. J. clin. Invest. **16**, 767 (1937). — KING, S. E., and D. S. BALDWIN: Renal hemodynamics during erect lordosis in normal man and subjects with orthostatic proteinuria. Proc. Soc. exp. Biol. (N.Y.) **86**, 634 (1954). — KINTER, W. B.: Renal tubular transport of Diodrast-I^{131} and PAH in Necturus: evidence for simultaneous reabsorption and secretion. Amer. J. Physiol. **196**, 1141 (1959). — KINTER, W. B., and J. R. PAPPENHEIMER: Renal extraction of PAH and of Diodrast-I^{131} as a function of arterial red cell concentration. Amer. J. Physiol. **185**, 391 (1956a). — Role of red blood corpuscles in regulation of renal blood flow and glomerular filtration rate. Amer. J. Physiol. **185**, 399 (1956b). — KIRKENDALL, W. M., and J. W. CULBERTSON: Some effects of hexamethonium on renal circulation. J. clin. Invest. **31**, 644 (1952) (abstract). — KIRKENDALL, W. M., J. W. CULBERTSON and J. W. ECKSTEIN: Renal hemodynamics in patients with coarctation of the aorta. J. Lab. clin. Med. **53**, 6 (1959). — KIVALO, E., P. MARJANEN and U. K. RINNE: Response of the hypothalamic neurosecretory substance to serotonin. Acta endocr. (Kbh.) **28**, 553 (1958). — KLEEMAN, C. R., D. A. ADAMS and M. H. MAXWELL: The defect in urinary dilution associated with chronic renal disease. Clin. Res. Proc. **7**, 77 (1959) (abstract). — KLEEMAN, C. R., D. ADAMS, M. MAXWELL and L. BERNSTEIN: The effect of increased renal hemodynamics on the parameters of maximal water diuresis. Clin. Res. Proc. **8**, 115 (1960) (abstract). — KLEEMAN, C. R., D. BERNSTEIN, M. H. MAXWELL and J. T. DOWLING: The effect of parathyroid function on serum phosphorus and phosphorus clearance during a calcium infusion. Clin. Res. Proc. 7, 247 (1959b) (abstract). — KLEEMAN, C. R., and R. E. COOKE: The acute effects of parathyroid hormone on the metabolism of endogenous phosphate. J. Lab. clin. Med. 38, 112 (1951). — KLEEMAN, C. R., and F. H. EPSTEIN: An illustrative case of chronic pyelonephritis with persistently hypotonic urine. Amer. J. Med. 23, 488 (1957). — KLEEMAN, C. R., F. H. EPSTEIN and C. WHITE: The effect of variations in solute excretion and glomerular filtration on water diuresis. J. clin. Invest. 35, 749 (1956). — KLEEMAN, C. R., J. KOPLOWITZ and M. H. MAXWELL: Acute effect of 6-methylprednisolone (Medrol) on impaired water excretion of adrenal and pituitary insufficiency. Proc. Soc. exp. Biol. (N.Y.) 100, 615 (1959). — KLEEMAN, C. R., J. KOPLOWITZ, M. H. MAXWELL and J. T. DOWLING: The effect of the acute and chronic administration of hydrocortisone on the release, inactivation and action of antidiuretic hormone. Clin. Res. Proc. 7, 111 (1959a) (abstract). — KLEEMAN, C. R., and M. H. MAXWELL: The role of nonhormonal factors in the impaired water diuresis associated with Addison's disease and anterior pituitary insufficiency. Clin. Res. Proc. 5, 191 (1957) (abstract). — Contributory role of extrarenal factors in the polyuria of potassium depletion. New Engl. J. Med. 260, 268 (1959). — KLEEMAN, C. R., M. H. MAXWELL and R. ROCKNEY: Production of hypertonic urine in humans in the probable absence of antidiuretic hormone (ADH). Proc. Soc. exp. Biol. (N.Y.) 96, 189 (1957). — Mechanisms of impaired water excretion in adrenal and pituitary insufficiency. I. The role of altered glomerular filtration rate and solute excretion. J. clin. Invest. 37, 1799 (1958). — KLEEMAN, C. R., M. H. MAXWELL and S. WITLIN: Functional isosthenuria. Arch. intern. Med. 101, 1023 (1958). — KLEEMAN, C. R., M. E. RUBINI, E. LAMDIN and F. H. EPSTEIN: Studies on alcohol diuresis. II. The evaluation of ethyl alcohol as an inhibitor of the neurohypophysis. J. clin. Invest. 34, 448 (1955a). — KLEEMAN, C. R., M. E. RUBINI, E. LAMDIN, R. F. KILEY and I. L. BENNETT jr.: Interrelationship of acute alkalosis and potassium metabolism. Metabolism 4, 238 (1955b). — KLEIN, R., and R. C. GOW: Interaction of parathyroid hormone and vitamin D on the renal excretion of phosphate. J. clin. Endocr. 13, 271 (1953). — KLEITMAN, N.: Studies on the physiology of sleep. I. The effects of prolonged sleeplessness on man. Amer. J. Physiol. 66, 67 (1923). — KLEMPERER, F., and W. BAUER: Influence of aspirin on urate excretion. J. clin. Invest. 23, 950 (1944) (abstract). — KLISIECKI, A., MARY PICKFORD, P. ROTHSCHILD and E. B. VERNEY: Absorption and excretion of water by mammal. I. Relation between absorption of water and its excretion by innervated and denervated kidney. Proc. roy. Soc. B 112, 496 (1933a). — II. Factors influencing the response of the kidney to water ingestion. Proc. roy. Soc. B 112, 521 (1933b). — KLOPP, C., N. F. YOUNG and H. C. TAYLOR: Probable errors in the simultaneous measurement of separate kidney functions. J. clin. Invest. 24, 117 (1944). — The effects of testosterone and of testosterone propionate on renal functions in man. J. clin. Invest. 24, 189 (1945). — KLOSTERMAN, A. M., J. E. HAINES, H. M. HAUCK and A. B. KLINE: Renal threshold for ascorbic acid; modified method for its estimation with results for 12 adult subjects. J. Nutr. 33, 505 (1947). — KLOTZ, H. P., et F. KAHN: A propos du controle central de la secrétion d'aldostérone. Ann. Endocr. (Paris) 18, 587 (1957). — KLÜMPER, J. D., K. J. ULLRICH u. H. H. HILGER: Das Verhalten des Harnstoffs in den Sammelrohren der Säugetierniere. Pflügers Arch. ges. Physiol. 267, 238 (1958). — KNIGHT jr., R. P., D. S. KORNFELD, G. H. GLASER and P. K. BONDY: Effects of intravenous hydrocortisone on electrolytes of serum and urine in man. J. clin. Endocr. 15, 176 (1955). — KNOEFEL, P. K., C. A. HANDLEY and R. A. HUGGINS: Renal functions during positive pressure respiration. Proc. Soc. exp. Biol. (N.Y.) 82, 430 (1953). — KNOEFEL, P. K., and K. C. HUANG: The biochemomorphology of renal tubular transport: Iodinated benzoic acids. J. Pharmacol. exp. Ther. 117, 307 (1956). — Biochemorphology of renal tubular transport: Hippuric acid and related substances. J. Pharmacol. exp. Ther. 126, 296 (1959). — KNOWLES jr., H. C.: Hypernatremia. Metabolism 5, 508 (1956). — KOCH, A. R., P. BRAZEAU and A. GILMAN: Role of renal tubular secretion in potassium homeostasis. Amer. J. Physiol. 186, 350 (1956). — KOEFOED, H.: Investigation of the kidneys of the kangaroo rat by the maceration-method. Scand. J. clin. Lab. Invest. 1, 340 (1949) (abstract). — KOEFOED- JOHNSEN, V., and H. H. USSING: The nature of the frog skin potential. Acta physiol. scand. 42, 298 (1958). — KOESTER, H. L., J. C. LOCKE and H. G. SWANN: Effluent constrictions in the renal vascular system. Tex. Rep. Biol. Med. 13, 251 (1955). — KOISHI, T.: Studies on renal tubular transport. I. Accumulation of p-aminohippurate by kidney slices. Jap. J. Pharmacol. 8, 101 (1959). — II. Effect of certain reagents on accumulation of p-aminohippurate by kidney slices. Jap. J. Pharmacol. 8, 124 (1959). — KOIWA, M.: Beeinflussung glomerularer Filtration und tubularer Rückresorption durch Infusion von Gummilösung und Bluttransfusion bei gesunden sowie Kantharidinkaninchen. Tôhoku J. exp. Med. 37, 139 (1939). — KOROBKOW, L.: Zur Frage der selbständigen Tätigkeit der Gefäße. Pflügers Arch. ges. Physiol. 219, 673 (1928). — KOTTKE, F. J., C. F. CODE and E. H. WOOD: Urine dilution and concentration tests in adrenalectomized dogs. Amer. J. Physiol. **136**, 229 (1942). — KOURILSKY, R., S. KOURILSKY, M. LAUDAT et J. REGAUD: La physiologie du diabète insipide humain doit être conçue en fonction de la soif beaucoup plus que de la polyurie. Bull. Soc. méd. Hôp. Paris **58**, 104 (1942). — KOVACS, K., and M. A. DAVID: Effect of cortisone on the morphological reactions of the adrenal cortex due to changes in the Na/K intake. Acta anat. (Basel) **36**, 169 (1959). — KOZA, D. W., F. J. KOTTKE and M. OLSON: Effects of epinephrine on the normal, hypertensive and denervated renal vascular systems in man. J. appl. Physiol. **3**, 610 (1951). — KRAKUSIN, J. S., and R. B. JENNINGS: Radioautographic localization of Na^{22} in the rat kidney. Arch. Path. (Chicago) **59**, 471 (1955). — KRAMER, K., G. A. SAXTON and D. E. TIMMONS: Further evidence of the existence of a kidney shunt circulation. XVIII. Internat. Physiol. Congr. **18**, 314 (1950). — KRAMER, K., u. K. J. ULLRICH: Bestimmung des O_2-Verbrauches der Nierenrinde in situ an Hunden. Pflügers Arch. ges. Physiol. **266**, 54 (1957) (abstract). — O_2-Sättigung und Hb-Gehalt des Capillarblutes der Nierenrinde. Pflügers Arch. ges. Physiol. **267**, 251 (1958). — KRANE, S. M., and R. K. CRANE: The accumulation of D-galactose against a concentration gradient by slices of rabbit kidney cortex. J. biol. Chem. **234**, 211 (1959). — KRISS, J. P., and P. H. FUTCHER: Renal excretion and tubular reabsorption of salt in Cushing's syndrome after intravenous administration of hypertonic sodium chloride. J. clin. Endocr. **9**, 13 (1949). — KRISS, J. P., P. H. FUTCHER and M. L. GOLDMAN: Unilateral adrenalectomy, unilateral splanchnic nerve resection and homolateral renal function. Amer. J. Physiol. **154** 229 (1948). — KRITZLER, R. A., and A. B. GUTMAN: "Alkaline" phosphatase activity of the proximal convoluted tubules and the mechanism of phlorizin glycuresis. Amer. J. Physiol. **134**, 94 (1941). — KROGH, A.: Studies on the physiology of capillaries. II. The reactions to local stimuli of the blood-vessels in the skin and web of the frog. J. Physiol. (Lond.) **55**, 412 (1921). — KROGSGAARD, A. R.: The effect of intravenously injected reserpine on blood pressure, renal function and sodium excretion. Acta med. scand. **154**, 41 (1956). — KRUHØFFER, P.: Determination of inulin in urine and plasma. Acta physiol. scand. **11**, 1 (1946). — Studies on water-electrolyte excretion and glomerular activity in the mammalian kidney. Copenhagen: Roenkilde and Bagger 1950. — KUBICEK, W. G., R. B. HARVEY and F. J. KOTTKE: The adrenalin sensitivity of the denervated dog kidney. Fed. Proc. **7**, 68 (1948) (abstract). — KUHN, W., u. K. RYFFEL: Herstellung konzentrierter Lösungen aus verdünnten durch bloße Membranwirkung; ein Modellversuch zur Funktion der Niere. Hoppe-Seylers Z. physiol. Chem. **276**, 145 (1942). — KUNIN, A. S., E. H. DEARBORN, B. A. BURROWS and A. S. RELMAN: Comparison of renal excretion of rubidium and potassium. Amer. J. Physiol. **197**, 1297 (1959). — KUNTZ, A.: The autonomic nervous system. Philadelphia: Lea and Febiger 1945. — KUNZ, H. W., E. L. PRATT, G. W. MELLIN and M. W. CHEUNG: Impairment of urinary concentration in sickle cell anemia. Pediatrics **13**, 352 (1954). — KUSCHINSKY, G., u. H. E. BUNDSCHUH: Über eine diuretische und Kochsalz ausschwemmende Substanz in Hypophysenhinterlappen-Präparaten. Naunyn-Schmiedeberg's Arch. exp. Path. Pharmak. **192**, 683 (1939). — KUWABARA, K.: Studies on renal tubular functions. I. Studies on the uptake of p-aminohippurate (PAH) by slices of the renal cortex of a rabbit. Folia pharmacol. jap. **53**, 1036 (1957). — KWAAN, H. C., and H. J. BARTELSTONE: Corticotropin release following injections of minute doses of arginine vasopressin into the third ventricle of the dog. Endocrinology **65**, 982 (1959).

LAAKE, H.: Experimental investigations of excretory and reabsorptive functions of renal tubules in normal and nephrotic rabbits. Acta med. scand. Suppl. **168**, 1 (1945). — Clinical investigations of certain functions of the renal tubules under normal and pathologic conditions and under the influence of carbonic anhydrase inhibitor. Acta med. scand. **155**, 27 (1956). — LABBE, M., P.-L. VIOLLE et E. AZERAD: Action de la rétropituitrine sur la diurèse chez l'homme en état de sommeil. C. R. Soc. Biol. (Paris) **94**, 848 (1926). — LADD, M.: Effect of prehydration on the response to saline infusion in man. J. appl. Physiol. **3**, 379 (1951a). — Effect of prehydration upon renal excretion of sodium in man. J. appl. Physiol. **3**, 603 (1951b). — Renal excretion of sodium and water in man as affected by prehydration, saline infusion, pitressin and thiomerin. J. appl. Physiol. **4**, 602 (1952). — LADD, M., LOIS LIDDLE and J. A. GAGNON: Renal excretion of inulin, creatinine and ferrocyanide, at normal and reduced clearance levels in the dog. Amer. J. Physiol. **184**, 505 (1956). — LADD, M., LOIS LIDDLE, J. A. GAGNON and R. W. CLARKE: Glomerular and tubular functions in sheep and goats. J. appl. Physiol. **10**, 249 (1957). — LAIDLAW, J. C., MAY COHEN and A. G. GORNALL: Studies on the origin of aldosterone during human pregnancy. J. clin. Endocr. **18**, 222 (1958). — LAIDLAW, J. C., J. F. DINGMAN, W. L. ARONS, J. T. FINKENSTAEDT and G. W. THORN: Comparison of the metabolic effects of cortisone and hydrocortisone in man. Ann. N.Y. Acad. Sci. **61**, 315 (1955). — LAIDLAW, C., D. JENKINS, W. J. REDDY and THEODOR JAKOBSON: The diurnal variation in adrenocortical secretion. J. clin. Invest. **33**, 950 (1954) (abstract). — LAMBERT, P.-P.: Étude comparée de l'élimination de l'inuline, de la créatinine et de l'uroselectan B par le rein des oiseaux. Arch. int. Pharmacodyn. 71, 313 (1945). — A study of the mechanism by which toxic tubular damage changes the renal threshold for glucose. The kidney, p. 79. Ciba Found. Symp. Boston: Little Brown & Co. 1954. — LAMBERT, P.-P., et F. GRÉGOIRE: Hormones cortico-surrénales et réabsorption rénale des protéines. Ann. Endocr. (Paris) 15, 957 (1954). — LAMBERT, P.-P., F. GREGOIRE et C. DE H. DE BRAUCOURT: Hémodynamique glomérulaire et excrétion de l'hémoglobine. Arch. int. Physiol. 60, 506 (1952). — LAMBERT, P.-P., F. GREGOIRE, C. MALMENDIER, F. VANDERVEIKEN et G. GUERITTE: Recherches sur le mécanisme de l'albuminurie. Bull. Acad. roy. Méd. Belg. 22, 524 (1957). — LAMBERT, P.-P., J. LEBRUN et C. DE H. DE BRAUCOURT: Influence du glucoside de désoxycorticosterone sur la résorption rénale du glucose. Acta clin. belg. 3, 529 (1948). — Acetate de désoxycorticosterone et réabsorption rénale du glucose. J. Urol. méd. Chir. 55, 789 (1949). — LAMBERT, P.-P., R. TAGNON et J. CORVILAIN: ACTH et seuils d'éxcretion du glucose. J. Urol. méd. chir. 57, 317 (1951). — LAMBERT, P.-P., R. TAGNON, J. CORVILAIN, C. H. DE BRAUCOURT and M. BRUNEEL: Hormone corticotrope hypophysaire et seuils d'éxcretion du glucose. Acta clin. belg. 6, 107 (1951). — LAMBERT, P.-P., R. TAGNON, J. CORVILAIN et C. COËRS: A propos de deux cas d'intoxication par le cyanure. Physiopathologie de leur glucosurie. Acta clin. belg. 5, 14 (1950). — LAMBERT, P.-P., E. VAN KESSEL et C. LEPLAT: Étude sur l'élimination des phosphates inorganiques chez l'homme. Acta med. scand. 128, 386 (1947). — LAMBIE, ANNE, T., A. S. RELMAN and W. B. SCHWARTZ: Electrolyte and acid-base balance during acute loading with rubidium chloride. J. clin. Invest. 38, 1538 (1959). — LAMBIOTTE, CLAUDINE, J. BLANCHARD and S. GRAFF: Thiosulphate clearance in pregnancy. J. clin. Invest. 29, 1207 (1950). — LAMBRECHTS, A.: Activité diabétogène de quelques dérivés de la phlorhizine. C. R. Soc. Biol. Paris 121, 870 (1936). — Nouvelles recherches sur le diabète phlorhizique, la phlorhizine et quelques substances apparentées. Arch. int. Physiol. 44, Suppl., 1 (1937). — LAMDIN, E., C. R. KLEEMAN, M. RUBINI and F. H. EPSTEIN: Studies on alcohol diuresis. III. The response to ethyl alcohol in certain disease states characterized by impaired water intolerance. J. clin. Invest. 35, 386 (1956). — LAMMERS, H.-J., et T. SMITHIUS: Étude d'une anastomose artérioveineuse au niveau interlobaire du rein humain. C. R. Ass. Anat. 42, 836 (1955). — LANDAU, R. L., D. M. BERGENSTAL, KATHLEEN LUGIBIHL, D. F. DIMICK and ERNESTINE RASHID: The relationship of estrogen and of pituitary hormones to the metabolic effects of progesterone. J. clin. Endocr. 17, 177 (1957). — LANDAU, R. L., D. M. BERGENSTAL, KATHLEEN LUGIBIHL and MARY E. KASCHT: The metabolic effects of progesterone in man. J. clin. Endocr. 15, 1194 (1955). — LANDAU, R. L., and KATHLEEN LUGIBIHL: Inhibition of the sodium-retaining influence of aldosterone by progesterone. J. clin. Endocr. 18, 1237 (1958). — LANDIS, E. M., K. A. ELSOM, PHYLLIS A. BOTT and E. H. SHIELS: Simultaneous plasma clearances of creatinine and certain organic compounds of iodine in relation to human kidney function. J. clin. Invest. 15, 397 (1936). — LANDOWNE, M., and A. S. ALVING: Method of determining specific renal functions of glomerular filtration, maximal tubular excretion (or reabsorption), and "effective blood flow" using single injection of single substance. J. Lab. clin. Med. 32, 931 (1947). — LANGERON, L., V. NOLF et J. LIEFOOGHE: Contribution à l'étude de l'effet bioclinique des hormones stéroides genito-surrénales sur le fonctionnement rénal. J. Urol. méd. chir. 57, 293 (1959). — LANGERON, L., M. PAGET, V. NOLF et J. DURIEZ: Le test de l'hyposulfite de sodium pour la mesure de la filtration glomerulaire. Presse méd. 57, 222 (1949). — LANGSTON, J. B., A. C. GUYTON and W. J. GILLESPIE jr.: Acute effect of changes in renal arterial pressure and sympathetic blockade on kidney function. Amer. J. Physiol. 197, 595 (1959). — Autoregulation of renal blood flow resulting from renal damage. Fed. Proc. 19, 360 (1960) (abstract). — LARAGH, J. H.: Some effects of chlorothiazide on electrolyte metabolism and its use in edematous states. Ann. N.Y. Acad. Sci. 71, 409 (1958). — LARAGH, J. H., H. B. VAN DYKE, J. JACOBSON, K. ADAMSONS jr. and S. L. ENGEL: The experimental production of ascites in the dog with diabetes insipidus. J. clin. Invest. 35, 897 (1956). — LARAGH, J. H., H. O. HEINEMANN and F. E. DEMARTINI: Effect of chlorothiazide on electrolyte transport in man. Its use in the treatment of edema of congestive heart failure, nephrosis, and cirrhosis. J. Amer. med. Ass. 166, 145 (1958). — LARAGH, J. H., and H. C. STOERK: A study of the mechanism of secretion of the sodium-retaining hormone (aldosterone). J. clin. Invest. 36, 383 (1957). — LARSON, E.: Tolerance and fate of the pressor principle of posterior pituitary extract in anesthetized animals. J. Pharmacol. exp. Ther. 62, 346 (1938). — LASCHÉ, EUNICE M., W. H. PERLOFF and T. M. DURANT: Some aspects of adrenocortical function in cardiac decompensation. Amer. J. med. Sci. 222, 465 (1951). — LASSEN, N. A., J. B. LONGLEY and L. S. LILIENFIELD: Concentration of albumin in renal papilla. Science 128, 720 (1958). — LASSITER, W. E., C. W. GOTTSCHALK and MARGARET MYLLE: Composition of loop of Henle and collecting duct fluids in the hamster papilla. Fed. Proc. 19, 369 (1960) (abstract). — LATHEM, W.: The urinary excretion of sodium and potassium during the pyrogenic reaction in man. J. clin. Invest. 35, 947 (1956). — Urinary hemoglobin excretion and renal circulatory dynamics: A study of the effect of l-norepinephrine in the dog. J. clin. Invest.

36, 89 (1957a). — Renal hemoglobin transport: Glomerular permeability and tubular reabsorption during infusions of *l*-norepinephrine. Amer. J. Physiol. 189, 177 (1957b). — The renal excretion of hemoglobin: Regulatory mechanisms and the differential excretion of free and protein-bound hemoglobin. J. clin. Invest. 38, 652 (1959). — LATHEM, W., BETTY S. ROOF, J. F. NICKEL and S. E. BRADLEY: Urinary protein excretion and renal hemodynamic adjustments during orthostasis in patients with acute and chronic renal diseases. J. clin. Invest. 33, 1457 (1954). — LATHEM, W., and W. E. WORLEY: The distribution of extracorpuscular hemoglobin in circulating plasma. J. clin. Invest. 38, 474 (1959). — LATTIMER, J. K.: The action of testosterone propionate upon the kidneys of rats, dogs and men. J. Urol. (Baltimore) 48, 778 (1942). — LAURELL, C.-B., and MARGARETA NYMAN: Studies on the serum haptoglobin level in hemoglobinemia and its influence on renal excretion of hemoglobin. Blood 12, 493 (1957). — LAUSON, H. D.: The problem of estimating the rate of secretion of antidiuretic hormone in man. Amer. J. Med. 11, 135 (1951a). — Sources of error in plasma creatinine determination. J. appl. Physiol. 4, 227 (1951b). — Vasopressin and oxytocin in the plasma of man and other mammals. In: Hormones in human plasma, p. 225. Boston: Little Brown & Co. 1960. — LAUSON, H. D., and M. BOCANEGRA: Metabolism of antidiuretic hormone in dogs. Fed. Proc. 19, 167 (1960) (abstract). — LAUSON, H. D., CAROLYN W. FORMAN, HELEN MCNAMARA, G. MATTAR and H. L. BARNETT: Effect of corticotropin (ACTH) on glomerular permeability to albumin and on blood antidiuretic hormone concentration in children with the nephrotic syndrome. Amer. J. Dis. Child. 83, 87 (1952). — The effect of corticotropin (ACTH) on glomerular permeability to albumin in children with the nephrotic syndrome. J. clin. Invest. 33, 657 (1954). — LAUSON, H. D., and D. D. THOMPSON: Effects in dogs of decrease in glomerular filtration rate on cation excretion during intravenous administration of unreabsorbable anions. Amer. J. Physiol. 192, 198 (1958). — LAVENDER, A. R., and T. N. PULLMAN: Effects of unilateral renal arterial infusion of chlorothiazide. Fed. Proc. 17, 93 (1958) (abstract). — LEAF, A.: Diabetes insipidus. Clin. Endocr. 1, 73 (1960). — LEAF, A., F. C. BARTTER, R. F. SANTOS and O. WRONG: Evidence in man that urinary electrolyte loss induced by pitressin is a function of water retention. J. clin. Invest. 32, 868 (1953). — LEAF, A., and A. A. CAMARA: Renal tubular secretion of potassium in man. J. clin. Invest. 28, 1526 (1949). — LEAF, A., and W. T. COUTER: Evidence that renal sodium excretion by normal human subjects is regulated by adrenal cortical activity. J. clin. Invest. 28, 1067 (1949). — LEAF, A., W. S. KERR jr., O. WRONG and J. Y. CHATILLON: Effect of graded compression of the renal artery on water and solute excretion. Amer. J. Physiol. 179, 191 (1954). — LEAF, A., and A. R. MAMBY: The normal antidiuretic mechanism in man and dog. Its regulation by extracellular fluid tonicity. J. clin. Invest. 31, 54 (1952a). — An antidiuretic mechanism not regulated by extracellular fluid tonicity. J. clin. Invest. 31, 60 (1952b). — LEAF, A., A. R. MAMBY, H. RASMUSSEN and JOAN P. MARASCO: Some hormonal aspects of water excretion in man. J. clin. Invest. 31, 914 (1952a). — LEAF, A., H. RASMUSSEN, A. R. MAMBY and M. S. RABEN: Some hormonal aspects of water excretion in man. J. clin. Invest. 31, 646 (1952) (abstract). — LeBRIE, S. J., and H. S. MAYERSON: Composition and significance of renal lymph. Fed. Proc. 18, 89 (1959) (abstract). — LEBRUN, J.: Étude de la cléarance de l'hyposulfite de soude chez l'homme à basse concentration sanguine. J. Urol. méd. chir. 55, 745 (1949). — LEE, C.-C., R. C. ANDERSON and K. K. CHEN: The effect of carbutamide on tubular glucose transport and glucose tolerance in dogs. Arch. int. Pharmacodyn. 113, 302 (1958). — LeFEVRE, P. G.: The evidence for active transport of monosaccharides across the red cell membrane. Symp. Soc. exp. Biol. 8, 118 (1954). — LeFEVRE, P. G., and J. K. MARSHALL: Conformational specificity in a biological sugar transport system. Amer. J. Physiol. 194, 333 (1958). — LEHMAN, R. A., E. E. KING and H. TAUBE: The pharmacology of thiomerin. J. Pharmacol. exp. Ther. 99, 149 (1950). — LEIBMAN, K. C., and D. ALFORD: Nature of the inhibition of carbonic anhydrase by acetazolamide. Fed. Proc. 19, 50 (1960) (abstract). — LEITER, L.: The role of sodium chloride in the mechanism and treatment of chronic heart failure. Bull. N.Y. Acad. Med. 24, 702 (1948). — LEONARD, E., and J. ORLOFF: The regulation of ammonia excretion in the rat. Amer. J. Physiol. 182, 131 (1955). — LEQUESNE, L. P., and A. A. G. LEWIS: Post-operative retention of water and sodium, p. 193. The kidney. Ciba Foundation Symp. Boston: Little, Brown & Co. 1954. — LESLIE, S. H., B. JOHNSTON and E. RALLI: Renal function in patients with cirrhosis of the liver. J. clin. Invest. 30, 1200 (1951). — LESSER, G. T., M. F. DUNNING, F. H. EPSTEIN and E. Y. BERGER: Mercurial diuresis in edematous individuals. Circulation 5, 85 (1952). — LEVIN, W. C., R. GREGORY and A. BENNETT: Effect of chronic anemia on renal function as measured by inulin and diodrast clearances. J. Lab. clin. Med. 32, 1433 (1947) (abstract). — LEVINE, R., and B. HUDDLESTUN: The mode of excretion of fructose by the dog. Fed. Proc. 6, 151 (1947) (abstract). — LEVINE, V. E., and W. W. BECKER: Determination of inulin in blood and urine by means of vanillin in acid medium. Fed. Proc. 17, 263 (1958) (abstract). — LEVINGER, E. L., and R. F. ESCAMILLA: Hereditary diabetes insipidus: Report of 20 cases in seven generations.

J. clin. Endocr. **15**, 547 (1955). — LEVINSKY, N. G., and R. W. BERLINER: Changes in composition of the urine in ureter and bladder at low urine flow. Amer. J. Physiol. **196**, 549 (1959a). — The role of urea in the urine concentrating mechanism. J. clin. Invest. **38**, 741 (1959b). — LEVINSKY, N. G., D. G. DAVIDSON and R. W. BERLINER: Changes in urine concentration during prolonged administration of vasopressin and water. Amer. J. Physiol. **196**, 451 (1959a). — Effects of reduced glomerular filtration on urine concentration in the presence of antidiuretic hormone. J. clin. Invest. **38**, 730 (1959b). — LEVITAN, B. A.: Effect in normal man of hyperglycemia and glycosuria on excretion and reabsorption of phosphate. J. appl. Physiol. **4**, 224 (1951/52). — LEVITIN, H., A. MANITIUS and F. H. EPSTEIN: Urinary dilution in potassium deficiency. Yale J. Biol. Med. **32**, 390 (1960). — LEVITT, M. F., and M. E. BADER: Effect of cortisone and ACTH on fluid and electrolyte distribution in man. Amer. J. Med. **11**, 715 (1951). — LEVITT, M. F., M. BELSKY and DEMETRA POLIMEROS: Serum hypertonicity secondary to cerebral disease. Ann. intern. Med. **50**, 788 (1959). — LEVITT, M. F., M. H. HALPERN, DEMETRA P. POLIMEROS, A. Y. SWEET and D. GRIBETZ: The effect of abrupt changes in plasma calcium concentrations on renal function and electrolyte excretion in man and monkey. J. clin. Invest. **37**, 294 (1958). — LEVITT, M. F., M. S. LEVY, A. D. HAUSER and DEMETRA POLIMEROS: The concentrating defect in sickle cell disease. Clin. Res. Proc. **7**, 281 (1959) (abstract). — LEVITT, M. F., M. S. LEVY and DEMETRA POLIMEROS: The effect of a fall in filtration rate on solute and water excretion in hydropenic man. J. clin. Invest. **38**, 463 (1959). — LEVITT, M. F., L. B. TURNER and A. Y. SWEET: The effect of experimental venous obstruction on salt and water distribution and excretion in man. J. clin. Invest. **31**, 885 (1952). — LEVKOFF, A. H., T. W. DEMUNBRUN and A. D. KELLER: Disparity between fluid intake and renal concentrating deficit in dogs with diabetes insipidus. Amer. J. Physiol. **176**, 25 (1954). — LEVKOFF, A. H., T. W. DEMUNBRUN, R. M. PURSER and P. GREENBERG: Renal concentrating ability in dogs with experimental diabetes insipidus. Amer. J. Physiol. **171**, 743 (1952) (abstract). — LEVY, M. H., and J. L. ANKENY: Influence of glomerular filtration rate upon the renal tubular reabsorption of sodium. Proc. Soc. exp. Biol. (N.Y.) **79**, 491 (1952). — LEVY, M. N., and G. SAUCEDA: Diffusion of oxygen from arterial to venous segments of renal capillaries. Amer. J. Physiol. **196**, 1336 (1959). — LEVY, M. S., MARSCHELLE H. POWER and E. J. KEPLER: The specificity of the "water test" as a diagnostic procedure in Addison's disease. J. clin. Endocr. **6**, 607 (1946). — LEVY, R. I., I. M. WEINER and G. H. MUDGE: The effects of acid-base balance on the diuresis produced by organic and inorganic mercurials. J. clin. Invest. **37**, 1016 (1958). — LEWIS, A. A. G.: The control of the renal excretion of water. Roy. Coll. Surg. Eng. Ann. **13**, 36 (1953). — LEWIS, A. A. G., and T. M. CHALMERS: A nicotine test for the investigation of diabetes insipidus. Clin. Sci. **10**, 137 (1951). — LEWIS, A. E., R. D. GOODMAN and E. A. SCHUCK: Organ blood volume measurements in normal rats. J. Lab. clin. Med. **39**, 704 (1952). — LEWIS, C. S., A. J. SAMUELS, M. C. DAINES and H. H. HECHT: Chronic lung disease, polycythemia and congestive heart failure. Cardiorespiratory, vascular and renal adjustments in cor pulmonale. Circulation **6**, 874 (1952). — LEWIS, J. M., R. M. BUIE, S. M. SEVIER and T. R. HARRISON: The effect of posture and of congestion of the head on sodium excretion in normal subjects. Circulation **2**, 822 (1950). — LEWIS, J. S., C. A. STORVICK and H. M. HAUCK: Renal threshold for ascorbic acid in 12 normal adults, with note on state of tissue reserves of subjects on intake of ascorbic acid approximating suggested daily allowance. J. Nutr. **25**, 185 (1943). — LEWIS, O. J.: The development of the blood vessels of the metanephros. J. Anat. (Lond.) **92**, 84 (1958a). — The vascular arrangement of the mammalian renal glomerulus as revealed by a study of its development. J. Anat. (Lond.) **92**, 433 (1958b). — LEWIS, P. R., and MARY C. LOBBAN: Patterns of electrolyte excretion in human subjects during a prolonged period of life on a 22 hour day. J. Physiol. (Lond.) **133**, 670 (1956). — The effects of prolonged periods of life on abnormal time routines upon excretory rhythms in human subjects. Quart. J. exp. Physiol. **42**, 356 (1957a). — Dissociation of diurnal rhythms in human subjects living on abnormal time routines. Quart. J. exp. Physiol. **42**, 371 (1957b). — LEWIS, P. R., MARY C. LOBBAN and T. I. SHAW: Patterns of urine flow in human subjects during a prolonged period of life on a 22-hour day. J. Physiol. (Lond.) **133**, 659 (1956). — L'HEUREUX, M. V., and L. E. REICHERT: Parathyroid hormone activity of human and rat plasma constituents. Fed. Proc. **19**, 151 (1960) (abstract). — L'HEUREUX, M. V., HELEN M. TEPPERMAN and A. E. WILHELMI: A new preparation of the parathyroid hormone. J. biol. Chem. **168**, 167 (1947). — LIANG, T. J.: Über die Harnbildung in der Froschniere. XVIII. Über die Bedingungen der sekretorischen Abscheidung in den 2. Abschnitten. Pflügers Arch. ges. Physiol. **222**, 271 (1929). — LIDDLE, G. W.: Sodium diuresis induced by steroidal antagonists of aldosterone. Science **126**, 1016 (1957). — LIDDLE, G. W., L. L. BENNETT and P. H. FORSHAM: The prevention of ACTH-induced sodium retention by the use of potassium salts: a quantitative study. J. clin. Invest. **32**, 1197 (1953). — LIDDLE, G. W., L. E. DUNCAN jr. and F. C. BARTTER: Dual mechanism regulating adrenocortical function in man. Amer. J. Med.

21, 380 (1956). — LIEBERMAN, A. H., R. CURTIS, B. B. JOHNSON and J. A. LUETSCHER jr.: An observation of some factors concerned with aldosterone output. Clin. Res. Proc. 4, 211 (1956) (abstract). — LIGHT, A., and V. DU VIGNEAUD: On the nature of oxytocin and vasopressin from human pituitary. Proc. Soc. exp. Biol. (N.Y.) 98, 692 (1958). — LILIENFIELD, L. S., H. C. MAGANZINI and M. H. BAUER: Vascular regulation of renal medullary osmolarity. Clin. Res. Proc. 8, 88 (1960a) (abstract). — Renal medullary blood flow. Fed. Proc. 19, 363 (1960b) (abstract). — LILIENFIELD, L. S., J. C. ROSE and N. A. LASSEN: Diverse distribution of red cells and albumin in the dog kidney. Circulat. Res. 6, 810 (1958). — LILIENFIELD, L. S., J. C. ROSE and F. A. PORFIDO: Evidence for a red cell shunting mechanism in the kidney. Circulat. Res. 5, 64 (1957). — LILJESTRAND, A., and B. SWEDIN: The urinary excretion of phosphate in the dog. Acta physiol. scand. 25, 168 (1952). — LINDAHL, O., and B. JOSEPHSON: The kidney function and the renal clearances of some sulfanilamide derivatives. Acta med. scand. 120, 195 (1945). — LINDEMANN, W.: Über die Wirkung der Gegendruckerhöhung auf die Harnsecretion. Beitr. path. Anat. 21, 500 (1897). — LINDER, G.: The effect of mineral acid on acid-base regulation in health and nephritis. Quart. J. Med. 20, 285 (1927). — LINNEWEH, F., E. BUCHBORN u. BRIGITTE DELBRÜCK: Familiärer renaler Diabetes insipidus. Klin. Wschr. 35, 321 (1957). — LIPPMAN, R. W.: Endogenous and exogenous creatinine clearances in rat. Amer. J. Physiol. 151, 211 (1947). — LIPSCHITZ, W. L., and E. BUEDING: Mechanism of the biological formation of conjugated glucuronic acids. J. biol. Chem. 129, 333 (1939). — LIPSCHITZ, W. L., and E. STOKEY: Mechanisms of anti-diuresis in dog and in rat. Amer. J. Physiol. 148, 259 (1947). — LIPSETT, M. B., J. P. MACLEAN, C. D. WEST, M. C. LI and O. H. PEARSON: An analysis of the polyuria induced by hypophysectomy in man. J. Clin. Endocr. 16, 183 (1956). — LIPSETT, M. B., and O. H. PEARSON: Sodium depletion in adrenalectomized humans. J. clin. Invest. 37, 1394 (1958). — LITTLE, J. M.: Diuretic factor present in normal dog, human, and dialyzed human urine. J. Pharmacol. exp. Ther. 91, 124 (1947). — LITTLE, J. M., W. M. KELSEY and E. H. YOUNT jr.: Influence of the adrenal cortex on renal hemodynamics in the dog. Effects of ACTH and adrenal atrophy induced by Rhothane. Amer. J. Physiol. 185, 159 (1956). — LITTLE, J. M., S. L. WALLACE, E. C. WHATLEY and G. A. ANDERSON: Effect of pitressin on urinary excretion of chloride and water in human. Amer. J. Physiol. 151, 174 (1947). — LJUNGBERG, E.: Reabsorption of chlorides in kidney of rabbit. Acta med. scand. Suppl. 186, 1 (1947). — Chlorides in the kidney, the blood and the urine in experimental nephritis. Scand. J. clin. Lab. Invest. 1, 266 (1949). — LLAURADO, J. G.: Aldosterone excretion following hypophysectomy in man: Relation to urinary Na/K ratio. Metabolism 6, 556 (1957). — LLOYD, C. W., and JULIA LOBOTSKY: Serum antidiuretic substances and urinary corticosteroid in the urine. J. clin. Endocr. 10, 318 (1954). — LOCHNER, W., u. B. OCHWADT: Über die Beziehungen zwischen arteriellen Druck, Durchblutung, Durchflußzeit und Blutfüllung an der isolierten Hundeniere. Pflügers Arch. ges. Physiol. 258, 275 (1954). — LOCKE, A., E. R. MAIN and R. R. MELLON: Carbonic anhydrase inactivation as the source of sulfanilamide "acidosis". Science 93, 66 (1941). — LOEB, R. F.: Effect of sodium chloride in treatment of a patient with Addison's disease. Proc. Soc. exp. Biol. (N.Y.) 30, 808 (1933). — LOEB, R. F., D. W. ATCHLEY, D. W. RICHARDS jr., ETHEL M. BENEDICT and MARY E. DRISCOLL: On the mechanism of nephrotic edema. J. clin. Invest. 11, 621 (1932). — LOEB, R. F., D. W. ATCHLEY and J. STAHL: The role of sodium in adrenal insufficiency. J. Amer. med. Ass. 104, 2149 (1935). — LOEB, R. F., and EMILY G. NICHOLS: Factors influencing the diffusibility of calcium in human blood serum. J. biol. Chem. 72, 687 (1927). — LOEWE, L., P. ROSENBLATT, ERNA ALTURE-WERBER and MARY KOZAK: The prolonging action of penicillin by para-aminohippuric acid. Proc. Soc. exp. Biol. (N.Y.) 58, 298 (1945). — LÖWGREN, E.: Studies on benign proteinuria with special reference to the renal lymphatic system. Acta med. scand. 151, Suppl. 300 (1955). — LOGAN, M. A.: The early effects of parathyroid hormone on the blood and urine. J. biol. Chem. 127, 711 (1939). — Recent advances in the chemistry of calcification. Physiol. Rev. 20, 522 (1940). — LOMBARDO, T. A.: The effect of posture on the excretion of water and sodium by patients with congestive heart failure. Circulation 7, 91 (1953). — LOMBARDO, T. A., and T. R. HARRISON: Effect of neck compression on sodium excretion in subjects with congestive heart failure. Circulation 7, 88 (1953). — LOMBARDO, T. A., S. ISENBERG, B. B. OLIVER, W. N. VIAR, E. E. EDDLEMAN and T. R. HARRISON: Effects of bleeding on electrolyte excretion and on glomerular filtration. Circulation 3, 260 (1951). — LONDON, F., and L. L. TERRY: The Soffer test in essential hypertension. J. clin. Invest. 31, 51 (1952). — LONGLEY, J. B., M. B. BURG and H. J. BURTNER: Functional discrimination between the straight and convoluted segments of the renal proximal tubule. Fed. Proc. 19, 369 (1960) (abstract). — LONGLEY, J. B., and M. S. BURSTONE: Observations on the renal medullary circulation. J. Histochem. Cytochem. 6, 89 (1958) (abstract). — LONGLEY, J. B., and E. R. FISHER: Alkaline phosphatase and the periodic acid Schiff reaction in the proximal tubule of the vertebrate kidney: A study in segmental differentiation. Anat. Rec. 120, 1 (1954). — LONGLEY, J. B., N. A. LASSEN and L. S. LILIENFIELD: Tracer studies on renal medullary circulation. Fed. Proc.

17, 99 (1958) (abstract). — LONGSON, D., J. N. MILLS, S. THOMAS and P. A. YATES: Handling of phosphate by the human kidney at high plasma concentrations. J. Physiol. 131, 555 (1956). — LOOMIS, T. A., G. F. KOEPF and R. S. HUBBARD: The excretion of sulfanilamide and acetylsulfanilamide by the human kidney. Amer. J. Physiol. 141, 158 (1944). — LOT-SPEICH, W. D.: Renal tubular reabsorption of inorganic sulfate in the normal dog. Amer. J. Physiol. 151, 311 (1947). — LOTSPEICH, W. D., and D. M. KELLER: A study of some effects of phlorizin on the metabolism of kidney tissue *in vitro*. J. biol. Chem. 222, 843 (1956). — LOTSPEICH, W. D., and R. F. PITTS: Role of amino acids in renal tubular secretion of ammonia. J. biol. Chem. 168, 611 (1947). — LOTSPEICH, W. D., R. C. SWAN and R. F. PITTS: Renal tubular reabsorption of chloride. Amer. J. Physiol. 148, 445 (1947). — LOTSPEICH, W. D., and S. WORONKOW: Some quantitative studies on phlorizin inhibition of glucose transport in the kidney. Amer. J. Physiol. 195, 331 (1958). — LOTZ, W. E., R. V. TALMAGE and C. L. COMAR: Effect of parathyroid extract administration in sheep. Proc. Soc. exp. Biol. (N.Y.) 85, 292 (1954). — LOVE, A. H. G., R. A. RODDIE, J. ROSENSWEIG and R. G. SHANKS: The effect of pressure changes in the respired air on the renal excretion of water and electrolytes. Clin. Sci. 16, 281 (1957). — LOVE, J. K., and N. LIFSON: Transtubular movements of urea in the doubly perfused bullfrog kidney. Amer. J. Physiol. 193, 662 (1958). — LOWRY, O. H., and JEANNE A. LOPEZ: The determination of inorganic phosphate in the presence of labile phosphate esters. J. biol. Chem. 162, 421 (1946). — LUDEMANN, H., L. G. RAISZ and H. WIRZ: Filtration rate and water diuresis in the dog. Amer. J. Physiol. 166, 416 (1951). — LUDWIG, K.: Nieren und Harnbereitung. In WAGNERS Handbuch der Physiologie, Bd. 2, S. 628. 1844. — LUEKEN, B.: Über die Harnsäureausscheidung durch die Froschniere. Pflügers Arch. ges. Physiol. 229, 557 (1932). — LUETSCHER jr., J. A.: Effect of single injection of concentrated human serum albumin on circulating proteins and proteinuria in nephrosis. J. clin. Invest. 23, 365 (1944). — Studies of aldosterone in relation to water and electrolyte balance in man. Recent Progr. Hormone Res. 12, 175 (1956). — LUETSCHER jr., J. A., and B. J. AXELRAD: Sodium-retaining corticoid in the urine of normal children and adults and of patients with hypoadrenalism or hypopituitarism. J. clin. Endocr. 14, 1086 (1954a). — Increased aldosterone output during sodium deprivation in normal man. Proc. Soc. exp. Biol. (N.Y.) 87, 650 (1954b). — LUETSCHER jr., J. A., and R. H. CURTIS: Observations of aldosterone in human urine. Fed. Proc. 14, 746 (1955a) (abstract). — Aldosterone: Observations on the regulation of sodium and potassium balance. Ann. intern. Med. 43, 658 (1955b). — Relationship of aldosterone in urine to sodium balance and to some other endocrine functions. J. clin. Invest. 34, 951 (1955c). — LUETSCHER jr., J. A., A. DOWDY, J. HARVEY, R. NEHER and A. WETTSTEIN: Isolation of crystalline aldosterone from the urine of a child with the nephrotic syndrome. J. biol. Chem. 217, 505 (1955). — LUETSCHER jr., J. A., A. D. HALL and VIRGINIA L. KREMER: Treatment of nephrosis with concentration human serum albumin. II. Effects on renal function and on excretion of water and some electrolytes. J. clin. Invest. 29, 896 (1950). — LUETSCHER jr., J. A., and B. B. JOHNSON: Chromatographic separation of the sodium-retaining corticoid from the urine of children with nephrosis, compared with observations on normal children. J. clin. Invest. 33, 276 (1954a). — Observations on the sodium-retaining corticoid (aldosterone) in children and adults in relation to sodium balance and edema. J. clin. Invest. 33, 1441 (1954b). — LUETSCHER jr., J. A., R. NEHER and A. WETTSTEIN: Isolation of crystalline aldosterone from the urine of a nephrotic patient. Experientia (Basel) 10, 456 (1954). — LUFT, R., and B. SJÖGREN: The effect of desoxycorticosterone acetate and sodium chloride thyroxin and testosterone propionate in a case of panhypoadenopituitarism (Simmonds' disease) with special reference to kidney function and blood pressure. Acta endocr. (Kbh.) 2, 44 (1949a). — The significance of renal function for the effect of desoxycorticosterone acetate (DCA) in ADDISON's disease. Acta endocr. (Kbh.) 2, 365 (1949b). — The effect of desoxycorticosterone acetate (DCA) and sodium chloride on blood pressure and renal function. Acta endocr. (Kbh.) 3, 56 (1949c). — The significance of the adenohypophysis, adrenal cortex and thyroid in renal function in man. Acta endocr. (Kbh.) 4, 351 (1950). — A comparative study of the metabolic effect of adrenocorticotrophic hormone (ACTH), cortisone, and desoxycorticosterone acetate (DCA). Stanf. med. Bull. 9, 218 (1951). — LUNDBAEK, K., and V. P. PETERSEN: Filtration and glucose Tm in late diabetes mellitus. Scand. J. clin. Lab. Invest. 1, 346 (1949). — LUNDQUIST, F.: Renal tubular secretion of sulfonamides and p-aminobenzoic acid. Acta pharmacol. (Kbh.) 1, 307 (1945). — LUNDSGAARD, E.: Hemmung von Esterifizierungsvorgängen als Ursache der Phlorrhizinwirkung. Biochem. Z. 264/265, 209 (1933). — LYONS, R. H., G. K. MOE, ROSALIE B. NELIGH, S. W. HOOBLER, K. N. CAMPBELL, R. L. BERRY and BARBARA R. RENNICK: The effects of blockade of the autonomic ganglia in man with tetraethylammonium. Preliminary observations on its clinical application. Amer. J. med. Sci. 213, 315 (1947).

MACCALLUM, D. B.: Bearing of degenerating glomeruli on problem of vascular supply of mammalian kidney. Amer. J. Anat. 65, 69 (1939). — MACDONALD, R. J., and V. C. KELLY: Effects of altitude anoxia on renal function. Amer. J. Physiol. 154, 201 (1948). —

MacDonald, W. B.: Congenital pitressin resistant diabetes insipidus of renal origin. Pediatrics 15, 298 (1955). — Mach, R. S.: Idiopathic oedema with hyperaldosteronuria. Aldosterone, p. 186. New York: Little, Brown & Co. 1958. — Mach, R. S., J. Fabre, A. F. Muller et R. Neher: Oedèmes par rétention de chlorure de sodium avec hyperaldostéronurie. Essai de classification des états d'hyperaldostéronisme. Schweiz. med. Wschr. 85, 1229 (1955). — Machella, T. E., J. D. Helm and F. W. Chornock: Relation of hippuric acid excretion to volume of urine. J. clin. Invest. 21, 763 (1942). — MacKay, E. M., and Lois L. MacKay: The relation between the blood urea concentration and the amount of functioning renal tissue. J. clin. Invest. 4, 127 (1927). — MacKeith, N., M. S. Pembrey, W. Spurrell, E. Warner and H. J. W. J. Westlake: Observations on the adjustment of the human body to muscular work. Proc. roy. Soc. B 95, 413 (1923/24). — MacLean, J. P., M. C. Li, M. B. Lipsett, B. Ray and O. H. Pearson: The physiological role of adrenal salt hormone (aldosterone) in man. J. clin. Invest. 34, 951 (1955). — MacLean, J. P., M. B. Lipsett, M. C. Li, C. D. West and O. H. Pearson: Regulation of salt metabolism after hypophysectomy in man. J. clin. Endocr. 17, 346 (1957). — MacPherson, C. R., M. D. Milne and Barbara M. Evans: The excretion of salicylate. Brit. J. Pharmacol. 10, 484 (1955). — Mader, I. J., and L. T. Iseri: Spontaneous hypopotassemia, hypomagnesemia, alkalosis and tetany due to hypersecretion of corticosterone-like mineralocorticoid. Amer. J. Med. 19, 976 (1955). — Madison, L. L., and D. W. Seldin: Adaptation of ammonia-producing enzymes in the human kidney during chronic acidosis as revealed by the administration of precursor amino acids. Clin. Res. Proc. 3, 136 (1955) (abstract). — Madsen, P. O.: Prolonged, heavy salt-loading in adrenalectomized dogs. Acta endocr. (Kbh.) 20, 169 (1955). — Maffly, L. H., and A. Leaf: Water activity of mammalian tissues. Nature (Lond.) 182, 60 (1958). — Magoun, H. W., C. Fisher and S. W. Ranson: The neurohypophysis and water exchange in the monkey. Endocrinology 25, 161 (1939). — Mahler, R. F., and S. W. Stanbury: Potassium-losing renal disease. Renal and metabolic observations on a patient sustaining renal wastage of potassium. Quart. J. Med. 25, 21 (1956). — Mahoney, W., and D. Sheehan: The effect of total thyroidectomy upon experimental diabetes insipidus in dogs. Amer. J. Physiol. 112, 250 (1935). — The pituitary-hypothalamic mechanism: experimental occlusion of the pituitary stalk. Brain 59, 61 (1936). — Malmendier, C., F. Gregoire et P. P. Lambert: Pathophysiologie de l'albuminurie dans la nephrose et l'amyloidose. Effets du traitment par les hormones du cortex surrénal. Rev. franç. Ét. clin. biol. 2, 145 (1957). — Malmendier, C., et P. P. Lambert: Étude sur la concentration en serum-albumine du filtrat glomérulaire chez le chien. J. Urol. méd. chir. 61, 327 (1955). — Maluf, N. S. R.: Role of renal innervation in renal tubular function. Amer. J. Physiol. 139, 103 (1943). — Malvin, R. L., and W. D. Lotspeich: Relation between tubular transport of inorganic phosphate and bicarbonate in the dog. Amer. J. Physiol. 187, 51 (1956). — Malvin, R. L., and W. S. Wilde: Washout of renal countercurrent Na gradient by osmotic diuresis. Amer. J. Physiol. 197, 177 (1959). — Malvin, R. L., W. S. Wilde and L. P. Sullivan: Localization of nephron transport by stop flow analysis. Amer. J. Physiol. 194, 135 (1958a). — Bicarbonate reabsorption along renal tubules. Proc. Soc. exp. Biol. (N.Y.) 98, 448 (1958b). — Malvin, R. L., W. S. Wilde, L. P. Sullivan and A. J. Vander: Stop flow analysis of sodium reabsorption. Fed. Proc. 17, 103 (1958a) (abstract). — Malvin, R. L., W. S. Wilde, A. J. Vander and L. P. Sullivan: Localization and characterization of sodium transport along the renal tubule. Amer. J. Physiol. 195, 549 (1958b). — Manchester, R. C.: Influence of posterior pituitary extracts on mineral and water exchange in children. Proc. Soc. exp. Biol. (N.Y.) 29, 717 (1931/32). — The diurnal rhythm in water and mineral exchange. J. clin. Invest. 12, 995 (1933). — Mandel, E. E., and Florence L. Jones: Evaluation of methods measuring creatinine. Fed. Proc. 11, 100 (1952) (abstract). — Manitius, A., H. Levitin, D. Beck and F. H. Epstein: On the mechanism of impairment of renal concentrating ability in potassium deficiency. J. clin. Invest. 39, 684 (1960a). — On the mechanism of impairment of renal concentrating ability in hypercalcemia. J. clin. Invest. 39, 693 (1960b). — Mann, T., and D. Keilin: Sulphanilamide as a specific inhibitor of carbonic anhydrase. Nature (Lond.) 146, 164 (1940). — Maren, T. H.: Carbonic anhydrase inhibition. IV. The effects of metabolic acidosis on the response to Diamox. Bull. Johns Hopk. Hosp. 98, 159 (1956). — Maren, T. H., O. A. Sorsdahl and A. J. Dickhaus: Reduction of renal effect of acetazolamide (A) in the extracellular alkalosis of K⁺ depletion. Fed. Proc. 19, 366 (1960) (abstract). — Maren, T. H., Barbara C. Wadsworth, Elaine K. Yale and Lillian G. Alonso: Carbonic anhydrase inhibition. III. Effects of Diamox on electrolyte metabolism. Bull. Johns Hopk. Hosp. 95, 277 (1954). — Markley, K., M. Bocanegra, G. Morales and M. Chiappori: Oral sodium loading in normal individuals. J. clin. Invest. 36, 303 (1957). — Marsh, J. B., and D. L. Drabkin: Kidney phosphatase in alimentary hyperglycemia and phlorhizin glycosuria. A dynamic mechanism for renal threshold for glucose. J. biol. Chem. 168, 61 (1947). — Marshall jr., E. K.: The secretion of urine. Physiol. Rev. 6, 440 (1926). — A comparison of the function of the glomerular and aglomerular kidney. Amer. J. Physiol. **94**, 1 (1930). — The secretion of phenol red by the mammalian kidney. Amer. J. Physiol. **99**, 77 (1931/32a). — Kidney secretion in reptiles. Proc. Soc. exp. Biol. (N.Y.) **29**, 971 (1931/32b). — The secretion of urea in the frog. Amer. J. cell. comp. Physiol. **2**, 349 (1932/33). — The comparative physiology of the kidney in relation to theories of renal function. Physiol. Rev. **14**, 133 (1934). — MARSHALL jr., E. K., and K. C. BLANCHARD: The antidiuretic effect of 3-hydroxy-cinchoninic acid derivatives. J. Pharmacol. exp. Ther. **95**, 185 (1949). — MARSHALL jr., E. K., and MARIAN M. CRANE: The secretory function of the renal tubules. Amer. J. Physiol. **70**, 465 (1924). — MARSHALL jr., E. K., K. EMERSON jr. and W. C. CUTTING: The renal excretion of sulfanilamide. J. Pharmacol. exp. Ther. **61**, 191 (1937). — MARSHALL jr., E. K., and A. L. GRAFFLIN: The structure and function of the kidney of Lophius piscatorius. Bull. Johns Hopk. Hosp. **43**, 205 (1928). — The function of the proximal convoluted segment of the renal tubule. J. cell. comp. Physiol. **1**, 161 (1932). — MARSON, F. G. W.: Total adrenalectomy in hepatic cirrhosis with ascites. Lancet **1954 II**, 847. — MARTIN, G. J.: The effect of various agents on the excretion of uric acid and allantoin. Exp. Med. Surg. **6**, 24 (1948). — MARTIN, HELEN E., and A. M. WICK: Quantitative relationships between blood and urine ketone levels in diabetic ketosis. J. clin. Invest. **22**, 235 (1943). — MARTIN, S. J., H. C. HERRLICH and J. F. FAZEKAS: Relation between electrolyte imbalance and excretion of an antidiuretic substance in adrenalectomized cats. Amer. J. Physiol. **127**, 51 (1939). — MARTINI, L., and A. DEPOLI: Neurohumoral control of the release of adrenocorticotrophic hormone. J. Endocr. **13**, 229 (1955/56). — MARTINI, L., A. DEPOLI and S. CURRI: Hypothalamic stimulation of ACTH secretion. Proc. Soc. exp. Biol. (N.Y.) **91**, 490 (1956). — MARTINI, L., and C. MORPURGO: Neurohumoral control of the release of adrenocorticotrophic hormone. Nature (Lond.) **175**, 1127 (1955). — MARX, H.: Untersuchungen über den Wasserhaushalt. II. Die psychische Beeinflussung des Wasserhaushaltes. Klin. Wschr. **5**, 92 (1926). — Diuresis by conditioned reflex. Amer. J. Physiol. **96**, 356 (1931). — MASON, A. S.: Metabolic response to total adrenalectomy and hypophysectomy. Lancet **1955 II**, 632. — MATHIESEN, E. Ø., and C. TROLLE-LASSEN: Renal elimination of penicillin by the aged. Scand. J. clin. Lab. Invest. **9**, 213 (1957). — MATTAR, G., H. L. BARNETT, HELEN McNAMARA and H. D. LAUSON: Measurement of glomerular filtration rate in children with kidney disease. J. clin. Invest. **31**, 938 (1952). — MATTOX, V. R., H. L. MASON, A. ALBERT and C. F. CODE: Properties of a sodium-retaining principle from beef adrenal extract. J. Amer. chem. Soc. **75**, 4869 (1953). — MAXWELL, M. H., and E. S. BREED: The effect of the intravenous administration of pitressin on renal function in man. J. Pharmacol. exp. Ther. **103**, 190 (1951). — MAXWELL, M. H., E. S. BREED and I. L. SCHWARTZ: Renal venous pressure in chronic congestive heart failure. J. clin. Invest. **29**, 342 (1950). — MAXWELL, M. H., E. S. BREED and H. W. SMITH: Significance of the renal juxtamedullary circulation in man. Amer. J. Med., **9**, 216 (1950). — MAXWELL, M. H., D. M. GOMEZ, A. P. FISHMAN and H. W. SMITH: Effects of epinephrine and typhoid vaccine on segmental vascular resistances in the human kidney. J. Pharmacol. exp. Ther. **109**, 276 (1953). — MAXWELL, M. H., P. MORALES and C. H. CROWDER jr.: Effect of therapeutic doses of ephedrine on renal clearances in normal man. Proc. Soc. exp. Biol. (N.Y.) **77**, 539 (1951). — McBRIDE, W. O., I. M. WEINER and G. H. MUDGE: Inhibition of potassium secretion by mercurial diuretics. Fed. Proc. **17**, 107 (1958) (abstract). — McCANCE, R. A.: Experimental sodium chloride deficiency in man. Proc. roy. Soc. B **119**, 245 (1936). — Excretion of urea, salts and water during periods of hydropenia in man. J. Physiol. (Lond.) **104**, 196 (1945). — McCANCE, R. A., and M. A. v. FINCK: Titratable acidity, pH, ammonia and phosphates in urines of very young infants. Arch. Dis. Child. **22**, 200 (1947). — McCANCE, R. A., and E. M. WIDDOWSON: The response of the kidney to an alkalosis during salt deficiency. Proc. roy. Soc. B **120**, 228 (1936). — The secretion of urine in man during experimental salt deficiency. J. Physiol. (Lond.) **91**, 222 (1937). — Normal renal function in the first two days of life. Arch. Dis. Childh. **29**, 488 (1954). — McCANCE, R. A., and W. F. YOUNG: Secretion of urine by newborn infants. J. Physiol. (Lond.) **99**, 265 (1941). — The secretion of urine during dehydration and rehydration. J. Physiol. (Lond.) **102**, 415 (1943/44). — McCANN, S. M.: Effect of posterior lobe extracts on ACTH release. Fed. Proc. **16**, 85 (1957) (abstract). — McCANN, S. M., and J. R. BROBECK: Evidence for a role of the supraopticohypophyseal system in regulation of adrenocorticotrophin secretion. Proc. Soc. exp. Biol. (N.Y.) **87**, 318 (1954). — McCONAHEY, W. M., F. R. KEATING and M. H. POWER: An estimation of the renal and extrarenal clearance of radioiodine in man. J. clin. Invest. **30**, 778 (1951). — McCRORY, W. W., CAROLYN W. FORMAN, HELEN McNAMARA and H. L. BARNETT: Renal excretion of inorganic phosphate in newborn infants. J. clin. Invest. **31**, 357 (1952). — McCRORY, W. W., N. GOREN and D. GORNFELD: Demonstration of impairment of urinary concentration ability, or "Pitressin-resistance", in children with sickle-cell anemia. Amer. J. Dis. Child. **86**, 512 (1953). — McCULLAGH, E. P., and E. J. RYAN: The use of desoxycorticosterone acetate in Addison's disease. J. Amer. med. Ass. **114**, 2530 (1940). —

McDANELL, L., and F. P. UNDERHILL: Studies in carbohydrate metabolism. XX. New experiments upon the mechanism of salt glycosuria. J. biol. Chem. **29**, 273 (1917). — McDONALD, R. K., and J. H. MILLER: Effect of mercury on renal tubular transfer of p-amino-hippurate and glucose in man. Proc. Soc. exp. Biol. (N.Y.) **72**, 408 (1949). — McDONALD, R. K., J. H. MILLER and ELEANORE B. ROACH: Human glomerular permeability and tubular recovery values for hemoglobin. J. clin. Invest. **30**, 1041 (1951). — McDONALD, R. K., N. W. SHOCK and M. J. YIENGST: Effect of lactate on renal tubular transfer of p-amino-hippurate in man. Proc. Soc. exp. Biol. (N.Y.) **77**, 686 (1951). — McDONALD, R. K., D. H. SOLOMON and N. W. SHOCK: Aging as a factor in the renal hemodynamic changes induced by a standardized pyrogen. J. clin. Invest. **30**, 457 (1951). — McDONALD, R. K., H. N. WAGNER jr. and VIRGINIA K. WEISE: Endogenous ADH production and hydrocortisone release. Fed. Proc. **16**, 86 (1957) (abstract). — McGARRY, E., A. H. SEHON and B. ROSE: The isolation and electrophoretic characterization of the proteins in the urine of normal subjects. J. clin. Invest. **34**, 832 (1955). — McGAVACK, T. H., ANDREA SACCONE, MILDRED VOGEL and R. HARRIS: Craniopharyngeoma with panhypituitarism: case report with clinical and pathological study. J. clin. Endocr. **6**, 776 (1946). — McINTOSH, B. J., P. K. KNOEFEL and T. G. SCHARFF: Absence of competition between PAH synthesis and tubular transport of PAH. Fed. Proc. **16**, 321 (1957) (abstract). — McINTYRE, A. R., and H. B. VAN DYKE: The distribution and concentrations of water and halides in the blood and urine during diuresis-inhibition by pituitary extract. J. Pharmacol. exp. Ther. **42**, 155 (1931). — McKEE, F. W., and W. B. HAWKINS: Phlorhizin glucosuria. Physiol. Rev. **25**, 255 (1945). — McNAMARA, HELEN, and H. L. BARNETT: Renal excretion of electrolytes in premature infants during administration of sodium salts of unreabsorbed anions. J. clin. Invest. **33**, 774 (1954). — McQUARRIE, I., R. M. JOHNSON and MILDRED R. ZIEGLER: Plasma electrolyte disturbance in patient with hypercorticoadrenal syndrome contrasted with that found in Addison's disease. Endocrinology **21**, 762 (1937). — McQUARRIE, I., and MILDRED R. ZIEGLER: Disturbances in electrolyte metabolism of patients with nephrotic syndrome. Postgrad. Med. **6**, 281 (1949). — McSWINEY, R. R., and H. E. DE WARDENER: Renal-tract delay time and dead space. Lancet **1950 II**, 845. — MEHRIZI, A., and W. F. HAMILTON: Effect of levarterenol on renal blood flow and vascular volume in dogs. Amer. J. Physiol. **197**, 1115 (1959). — MELVILLE, E. V., and K. HARE: Antidiuretic material in supraoptic nucleus. Endocrinology **36**, 332 (1945). — MENAKER, W.: Buffer equilibria and reabsorption in the production of urinary acidity. Amer. J. Physiol. **154**, 174 (1948). — MENDELSOHN, M. L.: A technique of measurement, and the effect of x-ray on the leakage of PAH out of the rabbit kidney slice. Amer. J. Physiol. **182**, 119 (1955). — MERING, I. v.: Über Diabetes mellitus. I. Z. klin. Med. **14/15**, 405 (1888/89). — II. Z. klin. Med. **16/17**, 431 (1889/90). — MERONEY, W. H., M. E. RUBINI and W. B. BLYTHE: The effect of antecedent diet on urine concentrating ability. Ann. intern. Med. **48**, 562 (1958). — MERRILL, A. J.: Edema and decreased renal blood flow in patients with chronic congestive heart failure: Evidence of "forward failure" as primary cause of edema. J. clin. Invest. **25**, 389 (1946). — MERRILL, A. J., and W. H. CARGILL: Effect of exercise on renal plasma flow and filtration rate of normal and cardiac subjects. J. clin. Invest. **27**, 272 (1948). — MERRILL, A. J., J. L. MORRISON and E. S. BRANNON: Concentration of renin in renal venous blood in patients with chronic heart failure. Amer. J. Med. **1**, 468 (1946). — METCOFF, J., J. A. JAMES, G. GORDILLO and I. ANTONOWICZ: Renal electrolyte transport in normal and nephrotic children. J. Lab. clin. Med. **46**, 333 (1955). — METCOFF, J., W. M. KELSEY and C. A. JANEWAY: The nephrotic syndrome in children. An interpretation of its clinical, biochemical and renal features as variations of a single type of nephron disease. J. clin. Invest. **30**, 471 (1951). — METCOFF, J., N. NAKASONE and C. P. RANCE: On the role of the kidney during nephrotic edema: Potassium excretion and sodium retention. J. clin. Invest. **33**, 665 (1954). — MICHEL, FRANCES Y.: Arbutin diabetes. Proc. Soc. exp. Biol. (N.Y.) **35**, 62 (1936/37). — MICHIE, A. J., N. GIMBEL, CECILIA RIEGEL and M. RAGNI: Opening of intrarenal arteriovenous shunts without cortical ischemia by sudden administration of salt-poor concentrated human serum albumin. J. appl. Physiol. **3**, 472 (1950/51). — MIGEON, C. J., F. H. TYLER, J. P. MAHONEY, A. A. FLORENTIN, H. CASTLE, E. L. BLISS and L. T. SAMUELS: The diurnal variation of plasma levels and urinary excretion of 17-hydroxycorticosteroids in normal subjects, night workers and blind subjects. J. clin. Endocr. **16**, 622 (1956). — MILES, B. E., A. PATON and H. E. DE WARDENER: Maximum urine concentration. Brit. med. J. **1954 II**, 901. — MILES, B. E., M. G. VENTOM and H. E. DE WARDENER: Observations on the mechanism of circulatory auto-regulation in the perfused dog's kidney. J. Physiol. (Lond.) **123**, 143 (1954). — MILES, B. E., and H. E. DE WARDENER: Effect of emotion on renal function in normotensive and hypertensive women. Lancet **1953 II**, 539. — Intrarenal pressure. J. Physiol. (Lond.) **123**, 131 (1954). — MILES, B. E., H. E. DE WARDENER, H. C. CHURCHILL-DAVIDSON and W. D. WYLIE: The effect on the renal circulation of pentamethonium bromide during anaesthesia. Clin. Sci. **11**, 73 (1952). — MILES, B. E., H. E. DE WARDENER and R. R. McSWINEY: Renal function during emotional diuresis. Amer. J. Med. 12, 659 (1952). — MILLER jr., A. T., and J. O. MILLER jr.: Renal excretion of lactic acid in exercise. J. appl. Physiol. 1, 614 (1948/49). — MILLER, B. F., A. S. ALVING and J. RUBIN: Renal excretion of inulin at low plasma concentrations of this compound, and its relationship to glomerular filtration rate in normal, nephritic and hypertensive individuals. J. clin. Invest. 19, 89 (1940). — MILLER, B. F., A. LEAF, A. R. MAMBY and ZELMA MILLER: Validity of the endogenous creatinine clearance as a measure of glomerular filtration rate in the diseased human kidney. J. clin. Invest. 31, 309 (1952a). — A comparison of the allantoin and inulin clearances for the measurement of filtration rate in the diseased human kidney. J. clin. Invest. 31, 314 (1952b). — MILLER, B. F., and A. WINKLER: The ferrocyanide clearance in man. J. clin. Invest. 15, 489 (1936). — The renal clearance of endogenous creatinine in man. Comparison with exogenous creatinine and inulin. J. clin. Invest. 17, 31 (1938). — MILLER, G. E., and C. E. TOWNSEND: The in vitro inactivation of Pitressin by normal and cirrhotic human liver. J. clin. Invest. 33, 549 (1954). — MILLER, J. H.: Effect of insulin on maximal rate of renal tubular uptake of glucose in non-diabetic humans. Proc. Soc. exp. Biol. (N.Y.) 84, 322 (1953a). — Changes in renal tubular transport maxima associates with renal vasodilatation. J. appl. Physiol. 6, 129 (1953/54b). — MILLER, J. H., R. K. McDONALD and N. W. SHOCK: The renal extraction of p-aminohippurate in the aged individual. J. Geront. 6, 213 (1951). — Age changes in the maximal rate of renal tubular reabsorption of glucose. J. Geront. 7, 195 (1952). — MILLER, T. B., and A. E. FARAH: Inhibition of mercurial diuresis by non-diuretic mercurials. Fed. Proc. 19, 363 (1960) (abstract). — MILLER, T. B., and D. S. RIGGS: Mercurial diuresis in dogs with diabetes insipidus. Fed. Proc. 17, 395 (1958) (abstract). — MILLS, I. H., A. CASPER and F. C. BARTTER: On the role of the vagus in the control of aldosterone secretion. Science 128, 1140 (1958). — MILLS, J. N.: Diurnal rhythm in urine flow. J. Physiol. (Lond.) 113, 528 (1951). — MILLS, J. N., and S. W. STANBURY: Intrinsic diurnal rhythm in urinary electrolyte output. J. Physiol. (Lond.) 115, 18P (1951) (abstract). — MILLS, J. N., S. THOMAS and P. A. YATES: Assessment of voluntary bladder emptying in man. J. Physiol. (Lond.) 129, 408 (1955). — MILLS, L. C., and J. H. MOYER: The acute effects of hexamethonium or renal hemodynamics in normotensive and hypertensive human subjects. Amer. J. med. Sci. 226, 1 (1953). — MILLS, L. C., J. H. MOYER and J. M. SKELTON: The effect of norepinephrine and epinephrine on renal hemodynamics. Amer. J. med. Sci. 226, 653 (1953). — MILNE, M. D.: Observations on the action of the parathyroid hormone. Clin. Sci. 10, 471 (1951). — MILNE, M. D., R. C. MUEHRCKE and I. AIRD: Primary aldosteronism. Quart. J. Med. 26, 317 (1957). — MILNE, M. D., R. C. MUEHRCKE and B. E. HEARD: Potassium deficiency and the kidney. Brit. med. Bull. 13, 15 (1957). — MILNE, M. D., G. G. ROWE, K. SOMERS, R. C. MUEHRCKE and M. A. CRAWFORD: Observations on the pharmacology of mecamylamine. Clin. Sci. 16, 599 (1957). — MILNE, M. D., B. H. SCRIBNER and M. A. CRAWFORD: Non-ionic diffusion and the excretion of weak acids and bases. Amer. J. Med. 24, 709 (1958). — MILNE, M. D., S. W. STANBURY and A. E. THOMSON: Observations on the Fanconi syndrome and renal hyperchloraemic acidosis in the adult. Quart. J. Med. 21, 61 (1952). — MIRSKY, I. A., G. PAULISCH and M. STEIN: The antidiuretic activity of the plasma of adrenalectomized, hypophysectomized and adrenalectomized-hypophysectomized rats. Endocrinology 54, 691 (1954). — MIRSKY, I. A., M. STEIN and G. PAULISCH: The secretion of an antidiuretic substance into the circulation of rats exposed to noxious stimuli. Endocrinology 54, 491 (1954). — MITCHELL, G. A. G.: Anatomy of the autonomic nervous system. Edinburg: E. & S. Livingstone 1952. — MITCHELL, H. D., R. OWENS and W. L. VOLK: Clinical value of urea, clearance and phenolsulfonephthalein test. J. Urol. (Baltimore) 71, 230 (1954). — MITCHELL, W., J. C. SEABURY, H. V. MURDAUGH jr. and H. O. SIEKER: Volume receptors and postprandial diuresis in the seal. Clin. Res. Proc. 8, 63 (1960) (abstract). — MITTELMAN, A., D. O. GORE and H. G. BARKER: Urinary aldosterone excretion before and after portacaval shunting in cirrhosis of the liver. Fed. Proc. 18, 105 (1959) (abstract). — MÖLLENDORFF, W. v.: Der Exkretionsapparat. In Handbuch der kimroskopischen Anatomie des Menschen. Berlin: Springer 1930. — MÖLLER, E., J. F. McINTOSH and D. D. VAN SLYKE: Studies of urea excretion. II. Relationship between urine volume and the rate of urea excretion by normal adults. J. clin. Invest. 6, 427 (1928). — MOKOTOFF, R., and G. ROSS: The effect of spinal anesthesia on the renal ischemia in congestive heart failure. J. clin. Invest. 27, 335 (1948). — MOKOTOFF, R., G. ROSS and L. LEITER: Renal plasma flow and sodium reabsorption and excretion in congestive heart failure. J. clin. Invest. 27, 1 (1948). — MOLLISON, P.: Observations on cases of starvation at Belsen. Brit. med. J. 1946 I, 4. — MONAHAN, E. P., and S. FREEMAN: Maintenance of normal serum calcium by parathyroid gland in nephrectomized dogs. Amer. J. Physiol. 142, 104 (1944). — MONGE, C. C., M. V. RAMIREZ, J. N. FERNANDEZ and EDDA C. HORNE: Relationship between serum creatinine, endogenous creatinine clearance and urinary creatinine. Acta physiol. lat.-amer. 9, 50 (1959). — MONKE, J. V., and C. L. YUILE: The renal clearance of hemoglobin in the dog. J. exp. Med. 72, 149 (1940). — MONTGOMERY, H.: Quantitative studies of the composition of glomerular urine. XII. The reaction of glomerular urine of frogs and necturi. J. biol. Chem. 110, 749 (1935). — MONTGOMERY, H., and J. A. PIERCE: The site of acidification of the urine within the renal tubule of amphibia. Amer. J. Physiol. 118, 144 (1937). — MORE, R. H., and G. L. DUFF: The renal arterial vasculature in man. Amer. J. Path. 27, 95 (1951). — MOREL, F.: Quelques aspects de la régulation endocrinienne de l'équilibre hydrominéral enregistrés chez le rat à l'aide du radio-sodium Na24. Bull. biol. France Belg. Suppl. 34 (1955a). — Les modalités de l'excrétion du potassium par le rein: Étude expérimentale à l'aide du radio-potassium chez le lapin. Helv. physiol. pharmacol. Acta 13, 276 (1955b). — MOREL, F., et A. FALBRIARD: Étude de la perméabilite des diverses parties du nephron pour les ions sodium et potassium. Rev. franç. Ét. clin. Biol. 4, 471 (1959). — MOREL, F., et M. GUINNEBAULT: Emploi du potassium 42 pour l'étude du fontionnement rénal. Proc. 1st (UNESCO) Internat. Conf. Sci. Res. 4, 108 (1958). — MORGAN, E. E., and T. F. WILLIAMS: Renal titration curve for reabsorption of phosphate in normal humans. Clin. Res. 8, 63 (1960) (abstract). — MORISON, D. M.: A study of the renal circulation, with special reference to its finer distribution. Amer. J. Anat. 37, 53 (1926). — MOUSTGAARD, J.: Öm proteinstoffernes indflydelse paa myrefunctionen hos hund. Kommission hos Ejvind Christensens Forlag, Copenhagen, 1948. — MOYER, J. H., R. FORD, E. DENNIS and C. A. HANDLEY: Laboratory and clinical observations on mecamylamine as a hypotensive agent. Proc. Soc. exp. Biol. (N.Y.) 90, 402 (1955). — MOYER, J. H., R. V. FORD and C. L. SPURR: Pharmacodynamics of chlorothiazide (Diuril), an orally effective nonmercurial diuretic agent. Proc. Soc. exp. Biol. (N.Y.) 95, 529 (1957). — MOYER, J. H., and C. A. HANDLEY: Norepinephrine and epinephrine effect on renal hemodynamics: With particular reference to the possibility of vascular shunting and decreasing the active glomeruli Circulation 5, 91 (1952). — MOYER, J. H., C. A. HANDLEY and R. A. HUGGINS: The effect of adrenergic blockade and norepinephrine on renal and cardiovascular hemodynamics following hemorrhage. Circulat. Res. 2, 441 (1954). — MOYER, J. H., C. A. HANDLEY and R. A. SEIBERT: An analysis of the excretory products of a mercurial diuretic (meralluride) by column chromatography. Ann. N.Y. Acad. Sci. 65, 511 (1957). — MOYER, J. H., W. HUGHES and R. HUGGINS: The cardiovascular and renal hemodynamic response to the administration of reserpine (Serpasil). Amer. J. med. Sci. 227, 640 (1954). — MOYER, J. H., and R. McCONN: Renal hemodynamics in hypertensive patients following administration of pendiomide. Anesthesiology 17, 9 (1956). — MOYER, J. H., and L. C. MILLS: Hexamethonium — its effect on glomerular filtration rate, maximal tubular function, and renal excretion of electrolytes. J. clin. Invest. 32, 172 (1953). — MOYER, J. H., G. MORRIS and H. L. BEAZLEY: Renal hemodynamic response to vasopressor agents in the treatment of shock. Circulation 12, 96 (1955). — MUDD, R. H., H. W. DODGE jr., E. C. CLARK and R. V. RANDALL: Experimental diabetes insipidus: A study of the normal interphase. Proc. Mayo Clin. 32, 99 (1957). — MUDGE, G. H.: The kidney and potassium. Bull. N.Y. Acad. Med. 34, 152 (1958). — MUDGE, G. H., A. AMES III, J. FOULKS and A. GILMAN: Effect of drugs on renal secretion of potassium in the dog. Amer. J. Physiol. 161, 151 (1950). — MUDGE, G. H., J. FOULKS and A. GILMAN: The renal excretion of potassium. Proc. Soc. exp. Biol. (N.Y.) 67, 545 (1948). — Effect of urea diuresis on renal excretion of electrolytes. Amer. J. Physiol. 158, 218 (1949). — Renal secretion of potassium in the dog during cellular dehydration. Amer. J. Physiol. 161, 159 (1950). — MUDGE, G. H., and B. HARDIN: Response to mercurial diuretics during alkalosis: A comparison of acute metabolic and chronic hypokalemic alkalosis in the dog. J. clin. Invest. 35, 155 (1956). — MUDGE, G. H., and J. V. TAGGART: Effect of 2,4-dinitrophenol on renal transport mechanisms in the dog. Amer. J. Physiol. 161, 173 (1950a). — Effect of acetate on the renal excretion of p-aminohippurate in the dog. Amer. J. Physiol. 161, 191 (1950b). — MUDGE, G. H., and I. M. WEINER: The mechanism of action of mercurial and xanthine diuretics. Ann. N.Y. Acad. Sci. 71, 344 (1958). — MUEHRCKE, R. C., and M. D. MILNE: Primary hyperaldosteronism, long-standing potassium depletion, and pyelonephritis. Clin. Res. Proc. 5, 190 (1957) (abstract). — MUELLER, C. B., A. D. MASON jr. and D. G. STOUT: Anatomy of the glomerulus. Amer. J. Med. 18, 267 (1955). — MÜLLER, O. H., and I. M. WEINER: Polarographic evidence for the existence of two excretion products of mercurials in the dog. J. Pharmacol. exp. Ther. 118, 461 (1956). — MULINOS, M. G., C. L. SPINGARN and M. E. LOJKIN: Diabetes insipiduslike condition produced by small doses of desoxycorticosterone acetate in dogs. Amer. J. Physiol. 135, 102 (1941). — MULLER, A. F., E. Mach and H. NAEGELI: Comparison of the effect of aldosterone and cortexone (desoxycorticosterone) on electrolyte excretion in man. Acta endocr. (Kbh.) 20, 113 (1955). — MULLER, A. F., ELIZABETH L. MANNING et ANNE M. RIONDEL: Étude de l'aldostéronurie chez le sujet normal et chez le cardiaque oedémateux. Schweiz. med. Wschr. 86, 1362 (1956). — L'excrétion de l'aldostérone chez le sujet normal pendant la déplétion et la réplétion en potassium. Helv. med. Acta 25, 547 (1958a). — Diurnal variation of aldosterone related to position and activity in normal subjects and patients with pituitary insufficiency, p. 111. Aldosterone. Boston: Little,

Brown & Co. 1958 b. — MULLER, A. F., ANNE M. RIONDEL and R. S. MACH: Control of aldosterone excretion by changes in volume of body-fluid. Lancet 1956 I, 831. — MULLER, A. F., ANNE M. RIONDEL et ELIZABETH L. MANNING: Influence de l'ACTH sur la sécrétion de l'aldostérone. Helv. med. Acta 23, 572 (1956 a). — Mecanismes regulateurs de l'aldostérone chez l'homme. Helv. med. Acta 23, 610 (1956 b). — L'excrétion de l'aldostérone au cours du nycthémère. Helv. med. Acta 24, 463 (1957). — MULROW, P. J., and W. F. GANONG: Aldosterone secretion following hemorrhage in hypophysectomized dogs. Fed. Proc. 19, 152 (1960) (abstract). — MUNCK, O.: Renal circulation in acute renal failure. Oxford: Blackwell Sci. Publ. 1958. — MUNSICK, R. A., W. H. SAWYER and H. B. VAN DYKE: The antidiuretic potency of arginine and lysine vasopressins in the pig with observations on porcine renal function. Endocrinology 63, 688 (1958). — Avian neurohypophysial hormones: Pharmacological properties and tentative identification. Endocrinology 66, 860 (1960). — MUNSON, P. L.: Studies on the role of the parathyroids in calcium and phosphorus metabolism. Ann. N.Y. Acad. Sci. 60, 776 (1955). — MUNTWYLER, E., M. IACOBELLIS and G. E. GRIFFIN: Kidney glutaminase and carbonic anhydrase activities and renal electrolyte excretion in rats. Amer. J. Physiol. 184, 83 (1956). — MURDAUGH jr., H. V., R. E. GALLOWAY and ELLEN H. HAYES: Stop-flow analysis performed during water diuresis. Clin. Res. Proc. 7, 273 (1959) (abstract). — MURDAUGH jr., H. V., and R. R. ROBINSON: Magnesium excretion in the dog studied by stop-flow analysis. Amer. J. Physiol. 198, 571 (1960). — MURDAUGH jr., H. V., BERTIL SCHMIDT-NIELSEN, ELEANOR M. DOYLE and ROBERTA O'DELL: Renal tubular regulation of urea excretion in man. J. appl. Physiol. 13, 263 (1958). — MURPHY, J. J., M. K. MYINT, W. H. RATTNER, R. KLAUS and J. SHALLOW: The lymphatic system of the kidney. J. Urol. (Baltimore) 80, 1 (1958). — MURPHY, R. J. F., and E. A. STEAD jr.: Effects of exogenous and endogenous posterior pituitary antidiuretic hormone on water and electrolyte excretion. J. clin. Invest. 30, 1055 (1951). — MUSTAKALLIO, K. K., and A. TELKKÄ: Histochemical localization of the mercurial inhibition of succinic dehydrogenase in rat kidney. Science 118, 320 (1953). — MYANT, N. B., E. E. POCHIN and E. A. G. GOLDIE: The plasma iodide clearance rate of the human thyroid. Clin. Sci. 8, 109 (1949). — MYHRE, J. R., and E. K. BRODWALL: Kidney function studies in myelomatosis. Scand. J. clin. Lab. Invest. 9, 80 (1957).

NADAL, J. W., S. PEDERSEN and W. G. MADDOCK: A comparison between dehydration from salt loss and from water deprivation. J. clin. Invest. 20, 691 (1941). — NADELL, JUDITH: The effects of the carbonic anhydrase inhibitor "6063" on electrolytes and acid-base balance in two normal subjects and two patients with respiratory acidosis. J. clin. Invest. 32, 622 (1953). — NASH jr., T. P., and S. R. BENEDICT: The ammonia content of the blood, and its bearing on the mechanism of acid neutralization in the animal organism. J. biol. Chem. 48, 463 (1921). — NASSIM, J. R., P. D. SAVILLE and LILY MULLIGAN: The effect of stilboestrol on urinary phosphate excretion. Clin. Sci. 15, 369 (1956). — NECHAY, B. R.: Additive nature of the renal effects of aminophylline and hydrochlorothiazide. Fed. Proc. 19, 366 (1960) (abstract). — NECHAY, B. R., and LARYSSA NECHAY: Effects of probenecid, sodium salicylate, 2,4-dinitrophenol and pyrazinamide on renal secretion of uric acid in chickens. J. Pharmacol. exp. Ther. 125/126, 291 (1959). — NEHER, R., and A. WETTSTEIN: Physicochemical estimation of aldosterone in urine. J. clin. Invest. 35, 800 (1956). — NELSON, E. E., and G. G. WOODS: The diuretic-antidiuretic activity of posterior pituitary extracts. J. Pharmacol. exp. Ther. 50, 241 (1934). — NELSON III, W. P., and L. G. WELT: The effects of pitressin on the metabolism and excretion of water and electrolytes in normal subjects and patients with cirrhosis and ascites. J. clin. Invest. 31, 392 (1952). — NESBITT, T. E.: Determination of function of the individual kidney. J. Urol. (Baltimore) 71, 407 (1954). — NETRAVISESH, V.: Effects of posture and of neck compression on outputs of water, sodium and creatinine. J. appl. Physiol. 5, 544 (1953). — NEUBERG, J.: Der Stoffwechsel der Benzoesäure im menschlichen Organismus. Biochem. Z. 145/146, 249 (1924). — NEUFELD, A. H., and J. B. COLLIP: The primary action of the parathyroid hormone. Endocrinology 30, 135 (1942). — NEUMAN, W. F.: The mechanism of parathyroid function. J. Lancet 78, 190 (1958). — NEWMAN, ANNA E., E. S. REDGATE and G. FARRELL: Aldosterone secretion following posterior diencephalic-mesencephalic lesions. Fed. Proc. 18, 113 (1959) (abstract). — NEWMAN, ANNA E., E. S. REDGATE, F. M. YATSU and G. L. FARRELL: Brain stem lesions affecting secretion of aldosterone and hydrocortisone. Fed. Proc. 17, 117 (1958) (abstract). — NEWMAN, E. V., J. BORDLEY and J. WINTERNITZ: The interrelationships of glomerular filtration rate (mannitol clearance), extracellular fluid volume, surface area of the body and plasma concentration of mannitol. Bull. Johns Hopk. Hosp. 75, 253 (1944). — NEWMAN, E. V., A. GILMAN and F. S. PHILIPS: Renal clearance of thiosulfate in man. Bull. Johns Hopk. Hosp. 79, 229 (1946). — NEWMAN, E. V., A. KATTUS, A. GENECIN, J. GENEST, E. CALKINS and J. MURPHY: Observations on the clearance method of determining renal plasma flow with diodrast, para-aminohippuric acid (PAH) and para-acetylaminohippuric acid (PACA). Bull. Johns Hopk. Hosp. 84, 135 (1949). — NI, T., and P. B. REHBERG: On the mechanism of sugar excretion. I. Glucose. Biochem. J. **24**, 1039 (1930). — Ni, T. G., and P. B. Rehberg: On the influence of posture on kidney function. J. Physiol. (Lond.) **71**, 331 (1931). — Nicholes, H. J., and R. C. Herrin: Tubular reabsorption of urea, thiourea and derivatives of thiourea in dog kidney. Amer. J. Physiol. **135**, 113 (1941). — Nichols, B., W. Dear, S. W. Robinson and R. Guillemin: Diabetes insipidus (D.I.) and inhibition of stress-induced ACTH-release after hypothalamic lesion. Fed. Proc. **18**, 113 (1959) (abstract). — Nichols jr., B., and R. Guillemin: Endogenous and exogenous vasopressin on ACTH release. Endocrinology **64**, 914 (1959). — Nichols jr., B., R. Guillemin and R. A. Seibert: Endogenous and exogenous vasopressin on ACTH release. Fed. Proc. **17**, 398 (1958) (abstract). — Nicholson, T. F.: Renal function as affected by experimental unilateral kidney lesion. II. The effect of cyanide. Biochem. J. **45**, 112 (1949). — The site of acidification of the urine in the dog's kidney. Canad. J. Biochem. **35**, 419 (1957a). — A comparison of the effects of proximal and distal tubular damage on the action of desoxycorticosterone and aldosterone. Canad. J. Biochem. **35**, 641 (1957b). — The mode and site of the renal action of parathyroid extract in the dog. Canad. J. Biochem. **37**, 113 (1959). — Nicholson, T. F., R. W. I. Urquhart and D. L. Selby: Renal function as affected by experimental unilateral kidney lesions. I. Nephrosis due to sodium tartrate. J. exp. Med. **68**, 439 (1938). — Nickel, J. F., and S. E. Bradley: Renal blood flow. I. Extraction and clearance methods. Meth. med. Res. **5**, 147 (1952). — Nickel, J. F., L. Levine and J. A. Gagnon: Effects of acute passive tilting on arterial pressure, renal hemodynamics and urinary electrolyte excretion in the dog. J. appl. Physiol. **9**, 176 (1956). — Nickel, J. F., P. Lowrance and E. Leifer: Effect of sodium depletion and repletion on renal function and body fluids during uremia. J. clin. Invest. **30**, 664 (1951) (abstract). — Nickel, J. F., C. M. Smythe, E. M. Papper and S. E. Bradley: A study of the mode of action of the adrenal medullary hormones on sodium, potassium and water excretion in man. J. clin. Invest. **33**, 1687 (1954). — Nielsen, A. L.: On the mechanism of glycosuria. I. Acta med. scand. **130**, 219 (1948). — Nielsen, A. L., and H. O. Bang: The protein content of the diet and the function of the kidneys in human beings. Scand. J. clin. Lab. Invest. **1**, 295 (1949). — Noble, R. L.: Physiology of the adrenal cortex. Hormones **2**, 65 (1950). — Noble, R. L., H. Rinderknecht and P. C. Williams: Apparent augmentation of pituitary antidiuretic action by various retarding substances. J. Physiol. (Lond.) **96**, 293 (1939). — Noble, S.: Diurnal variations in excretion of chloride in normal subjects. Proc. Soc. exp. Biol. (N.Y.) **95**, 679 (1957). — *Nomenclature and criteria* for diagnosis and diseases of the heart and blood vessels. New York Heart Assn. New York: Peter F. Mallon, 1953. — Norn, M.: Untersuchungen über das Verhalten des Kaliums im Organismus. II. Über Schwankungen der Kalium-, Natrium- und Chloridausscheidung durch die Niere im Laufe des Tages. Skand. Arch. Physiol. **55**, 184 (1929). — Notter, B.: Der Einfluß von 5-Hydroxytryptamin (Serotonin) auf die Nierenfunktion beim Menschen. Schweiz. med. Wschr. **86**, 481 (1956). — Nugent, C. A., and F. H. Tyler: The renal excretion of uric acid in patients with gout and in nongouty subjects. J. clin. Invest. **38**, 1890 (1959). — Nungesser, W. C., E. W. Pfeiffer, D. A. Iverson and J. F. Wallerius: Evaluation of renal countercurrent hypothesis in aplodontia. Fed. Proc. **19**, 362 (1960) (abstract). — Nussbaum, M.: Fortgesetzte Untersuchungen über die Secretion der Niere. Pflügers Arch. ges. Physiol. **17**, 580 (1878).

    Oberling, C., A. Gautier et W. Bernhard: La structure des capillaries glomerulaires vue au microscope electronique. Presse méd. **59**, 938 (1951). — Ochwadt, B.: Über Bicarbonatausscheidung und Kohlensäuresystem im Harn während akuter Hypoxie. Pflügers Arch. ges. Physiol. **249**, 452 (1947). — Über Rückresorption und Ausscheidung von Bicarbonat durch die Niere während der Hyperventilationsalkalose. Pflügers Arch. ges. Physiol. **252**, 529 (1950). — Zur Selbststeuerung des Nierenkreislaufes. Pflügers Arch. ges. Physiol. **262**, 207 (1956). — Durchflußzeiten von Plasma und Erythrocyten, intrarenaler Hämatokrit und Widerstandsregulation der isolierten Niere. Pflügers Arch. ges. Physiol. **265**, 112 (1957). — Ochwadt, B. K., and R. F. Pitts: Disparity between phenol red and diodrast clearances in the dog. Amer. J. Physiol. **187**, 318 (1956a). — Effects of intravenous influsion of carbonic anhydrase on carbon dioxide tension of alkaline urine. Amer. J. Physiol. **185**, 426 (1956b). — O'Connor, J. M., and E. J. Conway: The localisation of excretion in the uriniferous tubule. J. Physiol. (Lond.) **56**, 190 (1922). — O'Connor, W. J.: Effect of section of supraopticohypophyseal tracts on inhibition of water-diuresis by emotional stress. Quart. J. exp. Physiol. **33**, 149 (1946). — The control of urine secretion in mammals by the pars nervosa of the pituitary. Biol. Rev. **22**, 30 (1947). — The excretion of administered sodium chloride by the conscious dog, and the effect of occlusion of the carotid arteries. Quart. J. exp. Physiol. **40**, 237 (1955). — The effect on urinary volume and composition of the ingestion of 0.9 percent sodium chloride and of occlusion of the carotid arteries. Quart. J. exp. Physiol. **43**, 367 (1958a). — The effect on the volume and composition of the urine of the infusion of adrenaline and noradrenaline. Quart. J. exp. Physiol. **43**, 384 (1958b). — O'Connor, W. J., and E. B. VERNEY: The effect of removal of the posterior lobe of the pituitary on the inhibition of water-diuresis by emotional stress. Quart. J. exp. Physiol. 31, 393 (1941/42). — The effect of increased activity of the sympathetic system in the inhibition of water diuresis by emotional stress. Quart. J. exp. Physiol. 33, 77 (1945). — O'DELL, R., and B. SCHMIDT-NIELSEN: Concentrating ability and kidney structure. Fed. Proc. 19, 366 (1960) (abstract). — ÖSTLING, G., and R. V. GASSTRÖM: Renal excretion of radioactive phosphate in urological patients. Ann. Chir. Gynaec. Fenn. 41, 223 (1952). — ÖSTLING, G., and G. TÖTTERMAN: Specific activity of inorganic phosphorus in plasma and urine during constant infusion of radioactive phosphate in man. Arch. int. Pharmacodyn. 92, 362 (1953). — Extrinsic (P^{32})/intrinsic (P^{31}) phosphorus clearance ratio in man. Scand. J. Clin. Lab. Invest. 6, 25 (1954). — OKEN, D. E., G. WHITTEMBURY, E. E. WINDHAGER, H. J. SCHATZMANN and A. K. SOLOMON: Active sodium transport by the proximal tubule of Necturus kidney. J. Clin. Invest. 38, 1029 (1959) (abstract). — OLEESKY, S.: A specific water diuresis test for adrenocortical insufficiency. Lancet 1953 I, 769. — OLIVECRONA, H.: Paraventricular nucleus and pituitary gland. Acta physiol. scand. 40, Suppl., 136 (1957). — OLIVER, J.: Architecture of the kidney in chronic Bright's disease. New York: P. B. Hoeber 1939. — New directions in renal morphology: Method, its results and its future. Harvey Lect. 40, 102 (1944). — The structure of the metabolic process in the nephron. J. Mt Sinai Hosp. 15, 175 (1948). — An essay toward a dynamic morphology of the mammalian nephron. Seminars on Renal Physiology, Amer. J. Med., New York, 1950. — OLIVER, J., and MURIEL MacDoWELL: Cellular mechanisms of protein metabolism in the nephron. VII. The characteristics and significance of the protein absorption droplets (hyaline droplets) in epidemic hemorrhagic fever and other renal diseases. J. exp. Med. 107, 731 (1958). — OLIVER, J., and E. SHEVKY: A comparison of the manner of excretion of neutral red and phenol red by the frog's kidney. J. exp. Med. 50, 15 (1929). — The relation of particle size to mechanism of dye excretion by the kidney. Amer. J. Physiol. 93, 363 (1930). — OLIVER, J., W. STRAUS, N. KRETCHMER, Y. C. LEE, H. W. DICKERMAN and FRANCES CHEROT: The histochemical characteristics of absorption droplets in the nephron. J. Histochem. Cytochem. 3, 277 (1955). — OLLAYOS, R. W., and A. W. WINKLER: Urinary excretion and serum concentration of inorganic phosphate in man. J. clin. Invest. 22, 147 (1943). — OREN, B. G., M. RICH and M. S. BELLE: Chlorothiazide (Diuril) as a hyperuricacidemic agent. J. Amer. med. Ass. 168, 2128 (1958). — ORLOFF, J., L. ARONOW and R. W. BERLINER: The transport of priscoline by the renal tubules. J. Pharmacol. exp. Ther. 109, 214 (1953). — ORLOFF, J., and R. W. BERLINER: The mechanism of the excretion of ammonia in the dog. J. clin. Invest. 35, 223 (1956). — ORLOFF, J., and W. D. BLAKE: Effects of concentrated salt-poor human albumin on metabolism and excretion of water and electrolytes in dogs. Amer. J. Physiol. 164, 167 (1951). — ORLOFF, J., and M. BURG: A direct renal tubule effect of strophanthidin on electrolyte excretion in the chicken. Amer. J. Med. 25, 129 (1958) (abstract). — ORLOFF, J., and D. G. DAVIDSON: The mechanism of potassium excretion in the chicken. J. clin. Invest. 38, 21 (1959). — ORLOFF, J., and T. J. KENNEDY jr.: Effect of lithium on acidification of urine. Fed. Proc. 11, 115 (1952) (abstract). — ORLOFF, J., T. J. KENNEDY jr. and R. W. BERLINER: The effect of potassium in nephrectomized rats with hypokalemic alkalosis. J. clin. Invest. 32, 538 (1953). — ORLOFF, J., H. N. WAGNER jr. and D. G. DAVIDSON: The effect of variations in solute excretion and vasopressin dosage on the excretion of water in the dog. J. clin. Invest. 37, 458 (1958). — ORLOFF, J., L. G. WELT and L. STOWE: The effects of concentrated salt-poor albumin on the metabolism and excretion of water and electrolytes in nephrosis and toxemia of pregnancy. J. clin. Invest. 29, 770 (1950). — ORTI, E., B. LAKEN and ELAINE P. RALLI: Antidiuretic substances in normal and cirrhotic urines. Fed. Proc. 17, 120 (1958) (abstract). — ORZECHOWSKI, G.: Über den Mechanismus der Ausscheidung von Säuregerbstoffen. Pflügers Arch. ges. Physiol. 225, 104 (1930). — OSTBERG, O.: Studien über die Zitronensäureausscheidung der Menschenniere in normalen und pathologischen Zuständen. Skand. Arch. Physiol. 61/62, 81 (1931). — OWEN, E. E., J. F. FLANAGAN and M. P. TYOR: Kidney as a source of blood ammonia: Effect of chlorothiazide. Proc. Soc. exp. Biol. (N.Y.) 102, 696 (1959). — OWEN, E. E., and J. V. VERNER jr.: Renal tubular acidosis and a syndrome of muscle paralysis and hypokalemia. Clin. Res. 7, 165 (1959) (abstract). — OWEN jr., J. A., F. L. ENGEL and T. B. WESTER: 9-α-Fluorohydrocortisone-induced hypertension in a male infant with adrenogenitalism, and in 6 adults with Addison's disease. J. clin. Endocr. 17, 272 (1957). — OWEN, J. A., BETTY IGGO, F. J. SCANDRETT and C. P. STEWART: The determination of creatinine in plasma or serum, and in urine; a critical examination. Biochem. J. 58, 426 (1954).

PAGE, I.: The action of certain diuretics on the function of the kidney as measured by the urea clearance test. J. clin. Invest 12, 737 (1933). — PAGE, I. H.: Serotonin (5-hydroxytryptamine); the last four years. Physiol. Rev. 38, 277 (1958). — PAGE, I. H., and J. W. McCUBBIN: Renal vascular and systemic arterial pressure responses to nervous and chemical stimulation of the kidney. Amer. J. Physiol. **173**, 411 (1953). — PAGE, I. H., R. D. TAYLOR, A. C. CORCORAN and LILLIAN MUELLER: Correlation of clinical types with renal function in arterial hypertension. II. Effect of spinal anesthesia. J. Amer. med. Ass. **124**, 736 (1944). — PAGE, L. B.: Effects of hypothermia on renal function. Amer. J. Physiol. **181**, 171 (1955). — PAGE, L. B., C. F. BAXTER, GABRIELLE H. REEM, J. C. SCOTT-BAKER and H. W. SMITH: Effect of unilateral splanchnic nerve resection on the renal excretion of sodium. Amer. J. Physiol. **177**, 194 (1954a). — PAGE, L. B., and GABRIELLE H. RHEEM: Urinary concentrating mechanism in the dog. Amer. J. Physiol. **171**, 572 (1952). — PAGE, L. B., J. C. SCOTT-BAKER, G. A. ZAK, E. L. BECKER and C. F. BAXTER: The effect of variation in filtration rate on the urinary concentrating mechanism in the seal, *Phoca vitulina* L. J. cell. comp. Physiol. **43**, 257 (1954b). — PAI, H.-C.: Dissections of nephrons from the human kidney. J. Anat. (Lond.) **69**, 344 (1934). — PAK POY, R. K. F.: Electron microscopy of the mammalian renal glomerulus. The problems of intercapillary tissue and the capillary loop basement membrane. Amer. J. Path. **34**, 885 (1958). — PAPPENHEIMER, J. R.: Über die Permeabilität der Glomerulusmembranen in der Niere. Klin. Wschr. **33**, 362 (1955). — Role of the red blood corpuscles in the regulation of renal blood flow and glomerular filtration rate. Physiologist 1, 8 (1958). — PAPPENHEIMER, J. R., and W. B. KINTER: Hematocrit ratio of blood within mammalian kidney and its significance for renal hemodynamics. Amer. J. Physiol. **185**, 377 (1956). — PAPPENHEIMER, J. R., and J. P. MAES: A quantitative measure of the vasomotor tone in the hindlimb muscles of the dog. Amer. J. Physiol. **137**, 187 (1942). — PAPPENHEIMER, J. R., E. M. RENKIN and L. M. BORRERO: Filtration, diffusion and molecular sieving through peripheral capillary membranes. A contribution to the pore theory of capillary permeability. Amer. J. Physiol. **167**, 13 (1951). — PAPPER, E. M.: Renal function during general anesthesia. Bull. N.Y. Acad. Med. **31**, 446 (1955). — PAPPER, S., and J. D. ROSENBAUM: Diurnal variation in the diuretic response to ingested water. J. clin. Invest. **31**, 401 (1952). — PAPPER, S., L. SAXON, M. B. BURG, H. W. SEIFER and J. D. ROSENBAUM: The effect of morphine sulfate upon the renal excretion of water and solute in man. J. Lab. clin. Med. **50**, 692 (1957). — PAPPER, S., L. SAXON, J. D. ROSENBAUM and H. W. COHEN: The effects of isotonic and hypertonic salt solutions on the renal excretion of sodium. J. Lab. clin. Med. **47**, 776 (1956). — PARIS, J., ELIZABETH FORD, NONA LORENZ, F. R. KEATING jr. and A. ALBERT: Effect of hormones on renal clearance of radioiodine in the rat. Amer. J. Physiol. **183**, 163 (1955). — PASCALE, L. R.: Therapeutic value of probenecid (Benemid) in gout. J. Amer. med. Ass. **149**, 1188 (1952). — PASCALE, L. R., A. DUBIN and W. S. HOFFMAN: Influence of Benemid on urinary excretion of phosphate in hypoparathyroidism. Metabolism **3**, 462 (1954). — PASQUALINI, R. Q., and A. CODEVILLA: Thirst-suppressing ("antidipsetic") effect of pitressin in diabetes insipidus. Acta endocr. (Kbh.) **30**, 37 (1958). — PASQUALINI, R. Q., y E. ETALA: Hipofisis y excrecion de cloruro de sodio. Rev. Soc. argent. Biol. **17**, 198 (1941). — PATALANO, A., y F. R. VIVONE: La depuracion urinaria de la creatinina endogena como medida de la filtracion glomerular. An. Inst. fis. Pat. hum. (B. Aires) **4**, 339 (1942). — PATEK jr., A. J., H. MANKIN, H. COLCHER, ALICE LOWELL and D. P. EARLE jr.: Effects of intravenous injection of concentrated human serum albumin upon blood plasma, ascites and renal functions in 3 patients with cirrhosis of liver. J. clin. Invest. **27**, 135 (1948). — PEARCE, J. W.: The effect of vagotomy and denervation of the carotid sinus on diuresis following plasma volume expansion. Canad. J. Biochem. **37**, 81 (1959). — PEARCE, J. W., and R. W. ROBERTS: The effect of vagotomy on the diuretic response to isotonic infusions. Rev. canad. Biol. **13**, 492 (1954) (abstract). — PEARCE, M. L., and E. V. NEWMAN: Some postural adjustments of salt and water excretion. J. clin. Invest. **33**, 1089 (1954). — PEASE, D. C.: Fine structures of the kidney seen by electron microscopy. J. Histochem. Cytochem. **3**, 295 (1955a). — Electron microscopy of the vascular bed of the kidney cortex. Anat. Rec. **121**, 701 (1955b). — Electron microscopy of the tubular cells of the kidney cortex. Anat. Rec. **121**, 723 (1955c). — PEASE, D. C., and R. F. BAKER: Electron microscopy of the kidney. Amer. J. Anat. **87**, 349 (1950). — PECHET, M. M., B. BOWERS and F. C. BARTTER: Metabolic studies with a new series of 1,4-diene steroids. I. Effects in Addisonian subjects of prednisone, prednisolone, and the 1,2-dehydroanalogues of corticosterone, desoxy-corticosterone, 17-hydroxy-11-desoxycorticosterone, and 9-α-fluorocortisol. J. clin. Invest. **38**, 681 (1959a). — Metabolic studies with a new series of 1,4-diene steroids. II. Effects in normal subjects of prednisone, prednisolone, and 9-α-fluoroprednisolone. J. clin. Invest. **38**, 691 (1959b). — PEIRCE, E. C. (2nd.): Renal lymphatics. Anat. Rec. **90**, 315 (1944). — PENA, J. C., and R. L. MALVIN: Retrograde movement of some non-electrolytes across the renal tubular epithelium. Fed. Proc. **19**, 368 (1960) (abstract). — PENCHARZ, R. I., J. HOPPER jr. and E. H. RYNEARSON: Water metabolism of the rat following removal of the anterior lobe of the hypophysis. Proc. Soc. exp. Biol. (N.Y.) **34**, 14 (1936). — PEREZ-STABLE, M.: La Prueba de inulina en ninos normales. Arch. Med. infant. **16**, 89 (1947). — PERLMUTT, J. H., and D. A. OLEWINE: Alteration of renal response to carbonic anhydrase inhibitor by synthetic adrenal steroids. Amer. J. Physiol. **195**, 142 (1958). — PERRY, W. F., and

T. W. Fyles: Antidiuretic activity of the serum of normal and diseased subjects. J. clin. Endocr. 13, 64 (1953). — Peter, K.: Untersuchungen über Bau und Entwicklung der Niere. Jena: Gustav Fischer 1927. — Peters, G.: Nebennieren und renale Oxytocin-Wirkungen bei der Ratte. Naunyn-Schmiedeberg's Arch. exp. Path. Pharmak. 235, 335 (1959). — Peters, J. P.: Role of sodium in edema. New Engl. J. Med. 239, 353 (1948). — The problem of cardiac edema. Amer. J. Med. 12, 66 (1952). — Peters, L., K. J. Fenton, Mary L. Wolf and A. Kandel: Inhibition of the renal tubular excretion of N'-methylnicotinamide (NMN) by small doses of a basic cyanine dye. J. Pharmacol. exp. Ther. 113, 148 (1955). — Petersdorf, R. G., and L. G. Welt: The effect of an infusion of hyperoncotic albumin on the excretion of water and solutes. J. clin. Invest. 32, 283 (1953). — Peterson, N. A., and J. M. Crismon: Effect of pH on the ultrafiltrable calcium from rabbit serum. Fed. Proc. 19, 251 (1960) (abstract). — Phillips, D. M., and K. Hare: Antidiuretic potency of neurohypophysis of cat following pituitary stalk section. Endocrinology 37, 29 (1945). — Phillips, R. A., V. P. Dole, P. B. Hamilton, K. Emerson jr., R. M. Archibald, D. D. van Slyke, Emily G. Stanley and W. H. Becker: Effects of acute hemorrhagic and traumatic shock on renal function of dogs. Amer. J. Physiol. 145, 314 (1946). — Piantoni, C.: Mecanismo de eliminación renal del ácido ascórbico. Rev. Soc. argent. Biol. 16, 175 (1940). — Pickford, Mary: The inhibitory effect of acetylcholine on water diuresis in the dog and its pituitary transmission. J. Physiol. (Lond.) 95, 226 (1939). — Control of secretion of antidiuretic hormone from pars nervosa of pituitary gland. Physiol. Rev. 25, 573 (1945). — Pickford, Mary, and A. E. Ritchie: Experiments on hypothalamic-pituitary control of water excretion in dogs. J. Physiol. (Lond.) 104, 105 (1945). — Pickford, Mary, and J. A. Watt: Comparison of some of the actions of adrenaline and noradrenaline on the kidney. Quart. J. exp. Physiol. 36, 205 (1950). — A comparison of the effect of intravenous and intracarotid injections of acetylcholine in the dog. J. Physiol. (Lond.) 114, 333 (1951). — Pierce, J. A., and H. Montgomery: A microquinhydrone electrode: its application to the determination of the pH of glomerular urine of Necturus. J. biol. Chem. 110, 763 (1935). — Piiper, J., and E. Schürmeyer: Über den Nachweis von arterio-venösen Anastomosen in der Hundeniere. Pflügers Arch. ges. Physiol. 261, 543 (1955). — Pilsum, J. F. van, and E. L. Seljeskog: Long term endogenous creatinine clearance in man. Proc. Soc. exp. Biol. (N.Y.) 97, 270 (1958). — Pincus, G.: A diurnal rhythm in the excretion of urinary keto-steroids by young men. J. clin. Endocr. 3, 195 (1943). — Pincus, G., Louise P. Romanoff and J. Carlo: A diurnal rhythm in the excretion of neutral reducing lipids by man and its relation to the 17-ketosteroid rhythm. J. clin. Endocr. 8, 221 (1948). — Pincus, J. B., H. A. Peterson and B. Kramer: A study by means of ultrafiltration of the condition of several inorganic constituents of blood serum in disease. J. biol. Chem. 68, 601 (1926). — Pineles, F.: Die Epithelkörperchen (Glandulae parathyroideae). In Handbuch der normalen und pathologischen Physiologie Bd. 16, S. 346. 1930. — Pitesky, I., and J. H. Last: Effects of seasonal heat stress on glomerular and tubular functions in the dog. Amer. J. Physiol. 164, 497 (1951). — Pitts, R. F.: The excretion of urine in the dog. VII. Inorganic phosphate in relation to plasma phosphate level. Amer. J. Physiol. 106, 1 (1933). — Urinary composition in marine fish. J. cell. comp. Physiol. 4, 389 (1934). — Excretion of creatine by the marine teleost, the red grouper. Ann. Rep. Tortugas Lab. (Carnegie Inst.) 1935, 90. — The excretion of phenol red by the chicken. J. cell. comp. Physiol. 11, 99 (1938). — The excretion of creatine by the dogfish, Squalus acanthias. J. cell. comp. Physiol. 12, 151 (1939). — Renal reabsorptive mechanism in dog common to glycine and creatine. Amer. J. Physiol. 140, 156 (1943). — Comparison of renal reabsorptive processes for several amino acids. Amer. J. Physiol. 140, 535 (1944a). — Effects of infusing glycin and of varying dietary protein intake on renal hemodynamics of dog. Amer. J. Physiol. 142, 355 (1944b). — Renal regulation of acid-base balance with special reference to mechanism for acidifying urine. Science 102, 49 (1945). — Renal excretion of acid. Fed. Proc. 7, 418 (1948). — Acid-base regulation by the kidneys. Amer. J. Med. 9, 356 (1950). — Modern concepts of acid-base regulation. Arch. intern. Med. 89, 864 (1952). — Some reflections on mechanism of action of diuretics. Amer. J. Med. 17, 745 (1958). — Pitts, R. F., and R. S. Alexander: The renal reabsorption mechanism for inorganic phosphate in normal and acidotic dogs. Amer. J. Physiol. 142, 648 (1944). — Nature of renal tubular mechanism for acidifying urine. Amer. J. Physiol. 144, 239 (1945). — Pitts, R. F., J. L. Ayer and W. A. Schiess: The renal regulation of acid-base balance in man. III. The reabsorption and excretion of bicarbonate. J. clin. Invest. 28, 35 (1949). — Pitts, R. F., and J. J. Duggan: Studies in diuresis. II. The relationship between glomerular filtration rate, proximal tubular reabsorption of sodium and diuretic efficacy of mercurials. J. clin. Invest. 29, 372 (1950). — Pitts, R. F., Ruth S. Gurd, R. H. Kessler and K. Hierholzer: Localization of acidification of urine, potassium and ammonia secretion and phosphate reabsorption in the nephron of the dog. Amer. J. Physiol. 194, 125 (1958a). — Pitts, R. F., and I. M. Korr: The excretion of urea by the chicken. J. cell. comp. Physiol. 11, 117 (1938). — Pitts, R. F., F. Kruck, R. Lo-

ZANO, D. W. TAYLOR, O. P. A. HEIDENREICH and R. H. KESSLER: Studies on the mechanism of diuretic action of chlorothiazide. J. Pharmacol. exp. Ther. **123**, 89 (1958b). — PITTS, R. F., and W. D. LOTSPEICH: Bicarbonate and the renal regulation of acid-base balance. Amer. J. Physiol. **147**, 138 (1946a). — Factors governing rate of excretion of titratable acid in dog. Amer. J. Physiol. **147**, 481 (1946b). — Use of thiosulfate clearance as measure of glomerular filtration rate in acidotic dogs. Proc. Soc. exp. Biol. (N.Y.) **64**, 224 (1947). — PITTS, R. F., W. D. LOTSPEICH, W. A. SCHIESS and J. L. AYER: Renal regulation of acid-base balance in man; nature of mechanism for acidifying urine. J. clin. Invest. **27**, 48 (1948). — PLATT, R.: Sodium and potassium excretion in chronic renal failure. Clin. Sci. **9**, 367 (1950). — PLATTS, M. M., and G. H. MUDGE: The accumulation of uric acid by rabbit kidney slices in vitro. Fed. Proc. **19**, 367 (1960) (abstract). — POLICARD, A., A. COLLET et L. GILTAIRE-RALYTE: Récherches au microscope électronique sur la structure du glomérule rénal des mammifères. Arch. Anat. micr. Morph. exp. **44**, 1 (1955). — POLONOVSKI, M., G. BIZARD et P. BOULANGER: Influence de l'injection des sels ammoniacaux sur l'ammoniemie. C. R. Soc. Biol. (Paris) **112**, 193 (1933). — POLONOVSKI, M., P. BOULANGER et G. BIZARD: Formation d'ammoniaque aux dépens des acides aminés dans le rein du chien in vivo. C. R. Acad. Sci. (Paris) **198**, 1815 (1934). — POPENOE, E. A., H. C. LAWLER and V. DU VIGNEAUD: Partial purification and amino acid content of vasopressin from hog posterior pituitary glands. J. Amer. chem. Soc. **74**, 3713 (1952). — POPPELL, J. W., F. CUAJUNCO jr., J. S. HORSLEY III., H. T. RANDALL and KATHLEEN E. ROBERTS: Renal arteriovenous ammonium difference and total renal ammonia production in normal, acidotic and alkalotic dogs. Clin. Res. **4**, 137 (1956) (abstract). — PORTWOOD, R. M., D. W. SELDIN, F. C. RECTOR jr. and R. CADE: The relation of urinary CO_2 tension to bicarbonate excretion. J. clin. Invest. **38**, 770 (1959). — POTTS, A. M., and T. F. GALLAGHER: Cystine, tyrosine and arginine content of high potency pressor and oxytocic pituitary hormones. J. biol. Chem. **143**, 561 (1942). — Separation of oxytocic and pressor principles of posterior pituitary extracts. J. biol. Chem. **154**, 349 (1944). — POULOS, P. P.: The renal tubular reabsorption and urinary excretion of calcium by the dog. J. Lab. clin. Med. **49**, 253 (1957). — POULSEN, H., and E. PRAETORIUS: Tubular excretion of uric acid in rabbits. Acta pharmacol. (Kbh.) **10**, 371 (1954). — POULSSON, L. T.: On the mechanism of sugar elimination in phlorrhizin glycosuria. A contribution to the filtration-reabsorption theory on kidney function. J. Physiol. (Lond.) **69**, 411 (1930). — PRAETORIUS, E., and J. E. KIRK: Hypouricemia: with evidence for tubular elimination of uric acid. J. Lab. clin. Med. **35**, 865 (1950). — PRÁT, V.: Separate clearance. III. The effect of filling the urinary bladder on kidney hemodynamics and function in man. Physiol. Bohemosl. **5**, 401 (1956). — PRITCHARD, J. A., A. C. BARNES and R. H. BRIGHT: The effect of the supine position on renal function in the near-term pergnant woman. J. clin. Invest. **34**, 777 (1955). — PRONINA, N. N.: O mekhanizme izmereniya diureza pri vodnykh nagruzkakh. Bjull. eksp. Biol. Med. **39**, 12 (1955). — PUCK, T. T., K. WASSERMAN and A. P. FISHMAN: Some effects of inorganic ions on the active transport of phenol red by isolated kidney tubules of the flounder. J. cell. comp. Physiol. **40**, 73 (1952). — PULLMAN, T. N., A. S. ALVING, R. J. DERN and M. LANDOWNE: The influence of dietary protein intake on specific renal functions in normal man. J. Lab. clin. Med. **44**, 320 (1954). — PULLMAN, T. N., and W. W. MCCLURE: The effect of *l*-noradrenaline on electrolyte excretion in normal man. J. Lab. clin. Med. **39**, 711 (1952). — PULLMAN, T. N., and W. W. MCCLURE: The response of the renal circulation in man to constant speed infusion of *l*-noradrenaline. Circulation **9**, 600 (1954).

QUICK, A. J.: The conjugation of benzoic acid in man. J. biol. Chem. **92**, 65 (1931). — The site of the synthesis of hippuric acid and phenylaceturic acid in the dog. J. biol. Chem. **96**, 73 (1932a). — The relationship between chemical structure and physiological response. II. The conjugation of hydroxy- and methoxybenzoic acids. J. biol. Chem. **97**, 403 (1932b). — The relationship between chemical structure and physiological response. IV. Conjugation of salicylic acid with glycine and its action on uric acid excretion. J. biol. Chem. **101**, 475 (1933).

RAASCHOU, F.: Chronic pyelonephritis with special reference to the kidney function. Copenhagen: Ejnar Munksgaard 1948. — RABASA, S. L., and FRIDA BERGMANN: Nephrogenic diabetes insipidus induced by aminopterin. Acta physiol. lat.-amer. **4**, 42 (1954). — RADIGAN, L. R., and S. ROBINSON: Effects of environmental heat stress and exercise on renal blood flow and filtration rate. Amer. J. Physiol. **159**, 585 (1949). — RAGAZ, L.: Zur Pharmakologie der p-Aminosalicylsäure. Nachweis, Verteilung im Organismus und renale Elimination. Schweiz. med. Wschr. **78**, 1213 (1948). — RAISZ, L. G.: Dextran and oxypolygelatin as plasma volume expanders: renal excretion and effects on renal function. J. Lab. clin. Med. **40**, 880 (1952). — RAISZ, L. G., W. Y. W. AU and R. L. SCHEER: Studies on the renal concentrating mechanism. III. Effect of heavy exercise. J. clin. Invest. **38**, 8 (1959a). — Studies on the renal concentrating mechanism. IV. Osmotic diuresis. J. clin. Invest. **38**, 1725 (1959b). — RAISZ, L. G., W. F. MCNEELY and L. SAXON: Studies on the renal concentrating mechanism. I. Role of vasopressin. J. Lab. clin. Med. **52**, 437 (1958). — RAISZ, L. G., W. F. McNEELY, L. SAXON and J. D. ROSENBAUM: The effects of cortisone and hydrocortisone on water diuresis and renal function in man. J. clin. Invest. **36**, 767 (1957) (abstract). — RAISZ, L. G., and R. L. SCHEER: Studies on the renal concentrating mechanism. II. Effect of small acute changes in solute excretion. J. clin. Invest. **38**, 1 (1959). — RALLI, ELAINE P., G. J. FRIEDMAN and S. H. RUBIN: The mechanism of the excretion of vitamin C by the human kidney. J. clin. Invest. **17**, 765 (1938). — RALLI, ELAINE P., J. S. ROBSON, D. CLARKE and C. L. HOAGLAND: Factors influencing ascites in patients with cirrhosis of the liver. J. clin. Invest. **24**, 316 (1945). — RAMEY, ESTELLE R., and M. S. GOLDSTEIN: The adrenal cortex and the sympathetic nervous system. Physiol. Rev. **37**, 155 (1957). — RAMMELKAMP, C. H., and S. E. BRADLEY: Excretion of penicillin in man. Proc. Soc. exp. Biol. (N.Y.) **53**, 30 (1943). — RANDALL jr., R. E., and S. PAPPER: Mechanism of postoperative limitation in sodium excretion: the role of extracellular fluid volume and of adrenal cortical activity. J. clin. Invest. **37**, 1628 (1958). — RANGES, H. A., and S. A. BRADLEY: Systemic and renal circulatory changes following the administration of adrenin, ephedrine and pare-drinol to normal man. J. clin. Invest. **22**, 687 (1943). — RANNEY, HELEN M., and D. J. McCUNE: Photometric micromethod for determination of inulin in serum and urine. J. biol. Chem. **150**, 311 (1943). — Renal function in children. Amer. J. Dis. Child. **69**, 322 (1945) (abstract). — RANTZ, L. A., and W. M. M. KIRBY: The absorption and excretion of penicillin following continuous intravenous and subcutaneous administration. J. clin. Invest. **23**, 789 (1944). — RAPOPORT, S., W. A. BRODSKY, C. D. WEST and B. MACKLER: Urinary flow, excretion of solutes and osmotic work during diuresis of solute loading in hydropenia in man. Science **108**, 630 (1948). — RAPOPORT, S., N. NELSON, G. M. GUEST and I. A. MIRSKY: The turnover of acid-soluble phosphorus in the kidneys of rats. Science **93**, 88 (1941). — RAPOPORT, S., and C. D. WEST: Ionic antagonism: effect of various anions on chloride excretion during osmotic diuresis in the dog. Amer. J. Physiol. **162**, 668 (1950). — RAPOPORT, S., C. D. WEST and W. A. BRODSKY: Excretion of solutes and os-motic work during osmotic diuresis of hypropenic man. The ideal and the proximal and distal tubular work; the biological maximum of work. Amer. J. Physiol. **157**, 363 (1949). — Salt-losing conditions; the renal defect in tuberculous meningitis. J. Lab. clin. Med. **37**, 550 (1951). — RATHER, L. J.: Filtration, reabsorption, and excretion of protein by the kidney. Medicine (Baltimore) **31**, 357 (1952). — RAUSCHKOLB, ELIZABETH W., and G. L. FARRELL: Evidence for diencephalic regulation of aldosterone secretion. Endocrinology **59**, 526 (1956). — RAUSCHKOLB, ELIZABETH W., G. L. FARRELL and S. KOLETSKY: Aldosterone secretion after hypophysectomy. Amer. J. Physiol. **184**, 55 (1956). — RAWSON, A. J.: Distribution of the lymphatics of the human kidney as shown in a case of carcinomatous permeation. Arch. Path. (Chicago) **47**, 283 (1949). — RECTOR jr., F. C., and J. ORLOFF: The effect of the administration of sodium bicarbonate and ammonium chloride on the excretion and production of ammonia. The absence of alterations in the activity of renal ammonia-producing enzymes in the dog. J. clin. Invest. **38**, 366 (1959). — RECTOR jr., F. C., R. M. PORTWOOD and D. W. SELDIN: Examination of the mixing hypothesis as an explanation for elevated urinary CO_2 tensions. Amer. J. Physiol. **197**, 861 (1959). — RECTOR jr., F. C., D. W. SELDIN and J. H. COPENHAVER: The mechanism of ammonia excretion during ammonium chloride acidosis. J. clin. Invest. **34**, 20 (1955). — RECTOR jr., F. C., D. W. SELDIN, A. D. ROBERTS jr. and J. H. COPENHAVER: Relation of ammonia excretion to urine p_H. Amer. J. Physiol. **179**, 353 (1954). — REES, S. B., S. S. FRANKLIN, J. T. AUGUST, J. H. SMALL, A. R. KENDALL, J. P. MERRILL and J. G. GIBSON: Stop flow analysis of renal tubular potassium and phosphate flux. Fed. Proc. **18**, 126 (1959). — REES, V. L., and V. IOB: Effects of ether anesthesia on renal func-tion. Bull. Univ. Mich. Hosp. **9**, 70 (1943). — REFORZO-MEMBRIVES, J., M. H. POWER and E. J. KEPLER: Studies on the renal excretion of water and electrolytes in cases of Addison's disease. J. clin. Endocr. **5**, 76 (1945). — REHBERG, P. B.: Studies on kidney function. II. The excretion of urea and chlorine analysed according to a modified filtration-reabsorption theory. Biochem. J. **20**, 461 (1926). — REID, R. T.: Observations on the structure of the renal glomerulus of the mouse revealed by the electron microscope. Aust. J. exp. Biol. med. Sci. **32**, 235 (1954). — REIFENSTEIN jr., E. C., L. W. KINSELL and F. ALBRIGHT: Observa-tions on the use of the serum phosphorus level as an index of pituitary growth hormone activity; the effect of estrogen therapy in acromegaly. Endocrinology **39**, 71 (1946). — REIMER, ANN, H. K. SCHOCH and L. H. NEWBURGH: Certain aspects of potassium meta-bolism. J. Amer. diet. Ass. **27**, 1042 (1951). — REINHOLD, J. G., H. F. FLIPPIN, A. H. DOMM, J. J. ZIMMERMAN and L. SCHWARTZ: Renal clearance of sulfamerazine, sulfadiazine, sulfathiazole and sulfapyridine in man. J. Pharmacol. exp. Ther. **83**, 279 (1945). — RELMAN, A. S., B. ETSTEN and W. B. SCHWARTZ: The regulation of renal bicarbonate reabsorption by plasma carbon dioxide tension. J. clin. Invest. **32**, 972 (1953). — RELMAN, A. S., A. LEAF and W. B. SCHWARTZ: Oral administration of a potent carbonic anhydrase inhibitor ("Diamox"). II. Its use as a diuretic in patients with severe congestive heart failure. New

Engl. J. Med. **250**, 800 (1954). — RELMAN, A. S., ARLENE M. ROY and W. B. SCHWARTZ: Effect of rubidium on acid-base balance in potassium deficient and normal rats. J. clin. Invest. **32**, 597 (1953) (abstract). — RELMAN, A. S., and W. B. SCHWARTZ: The effect of DOCA on electrolyte balance in normal man and its relation to sodium chloride intake. Yale J. Biol. Med. **24**, 540 (1952). — The nephropathy of potassium depletion. A clinical and pathological entity. New Engl. J. Med. **255**, 195 (1956). — The kidney in potassium depletion. Amer. J. Med. **24**, 764 (1958). — RELMAN, A. S., S. K. STEWART and W. B. SCHWARTZ: A study of the adjustments to sodium- and water-retaining hormones in normal subjects. J. clin. Invest. **37**, 924 (1958) (abstract). — RENNELS, E. G., and G. A. DRAGER: The relation of pituicytes to neurosecretion. Anat. Rec. **122**, 193 (1955). — RENNICK, BARBARA R.: The renal tubular excretion of choline and thiamine in the chicken. J. Pharmacol. exp. Ther. **122**, 449 (1958). — RENNICK, BARBARA R., K. M. CALHOON, H. GANDIA and G. K. MOE: Renal tubular secretion of tetraethylammonium in the dog and the chicken. J. Pharmacol. exp. Ther. **110**, 309 (1954). — RENNICK, BARBARA R., R. W. EVANS and G. K. MOE: Stop-flow analysis of renal tubular excretion of tetraethylammonium. Fed. Proc. **18**, 435 (1959) (abstract). — RENNICK, BARBARA R., and A. FARAH: Studies on the renal tubular transport of tetraethylammonium ion in the dog. J. Pharmacol. exp. Ther. **116**, 287 (1956). — RENNICK, BARBARA R., A. KANDEL and L. PETERS: Inhibition of the renal tubular excretion of tetraethylammonium and N'-methylnicotinamide by the basic cyanine dyes. J. Pharmacol. exp. Ther. **118**, 204 (1956). — RENNICK, BARBARA R., G. K. MOE, R. H. LYONS, S. W. HOOBLER and ROSALIE NELIGH: Absorption and renal excretion of tetraethylammonium ion. J. Pharmacol. exp. Ther. **91**, 210 (1947). — RENNIE, E. W.: Localization of intrarenal oxygen tensions by stop-from. Fed. Proc. **19**, 369 (1960) (abstract). — RENNIE, E. W., R. B. REEVES and J. R. PAPPENHEIMER: Oxygen pressure in urine and its relation to intrarenal blood flow. Amer. J. Physiol. **195**, 120 (1958). — RENWICK, REATA, J. S. ROBSON and C. P. STEWART: Observations upon the withdrawal of sodium chloride from the diet in hypertensive and normotensive individuals. J. clin. Invest. **34**, 1037 (1955a). — Observations upon the withdrawal of sodium chloride from the diet in hypertensive and normotensive individuals. Acta endocr. (Kbh.) **20**, 173 (1955b). — RENZI, A. A., M. RENZI, J. J. CHART and R. GAUNT: The effects of aldosterone and other steroids on water intoxication and renal function. Acta endocr. (Kbh.) **21**, 47 (1956). — REUBI, F. C.: Recherches sur le diabète rénal. I. Le mecanisme de la glycosurie. Helv. med. Acta **18**, 69 (1951). — Objections à la théorie de la séparation intrarénale des hématies et du plasma (Pappenheimer). Helv. med. Acta **25**, 516 (1958). — Glucose titration in renal glycosuria. The kidney. Ciba Foundation Symposia. Boston: Little, Brown & Co. 1954. — REUBI, F. C., and P. H. FUTCHER: The effects of histamine on renal function in hypertensive and normotensive subjects. J. clin. Invest. **28**, 440 (1949). — REUBI, F. C., P. MÜLLER et P. STUCKI: Effets circulatoires de la réserpine (Serpasil). Helv. med. Acta **21**, 493 (1954). — REUBI, F. C., and H. A. SCHROEDER: Can vascular shunting be induced in the kidney by vasoactive drugs? J. clin. Invest. **28**, 114 (1949). — REUBI, M. F.: Étude des fonctions rénales dans 2 cas de maladie de Vaquez. J. Urol. méd. chir. **58**, 231 (1952). — RHOADS, C. P., D. D. VAN SLYKE, ALMA HILLER and A. S. ALVING: The effects of novocainization and total section of the nerves of the renal pedicle on renal blood flow and function. Amer. J. Physiol. **110**, 392 (1934). — RHODIN, J.: Correlation of ultrastructural organization and function in normal and experimentally changed proximal convoluted tubule cells of the mouse kidney. Karolinska Institutet, Stockholm, Aktiebolaget Godvil, 1954 (thesis). — Electron microscopy of the glomerular capillary wall. Exp. cell Res. **8**, 572 (1955). — Electron microscopy of the kidney. Amer. J. Med. **24**, 661 (1958). — RICE, L., J. FRIEDEN and M. SMITH: Tubular action of mercurial diuretics. Amer. J. Physiol. **175**, 47 (1953). — RICHARDS, A. N.: The nature and mode of regulation of glomerular function. Amer. J. med. Sci. **170**, 781 (1925). — Methods and results of direct investigations on the function of the kidney. Beaumont Foundation Lectures (series 8). Baltimore: Williams and Wilkins 1929. — Urine formation in the amphibian kidney. Harvey Lect. **98** (1934). — RICHARDS, A. N., and J. B. BARNWELL: Experiments concerning the question of secretion of phenolsulphonephthalein by the renal tubule. Proc. roy. Soc. B **102**, 72 (1927). — RICHARDS, A. N., P. A. BOTT and B. B. WESTFALL: Experiments concerning the possibility that inulin is secreted by the tubules. Amer. J. Physiol. **123**, 281 (1938). — RICHARDS, A. N., and O. H. PLANT: The action of minute doses of adrenalin and pituitrin on the kidney. Amer. J. Physiol. **59**, 191 (1922). — RICHARDS, A. N., and C. F. SCHMIDT: A description of the glomerular circulation in the frog's kidney and observations concerning the action of adrenalin and various other substances upon it. Amer. J. Physiol. **71**, 178 (1924/25). — RICHARDS, A. N., and A. M. WALKER: The accessibility of the glomerular vessels to fluid perfused through the renal portal system of the frog's kidney. Amer. J. Physiol. **79**, 419 (1926/27). — Quantitative studies of the glomerular elimination of phenol red and indigo carmine in frogs. J. biol. Chem. **87**, 479 (1930). — Methods of collecting fluid from known regions of the renal tubules of amphibia and of per-

fusing the lumen of a single tubule. Amer. J. Physiol. 118, 111 (1937). — RICHARDS, A. N.,
B. B. WESTFALL and PHYLLIS A. BOTT: Renal excretion of inulin, creatinine and xylose in
normal dogs. Proc. Soc. exp. Biol. (N.Y.) 32, 73 (1934/35). — Inulin and creatinine clearances in dogs, with notes on some late effects of uranium poisoning. J. biol. Chem. 116,
749 (1936). — RICHARDSON, J. A., and C. R. HOUCK: Renal tubular excretory mass and
the reabsorption of sodium, chloride and potassium in female dogs receiving testosterone
propionate or estradiol benzoate. Amer. J. Physiol. 165, 93 (1951). — RICHTER, C. P.:
Experimental diabetes insipidus: its relation to the anterior and posterior lobes of the hypophysis. Amer. J. Physiol. 110, 439 (1934/35). — RICHTERICH-VAN BAERLE, R., and L. GOLD-
STEIN: Renal ammonia production as a model for the study of enzyme adaptation in mammals.
Experientia (Basel) 13, 30 (1957). — Distribution of glutamine metabolizing enzymes and production of urinary ammonia in the mammalian kidney. Amer. J. Physiol. 195, 316 (1958). —
RICHTERICH-VAN BAERLE, R., L. GOLDSTEIN and E. H. DEARBORN: Relation of ammonia
excretion to urine p_H in the guinea pig. Science 124, 74 (1956a). — Ammonia production in
the collecting ducts of mammalian kidneys. Nature (Lond.) 178, 698 (1956b). — Ammonia
excretion of the guinea pig and rabbit. Amer. J. Physiol. 192, 392 (1958). — RIGAS, D. A.,
and C. G. HELLER: The amount and nature of urinary proteins in normal human subjects.
J. clin. Invest. 30, 853 (1951). — RIGGS, D. S.: Renal clearance of iodide in the dog. Fed.
Proc. 8, 328 (1949) (abstract). — RIGGS, D. S., and D. A. BERKSON: Effect of acetazolamide
on mercurial diuresis. Fed. Proc. 17, 405 (1958) (abstract). — RINEHART, J. F.: Fine structure
of renal glomerulus as revealed by electron microscopy. Arch. Path. (Chicago) 59, 439 (1955). —
RINEHART, J. F., Marilyn G. FARQUHAR, H. C. JUNG and S. K. ABUL-HAJ: The normal glomerulus and its basic reactions in disease. Amer. J. Path. 29, 21 (1953). — RINSLER, M. G.,
and B. RIGBY: Function of aldosterone in the metabolism of sodium and water in pregnancy.
Brit. med. J. 1957 I, 966. — RITTER, E. R.: Pressure/flow relations in the kidney. Alleged
effects of pulse pressure. Amer. J. Physiol. 168, 480 (1952). — ROBERTS, H. J.: The syndrome
of hyponatremia and renal sodium loss probably resulting from inappropriate secretion of
antidiuretic hormone. Ann. intern. Med. 51, 1420 (1959). — ROBERTS, KATHLEEN E.: Effects
of cortisone administration on renal tubular capacity for reabsorption of phosphate and
excretion of potassium and titratable acid. Fed. Proc. 11, 130 (1952) (abstract). — ROBERTS,
KATHLEEN E., M. G. MAGIDA and R. F. PITTS: Relationship between potassium and bicarbonate in blood and urine. Amer. J. Physiol. 172, 47 (1953). — ROBERTS, KATHLEEN E.,
and R. F. PITTS: The influence of cortisone on renal function and electrolyte excretion in
the adrenalectomized dog. Endocrinology 50, 51 (1952). — The effects of cortisone and
desoxycorticosterone on the renal tubular reabsorption of phosphate and the excretion of
titratable acid and potassium in dogs. Endocrinology 52, 324 (1953). — ROBERTS, KATH-
LEEN E., and H. T. RANDALL: The effect of adrenal steroids on renal mechanisms of electrolyte excretion. Ann. N.Y. Acad. Sci. 61, 306 (1955). — ROBERTS, KATHLEEN E., H. T.
RANDALL, H. L. SANDERS and MARGARET HOOD: Effects of potassium on renal tubular
reabsorption of bicarbonate. J. clin. Invest. 34, 666 (1955). — ROBERTS, KATHLEEN E.,
H. T. RANDALL, P. VANAMEE and J. W. POPPELL: Renal mechanisms involved in bicarbonate
absorption. Metabolism 5, 404 (1956). — ROBINSON, C. E., L. V. DILL, J. F. CADDEN and
C. E. ISENHOUR: Glomerular filtration and renal blood flow in hypertensive woman and
in post-toxemic hypertension. Amer. J. Obstet. Gynec. 44, 616 (1942). — ROBINSON, F. J.,
M. H. POWER and E. J. KEPLER: Two new procedures to assist in the recognition and ex-
clusion of Addison's disease. A preliminary report. Proc. Mayo Clin. 16, 577 (1941). —
ROBINSON, J. R.: Ammonia formation by surviving kidney slices without specific sub-
strates. J. Physiol. (Lond.) 124, 1 (1954). — Reflections on renal function. Springfield, Ill.:
Ch. C. Thomas 1954a. — ROBINSON, R. R., H. V. MURGAUGH jr., ELLEN H. HAYES and
R. E. GALLOWAY: Urea excretion by the dog studied by stop-flow analysis. Clin. Res. Proc.
7, 274 (1959) (abstract). — ROBINSON, S., J. R. NICHOLAS, J. H. SMITH, W. J. DALY and
M. PEAREY: Time relation of renal and sweat gland adjustments to salt deficiency in men.
J. appl. Physiol. 8, 159 (1955). — ROBSON, ELIZABETH B., and G. A. ROSE: The effect of
intravenous lysine on the renal clearances of cystine, arginine and ornithine in normal sub-
jects, in patients with cystinuria and Fanconi syndrome and in their relatives. Clin. Sci.
16, 75 (1957). — ROBSON, J. S.: Single injection technique in evaluation of renal function.
Meth. med. Res. 5, 139 (1952). — ROBSON, J. S., M. H. FERGUSON, O. OLBRICK and C. P.
STEWART: The determination of the renal clearance of diodone and the maximal tubular
excretory capacity for diodone in man. Quart. J. exp. Physiol. 35, 173 (1949). — ROBSON,
J. S., D. B. HORN, H. A. DUDLEY and C. P. STEWART: Metabolic response to adrenalectomy.
Lancet 1955 II, 325. — ROE, J. H., J. H. EPSTEIN and N. P. GOLDSTEIN: A photometric
method for the determination of inulin in plasma and urine. J. biol. Chem. 178, 839 (1949). —
ROEMMELT, J. C., O. W. SARTORIUS and R. F. PITTS: Excretion and reabsorption of sodium
and water in the adrenalectomized dog. Amer. J. Physiol. 159, 124 (1949). — ROJEL, K.:
Inulin clearance and determination of inulin in blood and urine. Nord. Med. 16, 2948 (1942). —

Romer, A. S.: The vertebrate body. Philadelphia and London: W. B. Saunders 1955. — Roscoe, M. H.: The biphasic response of solute excretion to changes in urine flow. Acta med. scand. 156, 277 (1956/57). — Rosenbaum, J. D.: The fate of ingested water. Yale J. Biol. Med. 29, 263 (1956). — Rosenbaum, J. D., B. C. Ferguson, R. K. Davis and Elsie C. Rossmeisl: The influence of cortisone upon the diurnal rhythm of renal excretory function. J. clin. Invest. 31, 507 (1952). — Rosenbaum, J. D., S. Papper and M. M. Ashley: Variations in renal excretion of sodium independent of change in adrenocortical hormone dosage in patients with Addison's disease. J. clin. Endocr. 15, 1459 (1955). — Rosenbaum, J. D., S. Papper, H. W. Cohen and Regina McLean: The influence of ethanol upon maintained water diuresis in man. J. clin. Invest. 36, 1202 (1957). — Rosenberg, T.: The concept and definition of active transport. Symp. Soc. exp. Biol. 8, 27 (1954). — Rosenberg, T., u. W. Wilbrandt: Strukturabhängigkeit der Hemmwirkung von Phlorizin und anderen Phloretinderivaten auf den Glukosetransport durch die Erythrocytenmembran. Helv. physiol. pharmacol. Acta 15, 168 (1957). — Rosenfeld, G., Eugenia Rosemberg, F. Ungar and R. I. Dorfman: Regulation of the secretion of aldosterone-like material. Endocrinology 58, 255 (1956). — Rosenfeld, S., and A. Sellers: Physiological studies on the isolated perfused mammalian kidney. Clin. Res. Proc. 8, 135 (1960). — Rosnagle, R. S., and G. L. Farrell: Alterations in electrolyte intake and adrenal steroid secretion. Amer. J. Physiol. 187, 7 (1956). — Ross, E. J., W. J. Reddy, A. Rivera and G. W. Thorn: Effects of intravenous infusions of d, l-aldosterone acetate on sodium and potassium excretion in man. J. clin. Endocr. 19, 289 (1959). — Ross, W. F., and T. R. Wood: The partial purification and some observations on the nature of the parathyroid hormone. J. biol. Chem. 146, 49 (1942). — Roston, S.: Mathematical representation of some endocrinological systems. Bull. math. Biophysics 21, 271 (1959). — Roughton, F. J. W.: The kinetics and rapid thermochemistry of carbonic acid. J. Amer. chem. Soc. 63, 2930 (1941). — Rowntree, L. G., and J. T. Geraghty: An experimental and clinical study of the functional activity of the kidneys by means of phenolsulphonephthalein. J. Pharmacol. exp. Ther. 1, 579 (1909/10). — Royce, P. C., and G. Sayers: Pitressin and blood ACTH. Fed. Proc. 17, 136 (1958) (abstract). — Rubin, M. I., Erika Bruck and M. Rapoport: Maturation of renal function in childhood: clearance studies. J. clin. Invest. 28, 1144 (1949). — Rubini, M. E.: The conservation of water in potassium deficiency. Clin. Res. 8, 64 (1960). — Rubini, M. E., C. R. Kleeman and E. Lamdin: Studies on alcohol diuresis. I. The effect of ethyl alcohol ingestion on water, electrolyte and acid-base metabolism. J. clin. Invest. 34, 439 (1955). — Ruska, H., D. H. Moore and J. Weinstock: The base of the proximal convoluted tubule cells of rat kidney. J. biophys. biochem. Cytol. 3, 249 (1957). — Russell, G. V., and G. A. Drager: Correlation of neurosecretion with the known cause of diabetes insipidus. Dis. nerv. Syst. 15, 163 (1954). — Russo, H. F., L. D. Wright, Helen R. Skeggs, Elizabeth K. Tillson and K. H. Beyer: Renal clearance of essential amino acids: threonine and phenylalanine. Proc. Soc. exp. Biol. (N.Y.) 65, 215 (1947). — Ryberg, C. T.: Physiological variations in reaction of human urine. Acta physiol. scand. 6, 271 (1943). — On the formation of ammonia in the kidneys during acidosis. Acta physiol. scand. 15, 114 (1948a). — Some investigations on the CO₂ tension of the urine in man. Acta physiol. scand. 15, 123 (1948b). — Importance of sodium ions for the excretion of ammonium and hydrogen ions in the urine. Acta physiol. scand. 15, 161 (1948c). — Rydin, H., and E. B. Verney: The inhibition of water-diuresis by emotional stress and by muscular exercise. Quart. J. exp. Physiol. 27, 343 (1937/38).

Saffran, M., and A. V. Schally: The release of corticotrophin by anterior pituitary tissue in vitro. Canad. J. Biochem. 33, 408 (1955). — Saffran, M., A. V. Schally and B. G. Benfey: Stimulation of the release of corticotropin from the adenohypophysis by a neurohypophyseal factor. Endocrinology 57, 439 (1955). — Sala, G., and J. A. Luetscher jr.: The effect of sodium-retaining corticoid, electrocortin, desoxycorticosterone and cortisone on renal function and excretion of sodium and water in adrenalectomized rats. Endocrinology 55, 516 (1954). — Samiy, A. H. E., J. L. Brown and D. L. Globus: Effects of magnesium and calcium loading on renal excretion of electrolytes in dogs. Amer. J. Physiol. 198, 595 (1960). — Samiy, A. H. E., J. L. Brown, D. L. Globus, R. H. Kessler and D. D. Thompson: Interrelationship between renal transport systems of magnesium and calcium. Amer. J. Physiol. 198, 599 (1960). — Sanderson, P. H.: Renal function in Addison's disease. Clin. Sci. 6, 197 (1948). — Renal response to massive alkali loading in the human subject. The Kidney, Ciba Foundation Symposia, p. 165. Boston: Little, Brown & Co. 1954. — Sartorius, O. W., and H. Burlington: Acute effects of denervation on kidney function in the dog. Amer. J. Physiol. 185, 407 (1956). — Sartorius, O. W., D. Calhoon and R. F. Pitts: The capacity of the adrenalectomized rat to secrete hydrogen and ammonium ions. Endocrinology 51, 444 (1952). — Studies on the interrelation ships of the adrenal cortex and renal ammonia excretion by the rat. Endocrinology 52, 256 (1953). — Sartorius, O. W., and K. Roberts: The effects of pitressin and desoxycorticosterone in low dosage on the excretion of sodium, potassium and water by the normal dog. Endocrinology 45, 273 (1949). — SARTORIUS, O. W., J. C. ROEMMELT and R. F. PITTS: The renal regulation of acid-base balance in man. IV. The nature of the renal compensations in ammonium chloride acidosis. J. clin. Invest. 28, 423 (1949). — SAWYER, W.: Differences in the antidiuretic responses of rats to the intravenous administration of lysine and arginine vasopressins. Endocrinology 63, 694 (1958). — SAWYER, W. H., R. A. MUNSICK and H. B. VAN DYKE: Pharmacological evidence for the presence of arginine vasotocin and oxytocin in neurohyphophseal extracts from cold-blooded vertebrates. Nature (Lond.) 184, 1463 (1959). — SAWYER, W. H., and W. D. ROTH: Neurohypophyseal function in dehydrated and adrenalectomized rats as indicated by hormone assay and neurosecretory activity. Fed. Proc. 12, 125 (1953) (abstract). — SAYERS, G.: The adrenal cortex and homeostasis. Physiol. Rev. 30, 241 (1950). — Regulation of the secretory activity of the adrenal cortex. Amer. J. Med. 10, 539 (1951). — SAYERS, G., E. M. GLENN, K. L. SYDNOR, M. LIPSCOMB, M. L. SWEAT, L. W. KELLY jr., R. P. LEVY and W. McK. JEFFERIES: Plasma and urinary steroids after hydrocortisone infusion. J. clin. Invest. 34, 1600 (1955). — SAYERS G., E. S. REDGATE and P. C. ROYCE: Hypothalamus, adenohypophysis and adrenal cortex. Ann. Rev. Physiol. 20, 243 (1958). — SCHACHTER, D.: The chemical estimation of acyl glucuronides and its application to studies on the metabolism of benzoate and salicylate in man. J. clin. Invest. 36, 297 (1957). — SCHACHTER, D., and N. FREINKEL: Self-depression of Tm-pah in the dog at high plasma PAH levels and its reversibility by acetate. Amer. J. Physiol. 167, 531 (1951). — SCHACHTER, D., and J. G. MANIS: Salicylate and salicyl conjugates; fluorimetric estimation, biosynthesis and renal excretion in man. J. clin. Invest. 37, 800 (1958). — SCHACHTER, D., J. G. MANIS and J. V. TAGGART: Renal synthesis, degradation and active transport of aliphatic acyl amino acids. Relationship to p-aminohippurate transport. Amer. J. Physiol. 182, 537 (1955). — SCHACHTER, D., and J. V. TAGGART: Benzoyl coenzyme A and hippurate synthesis. J. biol. Chem. 203, 925 (1953). — SCHAFFER, N. K., J. F. CADDEN and H. J. STANDER: Measurement of antidiuretic activity as applied to eclamptic urine and properties of antidiuretic substances in rat urine, pituitary and beef liver. Endocrinology 28, 701 (1941). — SCHAFFER, N. K., L. V. DILL and J. F. CADDEN: Uric acid clearance in normal pregnancy and pre-eclampsia. J. clin. Invest. 22, 201 (1943). — SCHAFFER, N. K., L. V. DILL and H. J. STANDER: The effect of renin on the uric acid metabolism of the pregnant and non-pregnant Dalmatian dog. Endocrinology 29, 243 (1941). — SCHATZMANN, H. J., E. E. WINDHAGER and A. K. SOLOMON: Single proximal tubules of the Necturus kidney. II. Effect of 2,4-dinitrophenol and ouabain on water reabsorption. Amer. J. Physiol. 195, 570 (1958). — SCHEDL, H. P., and F. C. BARTTER: An explanation for and experimental correction of the abnormal water diuresis in cirrhosis. J. clin. Invest. 39, 248 (1960). — SCHER, A. M.: Focal blood flow measurements in cortex and medulla of kidney. Amer. J. Physiol. 167, 539 (1951). — Mechanism of autoregulation of renal blood flow. Nature (Lond.) 184, Suppl. 17, 1322 (1959). — SCHIESS, W. A., J. L. AYER, W. D. LOTSPEICH and R. F. PITTS: The renal regulation of acid-base balance in man. II. Factors affecting the excretion of titratable acid by the normal human subject. J. clin. Invest. 27, 57 (1948). — SCHLEGEL, J. U.: Effect of adrenaline, nor-adrenaline and hemoglobin on the pH of the urine. Amer. J. Physiol. 168, 522 (1952). — SCHLOSS, G.: Der Regulationsapparat am Gefäßpol des Nierenkörperchens in der normalen menschlichen Niere. Acta anat. (Basel) 1, 365, Suppl. 1/2 (1945/46). — SCHMIDT, C. F., and J. M. HAYMAN jr.: A note upon lymph formation in the dog's kidney and the effect of certain diuretics upon it. Amer. J. Physiol. 91, 157 (1929). — SCHMIDT-NIELSEN, BERTIL: Renal tubular excretion of urea in kangaroo rats. Amer. J. Physiol. 170, 45 (1952). — Urea excretion in white rats and kangaroo rats as influenced by excitement and by diet. Amer. J. Physiol. 181, 131 (1955). — Urea excretion in mammals. Physiol. Rev. 38, 139 (1958). — SCHMIDT-NIELSEN, BERTIL, and ROBERTA O'DELL: Effect of diet on distribution of urea and electrolytes in kidneys of sheep. Amer. J. Physiol. 197, 856 (1959). — Functional distribution of solutes in the renal tissue of rodents. Fed. Proc. 19, 366 (1960) (abstract). — SCHMIDT-NIELSEN, BERTIL, and H. OSAKI: Renal response to changes in nitrogen metabolism in sheep. Amer. J. Physiol. 193, 657 (1958). — SCHMIDT-NIELSEN, BERTIL, H. OSAKI, H. V. MURDAUGH jr. and ROBERTA O'DELL: Renal regulation of urea excretion in sheep. Amer. J. Physiol. 194, 221 (1958). — SCHMIDT-NIELSEN, BERTIL, K. SCHMIDT-NIELSEN, T. R. HOUPT and S. A. JARNUM: Urea excretion in the camel. Amer. J. Physiol. 188, 477 (1957). — SCHMIDT-NIELSEN, K., BERTIL SCHMIDT-NIELSEN and H. SCHNEIDERMAN: Salt excretion in desert mammals. Amer. J. Physiol. 154, 163 (1948). — SCHMITZ, H. L.: Studies on the action of diuretics. I. The effect of euphyllin and salyrgan upon glomerular filtration and tubular reabsorption. J. clin. Invest. 11, 1075 (1932). — SCHNECKLOTH, R. E., I. H. PAGE and A. C. CORCORAN: Depressed renal function in the carcinoid syndrome: Effects of serotonin in normal subjects and of an antiserotonin (Bromo-LSD). Clin. Res. Proc. 5, 308 (1957) (abstract). — SCHNEEBERG, N. G.: Concentration test of renal function using posterior pituitary injection; evaluation. Arch.

intern. Med. 80, 193 (1947). — SCHNEIDER, R. W., and A. C. CORCORAN: Familial nephrogenic osteopathy due to excessive tubular reabsorption of inorganic phosphate: A new syndrome and a novel mode of relief. J. Lab. clin. Med. 36, 985 (1950) (abstract). — SCHOEN, E. J.: Minimum urine total solute concentration in response to water loading in normal men. J. appl. Physiol. 10, 267 (1957). — SCHOR, N. A., and J. FERRER: The neurosecretory material of the rat's infundibular process in the diabetes insipidus induced by aminopterin. Acta physiol. lat.-amer. 7, 201 (1957). — SCHOU, P.: Experimental studies on kidney function during sulphate diuresis; investigations on tubular function of rabbit kidneys during infusion of hypertonic sulphate-solution. Acta physiol. scand. 7, 183 (1944a). — Experimental studies on kidney function during sulphate diuresis; investigations on kidney function in rabbits with chronic tubular nephritis. Acta physiol. scand. 7, 200 (1944b). — SCHREINER, G. E.: Determination of inulin by means of resorcinol. Proc. Soc. exp. Biol. (N.Y.) 74, 117 (1950). — SCHREINER, G. E., L. G. WESSON and W. P. ANSLOW: Contamination of commercial p-aminohippuric acid with p-aminobenzoic acid. Proc. Soc. exp. Biol. (N.Y.) 70, 726 (1949). — SCHROEDER, H. A., and J. M. STEELE: The behavior of renal blood flow after partial constriction of the renal artery. J. exp. Med. 72, 707 (1940). — SCHÜCK, O., R. SMAHELOVA u. J. STRIBRNA: Die osmotische Funktion der Nieren bei chronischer Niereninsuffizienz. Klin. Wschr. 37, 293 (1959). — SCHULTEN, H.: Über die Harnbildung in der Froschniere. Die Ausscheidung von Säurefarbstoffen durch die überlebende Froschniere. Pflügers Arch. ges. Physiol. 208, 1 (1925). — SCHULTHESS-SALLMANN, BEATRICE: Der Einfluß experimenteller Acidose und Alkalose auf die Ultrafiltrierbarkeit des Plasmacalciums und die Calciumausscheidung im Urin beim Menschen. Helv. med. Acta 25, 601 (1958). — SCHULTZ jr., E. H., and J. COWEN: Abnormalities in urine concentration function in alcoholics. Quart. J. Stud. Alcohol. 15, 379 (1954). — SCHWAB, L., and W. D. LOTSPEICH: Renal tubular reabsorption of acetoacetate in the dog. Amer. J. Physiol. 176, 195 (1954). — SCHWARTZ, I. L., E. S. BREED and M. H. MAXWELL: Comparison of the volume of distribution, renal and extrarenal clearances of inulin and mannitol in man. J. clin. Invest. 29, 517 (1950). — SCHWARTZ, W. B., W. BENNETT, S. CURELOP and F. C. BARTTER: A syndrome of renal sodium loss and hyponatremia probably resulting from inappropriate secretion of antidiuretic hormone. Amer. J. Med. 23, 529 (1957). — SCHWARTZ, W. B., A. FALBRIARD and G. LEMIEUX: The kinetics of bicarbonate reabsorption during acute respiratory acidosis. J. clin. Invest. 38, 939 (1959). — SCHWARTZ, W. B., A. FALBRIARD and A. S. RELMAN: An analysis of bicarbonate reabsorption during partial inhibition of carbonic anhydrase. J. clin. Invest. 37, 744 (1958). — SCHWARTZ, W. B., P. W. HALL 3rd, R. M. HAYS and A. S. RELMAN: On the mechanism of acidosis in chronic renal disease. J. clin. Invest. 38, 39 (1959). — SCHWARTZ, W. B., R. L. JENSON and A. S. RELMAN: Acidification of the urine and increased ammonium excretion without change in acid-base equilibrium: sodium reabsorption as a stimulus to the acidifying process. J. clin. Invest. 34, 673 (1955). — SCHWARTZ, W. B., G. LEMIEUX and A. FALBRIARD: Renal reabsorption of bicarbonate during acute respiratory alkalosis. J. clin. Invest. 38, 2197 (1959). — SCHWARTZ, W. B., and A. S. RELMAN: Metabolic and renal studies in chronic potassium depletion resulting from overuse of laxatives. J. clin. Invest. 32, 258 (1953). — The dependence of renal sodium reabsorption on hydrogen exchange. J. clin. Invest. 33, 965 (1954) (abstract). — SCHWARTZ, W. B., A. S. RELMAN and A. LEAF: Oral administration of a potent carbonic anhydrase inhibitor (Diamox): Its use as a diuretic in patients with severe congestive heart failure due to cor pulmonale. Ann. intern. Med. 42, 79 (1955). — SCHWEIZER, M., R. GAUNT, N. ZINKEN and W. O. NELSON: Role of adrenal cortex and anterior pituitary in diabetes insipidus. Amer. J. Physiol. 132, 141 (1941). — SCIAN, L. F., C. D. WESTERMANN, O. R. KRUESI and J. G. HILTON: Effect of ACTH and vasopressin on aldosterone secretion. Fed. Proc. 18, 545 (1959) (abstract). — SCOTT jr., H. W., and S. R. ELLIOTT II: Renal hemodynamics in congenital cyanotic heart disease. Bull. Johns Hopk. Hosp. 86, 58 (1950). — SCRIBNER, B. H., M. A. CRAWFORD and W. J. DEMPSTER: Urinary excretion by nonionic diffusion. Amer. J. Physiol. 196, 1135 (1959). — SEGAR, W. E.: Effect of hypothermia on tubular transport mechanisms. Amer. J. Physiol. 195, 91 (1958). — SEGAR, W. E., P. A. RILEY and T. G. BARILA: Urinary composition during hypothermia. Amer. J. Physiol. 185, 528 (1956). — SELDIN, D. W., R. M. PORTWOOD, F. C. RECTOR jr. and R. CADE: Characteristics of renal bicarbonate reabsorption in man. J. clin. Invest. 38, 1663 (1959). — SELDIN, D. W., and R. TARAIL: Effect of hypertonic solutions on metabolism and excretion of electrolytes. Amer. J. Physiol. 159, 160 (1949). — SELDIN, D. W., L. G. WELT and J. H. CORT: The role of sodium salts and adrenal steroids in the production of hypokalemic alkalosis. Yale J. Biol. Med. 29, 229 (1956). — SELKURT, E. E.: Influence of glucose renal tubular reabsorption and p-aminohippuric acid tubular excretion on simultaneous clearance of ascorbic acid. Amer. J. Physiol. 142, 182 (1944). — The relation of renal blood flow to effective arterial pressure in the intact kidney of the dog. Amer. J. Physiol. 147, 537 1946). — Effect of pulse pressure and mean arterial pressure modification on renal hemodynamics and electrolyte and water excretion. Circulation 4, 541 (1951). — Der Nierenkreislauf. Klin. Wschr. 33, 359 (1955). — SELKURT, E. E., M. BRANDFONBRENNER and H. M. GELLER: Effects of ureteral pressure increase on renal hemodynamics and the handling of water and electrolytes. Amer. J. Physiol. 170, 61 (1952). — SELKURT, E. E., P. W. HALL and M. P. SPENCER: Response of renal blood flow and clearance to graded partial obstruction of the renal vein. Amer. J. Physiol. 157, 40 (1949a). — Influence of graded arterial pressure decrement on renal clearance of creatinine, p-aminohippurate and sodium. Amer. J. Physiol. 159, 369 (1949b). — SELKURT, E. E., and C. R. HOUCK: The effect of sodium and potassium chloride on the renal clearance of ascorbic acid. Amer. J. Physiol. 141, 423 (1943/44). — SELKURT, E. E., and R. S. POST: Renal clearance of sodium in the dog: Effect of increasing sodium load on reabsorptive mechanism. Amer. J. Physiol. 162, 639 (1950). — SELKURT, E. E., M. P. SCIBETTA and T. E. CULL: Hemodynamics of intestinal circulation. Circulat. Res. 6, 92 (1958). — SELKURT, E. E., L. J. TALBOT and C. R. HOUCK: Effect of administration of estrogen on mechanism of ascorbic acid excretion in dog. Amer. J. Physiol. 140, 260 (1943). — SELLERS, A. L., N. GRIGGS, J. MARMORSTON and H. C. GOODMAN: Filtration and reabsorption of protein by the kidney. J. exp. Med. 100, 1 (1954). — SELLWOOD, R. V., and E. B. VERNEY: The effect of water and of isotonic saline administration on the renal plasma and glomerular filtrate flows in the dog, with incidental observations of the effects on those flows of compression of the carotid and renal arteries. Phil. Trans. B 238, 361 (1955). — SELYE, H.: Mechanism of parathyroid hormone action. Arch. Path. (Chicago) 34, 625 (1942). — SEMPLE, S. J. G., and H. E. DE WARDENER: Effect of increased renal venous pressure on circulatory "autoregulation" of isolated dog kidneys. Circulat. Res. 7, 643 (1959). — SHANNON, J. A.: Absorption and excretion of water and salts by the Elasmobranch fishes. IV. The secretion of exogenous creatinine by the dogfish, Squalus acanthias. J. cell. comp. Physiol. 4, 211 (1933). — The excretion of inulin by the dogfish, Squalus acanthias. J. cell. comp. Physiol. 5, 301 (1934). — The excretion of inulin by the dog. Amer. J. Physiol. 112, 405 (1935a). — The excretion of inulin and creatinine at low urine flows by the normal dog. Amer. J. Physiol. 114, 362 (1935b). — The renal excretion of creatinine in man. J. clin. Invest. 14, 403 (1935c). — Glomerular filtration and urea excretion in relation to urine flow in the dog. Amer. J. Physiol. 117, 206 (1936). — Excretion of inulin, creatinine, xylose and urea in the sheep. Proc. Soc. exp. Biol. (N.Y.) 37, 379 (1937). — The tubular reabsorption of xylose in the normal dog. Amer. J. Physiol. 122, 775 (1938a). — Urea excretion in the normal dog during forced diuresis. Amer. J. Physiol. 122, 782 (1938b). — The excretion of exogenous creatinine by the chicken. J. cell. comp. Physiol. 11, 123 (1938c). — The excretion of uric acid by the chicken. J. cell. comp. Physiol. 11, 135 (1938d). — The renal excretion of phenol red by the aglomerular fishes, Opsanus tau and Lophius piscatorius. J. cell. comp. Physiol. 11, 315 (1938e). — Renal tubular excretion. Physiol. Rev. 19, 63 (1939). — On the mechanism of the renal tubular excretion of creatinine in the dogfish, Squalus acanthias. J. cell. comp. Physiol. 16, 285 (1940). — Control of renal excretion of water; effect of variations in state of hydration on water excretion in dogs with diabetes insipidus. J. exp. Med. 76, 371 (1942a). — Control of renal excretion of water; rate of liberation of posterior pituitary antidiuretic hormone in dog. J. exp. Med. 76, 387 (1942b). — SHANNON, J. A., S. FARBER and L. TROAST: The measurement of glucose Tm in the normal dog. Amer. J. Physiol. 133, 752 (1941). — SHANNON, J. A., and S. FISHER: The renal tubular reabsorption of glucose in the normal dog. Amer. J. Physiol. 122, 765 (1938). — SHANNON, J. A., N. JOLLIFFE and H. W. SMITH: The excretion of urine in the dog. IV. The effect of maintenance diet upon the quantity of glomerular filtrate. Amer. J. Physiol. 101, 625 (1932a). — The excretion of urine in the dog. VI. The filtration and secretion of exogenous creatinine. Amer. J. Physiol. 102, 534 (1932b). — SHANNON, J. A., and H. A. RANGES: On renal tubular excretion of creatinine in normal man. J. clin. Invest. 20, 169 (1941). — SHANNON, J. A., and H. W. SMITH: The excretion of inulin, xylose and urea by normal and phlorizinized man. J. clin. Invest. 14, 393 (1935). — SHANNON, J. A., and F. R. WINTON: Renal excretion of inulin and creatinine by anaesthetized dog and pump-lung-kidney preparation. J. Physiol. (Lond.) 98, 97 (1940). — SHAPIRO, B.: The mechanism of phloridzin glucosuria. Biochem. J. 41, 151 (1947). — SHARE, L.: Effect of increased ureteral pressure on renal function. Amer. J. Physiol. 168, 97 (1952). — SHARE, L., and P. W. HALL III: Excretion of electrolytes and water by the salt-loaded adrenalectomized dog. Amer. J. Physiol. 183, 291 (1955). — SHARE, L., and J. B. STADLER: Alterations in sodium and potassium metabolism following hind leg fracture in the rat: Role of the adrenal cortex. Endocrinology 62, 119 (1958). — SHAW, C. C., W. P. BOGER, J. W. CROSSON, W. W. KEMP, W. S. M. LING and G. G. DUNCAN: Enhancement of penicillin blood levels in man by means of a new compound, caronamide. Amer. J. Med. 3, 206 (1947). — SHAW, E. C.: A study of the curve of elimination of phenolsulphonphthalein by the normal and diseased kidneys. J. Urol. (Baltimore) 13, 575 (1925). — SHERLOCK, SHEILA, A. E. READ, J. L. LAIDLAW and R. HASLAM: Chlorothiazide in liver disease. Ann. N.Y. Acad. Sci. 71, 430 (1958). —

SHERRY, S., G. J. FRIEDMAN, K. PALEY, J. BERKMAN and ELAINE P. RALLI: Mechanism of excretion of vitamin C by dog kidney. Amer. J. Physiol. **130**, 276 (1940). — SHIDEMAN, F. E., R. C. RATHBUN and FERNLEY STONEMAN: Inhibition of the renal tubular transport of p-aminohippurate and phenolsulfonphthalein as affected by acetate. Amer. J. Physiol. **170**, 31 (1952). — SHIDEMAN, F. E., and R. M. RENE: Succinate oxidation and Krebs cycle as an energy source for renal tubular transport mechanisms. Amer. J. Physiol. **166**, 104 (1951). — SHIPLEY, R. E., and R. S. STUDY: Changes in renal blood flow, extraction of inulin, glomerular filtration rate, tissue pressure and urine flow with acute alterations of renal artery blood pressure. Amer. J. Physiol. **167**, 676 (1951). — SHIPP, J. C., I. B. HANEN-SON, E. E. WINDHAGER, H. J. SCHATZMANN, G. WHITTEMBURY, H. YOSHIMURA and A. K. SOLOMON: Single proximal tubules of the Necturus kidney. Methods for micropuncture and microperfusion. Amer. J. Physiol. **195**, 563 (1958). — SHORE, V., and B. SHORE: Effect of mercuric chloride on some kidney enzymes in chow-fed and sucrose-fed rats. Amer. J. Physiol. **198**, 187 (1960). — SHORR, E., ALICE R. BERNHEIM and HERTHA TAUSSKY: The relation of urinary citric acid excretion to the menstrual cycle and the steroidal reproductive hormones. Science **95**, 606 (1942). — SHORR, E., R. O. LOEBEL and H. B. RICHARDSON: Tissue metabolism. I. The nature of phlorhizin diabetes. J. biol. Chem. **86**, 529 (1930). — SHORR, E., B. W. ZWEIFACH, R. F. FURCHGOTT and S. BAEZ: Hepatorenal factors in circulatory homeostasis. IV. Tissue origins of the vasotropic principles, VEM and VDM, which appear during evolution of hemorrhagic and tourniquet shock. Circulation **3**, 42 (1951). — SHÜCK, O., and J. STŘÍBRNÁ: Changes in renal sodium excretion after filling of the urinary bladder. Physiol. Bohemosl. **8**, 378 (1959). — SIEBENMANN, R. E.: Über eine tödlich verlaufende Anorexia nervosa mit Hypokaliämie. Schweiz. med. Wschr. **85**, 354 (1955). — SIEKER, H. O., O. H. GAUER and J. P. HENRY: The effect of continuous negative pressure breathing on water and electrolyte excretion by the human kidney. J. clin. Invest. **33**, 572 (1954). — SILVETTE, H.: Influence of post-pituitary extract on excretion of water and chlorides by renal tubules. Amer. J. Physiol. **128**, 747 (1940a). — Effect of diminishing doses of post-pituitary extract on urinary excretion of water and chlorides. Proc. Soc. exp. Biol. (N.Y.) **45**, 599 (1940b). — Mechanism of pentothal sodium antidiuresis. Arch. intern. Med. **70**, 567 (1942). — Some effects of low barometric pressures on kidney function in white rat. Amer. J. Physiol. **140**, 374 (1943). — SILVETTE, H., and S. W. BRITTON: Renal function in the opossum and the mechanism of corticoadrenal and post pituitary action. Amer. J. Physiol. **123**, 630 (1938). — SIMMONS, D. H., N. A. ASSALI and M. AVEDON: Relative influence of respiratory and metabolic acid-base changes on renal acid excretion. Amer. J. Physiol. **198**, 237 (1960). — SIMMONS, D. H., R. B. HARVEY and T. HOSHIKO: Role of adrenal and hypophysis in regulation of sodium excretion. Amer. J. Physiol. **181**, 379 (1955). — SIMPSON, G. E.: Diurnal variations in the rate of urine excretion for two hour intervals: Some associated factors. J. biol. Chem. **59**, 107 (1924). — The effect of sleep on urinary chlorides and pH. J. biol. Chem. **67**, 505 (1925). — Changes in the composition of urine brought about by sleep and other factors. J. biol. Chem. **84**, 393 (1929). — SIMPSON, S. A., J. F. TAIT, A. WETTSTEIN, R. NEHER, J. v. EUW u. T. REICHSTEIN: Isolierung eines neuen kristallisierten Hormons aus Nebennieren mit besonders hoher Wirksamkeit auf den Mineralstoffwechsel. Experientia (Basel) **9**, 333 (1953). — SIMPSON, S. A., J. F. TAIT, A. WETTSTEIN, R. NEHER, J. v. EUW, O. SCHINDLER u. T. REICHSTEIN: Konstitution des Aldosterons, des neuen Mineralocorticoids. Experientia (Basel) **10**, 132 (1954a). — Aldosteron. Isolierung und Eigenschaften. Über Bestandteile der Nebennierenrinde und verwandte Stoffe. Helv. chim. Acta **37**, 1163 (1954b). — Die Konstitution des Aldosterons. Über Bestandteile der Nebennierenrinde und verwandter Stoffe. Helv. chim. Acta **37**, 1200 (1954c). — SIMS, E. A. H., and K. E. KRANTZ: Serial studies of renal function during pregnancy and the puerperium in normal women. J. clin. Invest. **37**, 1764 (1958). — SINCLAIR-SMITH, B., A. A. KATTUS, J. GENEST and E. V. NEWMAN: The renal mechanism of electrolyte excretion and the metabolic balances of electrolytes and nitrogen in congestive cardiac failure; the effects of exercise, rest and aminophyllin. Bull. Johns Hopk. Hosp. **84**, 369 (1949). — SINGER, BERTHA: Aldosterone in the adrenal vein blood of nephrotic rats. Endocrinology **60**, 420 (1957). — Effect of aldosterone-antagonist, SC 8109, on the secretion of aldosterone in normal rats. Endocrinology **65**, 512 (1959). — SINGER, BERTHA, and M. P. STACK-DUNNE: The secretion of aldosterone and corticosterone by the rat adrenal. J. Endocr. **12**, 130 (1955). — SIROTA, J. G.: Renal tubule reabsorption of phosphate in hyperparathyroidism before and after removal of parathyroid adenoma. Fed. Proc. **12**, 133 (1953) (abstract). — SIROTA, J. H., D. S. BALDWIN and H. VILLARREAL: Diurnal variations in renal function in man. J. clin. Invest. **29**, 187 (1950). — SIROTA, J. H., and D. HAMERMAN: Renal function studies in an adult subject with the Fanconi syndrome. Amer. J. Med. **16**, 138 (1954). — SIROTA, J. H., and I. G. KROOP: Evidence suggesting renal tubular excretion of potassium in man during recovery from acute renal insufficiency. J. clin. Invest. **30**, 1082 (1951). — SIROTA, J. H., TSAI F. YÜ and A. B. GUTMAN: The effect of Benemid (p-(di-n-propylsulfamyl)-benzoic acid) on urate clearance and other discrete renal functions in gouty subjects. J. clin. Invest. **31**, 692 (1952). — SJÖSTRAND, F.: Über die Eigenfluoreszenz tierischer Gewebe mit besonderer Berücksichtigung der Säugetierniere. Acta anat. (Basel) **1**, Suppl., 1—2 (1945/46). — SJÖSTRAND, F., and J. RHODIN: The ultrastructure of the proximal convoluted tubules of the mouse kidney as revealed by high resolution electron microscopy. Exp. cell. Res. **4**, 426 (1953). — SKILLERN, P. G., A. C. CORCORAN and HAR-RIET DUSTAN: A study of diabetes insipidus and primary adrenal cortical failure in the same patient. J. Lab. clin. Med. **44**, 931 (1954). — SKILLERN, P. G., A. C. CORCORAN and A. L. SCHERBEL: Renal mechanisms in coincident Addison's disease and diabetes insipidus: Effects of vasopressin and hydrocortisone. J. clin. Endocr. **16**, 171 (1956). — SKULAN, T. W., H. E. WILLIAMSON and F. E. SHIDEMAN: Localization of renal tubular functions in the rat by stop flow analysis. Fed. Proc. **18**, 445 (1959) (abstract). — SLESSOR, A.: Studies concerning the mechanism of water retention in Addison's disease and in hypopituitarism. J. clin. Endocr. **11**, 700 (1951). — SLYKE, D. D. VAN: Effect of urine volume on urea excretion. J. clin. Invest. **26**, 1159 (1947). — SLYKE, D. D. VAN, ALMA HILLER and B. F. MILLER: The clearance, extraction percentage and estimated filtration of sodium ferrocyanide in the mammalian kidney. Comparison with inulin, creatinine and urea. Amer. J. Physiol. **113**, 611 (1935). — SLYKE, D. D. VAN, G. LINDER, ALMA HILLER, L. LEITER and F. J. MAC-INTOSH: The excretion of ammonia and titratable acid in nephritis. J. clin. Invest. **2**, 255 (1926). — SLYKE, D. D. VAN, R. A. PHILLIPS, P. B. HAMILTON, R. M. ARCHIBALD, P. H. FUTCHER and ALMA HILLER: Glutamine as source material of urinary ammonia. J. biol. Chem. **150**, 481 (1943). — SLYKE, D. D. VAN, C. P. RHOADS, ALMA HILLER and A. S. AL-VING: Relationships between urea excretion, renal blood flow, renal oxygen consumption and diuresis. The mechanism of urea excretion. Amer. J. Physiol. **109**, 336 (1934). — SMETANA, H.: Permeability of the renal glomeruli of several mammalian species to labelled proteins. Amer. J. Path. **23**, 255 (1947). — SMETANA, H., and F. R. JOHNSON: The origin of colloid and lipoid droplets in the epithelial cells of the renal tubules. Amer. J. Path. **18**, 1029 (1942). — SMITH, F. M., and E. M. MACKAY: Influence of posterior pituitary extracts on sodium balance in normal subject and in patient with diabetes insipidus. Proc. Soc. exp. Biol. (N.Y.) **34**, 116 (1936). — SMITH, H. W.: The absorption and excretion of water and salts by the Elasmobranch fishes. I. Fresh water Elasmobranchs. Amer. J. Physiol. **98**, 279 (1931). — The composition of urine in the seal. J. cell. comp. Physiol. **7**, 465 (1935). — The retention of physiological role of urea in the Elasmobranchii. Biol. Rev. **11**, 49 (1936). — The physiology of the kidney. New York: Oxford University Press 1937. — Physiology of the renal circulation. Harvey Lectures **35**, 166 (1939). — Excretion of water. Bull. N.Y. Acad. Med. **23**, 177 (1947). — The kidney. Structure and function in health and disease. New York: Oxford University Press 1951. — Principles of renal physiology. New York: Oxford University Press 1956. — Salt and water volume receptors. An exercise in physiologic apologetics. Amer. J. Med. **23**, 623 (1957). — SMITH, H. W., H. CHASIS, W. GOLDRING and H. A. RANGES: Glomerular dynamics in normal human kidney. J. clin. Invest. **19**, 751 (1940). — SMITH, H. W., H. CHASIS and H. A. RANGES: Suitability of inulin for intravenous administration to man. Proc. Soc. exp. Biol. (N.Y.) **37**, 726 (1937/38). — SMITH, H. W., and R. W. CLARKE: The excretion of inulin and creatinine by the anthropoid apes and other infrahuman primates. Amer. J. Physiol. **122**, 132 (1938). — SMITH, H. W., NORMA FINKEL-STEIN, LUCY ALIMINOSA, BETTY CRAWFORD and MARTHA GRABER: Renal clearances of substituted hippuric acid derivatives and other aromatic acids in dog and man. J. clin. Invest. **24**, 388 (1945). — SMITH, H. W., W. GOLDRING and H. CHASIS: The measurement of the tubular excretory mass, effective blood flow and filtration rate in the normal human kidney. J. clin. Invest. **17**, 263 (1938). — SMITH, H. W., W. GOLDRING, H. CHASIS, H. A. RANGES and S. E. BRADLEY: The application of saturation methods to the study of glome-rular and tubular function in the human kidney. J. Mt Sinai Hosp. **10**, 59 (1943). — SMITH, H. W., E. A. ROVENSTINE, W. GOLDRING, H. CHASIS and H. A. RANGES: The effects of spinal anesthesia on the circulation in normal unoperated man with reference to autonomy of the arterioles and especially those of the renal circulation. J. clin. Invest. **18**, 319 (1939). — SMITH, J. F.: Anatomical features of the human renal glomerular efferent vessel. J. Anat. (Lond.) **90**, 290 (1956). — SMITH, P. K., HELEN L. GLEASON, C. G. STOLL and S. OGOR-ZALEK: Studies on the pharmacology of salicylates. J. Pharmacol. exp. Ther. **87**, 237 (1946). — SMITH, P. K., R. W. OLLAYOS and A. W. WINKLER: Tubular reabsorption of phosphate in dog. J. clin. Invest. **22**, 143 (1943). — SMITH, W. O., A. KYRIAKOPOULOS, D. C. MOCK and J. F. HAMMARSTEN: The influence of various diuretic agents on the urinary excretion of magnesium in nonedematous subjects. Clin. Res. Proc. **7**, 162 (1959) (abstract). — SMITH, W. P., S. PAPPER and J. D. ROSENBAUM: Inhibition of antidiuretic hormone activity as the mechanism of promazine-induced diuresis. Clin. Res. Proc. **6**, 289 (1958) (abstract). — SMITH, WILLIE W.: Glomerular filtration and renal blood flow in the rabbit. Amer. J. Physiol. **133**, P452 (1941) (abstract). — SMITH, WILLIE W., NORMA FINKELSTEIN and H. W. SMITH: Renal

374 Laurence G. Wesson:

excretion of hexitols (sorbitol, mannitol, and dulcitol) and their derivatives (sorbitan, iso-mannide, and sorbide) and of endogenous creatinine-like chromogen in dog and man. J. biol. Chem. **135**, 231 (1940). — Smith, Willie W., and H. A. Ranges: Renal clearances of iopax, neoiopax and skiodan in man. Amer. J. Physiol. **123**, 720 (1938). — Smith, Willie W., and H. W. Smith: Protein binding of phenol red, diodrast, and other substances in plasma. J. biol. Chem. **124**, 107 (1938). — Smulyan, H., and L. G. Raisz: Pseudo-pseudohypopara-thyroidism with unusual features. J. clin. Endocr. **19**, 478 (1959). — Smythe, C. M., J. F. Nickel and S. E. Bradley: The effect of epinephrine (USP), l-epinephrine and l-norepi-nephrine on glomerular filtration rate, renal plasma flow, and the urinary excretion of sodium, potassium and water in normal man. J. clin. Invest. **31**, 499 (1952). — Snapper, I., u. E. Laqueur: Bestimmung der Hippursäure im Harn. Biochem. Z. **145/146**, 32 (1924). — Sobel, H., R. S. Levy, J. Marmorston, S. Schapiro and S. Rosenfeld: Increased excretion of urinary corticoids by guinea pigs following administration of Pitressin. Proc. Soc. exp. Biol. (N.Y.) **89**, 10 (1955). — Sodeman, W. A., and H. T. Engelhardt: Renal concentration test employing use of pituitary extracts. Response of normal subjects. Proc. Soc. exp. Biol. (N.Y.) **46**, 688 (1941). — Soffer, L. J., and J. L. Gabrilove: A simplified water-loading test for the diagnosis of Addison's disease. Metabolism **1**, 504 (1952). — Soffer, L. J., J. L. Gabrilove and M. D. Jacobs: Further studies with the salt tolerance test in normal individuals and in patients with adrenal cortical hyperfunction. J. clin. Invest. **28**, 1091 (1949). — Soffer, L. J., G. Lesnick, S. Z. Sorkin, H. H. Sobotka and Mildred Jacobs: The utilization of intravenously injected salt in normals and in patients with Cushing's syndrome before and after administration of desoxycorticosterone acetate. J. clin. Invest. **23**, 51 (1944). — Sohar, E., E. Scadron and M. F. Levitt: Changes in renal hemodynamics during normal pregnancy. Clin. Res. Proc. **4**, 142 (1956) (abstract). — Solomon, A. K., I. B. Hanenson, J. C. Shipp, E. E. Windhager and H. J. Schatzmann: In vivo perfusion of proximal tubule of Necturus kidney. Fed. Proc. **16**, 121 (1957) (ab-stract). — Solomon, S.: Transtubular potential differences of rat kidney. J. cell. comp. Physiol. **49**, 351 (1957). — Solomon, S., Betty J. Davis and O. R. Boone: Effect of atropine and choline on urinary electrolytes. Amer. J. Physiol. **198**, 233 (1960). — Spanner, R.: Über Gefäßkurzschlüsse in der Niere. Anat. Anz. **45**, 81 (1937). — Spencer, Herta, Vernice Vankinscott, I. Lewin and D. Laszlo: Removal of calcium in man by ethylene-diamine tetra-acetic acid. J. clin. Invest. **31**, 1023 (1952). — Spencer, M. P.: Renal dynamics in experimental polycythemia. Amer. J. Physiol. **165**, 399 (1951). — Acute effects of moderate increases in the hematocrit on the hemodynamics of the normal and denervated kidney. Amer. J. Physiol. **178**, 462 (1954). — Sperber, Christine, and I. Sperber: Observa-tions on creatinine excretion in ruminants. Kgl. Lantbrukshögskolans Ann. **22**, 125 (1956). — Sperber, I.: Studies on the mammalian kidney. Zool. Bidr. Uppsala **22**, 249 (1944). — The excretion of some glucuronic acid derivitives and phenol sulfuric esters in the chicken. Ann. roy. agric. Coll. Sweden **13**, 317 (1946). — Specific and nonspecific competition in tubu-lar excretion. Nature (Lond.) **161**, 236 (1948). — Investigations on the circulatory system of the avian kidney. Zool. Bidr. Uppsala **27**, 429 (1949a). — The excretion of piperidine, guanidine, methylguanidine and N'-methylnicotinamide in the chicken. Ann. roy. agric. Coll. Sweden **16**, 49 (1949b). — Competitive inhibition and specificity of renal tubular trans-port mechanisms. Arch. int. Pharmacodyn. **97**, 221 (1954). — Spinazzola, A. J., and T. R. Sherrod: The effects of serotonin (5-hydroxytryptamine) on renal hemodynamics. J. Pharmacol. exp. Ther. **119**, 114 (1957). — Spingarn, C., M. G. Mulinos and E. Maculla: Effects of pitressin tannate and water restriction on water exchange and renal function of normal dogs. Endocrinology **35**, 249 (1944). — Sprague, J. M.: The chemistry of diuretics. Ann. N.Y. Acad. Sci. **71**, 328 (1958). — Sprague, R. G., M. H. Power, H. L. Mason, A. Albert, D. R. Mathieson, P. S. Rech, E. C. Kendall, C. H. Slocumb and H. F. Pol-ley: Observations on the physiologic effects of cortisone and ACTH in man. Arch. intern. Med. **85**, 199 (1950). — Spritz, N., G. W. Frimpter, W. S. Braveman and A. L. Rubin: Osmole and water excretion in mercurial diuresis in congestive heart failure. Circulation **19**, 600 (1959). — Spurr, C. L., and R. V. Ford: The influence of pitocin on renal function in patients with pituitary insufficiency, renal disease and hypertension, and in normal patients. J. Lab. clin. Med. **48**, 946 (1956) (abstract). — Spurr, C. L., R. V. Ford and J. H. Moyer: The effect of probenecid (Benemid) on phosphate excretion and other meta-bolic processes. Amer. J. med. Sci. **228**, 256 (1954). — Squires, R. D., P. Han and Mary Zemach: Osmoreceptors in the cat. Fed. Proc. **18**, 151 (1959) (abstract). — Squires, R. D., and E. J. Huth: Experimental potassium depletion in normal human subjects. I. Rela-tion of ionic intakes to the renal conservation of potassium. J. clin. Invest. **38**, 1134 (1959). — Stahl, J., F. Stephan, H. Jahn, M. Urban and M. Jahn: Experimental cortexone poly-uria and cortexone oedema in dogs. Aldosterone, p. 167. Boston: Little, Brown & Co. 1958). — Stalder, G., R. Schmid u. I. Gerstner: Die maximale tubuläre Phosphat-Rückresorp-tion (Tm_p) in den Nieren des gesunden Kindes. Ann. Paediat. **189**, 293 (1957). — Stam-

LER, J.: Failure of tubular reabsorption loads of ascorbic acid or amino acids to affect renal handling of sodium and potassium. Amer. J. Physiol. 165, 109 (1951). — STAMLER, J., L. DREIFUS, L. N. KATZ and I. J. LICHTON: Response to rapid water, sodium and dextran loads of intact Ringer's-infused unanesthetized dogs. Amer. J. Physiol. 195, 362 (1958). — STANBURY, S. W.: In: Aldosterone, p. 221. Boston: Little, Brown & Co. 1958a. — Some aspects of disordered renal tubular function. Advanc. intern. Med. 9, 231 (1958b). — STANBURY, S. W., and A. E. THOMSON: Diurnal variations in electrolyte excretion. Clin. Sci. 10, 267 (1951). — The renal response to respiratory alkalosis. Clin. Sci. 11, 357 (1952). — STARK, IRENE, and M. SOMOGYI: Quantitative relationship between beta-hydroxybutyric acid and acetoacetic acid in blood and urine. J. biol. Chem. 147, 319 (1943). — STARLING, E. H., and E. B. VERNEY: The secretion of urine as studied on the isolated kidney. Proc. roy. Soc. B 97, 321 (1925). — STEAD jr., E. A.: Edema and dyspnea of heart failure. Bull. N.Y. Acad. Med. 28, 159 (1952). — STEHLE, R. L.: The diuretic-antidiuretic action of pituitary extract. Amer. J. Physiol. 79, 289 (1926/27). — Der antidiuretisch wirkende Anteil des Hypophysenhinterlappens. Naunyn-Schmiedeberg's Arch. exp. Path. Pharmak. 175, 471 (1934). — STEHLE, R. L., and W. J. BOURNE: The effect of pituitary extract on the secretion and composition of the urine. J. Physiol. (Lond.) 60, 229 (1925). — STEIGER, M., u. E. STREHLER: Atmung und Ammoniakbildung der Niere bei sublimatvergifteten Kaninchen. Klin. Wschr. 25, 171 (1946). — STEIN, M., R. SCHWARTZ and I. A. MIRSKY: The antidiuretic activity of plasma of patients with hepatic cirrhosis, congestive heart failure, hypertension and other clinical disorders. J. clin. Invest. 33, 77 (1954). — STEIN, W. H., A. G. BEARN and S. MOORE: The amino acid content of the blood and urine in Wilson's disease. J. clin. Invest. 33, 410 (1954). — STEINITZ, K.: A colorimetric method for the determination of inulin in blood plasma and urine. J. biol. Chem. 126, 589 (1938). — Studies on conditions of glucose excretion in man. J. clin. Invest. 19, 299 (1940a). — Renal excretion of sucrose in normal man; comparison with inulin. Amer. J. Physiol. 129, 252 (1940b). — STEINITZ, K., and H. TURKAND: Determination of glomerular filtration by endogenous creatinine clearance. J. clin. Invest. 19, 285 (1940). — STEWART, G. S., and H. F. BOWEN: The parathyroid control of serum calcium independent of renal mediation. Endocrinology 48, 568 (1951). — The urinary phosphate excretion factor of parathyroid gland extracts: a hormone or an artefact. Endocrinology 51, 80 (1952). — STEWART, J. D., and G. MARGARET ROURKE: The effects of large intravenous infusions on body fluid. J. clin. Invest. 21, 197 (1942). — STOCK, R. J., G. H. MUDGE and MIRIAM J. NURNBERG: Congestive heart failure variations in electrolyte metabolism with salt restriction and mercurial diuretics. Circulation 4, 54 (1951). — STOERK, H. C.: Activity of parathyroid hormone in the nephrectomized rat. Proc. Soc. exp. Biol. (N.Y.) 54, 50 (1943). — STOERK, H. C., and W. H. CARNES: The relation of the dietary Ca:P ratio to serum Ca and to parathyroid volume. J. Nutr. 29, 43 (1945). — STOERK, H. C., and R. H. SILBER: Parathormone in renal reabsorption of phosphate. Lab. Invest. 5, 213 (1956). — STOLOFF, I. L., D. M. WATKIN and N. W. SHOCK: The ratio Tm-pah/ Tm-diodrast in man at different levels of Tm. Clin. Res. Proc. 3, 134 (1955) (abstract). — STONER, H. B., and D. DEXTER: Glomerular filtration rate after adrenal medullectomy in the rat. Endocrinology 54, 708 (1954). — STØREN, E. J.: Effect of pentobarbital anesthesia on Tm-pah in the dog. Amer. J. Physiol. 192, 387 (1958a). — Effect of pentobarbital sodium on uptake of PAH by rat kidney cortex slices in vitro. Amer. J. Physiol. 195, 343 (1958b). — STOVER, J. W., R. W. GRIFFIN and R. V. FORD: Effects of chronic pentapyrrolidinium-induced hypotension on renal hemodynamics and on the excretion of water and electrolytes in hypertension. Ann. intern. Med. 44, 893 (1956). — STRAUS, F., and B. SPARGO: Ultrastructural changes in the renal papillary tip with K depletion. Fed. Proc. 19, 367 (1960) (abstract). — STRAUS, W., and J. OLIVER: Cellular mechanisms of protein metabolism in the nephron. VI. The immunological demonstration of egg white in droplets and other cellular fractions of the rat kidney after intraperitoneal injection. J. exp. Med. 102, 1 (1955). — STRAUSS, M. B., W. H. BIRCHARD and L. SAXON: Correction of impaired water excretion in cirrhosis of the liver by alcohol ingestion or expansion of extracellular fluid volume: the role of the antidiuretic hormone. Trans. Ass. Amer. Phycns 49, 222 (1956). — STRAUSS, M. B., R. K. DAVIS, J. D. ROSENBAUM and ELSIE C. ROSSMEISL: "Water diuresis" produced during recumbency by the intravenous infusion of isotonic saline. J. clin. Invest. 30, 862 (1951). — Production of increased renal sodium excretion by the hypotonic expansion of extracellular fluid volume in recumbent subjects. J. clin. Invest. 31, 80 (1952). — STRAUSS, M. B., and L. E. EARLEY: An inquiry into the role of "sodium-retaining" steroids in the homeostasis of body sodium in man. Trans. Ass. Amer. Phycns 23, 200 (1959). — STRAUSS, M. B., E. LAMDIN, W. P. SMITH and D. J. BLEIFER: Surfeit and deficit of sodium. Arch. intern. Med. 102, 527 (1958). — STRAUSS, M. B., and J. D. ROSENBAUM: The dependence of water diuresis upon electrolyte excretion. J. clin. Invest. 29, 841 (1950). — STRAUSS, M. B., J. D. ROSENBAUM and W. P. NELSON: The effect of alcohol on the renal excretion of water and electrolyte. J. clin. Invest. 29, 1053 (1950). — STRICKLER, J. C., R. H.

KESSLER and R. F. PITTS: Direct renal action of cardiac glycosides and structurally related compounds. Fed. Proc. 19, 365 (1960) (abstract). — STRÖM, L.: Studies on the renal excretion of P^{32} in infancy and childhood. Acta paediat. (Uppsala) Suppl. 82 (1951). — STUDY, R. S., and R. E. SHIPLEY: Comparison of direct with indirect renal blood flow, extraction of inulin and diodrast, before and during acute renal nerve stimulation. Amer. J. Physiol. 163, 442 (1950). — SUGARMAN, J., M. FRIEDMAN, EVALYN BARRETT and T. ADDIS: Distribution, flow, protein and urea content of renal lymph. Amer. J. Physiol. 138, 108 (1942). — SULLIVAN, L. P., W. S. WILDE and R. L. MALVIN: Renal transport sites for K, H and NH$_3$. Effect of impermeant anions on their transport. Amer. J. Physiol. 198, 244 (1960). — SULLIVAN, L. P., W. S. WILDE, R. L. MALVIN and A. J. VANDER: Site of renal transport of potassium as revealed by stop flow analysis. Fed. Proc. 17, 158 (1958) (abstract). — SULLIVAN, M. X., and F. IRREVERRE: A highly specific test for creatinine. J. Biol. Chem. 233, 530 (1958). — SULLIVAN, W. J., and P. J. DORMAN: The renal response to chronic respiratory acidosis. J. clin. Invest. 34, 268 (1955). — SUNDIN, T.: The influence of body posture on the urinary excretion of adrenaline and noradrenaline. Acta med. scand. Suppl. 311—313 (1956). — SURTSHIN, A., J. HOELTZENBEIN and H. L. WHITE: Some effects of negative pressure breathing on urine excretion. Amer. J. Physiol. 180, 612 (1955). — SURTSHIN, A., C. B. MUELLER and H. L. WHITE: Effect of acute changes in glomerular filtration rate on water and electrolyte excretion: mechanism of denervation diuresis. Amer. J. Physiol. 169, 159 (1952). — SURTSHIN, A., and A. G. PARELMAN: Renal localization, excretion and toxicity of mercuric chloride in normal and "nephrotic" rats. Proc. Soc. exp. Biol. (N.Y.) 95, 628 (1957). — SURTSHIN, A., DORIS ROLF and H. L. WHITE: Constancy of sodium excretion in the presence of chronically altered filtration rate. Amer. J. Physiol. 165, 429 (1951). — SURTSHIN, A., and W. P. SCHMANDT: Comparison of continuously collected urines from the two normal kidneys and some effects of unilateral denervation. Amer. J. Physiol. 185, 418 (1956). — SURTSHIN, A., and H. L. WHITE: Postural effects on renal tubular activity. J. clin. Invest. 35, 267 (1956). — SURTSHIN, A., and K. YAGI: Distribution in renal cell fractions of sulfhydryl groups in rats on normal and sucrose diets and its relation to renal mercury distribution after mercuric chloride injection. Amer. J. Physiol. 192, 405 (1958). — SWANN, H. G., F. W. FEIST and H. J. LOWE: Fluid draining from functionally distended kidney. Proc. Soc. exp. Biol. (N.Y.) 88, 218 (1955). — SWANN, H. G., B. W. HINK, H. KOESTER, V. MOORE and J. M. PRINE: The intrarenal pressure. Science 115, 64 (1952). — SWANN, H. G., A. V. MONTGOMERY and J. S. LOWRY: Effect of renal venous occlusion on intrarenal pressure. Proc. Soc. exp. Biol. (N.Y.) 76, 773 (1951). — SWANN, H. G., and J. M. PRINE: Relation of intrarenal pressure to blood pressure and to perinephritic hypertension. Fed. Proc. 10, 134 (1951) (abstract). — SWANN, H. G., J. G. SINCLAIR and M. V. PARKER: Attempt to visualize a renal interstitial space. Fed. Proc. 17, 159 (1958) (abstract). — SWANSON, R. E.: Creatinine secretion by the frog renal tubule. Amer. J. Physiol. 84, 527 (1956). — SWANSON, R. E., and M. B. VISSCHER: Transtubular water movement in the isolated doubly-perfused bullfrog kidney. Amer. J. Physiol. 184, 535 (1956). — SWINGLE, W. W., M. BEN, R. MAXWELL, C. BAKER, E. FEDOR and G. BARLOW: Effect of the sodium-retaining factor of the adrenal cortex upon the serum electrolytes of adrenalectomized dogs. Endocrinology 54, 698 (1954). — SWINGLE, W. W., R. MAXWELL, M. BEN, C. BAKER, S. J. LeBRIE and M. EISLER: A comparative study of aldosterone and other adrenal steroids in adrenalectomized dogs. Endocrinology 55, 813 (1954a). — Effect of aldosterone and desoxycorticosterone (DOC) on adrenalectomized dogs. Proc. Soc. exp. Biol. (N.Y.) 86, 147 (1954b).

TAGGART, J. V.: Protein binding of p-aminohippurate in human and dog plasma. Amer. J. Physiol. 167, 248 (1951). — Renal transport of p-aminohippurate labelled with oxygen-18. Science 124, 401 (1956). — Mechanisms of renal tubular transport. Amer. J. Med. 24, 774 (1958). — TAGGART, J. V., and R. P. FORSTER: Renal tubular transport: effect of 2,4-dinitrophenol and related compounds on phenol red transport in the isolated tubules of the flounder. Amer. J. Physiol. 161, 167 (1950). — TAGGART, J. V., L. SILVERMAN and E. M. TRAYNER: Influence of renal electrolyte composition on the tubular excretion of p-aminohippurate. Amer. J. Physiol. 173, 345 (1953). — TALBOTT, J. H.: Gout. Oxford Med. 4, 79 (1943). — TALBOTT, J. H.: Hypothermia. Josiah Macy Conf. on cold injury, 1951. — TALBOTT, J. H., B. CASTLEMAN, R. H. SMITHWICK, R. S. MELVILLE and L. J. PECORA: Renal biopsy studies correlated with renal clearance observations in hypertensive patients treated by radical sympathectomy. J. clin. Invest. 22, 387 (1943). — TALBOTT, J. H., L. J. PECORA, R. S. MELVILLE and W. V. CONSOLAZIO: Renal function in patients with Addison's disease and in patients with adrenal insufficiency secondary to pituitary panhypofunction. J. clin. Invest. 21, 107 (1942). — TALMAGE, R. V., and F. W. KRAINTZ: Immediate changes in phosphate excretion following parathyroidectomy in the rat. Proc. Soc. exp. Biol. (N.Y.) 85, 416 (1954a). — TALMAGE, R. V., and F. W. KRAINTZ: Progressive changes in renal phosphate and calcium excretion in rate following parathyroidectomy or parathyroid administration. Proc. Soc. exp. Biol. (N.Y.) 87, 263 (1954b). — TALMAGE, R. V., F. W. KRAINTZ and G. D. BUCHANAN: Effect of parathyroid extract and phosphate salts on renal calcium and phosphate excretion after parathyroidectomy. Proc. Soc. exp. Biol. (N.Y.) 88, 600 (1955). — Renal calcium and phosphate excretion in parathyroidectomized mice. Fed. Proc. 18, 155 (1959) (abstract). — TALMAGE, R. V., F. W. KRAINTZ, R. C. FROST and L. KRAINTZ: Evidence for a dual action of parathyroid extract in maintaining serum calcium and phosphate levels. Endocrinology 52, 318 (1953). — TALPERS, S. J., and J. D. STEIN jr.: Tubular reabsorption of phosphorus as a measure of parathyroid activity. Metabolism 8, 170 (1959). — TALSO, P. J., A. P. CROSLEY jr. and R. W. CLARKE: Effects of cold pressor test on glomerular filtration and effective renal plasma flow. J. Lab. clin. Med. 33, 430 (1948). — TAMURA, K., G. KIHARA and S. KUKI: Artificial perfusion of the frog's or toad's kidney with special reference to abnormal reflux of the renal-portal fluid into the glomerular capillaries. Jap. J. med. Sci., IV. Pharmacol. 2, 18P (1927/28). — TANK, G. W., and R. C. HERRIN: Effect of protein and amino acids upon renal function in the dog. Amer. J. Physiol. 178, 165 (1954). — TARAIL, R., and F. M. MATEER: Pitressin and mercuhydrin in relation to electrolyte excretion of patients with diabetes insipidus. Fed. Proc. 10, 135 (1951) (abstract).- TAYLOR jr., H. C., I. WELLEN and CATHERINE A. WELSH: Renal function studies in normal pregnancy and in toxemia based on clearances of inulin, phenol red and diodrast. Amer. J. Obstet. Gynec. 43, 567 (1942). — TAYLOR, R. D., A. C. CORCORAN, J. C. SHRADER, W. C. YOUNG and I. H. PAGE: Effects of large doses of a vitamin A concentrate in normal and hypertensive patients. Amer. J. med. Sci. 206, 659 (1943). — TAYLOR, W. H.: Water diuresis in chronic hypochromic anaemia. Clin. Sci. 14, 731 (1955). — TAYMOR, R. C., J. B. MINOR and C. K. FRIEDBERG: Influence of carbonic anhydrase inhibition on renal effects of acute respiratory alkalosis and acidosis in human subjects. J. appl. Physiol. 7, 43 (1954). — TEABEAUT, R., F. L. ENGEL and H. TAYLOR: Hypokalemic, hypochloremic alkalosis in Cushing's syndrome. Observations on the effects of treatment with potassium chloride and testosterone. J. clin. Endocr. 10, 399 (1950). — TELKKA, A., and K. K. MUSTAKALLIO: Proximal or distal mercurial inhibition of succinic dehydrogenase in the kidney tubules of rat. Science 121, 146 (1955). — TERP, P.: Studies on elimination of procaine. III. Determination of the renal clearance of procaine and p-aminobenzoic acid in dog and rabbit. Acta pharmacol. 7, 259 (1951). — TERRY, R., D. R. HAWKINS, E. H. CHURCH and G. H. WHIPPLE: Proteinuria related to hyperproteinemia in dogs following plasma given parenterally. A renal threshold for plasma proteins. J. exp. Med. 87, 561 (1948). — TERUI, M.: Über die Harnstoffausscheidung in der isolierten überlebenden Niere im normalen sowie pathologischen Zustand bei Durchströmung mit harnstoffhaltiger Ringerlösung von verschieden starker Konzentration. Tôhoku J. exp. Med. 41, 208 (1941). — THEOBALD, G. W., and E. B. VERNEY: The inhibition of water diuresis by afferent nerve stimuli after complete denervation of the kidney. J. Physiol. (Lond.) 83, 341 (1935). — THOMAS jr., C. A.: New scheme for performance of osmotic work by membranes. Science 123, 60 (1956). — THOMPSON, D. D., and MARTHA J. BARRETT: Urine flow and solute excretion during osmotic diuresis. Amer. J. Physiol. 176, 33 (1954). — Renal reabsorption of bicarbonate. Amer. J. Physiol. 176, 201 (1954b). — THOMPSON, D. D., MARTHA J. BARRETT and R. F. PITTS: Significance of glomerular perfusion in relation to variability of filtration rate. Amer. J. Physiol. 167, 546 (1951). — THOMPSON, D. D., and H. H. HIATT: Renal reabsorption of phosphate in normal human subjects and in patients with parathyroid disease. J. clin. Invest. 36, 550 (1957a). — Effects of phosphate loading and depletion on the renal excretion of inorganic phosphate. J. clin. Invest. 36, 566 (1957b). — THOMPSON, D. D., F. KAVALER, R. LOZANO and R. F. PITTS: Evaluation of the cell separation hypothesis of autoregulation of renal blood flow and filtration rate. Blood flow, filtration rate and PAH extraction as functions of arterial pressure in normal and anemic dogs. Amer. J. Physiol. 191, 493 (1957). — THOMPSON, D. D., and R. F. PITTS: Effects of alterations of renal arterial pressure on sodium and water excretion. Amer. J. Physiol. 168, 490 (1952). — THOMPSON, J. E., T. F. SILVA, D. KINSEY and R. H. SMITHWICK: The effect of acute salt loads on the urinary sodium output of normotensive and hypertensive patients before and after surgery. Circulation 10, 912 (1954). — THOMSON, A. E., E. G. BROWNELL and G. R. CUMMING: Water diuresis in adrenal cortical insufficiency. Ann. intern. Med. 52, 949 (1960). — THOMSON, D. L., and J. B. COLLIP: The parathyroid glands. Physiol. Rev. 12, 309 (1932). — THORN, G. W., S. S. DORRANCE and E. DAY: Addison's disease: evaluation of synthetic desoxycorticosterone acetate therapy in 158 patients. Ann. intern. Med. 16, 1063 (1942). — THORN, G. W., L. L. ENGEL and R. A. LEWIS: Effect of 17-hydroxycorticosterone and related adrenal cortical steroids on sodium and chloride excretion. Science 94, 348 (1941). — THORN, G. W., J. H. HARRISON, J. P. MERRILL, M. G. CRISCITIELLO, T. F. FRAWLEY and J. T. FINKENSTAEDT: Clinical studies on bilateral complete adrenalectomy in patients with severe hypertensive vascular disease. Ann. intern. Med. 37, 972 (1952). — THORN, N. A.: Mammalian antidiuretic hormone. Physiol. Rev. 38, 169

(1958). — Thorn, N. A., and L. Silver: Chemical form of circulating antidiuretic hormone in rats. J. exp. Med. 105, 575 (1957). — Threefoot, S. A., G. E. Burch and C. T. Ray: Studies of excretion of radiorubidium (Rb[86]) and potassium in man with and without congestive heart failure. J. Lab. clin. Med. 44, 941 (1954). — Thurau, K., K. Kramer, P. Deetjen and H. Brechtelsbauer: Renal medullary blood flow and its relation to renal function. Fed. Proc. 19, 360 (1960) (abstract). — Tibbetts, Dorothy M., and J. C. Aub: Magnesium metabolism in health and disease. I. The magnesium and calcium excretion of normal individuals, also the effects of magnesium, chloride and phosphate ions. J. clin. Invest. 16, 491 (1937a). — Magnesium metabolism in health and disease. II. The effect of the parathyroid hormone. J. clin. Invest. 16, 503 (1937b). — Tobian, L.: Physiology of the juxtglomerular cells. Ann. intern. Med. 52, 395 (1960). — Törnblom, N.: On the functional relationship between the pituitary gland and the parathyroids. Acta endocr. 2, Suppl. 4 (1949). — Toft, R. J., and R. V. Talmage: Parathyroid activity after nephrectomy as indicated by changes in osteoclast count in femur. Fed. Proc. 19, 51 (1960) (abstract). — Tomsett, R., Selma Shultz and W. McDermott: The relation of protein binding to the pharmacology and antibacterial activity of penicillins X, G, dihydro F, and K. J. Bact. 53, 581 (1947). — Toribara, T. Y., A. R. Terepka and Priscilla A. Dewey: The ultrafiltrable calcium of human serum. I. Ultrafiltration methods and normal values. J. clin. Invest. 36, 738 (1957). — Tosteson, D. C., and H. L. White: Permeability of different segments of the renal tubule to water. Fed. Proc. 18, 160 (1959) (abstract). — Toussaint, C., M. Telerman and P. Vereerstraeten: Effects of acute hypochloremia on glomerular filtration rate and electrolyte excretion in the dog. Experientia (Basel) 14, 417 (1958). — Effect of potassium salts administration on the renal excretion of bicarbonate during acute respiratory acidosis and hypochloremic alkalosis in the dog. Experientia (Basel) 15, 232 (1959a). — Bicarbonate excretion after prolonged exposure to carbon dioxide in the normal dog. Experientia (Basel) 15, 434 (1959b). — Trager, W., and M. C. Hutchinson: The influence of ammonium ion on the plasma atabrine level and on the urinary excretion of atabrine. J. clin. Invest. 25, 694 (1946). — Trautner, E. M., R. Morris, C. H. Noack and S. Gershon: The excretion and retention of ingested lithium and its effect on the ionic balance of man. Med. J. Aust. 42, 280 (1955). — Tronchetti, F., G. Mucio et R. Romanelli: Influence de quelques stimulines hypophysaires sur l'excrétion urinaire de substances douées d'action aldostéronique. Ann. Endocr. (Paris) 18, 658 (1957). — Trueta, J., A. E. Barclay, P. M. Daniel, K. J. Franklin and M. M. L. Pritchard: Studies of the renal circulation. Springfield, Ill.: Ch. C. Thomas 1947. — Tudvad, F.: Sugar reabsorption in prematures and full term babies. Scand. J. clin. Lab. Invest. 1, 281 (1949). — Tudvad, F., and J. Vesterdal: Inulin and PAH clearances in newborn infants. Scand. J. clin. Lab. Invest. 1, 345 (1949). — Tweedy, W. R., and W. W. Campbell: The effect of parathyroid extract upon the distribution, retention and excretion of labeled phosphorus. J. biol. Chem. 154 (1944). — Tyler, F. H., C. Migeon, A. A. Florentin and L. T. Samuels: The diurnal variation of 17-hydroxycorticosteroid levels in plasma. J. clin. Endocr. 14, 774 (1954) (abstract). — Tyer, M. P., and J. S. Eldridge: A comparison of the metabolism of rubidium 86 and potassium 42 following simultaneous injection into man. Amer. J. med. Sci. 232, 186 (1956).

Ulick, S., J. H. Larah and S. Lieberman: The isolation of a urinary metabolite of aldosterone and its use to measure the rate of secretion of aldosterone by the adrenal cortex of man. Trans. Ass. Amer. Phycns 71, 225 (1958). — Ullman, T. D.: Hyperosmolarity of the extracellular fluid in encephalitis. Amer. J. Med. 15, 885 (1953). — Ullman, T. D., S. H. Blondheim, S. Dikstein and D. Ben-Ishay: Water and salt excretion after intravenous salt load in hypertensive subjects. Circulation 19, 729 (1959). — Ullrick, K. J.: Über das Vorkommen von Phosphorverbindungen in verschiedenen Nierenabschnitten und Änderungen ihrer Konzentration in Abhängigkeit vom Diuresezustand. Pflügers Arch. ges. Physiol. 262, 551 (1956). — Ullrich, K. J., F. O. Drenckhahn u. K. H. Jarausch: Untersuchungen zum Problem der Harnkonzentrierung und -verdünnung. Über das osmotische Verhalten von Nierenzellen und die begleitende Elektrolytanhäufung im Nierengewebe bei verschiedenen Diuresezuständen. Pflügers Arch. ges. Physiol. 261, 62 (1955). — Ullrich, K. J., H. H. Hilger u. J. D. Klümper: Sekretion von Ammoniumionen in den Sammelrohren der Säugetierniere. Pflügers Arch. ges. Physiol. 267, 244 (1958). — Ullrich, K. J., H. H. Hilger, J. D. Klümper u. F. W. Eigler: Über die Regulation des Säure-Basenhaushaltes durch Ionenaustausch in den Sammelrohren der Säugetierniere. Pflügers Arch. ges. Physiol. 268, 42 (1958/59) (abstract). — Ullrich, K. J., u. K. H. Jarausch: Untersuchungen zum Problem der Harnkonzentrierung und Harnverdünnung. Über die Verteilung von Elektrolyten (Na, K, Ca, Mg, Cl, anorganischem Phosphat), Harnstoff, Aminosäuren und exogenem Kreatinin in Rinde und Mark der Hundenniere bei verschiedenen Diuresezuständen. Pflügers Arch. ges. Physiol. 262, 537 (1956). — Ullrich, K. J., K. H. Jarausch u. W. Overbeck: Verteilung von Na, K, Ca, Mg, Cl, PO_4 und Harnstoff in Rinde und Mark der Hundeniere bei verschiedenen Funktionszuständen. Ber. ges. Physiol. 179/180, 131 (1956) (abstract). — UNGER, A. M., J. H. MAGEE, D. W. RICHARDSON and E. M. WYSO: Studies of renal function before and after 1 year of hypotensive drug therapy. Clin. Res. 7, 281 (1959) (abstract). — UNNA, K.: Arterieller Druck und Nierendurchblutung. Pflügers Arch. ges. Physiol. 235, 515 (1934/35). — UNNA, K., u. L. WALLERSKIRCHEN: Über den Zusammenhang zwischen Chlorid- und Wasserausscheidung nach Pituitrin. Naunyn-Schmiedeberg's Arch. exp. Path. Pharmak. 181, 681 (1936). — URBACH, J. R., M. D. PHELPS, W. S. STEIGER and S. BELLET: Effect of water diuresis on renal excretion of certain urinary solutes in normal man. J. appl. Physiol. 6, 243 (1953).

VALTIN, H., I. D. WILSON and S. M. TENNEY: CO_2 diuresis, with special reference to the role of the left atrial stretch receptor mechanism. J. appl. Physiol. 14, 844 (1959). — VANAMEE, P., F. CUAJUNCO jr., H. T. RANDALL and KATHLEEN E. ROBERTS: Additive effects of respiratory alkalosis, carbonic anhydrase inhibition and potassium on renal tubular reabsorption of bicarbonate. Fed. Proc. 15, 190 (1956) (abstract). — VANDER, A. J., R. L. MALVIN, W. S. WILDE, J. LAPIDES, L. P. SULLIVAN and VIRGINIA M. McMURRAY: Effects of adrenalectomy and aldosterone on proximal and distal tubular sodium reabsorption. Proc. Soc. exp. Biol. (N.Y.) 99, 323 (1958a). — VANDER, A. J., R. L. MALVIN, W. S. WILDE and L. P. SULLIVAN: Localization of the site of action of mercurial diuretics by stop flow analysis. Amer. J. Physiol. 195, 558 (1958b). — Localization of the site of action of chlorothiazide by stop flow analysis. J. Pharmacol. exp. Ther. 125, 19 (1959). — VANDER, A. J., W. S. WILDE and R. L. MALVIN: Stop flow analysis of aldosterone influence on distal tubular sodium transport kinetics. Fed. Proc. 18, 162 (1959) (abstract). — VARGAS, R., and E. J. CAFRUNY: Effects of p-chloromercuribenzoate on urine flow and sodium excretion of perfused dog kidney. Fed. Proc. 18, 455 (1959) (abstract). — VENNING, ELEANOR H., and INGE DYRENFURTH: Aldosterone excretion in pregnancy. J. clin. Endocr. 16, 426 (1956). — VENNING, ELEANOR H., INGE DYRENFURTH and J. C. BECK: Effect of corticotropin and prednisone on the excretion of aldosterone in man. J. clin. Endocr. 16, 1541 (1957). — VENNING, ELEANOR H., INGE DYRENFURTH and C. GIROUD: Diurnal variation in excretion of a sodium-retaining substance. Fed. Proc. 14, 297 (1955) (abstract). — Aldosterone excretion in healthy persons. J. clin. Endocr. 16, 1326 (1956). — VENNING, ELEANOR H., INGE DYRENFURTH, C. J. P. GIROUD and J. C. BECK: Effect of growth hormone on aldosterone excretion. Metabolism 5, 697 (1956). — VENNING, ELEANOR H., C. J. P. GIROUD, INGE DYRENFURTH and J. C. BECK: Studies with aldosterone. Canad. J. Biochem. 33, 605 (1955). — VENNING, ELEANOR H., J. R. McCORRISTON, INGE DYRENFURTH and J. C. BECK: Aldosterone excretion following trauma. Metabolism 7, 293 (1958). — VENNING, ELEANOR H., T. PRIMROSE, L. C. S. CALIGARIS and INGE DYRENFURTH: Aldosterone excretion in pregnancy. J. clin. Endocr. 17, 473 (1957). — VENNING, ELEANOR H., BERTHA SINGER, A. CARBALLEIRA, INGE DYRENFURTH, J. C. BECK and C. P. GIROUD: The excretion of sodium-retaining substances in human beings. Ciba Found. Symp. 8, 190 (1955). — VERA, RUTH, and H. CROXATTO: Muscular work and antidiuretic substances of the blood. J. appl. Physiol. 7, 172 (1954/55). — VERMET, A., A. DUCKERT et A. F. MULLER: Hypokaliemie et oedèmes par déperdition intestinale de potassium. Helv. med. Acta 23, 490 (1956). — VERNEY, E. B.: Absorption and excretion of water; antidiuretic hormone. Lancet 1946 II, 739. — Antidiuretic hormone and factors which determine its release. Proc. roy. Soc. B 135, 25 (1947). — Agents determining and influencing the functions of the pars nervosa of the pituitary. Brit. med. J. 1948 II, 119. — Water diuresis. Irish J. med. Sci. 6, 377 (1954). — Renal excretion of water and salt. Lancet 1957 II, 1237. — VESTERDAL, J., and F. TUDVAD: Studies on the kidney function in premature and full-term infants by estimation of the inulin and para-aminohippurate clearances. Acta paediat. (Uppsala) 37, 429 (1949). — VEYRAT, R., A. F. MULLER, A. DUCKERT et ANNE M. RIONDEL: Étude des conditions de non-résponse aux diurétiques. Helv. med. Acta 26, 666 (1959). — VIAR, W. N., B. V. OLIVER, S. EISENBERG, T. A. LOMBARDO, K. W. HARRISON and T. R. HARRISON: The effect of posture and of compression of the neck on excretion of electrolytes and glomerular filtration: further studies. Circulation 3, 105 (1951). — VIGNEAUD, V. DU, D. T. GISH and P. G. KATSOYANNIS: A synthetic preparation possessing biological properties associated with arginine-vasopressin. J. Amer. chem. Soc. 76, 4751 (1954). — VIGNEAUD, V. DU, H. C. LAWLER and E. A. POPENOE: Enzymatic cleavage of glycinamide from vasopressin and a proposed structure for this pressor-antidiuretic hormone of the posterior pituitary. J. Amer. chem. Soc. 75, 4880 (1953). — VIGNEAUD, V. DU, CHARLOTTE RESSLER, J. M. SWAN, C. W. ROBERTS and P. G. KATSOYANNIS: The synthesis of oxytocin. J. Amer. chem. Soc. 76, 3115 (1954). — VIMTRUP, B. J.: On the number, shape, structure and surface area of the glomeruli in the kidneys of man and mammals. Amer. J. Anat. 41, 123 (1928). — Histological examinations of kidneys of heteromyidae. Scand. J. clin. Lab. Invest. 1, 339 (1949) (abstract). — VIRCHOW, R.: Einige Bemerkungen über die Circulationsverhältnisse in den Nieren. Virchows Arch. path. Anat. 12, 310 (1857). — VISHWAKARMA, P.: Excretion of malic acid in relation

380   LAURENCE G. WESSON:

to tricarboxylic acid cycle in kidney. Fed. Proc. **16**, 132 (1957) (abstract). — VISHWA-
KARMA, P., and W. D. LOTSPEICH: Excretion of *l*-malic acid in the chicken. Amer. J. Physiol.
198, 819 (1960a). — Excretion of *d*-malic acid in the chicken. Amer. J. Physiol. **198**, 824
(1960b). — VISSCHER, F. E.: Renal clearance of beta-hydroxybutyric acid in a dog. Proc.
Soc. exp. Biol. (N.Y.) **60**, 296 (1954). — VÖLKER, H.: Über die tagesperiodischen Schwankungen einiger Lebensvorgänge des Menschen. Pflügers Arch. ges. Physiol. **215**, 43 (1927). —
VOGEL, G., ELIZABETH KRÄMER u. E. HEYM: Untersuchungen zum Mechanismus der
Kalium-Ausscheidung durch die künstlich perfundierte Amphibienniere. Pflügers Arch.
ges. Physiol. **263**, 357 (1956). — VOLLE, R. L., R. E. GREEN and L. PETERS: Inhibition of
renal tubular excretion of N'-methylnicotinamide (NMN) by other organic bases in the
chicken. Fed. Proc. **16**, 342 (1957) (abstract). — VOLLE, R. L., C. G. HUGGINS, G. A. RODRI-
GUEZ and L. PETERS: Inhibition of the renal tubular transport of N'-methylnicotinamide
(NMN) by 1,1-dialkylpiperidinium compounds in the avian kidney. J. Pharmacol. exp.
Ther. **125/126**, 190 (1959). — VOLLE, R. L., and L. PETERS: Renal tubular transport charac-
teristics of mecamylamine and quinine in the chicken. Fed. Proc. **18**, 455 (1959) (abstract).
WACHSTEIN, M., and E. MEISEL: Enzymatic staining reactions in the kidneys of potas-
sium- depleted rats. Amer. J. Path. **35**, 1189 (1959). — WADDELL, W. J., and T. C. BUTLER:
The distribution and excretion of phenobarbital. J. clin. Invest. **36**, 1217 (1957). — WAKIM,
K. G., J. F. HERRICK, E. J. BALDES and F. C. MANN: Effect of pitressin on renal circulation
and urine secretion. J. Lab. clin. Med. **27**, 1013 (1942). — WALKER, A. M.: Comparisons
of total molecular concentration of glomerular urine and blood plasma from the frog and from
necturus. J. biol. Chem. **87**, 499 (1930). — Quantitative studies of the composition of
glomerular urine. X. The concentration of inorganic phosphate in glomerular urine from
frogs and necturi determined by an ultramicromodification of the Bell-Doisy method. J.
biol. Chem. **101**, 239 (1933). — Experiments upon the relation between the pituitary gland
and water diuresis. Amer. J. Physiol. **127**, 519 (1939). — Ammonia formation in the amphibian kidney. Amer. J. Physiol. **131**, 187 (1940). — WALKER, A. M., PHYLLIS A. BOTT, J. OLIVER
and MURIEL C. MACDOWELL: Collection and analysis of fluid from single nephrons of mammalian kidney. Amer. J. Physiol. **134**, 580 (1941). — WALKER, A. M., and K. A. ELSOM: A quantitative study of the glomerular elimination of urea in frogs. J. biol. Chem. **91**, 593 (1931). —
WALKER, A. M., and C. L. HUDSON: The reabsorption of glucose from the renal tubule of
amphibia and the action of phlorhizin upon it. Amer. J. Physiol. **118**, 130 (1937a). — The
role of the tubule in the excretion of urea by the amphibian kidney. Amer. J. Physiol. **118**,
153 (1937b). — The role of the tubule in the excretion of inorganic phosphates by the
amphibian kidney. Amer. J. Physiol. **118**, 167 (1937c). — WALKER, A. M., C. L. HUDSON,
T. FINDLEY jr. and A. N. RICHARDS: The total molecular concentration and the chloride
concentration of fluid from different segments of the renal tubule of amphibia. Amer. J.
Physiol. **118**, 125 (1937b). — WALKER, A. M., and J. OLIVER: Methods for collection of
fluid from single glomeruli and tubules of mammalian kidney. Amer. J. Physiol. **134**, 562
(1941). — WALKER, A. M., and J. A. REISINGER: Quantitative studies of the composition
of glomerular urine. IX. The concentration of reducing substances in glomerular urine
from frogs and Necturi determined by an ultramicroadaptation of the method of Sumner.
Observations on the action of phlorhizin. J. biol. Chem. **101**, 223 (1933). — WALKER, A. M.,
C. F. SCHMIDT, K. A. ELSOM and C. G. JOHNSTON: Renal blood flow of unaenesthetized
rabbits and dogs in diuresis and antidiuresis. Amer. J. Physiol. **118**, 95 (1937a). —
WALKER, J. M.: The effect of smoking on water diuresis in man. Quart. J. Med. **18**, 51
(1949). — WALKER, W. F., M. S. SILELI, F. W. REUTTER, W. C. SHOEMAKER, D. FRIEND
and F. D. MOORE: Adrenal medullary secretion in hemorrhagic shock. Amer. J. Physiol.
197, 773 (1959a). — WALKER, W. F., M. S. ZILELI, F. W. REUTTER, W. C. SHOEMAKER and
F. D. MOORE: Factors influencing the "resting" secretion of the adrenal medulla. Amer.
J. Physiol. **197**, 765 (1959b). — WALKER, W. G., and C. C. J. CARPENTER: The effects of
hypokalemia and hypercalcemia on the renal-concentrating mechanism. Clin. Res. Proc.
6, 285 (1958) (abstract). — WALLENIUS, G.: Renal clearance of Dextran as a measure of
glomerular permeability. Acta Soc. Med. Upsaliensis **59**, Suppl. 4 (1954). — WALSER, M.,
and ANN A. BROWDER: Ion association. III. The effect of sulfate infusion on calcium excretion. J. clin. Invest. **38**, 1404 (1959). — WALSER, M., D. G. DAVIDSON and J. ORLOFF: The
renal clearance of alkali-stable inulin. J. clin. Invest. **34**, 1520 (1955). — WANG, C. Y., and
M. NICKERSON: Effect of dibenamine on renal function. Proc. Soc. exp. Biol. (N.Y.) **70**,
92 (1949). — WARDENER, H. E. DE, and F. DEL GRECO: The influence of solute excretion
rate on the production of a hypotonic urine in man. Clin. Sci. **14**, 715 (1955). — WARDENER,
H. E. DE, and A. HERXHEIMER: The effect of a high water intake on the kidney's ability
to concentrate the urine in man. J. Physiol. (Lond.) **139**, 42 (1957). — WARDENER, H. E. DE,
and R. R. MCSWINEY: Renal haemodynamics in vaso-vagal fainting due to haemorrhage.
Clin. Sci. **10**, 209 (1951). — WARDENER, H. E. DE, R. R. MCSWINEY and B. E. MILES: Renal
haemodynamics in primary polycythaemia. Lancet **1951**II, 204. — WARDENER, H. E. DE,

and B. E. MILES: The effect of haemorrhage on the circulatory autoregulation of the dog's kidney perfused in situ. Clin. Sci. 11, 267 (1952). — WARING, A. J., L. KAJDI and V. TAPPAN: A congenital defect of water metabolism. Amer. J. Dis. Child. 69, 323 (1945) (abstract). — WARREN, J. V., E. S. BRANNAN and A. J. MERRILL: A method of obtaining renal venous blood in unanesthetized persons with observations on the extraction of oxygen and sodium para-aminohippurate. Science 100, 108 (1944). — WASHINGTON II, J. A., I. M. WEINER and G. H. MUDGE: Effect of acetazolamide on the renal mechanism of salicylate excretion in dogs. Fed. Proc. 18, 166 (1959) (abstract). — WASSERMAN, K., E. L. BECKER and A. P. FISHMAN: Transport of phenol red in the flounder renal tubule. J. cell. comp. Physiol. 42, 385 (1953). — WATERHOUSE, CHRISTINE, and E. H. KEUTMAN: Kidney function in adrenal insufficiency. J. clin. Invest. 27, 372 (1948). — WATKIN, D. M., H. F. FROEB, F. T. HATCH and A. B. GUTMAN: Effects of diet in essential hypertension. II. Results with unmodified Kempner rice diet in 50 hospitalized patients. Amer. J. Med. 9, 441 (1950). — WATTS, D. T.: Arterial blood epinephrine levels during hemorrhagic hypotension in dogs. Amer. J. Physiol. 184, 271 (1956). — WAUGH, W. H.: Flow as a function of arterial pressure in the oil-perfused kidney. Circulat. Res. 6, 107 (1958a). — Myogenic nature of autoregulation of renal flow in the absence of blood corpuscles. Circulat. Res. 6, 363 (1958b). — WAUGH, W. H., and W. F. HAMILTON: Physical effects of increased venous and extrarenal pressure on renal vascular resistance. Circulat. Res. 6, 116 (1958). — WAY, E. L., P. K. SMITH, D. L. HOWIE, ROWENA WEISS and R. SWANSON: The absorption, distribution, excretion and fate of para-aminosalicylic acid. J. Pharmacol. exp. Ther. 93, 368 (1948). — WEARN, J. T.: Observations upon the composition of glomerular urine. Amer. J. Physiol. 59, 490 (1922) (abstract). — WEAVER, A. N., C. T. MCCARVER and H. G. SWANN: Distribution of blood in the functional kidney. J. exp. Med. 104, 41 (1956). — WEGRIA, R., N. E. CAPECI, M. R. BLUMENTHAL, P. KORNFELD, D. R. HAYS, R. A. ELIAS and J. G. HILTON: The pathogenesis of proteinuria in the acutely congested kidney. J. clin. Invest. 34, 737 (1955). — WEINER, I. M., ADALEEN E. BURNETT and BARBARA R. RENNICK: The renal tubular secretion of mersalyl (salyrgan) in the chicken. J. Pharmacol. exp. Ther. 118, 470 (1956). — WEINER, I. M., K. GARLID, D. SAPIR and G. H. MUDGE: The effects of dimercaprol (BAL) on the renal excretion of mercurials. J. Pharmacol. exp. Ther. 127, 325 (1959). — WEINER, I. M., R. I. LEVY and G. H. MUDGE: Excretory products of various mercury compounds in acidosis and alkalosis. Fed. Proc. 16, 345 (1957) (abstract). — WEINER, I. M., and O. H. MÜLLER: A polarographic study of mersalyl (Salyrgan)-thiol complexes and of the excreted products of mersalyl. J. Pharmacol. exp. Ther. 113, 241 (1955). — WEINER, I. M., J. A. WASHINGTON II and G. H. MUDGE: Studies on the renal excretion of salicylate in the dog. Bull. Johns Hopk. Hosp. 105, 284 (1959). — WEINSTEIN, H., R. M. BERNE and H. SACHS: Vasopressin in blood: Effect of hemorrhage. Endocrinology 66, 712 (1960). — WEISS, C., H. PASSOW and A. ROTHSTEIN: Autoregulation of flow in isolated rat kidney in the absence of red cells. Amer. J. Physiol. 196, 1115 (1959). — WEISS, M. B., and J. B. LONGLEY: Renal glutaminase I distribution and ammonia excretion in the rat. Amer. J. Physiol. 198, 223 (1960). — WEISSBERGER, LOUISE H.: Phosphorus metabolism in phlorhizin diabetes, with radioactive phosphorus as an indicator. J. biol. Chem. 139, 543 (1941). — WELLEN, I., CATHERINE A. WELSH and H. C. TAYLOR jr.: Filtration rate, effective renal blood flow, tubular excretory mass and phenol red clearance in specific toxemia of pregnancy. J. clin. Invest. 21, 63 (1942). — WELLER, J. M., and S. W. HOOBLER: Salt metabolism in hypertension. Ann. intern. Med. 50, 106 (1959). — WELSH, CATHERINE A., A. ROSENTHAL, M. T. DUNCAN and H. C. TAYLOR: The effects of testosterone propionate on renal function in the dog, as measured by the creatinine and diodrast clearance and diodrast Tm. Amer. J. Physiol. 137, 338 (1942a). — WELSH, CATHERINE A., I. WELLEN and H. C. TAYLOR jr.: Filtration rate, effective renal blood flow, tubular excretory mass and phenol red clearance in normal pregnancy. J. clin. Invest. 21, 57 (1942b). — WELSH III, G. W., and E. A. H. SIMS: Renal tubular reabsorption of glucose and the mechanism of glucosuria in pregnancy. Clin. Res. Proc. 6, 287 (1958) (abstract). — WELT, L. G.: Edema and hyponatremia. Arch. intern. Med. 89, 931 (1952). — Renal factors in regulation of electrolyte balance. Arch. intern. Med. 95, 365 (1955). — Volume receptors. Circulation 21, 1002 (1960). — WELT, L. G., A. V. N. GOODYER, J. H. DARRAGH, W. A. ABELE and W. H. MERONEY: Site of saluretic action of an organic mercurial compound. J. appl. Physiol. 6, 134 (1953). — WELT, L. G., W. HOLLANDER jr. and W. B. BLYTHE: The consequences of potassium depletion. J. chron. Dis. 11, 213 (1960). — WELT, L. G., and W. P. NELSON III: Excretion of water by normal subjects. J. appl. Physiol. 4, 709 (1952). — WELT, L. G., and J. ORLOFF: The effects of an increase in plasma volume on the metabolism and excretion of water and electrolytes by normal subjects. J. clin. Invest. 30, 751 (1951). — WELT, L. G., D. W. SELDIN, W. P. NELSON III, W. J. GERMAN and J. P. PETERS: Role of the central nervous system in metabolism of electrolytes and water. Arch. intern. Med. 90, 355 (1952). — WELT, L. G., D. T. YOUNG, O. A. THORUP jr. and C. H. BURNETT: Renal tubular phenomena under the influence of a carbonic anhydrase inhibitor. Amer. J. Med. 16, 612 (1954) (abstract). — WERKO, L., H. BUCHT, J. EK and E. VARNAUSKAS: Studies of the renal circulation and renal function in mitral valvular disease. IV. The effect of a single intravenous injection of lanatoside C. Cardiologia (Basel) 29, 305 (1956a). — WERKO, L., H. BUCHT and B. JOSEPHSON: The renal extraction of para-amino-hippuric acid and oxygen in man during postural changes of the circulation. Scand. J. clin. Lab. Invest. 1, 321 (9491). — WERKO, L., H. BUCHT, B. JOSEPHSON and J. EK: The effect of noradrenalin and adrenalin on renal hemodynamics and renal function in man. Scand. J. clin. Lab. Invest. 3, 255 (1951). — WERKO, L., J. EK, H. BUCHT and H. ELIASCH: Correlation between renal dynamics, cardiac output and right heart pressures in mitral valvular disease. Scand. J. clin. Lab. Invest. 4, 15 (1952). — WERKO, L., J. EK, H. BUCHT and J. KARNELL: Cardia ouput, blood pressures and renal dynamics in coarctation of the aorta. Scand. J. clin. Lab. Invest. 8, 193 (1956b). — WERKO, L., J. EK, E. VARNAUSKAS, H. BUCHT, B. THO-MASSON and H. ELIASCH: The relationship between renal blood flow, glomerular filtration rate and sodium excretion, cardiac output and pulmonary and systemic blood pressures in various heart disorders. Amer. Heart J. 49, 823 (1955). — WERKO, L., E. VARNAUSKAS, J. EK, H. BUCHT, B. THOMASSON, J. BERGSTROM and H. ELIASCH: Studies on the renal circulation and renal function in mitral valvular disease. II. Effect of apresoline. Circulation 9, 700 (1954b). — WERKO, L., E. VARNAUSKAS, H. ELIASCH, J. EK, H. BUCHT, B. THO-MASSON and J. BERGSTROM: Studies on the renal circulation and renal function in mitral valvular disease. I. Effect of exercise. Circulation 9, 687 (1954a). — WESSON jr., L. G.: Electrolyte excretion studies in the dog. Meth. med. Res. 5, 175 (1952). — A theoretical analysis of urea excretion by the mammalian kidney. Amer. J. Physiol. 179, 364 (1954). — Glomerular and tubular factors in the renal excretion of sodium chloride. Medicine (Balti-more) 36, 281 (1957). — Renal tubular chloride reabsorption in the dog during rapidly changing plasma chloride concentration. Amer. J. Physiol. 195, 133 (1958). — Effects of acute elevation of blood CO_2 tension on renal excretion of chloride and sodium by the anesthetized dog. Amer. J. Physiol. 196, 529 (1959). — WESSON jr., L. G., and W. P. ANS-LOW: Excretion of sodium and water during osmotic diuresis in the dog. Amer. J. Physiol. 153, 465 (1948). — Effect of osmotic and mercurial diuresis on simultaneous water diuresis. Amer. J. Physiol. 170, 255 (1952). — Relationship of changes in glomerular filtration, plasma chloride and bicarbonate concentrations and urinary osmotic load to renal excretion of chloride. Amer. J. Physiol. 180, 237 (1955). — WESSON jr., L. G., W. P. ANSLOW, L. G. RAISZ, A. A. BOLOMEY and M. LADD: Effect of sustained expansion of extracellular fluid volume upon filtration rate, renal plasma flow and electrolyte and water excretion in the dog. Amer. J. Physiol. 162, 677 (1950). — WESSON jr., L. G., W. P. ANSLOW and H. W. SMITH: The renal excretion of strong electrolytes. Bull. N.Y. Acad. Med. 24, 586 (1948). — WES-SON jr., L. G., and D. P. LAULER: Nephron reabsorption site for calcium and magnesium in the dog. Proc. Soc. exp. Biol. (N.Y.) 101, 235 (1959). — WESSON jr., L. G., A. SUNSHINE and JEANNE A. EPSTEIN: Chloride, potassium and aldosterone excretion in a sodium-retaining patient (hepatic cirrhosis) during forced natriuresis. J. Lab. clin. Med. 52, 78 (1958). — WEST, C. D., and RUTH K. BAYLESS: Relation of the saluresis of urea and mannitol loading to the normal excretion of electrolyte. Amer. J. Physiol. 191, 512 (1957). — WEST, C. D., S. A. KAPLAN, S. J. FOMON and S. RAPOPORT: Urine flow and solute excretion during osmotic diuresis in hydrated dogs: role of distal tubule in the production of hypotonic urine. Amer. J. Physiol. 170, 239 (1952). — WEST, C. D., and S. RAPOPORT: Urine flow and solute excretion of hydropenic dog under 'resting' conditions and during osmotic diuresis. Amer. J. Physiol. 163, 159 (1950). — WEST, C. D., J. TRAEGER and S. A. KAPLAN: A comparison of the relative effectiveness of hydropenia and of Pitressin in producing a concentrated urine. J. clin. Invest. 34, 887 (1955). — WEST, J. R., and J. G. KRAMER: Nephrogenic diabetes insipidus. Pediatrics 15, 424 (1955). — WEST, J. R., H. W. SMITH and H. CHASIS: Glomerular filtration rate, effective renal plasma flow, and maximal tubular excretory capacity in infancy. J. Pediat. 32, 10 (1948). — WESTFALL, B. B., T. FINDLEY and A. N. RICHARDS: Quantitative studies of the composition of glomerular urine. XII. The concen-tration of chloride in glomerular urine of frogs and necturi. J. biol. Chem. 107, 661 (1934). — WESTFALL, B. B., and E. M. LANDIS: The molecular weight of inulin. J. biol. Chem. 116, 727 (1936). — WESTON, R. E., DORIS J. W. ESCHER, J. GROSSMAN and L. LEITER: Mecha-nisms contributing to unresponsiveness to mercurial diuretics in congestive heart failure. J. clin. Invest. 31, 901 (1952). — WESTON, R. E., J. GROSSMAN, I. S. EDELMAN, DORIS J. W. ESCHER, L. LEITER and LILLIAN HELLMAN: Renal tubular action of diuretics. II. Effects of mercurial diuresis on glucose reabsorption. Fed. Proc. 8, 164 (1949) (abstract). — WESTON, R. E., J. GROSSMAN, A. ESSIG, MARIAN C. ISAACS, I. B. HANENSON and HELEN B. HOROWITZ: Homeostatic regulation of body fluid volume in nonedematous subjects. Metabolism 9, 157 (1960). — WESTON, R. E., J. GROSSMAN and L. LEITER: The effect of mercurial diuretics on renal ammonia and titrable acidity production in acidotic human subjects with reference to site of diuretic action. J. clin. Invest. 30, 1262 (1951). — WESTON, R. E., LILLIAN HELLMAN,

DORIS J. W. ESCHER, I. S. EDELMAN, J. GROSSMAN and L. LEITER: Studies on the influence of the low sodium cardiac diet and the Kempner regimen on renal hemodynamics and electrolyte excretion in hypertensive subjects. J. clin. Invest. 29, 639 (1950). — WESTON, R. E., HELEN B. HOROWITZ, J. GROSSMAN, I. B. HANENSON and L. LEITER: Decreased antidiuretic response to beta-hypophamine in hyperthyroidism. J. clin. Endocr. 16, 322 (1956). — WHITE, A. G.: Diabetes insipidus associated with edema. Report of a case with discussion of the physiologic implications. New Engl. J. Med. 250, 633 (1954). — Mechanisms regulating the renal transport of p-aminohippurate: relative velocities and energy dependence of uptake and secretion. Amer. J. Physiol. 191, 50 (1957). — WHITE, A. G., M. KURTZ and G. RUBIN: Comparative renal responses to water and the antidiuretic hormone in diabetes insipidus and in chronic renal disease. Amer. J. Med. 16, 220 (1954). — WHITE, A. G., and G. RUBIN: Physiological mechanisms regulating rate of urinary flow in renal disease. Proc. Soc. exp. Biol. (N.Y.) 86, 30 (1954). — WHITE, A. G., G. RUBIN and L. LEITER: Studies in edema. III. The effect of pitressin on the renal excretion of water and electrolytes in patients with and without liver disease. J. clin. Invest. 30, 1287 (1951). — Studies in edema. IV. Water retention and the antidiuretic hormone in hepatic and cardiac disease. J. clin. Invest. 32, 931 (1953). — WHITE, H. L.: Studies on renal tubule function. I. A comparison of the concentration ratios of various urinary constituents. Amer. J. Physiol. 65, 200 (1923). — Observations on the nature of glomerular activity. Amer. J. Physiol. 90, 689 (1929). — Observations indicating absence of glomerular intermittence in normal dogs and rabbits. Amer. J. Physiol. 128, 159 (1939). — Observations on behavior of diodrast in dog. Amer. J. Physiol. 130, 454 (1940a). — The effects of phlorhizin on renal plasma flow, on glomerular filtration and on the tubular excretion of diodrast in the dog. Amer. J. Physiol. 130, 582 (1940b). — WHITE, H. L., T. FINDLEY jr. and J. C. EDWARDS: Interpretation of diodrast clearances in man. Proc. Soc. exp. Biol. (N.Y.) 43, 11 (1940). — WHITE, H. L., and P. HEINBECKER: Pituitary regulation of water exchange in the dog and monkey. Amer. J. Physiol. 118, 276 (1937). — Observations on inulin and diodrast clearances and on renal plasma flow in normal and hypophysectomized dogs. Amer. J. Physiol. 130, 464 (1940). — WHITE, H. L., P. HEINBECKER and DORIS ROLF: Effects of hypophysectomy on some renal functions. Proc. Soc. exp. Biol. (N.Y.) 46, 44 (1941). — Effects of the removal of the anterior lobe of the hypophysis on some renal functions. Amer. J. Physiol. 136, 584 (1942). — Some endocrine influences on renal function and cardiac output. Amer. J. Physiol. 149, 404 (1947). — Further observations on the depression of renal function following hypophysectomy. Amer. J. Physiol. 156, 67 (1949a). — Enhancing effects of growth hormone on renal function. Amer. J. Physiol. 157, 47 (1949b). — Renotropic effects of growth hormone preparations. Amer. J. Physiol. 165, 442 (1951). — WHITE, H. L., and BETTY MONAGHAN: A comparison of the clearances of creatinine and of various sugars. Amer. J. Physiol. 106, 16 (1933). — WHITE, H. L., and DORIS ROLF: Effects of exercise and of some other influences on renal circulation in man. Amer. J. Physiol. 152, 505 (1948). — Renal glutaminase in adrenalectomized and in hypophysectomized rats, and plasma glutamine levels in normal and adrenalectomized rats. Amer. J. Physiol. 174, 27 (1953). — WHITE, H. L., I. T. ROSEN, S. S. FISCHER and G. H. WOOD: The influence of posture on renal activity. Amer. J. Physiol. 78, 185 (1926). — WHITE, H. L., and F. O. SCHMITT: The site of reabsorption in the kidney tubule of Necturus. Amer. J. Physiol. 76, 483 (1926). — WHITE, H. L., D. C. TOSTESON and DORIS ROLF: Roles of blood and urine flows in distributing THO and Na^{22} within the kidney. Fed. Proc. 19, 365 (1960) (abstract). — WHITNEY, J., S. SMITH III, J. MARMORSTON, H. GOODMAN and A. SELLERS: Antidiuretic effect of renin in the dog. Amer. J. Physiol. 176, 419 (1954). — WHITTAKER, S. R. F., and F. R. WINTON: The apparent viscosity of blood flowing in the isolated hindlimb of the dog, and its variation with corpuscular concentration. J. Physiol. (Lond.) 78, 22 (1933). — WHITTEMBURY, G., D. E. OKEN, E. E. WINDHAGER and A. K. SOLOMON: Single proximal tubules of Necturus kidney. IV. Dependence of H$_2$O movement on osmotic gradients. Amer. J. Physiol. 197, 1121 (1959a). — Perfusion of single proximal tubules of Necturus kidney: dependence of water flux upon solute movement. Fed. Proc. 18, 170 (1959b) (abstract). — WIDMARK, E. M. P.: Studies in the acetone concentration in blood, urine and alveolar air. II. The passage of acetone and acetoacetic acid into the urine. Biochem. J. 14, 364 (1920). — WIGGINS, W. S., C. H. MANRY, R. H. LYONS and R. F. PITTS: The effect of salt loading and salt depletion on renal function and electrolyte excretion in man. Circulation 3, 275 (1951). — WILBRANDT, W.: Electrical potential differences across the wall of kidney tubules of Necturus. J. cell. comp. Physiol. 11, 425 (1938). — Secretion and transport of non-electrolytes. Symp. Soc. exp. Biol. 8, 136 (1954). — The relation between rate and affinity in carrier transports. J. cell. comp. Physiol. 47, 137 (1956). — WILDE, W. S., and R. L. MALVIN: Graphical placement of transport segments along the nephron from urine concentration pattern developed from stop flow technique. Amer. J. Physiol. 195, 153 (1958). — Movement of peritubular Na^{24} across the nephron wall during stop flow. Fed. Proc. 18, 170 (1959) (abstract). — WILKINS, R. W.,

S. E. Bradley and C. K. Friedland: The acute circulatory effects of the head-down position (negative G) in normal man, with a note on some measures designed to relieve cranial congestion in this position. J. clin. Invest. **29**, 940 (1950). — Wilkins, R. W., C. M. Tinsley, J. W. Culbertson, B. A. Burrows, W. E. Judson and C. E. Burnett: Effects of venous congestion of the limbs upon renal clearances and the excretion of water and salt. I. Studies in normal subjects and in hypertensive patients before and after splanchnicectomy. J. clin. Invest. **32**, 1101 (1953). — Wilkinson, A. W.: Adrenalectomy and the metabolic response to injury. Lancet **1956I**, 184. — Wilkinson, E. L., H. Backman and H. H. Hecht: Cardiovascular and renal adjustments to a new hypotensive agent. Amer. J. Med. **13**, 101 (1952) (abstract). — Williams, Florence, and J. R. Leonards: The effect of sodium bicarbonate on the renal excretion of salicylate. J. Pharmacol. exp. Ther. **93**, 401 (1948). — Williams, Jeannine, F. C. Rector jr., N. W. Carter and D. W. Seldin: Effect of anions on NH_3 excretion in hypokalemic alkalosis. Clin. Res. Proc. 8, 65 (1960) (abstract). — Williams, R. H., and C. Henry: Nephrogenic diabetes insipidus: transmitted by females and appearing during infancy in males. Ann. intern. Med. **27**, 84 (1947). — Williams, T. F.: Urinary pH in relation to availability of sodium. Clin. Res. Proc. 8, 90 (1960) (abstract). — Williamson, H. E., F. E. Shideman and D. A. LeSher: Antagonism of the effect of certain steroids on the renal excretion of water and electrolytes by 2-amino-4-(p-chloro-anilino)-s-triazine. J. Pharmacol. exp. Ther. **126**, 82 (1959). — Williamson, H. E., T. W. Skulan and F. E. Shideman: Effect of adrenalectomy on the pattern of sodium and potassium exchange in the renal tubule of the rat. Fed. Proc. **18**, 459 (1959). — Willis, M. J., and F. W. Sunderman: Studies in serum electrolytes. XIX. Nomograms for calculating magnesium ion in serum and ultrafiltrates. J. biol. Chem. **197**, 343 (1952). — Willoughby, L.: The binding of myoglobin by plasma protein. J. exp. Med. **111**, 65 (1960). — Wills, J. H., and Edna Main: Renal function in normal rabbits and dogs and the effect of uranyl salts. Amer. J. Physiol. **154**, 220 (1948). — Wilmer, H. A.: Arrangement of capillary tuft of human glomerulus; injection study. Anat. Rec. **80**, 507 (1941). — Wilson, D. M., E. H. Rynearson and T. J. Dry: Cardiac failure following treatment of Addison's disease with desoxycorticosterone acetate. Proc. Mayo Clin. **16**, 168 (1941). — Wilson, D. W., W. L. Long, H. C. Thompson and Sylva Thurlow: Changes in the composition of the urine after muscular exercise. J. biol. Chem. **65**, 755 (1925). — Wilson, H. E. C., and Audrey Muirhead: Evidence of the presence of a pitressin like substance in the tissue fluids in nephrosis. Acta paediat. **45**, 77 (1956). — Wilson, Jean D., and D. W. Seldin: Effect of adrenalectomy on production and excretion of ammonia by the kidney. Amer. J. Physiol. **188**, 524 (1957). — Wilson jr., J. R., and C. R. Harrison: Cardiovascular, renal and general effects of large rapid plasma infusions in convalescent men. J. clin. Invest. **29**, 251 (1950). — Windhager, E. E., and G. Giebisch: Micropuncture study in the rat during osmotic diuresis. Fed. Proc. **18**, 171 (1959) (abstract). — Micropuncture study of renal tubular acidification in the rat. Fed. Proc. **19**, 369 (1960) (abstract). — Windhager, E. E., G. Whittembury, D. E. Oken, H. J. Schatzmann and A. K. Solomon: Single proximal tubules of the Necturus kidney. III. Dependence of H_2O movement on NaCl concentration. Amer. J. Physiol. **197**, 313 (1959). — Winer, N. J.: Renal function in diabetes insipidus. Arch. intern. Med. **70**, 61 (1942). — Winkler, A. W., and J. Parra: The measurement of glomerular filtration. Creatinine, sucrose and urea clearances in subjects without renal disease. J. clin. Invest. **16**, 859 (1937a). — The measurement of glomerular filtration. The creatinine, sucrose and urea clearances in subjects with renal disease. J. clin. Invest. **16**, 869 (1937b). — Winkler, A. W., and P. K. Smith: Renal excretion of potassium salts. Amer. J. Physiol. **138**, 94 (1942). — Winter, C. A., C. Elizabeth Gaffney and L. Flataker: The effect of N-allylnormorphine upon the antidiuretic action of morphine. J. Pharmacol. exp. Ther. **111**, 360 (1954). — Winter, C. A., W. R. Ingram and R. C. Eaton: Effect of dietary changes upon urine volume and renal function in experimental diabetes insipidus. Amer. J. Physiol. **139**, 700 (1943). — Winton, F. R.: The influence of increase of ureter pressure on the isolated mammalian kidney. J. Physiol. (Lond.) **71**, 381 (1931a). — The glomerular pressure in the isolated mammalian kidney. J. Physiol. (Lond.) **72**, 361 (1931b). — The control of the glomerular pressure by vascular changes within the isolated mammalian kidney, demonstrated by the actions of adrenaline. J. Physiol. (Lond.) **73**, 151 (1931c). — The influence of venous pressure on the isolated mammalian kidney. J. Physiol. (Lond.) **72**, 49 (1931d). — Intrarenal pressure. J. Physiol. (Lond.) **78**, 9P (1933) (abstract). — Intrarenal pressure and its variations due to cooling and "reducing" the isolated kidney of the dog. J. Physiol. (Lond.) **82**, 27P (1934a) (abstract). — The relation between diuresis and maximum ureter pressure, and its bearing on current methods of estimating the rate of glomerular filtration. J. Physiol. (Lond.) **83**, 38P (1934) (abstract). — The influence of changes in arterial pressure on the intrarenal pressure in the isolated mammalian kidney. J. Physiol. (Lond.) **87**, 18P (1936) (abstract). — Physical factors involved in the activities of the mammalian kidney. Physiol. Rev. **17**, 408 (1937). — Hydrostatic pressures affecting the flow of urine and blood in the kidney. Harvey Lect. **47**, 21 (1951). — The pressures and flows of blood and urine within the kidney. In: Modern views on the secretion of urine. Boston: Little, Brown & Co. 1956. — WIRZ, H.: Der osmotische Druck des Blutes in der Nierenpapille. Helv. physiol. pharmacol. Acta **11**, 20 (1953). — Der Einfluß des antidiuretischen Hormons auf den intra-tubulären Druck der Rattenniere. Helv. physiol. pharmacol. Acta **13**, C42 (1955a) (abstract). — Druckmessung in Kapillaren und Tubuli der Niere durch Micropunktion. Helv. physiol. pharmacol. Acta **13**, 42 (1955b). — Der osmotische Druck in der corticalen Tubuli der Rattenniere. Helv. physiol. pharmacol. Acta **14**, 353 (1956). — WIRZ, H., and PHYLLIS A. BOTT: Potassium and reducing substances in proximal tubule fluid of the rat kidney. Proc. Soc. exp. Biol. (N.Y.) **87**, 405 (1954). — WIRZ, H., B. HARGITAY and W. KUHN: Lokalization des Konzentrierungsprozesses in der Niere durch direkte Kryoskopie. Helv. physiol. pharmacol. Acta **9**, 196 (1951). — WOLBACH, R. A.: Renal regulation of acid-base balance in the chicken. Amer. J. Physiol. **181**, 149 (1955). — WOLF, A. V.: Renal regulation of water and some electrolytes in man, with special reference to their relative retention and excretion. Amer. J. Physiol. **148**, 54 (1947). — WOLF, A. V., and S. M. BALL: Effect of intravenous calcium salts on renal excretion in the dog. Amer. J. Physiol. **158**, 205 (1949). — WOLF, G. A.: The effect of pain on renal function. Proc. Soc. Res. nerv. ment. Dis. **23**, 358 (1943). — WOLF, R. L., and G. S. EADIE: Reabsorption of bromide by the kidney. Amer. J. Physiol. **163**, 436 (1950). — WOLF, S., J. B. PFEIFFER, H. S. RIPLEY, O. S. WINTER and H. G. WOLFF: Hypertension as a reaction pattern to stress; summary of experimental data on variations in blood pressure and renal blood flow. Ann. intern. Med. **29**, 1056 (1948). — WOLFF, H. P., K. R. KOCZOREK and E. BUCHBORN: Aldosteronuria in oedema. In: Aldo-sterone. Boston: Little, Brown & Co. 1958. — WOLFF, H. P., K. R. KOCZOREK, E. BUCH-BORN and G. RIEKER: Endocrine factors. J. chron. Dis. **9**, 554 (1959). — WOLFSON, W. Q., C. COHN, R. LEVINE and B. HUDDLESTUN: Transport and excretion of uric acid in man. III. Physiologic significance of the uricosuric effect of caronamide. Amer. J. Med. **4**, 774 (1948) (abstract). — WOMERSLEY, R. A.: Studies on the renal excretion of magnesium and other electrolytes. Clin. Sci. **15**, 465 (1956). — WOMERSLEY, R. A., and J. H. DARRAGH: Potassium and sodium restriction in the normal human. J. clin. Invest. **34**, 456 (1955). — WOMERSLEY, R. A., O. A. THORUP and L. G. WELT: The influence of enhanced sodium re-absorption by DOCA and compounds E and F on the rates of excretion of water, potassium and ammonia. J. clin. Invest. **32**, 613 (1953). — WOOD, E. H.: Glucose reabsorption in the amphibian kidney. Amer. J. Physiol. **133**, P497 (1941) (abstract). — WOOD, T. R., and W. F. ROSS: The ketene acetylation of the parathyroid hormone. J. biol. Chem. **146**, 59 (1942). — WOODSON, H. W., S. W. HIER, J. D. SOLOMON and O. BERGEIM: Urinary excre-tion of amino acids by human subjects on normal diets. J. biol. Chem. **172**, 613 (1948). — WRIGHT, L. D., H. F. RUSSO, HELEN R. SKEGGS, ELIZABETH A. PATCH and K. H. BEYER: Renal clearance of essential amino acids; arginine, histidine lysine and methionine. Amer. J. Physiol. **149**, 130 (1947). — WRONG, O.: The relationship between water retention and electrolyte excretion following administration of antidiuretic hormone. Clin. Sci. **15**, 401 (1956). — The volume control of body fluids. Brit. med. Bull. **13**, 10 (1957).

    YAGI, K., and H. L. WHITE: Comparison of ammonium sulfate fractionation of proteins and of protein-bound mercury in kidney soluble fraction of chow-fed and sucrose-fed rats. Amer. J. Physiol. **194**, 547 (1958). — YAMADA, E.: The fine structure of the renal glomerulus of the mouse. J. biophys. biochem. Cytol. **1**, 551 (1955). — YANKOPOULOS, N. A., J. O. DAVIS, B. KLIMAN and R. E. PETERSON: Increased aldosterone secretion following acute constriction of thoracic and of abdominal inferior vena cava. Fed. Proc. **17**, 173 (1958) (abstract). — Evidence that a humoral agent stimulates the adrenal cortex to secrete aldo-sterone in experimental secondary hyperaldosteronism. J. clin. Invest. **38**, 1278 (1959). — YOFFEE, H. F., and J. F. DINGMAN: Studies of the effect of calcium on the antidiuretic action of vasopressin. Clin. Res. Proc. **7**, 272 (1959) (abstract). — YOSHIDA, H.: Über die Harnbildung in der Froschniere. Pflügers Arch. ges. Physiol. **206**, 274 (1924). — YOSHIMURA, H., O. OKUMURA, K. NISHIKAWA, M. YUASA, M. YADA and J. SUGIMOTO: Studies on mechanism of ammonia excretion by the kidney. J. Physiol. Soc. Jap. **20**, 988 (1958). — YOUNG, I. MAUREEN, H. E. DE WARDENER and B. E. MILES: Mechanism of the renal excretion of methonium compounds. Brit. med. J. **1951** II, 1500. — YOUNG jr., M. K., and L. G. RAISZ: An anthrone procedure for determination of inulin in biological fluids. Proc. Soc. exp. Biol. (N.Y.) **80**, 771 (1952). — YOUNG, W. F., and R. A. McCANCE: Secretion of urine by dehydrated and normal infants. Arch. Dis. Child. **17**, 65 (1942). — YOUNT, E., and J. M. LITTLE: Renal clearance in patients with myxedema. J. clin. Endocr. **15**, 343 (1955). — YÜ, TSAI F., L. BERGER, D. J. STONE, J. WOLF and A. B. GUTMAN: Effect of pyrazinamide and pyrazinoic acid on urate clearance and other discrete renal functions. Proc. Soc. exp. Biol. (N.Y.) **96**, 264 (1957a). — YÜ, TSAI F., J. J. BURNS, P. G. DAYTON, A. B. GUTMAN and B. B. BRODIE: A p-nitro analogue of phenyl-butazone possessing potent antirheumatic, sodium retaining and uricosuric properties. J. Pharmacol. exp. Ther. **126**, 185 (1959). — YÜ, TSAI F., and A. B. GUTMAN: Ultrafiltrability of plasma urate in man. Proc. Soc. exp. Biol. (N.Y.) **84**, 21 (1953). — Paradoxical retention of uric acid by uricosuric drugs in low dosage. Proc. Soc. exp. Biol. (N.Y.) **90**, 542 (1955). — Renal regulation of uric acid excretion in normal and gouty man: modification by uricosuric agents. Bull. N.Y. Acad. Med. **34**, 287 (1958). — A consideration of the mechanisms of presumptive tubular excretion of urate in man. Fed. Proc. **18**, 175 (1959) (abstract). — YÜ, TSAI F., B. C. PATON, T. CHENKIN, J. J. BURNS, B. B. BRODIE and A. B. GUTMAN: Effect of a phenylbutazone analog (4-(phenylthioethyl)-1,2-diphenyl 3,5-pyrazolidinedione) on urate clearance and other discrete renal functions in gouty subjects. Evaluation as uricosuric agent. J. clin. Invest. **35**, 374 (1956). — YÜ, TSAI F., J. H. SIROTA, L. BERGER, M. HALPERN and A. B. GUTMAN: Effect of sodium lactate infusion on urate clearance in man. Proc. Soc. exp. Biol. (N.Y.) **96**, 809 (1957b). — YÜ, TSAI F., J. H. SIROTA and A. B. GUTMAN: Effect of phenylbutazone (3,5-dioxo-1,2-diphenyl-4-N-butylpyrazolidene) on renal clearance of urate and other discrete renal functions in gouty subjects. J. clin. Invest. **32**, 1121 (1953). — YUILE, C. L., and W. F. CLARK: Myohemoglobinuria; study of renal clearance of myohemoglobin in dogs. J. exp. Med. **74**, 187 (1941). — YUILE, C. L., J. F. STEINMAN, P. F. HAHN and W. F. CLARK: Tubular factor in renal hemoglobin excretion. J. exp. Med. **74**, 197 (1941).

ZAK, G. A., C. BRUN and H. W. SMITH: The mechanism of formation of osmotically concentrated urine during the antidiuretic state. J. clin. Invest. **33**, 1064 (1954). — ZARAFONETIS, C. J. D., W. A. STEIGER, L. MOLTHAN, J. MCMASTER and V. F. COLVILLE: Renal defect associated with sickle cell trait and sickle cell disease. J. Lab. clin. Med. **44**, 959 (1954) (abstract). — ZIERLER, K. L., and J. L. LILIENTHAL jr.: Sodium loss in man induced by desoxycorticosterone acetate. Amer. J. Med. **4**, 186 (1948). — ZIMMERMANN, K. W.: Über den Bau des Glomerulus der Säugetiere. Z. mikr.-anat. Forsch. **32**, 176 (1933). — ZUIDEMA, G. D., and N. P. CLARKE: Central localization of the osmotic control center. Amer. J. Physiol. **188**, 616 (1957). — ZUIDEMA, G. D., N. P. CLARKE and MARY F. MINTON: Osmotic regulation of body fluids. Amer. J. Physiol. **187**, 85 (1956). — ZUIDEMA, G. D., N. P. CLARKE. J. L. REEVES, O. H. GAUER and J. P. HENRY: Influence of moderate changes in blood volume on urine flow. Amer. J. Physiol. **186**, 89 (1956). — ZUNTZ, H. N.: Zur Kenntnis des Phlorhizindiabetes. Arch. Physiol. **19**, 570 (1895).

Disorders of renal function

By

CLIFFORD WILSON[1]

With 1 figure

A. Introduction

The function of the kidneys is to elaborate a urine appropriate in volume and composition to the needs of the body. A consideration of disordered renal function must therefore include, the circumstances in which the kidneys fail in this objective, the disordered mechanism of urine formation under these circumstances, and the results on the body processes as a whole.

In the previous chapter the physiological aspects of these problems have been considered in detail. In the present chapter an attempt will be made to give an account of disordered renal function with a clinical approach. When the kidneys are structurally disorganised the application of methods and reasoning appropriate to normally functioning kidneys may be uncertain or even impossible. Frequently multiple factors operate in disturbing renal function, and the resulting disorders may be so complex as to defy analysis on physiological grounds. The more simple and relatively crude tests of renal function may in these circumstances be the most reliable for diagnosis and prognosis.

Disorders of glomerular and tubular function will first be considered from the point view of their clinical incidence and their separate contribution to renal failure in disease. Secondly the effects of renal dysfunction on the bodily processes as a whole be discussed, i.e. disturbances of renal homeostasis. The classical studies of HOMER SMITH established the theoretical basis of this concept and for an account of the detailed mechanisms, reference should be made to the foregoing section on renal physiology. In this homeostatic control, the purely excretory function of the kidney — i.e. elimination of the waste products of metabolism — plays only a minor part. Of much greater significance is the maintenance of the various body equilibria, especially in relation to the volume of body water, electrolyte conservation and acid base regulation. In this vital activity — the maintenance of what CLAUDE BERNARD called the "milieu interieur" — the kidney acts largely under the influence of the endocrine system, particularly the pituitary and suprarenal glands. A special complication is the fact that disorders of the various body equilibria, whether of body water, electrolytes or acid-base balance, themselves interfere with renal function, and such reciprocal action may lead to a vicious circle of homeostatic breakdown which is of great clinical importance. In this section also must be considered the relationship of the kidney to high blood pressure. Although the nature of renal hypertension is still obscure,

---

[1] This chapter nas been written in collaboration with the following members of the Medical Unit of the London Hospital, J. M. LEDINGHAM, M. A. FLOYER, D. W. VERE, R. H. BALME.

25*

high blood pressure is such a frequent and important manifestation of renal disease that it seems justifiable to regard blood pressure regulation as one of the homeostatic functions of the kidney.

The third section of this chapter will deal with the particular patterns of disordered renal physiology which are found in various types of kidney disease. This will provide a description of the various syndromes of uraemia with which the patient may present. Of particular importance in this discussion will be the relative contributions which renal and extra-renal factors make to the clinical picture of uraemia in different froms of renal disease, and their practical implications in treatment.

B. Disorders of the mechanism of urine formation
I. Changes in glomerular filtration

Since glomerular filtration is a purely physical process dependent on filtration pressure and blood flow, deviations from the normal will be expected when these factors are altered by disease. This alteration may take the form of structural damage to the glomeruli, or of circulatory changes affecting glomerular capillary pressure and flow. In addition, both structural and circulatory changes may damage the capillary walls leading to abnormal permeability. Thus disorders of glomerular filtration will include reduction in filtration rate, which is common, and increase in filtration which is rare, together with qualitative changes in the filtrate due to the leakage of excessive amounts of protein and the passage of red blood cells and leucocytes through the capillary membranes. The most serious effects are those which result from reduction in glomerular filtration and increased membrane permeability. The former leads to diminished clearance from the blood of normally diffusible substances, i.e. the waste products of protein catabolism and other electrolytes; the latter causes protein loss with eventual depletion of blood and tissue proteins, whilst leakage of erythrocytes if continuous is one of the several causes of anaemia in renal disease. Tubular reabsorption can to some extent compensate for variations in glomerular filtration, but when the latter is severely restricted by disease there is no adequate compensatory mechanism and metabolic waste products accumulate in the blood, a condition usually referred to as "nitrogen retention". This is however an imperfect description since the more serious effects of glomerular failure on the patient may be due to retention of non-nitrogenous substances such as sodium or potassium, or to failure of excretion of anions leading to severe acidosis, or to some "toxic" substance or substances as yet unknown.

1. Reduced glomerular filtration
a) Causation

Structural damage to the glomeruli occurs in almost all forms of organic renal disease but is most pronounced in glomerulo-nephritis. In acute glomerulo-nephritis, where the glomeruli are diffusely involved (Type I nephritis, ELLIS), glomerular filtration may be so much reduced that anuria or severe oliguria results. In most cases however there is reduction in urine volume which is primarily due to diminished glomerular filtration rate. The renal blood flow is usually normal or slightly reduced, but may be on occasions increased, e.g. BRADLEY (1949) showed increased P.A.H. recovery from renal vein blood. SMITH (1951) suggests that reduced filtration may be due to reduction of filtration surface.

There is on the other hand evidence that glomerular capillary pressure may be reduced by excessive constriction of the afferent arterioles (EARLE, TAGGART and SHANNON; BLACK et al.; BRADLEY et al.) and support for such excessive vasoconstriction may be found in the occurrence of necrosis of these vessels in severe cases. In chronic glomerulo-nephritis, and in other forms of chronic renal disease including pyelonephritis, ischaemic atrophy due to arterial disease or urinary obstruction, diabetic nephrosclerosis, and amyloid disease, glomerular filtration is restricted by progressive reduction in the number of functioning nephrons. It is difficult to interpret clearance tests when much disorganisation of renal architecture has occurred (BRADLEY 1948a) but there is in advanced cases evidence of reduction both in glomerular filtration rate and renal blood flow.

Extra-renal factors leading to impaired circulation through the renal glomeruli frequently cause diminished glomerular filtration, and may act by reducing the rate glomerular blood flow or filtration pressure or both factors together. When filtration pressure is reduced the filtration fraction is diminished to a greater extent than filtration rate. In general the extra-renal states with reduced glomerular filtration are those in which 1. the blood volume is diminished or 2. the blood pressure is considerably reduced or 3. cardiac failure is present. The most severe reduction in glomerular filtration occurs with acute rise in intrapelvic pressure due to urinary tract obstruction, and in acute cortical ischaemia, both of which may lead to total suppression of urine formation. These circulatory factors will be now discussed in further detail.

Diminished blood volume (hypovolaemia). The common causes are loss of blood, particularly gastro-intestinal haemorrhage, sodium and water depletion (for example due to vomiting, diarrhoea, gastric aspiration) and prolonged urinary electrolyte depletion such as may follow the use of diuretics or in severe diabetic ketosis or adrenal cortical failure. In all these states of depressed circulating blood volume, cardiac output is diminished and in addition the blood flow through the less vital organs, including the kidneys, is disproportionately reduced by increased arteriolar constriction. Thus renal blood flow may diminish while the arterial blood pressure is still maintained (VAN SLYKE). Diminished renal blood flow with reduction of glomerular filtration has been demonstrated in vomiting due to pyloric obstruction (BURNETT, BURROWS and COMMONS), in diabetic ketosis (BERNSTEIN, FOLEY and HOFFMAN) and in Addison's disease (TALBOT et al.; WATERHOUSE and KEUTMANN).

Fall in arterial pressure. Hypotension occurs when compensatory vaso-constriction fails in hypovolaemia, i.e. in states of shock with so-called peripheral circulatory failure. Renal arteriolar constriction may produce disproportionate reduction in glomerular blood flow (LAUSON, BRADLEY and COURNAND), in shock due to haemorrhage, trauma or burns. In these cases a low filtration fraction indicates excessive afferent arteriolar constriction leading to fall in filtration pressure out of proportion to reduction in blood flow. Anaesthesia may contribute to reduction in renal blood flow and further impair filtration rate (PAPPER). Hypotension may also be a contributory factor to impaired glomerular filtration in Addision's disease. In acute hypotension caused by hexamethonium, the glomerular filtration rate falls (MOYER and MILLS) and with prolonged hypotension anuria may occur.

Heart failure. Acute left ventricular failure, particularly following coronary thrombosis, may lead to hypotension with consequent reduction in glomerular filtration rate. In chronic congestive failure, reduction in glomerular filtration rate was demonstrated by SEYMOUR et al., whilst MERRILL (1946) and MERRILL and CARGILL showed that in patients with cardiac oedema, decrease in filtration rate was proportionately less than the reduction in renal blood flow i.e. the filtration fraction was increased, presumably due to efferent arteriolar constriction.

Urinary tract obstruction. Rise in renal pelvic pressure will obviously increase the resistance to glomerular filtration and may lead eventually to suppression of urine. Conversely sudden release of obstruction may be followed by a large osmotic diuresis which will cause severe water and electrolyte depletion leading to hypovolaemia and circulatory renal failure (Bull 1955). Obstructive lesions of the urinary tract will reduce glomerular filtration both by reducing the effective filtration pressure and by reducing glomerular blood flow.

Acute cortical ischaemia. A particularly severe form of circulatory glomerular failure is that which is described by various terms, including lower nephron nephrosis, traumatic anuria and acute tubular necrosis. The micro-dissection studies of Oliver, MacDowell and Tracy provide convincing evidence of diffuse cortical ischaemia as the cause of suppression of glomerular filtration in these patients although the mechanism of production of the ischaemia is obscure. Since the functional disturbance is manifestly glomerular and tubular, and on the available evidence is caused by acute renal circulatory insufficiency, the term acute cortical ischaemia appears to be less objectionable than those which suggest a primary or predominant tubular lesion. Furthermore histological evidence of organic tubular damage is always focal, often inconspicuous and sometimes absent. Widely diverse factors such as crush injuries of the limbs, surgical operations, obstetric shock, incompatible blood transfusion, idiosyncray to drugs, and operations on the urinary tract may be responsible for this syndrome, which will be discussed in detail later. Clearance studies have suggested a gross reduction in renal blood flow and filtration rate (Sirota; Bull, Joekes and Lowe), but direct methods indicate that renal blood flow may be 30—50% of normal (Munck). Studies of the renal arteriovenous oxygen differences and PAH recoveries from renal vein blood have revealed no evidence of the existence in man of an intra-renal shunt mechanism such as was observed in rabbits by Trueta et al. after application of a tourniquet to the limb. In haemorrhage and shock, the increased constriction of the renal arterioles may persist after the blood pressure returns to the normal level (Philips et al.).

Metabolic factors. Although rarely of serious clinical importance, it appears that, apart from disturbances of blood volume, certain metabolic factors may have a direct effect on glomerular filtration rate. Thus potassium depletion (Schwartz and Relman), adrenal insufficiency, and hypercalcaemia (Scholz; Ottolander et al.; Fourman), all appear to have a depressant effect on glomerular filtration.

b) Results

Reduced glomerular filtration results in failure of clearance from the blood of diffusible substances. Some of these, such as urea, are relatively inert, others such as sodium and potassium, whilst physiologically useful, may cause serious effects when their concentration in the extracellular fluid increases above physiological levels. Nevertheless all solutes will contribute to the increased osmolarity of the glomerular filtrate.

Although in the above circumstances we can be reasonably certain when glomerular filtration is reduced, and the degree of reduction can be roughly estimated, the effects on the body fluids can be foretold with much less certainty owing to the influence of tubular activity. For the tubules determine how much of any particular constituent of glomerular filtrate is excreted, and this tubular activity depends on extra-renal regulating mechanisms which in disease are modified by tubular damage. In general however tubular compensation is remarkably effective for those substances which in health are in greater part reabsorbed by the tubules; i.e. water, glucose, and the anions and cations which are the normal components of extra-cellular and intra-cellular fluid. We can be more certain about the effects of reduced glomerular filtration on metabolic waste products derived from protein catabolism, which are not actively reabsorbed by the renal tubules. Impairment of glomerular filtration will result in a proportionate failure of clearance of these substances, particularly urea, and the blood levels will rise. Thus the level of blood non-protein nitrogen provides an approximate measure of failure of glomerular filtration. With progressive reduction in nephrons this measure becomes less accurate owing to increasing back diffusion of urea in the surviving tubules. The increased filtration load may however be sufficient to maintain adequate clearance for many years with the blood urea at a constant high level (PLATT 1952); this is particularly true of uraemia due to urinary tract obstruction, or to renal atrophy and fibrosis due to calculus formation, or healed renal tuberculosis, i.e. wherever organic disease is only slowly progressive. Nevertheless this increased filtration load produces osmotic diuresis which may be harmful when it leads to polyuria, isosthenuria and loss of electrolytes.

When excretion of any substance is determined entirely or largely by glomerular filtration, it will be affected by glomerular failure according to the blood level. This in turn depends on the amount ingested or produced by catabolism. Some of the conditions described above which reduce glomerular filtration are accompanied by an increase in endogenous protein breakdown, and failure of glomerular excretion will be aggravated. This is the case for example when intake of carbohydrate is reduced by anorexia, vomiting or diarrhoea, or where protein breakdown is increased by fever or tissue destruction. Not only urea, but also potassium and anions derived from metabolic oxidation, may be increased in the blood and interstitial fluid under these circumstances. A similar aggravation of defective filtration is seen after gastro-intestinal haemorrhage, when the elevation of blood urea can be partly attributed to increased protein absorption from the gut (BLACK).

An unequivocal picture of the effects of failure of glomerular filtration is provided by acute cortical ischaemia in which extreme oliguria or anuria develop. The structural and functional pathology of this condition have been greatly clarified by the studies of MUIRHEAD et al.; BULL, JOEKES and LOWE; OLIVER, MACDOWELL and TRACY; BULL 1955; and MERRILL 1955. In the anuria phase, the blood urea rises rapidly, and even on a low protein high carbohydrate intake, often continue to do so by 30 mgm./100 ml. per day. The occurrence of vomiting or infection may cause a much more rapid rise for the reasons given above. Of more serious importance is the rise in serum potassium, which is largely due to liberation of potassium from the cells, aggravated by increased protein breakdown. Hyperkalaemia may be detected by changes in the electrocardiogram and if uncorrected may lead to death from cardiac arrest. This result of depressed glomerular filtration underlines the danger of administering potassium salts to patients with impaired renal function. Accumulation of water as a result of failure of filtration results not only from administered fluids but also from "metabolic water" derived from increased protein catabolism and oxidation of fat and carbohydrate (SWANN and MERRILL; HAMBURGER and MATHÉ). This may lead to overhydration and hypotonicity of the extra-cellular fluid, followed by passage of sodium and water into the cells leading to cellular overhydration. Retention of anions (phosphate, sulphate, chloride) leads to "metabolic" acidosis with reduction of plasma bicarbonate. Phosphate retention may cause depression of serum calcium. Even after urine flow is re-established in acute cortical ischaemia, the depression of renal blood flow may take three to nine months to recover (MARSHALL and HOFFMAN; BULL, JOEKES and LOWE). During the recovery phase the effects of tubular dysfunction are more important than those of impaired glomerular filtration and will be discussed later. It seems likely that where hypovolaemia or hypotension are responsible for depression of glomerular filtration (e.g. in shock), the associated focal tubular damage is due to reduced renal blood flow, in contrast to other forms of suppression of urine where toxic substances lead to diffuse tubular degeneration (OLIVER, MACDOWELL and TRACY). Less severe forms of glomerular circulatory deficit, e.g. in dehydration due to repeated vomiting, may if prolonged, lead to tubular dysfunction and epithelial cell necrosis with subsequent calcification.

It is apparent that severe and extensive damage to the glomeruli, either organic or circulatory, is necessary before impaired filtration leads to complete suppression of urine with the results described above. Acute cortical ischaemia, severe acute diffuse glomerulo-nephritis and bilateral urinary tract obstruction are almost the only conditions which produce this major disturbance. Other forms of organic renal disease and extra-renal uraemia rarely present such a marked degree of metabolite retention; in these conditions, until renal disorganisation becomes gross and the condition is pre-terminal, diminished glomerular filtration produces little more than elevation of the blood urea. When chronic renal disease reaches its terminal stages however, various manifestations occur which are unexplained either by elevation of blood urea or by electrolyte disturbance. Gastro-intestinal disorders, cerebral symptoms including coma and convulsions, pericarditis, and a haemorrhagic tendency, are late symptoms of uraemia which suggest the retention of some "toxic" metabolite. Some workers have expressed the view that phenol derivatives, resulting from intestinal putrefaction of protein breakdown products may play such a role, but the evidence for this is not convincing (FISHBERG; HARRISON and MASON). It is of interest that treatment of uraemia by dialysis with the artificial kidney may lead to relief of cerebral and digestive symptoms without any consistent change in the known biochemical abnormalities of the blood.

The question whether sodium retention in heart failure can be attributed to depressed glomerular filtration is a controversial one (see SMITH 1951; MARRIOTT). There is much impressive evidence against this view which will be discussed later.

2. Increased glomerular filtration

Increased glomerular filtration can never be regarded as a pathological state, but certain factors can be shown to increase the rate (apart from any blood volume changes), presumably by increasing renal blood flow. Thus fever reduces efferent arteriolar constriction and causes a rise in glomerular filtration rate. A.C.T.H. and glutocorticoids also cause a rise in glomerular filtration rate (ALEXANDER et al. 1951 and BURNETT) and increased inulin clearance has been reported in acromegaly and after administration of growth hormone (SURTSHIN, ROLF and WHITE).

3. Increased glomerular permeability

The concept of the glomerulus as a filter or sieve, which plays a purely passive role in sorting large from small molecules (CUSHNY) remains essentially correct. Nevertheless it requires some modification since the filtering surface is a complex living tissue with a basement membrane, endothelium, and epithelium forming a delicate network (VERNIER). The "pores" in this structure have a functional and not merely a gross structural existence. Their "size" is probably determined by electrical charges near their surface, the types of ions lining them, the affinity of their surface for water, and the degree to which the membrane is stretched or relaxed. The permeability of collodion membranes for proteins varies markedly after treatment with electrolytes, amino acids or proteins (DAVSON and DANIELLI). Other factors complicating membrane permeability are the degree of association, the shapes, and the hydration of molecules. Against this background proteinuria is seen as a potentially reversible and functional abnormality where structural glomerular damage is slight, but it becomes irreversible when extensive lesions are present. Abnormal glomerular permeability does not affect small molecules and ions which normally pass the filter, save for small Donnan effects. In general, proteins with molecular weight above 60,000 are retained by the glomeruli but this is not a sharp boundary. When egg albumin is injected into animals, much protein appears in the urine which includes not only the injected protein but also plasma albumin (RATHER). Haemoglobin enters the urine from the plasma as if there were a variable "threshold". The explanation appears to be that haemoglobin is bound to haptoglobin in blood and is not excreted until the circulating haptoglobin becomes saturated (POLONOVSKI and JAYLE). Small amounts of albumin pass the glomerular filter in health (RATHER) and normally all but about 10 mgm. daily is reabsorbed in the proximal tubule.

In renal disease the pattern of proteinuria depends on the type of lesion. In the majority of diseases there is no diagnostic pattern, i.e. the urine protein differs quantitatively from plasma protein only as might be expected on the basis of ultra-filtration and non-preferential tubular reabsorption (HARDWICKE and SQUIRE). BUTLER and FLYNN have reviewed this problem and investigated proteinuria by electrophoresis in many forms of renal disease, with special reference to specific renal tubular disorders. In the latter a distinctive pattern was seen characterised by high α_2- and β-globulin fractions. This "tubular proteinuria pattern" is present only when excretion exceeds 15 mgm./100 ml., and in the opinion of the authors may be due to failure of the tubules to absorb high molecular weight proteins leaking through the normal (or abnormal) glomerular filter. In multiple myeloma the electrophoretic pattern usually shows a solitary peak between the β- and γ-globulin regions, although albuminuria may also be present. Increase in the α globulin fractions has also been reported in the urine of patients with renal calculi, independent of abnormalities due to urinary tract infection (BOYCE, GARVEY and NORFLEET).

Abnormal glomerular permeability for proteins may be investigated in two ways. Single proteins may be studied, and their excretion is then found to depend upon their concentration in the plasma, the glomerular filtration rate, the degree of tubular reabsorption, and a quantity called the "sieving" or permeability coefficient which measures glomerular permeability for that protein (BING). From these investigations, permeability appears to be related to the molecular size of the filtered proteins and their diffusion constants (HARDWICKE and SOOTHILL). A second method studies the degree to which small molecules are filtered in preference to large, i.e. the permeabilities for large and small molecules are compared. The result is a measure of "selective permeability" (PAPPENHEIMER) or "restrictive" permeability (MOVAT, STEINER and SLATER) of the glomeruli. It has been shown (BLAINEY et al.) that slight variations in selective permeability characterise the different histological varieties of nephritis. Thus, where extensive membraneous damage is seen in the glomeruli, relatively more of the larger proteins escape into the urine than when histological changes are minimal.

Proteinuria may occur in the absence of organic renal disease, and chronic venous congestion appears to be the most important cause, for example in cardiac failure or constrictive pericarditis. It seems unlikely that the distending effect of high venous pressure can extend beyond the efferent glomerular arteriole, and CUSHNY explained this type of proteinuria as due to renal anoxia. Raised renal venous pressure may also operate in postural proteinuria since there is evidence that the inferior vena cava may be compressed by the liver in certain abnormal postures (BULL 1948). Bacterial infection anywhere in the urinary tract will cause proteinuria and it is essential to exclude this complication before assuming the presence of abnormal glomerular permeability.

Erythrocytes and leucocytes pass the glomerular filter when the membrane is grossly damaged. In patients with unexplained haematuria the urine deposit should be freshly examined for blood casts to distinguish glomerular haemorrhage from bleeding in the lower urinary tract. Recurrent focal nephritis is a common cause of unexplained haematuria in young subjects and granular casts are commonly found in the urine deposit. Hyaline casts are formed by the combination of a protein, present in normal urine in small amounts, with albumin which is filtered through damaged glomeruli (McQUEEN). Hyaline casts have therefore no more significance than proteinuria alone, whereas granular casts indicate active nephron damage. Bacteria have been shown to pass BOWMAN'S membrane and fat droplets may enter the urine in fat embolism.

The results of abnormal glomerular permeability are hypoproteinaemic oedema (see section on Nephrotic Syndrome) with consequent increase in endogenous protein breakdown. Occasionally haematuria may be sufficiently severe and prolonged to cause haemorrhagic anaemia. The only therapeutic agents which appear to modify abnormal glomerular permeability are the glucocorticoid steroid hormones. Unfortunately their action is unpredictable and almost confined to cases of nephrotic syndrome with minimal glomerular structural changes. The relief of renal venous congestion will naturally reverse proteinuria due to this cause.

II. Disorders of tubular function

1. Defective tubular reabsorption

a) Unselective

One of the most remarkable features of chronic renal failure, such as results from glomerulo-nephritis or pyelonephritis, is the ability of the kidney to maintain homeostasis in the body fluids so well and to so late a stage (PLATT 1950, 1952). The tendency is for the kidney to excrete a urine which becomes fixed both in volume and composition, thus progressively narrowing its useful range of function. In such a state the patient may remain in water and electrolyte balance providing intake lies within this narrowing range of adaptability. Intake above or below this range, either of water or electrolytes, results in retention or depletion respectively. The mechanisms underlying this narrowing range of renal adaptability are complex. Probably the most important one is that known as osmotic diuresis. In a condition of hydropenia the actual rate of urine flow is correlated with the rate of excretion of all solutes (RAPOPORT et al.). When the rate of excretion of solutes rises, so does the rate of urine flow, i.e. osmotic diuresis occurs. An important example of this is the diuresis which results from hyperglycaemia and glycosuria in diabetes mellitus. Elevation of the blood urea either by its administration or in disease acts in a similar manner. During an osmotic diuresis certain solutes are excreted to a greater extent than others. Thus, sodium and chloride, hydrogen ion and ammonium in particular are lost, even when sodium chloride depletion is present (SIMMONS, HARVEY and HOSHIKO), whereas potassium (RAPOPORT, WEST and BRODSKY), phosphate (RAPOPORT, WEST and BRODSKY), glucose and amino-acids (LOWE, MOODIE and THOMSON) are conserved during osmotic diuresis. In organic renal disease the number of nephrons is likely to be reduced, and even when there is no change in the excreted solute load the excreted load per nephron must be increased and this will cause osmotic diuresis. If in addition there is urea retention, the increased urea filtered will promote a still greater diuresis. To counter this reduction in tubular reabsorption, various corrective humoral influences will operate, but ultimately these too will fail and depletion of body water and electrolytes, especially salt depletion, will occur.

Although osmotic diuresis is probably the most important factor leading to non-selective impairment of tubular absorption in organic renal disease, other mechanisms frequently play a part. These vary according to the nature of the disease. Patients suffering from *progressive nephritis* tend to pass through stages, firstly of nocturnal frequency due to failure to concentrate the night urine, secondly diurnal polyuria and terminally oliguria. It is probable that the mechanism underlying the polyuria is osmotic diuresis resulting from a reduction in the number of functioning nephrons and the increase of excreted solute load per nephron (PLATT 1952; BRICKER, MORRIN and KIME). The increased concentration of urea and other solutes in the blood in renal failure cannot however wholly account for the diuresis, since impairment of the renal concentrating power persists when the filtered load is reduced by haemodialysis (FRANKLIN, NIALL and MERRILL). Furthermore, in experimental unilateral renal disease, concentrating power is impaired despite maintenance of the normal solute concentration in the plasma (BRICKER et al. 1959). Hypertrophy of the remaining nephrons is often seen in chronic nephritis and pyelonephritis, and it is possible that this is a compensatory mechanism to maintain as high a glomerular filtration rate as possible. The slower rate of flow through the dilated and hypertrophied tubules of these nephrons may to some extent diminish the degree of the osmotic diuresis, but cannot entirely overcome it. Accompanying this water loss there may also be an obligatory loss of sodium chloride which will result in salt depletion should the intake of salt be restricted.

Another aspect of tubular failure in chronic glomerulo-nephritis or pyelonephritis is the inability to handle the predominantly acid end products of normal metabolism. Although the kidney can still acidify the urine to a p_H of below 5.5, it does so only after the plasma bicarbonate level has fallen below 20 mEq/l. Furthermore there is great reduction in ammonium ion secretion, and bicarbonate excretion continues even after systemic acidosis has developed, until the plasma bicarbonate level falls to 15—20 mEq/l. (SCHWARTZ et al. 1959). Both these abnormalities predispose to failure of cation reabsorption, particularly of sodium. The loss of sodium causes shrinkage of the extracellular space and adds an extra-renal component to the already present uraemia; potassium loss (which is however unusual) may produce muscular weakness and cardiac failure, whilst calcium depletion leads to renal osteodystrophy. These forms of defective tubular reabsorption are usually seen only in the terminal stages of uraemia in chronic glomerulo-nephritis, but in chronic pyelonephritis, where the lesion is predominantly tubular, they may arise before the glomerular filtration rate is seriously affected. In rare cases more selective loss of sodium or potassium may occur, leading to clinical deficiency states which will be discussed in the next section.

In *acute anuria* there is evidence that the number of functioning nephrons is greatly reduced (BULL, JOEKES and LOWE). The tubules of the surviving nephrons are yet capable of some function and are not simply acting as inert channels conducting glomerular filtrate to the collecting tubules. Thus the dilute urine passed in the oliguric and the later diuretic phases is partly due to osmotic diuresis produced by the high blood urea which directly increases the excreted load per nephron. However, osmotic diuresis alone will not entirely explain defects of tubular reabsorption. Thus, in the oliguric phase, glycosuria and amino-aciduria may occur, and in the diuretic phases, potassium and magnesium may be lost in excess (LOWE, MOODIE and THOMSON). The former indicates impaired absorption in the proximal tubules, and the latter could also arise from this cause. The loss of sodium in the diuretic phase, which can be very gross, is probably due partly to an osmotic diuresis and partly to distal tubular damage.

Experimental partial nephrectomy in animals, in which five sixths of the renal substance has been removed, is rapidly followed by hypertrophy of glomeruli and dilatation of tubules with hyperplasia of the epithelium (CHANUTIN and FERRIS: WOOD and ETHRIDGE). These changes are accompanied by progressive polyuria and urea retention, the polyuria presumably being due to osmotic diuresis, which the remaining hypertrophied nephrons have not been able to overcome. It is probable that a similar state of affairs accounts for polyuria in man after removal of a large proportion of the renal substance.

b) Selective tubular reabsorption defects

It is possible for one or more specific functions of the renal tubules to be impaired or absent even though the glomerular and the remaining tubular functions are completely normal. This picture is best seen in congenital defects in which renal function may be completely normal in all aspects save one; such an example is renal glycosuria, in which there is failure of complete glucose reabsorption at normal blood sugar levels. Sometimes the tubular disorder causes metabolic disturbances which in turn may lead to further damage to the kidney; renal tubular acidosis, in which there is failure of excretion of acid, may result in renal damage by calcification and by stone formation.

When certain substances accumulate in the tissues it is possible for their presence in the tubular epithelium to interference with function. This may occur after ingestion of poisons, e.g. lead, producing impaired tubular reabsorption of amino-acids and amino-aciduria. Sometimes a specific metabolic defect results in such a "toxic" accummulation, e.g. in galactosaemia, galactose is not metabolised and accumulates in the blood and tissues. This causes failure of tubular absorption of aminoacids, phosphate, and glucose; tubular function returns to normal when a galactose free diet is given. Finally, organic renal disease such as chronic nephritis or pyelonephritis occasionally produces selective impairment of one or more tubular functions. These conditions will be first described.

α) Tubular disorders in primary organic renal disease

Generalised organic renal disease never causes such specific loss of tubular function as is seen in congenital abnormalities but sometimes impairment of one particular function may dominate the clinical picture. This has led to such terms as "salt-losing nephritis". This merely indicates the dominant disorder in a kidney damaged by generalised disease, and does not imply that the process exclusively affects one specific tubular function.

"Salt-losing nephritis" was first described by THORN, KOEPF and CLINTON and other cases have been reported by SAWYER and SOLEZ; BORST; NUSSBAUM, BERNHARD and MATTIA; JOINER and THORNE; MURPHY, SETTIMI and KOZOKOFF; MURPHY et al.; KNOWLES, LEVITIN and BRIDGES. The pathology has been reviewed by ENTICKNAP. The syndrome usually occurs in patients suffering from chronic pyelonephritis with renal failure, but the condition has been observed following excessive alkali therapy for peptic ulcer (ROSENHEIM; CHEYNE and WHITBREAD). Excessive sodium is lost in the urine with consequent dehydration and hyponatraemia. The blood pressure is normal or low and there may be excessive pigmentation of the skin, accompanied by increasing weakness and vomiting. This disorder has been mistaken for Addison's disease but can be distinguished by failure to respond to steroid therapy, although improvement occurs when large amounts of salt are administered. Spontaneous development of this syndrome is rare, but since the ability of the failing kidney to maintain homeostasis is impaired, prolonged salt restriction or the use of diuretics or cation exchange resins may well cause severe sodium depletion.

"Potassium-losing nephritis". There have been many reports of chronic renal disease leading to potassium deficiency (EARLE et al. 1951 b, EVANS and MILNE). Although the term potassium-losing nephritis has been frequently used, the underlying pathology and the mechanism of potassium loss is uncertain in the majority of cases. Following the description by CONN (1956 b) of potassium deficiency due to an aldosterone secreting adenoma of the adrenal cortex, cases previously diagnosed as "potassium-losing nephritis" have on reinvestigation been recognised as examples of Conn's syndrome, i.e. primary aldosteronism (MILNE, MUEHRCKE and AIRD). This condition usually presents with thirst, polyuria and attacks of muscle weakness, associated with hypertension, hypokalaemic alkalosis, and only moderate impairment of renal function. In other instances described as "potassium-losing nephritis" there is acidosis and a moderate degree of renal impairment, but no hypertension (MAHLER and STANBURY, BROOKS et al.). It is well known that specific tubular anomalies such as renal tubular acidosis or Fanconi syndrome (vide infra) may give rise to potassium deficiency and renal failure. Some cases described as "potassium-losing nephritis" may therefore be examples of renal tubular acidosis without bone disease or renal calcification (PLATT 1959). The confusion with primary organic renal disease is increased by the fact that potassium depletion may give rise to changes in the kidney closely resembling chronic pyelopnephritis (see section on potassium deficiency). Other renal conditions may also result in excessive loss of potassium: BROOKS et al. described a patient with renal sarcoidosis and hypokalaemia. Glomerulo-nephritis in the nephrotic stage may also be associated with excessive potassium loss (TEGELAERS and TIDDENS; STANBURY and MACAULAY) and hypokalaemia sometimes follows uretero-colic anastomosis. Patients with chronic renal failure may also be rendered potassium deficient by prolonged treatment with diuretics, especially those which inhibit carbonic anhydrase such as acetazolamide and chlorothiazide. Furthermore, low protein diet, commonly prescribed in uraemia, is poor in potassium, and this may aggravate potassium depletion.

"Water-losing nephritis". Polyuria and thirst are common symptoms in renal failure and, as stated above, the most important cause is osmotic overloading of the remaining tubules in the diseased kidney. In these circumstances the patient passes copious urine of specifity 1010. Severe polyuria of a different origin has been described in chronic renal disease (ROUSSAK and OLESKY). In these cases the specific gravity of the urine remains below 1005. The condition resembles diabetes insipidus in that after water deprivation the rate of urine flow is undiminished and concentration does not rise; it differs, however, in failure to respond to pitressin. This condition, which is very rare, must not be confused with congenital renal diabetes insipidus (vide infra) which usually appears in infancy.

Disorders of calcium and phosphate excretion. Chronic renal failure is frequently associated with high phosphate and low calcium levels in the blood. The serum phosphate rises as glomerular filtration falls (GOLDMAN and BASSETT); low serum calcium may be partly due to excessive calcium excretion in compensation for lack of tubular secretion of hydrogen ions and ammonia (ALBRIGHT and REIFENSTEIN 1948). Various types of osteodystrophy may result, especially in children and adolescents with longstanding renal impairment. Recent studies have shown that both the renal handling of calcium and phosphate and the osteodystrophy associated with organic renal disease are complex (STANBURY 1957). In general, organic renal disease causes phosphate retention whereas congenital tubular defects cause excessive phosphate loss, but there are many exceptions to this. The question is discussed further in the sections on renal hyperphosphaturia and specific disturbances of electrolyte control in renal failure.

Nephrotic syndrome. In children with the nephrotic syndrome tubular defects have been described somewhat similar to those seen in the Fanconi syndrome. Amino-aciduria (BLAINEY 1954), glycosuria, failure of urinary acidification in the absence of raised blood urea, and excessive loss of potassium may occur (TEGELAERS and TIDDENS 1955; STANBURY and MACULEY 1957). Treatment with diuretics and cortisone may produce potassium depletion and this may be a factor in the maintenance of persistent oedema.

β) Specific functional tubular anomalies

The combination of amino-aciduria, glycosuria, hyperphosphaturia and rickets has long been known and was originally described by LIGNAC (1924), DE TONI (1933), and FANCONI (1936a); it is usually referred to as the Fanconi syndrome. Recently it has been demonstrated that this combination of renal tubular abnormalities may be the result of many different disorders which damage or interfere with the function of the renal tubular cells. It occurs in cystine storage disease, galactosaemia, Wilson's disease (hepato-lenticular degeneration), multiple myelomatosis, scurvy, and in poisoning with lysol and with heavy metals such as lead and cadmium. There is however a group of patients in whom these abnormalities are not caused by exogenous poisons or extra-renal metabolic disorders. In this group (sometimes referred to as the "adult" Fanconi syndrome), the most certain aetiological factor appears to be genetic. In addition to the fully developed syndrome with the multiple anomalies described above, isolated tubular defects may sometimes be inherited, but these are not usually related genetically to the full syndrome. These isolated tubular defects are described under renal tubular acidosis, hypophosphataemia and renal glycosuria. Finally there are other congenital or hereditary tubular anomalies which do not occur as part of the Fanconi syndrome, namely cystinuria, renal diabetes insipidus, pseudo-hypoparathyroidism, idiopathic hypercalcaemia and glycinuria.

In the *"adult" Fanconi syndrome* there is impaired tubular reabsorption of amino-acids, phosphate and glucose, failure to acidify the urine, and excessive loss of potassium. The condition may occur in adults or in children, and in the latter it may be difficult to differentiate from cystine storage disease (vide infra).

The presenting symptoms may be those of osteomalacia or rickets, or attacks of weakness due to potassium deficiency. When a careful history is taken it is usually evident that the disease has been present for a considerable time. The osteomalacia is presumably due to excessive loss of phosphate through the kidney; although in addition there is evidence of impaired absorption of phosphate by the gut (DAVIES et al. 1958). The plasma phosphate is usually low (1 to 2 mgm. per 100 ml.) and the calcium normal or slightly low. The skeletal abnormality is typical of osteomalacia or vitamin D resistant rickets (STOWERS and DENT 1947; DENT and HODSON 1954; ANDERSON, MILLER and KENNY 1952; DENT and HARRIS 1956). A large number of amino-acids appear in the urine and the excretion pattern does not vary much from patient to patient; the blood level of amino-acids is normal. Cirrhosis of the liver occasionally occurs (STOWERS and DENT 1947) but is probably not secondary to amino-acid loss (DENT and HARRIS 1956). The glycosuria is usually associated with a normal blood sugar although the glucose tolerance test may show a curve resembling mild diabetes. Failure of urinary acidification is very similar to that seen in renal tubular acidosis; there is a systemic acidosis with urine p_H about 7.0 which shows little fall when an acid load is given (MILNE, STANBURY and THOMSON 1952). The excretion of ammonia tends to be higher than in renal tubular acidosis, possibly due to ammonia formation from the amino-acids in the tubular lumen. Potassium loss is not infrequently severe and may then be responsible for the presenting symptoms: furthermore, changes in renal function secondary to potassium deficiency may be superimposed on the primary disorder. The occasionally abnormal glucose tolerance test may also be due to potassium depletion, since the formation of glycogen from glucose is associated with the passage of potassium into cells, hence the rate of disappearance of glucose from the blood may be delayed when the serum potassium is low. Deaths have been reported during glucose tolerance tests in this condition, possibly from a sudden fall in serum potassium (STOWERS and DENT).

Post-mortem the kidneys are usually normal in size and show little macroscopic change; there is no calcification and stone formation is rare. Cystine deposits are not found in the "adult" Fanconi syndrome. There may be severe vacuolization of the proximal tubule (STOWERS and DENT) which is probably due to potassium deficiency. Microdissection shows marked atrophy of the part of the proximal tubule next to the glomerulus giving the so-called "swan neck" deformity (CLAY, DARMADY and HAWKINS). This may be of aetiological significance since it has been shown that glucose, phosphate and amino-acids are reabsorbed in the proximal tubule.

The adult Fanconi syndrome may occur in siblings (STOWERS and DENT: LINDER, BULL and GRAYCE; DENT and HARRIS) and its thought to be transmitted as a simple recessive gene (DENT and HARRIS). In some instances siblings of patients with the complete syndrome are found to have asymptomatic glycosuria, amino-aciduria and hypophosphataemia without rickets or potassium loss (DENT 1952). There appears to be no genetic connection between the adult Fanconi syndrome and cystine storage disease, cystinuria, renal tubular acidosis, or renal hyperphosphaturia without amino-aciduria. Since many poisons and metabolic abnormalities, especially those in which there is excessive intracellular storage of specific substances, cause a similar pattern of renal tubular dysfunction to that described above, it is possible that the adult Fanconi syndrome may be caused either by undetected poisoning or by undiscovered metabolic abnormalitis which are themselves hereditary. A review of all published cases of the adult Fanconi syndrome has been made by WALLIS and ENGLE.

Renal tubular acidosis. BUTLER, WILSON and FARBER described, in infants
under six months of age, a syndrome characterised by persistent dehydration
(in spite of normal food and fluid intake), hyperpnoea, low plasma bicarbonate,
and hyperchloraemia. Post-mortem examination revealed calcification in and
around the renal tubules. LIGHTWOOD (1935) described similar post-mortem changes
in this condition. Since then there have been many reports of the syndrome, occurring during the first year of life. Following adequate and persistent alkali therapy
the great majority of infants recover by the age of two years and there is at
present no evidence that the disorder recurs during later life (HARTMANN; STAP-
LETON; LIGHTWOOD, PAYNE and BLACK).

BAINES, BARCLAY and COOK reported the occurrence of hyperchloraemia,
low plasma bicarbonate and nephrocalcinosis in an adult, and ALBRIGHT et al. (1946)
observed patients in whom this syndrome was associated with osteomalacia.
Describing the disorder as "tubular insufficiency without glomerular insufficiency", they postulated a failure of the renal tubules to secrete sufficient acid
to maintain normal blood, p_H, leading to resorption of calcium from the bones,
osteomalacia and renal calcification. Further examples have been described
by many authors (PINES and MUDGE; MILNE, STANBURY and THOMSON; FOSS,
PERRY and WOOD; REYNOLDS). The syndrome usually presents with recurrent
renal calculi, with osteomalacia, or with recurrent attacks of muscle weakness
due to potassium deficiency, associated with low plasma bicarbonate, hyperchloraemia, hypokalaemia, but normal blood urea. In some patients the biochemical abnormalities are found in the absence of renal calculi, renal calcification,
and osteomalacia. The disorder of renal tubular function appears to be the same
in both the adult and the infantile group. Glomerular filtration rate and blood
urea remain normal unless there is secondary damage from nephrocalcinosis or
renal stones, or unless fibrotic changes resembling pyelonephritis develop
(presumably secondary to long standing potassium deficiency). There is no
excessive loss of glucose or of amino acids in the urine. Polyuria (two to four
litres a day) usually occurs with urine specific gravity of 1001 to 1010 and
p_H 6 to 7.5. Notwithstanding the hypokalaemia, the urine contains a large
amount of potassium. Serum calcium is usually normal but the phosphate tends
to be low. In spite of detailed studies the cause of the disorder is still not clear.
LATNER and BERNARD reported primary inadequacy of bicarbonate reabsorption;
FRICK, RUBINI and MERONEY suggested that carbonic anhydrase was deficient.
MILNE, STANBURY and THOMSON, and REYNOLDS showed that the renal tubules
were able to secrete a large amount of acid provided there was sufficient buffer
to prevent the urine p_H from falling below 6; thus the tubules were unable to
maintain a high hydrogen ion gradient between plasma and urine; ammonia
excretion was normal or high for the urinary p_H.

This disorder has recently been studied in detail by ELKINTON et al., who
compared the response of patients with renal tubular acidosis and normal subjects
to a large acid load (ammonium chloride) given for periods up to five days. There
was no clear cut difference in ability to increase the rate of acid excretion.
However, when acid excretion rate was related to the disturbance in the blood
buffer mechanism by calculating the "clearance" of acid by the kidney (acid
excretion rate divided by the reciprocal of blood CO_2 content) there was a clear
separation between the patients and the normal subjects. This measurement also
showed up difference in response to acid load between normal subjects and
relatives, themselves symptomless, of patients with renal tubular acidosis (HUTH.
WEBSTER and ELKINTON). There appeared to be at least two different disorders.
In three cases the tubules could not maintain a high hydrogen ion gradient

between plasma and blood, but there was no impairment of total acid secretion provided sufficient urinary buffer was present. In two cases urinary p_H could be lowered to near normal levels but there appeared to be a primary deficiency of urinary phosphate and thus deficiency of total acid excretion. WEBSTER et al. investigated the role of carbonic anhydrase by measuring the changes in the excretion of bicarbonate and of acid after giving acetazolamide to normal subjects and to patients with renal tubular acidosis. The results were compatible with, but not conclusively in favour of the hypothesis that the primary disorder in renal tubular acidosis is lack of carbonic anhydrase.

Further evidence on the genetic relationship of renal tubular acidosis has been obtained by HUTH, WEBSTER and ELKINTON who investigated the relatives of a patient with renal tubular acidosis by measuring "acid clearance" following ammonium chloride. Reviewing the family histories of 162 examples of renal tubular acidosis described in the literature, they concluded that genetically, these were separable into two groups. 87 cases presented in the first year of life and showed a high rate of recovery following alkali therapy. In this group the disorder could be attributed to delay in development of tubular acid secretion which is normally acquired during the first year of life (McCANCE and HATEMI). If there is a genetic factor in this group it must be recessive since no parents and only three siblings were affected. Two thirds of the patients were male. In the other 75 cases the onset was in late childhood or early adult life, and in this group recovery was not recorded. Two thirds of the patients were female and the family incidence was high, suggesting transmission by a dominant gene.

The relationship between defective urinary acidification and calcium metabolism is not fully understood. In the above analysis of published cases it was found that, of 75 patients with renal tubular acidosis of late onset, 45% had rickets or osteomalacia and 77% suffered from nephrocalcinosis or nephrolithiasis. ALBRIGHT and REIFENSTEIN (1948) suggested that increased mobilisation of calcium from bone is due to systemic acidosis, but there has been little further evidence in support of this. DEDMON and WRONG observed low rates of citrate excretion in renal tubular acidosis, and it is possible that this is related to precipitation of calcium in the renal cells or renal pelvis.

The cause of excessive renal potassium loss is also unknown. It is not due to increased tubular secretion of potassium in exchange for sodium owing to reduced hydrogen ion excretion, since there is little change in the excretion of potassium when the systemic acidosis is corrected by giving sodium bicarbonate (REYNOLDS). Further work is necessary to determine the primary cause of impaired urinary acidification in these syndromes and to clarify the mechanism of other disorders such as osteomalacia and potassium loss.

Lowe's Syndrome. Another form of impaired renal acid excretion was described by LOWE, TERREY and MacLACHLAN. They described a primary deficiency of ammonia production by the kidney, associated with hydrophthalmos and mental retardation. This disorder has been termed the "cerebro-oculorenal" syndrome.

Renal hyperphosphaturia (renal hypophosphataemia, vitamin D resistant rickets, phosphate diabetes). This tubular anomaly is due to impaired reabsorption of phosphate, resulting in excessive renal loss and depression of the serum phosphate level. Severe bone disease develops, in children as rickets which fails to respond to ordinary doses of vitamin D, and in adults as osteomalacia. Glycosuria may be present, but impairment of urinary acidication, potassium depletion and amino-aciduria are absent (DENT 1952). Histologically the kidneys appear normal but the proximal tubules are found to be deficient in the enzyme phosphatase. The bones show changes of rickets or osteomalacia, indistinguishable from

those due to vitamin D deficiency (ALBRIGHT and REIFENSTEIN). Administration
of large amounts of vitamin D (up to 400,000 units a day) increases the levels
of serum calcium and phosphorus, while calcium and phosphorus balance becomes
positive due not only to reduction in the urinary loss of phosphorus, but also to
increased absorption of both calcium and phosphorus from the intestine (ROBERT-
SON, HARRIS and McCUNE; DENT and HARRIS). DAVIES et al. have suggested that
vitamin D has a similar action in the Fanconi syndrome, i.e. it is possible that
intestinal absorption is defective, as well as tubular reabsorption, in this condition.
The disease is hereditary and may be transmitted as an incompletely manifested
Mendelian dominant (DENT and HARRIS; WINTERS et al.). There are apparently
two types, one severe and another mild, which are inherited independently (DENT
and HARRIS). A similar but rarer condition, which does not appear to be hereditary, has been described in adolescents and young adults (McCANCE 1947; DENT
and HARRIS). This may be different in pathogenesis since acidosis is sometimes
present. The osteomalacia which is occasionally associated with neurofibromatosis
(von Recklinghausen's disease) may be due to renal hyperphosphaturia, the neurofibromatosis and the renal lesion being inherited together (SWANN).

   Renal glycosuria is one of the commonest renal tubular defects, and like
other anomalies may be inherited. Glucose appears in the urine at normal blood
sugar levels without any other renal abnormality. It has been claimed that
diabetes mellitus may eventually develop, but since both disorders are common,
this may well be coincidence (TAGGART; MUDGE).

   Congenital cystinuria presents with a high urinary excretion of cystine and
liability to cystine stone formation. Originally thought to be a metabolic disorder
involving excessive production of cystine, it is now recognised as a tubular
reabsorption defect, the blood level of cystine being normal (DENT and ROSE;
FOWLER, HARRIS and WARREN). Studies by YEH et al., DENT and ROSE; STEIN;
DENT, SENIOR and WALSHE, and DENT and SENIOR have shown that there is
also excessive renal loss of lysine, arginine and ornithine, which persists at a
steady level throughout life (daily loss approximately, lysine 1.8 g., arginine
0.8 g., cystine 0.75 g., ornithine 0.4 g.). The kidney is otherwise normal unless
structural damage results from the formation of calculi. The latter consist of
cystine alone since lysine, arginine, and ornithine are freely soluble while cystine
precipitates readily in the concentrated acid night urine. Congenital cystinuria
differs from the "adult" Fanconi syndrome and from cystine storage disease in
that the absorption defect is restricted to these four amino-acids, which suggests
a common mechanism for their reabsorption (DENT and ROSE). In support of
this it has been shown that an intravenous infusion of lysine in a normal subject
leads to excretion also of cystine, ornithine and arginine, presumably due to
saturation of the common reabsorption mechanism (ROBSON and ROSE). The
condition is hereditary (HARRIS et al. 1955a, b) and it has been shown that patients
suffering from cystine stone formation may have apparently healthy relatives
who excrete either all four amino-acids, or cystine and lysine alone (HARRIS and
WARREN).

   Renal diabetes insipidus usually presents in childhood with the excretion of
copious amounts of very dilute urine, and failure to concentrate either on water
deprivation or after administration of pitressin. In all other respects the kidney
is normal, although later in life hydronephrosis may develop, possibly secondary
to over-distension of the bladder. Impairment of renal function may then occur.
Physical retardation may be a feature, and has been attributed to anorexia
caused by continual thirst (FLAX and GERSH). The condition appears chiefly in
males and may be due to a sex-linked recessive gene transmitted by the female

(WILLIAMS and HENRY). Carrier females may however show slight impairment of urine concentration (CARTER and SIMPKISS). Post-mortem, the kidney is normal both to the naked eye and histologically, provided there is no hydronephrosis. Micro-disseaction of the kidney has shown no abnormality of the distal tubule (MACDONALD).

Pseudo-hypoparathyroidism. A few patients have been described with normal parathyroid glands but with clinical and biochemical evidence of hypoparathyroidism. There is no response to parathyroid hormone administration. It has been suggested that the renal tubules are insensitive to parathyroid hormone so that phosphate reabsorption is excessive (ALBRIGHT and REIFENSTEIN). Clinically the patient tends to be of small, thick set stature with a plump, round face; the fingers are stumpy due to shortening of the metacarpals; tetany or latent tetany is common. The bones are denser than normal and there may be calcification of soft tissues, especially round the joints. The calcium level in the blood is very low and the phosphate level high.

Idiopathic hypercalciuria, described by ALBRIGHT and REIFENSTEIN, is extremely rare. The urinary excretion of calcium is high but there is no evidence of parathyroid hyper-function, and the blood level of both calcium and phosphate is normal. Osteomalacia develops and renal calculi may form. The cause of the condition is unknown but there may be a specific calcium reabsorption defect.

Idiopathic hypercalcaemia in infants (LIGHTWOOD 1952) is probably due to vitamin D overdose or to increased sensitivity to the vitamin; there is no evidence of renal dysfunction.

Glycinuria. DENT and HARRIS have described severe osteomalacia associated with excessive loss of glycine alone, the excretion of all other amino-acids being normal. DE VRIES et al. have reported the occurrence of glycinuria without osteomalacia and in one case an oxalate stone was present.

γ) Tubular dysfunction associated with general metabolic disorders or chemical poisons

Potassium deficiency. Excessive loss of potassium may occur from the gastrointestinal tract or in the urine. Chronic diarrhoea from any cause, especially steatorrhoea, or prolonged abuse of irritant aperients, can produce serious depletion of body potassium. Renal loss occurs in chronic renal failure, in tubular disorders such as renal tubular acidosis or Fanconi syndrome as already described, and in endocrine disorders in which the kidney excretes potassium in response to hypersecretion of electrolyte active hormones. Potassium deficiency from any cause produces both specific changes in renal function and microscopical lesions. In most instances both functional and structural changes are reversed on potassium repletion. When the deficiency is due to excessive renal potassium loss these secondary changes will be superimposed upon the primary renal disorder and may modify the functional and structural picture of the latter. *Renal structural changes* in potassium deficiency states have been studied extensively both in patients and in experimental animals. In man the most constant finding is vacuolization of the epithelial cells of the convoluted tubules (PERKINS, PETERSEN and RILEY; SCHWARTZ and RELMAN; MILNE, MUEHRCKE and HEARD). These vacuoles may be large, numerous, and do not stain for fat, glucose, or protein. In addition, granularity of the tubular cells, and, in severe cases, necrosis and sloughing, have also been reported (RELMAN and SCHWARTZ 1956, 1958). Similar abnormalities were first described in association with chronic diarrhoea (JAFFE and STEINBERG) but have only recently been ascribed to potassium deficiency. In the rat rendered potassium deficient, tubular degeneration is found, but in addition there is marked hyperplasia of the epithelium of the (collecting) tubules in the innermost zone of the medulla; this may cause blockage and dilatation of the tubules (Oliver et al.; Craig and Schwartz). In cases studied by repeated renal biopsy and in experimental animals, the lesions usually disappear when potassium depletion is corrected (Relman and Schwartz 1956; Tauxe, Wakim and Baggenstoss). Following prolonged deficiency in rats and mice, irreversible interstitial fibrosis and glomerular hyalinisation have been observed (Liebow, McFarland and Tennant; Fourman, McCance and Parker) and in some patients with prolonged potassium deficiency a histological picture very similar to chronic pyelonephritis has been described. This occurs most often with potassium deficiency due to tubular dysfunction, so that it may be difficult to determine whether the structural changes are due to primary renal disease or to the potassium deficiency. Similar changes have been described however in potassium depletion of extra-renal origin, e.g. in chronic diarrhoea (Jensen, Baggenstoss and Bargen; Milne, Muehrcke and Heard) and in primary aldosteronism (Milne, Muehrcke and Aird). *Changes in renal function* produced by potassium depletion have been studied both in patients (Schwartz and Relman), and in normal subjects rendered deficient by low potassium diet and by cation exchange resins (Black and Milne; Evans et al.; Fourman 1954). The specific changes in renal function, which can nearly always be reversed when the potassium deficiency is corrected, affect both glomerular and tubular function. Glomerular filtration is often reduced (Schwartz and Relman) but this may also be due to primary renal disease or to dehydration secondary to diarrhoea; in primary aldosteronism (Dustan, Corcoran and Page) there may be little change. A rise in blood urea occurs if filtration is moderately impaired. Loss of concentrating power is one of the earliest abnormalities to appear in potassium deficiency; up to five litres a day of urine of low specific gravity (1002—1010) may be passed and thirst may be severe (Schwartz and Relman). As in organic renal failure, ability to concentrate the night urine may first he impaired. On a low potassium diet the kidney continues to excrete potassium for several weeks, whereas the healthy kidney conserves potassium very efficiently provided there is no excessive hormonal stimulus to potassium excretion (Black and Milne). Thus continued renal potassium loss in the presence of deficiency always indicates a renal tubular lesion or excessive hormonal stimulus to K elimination. Substances which usually increase potassium excretion such as acetazolamide, sodium bicarbonate, or ammonium chloride have much less effect in established deficiency (Evans et al.; Clarke et al.). Sodium is retained and expansion of extracellular fluid may lead to oedema in potassium depleted subjects. There is also delayed excretion of sodium after a salt load (Black and Milne; Fourman and Hervey). Acid base balance is also disturbed, extracellular alkalosis with raised plasma bicarbonate being associated with intracellular acidosis (Clarke et al.). The urinary pH is usually about 7 and rarely falls below 6. The urine contains bicarbonate but less than might be expected for the level of plasma bicarbonate, indicating increased reabsorption; "titratable" acidity is low but urinary ammonium is relatively high. When an acid load is given hydrogen ions are excreted mainly as ammonium (NH_4) and little fall in pH occurs (Schwartz and Relman; Milne, Muehrcke and Heard). Phosphate clearance is increased and the serum level may be low; calcium levels are usually unchanged. In some patients with long standing potassium loss, permanent impairment of renal function has been described (Milne, Muehrcke and Heard). Since chronic K deficiency is most commonly due to primary renal disorders it is often uncertain whether the renal impairment is due to primary organic disease or to the effects of prolonged potassium deficiency.

Cystine storage disease (Lignac-Fanconi syndrome, cystinosis). LIGNAC, and DE TONI, described in children rickets, dwarfism and renal disease, with extensive deposits of cystine in the tissues. FANCONI (1931, 1936 a, b) reported hyperphosphaturia, amino-aciduria, and glycosuria in such patients. The disease always presents in early life. The child appears normal for the first few months after birth but then suffers from polydipsia, polyuria and anorexia. Signs of rickets appear, which fail to respond to normal doses of vitamin D. Tetany and attacks of muscular weakness may be present. Cystine deposits can usually be seen in the cornea. There is mental and physical retardation and death usually occurs before puberty from infection or renal failure. Affected children are often described as fair, plump, and of a happy and contented disposition in spite of mental retardation (BICKEL et al.; BICKEL and SMELLIE; DENT 1952; BICKEL and THURSBY PELHAM; BICKEL). Renal tubular dysfunction is similar to that found in the "adult" Fanconi syndrome. There is glycosuria and marked amino-aciduria (up to twenty amino-acids may be found) with normal levels of blood glucose and amino-nitrogen, hyperphosphaturia with hypophosphataemia, hypokalaemia and systemic acidosis. The urine is copious and dilute, specific gravity being below 1010, and pH fixed at about 7.0. The renal tubular disorder may be caused by deposition of cystine. By following from birth the siblings of affected members of a family, it has been shown that renal function is normal for the first five months of life, at which time glycosuria, amino-aciduria, and cystine deposits in the cornea appear simultaneously (BICKEL et al.; BICKEL and THURSBY PELHAM). Post-mortem, the kidneys and other tissues are found to contain a large amount of cystine (GATZIMOS, SCHULZ and NEWNUM). There may also be vacuolisation of proximal tubule, probably due to chronic potassium depletion. Flattening of the epithelium in the proximal convoluted tubule adjacent to the glomerulus ("swan neck" deformity) is seen as in the "adult" Fanconi syndrome (CLAY, DARMADY and HAWKINS). CLAYTON and PATRICK have suggested that excessive cystine in the tissues may reduce the availability of free thiol groups which are necessary for the proper function of many enzyme systems, especially for the enzymes of the citric acid cycle. They demonstrated that in cystinosis the activity of liver succinic dehydrogenase is very low but can be raised by incubation with cysteine (which contains thiol groups). In addition blood pyruvate levels were found to be high in cystinosis. In order to increase the number of available thiol groups and thus improve enzyme function, CLAYTON and PATRICK gave dimercaptol (BAL) and penicillamine to three children with cystinosis. There was rapid clinical improvement in all, and immediate weight gain in two cases. Blood pyruvate levels fell, renal loss of amino acids was reduced, and acidosis improved. This preliminary report gives promise that the metabolic disorders in cystinosis will soon be better understood and that effective treatment may be possible.

Galactosaemia also presents in infancy; the child fails to thrive on a normal milk diet, loses weight, develops cataracts, and may die with cirrhosis of the liver. The disorder is due to failure to metabolise galactose which accumulates in the blood and is excreted in large amounts in the urine. The enzyme which catalyses the conversion of galactose-1-phosphate to glucose-1-phosphate has been shown to be absent from erythrocytes (SCHWARTZ et al. 1955; KALCKAR, ANDERSON and ISSELBACHER) suggesting that this enzyme may be lacking in other tissues. The resulting accumulation of galactose-1-phosphate may cause specific cell damage. Aminoaciduria occurs (HOLZEL, KOMROWER and WILSON; BICKEL and HICKMANS; CUSHWORTH, DENT and FLYNN), though the plasma level of amino-nitrogen is normal, indicating failure of reabsorption of amino-acids by the renal tubules (KOMROWER; HSIA et al.; CUSHWORTH, DENT and FLYNN). When given a galactose free diet the child thrives and the blood level of galactose falls rapidly to normal, although the amino-aciduria persists for a few days; there is a similar interval before amino-aciduria reappears following administration of galactose (CUSH-WORTH, DENT and FLYNN) suggesting that accumulation of galactose in the tubular cells impairs reabsorption of amino-acids (HARRIS). In some patients there is glycosuria and excessive loss of phosphate, but other tubular defects have not been reported.

Hepato-lenticular degeneration (Wilson's disease) is an inborn error of metabolism in which cirrhosis of the liver and degeneration of the lenticular nucleus result from deposition of copper in the tissues. The primary metabolic fault appears to be deficient synthesis of caeruloplasmin (BEARN 1953; EARL, MOULTON and SELVERSTONE), a γ-globulin to which most of the copper is bound in plasma. Since the blood level of this substance is greatly reduced, copper is loosely bound to albumin and appears to be more readily deposited in the tissues. There is also an unexplained increase in copper absorption from the bowel. Urinary copper output is excessive (200—700 ug. daily) and tubular defects arise, probably from deposition of copper in the tubular epithelium. Aminoaciduria occurs (UZMAN and DENNY-BROWN; STEIN, BEARN and MOORE) and may be accompanied by glycosuria, hyperphosphaturia and hyperuricosuria (COOPER et al.; UZMAN and HOOD; MAHONEY et al.; BEARN 1957). Since these features are usually absent in early life but increase as the condition progresses it seems probable that the tubular dysfunction is a secondary effect and not an inherited abnormality. The pattern of amino-acid excretion is very similar to that seen in lead poisoning. No other tubular anomalies have been reported.

Other causes of amino-aciduria. Amino-aciduria occurs in patients with lead poisoning; renal function returns to normal when the lead poisoning is treated (WILSON, THOMSON and DENT); rickets has also been reported in this condition (CAFFEY). Amino-aciduria has also been reported in cadmium, mercury, uranium (CLARKSON and KENCH 1956) and lysol poisoning (SPENCER and FRANGLEN); in multiple myelomatosis (ENGLE and WALLIS), scurvy (JONXIS and HUISMAN), and vitamin D deficiency rickets (JONXIS). Osteomalacia has been reported in cadmium poisoning (NICAUD et al.).

Summary. In the light of present knowledge it appears that there are two main types of defect giving rise to selective functional tubular abnormalities. One is associated with flattening of the epithelium of the first part of the proximal convoluted tubules and is characterised by faulty reabsorption of glucose, amino-acids, and phosphate. The other is not apparently associated with any specific structural lesion and gives rise to failure of acidification of the urine and loss of potassium. These patterns of tubular dysfunction may occur together or separately. They may be due to primary renal disease or to a variety of nephrotoxic agents; in the absence of any such environmental cause, they are usually of genetic origin.

δ) Endocrine disorders

Addison's disease. The main features of the renal abnormality in Addison's disease are the increased excretion of sodium (LOEB et al. 1933) and the delayed excretion of a water load (ROWNTREE and SNELL). These phenomena were noted early in the study of the renal function in this condition, and much subsequent work has helped to elucidate, albeit incompletely, the underlying mechanism. The increased sodium excretion leads to sodium depletion with contraction of the extracellular and plasma volumes, and therefore to circulatory failure and extrarenal uraemia. The delayed ability to excrete a water load makes these patients particularly intolerant of an excessive fluid intake and exposes them to the danger of water intoxication. Clearance studies in adrenal insufficiency have demonstrated a moderate fall in the renal plasma flow, a greater fall in the glomerular filtration rate with a correspondingly reduced filtration fraction, and reduction of the maximum absorptive power of the tubules for glucose (TALBOT et al.). The fall in glomerular filtration rate is partly due to the fall in extracellular fluid volume, but not entirely so, since sudden withdrawal of replacement therapy in Addison's disease results in a fall in glomerular filtration rate before the extracellular space, as measured by inulin, is decreased (MENDELSOHN and PEARSON). There is experimental evidence that the glucocorticoids, cortisone and hydrocortisone, are capable of restoring the glomerular filtration rate to normal without any alteration in the extracellular space, and it has been suggested that these steroids raise the efferent and lower the afferent arteriolar tone in the renal cortex. This would have the effect of raising the filtration fraction and increasing the glomerular filtration rate. Aldosterone has little effect on the glomerular filtration rate (GAUNT, RENZI and CHART).

The increased excretion of sodium is probably due to decreased tubular reabsorption (ROEMMELT, SARTORIUS and PITTS), and reduction of circulating aldosterone is almost certainly mainly responsible for this. There is evidence from "stopflow" analysis that this action of aldosterone is sited in the distal tubule (VANDER et al.). The glucocorticoid hormones have in this respect a very weak action compared with aldosterone. The reduction of the glomerular filtration rate in Addison's disease tends to conserve sodium, and it is possible that the administration of cortisone, which raises the glomerular filtration rate but has very little action on tubular reabsorption of sodium, may further increase sodium depletion. This may account for the liability to sodium depletion shown by patients treated with cortisone, who are not receiving salt supplements or a more powerful sodium retaining corticoid such as deoxycortone or the synthetic fluorohydrocortisone. Potassium retention in adrenocortical failure is partly due to the fall in glomerular filtration rate and partly to the absence of the direct effect of the adrenal corticoids, probably mainly aldosterone, on the tubular excretion of potassium.

The uraemia observed in the Addisonian crisis is again partly due to the fall in the glomerular filtration rate, but there is evidence that urea retention commences before the glomerular filtration rate falls in experimental adrenal insufficiency (GAUDINO and LEVITT). This suggests that endogenous protein catabolism is accelerated.

The failure of normal water diuresis following ingestion or injection of water is not corrected by the administration of sodium chloride or of steroids, such as deoxycortone or aldosterone, with powerful electrolyte action. Cortisone and hydrocortisone, on the other hand, quickly correct this disability; the improvement in water excretion is not directly related to increase in the glomerular filtration rate and the mechanism is not yet understood (RAMEY and GOLDSTEIN). A further alteration in renal function in adrenocortical failure is the loss of the normal diurnal rhythm in which water, sodium and potassium excretion are increased by day (STANBURY and THOMPSON). This rhythm is restored by the administration of glucocorticoids, but not by deoxycortone or aldosterone.

The evidence at present suggests that aldosterone output by the adrenal is not under the influence of the adrenocorticotrophic hormone. Hence in hypopituitarism the sodium losing state with consequent dehydration does not occur. On the other hand the output of glucocorticoids is greatly reduced in the absence of ACTH and this leads to a failure of water diuresis. Such patients are very prone to water intoxication particularly during performance of water tolerance tests (WYNN and GARROD).

Aldosteronism. Aldosterone depresses the tubular reabsorption of potassium and leads to depletion of potassium, provided sodium is available in the diet. Its primary action is to increase sodium reabsorption, and primary and secondary aldosteronism will be discussed under this heading. The reverse situation of spontaneous isolated hypoaldosteronism has been invoked to explain rare cases presenting in a variety of ways, which include hypotension, hyperkalaemia and Stokes-Adams attacks (HUDSON, CHOBANIAN and RELMAN; SKANSE and HOCKFELT; LAMBREW et al.; HILL et al.).

Hyperparathyroidism. The mode of action of the parathyroid hormone in the body is still uncertain. There seems no doubt that it has a local action on bone resulting in osteoclastic resorption. This action alone appears insufficient to account for the observed rise in serum calcium and fall in phosphate. There is evidence that parathyroid hormone raises the renal clearance of phosphate (ALBRIGHT et al. 1929; TWEEDY and CAMPBELL; MILNE). This action is more marked in patients with hypoparathyroidism than in normal subjects. Studies of the phosphate clearance in relation to the inulin or creatinine clearance have shown that the ratio of phosphate to inulin or creatinine depends on the level of serum phosphate. In hyperparathyroidism this ratio is usually increased (McGEOWN; NORDIN and FRASER; HODGKINSON), and after removal of the parathyroid tumour the ratio falls within the normal range. This would indicate that parathyroid hormone decreases the tubular reabsorption of phosphate. Thus it seems probable that parathyroid hormone acts at more than one site in the body.

Apart from the increased renal excretion of phosphate and calcium in hyperparathyroidism, polyuria with hypotonic urine has been frequently observed (GUTMAN, SWENSON and PARSONS; ALEXANDER et al. 1944; FOURMAN, McCONKEY and SMITH). This may be of such severity as to mimic diabetes insipidus, particularly in the absence of radiological evidence of renal calcification (SNAPPER). The polyuria is resistant to dehydration and to pitressin, but disappears after removal of the parathyroid tumour, when the ability of the kidney to excrete urine more concentrated than plasma is immediately restored. The suggestion has been made that the increased urine volume is due to failure of the second part of distal tubule to concentrate hypotonic urine from the first part of the distal tubule (COHEN et al.). The renal excretion of hydrogen ion may be impaired in hyperparathyroidism and this may lead to systemic acidosis (COHEN et al.; FANCONI and ROSE; WRONG and DAVIES; FOURMAN, McCONKEY and SMITH).

Diabetes insipidus. Diabetes insipidus is caused by structural or functional derangement of the posterior pituitary or the supra-optic nucleus of the hypothalamus, resulting in failure of secretion of antidiuretic hormone in response to increasing osmotic pressure of the plasma. The control of extracellular fluid osmotic pressure by osmoreceptors situated in the supra-optic nucleus has been investigated by JEWELL and VERNEY and will be discussed later.

The average glomerular filtration rate in man of 120 ml./min. is converted by a process of tubular water reabsorption to about 1—4 ml./min. of urine flow. Tubular reabsorption is believed to take place both passively and actively, the former in the proximal and the latter in the distal tubule (SMITH 1951). In the proximal tubule some seven eighths of the filtered water diffuses out of the tubular lumen, together with electrolytes, glucose and certain other constituents, leaving an isotonic or slightly hypotonic fluid. This passive reabsorption of water is not under physiological control and can only be diminished as a result of excretion of an excessive amount of osmotically active substance, in other words an osmotic diuresis. The amount of 'active' reabsorption of water in the distal tubule is under physiological control and is varied through the action of the antidiuretic hormone in order to maintain osmotic homeostasis in the extracellular fluid. In the absence of antidiuretic hormone, what remains of the glomerular filtrate after passive reabsorption in the proximal tubule, passes out in the urine and may amount to more than 20 litres per day. Owing to further reabsorption of sodium and chloride in the distal tubule, however, the osmotic pressure of the final urine is very much less than that of plasma, hence the specific gravity falls to around 1001.

Apart from this failure of distal tubular reabsorption of water, renal function is normal in diabetes insipidus providing the patient is maintained in a satisfactory state of hydration by replacement therapy (WINER). When the diuresis is uncontrolled, the diodone clearance falls, indicating reduction in the renal blood flow, which is probably attributable to dehydration. The glomerular filtration rate and maximum excretory power of the tubules for diodone $(T_M D)$ remain unaltered (WHITE, HEINBECKER and ROLF 1942, 1947). The severity of diabetes insipidus can to some extent be modified by altering the excreted solute load as mentioned above. Thus a diet high in sodium chloride will increase the urine volume and vice versa. The urine output may fall and the specific gravity rise when there is concurrent heart failure, due to reduction of the glomerular filtration rate. Diuretics, particularly of the chlorothiazide group, may diminish flow in diabetes insipidus, again probably by reducing glomerular filtration rate (HAVARD and WOOD).

In normal subjects a high water intake impairs the ability of the kidney to concentrate the urine (DE WARDENER and HERXHEIMER). Thus, the clinician may sometimes be in doubt whether a patient exhibiting gross polyuria with hypotonic urine is suffering from true diabetes insipidus or from some obsessional desire to drink leading to secondary polyuria. The term "compulsive water drinking" has been given to the latter group of patients (BARLOW and DE WARDENER). The differentiation may be most difficult and these authors have suggested a diagnostic test based on measurement of serum osmolarity and on the comparison of the response to pitressin and fluid deprivation.

ε) Action of diuretics

The physiological aspects of this subject have been discussed in detail in the previous chapter. Reference is made here to the mode of action and limitations of the common diuretics used in the treatment of renal oedema, particularly in the nephrotic syndrome.

Diuretic therapy aims to increase the excretion of sodium and water and this is usually effected by reducing tubular reabsorption of sodium. In the process, tubular reabsorption or secretion of other electrolytes is almost always modified and these "side effects" have to be compensated by appropriate substitution therapy.

Diuretics may act by increasing the osmotic pressure of the glomerular filtrate, by blocking sodium reabsorption directly, or by counteracting the physiological control of sodium reabsorption, for example by use of the aldosterone antagonists.

Osmotic diuresis may be produced by urea, dextrose or mannitol. Some sugars (e.g. sucrose) are to be avoided since they may produce tubular damage (ANDERSON and BETHEA). The high-concentration of a nonabsorbable solute reduces reabsorption of water in the proximal tubule, hence the volume of the tubular fluid is excessive and the sodium concentration subnormal. Sodium reabsorption is therefore reduced even in the presence of marked dehydration (HERVEY,

McCANCE and TAYLOR). This is the reason for the severe sodium and water depletion which may occur in the diabetic with heavy glycosuria. Acidifying diuretics such as ammonium chloride present the kidney with an increased load of anion which must be excreted with an equivalent amount of cation (SARTORIUS, ROEMMELT and PITTS). This increases the excretion of metallic cations, chiefly sodium, until the tubules can increase the output of ammonium.

Direct inhibition of sodium reabsorption may be brought about in various ways and is not fully understood. Tubular transport of sodium (and other electrolytes) may be blocked e.g. by xanthines, aminometradine, chlorothiazide; or anion reabsorption may be inhibited, e.g. by organic mercurials, acetazolamide, chlorothiazide (MUDGE and WEINER; LARAGH 1958). The organic mercurials form complex ions which may block chloride reabsorption in the proximal or distal tubules. As chloride depletion increases, the resulting mild alkalosis renders the action of the drug less effective, hence ammonium chloride should be given to maintain adequate diuresis. It is doubtful whether organic mercurials produce tubular damage apart from the above action (GOODWIN). Prolonged use may lead to severe sodium depletion, especially on a low sodium diet (LUETSCHER 1955). Acetazolamide ("Diamox") inhibits carbonic anhydrase and thus prevents bicarbonate reabsorption. Sodium bicarbonate is excreted in excess and hydrogen ion secretion reduced, as also is secretion of ammonium. Since potassium competes against hydrion for tubular exchange with sodium (BERLINER), potassium secretion increases in these circumstances as well as sodium excretion. Thus potassium depletion and acidosis are the disadvantages of acetazolamide as a diuretic; moreover, as acidosis increases, the filtered load of bicarbonate falls and the drug loses its effectiveness (COUNIHAN, EVANS and MILNE). Chlorothiazide inhibits carbonic anhydrase to some extent (MUDGE and WEINER) but its chief disadvantage is potassium depletion, which must be corrected by giving potassium supplements.

Aldosterone antagonists may be of value in nephrotic, cardiac or cirrhotic oedema of long duration when secondary aldosteronism has developed (LIDDLE 1957, 1958, BOLTE et al.). The spironolactones block the action of aldosterone peripherally, i.e. in the tubule cell by substrate competition (MILLS) but their effectiveness has been found to bear little relationship to the degree of estimated enhanced aldosterone secretion (SLATER et al.). These substances are most successful in combination with other diuretic agents such as urea or chlorothiazide which increase the tubular content of sodium (EDMONDS and WILSON; EDMONDS). Secondary aldosteronism occurs in hypoproteinaemic oedema in response to hypovolaemia. This can be temporarily corrected by salt-free albumen infusions (ORLOFF, WELT and STOWE) or dextran (JAMES, CORDILLO and METCAFF). These plasma expanders may initiate a diuresis, partly by increasing glomerular filtration, but their effect is temporary as they themselves are rapidly excreted. In advanced renal disease hyponatraemia may so reduce the filtered load of sodium that none of these various diuretic agents is effective.

2. Increased tubular reabsorption

There is no pathological condition in which generalised tubular reabsorption is excessive, comparable with the unselective defective reabsorption caused by osmotic diuresis and other conditions referred to above. Excessive reabsorption takes place purely selectively, mainly as a result disturbances in the hormonal control of tubular function. These are for the most part the converse of specific (hormonal) absorption defects and will be dealt with on the basis of selective reabsorption of specific substances.

Sodium and chloride. Sodium (and secondarily chloride) reabsorption by the tubule is controlled mainly by the adrenal cortical steroid, aldosterone (SIMPSON, TAIT and BUSH; SIMPSON et al.; GAUNT, RENZI and CHART; LUETSCHER 1956). Other steroids, derived from the adrenal and elsewhere, possess sodium retaining activity to a very much smaller degree than aldosterone, although they may be of importance in certain conditions. Excessive secretion of aldosterone induces sodium retention which may or may not be accompanied by simultaneous water retention; in the former case oedema results, and in the latter, hypernatraemia. All oedematous states, including congestive heart failure, cirrhosis of the liver and the nephrotic syndrome, are now known to be associated with an excessive output of aldosterone (LUETSCHER and JOHNSON 1954a). The condition has been termed secondary aldosteronism (CONN 1956). Whether the increased tubular reabsorption of sodium is entirely due to the increased aldosterone is uncertain. The possibility remains that when the glomerular filtrate falls, as it may do in certain of these conditions, the amount of filtered sodium presented to the distal tubule is so much less than normal that it is almost completely reabsorbed. The stimulus to aldosterone excretion in these conditions is very much the subject of current thought and experiment, and is considered in detail in the section dealing with disturbances in body water. Briefly, most of the evidence points to control by some hypothetical receptor, sensitive to changes in volume or more probably pressure in the extracellular compartment, possibly in the plasma fraction (BARTTER). Various sites of such a pressor receptor or receptors have been postulated, in the right atrium and at the junction of the thyroid and carotid arteries (MILLS, CASPER and BARTTER: BARTTER, MILLS and GANN) and in the renal vessels (CARPENTER, DAVIS, AYERS 1961a; DAVIS et al.; DAVIS, AYERS and CARPENTER). There is increasing evidence that the renin-angiotensin mechanism in the kidney may be involved (LARAGH 1960). Retention of sodium resulting from increased secretion of aldosterone would tend to raise the extracellular sodium concentration were it not that in oedematous states, water is reabsorbed in parallel with sodium, so maintaining isotonicity of the body fluids. At first sight this increased water reabsorption would appear to be the natural response of the hypothalamic osmoreceptors (VERNEY 1947) to increased osmotic perssure, and such may indeed be the case. Thus there have been many reports of increased antidiuretic activity in the urine in the oedematous states (LEAF and MAMBY 1952b), and this may be due to posterior pituitary hormone. However, the sodium retention of primary aldosteronism is not accompanied by water retention, and a moderate degree of hypernatraemia does take place. Why there should be water retention under some circumstances and not others is problematical. One possibility is that the stimulus giving rise to sencondary aldosteronism also operates the pituitary antidiuretic mechanism. It is interesting to note that the administration of aldosterone to normal subjects results in a situation identical with primary aldosteronism (AUGUST, NELSON and THORN), i. e. there is initial retention of sodium with mild hypernatraemia but no oedema, followed by an escape from the renal sodium conservation, despite continuation of renal potassium loss.

It is possible that steroids other than aldosterone may play a part in the maintenance of chronic oedema. There is now good evidence that in cirrhosis of the liver, detoxication of circulating oestrogens may be defective. Oestrogens are known to have a weak sodium retaining action on the kidney, and an increase in circulating oestrogens may well be a factor in the causation of oedema in hepatic cirrhosis (PREEDY and AITKEN). Aldosterone not only causes the renal tubules to retain sodium, but also depresses their reabsorption of potassium, which may, if prolonged, bring about depletion of intracellular potassium. Potassium depletion is known to occur in chronic oedema, although other factors than aldosterone, e.g. increased tissue catabolism probably play a part.

Primary aldosteronism, first described by CONN (1955a), results from the apparently autonomous overproduction of aldosterone by the adrenal cortex. The usual cause is adrenal cortical adenoma, although cases have also been described in association with carcinoma and with bilateral adrenal cortical hyperplasia (FOYE and FEICHTMEIR; VAN BUCHEM, DUORENBOS and ELINGS; MILNE, MUEHRCKE and AIRD; CONN 1961). In primary aldosteronism there is excessive renal reabsorption of sodium and excretion of potassium. The former is unaccompanied by simultaneous water retention and so results in a slight to moderate rise in the level of serum sodium, but no oedema. Potassium loss results in hypokalaemia and extreme depletion of cellular potassium with consequent impairment of skeletal, cardiac and smooth muscle function. Two important diagnostic difficulties may arise. Firstly primary aldosteronism may be mistaken for chronic pyelonephritis for two reasons. Rare cases of chronic pyelonephritis are associated with a selective failure of the tubules to reabsorb potassium, and so may present with potassium depletion (MAHLER and STANBURY). Furthermore the incidence of pyelonephritis (or at any rate a similar structural lesion) in primary aldosteronism is greater than would be likely to occur by chance. Hence differentiation may be extremely difficult in the established case of primary aldosteronism with secondary renal damage, and the reader is referred to special papers on this subject (MILNE, MUEHRCKE and AIRD; BARTTER and BIGLIERI). The second important diagnostic point is that primary aldosteronism has been discovered by the chance finding of hypokalaemia in cases of asymptomatic hypertension. Secondary aldosteronism also occurs in malignant hypertension (LARAGH 1961). Hence it is a wise course to estimate the serum electrolytes in all cases of hypertension of uncertain aetiology, especially in the presence of polyuria.

Potassium. As mentioned above, aldosterone suppresses the tubular reabsorption of potassium, hence conversely in the absence of aldosterone, potassium is retained. The latter is the situation in adrenal cortical failure where potassium excretion is depressed and hyperkalaemia occurs. Although most work points to the control of aldosterone secretion by some hypothetical pressor-receptor in the extracellular compartment, there is some evidence that the level of serum potassium also influences aldosterone production (LARAGH and STOERK; JOHNSON, LIEBERMAN and MULROW) and the whole problem is still under investigation.

Phosphate and calcium. The action of the parathyroid hormone has been considered in an earlier section (see Defective Tubular Reabsorption due to Endocrine Disease). In hypoparathyroidism there is reduction of the renal phosphate clearance which can be corrected by the administration of parathyroid hormone. This lowered clearance must be due to increased tubular reabsorption of phosphate. The renal handling of calcium is very difficult to investigate and is little understood. It is probable that the parathyroid hormone has no direct action on the tubular reabsorption of calcium.

Water. The tubular reabsorption of water is under the influence of the antidiuretic hormone of the posterior pituitary. The mechanism controlling the release of ADH has been investigated by VERNEY (1947) who has provided evidence for the existence of osmoreceptors linked with the neurohypophysis. These neuro-receptors respond to small changes (of the order of 2%) in the osmotic pressure of the plasma, brought about by alterations in the concentration of sodium chloride but not of dextrose or urea. Dehydration raises the concentration of sodium chloride in the plasma and so excites this mechanism for the tubular retention of water. There is also evidence that other conditions than osmolarity of the body fluids influence antidiuretic hormone release, and these may have a common factor in some circulatory disturbance. In disease processes there is no certain evidence that excessive reabsorption of water occurs selectively. It does however take place in conjunction with sodium chloride during oedema formation, and it is very probable, though unproved, that the antidiuretic hormone is implicated. A syndrome of hyponatraemia which may be due to excessive secretion of pituitary (or some other) antidiuretic hormone has recently been described (SCHWARTZ et al. 1957; SCHWARTZ, TASSEL and BARTTER; GOLDBERG and HANDLER; ROBERTS; EPSTEIN and LEVITIN; CARTER, RECTOR and SELDIN). It has peen shown that the administration of vasopression to normal subjects over a brolonged period results in a new steady state of overhydration and hyponatraemia with "escape" from the antidiuretic action of vasopressin on the kidney (LEAF et al.; LEAF and MAMBY 1952b; JAENIKE and WATERHOUSE).

3. Abnormalities of tubular secretion

Tubular secretion is largely a function of the distal tubule and chiefly concerns the excretion of hydrion, ammonium and potassium. Certain foreign substances used in diagnosis (e.g. iodine-containing contrast media) or treatment (e.g. mecamylamine) are secreted by the tubules and finally, important enzymes or humoral factors such as renin and erythropoietin are formed by a specialised form of tubular secretory activity.

Abnormalities in secretion of hydrogen ion and ammonium are fully discussed in the sections on renal tubular acidosis and disorders of acid-base regulation. Since potassium and hydrogen compete in tubular cation exchange (BERLINER) secretion of the two ions will be affected reciprocally. Thus increase in hydrion secretion in respiratory or metabolic acidosis carries the risk of potassium intoxication, an effect which is exaggerated by potassium release from the tissue cells in acidosis (BARKER et al.; ORLOFF and DAVIDSON). Conversely potassium depletion may result when hydrion secretion is reduced, for example by carbonic anhydrase inhibitors such as azetazolamide. Potassium secretion is increased and hydrion secretion diminished in adrenocortical hyperfunction (primary or secondary aldosteronism). In the selective tubular anomalies such as Fanconi syndrome, in which renal tubular acidosis is a feature, impaired acid secretion may be partly dependent on the potassium depletion which is present as a primary defect (WRONG and DAVIES). In these conditions there is failure to secrete both hydrion and ammonium, whereas in pure potassium depletion (e.g. in steatorrhoea) there is marked inability to acidify the urine normally, yet ammonium secretion is well maintained (CLARKE et al.). Potassium secretion is reduced in Addison's disease due to failure of normal mineralo-corticoid action (WINKLER, SMITH and HOLT). In chronic renal failure effective potassium secretion is maintained until the late stages (LEAF and CAMARA; PLATT 1950) so that dangerous hyperkalaemia is rarely seen, even though various factors such as acidosis, vomiting and proteinuria may increase the mobilisation of potassium from the tissue cells. In acute oliguric uraemia on the other hand, tubular function is in abeyance and serious potassium retention may occur, aggravated by the effects of increased protein catabolism.

Various foreign substances are eliminated in the urine by tubular secretion and this may be impaired in renal disease. Mecamylamine is partly filtered, partly secreted as a weak base, and its subsequent behaviour depends on the urine pH (MILNE et al.). If the tubular fluid is acid it is excreted, but if alkaline, it diffuses back into the blood stream. Radio-opaque iodinated compounds used as contrast media in intravenous pyelography, are secreted by the proximal tubule; failure to visualise the substance is due to lack of secretion in adequate amount and not only to lack of renal concentrating power. The cause may be gross reduction of functioning nephrons as in chronic renal disease or temporary inhibition of secretion by some extraneous factor. Thus lack of visualisation of the medium on one side does not necessarily indicate a "non-functioning kidney", and at times excretion may not be seen on either side although other renal function tests are unimpaired. Different substances e.g. aromatic acids, may compete for a single secretion pathway. This is the basis for blockage of penicillin secretion by carinamide (SHAW).

III. Interpretation of renal function tests in disease

The principles underlying and techniques employed in tests of renal function are described in the previous chapter. The following section deals with the clinical application and appraisal of such tests.

It has already been pointed out that kidney function may be impaired by circulatory disturbances within the body, such as those arising in cardiac or peripheral circulatory failure, the latter being commonly due to such conditions as acute haemorrhage or dehydration. Under these circumstances the renal blood flow, and to a lesser extent the glomerular filtration rate are markedly reduced. This phenomenon has been referred to as extra-renal or pre-renal uraemia, with the implication that diminished filtration rate leading to urea retention does not necessarily imply organic renal damage. Since uraemia from any cause may give rise to vomiting, an element of pre-renal nitrogen retention is frequently superimposed on the renal failure of organic renal disease; in fact the uraemic state is likely to lead to a vicious circle, the vomiting increasing dehydration and thus producing a further rise in blood urea. Recognition of such a state of affairs and its correlation by intravenous fluid therapy may result in great improvement both in renal function and in the clinical state (BLACK and WILLIAMS). A more insidious example of pre-renal uraemia complicating organic renal disease occurs when the dehydration is brought about by the excessive loss of sodium chloride through the kidney itself. When severe, this may lead to a state closely resembling an Addisonian crisis ("salt-losing nephritis"), but milder degrees of impaired tubular reabsorption of sodium chloride are very common in chronic structural disease of the kidneys (particularly in ascending pyelonephritis) and the clinician must be aware of the possibility of dehydration from this cause. Thus tests of renal function are unreliable in patients who are dehydrated or in heart failure. The measurement of the blood urea level is usually sufficient at this stage, and the other tests should be left until the circulatory disturbances have as far as possible been rectified.

1. Individual tests of renal function

It is now proposed to consider the various tests of renal function and their interpretation in disease.

a) Estimations of blood or plasma concentrations of metabolites

The blood urea concentration. This estimation is usually performed routinely and is a most valuable indication of the extent of retention within the body of products of protein catabolism, some of which are known to be toxic. The height of the blood urea depends on the rate of urea production and the urea clearance rate. Urea production is increased with a rise in dietary protein, in gastro-intestinal haemorrhage, and with accelerated tissue protein catabolism in fevers, infections and after trauma (including surgical operations). Urea clearance may be decreased by circulatory disturbances, as mentioned above, or by structural renal damage. Thus the bare measurement of the blood urea level provides no certain evidence of the extent or even of the existence of organic renal damage. This is particularly so when the blood urea is at the upper limit of normal. Although it is possible to express the "normal" range of blood urea in a healthy population of known dietetic habits, the finding of a blood urea level within this range in a particular subject is no guarantee of normal renal function. Thus an individual on a low protein diet may have a blood urea level around 20 mg. per 100 ml., which only rises to 40 mg. per 100 ml. — still within the commonly accepted "normal" range — when the glomerular filtration rate is halved by disease. Conversely, a patient placed on a high protein diet may show a rise in blood urea beyond the "normal" range even though renal function is unchanged. This relationship between dietary protein intake and blood urea level has been studied by ADDIS et al. (1947).

The plasma creatinine concentration. The rate of formation of creatinine in the body is related to the bulk of muscle tissue and is much less influenced, as compared with urea, by fluctuations in the dietary protein and the rate of endo-genous protein catabolism. Thus the level of plasma creatinine is a somewhat more precise indicator of renal function than is the level of blood urea; nevertheless the creatinine clearance may be reduced by half while the plasma creatinine level remains within the generally accepted normal range of $1.0 \pm$ S.D. 0.2 mg. per 100 ml. (ADDIS 1949, ADDIS et al. 1951).

b) Renal blood flow

The application of the FICK principle to the measurement of renal blood flow has been dealt with elswhere (see Normal Physiology of Kidney). The method requires measurement of the arterial and renal-venous concentrations, and the urinary excretion of any substance which is removed partly or wholly from the blood as it passes through the kidney. Renal venous blood for this purpose is obtained by catheterisation of the renal vein, and if this technique is employed the significance of the result must be beyond question (WARREN, BRANNAN and MERRILL; BRADLEY 1948a). However, catheterisation of the renal vein is laborious and it has been customary to use a substance, such as PAH or Diodone, which is known to be almost completely extracted from the blood during passage through the kidneys (SMITH, GOLDRING and CHASIS; SMITH 1943). This more convenient technique has been widely employed in renal disease. The results are only valid so long as the extracted fraction does not fall below normal, otherwise false low values of renal blood flow will be obtained. Thus in both early and late glomerulo-nephritis it has been shown that the extracted fraction may fall (BRADLEY 1948a), and in acute anuria with tubular injury as little as 2% may be extracted.

c) Glomerular filtration rate

Substances and techniques used in the measurement of this rate have been described elswhere, and it is only necessary to refer to them briefly here. The urea clearance, although still widely used, is a most unsatisfactory test, since it is affected by the degree of back diffusion of urea from the tubular lumen to the bloodstream which occurs both in health and disease. This back diffusion is variable and depends on the relative concentration of urea in the urine and the body fluids. The endogenous creatinine clearance has now largely superceded it in routine hospital work. In normal subjects this clearance closely approximates that of inulin and is comparatively simple to perform since it does not involve introducing a foreign substance into the body and maintaining its concentration constant over the period of urine collection. Clearance measurements are customarily expressed in relation to surface area since they correlate better with this than with body weight in normal subjects. However, there is no valid reason for the use of surface area in this respect, and there is some evidence that over extremes of weight, the glomerular filtration rate correlates better with total body water. It is most important that some correction for body size be applied to clearance measurements so that minor departures from normal can be detected. Certain practical difficulties are encountered in the routine estimation of renal clearance, chief amongst which are incomplete emptying of the bladder and inaccurate timing in the colletion of urinary samples. The former is all too common in patients with genito-urinary disorders, who suffer from disturbances of micturition, and in women and small children. It also occurs in hypertensive patients under treatment with ganglion blocking drugs. Under these circumstances clearance tests must be performed with a catheter in the bladder, although as an alternative to this, the creatinine clearance may be measured over an extended period (e.g. 12—24 hours) when timing errors become less important.

Interpretation of clearance tests in disease. Although in normal subjects inulin and creatinine clearances are in close agreement, and are assumed to represent the glomerular filtration rate, this assumption does not necessarily hold good in disease. Both inulin and creatinine may diffuse back passively from the tubules when the latter are damaged, so giving a false low value for the glomerular filtration rate. This possibility is however a theoretical rather than a practical disadvantage, since the clinican is interested more in the actual clearance of these and related substances than with the glomerular filtration rate itself. It is furthermore possible that creatinine may be actively reabsorbed or excreted by the tubules. Active tubular reabsorption is probably the explanation of the decreased creatinine clearance compared with inulin clearance observed in diabetic acidosis (McCANCE and WIDDOWSON 1939), whilst tubular excretion is probably responsible for the reverse finding in renal disease (HARE et al.).

As already mentioned, the glomerular filtration rate may be depressed in heart failure and peripheral circulatory failure, and shows recovery if these can be overcome. In organic renal disease, the glomerular filtration rate usually falls parallel with the renal blood flow and impairment of tubular function, but there are two exceptions to this relationship. In acute glomerulo-nephritis glomerular filtration may be selectively impaired in the presence of normal renal blood flow and normal tubular function (EARLE, TAGGART and SHANNON; BLACK et al.). Thus in this condition there may be urea retention with a high urine specific gravity and urea concentration. Later in the course of chronic nephritis when renal blood flow is reduced, the glomerular filtration rate is still proportionately more affected. On the other hand, in essential hypertension, renal blood flow and tubular function are depressed before the glomerular filtration rate, which is maintained as a consequence of the high filtration fraction (GOLD-RING et al.).

d) Tubular function tests
α) General

Tests of tubular function vary from the roughly quantitative to the more precise. In the former class are the concentration tests, based either on specific gravity measurements (VOLHARD) or on urine urea concentration (MACLEAN and

DE WESSELOW). Whilst urine concentration is not exclusively a tubular function as was at one time believed, the counter-current mechanism utilises the energy provided by the enzymes of the Krebs tricarbocylic-acid cycle to maintain the sodium pump. Integrity of tubular function is therefore essential for water reabsorption. Of more precise value are the saturation tests used in determining the maximum power of the tubules to reabsorb glucose or excrete Diodone or para-amino-hippuric acid. These are rarely employed in routine hospital work and the reader is referred to more specialised books on the subject (SMITH 1951). The phenolsulphonphthalein (P.S.P.) test is also mainly one of tubular function; in its original form it is not very sensitive, and a more sensitive technique, based on the excretion of P.S.P. in the first 15 min. after intravenous injection, has been employed (FISHBERG).

The simple concentration tests are fairly readily carried out in hospital patients under ward supervision, since accurately timed collections of urine are not required. Close observance however to the control of fluid intake before and during the tests in important. A more convenient simple concentration test, which does not require prolonged water deprivation, involves the injection of vasopressin tannate in oil (DE WARDENER 1956).

β) Specific tubular function tests

In the differential diagnosis of *severe polyuria*, it is customary to employ a water deprivation test which is continued until either the urinary specific gravity rises above 1020 or the patient loses 5% of body weight, whichever is the earlier. Failure to concentrate the urine is followed by further investigation by the injection of 5 units of vasopressin tanate in oil. If, under these circumstances, renal concentrating power is till inadequate, the condition is probably due either to nephrogenic diabetes insipidus or compulsive water drinking (see under diabetes insipidus).

Hydrogen ion excretion: a test of the ability of the kidney to excrete hydrogen ion is of value in the investigation of nephrocalcinosis and systemic acidosis of renal origin. A convenient and well standardised test involving the administration of a single dose of ammonium chloride has been described by WRONG and DAVIES. In renal tubular acidosis, the kidney is unable to acidify the urine to the normal extent following the administration of ammonium chloride, but excretion of ammonium ion is either normal or above normal for the pH of the urine. This test is particularly valuable for the detection of early cases before systemic acidosis has developed. In renal failure with systemic acidosis due to chronic nephritis or pyelonephritis, acidification of the urine is usually normal.

Phosphate excretion: when the serum level of phosphate is depressed, the possibility of excessive renal phosphaturia may be investigated by measuring the clearance rate of phosphate relative to creatinine in the fasting state. This clearance ratio depends on the level of serum phosphate, and normal ranges have been published (McGEOWN and BULL). Another technique involves the measurement of the renal phosphate threshold by means of an intravenous infusion of neutral phosphate (HYDE et al.). These tests are of particular value in the investigation of Vitamin D resistant rickets and hyperparathyroidism.

Calcium excretion: excessive renal loss of calcium is nearly always due to hypercalcaemia. In the absence of hypercalcaemia it may be due to a high calcium intake, immobilisation, renal tubular acidosis or so-called idiopathic hypercalcuria. The latter may itself be a primary disturbance of intestinal function resulting in excessive calcium absorption. The investigation of hypercalcuria of obscure origin is best achieved by performing a full calcium balance on a diet containing less than 150 mgm. of calcium a day.

Glucose reabsorption: This may fail as an isolated phenomenon in renal glycosuria or as one of the multiple tubular defects seen in the Fanconi syndrome. The presence of a lowered renal threshold for glucose is simply detected by simultaneous measurement of blood and urinary glucose concentrations or by a glucose tolerance test.

Amino-acid excretion: abnormalities of amino-acid excretion such as occur in xanthinuria, cystinuria and in the Fanconi syndrome are detected by paper chromatographic techniques.

Interpretation of tubular function tests in disease states. Many factors play a part in determining the maximum attainable specific gravity or urine urea concentration. Firstly there may be a direct failure to produce urine of osmotic pressure higher than that of plasma. This may be due to organic damage to the tubules or to reversible functional changes secondary to ischaemia, depression by drugs, potassium depletion, or hypercalcaemia. Secondly, the excretion of large amounts of osmotically active substances (e.g. sodium chloride, urea, mannitol) results in the passage of urine of osmolarity approaching that of plasma even in a state of hydropenia (Rapoport et al.). This osmotic diuresis may account for the low maximum specific gravity attainable in patients after subtotal nephrectomy who have only a quarter or less of residual normal renal tissue; in these patients the blood urea is raised and the total osmolarity of urine passing through individual nephrons is raised to an even greater extent. The same considerations apply to any organic renal disease which has resulted in a diminution of the total number of functioning nephrons (Platt 1952; Franklin and Merrill 1960a); under these circumstances the remaining nephrons undergo hypertrophy and probably pass a larger individual filtrate volume. With only moderate reduction in the number of functioning nephrons, hypertrophy may result in the passage of a normal total volume of glomerular filtrate; an individual tubule under these circumstances has to deal with a total increase of solutes, and osmotic diuresis may result in the passage of urine of lowered maximum specific gravity. The term *glomerulo-tubular imbalance* has been suggested for this state of affairs. In all the above circumstances the maximum attainable osmolarity of the urine approximates to that of plasma, while the urine specific gravity approaches and eventually becomes fixed around 1010. These and other considerations will seriously affect the interpretation of the more complex tubular saturation tests, eg. T_m Diodone ov P.A.H., in renal disease. Nevertheless the latter are the most sensitive indices of impaired tubular function. With such tests, impaired tubular excretory function has been shown to occur early in essential hypertension and before any reduction in glomerular filtration rate (Smith 1943; Goldring et al.). In chronic nephritis tubular function is impaired but, at least in the early stages, to a lesser degree than the filtration rate (Earle, Taggart and Shannon). In chronic pyelonephritis, as in essential hypertension, tubular excretory power is more affected than filtration rate, but the ratio of the clearance to the maximum tubular excretion of Diodone tends to be in the normal range rather than reduced (Raaschou). The significance of these latter changes is most difficult to interpret (Smith 1943).

2. Choice of renal function tests for routine use

For detecting the presence of early functional impairment, the simply applied concentration tests, i.e. the measurement of maximum specific gravity or urea concentration of the urine, are the most valuable. A urinary specific gravity greater than 1.025 or a maximum urine urea concentration greater than 25 G/l. is strong evidence against renal functional impairment. Two warnings must however be given. First, in the presence of circulatory disturbances mentioned earlier, and in acute glomerulo-nephritis, these tests may be normal yet the glomerular filtration rate may be impaired and urea retention may be present. Thus it is advisable to estimate blood urea and creatinine clearance as part of routine investigation. Secondly, despite adequate preceding water deprivation, the tests may be invalidated in oedematous patients if diuresis is occurring at the time. The modified test using vasopressin tannate (DE WARDENER) overcomes this difficulty.

For assessing the progress of functional impairment, measurement of urine specific gravity has little value since it becomes fixed at a relatively early stage. Subsequent deterioration may then be assessed by estimation of the creatinine clearance, 15 min. PSP excretion, and the blood urea level. When renal function is grossly impaired, change in the blood urea is a more reliable quantitative indicator of further deterioration than the creatinine clearance, providing the protein intake remains constant.

Differential renal function tests. The problem of hypertension in the presence of apparently unilateral renal disease frequently confronts the surgeon. Removal of the abnormal kidney results in permanent lowering of the blood pressure in the minority of patients so treated. The explanation of this disappointing result may lie in the fact that the apparently normal kidney has itself been damaged either by the same processes as has affected the other, or as a consequence of being exposed to hypertension (WILSON and BYROM 1941). A further possibility, particularly in older patients, is that the high blood pressure may be due to essential hypertension rather than to the unilateral renal disease so that nephrectomy could not be expected to bring relief. This probably explains the greater likelihood of success from nephrectomy in younger people, and emphasises the need for a careful investigation of the family history for evidence of hypertension.

The most dramatic and consistent successes following surgical treatment for hypertension have been in cases of renal artery stenosis. Experimental narrowing of one renal artery results in the excretion of urine of smaller volume and containing a lower concentration of sodium in comparison with the urine from the opposite kidney (SELKURT, HALL and SPENCER; BLAKE et al.; and MUELLER et al.). On this basis, a number of differential renal function tests have been devised for the detection of renal artery stenosis in man. These are described in detail under unilateral renal disease (pp. 448).

Differential renal function tests have been mainly successful in the detection of main or branch renal artery stenosis as a cause of hypertension. Another problem is that of predicting the result of nephrectomy in other forms of unilateral renal lesion, in particular unilateral pyelonephritis. It is possible that when nephrectomy is successful in this group, the same functional disorder in regard to water and sodium excretion may be present as in renal artery stenosis, but the evidence at present is inadequate (SPENCER; STAMEY et al.).

Whenever unilateral nephrectomy is under consideration for the treatment of hypertension, it is important that the overall renal function should be good. GRABER and SHACKMAN consider that before nephrectomy is undertaken the function of the contralateral kidney should be shown to be normal. It is probably sufficient however to ensure that the overall clearance of creatinine or inulin is within the normal range. There is some evidence that in acutely developing hypertension due to unilateral renal disease, depression of overall renal function may improve after nephrectomy. This could be explained by lack of time for compensatory hypertrophy or by some reversible circulatory change in the opposite kidney.

3. Changes in renal function with age

In paediatric practice, difficulties often arise in relating measurements of renal function in infants and children to the adult normal standards. In fact when comparisons of clearance rates are made at different ages, the results must be corrected for some parameter related to the size of the individual. McINTOSH, MOLLER and vanSLYKE suggested an appropriate parameter was body surface area rather than weight. Using this as a basis for comparison, the urea clearance is the same for normal children over the age of two as for adults. However, below the age of two the urea clearance falls progressively until at the age of a few days it is only about one quarter of the adult figure. McCANCE and WIDDOWSON (1952) suggest that a more appropriate parameter than body surface area is total body water. When urea clearance and GFR are related to this parameter there is much less difference between adults and infants, but on the other hand, adolescents show clearances actually exceeding the adult figure. McCANCE (1950) suggests that this represents a true increase in renal clearance in adolescents, which may be due to the increased protein intake and catabolism occurring in this age group. There is experimental evidence in animals that large changes in protein intake induce parallel changes in filtration rate. Problems of renal function in infancy have been dealt with by McCANCE (1950); McCANCE and HATEMI; ROBIN, BRUCK and RAPOPORT and EDELMAN, BARNETT and TROUPKOU.

At the other end of the age range, DAVIES and SHOCK have demonstrated in male subjects progressive diminution of inulin and diodone clearances with increasing age from 24 to 89 years. The concentrating ability also declines (LEWIS and ALVING; MILLER and SHOCK).

C. Disorders of homeostasis in renal disease

In the preceding section an attempt has been made to separate the biochemical disorders which result from impairment of glomerular and tubular function. Such a separation can be made with fair success where specific lesions of tubular reabsorption or secretion occur independently of glomerular function, but even so these frequently produce secondary effects on glomerular filtration. Or again it may be possible to recognise the separate effects of glomerular failure where this is extreme as in acute anuria. Nevertheless in general the clinical manifestations of renal failure can be explained only with reference to combined glomerulo-tubular dysfunction and the effects of this on the organism as a whole. Thus an understanding of the various mechanisms of disturbed homeostasis is necessary before the clinical picture in renal disease can be accurately interpreted and correct treatment decided upon. Of these, regulation of fluid volume, osmolality, the levels of individual electrolytes particularly sodium and potassium, and acid-base balance have been most fully investigated. Less well understood are the regulation of arterial pressure, calcium metabolism, and erythropoiesis. In attempting to understand how these complex processes are affected by renal disease certain general relationships must be recognised.

1. Although it is possible to describe the changes in individual forms of homeostasis separately, this is an artificial approach since they are interrelated and are subject to a variety of adaptations to one another.

2. The endocrine system plays a vital role in determining the renal response to environmental change, and the interaction between hormones such as ADH or aldosterone and the kidney is apparently in the nature of a feed back mechanism. Renal disease will influence the responsiveness of the kidney to hormonal action and will impair the efficiency of these feed back mechanisms.

3. Disorders of homeostasis all produce secondary effects on renal function hence, on the one hand renal failure may give rise to "vicious circles" which prolong and intensify its course, and on the other, extrarenal factors disturbing homeostasis will adversely affect renal function, giving rise to difficulties in diagnosis between primary renal and extrarenal failure. This is aggravated by the fact that some extra-renal disturbances, e.g. potassium deficiency, hypertension and circulatory insufficiency may themselves produce structural renal damage.

4. The correlation of disorders of homeostasis with structural renal damage varies extremely widely, for example total suppression of renal function may be unassociated with any obvious histological abnormality of the kidney: hypertension may result from unilateral renal damage; gross proteinuria, leading to the complex homeostatic disturbances of the nephrotic syndrome may occur with minimal histological glomerular lesions; specific tubular anomalies may be due to inherited enzyme deficiencies unassociated with structural tubular damage.

Before the separate disorders of homeostasis are discussed it is necessary to describe the syndromes of renal failure and in particular to outline the various features of fully developed uraemia. Whilst many of these correlate well with biochemical changes, there are others which still remain unexplained, so that without this clinical background, a description of the "pathological physiology" of renal disease is both incomplete and lacking in perspective.

I. Syndromes of renal failure

Renal failure may present with a number of diverse clinical patterns according to the nature of the cause. The most distinct patterns are 1. acute uraemia due to sudden suppression of glomerular and tubular function; 2. chronic uraemia resulting from progressive organic renal disease; and 3. extra-renal uraemia due to circulatory impairment of the kidney, usually associated with reduction in blood volume, blood pressure or cardiac output. When such circulatory impairment is superimposed on either of the other uraemic syndromes, the extra-renal component is usually reversible when the cause is recognised and removed. In addition to these varieties of uraemia in which there is combined glomerular and tubular dysfunction due to organic kidney disease, renal failure may arise from the specific functional tubular anomalies already described. These when severe may lead to secondary structural changes, hence in their later stages a picture of uraemia may emerge which is difficult to distinguish from that due to chronic glomerulonephritis or pyelonephritis.

So far the emphasis has been on biochemical changes. The majority of uraemic patients however suffer from high blood pressure and with this are associated cerebral, retinal, cardiac and visceral manifestations which may be prominent features in the development of uraemia. In addition, loss of protein in the urine leads to a complex series of physiological changes which has been termed the nephrotic syndrome. Finally anaemia is often a prominent feature, and although a variety of factors may contribute, the basic cause is hypoplasia of the bone marrow due to deficiency of a renal haemopoietic factor. Thus the clinical picture of uraemia will depend on the type of renal lesion, the pattern of biochemical disturbance, and the cardiovascular complications of which hypertension is the most important.

Clinical picture of uraemia

It is surprising how few of the clinical manifestations of uraemia can be attributed with certainty to accumulation in the blood and tissues of breakdown products of metabolism. Acidosis is most clearly an example of excretory failure and its effects are described below. Urea retention is undoubtedly a cause of osmotic diuresis and is responsible for the polyuria of chronic renal failure. Nevertheless this symptom is rarely extreme, since in most patients with advanced renal disease the glomerular filtrate volume is greatly reduced owing to the reduction in the actual number of nephrons. There is moreover in these patients inability to form a dilute urine after water drinking, hance isosthenuria with fixation of urine specific gravity at around 1010 is the rule. This restricted water excretion may account for the ease with which patients in chronic uraemia develop oedema and heart failure, especially if excessive fluids are administered parenterally.

Apart from osmotic diuresis it is difficult to attribute with certainty any clinical effects to urea retention. The urea content of the saliva and of the gastric and intestinal secretions is increased, and ammonia formation in the mouth, stomach or intestines may be a contributory factor in the production of *gastrointestinal symptoms* such as stomatitis, anorexia, hiccough, nausea, vomiting and diarrhoea (HARRISON and MASON 1937). Nevertheless these symptoms are often transient and may respond to symptomatic therapy even while the blood urea remains elevated or continues to rise. Although the term "uraemic colitis" is frequently quoted as a clinical manifestation of uraemia, diarrhoea is a rare symptom and is in ho way related to the level of blood urea (MASON 1952; NEWBURGH and CAMARA 1951; OLSEN and BASSETT 1951). When they do occur, these gastrointestinal symptoms are of importance in that they may aggravate the effects of renal failure. Thus impairment of appetite results in low calorie intake which leads to increased endogenous protein breakdown; vomiting and diarrhoea produce loss of water and sodium which adds to dehydration. Hypochlorhydria or achlorhydria is usually present in the chronic uraemic state, hence alkalosis due to chloride loss rarely occurs. Iron intake may be inadequate due to anorexia or vomiting, or absorption may be interfered with, thereby increasing the tendency to anaemia.

The neuro-muscular symptoms of uraemia are again difficult to explain in terms of metabolite retention. Muscular twitchings, muscle cramps and latent tetany are common manifestations. Alkalosis and diminished blood level of ionised calcium increase neuromuscular irritability, whilst increased levels of potassium and magnesium diminish it. Thus a balance of factors is involved, but the relation of this to neuro-muscular manifestations in uraemia is quite obscure. There is no evidence that muscle tremors in uraemic patients are associated with low serum magnesium levels, indeed in azotaemia the level tends to be high (SMITH and HAMMARSTEN 1958). Calcium administration may relieve these symptoms even though hypocalcaemia is not demonstrable. Acidosis increases the ionisation of calcium in the blood, which may protect agaits hypocalcaemia (BULL 1955). Convulsions in uraemia are usually attributable to hypertensive encephalopathy, but in patients without hypertension, may be due to fluid retention or to the same factors as produce localized muscle twitchings. Attacks of muscular weakness should always suggest potassium depletion, and with more frequent estimation of serum electrolytes this condition is being diagnosed with increasing frequency in patients with renal disease. It is however less often a feature of chronic uraemia than a manifestation of selective tubular deficiency leading to potassium depletion, either genetically determined or, more rarely, due to nephrotoxic chemicals or chronic pyelonephritis. Potassium depletion may also result from excessive use of diuretics.

Cerebral depression, apathy, disorientation and finally coma, cannot yet with certainty be correlated with any specific biochemical derangement. Sodium depletion with cellular overhydration may cause lassitude, mental confusion and coma; acidosis and anaemia may be contributory factors, as may cerebral arterial disease, increased intracranial pressure and cerebral oedema.

Anaemia in renal disease. When the hypoplastic character of anaemia in patients with uraemia was established (DAMESHEK 1935; NORDENSON 1938), it was assumed that depression of erythropoiesis was due to the toxic effect of retained metabolites on the bone marrow. There are obviously several other factors which may contribute to anaemia in chronic renal disease. These include haemodilution in oedematous patients, infection, haematuria, and possibly haemolysis. The latter has been investigated by red cell survival studies (CHAPLIN and MOLLISON 1953; JOSKE, McALISTER and PRANKERD 1956), and the evidence suggests that haemolysis is rarely responsible for severe anaemia. It may be more important in uraemia associated with malignant hypertension (CHAPLIN and MOLLISON 1953; VEREL et al. 1959). By far the most important cause of anaemia in chronic renal disease is however depression of red cell formation, apparently due to failure of the kidneys to produce erythropoietin, a relatively heat stable, non-dialysable mucoprotein (JACOBSON et al. 1957; RAMBACH, COOPER and ALT 1958; GOLDWASSER and WHITE 1959). Biological assay of the active principle has been attempted by variety of methods. Using for assay, rats rendered artificially polycythaemic by transfusion, increase in erythropoietic activity in plasma has been demonstrated in a wide range of anaemias, but no such activity appears to be present in plasma from patients with hypoplastic anaemia of comparable severity due to chronic renal disease (PENINGTON 1960). This deficiency in erythropoietin production by the kidney appears to be independent of the degree of metabolite retention, since hypoplastic anaemia is occasionally observed before the development of nitrogen retention, and on the other hand may be absent in patients with long standing uraemia. Polycythaemia may occur in association with renal carcinoma (DAMON et al. 1958), and it has been claimed that high plasma erythropoietin levels may be found in such cases. Extracts from the tumours may contain abnormal amounts of erythropoietin (HEWLETT et al. 1960), and surgical removal of the abnormal kidney is usually followed by return of the red cell count to normal.

Owing to the considerable difficulties of biological assay, and the failure to obtain active extracts which stimulate erythropoiesis in man, there are still many aspects of this problem which need further clarification. In particular we cannot be certain that failure of erythropoietin production by the kidney is not due to some form of metabolite retention as yet unrecognised, or to ischaemic changes similar to those which lead to overproduction of renin.

Cardiovascular disorders in the uraemic patient are of a varied character, and hypertensive manifestations predominate. Heart failure may be caused or aggravated by a number of factors, including sodium and water retention, anaemia and infection. Some cardiovascular changes are however metabolic in origin. Potassium retention as a cause of cardiac arrest has been already discussed. It occurs principally in acute oliguric states such as acute cortical ischaemia, glomerulonephritis and obstructive anuria; it may however occur in chronic uraemia, producing muscular paralysis as its main manifestation (KEITH and BURCHELL 1949; MARCHAND and FINCH 1944; BULL, CARTER and LOWE 1953). The general effects of potassium depletion have already been discussed. Characteristic changes in the electrocardiogram are produced by both hypo- and hyper-kalaemia. Pericarditis is a common pre-terminal manifestation of uraemia. It is usually sterile, fibrinous or with effusion, and may be haemorrhagic; the aetiology is unknown. Uraemic patients have a reduced tolerance for digitalis which may give rise to arrhythmia, nausea and vomiting.

Respiratory changes in uraemia are usually incidental to hypertensive heart failure or infection. Chronic bilateral opacities in the x-ray picture may develop in patients with protracted left ventricular failure, and the term "uraemic lung" has been applied to this condition (DONIACH 1947). The deep sighing respiration due to chronic acidosis is a rare manifestation and is usually pre-terminal.

Cutaneous manifestations in uraemia include laxity and dryness of the skin due to dehydration; pruritus, for which no satisfactory explanation is forthcoming; and various skin rashes which may include purpuric, papular, urticarial or eczematoid eruptions. These may sometimes be attributed to drug hypersensitivity or to secondary infection, but usually their causation is obscure. There is certainly increased urea excretion in the sweat and "urea frost" may be seen as white deposit on the skin. This is not however necessarily associated with pruritus and skin rashes.

Haemorrhage into the skin may take the form of purpura or large ecchymoses. Haemorrhages from the buccal mucous membrane and gastrointestinal tract, and haemarthroses are also encountered. There is no correlation between anaemia or platelet deficiency and these haemorrhagic manifestations, which appear to be due to increased capillary fragility.

In summary, retention of specific metabolic waste produces provides an imperfect explanation for many of the clinical features of uraemia which are associated with excretory failure. Elevation of blood urea (or of non-protein nitrogen in the blood) is a useful chemical index of the degree of excretory failure, and a few manifestations of advanced uraemia may be partly explained on the basis of urea or electrolyte retention. For the most part however the majority of symptoms in late uraemia have yet no known chemical basis. It may be that the relief of these symptoms by dialysis with the artificial kidney will throw further light on this problem.

II. Disorders of electrolyte homeostasis

It is not possible to separate disturbances of electrolyte homeostasis from those of body water, acid-base balance, and probably hypertension, since all these variables are interrelated. At the risk of some repetition these questions will however be dealth with seriatim. In spite of gross damage and rising blood urea the failing kidney is able to maintain electrolytic homeostasis until a very late stage (PLATT 1950). However, as renal failure progresses the kidney becomes progressively less adaptable and is less able to compensate for excess or depletion of electrolytes (CRAWFORD et al. 1954). With progressive nephron damage the glomerular filtration rate diminishes, and at a level of creatinine clearance of 10—20 ml./min., urine volume falls. PLATT, ROSCOE and SMITH (1952) suggested that in advanced renal disease the urine was formed by a small number of intact nephrons and this view been confirmed by BRICKER, MORRIN and KIME (1960). Thus each surviving nephron must handle an increased solute load relative to the filtrate volume, i.e. continuous osmotic diuresis will lead to increased loss of sodium and water in the urine as the urine osmolarity approaches that of plasma. When the urine volume falls due to severe nephron destruction, further dehydration cannot occur but the patient is now vulnerable to an increased load of water, electrolytes or organic metabolites, since no mechanism exists for increasing solute excretion.

a) Sodium

Since the extra-cellular fluid is largely isotonic salt solution and is so maintained by the osmolar control of ADH, variations of sodium are inseparable from those of body water, i.e. sodium depletion and retention are in general manifested by "dehydration" and oedema. The latter is dealt with in detail under "Nephrotic Syndrome".

Retention of sodium in renal disease may be renal or extra-renal in origin. Renal sodium retention follows reduction in glomerular filtration due to disease or destruction of glomeruli. It is seen characteristically in acute nephritis and in the syndrome of anuria when sodium and water are administered over and above the amounts eliminated by extra-renal routes. Extra-renal causes may act on the glomeruli or tubules. Reduction in renal blood flow due to heart failure, reduction in plasma volume, or acute hypotension in haemorrhage or shock will reduce the filtered load of sodium. Excessive tubular reabsorption of sodium occurs only as a result of increased aldosterone secretion, for example in chronic hypovolaemic states such as the nephrotic syndrome, and in primary aldosteronism due to adrenal tumours. In chronic uraemia sodium retention is obviated by osmotic diuresis in the surviving nephrons and will only occur if glomerular filtration is excessively reduced by heart failure, or when other contributory factors develop such as hypoproteinaemia, anaemia or secondary aldosteronism.

Sodium depletion is much commoner than sodium retention and again may be renal or extra-renal in origin. Renal salt loss results from tubular dysfunction, either in the form of osmotic diuresis or specific impairment of the reabsorptive mechanism, e.g. in diseases such as pyelonephritis which selectively damage the distal tubules leading to so-called "sodium losing nephritis" already discussed. Extra-renal causes include vomiting, diarrhoea and sweating which frequently occur in renal disease and, of very great importance, therapeutic measures for the relief of oedema such as restricted salt intake, diuretics, ion-exchange resins and subcutaneous drainage. In Addison's disease sodium depletion is due to aldosterone deficiency. Whatever the cause of the sodium depletion, the effects on renal function may be serious in the patient with renal disease since glomerular filtration is further reduced (NICKEL et al. 1953) owing to impairment of renal blood flow, and in severe cases, as a result of the hypotension associated with hypovolaemia. The uraemia caused by sodium depletion is however reversible if the cause is corrected or, in salt losing states, by administration of sodium. If however the condition is not relieved, a shock like state may ensue which is often fatal. This may even occur in the presence of oedema, as in the nephrotic syndrome when chronically sodium depleted patients are subjected to subcutaneous drainage. The clinical manifestations by which sodium depletion may be recognised include weakness, loss of tissue elasticity, thirst, polyuria, fixation of urinary specific gravity and low blood pressure.

b) Potassium

Clinical manifestations due to retension of potassium are rare in the common forms of chronic renal disease, largely as a result of glomerular-tubular imbalance in the surviving nephrons in which osmotic diuresis compensates for reduced glomerular filtration. Tubular secretion which is the important mechanism for excretion of potassium, appears to be little affected except in those rare diseases characterised by specific tubular defects (BLACK and EMERY 1957).

Potassium retention like sodium retention is confined to those conditions where glomerular filtration is grossly impaired, such as acute nephritis and other types of acute oliguric uraemia. Extra-renal factors are however of special importance in producing the high blood levels which are the cause of cardiac arrest and muscle paralysis. Increased cell breakdown due to infection, fever, starvation and catabolic steroids will lead to hyperkalaemia when glomerular filtration is reduced, and in acidosis potassium will move from the intra-cellular to the extra-cellular fluid. The latter is an important factor in acute uraemia. Reversal of this leakage is promptly brought about by insulin and glucose which moves potassium back into the cells.

Potassium depletion may again be of renal or extra-renal origin. Hypokalaemia occurring during the recovery phase of anuric states is a typical example of potassium depletion due to massive osmotic diuresis and to a lesser extent this may occur after the relief of chronic urinary retention and in chronic nephritis with azotaemia. The other and rarer renal cause is a specific disturbance of the ion-exchange mechanism in the distal tubule and has been previously described in the section on specific tubular defects. Both types of renal potassium loss may be present, e.g. in chronic hydronephrosis (BERLYNE 1961). Extra-renal causes may operate via the kidney, such as primary and secondary aldosteronism, the latter being particularly important in the nephrotic syndrome and in severe sodium depletion; or the potassium loss may be extra-renal as in chronic diarrhoea. Therapeutic agents such as chlorthiazide which provoke potassium diuresis, or adrenal steroids which in addition increase tissue breakdown will, if long continued, lead to severe potassium loss. The effects of potassium depletion on the kidney are both structural and functional. Structural damage is primarily tubular but may lead to severe disorganisation of the kidney resembling chronic pyelonephritis. Functional changes include reduction in GFR, impaired concentration of the urine and reduced ability to form an acid urine (see p. 403). Nocturia and polyuria develop which are not responsive to ADH administration, thirst is a prominent symptom, and uraemia will appear or be aggravated as structural damage to the kidney develops.

c) Magnesium

The normal kidney is capable of good conservation of magnesium when dietary intake is deficient. Thus on a fluid diet containing less magnesium than 0.12 mEq/l. the renal loss may be reduced to less than 1 mEq per day (BARNES, COPE and HARRISON 1958). When the serum magnesium fell below 0.25 mEq/l. in a patient after massive intestinal resection the renal loss was as little as 0.1 mEq daily (FLETCHER et al. 1960). In chronic renal disease, disturbances in magnesium metabolism may arise and their character depends on the stage of the disease. In the absence of azotaemia, occasionally a very low level of serum magnesium may occur, whereas in the presence of azotaemia the level may be raised and correlated with the serum potassium level (SMITH and HAMMARSTEN 1958). It is possible that magnesium depletion in the former case may occur as a consequence of osmotic diuresis, as in the magnesium depletion during diabetic coma. Magnesium depletion through renal loss, may be a feature of primary aldosteronism (MADER and ISERI 1955), and there is some collateral evidence that aldosterone promotes magnesium excretion both in the urine and faeces experimentally (HANNA and McINTYRE 1960). A negative magnesium balance through increased urinary loss also occurs in primary hyperparathyroidism and here the action may be related to the increased filtered load of calcium (HANNA et al. 1961).

d) Calcium

The role of the kidney in the regulation of calcium metabolism is obscure and there is considerable evidence that abnormalities of calcium homeostasis in kidney disease may be due to the effects of renal failure on extra-renal processes rather than to abnormal handling of calcium by the kidney. For a detailed discussion of this complex problem the reader is referred to papers by STANBURY (1960), STANBURY and LUMB (1962), DENT and HARRIS (1956) and DENT (1960).

Disordered calcium metabolism in renal disease is manifested by various types of osteodystrophy, although there is good evidence from metabolic studies that biochemical changes are present in many patients in the absence of clinical or radiological evidence of bone disease (FOLLIS and JACKSON 1943, BERNER 1944, FOLLIS 1950). The variety of structural changes in the skeleton indicates the multiplicity of different processes involved. The two main types of osteodystrophy are rickets or osteomalacia (COCKAYNE and LEE LANDER 1932), and osteitis fibrosa due to secondary hyperparathyroidism (ALBRIGHT and REIFENSTEIN 1948). Other changes, including osteosclerosis may be present (STANBURY 1957). In terms of the varieties of renal disease giving rise to osteodystrophy there are two main and probably distinct types, azotaemic or glomerular osteodystrophy (STANBURY 1957) and the renal rickets associated with primary tubular anomalies of which the Fanconi syndrome is the outstanding example. When renal tubular acidosis is present, deposition of calcium in the kidney (nephrocalcinosis) occurs and leads to progressive renal damage and uraemia. The various factors which may be involved in the pathogenesis of renal osteodystrophy include intestinal mal-absorption of calcium and phosphorus, resistance to vitamin D, depression of the level of serum calcium, elevated serum phosphorus, altered ionic product of these two factors, secondary hyperparathyroidism, interference with deposition of calcium in bone and abnormal mobilisation of calcium from bone, acidosis, disturbed formation of citrate and handling by the kidney of phosphate, either by reduced clearance or by defective tubular reabsorption. The extreme variability of the biochemical findings in clinically similar cases makes it difficult to formulate any clear concept of pathogenesis. Nevertheless metabolic studies, especially of external calcium balances and the effects of different forms of therapy, have made possible a critical assessment of the causal significance of some of these variables.

Renal osteodystrophy occurs in chronic renal diseases, including chronic pyelonephritis, chronic glomerulonephritis and congenital renal disease, and the severity of the bone lesion is proportionate to the chronicity of the renal disease, which is usually determined by the absence or slight degree of hypertension. Phosphate retention (MITCHELL 1930) or metabolic acidosis (ALBRIGHT et al. 1946) have been postulated as the reasons for depression of serum calcium, through the promotion of excessive faecal or urinary loss of calcium respectively. There is however no consistency in the serum levels of calcium or phosphate, which may be raised, normal or low in different cases, nor is the calcium and phosphorus product regularly depressed. Whilst a reciprocal relationship may exist between serum calcium and phosphorus this is not regularly the case. External mineral balances performed by a number of observers (LIU and CHU 1943; STANBURY 1960; DENT, HARPER and PHILPOT 1961) suggest indeed that the essential abnormality is a failure to absorb and utilise ingested calcium and phosphorus as in the case of nutritional vitamin D deficiency. The conclusion is, that in some way not yet understood, renal failure increases resistance to vitamin D, and this hypothesis is supported by the evidence that administration of vitamin D in large amounts may lead to considerable improvement. Secondary hyperparathyroidism appears to be a response to the deficiency in ionised blood calcium and will tend to maintain normal or even high levels of serum calcium. In individual cases the change from osteomalacia to osteitis fibrosa has been described and corresponds to the degree of parathyroid hyperplasia (GILMOUR 1947). In the case of primary tubular defects (Fanconi syndrome) multiple factors appear to be involved in the production of osteomalacia. Evidence of defective intestinal absorption of calcium and phosphorus has been obtained and may be corrected by vitamin D administration (SAVILLE et al. 1955; DAVIES et al. 1958); renal tubular acidosis, hyperphosphaturia and hypercalcuria may play a contributory role, although there is at present no convincing evidence for this.

III. Disorders of body water

Disturbances of body water in renal disease are manifestations of defective volume control. In most circumstances, variations in sodium and water excretion will be closely linked, but there are some exceptions. Water intoxication and depletion may occur independently of body sodium, and salt depletion may coexist with oedema. In so far as the glomerular filtration rate varies with plasma volume, changes in the latter will be self-correcting until the limits of variation of GFR are restricted by structural glomerular damage; but the finer adjustments are made by changes in tubular reabsorption of sodium. There appear to be a number of physiological mechanisms controlling sodium reabsorption; one of these is the renin-aldosterone mechanism, by which pressor receptors stimulate renin production in the juxtaglomerular apparatus, thereby regulating aldosterone secretion and tubular reabsorption of sodium. In renal disease both glomerular filtration and tubular response to aldosterone may be affected, but in addition, disturbance in water excretion may result from defects in the tubular response to ADH, or in the counter-current mechanism for urine concentration, or from sequestration of water in the tissues due to hypoproteinaemia. Thus, as in the case of electrolyte homeostasis, volume control in renal disease will be affected by both renal and extra-renal factors.

a) Water retention

The role of sodium retention in the pathogenesis of renal oedema has already been discussed in detail, and it remains to supplement this in terms of contributory factors. In acute nephritis water retention is due to reduced GFR, but raised capillary pressure (MACLEOD 1960) may be important in producing the generalised distribution of the oedema. Heart failure is also a frequent complication (SHARPEY-SCHAFER 1955) particularly in cases with severe hypertension. Hypoproteinuria may also contribute even when the nephritis is of short duration (ELLIS 1942). Haemodilution is present in acute nephritis (ROSCOE 1950) and the hypervolaemia may be contributory in the production of both hypertension and heart failure. In acute nephritis and anuria the patient is therefore prone to water retention which may lead to acute pulmonary oedema (BLUEMLE, POTTER and ELKINGTON 1955) or cerebral oedema (SHACKMAN et al. 1962). The nephrotic syndrome is discussed in a later section. A variety of factors operate in this condition; although reduced osmotic pressure of the plasma protein is the primary cause of the oedema, increased secretion of aldosterone and ADH are known to occur and may be contributory. In chronic nephritis oedema may be absent even in the azotaemic stage. This is probably the result of osmotic diuresis and sodium depletion. With progressive reduction in glomerular filtration however oedema returns and may be precipitated or aggravated by heart failure, anaemia and hypoproteinaemia. The inability of patients with renal disease to excrete a water load is used as a test of renal function; sometimes administration of water may however produce water intoxication in the presence of hyponatraemia, muscle cramps and convulsions being the prominent symptoms.

b) Water depletion

Water depletion is usually synonymous with sodium depletion, the extracellular fluid remaining isotonic. The causes have been already described under this heading. Polyuria is one of the earliest symptoms of renal disease and usually starts with nocturia due to failure of nocturnal urine concentration. A later manifestation of impairment in the concentrating mechanism is osmotic diuresis, and with progressive sodium depletion the counter-current mechanism may become less efficient owing to loss of medullary hyperosmolarity (ORLOFF, WAGNER and DAVIDSON 1958). Further water loss may be due to impaired response to ADH. Both may cause the polyuria in nephrogenic diabetes insipidus (ROUSSAK and OLEESKY 1954) especially seen in cases of pyelonephritis. Potassium depletion produces a functional tubular unresponsiveness to ADH which is reversible, for example in urinary tract obstruction (BERLYNE 1961). The polyuria of primary aldosteronism is of this nature. Thirst is the natural response to fluid loss and fluid intake should not be restricted except in oliguric renal failure. The role of the dietary content in increasing the solute load should be taken into account; high protein diets aggravate osmotic diuresis as do conditions which increase the metabolic rate such as infection and fever. The correction of water depletion in the great majority of patients requires repletion of body sodium, and this will often bring about a prompt improvement in renal function with fall in blood urea and relief of symptoms.

IV. Disturbances of acid-base balance

Acid-base balance is maintained by elimination of carbon dioxide at the lungs and excretion of hydrion by the distal tubules. The renal contribution depends on ammonia formation, availability of bicarbonate, and on the acceptance of hydrion by phosphate buffer in the tubular fluid. In renal failure the disturbance of acid-base balance is almost invariably in the direction of defective ammonia excretion, although titratable acidity also is lowered by reduction of available phosphate (WRONG and DAVIES 1959). The urine achieves a high acidity however since there is no defect of hydrion excretion (BRICKER, MORRIN and KIME 1960). In renal tubular acidosis on the other hand, excretion of hydrion is impaired and the urine pH remains high. Ammonia secretion is still possible however and may prevent acidosis for a time (see p. 400). The accumulation of fixed anions occurs when glomerular filtration is greatly reduced as in anuria (MERRILL 1955). These cause a reduction in plasma bicarbonate but it is doubtful how much they contribute to the acute acidosis which may develop in such patients. Hyperchloraemic acidosis occurs in a variety of conditions, in particular after uretero-colic anastomosis due to excessive chloride reabsorption from the bowel. The situation is however complicated by distal tubular damage due to ascending pyelonephritis.

The effects of renal acidosis on the body processes depend on its severity. The classical symptom is hyperpnea, so-called KUSSMAUL breathing. This leads to loss of carbonic acid which partly compensates for the acidosis. The net acid-base disturbance can be measured only by blood p_H estimation, since renal acidosis due to hydrogen ion retention and respiratory alkalosis due to over-breathing both lower the plasma bicarbonate, but have opposite effects on the blood p_H. Acidosis also has a direct effect on cell permeability for electrolytes and impairs the efficacy of the sodium pump. Sodium therefore enters and potassium leaves the cells — an important factor in the hyperkalaemia of renal failure (KEATING et al. 1953). Correction of renal acidosis by infusions of sodium lactate or bicarbonate is an urgent indication in uraemia, particularly in acute oliguric states. Prompt treatment will often improve the mental state and lower the blood potassium. Since acidosis increases the ionisation of serum calcium this treatment may precipitate tetany, necessitating administration of calcium for its relief.

Alkalosis in renal disease is usually the result of the misguided administration of potassium salts. Since gastric acidity is low in uraemia, vomiting rarely produces alkalosis. Alkalosis and uraemia may be associated in the "milk alkali syndrome" but again the alkalosis is due to the prolonged administration of alkalis. The uraemia in this condition is probably due to renal damage resulting from hypercalcaemia. Administration of alkalis for long periods has been shown to have little effect on renal function. The nitrogen retention which is seen in various alkalotic states (e.g. in pyloric stenosis) is probably attributable to the associated electrolyte disturbance, particularly sodium and water depletion.

V. Hypertension in renal disease

When RICHARD BRIGHT (1836) first described the occurrence of cardiac hypertrophy without valvular abnormality in patients with renal disease, the connection of high blood pressure with the kidney was established. In explanation of this relationship he suggested that "the two most ready solutions appear to be either that the altered quality of the blood affords irregular and unwonted stimulus to the organ immediately, or that it so affects the minute and capillary circulation as to render greater action necessary to force the blood through the distant subdivisions of the vascular system". Thus BRIGHT formulated what is still the most complex problem of renal disease and indeed anticipated the conclusions which, though still controversial, are beginning to emerge; i.e. a humoral factor or factors either increase the peripheral resistance or stimulate the heart to greater activity.

The next step in clarifying the relationship of renal disease to high blood pressure was the recognition of essential hypertension through the clinical observations of ALLBUTT (1895) and HUCHARD (1899). The discovery that high blood pressure could run a protracted course without at any time producing evidence of renal involvement led, like many major discoveries, to an over-simplification, namely that essential hypertension was never complicated by renal damage. The correction of this misconception was a long and controversial process. VOLHARD and FAHR (1914) in their monograph on Bright's disease firmly established the concept of malignant nephrosclerosis as a form of primary hypertensive vascular disease which led to rapidly progressive renal damage, although they considered this to be a combination of hypertensive disease and nephritis. Further elucidation of the problem came from experimental evidence following the discovery by GOLDBLATT et al. (1934) that persistent hypertension could be produced in dogs by renal artery constriction. Applying GOLDBLATT's technique to rats, WILSON and BYROM (1939) found that in this animal, persistent hypertension followed unilateral renal artery constriction. They were thereby able to study the effect of hypertension on the opposite kidney, which, in severe cases, they found to show structural lesions of malignant nephrosclerosis. Since these lesions were absent from the clamped kidney (which was shown to be protected from the hypertention) they concluded that the structural changes of malignant nephrosclerosis were determined by the severity of the hypertension. This work first clearly established that essential hypertension could lead to severe renal damage, i.e. that "malignant nephrosclerosis" was the end result of malignant hypertension and not its cause. It also explained the confusing similarity of the terminal structural changes in hypertension of differing aetiology.

The humoral basis of renal hypertension was soon established when it became apparent (see GOLDBLATT 1947) that renal denervation and extensive sympathectomy failed to abolish or prevent experimental renal hypertension in animals.

This led to a revival of interest in the pressor substance obtained from renal extracts by TIGERSTEDT and BERGMAN (1898). The discovery of the renin-angiotensin system quickly followed, and appeared to provide an appropriate humoral basis for renal hypertension. Repeated efforts have been made to prove this thesis; these have led to a number of important discoveries relating to renal homeostatic function, but still leave the problem of renal hypertension unsolved. The main aspects of this subject will now be discussed.

1. Renal diseases leading to hypertension

High blood pressure is a feature of most renal diseases. Its early development is clearly seen in acute nephritis and this is one of the few instances where reversal of hypertension is observed following resolution of the structural lesion. The chronic renal diseases leading to hypertension include glomerulo-nephritis, pyelonephritis, diabetic glomerulo-sclerosis, the collagen diseases with renal involvement, especially disseminated lupus and polyarteritis nodosa, congenital polycystic kidney and irradiation nephritis. Of special interest is the parallel with experimental hypertension provided by unilateral renal disease in man, in which high blood pressure may be caused by unilateral renal artery stenosis, pyelonephritis, tuberculosis, tumours and unilateral renal injury. The special features of hypertension in various renal diseases will be described in a later section. In unilateral renal disease the blood pressure may be restored to normal if the cause can be removed, e.g. by the correction of renal artery stenosis or by nephrectomy. In bilateral chronic renal disease however hypertension is permanent and progressive. In its early stages it may be labile and intermittent, but in the course of time the diastolic pressure becomes fixed at a higher level than normal, and in a proportion of cases malignant hypertension, characterised by the appearance of papilloedema, develops. In its natural history therefore chronic renal hypertension closely resembles essential hypertension, and indeed the clinical, haemodynamic and structural characteristics of the hypertensive state itself are indistinguishable in both types. There is however an important difference; the malignant phase develops in onyl a small proportion of cases of essential hypertension — probably less than 1%, whereas in renal hypertension a malignant termination is observed in one third to half the cases (WILSON 1953).

2. Circulatory dynamics in hypertension

This subject has been well reviewed by FREIS (1960). Most authors agree that cardiac output in established hypertension is within normal limits (GOLD-RING and CHASSIS 1944; BOLOMEY et al. 1949, WERKO and LAGERLOF 1949; BROD et al. 1962). Some have claimed however that cardiac output may be raised, especially in early hypertension in young subjects (WIDIMSKY, FEJFAROUA and FEJFAR 1957). Capillary pressure is normal (ELLIS and WEISS 1929). The pressure gradient between brachial and digital arteries is normal (OPPENHEIMER and PRINZMETAL 1937). This suggests that the blood pressure is raised as a result of increased peripheral resistance, chiefly in the arterioles. Arteriolar narrowing appears to be due to reversible muscular constriction rather than to organic changes. Reflex vasodilatation can occur and blood flow can be increased to the same extent as in normal subjects (PRINZMETAL and WILSON 1936; PICKERING 1936). The arteriolar constriction is not due to excessive sympathetic vasomotor tone since sympathetic block to a limb increases blood flow no more in hypertensive than in normal subjects (PRINZMETAL and WILSON 1936; PICKERING 1936). Peripheral resistance appears to be increased in all parts of the circulation. Renal blood flow is however reduced, indicating that the rise in renal arterial resistance is proportionately greater than in other vascular territories. The peripheral resistance in muscles may be slightly less elevated than in the rest of the circulation (PICKERING 1955; BROD et al. 1962). Although, as stated above, it is generally agreed that there is no difference in circulatory haemodynamics between essential hypertension and long established renal hypertension, BROD (1961) has suggested that in chronic renal hypertension blood flow through muscle is normal, whereas it may be slightly increased in essential hypertension. Most authors have hitherto accepted these various haemodynamic features as compatible with the hypothesis that chronic renal hypertension is due to a circulating pressor agent constricting arterioles in all parts of the circulation, but having rather more effect on the renal vessels and perhaps less on arterioles in skeletal muscles. In acute nephritis circulatory dynamics are different. Blood volume, central venous pressure, capillary pressure and cardiac output are all increased, whilst peripheral resistance is said to be within normal limits (DE FAZIO et al. 1959).

3. Pathogenesis of renal hypertension

Renin-angiotensin mechanism. TIGERSTEDT and BERGMAN (1898) prepared an extract from the kidney, which caused a transient rise of blood pressure when injected into rabbits; this they termed renin. No further advance was made however until GOLDBLATT et al. (1934), by partial constriction of one renal artery with an adjustable clamp and removal of the other kidney, observed persistent elevation of blood pressure in the absence of uraemia. In the following years, hypertension was produced by other experimental procedures. PAGE (1939) surrounded the kidney with cellophane which induced perinephritis and fibrosis; GROLLMAN (1944) obtained hypertension after renal compression with a broad ligature tied in a "figure of eight". Renal artery constriction was also shown to induce hypertension in the monkey (GOLDBLATT 1937a), in sheep and goats (GOLDBLATT, KAHN and LEWIS 1943) and in rabbits (PICKERING and PRINZMETAL 1938).

In all these experiments it was necessary either to constrict both renal arteries or to constrict one renal artery and remove the opposite kidney; constriction of one renal artery without contralateral nephrectomy resulted in a transient rise of blood pressure only. In animals with severe hypertension, arterial lesions similar to those found in malignant hypertension in man, i.e. fibrinoid necrosis, could be demonstrated in various organs, but were absent from the kidney, presumably because it was protected by the constricting clamp from the effects of the high blood pressure (WILSON and PICKERING 1938; GOLDBLATT 1938). The application of the GOLDBLATT technique to the rat by WILSON and BYROM (1939) produced results, already described, which finally clarified the relationship of malignant hypertension to renal vascular damage. In a later paper (WILSON and BYROM 1941) these authors published the results of further experiments on the reversibility of renal hypertension in the rat. When the clipped kidney was excised after a short period of hypertension, before vascular damage had occurred in the untouched kidney, blood pressure returned to normal. If, however, the hypertension was allowed to persist for many weeks so that arterial lesions occurred in the untouched kidney, removal of the clipped kidney did not restore the blood pressure to normal. WILSON and BYROM concluded that secondary vascular damage in the opposite kidney enabled it to maintain the hypertension following excision of the clipped kidney. They put forward the concept of the "vicious circle" in which severe hypertension caused renal damage, which in turn resulted in further elevation of the blood pressure. These various studies in experimental hypertension led to an intensive search for a humoral pressure substance. BRAUN-MENENDEZ et al. (1940) obtained from the venous blood of a clamped kidney in dogs an extract which raised the blood pressure. Later they found that this extract acted on plasma to produce a dialysable pressor substance of small molecular weight which they named hypertensin. At the same time, KOHLSTAEDT, PAGE and HELMER (1940) obtained renal pressor extracts similar to the renin described by TIGERSTEDT and BERGMAN. They showed that renin is an enzyme and suggested that it reacted with a substance in the plasma to produce a pressor substance which they called angiotonin. Angiotonin and hypertensin were shown to be the same substance and in a joint communication BRAUN-MENENDEZ and PAGE (1958) suggested that the name angiotensin should be generally accepted. Recent work (PEART 1956; ELLIOT and PEART 1957; SKEGGS, KAHN and SHUMWAY 1956a and b) has shown angiotensin to be a decapeptide which is converted in plasma to the active octopeptide. Both have now been synthesised (SCHWYZE and SIEBER 1956; BURPUS, SCHWARZ and PAGE 1956).

The proof that renal hypertension is due to the renin-angiotensin system is however still lacking. Although circulating renin or angiotensin has been identified soon after renal artery constriction, this is not the case in long-standing hypertension. TAQUINI and FASCIOLO (1946, 1947) were able to demonstrate a pressor substance in the renal venous blood of dogs a short time after renal artery constriction, but failed to do so in hypertension of long duration. HAYNES and DEXTER (1947) recorded similar findings. KAHN et al. (1952) reported an increase of circulating angiotensin in patients with malignant hypertension but not in those with benign essential or with chronic renal hypertension. PEART (1959) succeeded in demonstrating angiotensin in the blood of a rabbit with hypertension maintained by an angiotensin infusion, but was unable to find it in renal venous blood from a rabbit with hypertension following renal artery constriction. HELMER (1961) claimed to have demonstrated angiotensin in the renal venous blood of patients with renal artery stenosis, whilst none could be found after surgical restoration of normal blood flow to the kidney.

Other workers have studied the effect of neutralising circulating renin with "anti-renin". After injection of dog renin into hogs, plasma globulin concentrates from the hog will restore the blood pressure to normal for a short period when injected into a dog with renal hypertension, but have no effect when injected into a normal animal. WAKERLIN et al. (1953) claim that in dogs anti-renin causes reduction in blood pressure even in long standing renal hypertension and regard this as evidence that circulating renin is the cause of the raised blood pressure at all stages.

If arteriolar constriction due to circulating angiotensin is the sole mechanism by which renal hypertension is maintained, both in experimental animals and in man, it should be possible to demonstrate angiotensin in the blood in concentrations which produce hypertension in normal animals after angiotensin infusion. Since this has not yet been accomplished it seems probable that other aetiological factors are involved in the production of renal hypertension. It is possible that when the blood pressure has been raised and maintained for a short time by the renin-angiotensin mechanism, permanent changes occur in the peripheral circulation which will maintain the hypertension even though the initial cause ceases to operate. A second possibility (OGDEN 1947) is that after hypertension is established, the buffer nerve mechanism becomes "reset" at a higher level after which the sympathetic system maintains the hypertension. The evidence against this is the prompt reversal of chronic renal hypertension when the constriction of the renal artery is removed, indicating that the provoking cause still resides in the kidney. BYROM and DODSON (1949) were able in this way to abolish hypertension of three months duration in rats by removal of the renal artery clip. FLOYER (1951) restored blood pressure to normal in rats which had been hypertensive for one year by removal of the renal artery clip and excision of the opposite kidney. MURRAY, MERRILL and HARRISON (1958) transplanted a normal kidney from one member of a pair of identical twins to the other who was suffering from chronic renal disease and hypertension. After excision of both diseased kidneys the blood pressure, which had been raised for a number of years, was immediately restored to normal. This indicates that in man the kidney maintains the hypertension even in the chronic stages of renal disease.

As an alternative to the production of a vasoconstrictor agent, it is possible that renal artery constriction maintains hypertension by another mechanism. One such possibility is that it inhibits a physiological depressor activity of the kidney; a second is by stimulation of the adrenal cortex leading to increased production of aldosterone. These possibilities will now be discussed.

Renoprival hypertension: evidence for a renal depressor mechanism. GROLLMAN and RULE (1943) described the development of hypertension following removal of both kidneys from one member of a pair of parabiotic rats. There is sufficient exchange across the parabiotic union to maintain relatively normal levels of urea, potassium, and other substances. This observation was confirmed by LEDINGHAM (1951) who (1954a) suggested that the name "renoprival" hypertension be used to describe high blood pressure following total nephrectomy. GROLLMAN, MUIRHEAD and VANATTA (1949) obtained renoprival hypertension in dogs kept alive by peritoneal dialysis or with the artificial kidney for several weeks after total nephrectomy. The blood pressure rose to high levels and the production of acute hypertensive arterial lesions was observed. FLOYER (1951, 1955) studied renoprival hypertension in rats, keeping them alive for five days after nephrectomy by peritoneal dialysis or by glucose feeding. These various observations suggest that the normal kidney has a blood pressure lowering function, the loss of which after total nephrectomy causes hypertension. Evidence of a similar nature is obtained by transplanting a normal kidney into animals with hypertension. KOLFF and PAGE (1954b) showed that the blood pressure of dogs with renoprival hypertension could be lowered in a few hours by transplanting a normal kidney. A similar effect was demonstrated (KOLFF 1958) in dogs with renal hypertension. MURRAY, MERRILL and HARRISON (1958) showed that implantation of a normal kidney into a hypertensive twin lowered the blood pressure rapidly though it did not remain at normal levels until the abnormal kidneys were excised.

It has been claimed that renoprival hypertension is solely the result of overhydration in animals which have access to water but which cannot excrete. KOLFF and PAGE (1954a) and KOLFF, PAGE and CORCORAN (1954), in a careful study, showed that overhydration is not necessary for the development of renoprival hypertension, although it may increase the rate of rise. They also confirmed an observation made previously by GROLLMAN, MUIRHEAD and VANATTA (1959) that if one kidney is excised and the other ureter inserted into the vena cava, the animal becomes uraemic but does not develop hypertension. Overhydration in these animals does not affect the blood pressure. MERRILL, GIORDANO and HEETDERKS (1961) showed that in patients with acute renal failure, due either to cortical necrosis or to accidental removal of a single kidney, the blood pressure remains normal so long as strict fluid balance is maintained. The infusion of a small amount of saline however produced a marked rise in blood pressure. It thus appears that the normal kidney, by some mechanism unconnected with excretion, maintains the blood pressure at normal levels, and furthermore that it prevents the development of hypertension in states of acute overhydration. Evidence of a renal depressor mechanism has also been derived from the results of nephrectomy in renal hypertension. PICKERING (1945) induced hypertension in rabbits by renal artery constriction and removal of the opposite kidney. If the clipped kidney was excised one week later, the blood pressure returned to normal in a few hours; if however hypertension had been present for eight weeks the blood pressure remained high after total nephrectomy until a short time before the animal died of uraemia. FLOYER (1951, 1955) reported similar results in rats. In the single clipped kidney (the opposite kidney having been removed), the contrast between the dramatic fall of blood pressure to normal in a few hours following removal of the renal artery constriction, and the persistence of hypertension following excision of the clipped kidney, is most striking. It is strong evidence against the hypothesis that the kidney maintains hypertension directly by secretion of a renal pressor substance; if this were so it would be expected that the blood pressure would fall at the same rate whether the kidney was excised or whether the renal artery constriction were removed. These observations suggest that a similar mechanism to that of renoprival hypertension is operating in the later stages of hypertension due to renal artery constriction. FLOYER (1955) confirmed the observation of WILSON and BYROM (1939) that excision of the clipped kidney restores the blood pressure to normal in rats with hypertension of a few weeks duration before vascular damage has occurred in the opposite kidney. After bilateral nephrectomy in similar animals, the blood pressure remained raised. As a possible explanation, FLOYER (1957) suggested that renin from the clipped kidney, in amounts insufficient to affect the blood pressure by generalised arteriolar constriction, might nevertheless inhibit the blood pressure reducing function of the opposite kidney. The effects of anti-renin provide some support for this hypothesis. SHIPLEY (cited by PAGE 1960) and KOLFF and PAGE (1955a and b) demonstrated that anti-renin lowers the blood pressure of a dog with chronic renal hypertension for a few hours. Following total nephrectomy the hypertension persisted and was no longer affected by anti-renin.

28*

Relationship of adrenal cortex to renal hypertension. Goldblatt (1937 b) and Blalock and Levy (1937) showed that adrenalectomy would prevent or abolish hypertension following renal artery constriction. Page (1938) demonstrated that replacement therapy with salt or cortical extract could counteract this. Similar results were obtained in rats by Floyer (1951) and Gross (1960). Renoprival hypertension is also affected by the adrenals; Ledingham (1951) showed that adrenalectomy would prevent or abolish hypertension in a nephrectomised member of a pair of parabiotic rats. The synthetic saltretaining steroid desoxycorticosterone acetate (DOCA) will cause hypertension only if given with an excess of salt. Ledingham (1954 b) showed that D.O.C.A. hypertension is not prevented by removal of the adrenals. Aldosterone similarly produces hypertension only when given with excess of salt (Gross and Dettbarn 1956; Gross, Loustalot and Meier 1957). It is possible to produce hypertension in animals by giving large amounts of salt (Meneely et al. 1953; Tobian, Janecek and Tomboulian 1959). Hypertension has been reported in a boy with an abnormal craving for salt (McQuarrie, Thompson and Anderson 1936); while taking about 80 grams of salt a day his blood pressure was 170/110; reduction of his salt intake resulted in a fall to normal. Dahl (1960) has drawn attention to the increased incidence of hypertension in areas of Japan where large amounts of salt are consumed.

Dean and Masson (1951) observed in rats that following injection of renin or the production of renal encapsulation hypertension, hyperplasia of the zona glomerulosa of the adrenal cortex occurred. Davis, Ayers and Carpenter (1961) showed that the kidney was the source of an aldosterone stimulating hormone, and Laragh et al. (1960a) and Genest et al. (1961 b) demonstrated that an infusion of angiotensin stimulated aldosterone secretion. Carpenter, Davis and Ayers (1961 b) found an increased concentration of aldosterone in the adrenal vein blood after injection of renin or angiotensin in dogs and also after renal artery constriction. In the latter case aldosterone secretion was increased in dogs with malignant hypertension but was within normal limits in those with benign hypertesnion. Larach et al. (1960 b) have reported increased secretion of aldosterone in human malignant hypertension.

Wakerlin, Marshall and Minatova (1948) showed than in dogs, clamping of one renal artery led to an increase in the renin content of the clamped kidney with a decrease in that of the untouched kidney. Gross (1960) reported similar findings in the rat. He also observed that the renin content of the kidneys in normal animals is inversely proportional to the degree of sodium retention. High salt intake, D.O.C.A. or aldosterone and salt, decrease the renin content, whereas salt depletion or adrenalectomy increase it. Ruyter (1925) first described granules in the cells of juxtaglomerular apparatus of the kidney and Goormaghtigh (1939) suggested that these may contain renin. Recently it has been shown that nearly all the renin in the kidney is localised near the juxtaglomerular apparatus (Cook and Pickering 1958). Hartroft and Edelman (1959) reported that fluorescent antibodies prepared against renin become bound to the granules in the juxtaglomerular cells. Tobian et al. (1958) and Hartroft and Edelman (1959) showed that there is a correlation between the renin content of the kidney and the number of granules in the juxtaglomerular apparatus; both are increased on a low, and reduced on a high, salt intake. The relationship between tissue electrolytes, juxtaglomerular cells and hypertension has been reviewed by Tobian (1960). These varied observations appear to have established a direct relationship between renal artery constriction, renin production and aldosterone secretion. The biological significance of this relationship has been studied by Tobian, Winn and Janecek

(1961) who demonstrated that the ability of a normal kidney to reduce the blood pressure in a rat with renal hypertension varies with the renal perfusion pressure. It appears probable therefore that the juxtaglomerular apparatus acts in the role of a pressure receptor which responds to the fall in blood pressure produced by constriction of the renal artery in the same way as, in the normal kidney, it might be expected to respond to a reduction in blood volume. Increased renin production and the consequent increased aldosterone secretion may thus act as part of a homeostatic mechanism directed towards sodium and water retention and restoration of renal perfusion pressure. There is so far no evidence that this mechanism causes renal hypertension. It could conceivably cause or contribute to acute rise in blood pressure after renal artery constriction or in acute nephritis, but there is so far no evidence that it plays a part in the maintenance of chronic renal hypertension. Nevertheless, the relationship between high blood pressure on the one hand and body sodium and adrenal cortical activity on the other, indicates that there is a close connection between the homeostatic mechanisms for blood pressure regulation and volume control, and the focal point of this correlation appears to be the renal artery perfusion pressure. Further clarification of the mechanism of renal hypertension will depend therefore on a clearer under-standing of circulatory volume — pressure relationships. It seems improbable that increased aldosterone secretion causes renal hypertension; in fact at the present time the former has been demonstrable only when severe hypertensive renal damage is present as in malignant hypertension or in the special case of unilateral renal artery stenosis. The evidence that angiotensin produces renal hypertension directly by its general vasoconstrictor action on the arterioles is still lacking; and the possibility remains that the kidney regulates blood pressure by a depressor mechanism which is impaired in a similar manner by both renal artery constriction and by nephrectomy.

D. Disorders of renal function in specific diseases

The disorders of renal function described in the foregoing sections present a great variety of patterns in different diseases of the kidney. The extent to which retention of metabolic waste products and other derangements of the homeostatic mechanism become manifest depends on a number of factors; these include, the type and extent of the structural lesion in the glomeruli and tubules, the stage in the natural development of the disease, the incidence of extra-renal factors reacting adversely on renal function and, not least in importance, the influence of treatment. From the clinical viewpoint there are several clear cut different forms of renal disease which have fairly well defined functional patterns, for example acute uraemia due to suppression of urine and the milder variants of this in acute diffuse nephritis; the nephrotic syndrome; chronic pyelonephritis; urinary tract obstruction; the chronic uraemia common to all forms of chronic renal disease, and the syndrome of malignant hypertension. Throughout the course of any type of renal disease the patient may present a sequence of quite dissimilar clinical and functional disorders. In this section an attempt will be made to describe these patterns of disordered function occurring in the common renal diseases.

I. Glomerulonephritis

This condition in its early stages is characterised by extensive, usually diffuse, inflammation of the kidney with glomerular, tubular, interstitial and vascular damage. There is convincing evidence that these result from an abnormal antigen-antibody reaction and this concept brings the common forms of glomerulo-nephritis into relation with the generalised collagen diseases, such as polyarteritis nodosa and disseminated lupus erythematosus, of which glomerulo-nephritis is often a prominent feature. Whether occurring alone or as part of generalised collagen disease, glomerulo-nephritis may be diffuse, or more rarely focal, in terms of glomerular involvement. Focal nephritis is not usually associated with renal failure, oedema or hypertension, but in disseminated lupus and other conditions there is evidence from repeated renal biopsy that focal nephritis may be followed by diffuse nephritis (MUEHRCKE et al. 1957; RUSBY and WILSON 1960). Moreover repeated attacks of acute focal nephritis will lead to disordered renal function as nephron damage becomes more extensive. Of the variety of courses which diffuse glomerulonephritis may take, it is now commonly accepted that two main types justify separation on the grounds of their clinical and histological differences and particularly of their distinct natural histories. The most satisfactory definition of these was made by ELLIS (1942) who introduced the terms Type I and Type II nephritis. This terminology has proved less exceptionable than nomenclatures based on clinical or histological features which are often transient or inconstant.

1. Type I nephritis

(Acute diffuse nephritis)

In the acute stage Type I nephritis presents one of the most characteristic syndromes of Bright's disease. The outstanding disorders of function are generalised oedema, hypertension and haematuria. Renal function is not seriously impaired except in the most severe cases when oliguria or anuria develops. In these, severe diffuse glomerulitis causes complete, or near complete, failure of glomerular filtration and uraemia develops with the functional pattern des-cribed later under "acute anuria". The most serious difference from other causes of acute anuria is the frequent irreversibility of the lesion. In the great majority of patients with acute nephritis however renal functional impairment takes the form of slight or moderate nitrogen retention (up to 100 mgm./100 ml.) with relatively well preserved renal concentrating power; i.e. glomerular filtration is predominantly affected and the urine is diminished in amount and concentrated, with a high normal specific gravity. Measurements of diodone or PAH clearance show the renal blood flow to be normal or reduced and occasionally even increased above normal (EARLE, TAGGART and SHANNON 1944; HILDEN 1943; BLACK et al. 1948; EARLE et al. 1951a, BRADLEY 1948a and b). Inulin clearance studies show that glomerular filtration is depressed more than renal blood flow, indicating a diminished filtration fraction. This would be consistent with excessive afferent arteriolar constriction (BLACK et al. 1948) or diminished effective filtering surface, or both. The former has some support from the finding of necrosis of the afferent arterioles in severe cases of acute nephritis dying in acute uraemia (ELLIS 1942). In spite of the usual finding of a concentrated urine in acute nephritis, tests of tubular function often show impairment, including reduction of limits of specific gravity and urine urea concentration. BRADLEY (1949) by renal vein catheterisa-tion found reduced PAH extraction. It is important to bear in mind that extra-renal factors, particularly vomiting and heart failure may greatly aggravate glomerular dysfunction in acute nephritis and in these circumstances the rise in blood urea may exceed 300 mgm./100 ml., with rapid reversal when dehydration or heart failure are treated.

The oedema of acute nephritis is usually generalised, moderate in degree and transient. The cause of sodium and water retention is obscure. In rare cases heart failure may contribute but is unlikely to be the main cause as PETERS (1953) has suggested, since the generalised distribution of oedema is unlike that of heart failure. Moreover heart failure is more common in patients with severe hypertension whereas nephritic oedema may be severe in the absence of hypertension. It is difficult to attribute the sodium retention exclusively to impaired glomerular filtration since oedema is often absent in cases where oliguria is extreme or nitrogen retention most marked. The plasma proteins are considerably depressed in about one third of the cases of acute nephritis and this may well aggravate and prolong the oedema. There is no evidence of secondary aldosteronism in acute nephritis, as there is in the nephrotic syndrome. For the present we must accept the oedema of acute nephritis as a specific but unexplained disorder of extra-cellular fluid volume control and leave open the possibility that it may be partly extra-renal in origin. It is interesting that cases of generalised oedema and hypertension of acute onset have been described without albuminuria (CROFTON and TRUELOVE 1948; FISHBERG 1954) and renal biopsy findings (HUTT, PINNIGER and DE WARDENER 1958) suggest that the fluid retention characteristic of acute nephritis may be associated with minimal structural changes in the glomeruli. A well established feature of sodium retention in acute nephritis is the increased plasma volume, which partially explains the low haemoglobin and low plasma protein concentration of the blood. The hypervolaemia may be sufficient to increase the jugular venous pressure, and undoubtedly contributes to the acute heart failure which complicates acute nephritis in about 10% of cases. Nevertheless, heart failure in acute nephritis is predominantly left ventricular and is almost invariably associated with marked hypertension (ELLIS 1942). It seems likely that myocardial damage may occur in acute nephritis and electrocardiographic changes have been described in a high proportion of cases (MASTER, JAFFE and DACK 1937). Although acute vascular lesions are rarely found in the heart, unexplained bradycardia and tachycardia are observed, and myocardial lesions are a common feature of other collagen diseases. Apart from sodium retention, electrolyte disorders and acid-base disturbances are uncommon in acute nephritis. In anuric or oliguric cases potassium retention occurs and for this reason potassium salts should not be administered in this disease. Hypoproteinaemia may be severe and is always accompanied by heavy albuminuria, but the short duration of proteinuria makes it unlikely that this is the sole cause of the low blood levels. In cases with acute anuria, plasma albumin may fall to 1.0 G/100 ml. and although haemodilution may be a contributory factor it seems inescapable that protein synthesis is depressed in such cases.

The cause of hypertension in acute nephritis is not known. The finding of a reduced filtration fraction suggests excessive constriction of the afferent arterioles and provides a possible analogy with experimental renal hypertension produced by partial occlusion of the renal arteries. An increase in renin activity of the blood has been reported in acute nephritis (DEXTER and HAYNES 1944). On the other hand clinical observation suggests that hypertension and oedema are closely related (see EARLE, FARBER and ALEXANDER 1950 for possible evidence) and both may be dependent on changes in the hormonal regulation of tissue electrolyte distribution. Of considerable interest are attacks of hypertensive encephalopathy in acute nephritis. Headache, convulsions, blindness and coma may be preceded by sudden rise in blood pressure and may occasionally result in organic cerebral vascular lesions. In general however the encephalopathy is transient and leaves no permanent disability. Attacks can be rapidly relieved by lowering the blood pressure with hypotensive drugs. It seems likely that this type of hypertensive encephalopathy is due to excessive vasoconstriction of the cerebral arteries associated with sudden elevation of arterial pressure and possibly with fluid retention. BYROM (1954) demonstrated photographically the occurrence of local cerebral arterial constriction during attacks of hypertensive encephalopathy produced experimentally in rats, with relief of the constriction when the hypertension was abolished. Anaemia in the early stages of Type I nephritis is more apparent than real, the depression of haemoglobin being due to blood dilution (ROSCOE 1950). A true anaemia may however develop after severe primary infection or if the nephritis is prolonged. In the latter case persistent haematuria is only a minor factor, and depression of haemopoiesis due to defective erythropoietin production is the probable cause (see p. 423).

When acute nephritis fails to recover, the pattern of disordered renal function depends on the subsequent course of the disease. If it follows the rapidly progressive course (subacute nephritis of VOLHARD) hypertension and haematuria persist, renal function deteriorates and oedema often increases. Heavy proteinuria may give rise to severe hypoproteinaemia so that all the features of the nephrotic syndrome may be present. There is often a rapidly progressive anaemia of the hypoplastic type and heart failure is an almost constant feature in the late stages. In about half of the cases malignant hypertension develops and leads to rapid deterioration of renal failure. In the chronic course of Type I nephritis all the functional abnormalities may disappear except albuminuria. This may persist for decades unaccompanied by symptoms but eventually hypertension appears, at first slight or moderate and labile, later rising to high levels and passing into the malignant phase in about one third of the cases (WILSON 1953). Sooner or later renal function fails. Chronic nephritis is, after chronic pyelonephritis, the commonest cause of *chronic renal failure*. This type of disordered renal function occurs in the later stages of all bilateral forms of chronic renal disease, including chronic pyelonephritis, renal tuberculosis, calculus pyelonephritis, chronic urinary tract obstruction, amyloid disease, polycystic kidney and other forms of congenital renal disease. The sequence of functional changes is determined by the progressive destruction of nephrons in which diminished concentrating power precedes failure of glomerular filtration — often for many years. The first clinical manifestation is usually nocturia, due to loss of the diurnal rhythm of tubular water and electrolyte reabsorption (STANBURY and THOMSON 1951). Narrowing of the limits of urine specific gravity then occurs and diminished urine urea concentration may be observed long before the blood urea rises. Although the interpretation of clearance tests is uncertain in advanced chronic renal disease, creatinine clearance and inulin clearance may be similarly reduced at this stage. When however nephron destruction is such that the blood urea rises, a moderate degree of polyuria, both by day and by night, results from osmotic diuresis. Thirst is now a common symptom but the daily fluid intake and output rarely exceed three to four litres owing to the marked reduction in glomerular filtration. The urine specific gravity is now fixed about 1010 — i.e. the urine is isotonic with the glomerular filtrate (isosthenuria) or slightly hypotonic, although of course the composition is still different, urea diffusing back at the tubules in increased amounts and sodium still being reabsorbed. The failure to form a markedly hypotonic urine, even after water drinking, implies that patients with chronic renal failure may become easily and dangerously overhydrated, and conversely they may rapidly pass into severe dehydration if they are suddenly deprived of fluid or if attacks of vomiting and diarrhoea occur. In spite of this limitation of response to varying water and solute loads, the patient with chronic uraemia may remain for a considerable time in both water and electrolyte equilibrium and the elimination of urea may keep pace with its production. There is good evidence that potassium equilibrium is maintained by tubular excretion since the amount in the urine at low levels of clearance is much greater than could be filtered as measured by creatinine and inulin clearance (LEAF and CAMARA 1949; PLATT 1950; BERLINER, KENNEDY and ORLOFF 1951; BLACK and EMERY 1957). In very rare cases however this water and electrolyte balance is not maintained and excessive loss of sodium or potassium or water may occur. In other cases there is excessive retention of sodium and water which is unexplained by heart failure or hypoproteinaemia; rarer still potassium retention may lead to hyperkalaemia. Acidosis is a constant feature of chronic uraemia in the late stages and gives rise to the typical acidotic (KUSSMAUL) respiration. There is failure of excretion of phosphate, sulphate and organic acids and the alkali reserve is further depleted by failure of tubular excretion of hydrion and ammonia. The plasma bicarbonate level is correspondingly reduced and the pH falls. These clinical manifestations of disordered metabolism are late to develop in chronic nephritis. Hypertensive manifestations, especially breathlessness on exertion or at night, due to heart failure, early morning headaches with nausea or vomiting, and visual disturbance due to retinopathy, may precede true uraemic symptoms by months or years.

In a few patients with chronic nephritis severe disturbances of calcium metabolism lead to osteodystrophy. These are usually patients in whom hypertension is slight or absent so that uraemia runs a very chronic course. The factors underlying these disturbances are discussed in a previous section. They include phosphate retention, depression of calcium absorption from the intestine, chronic acidosis and secondary hyperparathyroidism. The commonly resulting bone lesions are osteomalacia and osteitis fibrosa. Excessive mobilisation of calcium from bone may lead to metastatic calcification in other tissues especially in the arterial walls, and depression of the ionised blood calcium may lead to tetany.

Again the importance of extra-renal factors on renal function must be emphasised. They include anaemia and heart failure, but more particularly water and sodium depletion due to vomiting, diarrhoea, polyuria and use of diuretics. Recognition of these factors may indicate therapeutic measures which will lead to temporary recovery. On the other hand they may be the precipitating cause of fatal uraemia, signalised by sudden reduction in urine output, even anuria, with steep elevation in blood urea and a deterioration in the patient's condition leading to terminal coma.

2. Type II nephritis

(Subchronic nephritis of VOLHARD; membranous glomerulonephritis)

In this form of glomerulonephritis the onset is usually insidious with generalised oedema; proteinuria is heavy (10—30 grammes daily), the plasma albumin is severely depleted and the blood cholesterol raised; i.e. this is the form of Bright's disease in which the nephrotic syndrome is most constantly present. The structural lesion is that of a progressive, slowly developing glomerulonephritis, which leads to hyalinisation of the tufts by way of diffuse or focal thickening of the capillary basement membranes. Interstitial inflammation and fibrosis is very variable; it may be minimal and focal when glomerular damage is diffuse and severe. Tubular atrophy is roughly proportional in degree and extent to interstitial fibrosis but lipoid deposition both in tubular epithelium and interstitial tissue is independent of the severity of the nephritis and is more closely related to the lipaemia which forms a characteristic feature of the nephrotic syndrome. In many cases albuminuria precedes the onset of oedema for months or years (ELLIS 1942). Very occasionally a patient may present in the late stages of uraemia, and post-mortem the kidney may show the fully developed picture of Type II nephritis, yet oedema may not have been noted at any time during the course of the disease. These observations, and recent information obtained by renal biopsy studies emphasise that the nephrotic syndrome is not causally related to the degree of structural glomerular damage in Type II nephritis.

Hypertension is one of the most variable factors in Type II nephritis. It is only moderate in most cases, and in some the blood pressure is normal; in others, the blood pressure is high and renal function is impaired from the early stages of the disease. In the majority the blood pressure tends to rise as the structural lesion progresses and in more than half there is terminal malignant hypertension (WILSON 1953). Renal biopsy studies have shown that in general, hypertension is related to the severity of the glomerulitis. The blood pressure tends to be higher and the course of the disease more rapid in adults than in children, and in men than in women. This relationship of hypertension to the severity of the glome-rulitis probably explains the absence of hypertension in those cases where clinical and histological evidence of glomerulonephritis is minimal. Such patients are still considered by some writers to be suffering from a distinct disease (lipoid nephrosis). As ELLIS (1942) pointed out, however, there is no convincing evidence for this nor is there any particular value in making the distinction so long as the difference between Type I and Type II nephritis is recognised.

An important aspect of the close correlation between structural glomerular changes and hypertension, and their lack of correlation with the nephrotic syndrome is the relevance of these relationships to recovery and the response to therapy. Those patients without hypertension, with little or no clinical evidence of nephritis (absence of granular casts, erythrocytes and leucocytes in the urinary deposit) and with minimal glomerular lesions revealed on renal biopsy, may respond well to steroid therapy (ROSS and SMITH 1963). These are also the cases which most frequently recover spontaneously. On the other hand, when hyper-tension and signs of severe glomerular damage, such as haematuria and renal failure, are present, spontaneous recovery rarely occurs and steroid therapy has not been shown to improve the prognosis, although it may produce some temporary relief of oedema.

The development of uraemia in Type II nephritis may be renal or extra-renal in origin. Episodes of nitrogen retention and even of tubular functional impair-ment may occur when gross anasarca develops (causing sudden reduction in plasma volume), or when electrolyte disturbances, especially sodium and potassium depletion, are provoked, for example by removal of oedema fluid, by excessive salt restriction, continued use of diuretics, paracentesis of serous effusions or subcutaneous drainage. These are the usual circumstances in which extra-renal factors may embarrass kidney function in Type II nephritis. Structural renal failure is as a rule insidious in dvelopment and closely parallels the degree of hypertension. If the blood pressure is only moderately elevated, impaired concentrating power may ante-date nitrogen retension by many years. This slowly developing uraemia is most commonly observed in women since the disease tends to run a more protracted course and the effects of hypertension are better tolerated than in men. In the latter, the course is usually more rapidly progressive to renal failure in two to six years, and uraemia is often accelerated by malignant hypertension, with its distressing train of symptoms due to hyper-tensive retinopathy, encephalopathy and left ventricular failure. During this rap-id course oedema may persist or even increase as renal failure develops. In more slowly progressive cases the degree of proteinuria gradually diminishes and the plasma proteins may return to normal levels in one to two years after the onset. Such patients may then continue for many years with minimal oedema, although the nephrotic syndrome may recur during the course of the disease. As nitrogen retention develops, osmotic diuresis may lead to sodium depletion so that the patient becomes oedema free in the later stages; but even so, terminal heart failure may bring it back in severe degree, particularly if the plasma protein level is depressed and anaemia is present.

Urinary abnormalities in glomerulonephritis

Proteinuria may be regarded as a constant feature of glomerulonephritis in all its stages. Although cases of acute nephritis without proteinuria have been described, they are excessively rare. In chronic nephritis the amount of protein excreted may be greatly diminished owing to reduction of functioning nephrons and the urine may be greatly diluted by osmotic diuresis, so that only slight proteinuria may be detected by the usual tests. When proteinuria is severe, as in Type II nephritis, there may be wide variations during the day and from day to day. At all stages there may be a large postural element, and this is particularly true in young subjects after acute nephritis, in whom orthostatic albuminuria may persist long after the nephritis has resolved. In chronic renal failure the urine is colourless, and precipitated albumin is white instead of the usual buff colour, owing to the absence of urochromogens.

Increase in proteinuria in chronic nephritis may be due to a further attack of nephritis (which is rare), to venous congestion of the kidney as a result of heart failure or to sudden concentration of the urine due to fluid restriction or dehydration from some extra-renal cause. It may also be caused by superimposed ascending pyelonephritis, a common complication of all forms of chronic renal disease. In Type II nephritis it may be the result of renal vein thrombosis.

Haematuria is a usual feature of acute glomerulonephritis. Recurrent attacks are extremely rare in chronic Type I nephritis but are not uncommon during the course of Type II nephritis when they may cause a return of or increase in oedema. Malignant hypertension may cause frank haematuria in any patient with chronic nephritis, due to acute arteriolar or glomerular necrosis. Uraemic patients may also bleed spontaneously from the urinary tract owing to increased capillary fragility.

From the diagnostic point of view the most important urinary constituents are granular casts together with excess of erythrocytes and leucocytes. Examination for casts should always be made in the deposit from a fresh, uncentrifuged specimen of urine. Granular casts are derived from degenerated tubular epithelium, and their presence almost invariably signifies active nephritis. Occasional casts may appear in the urine as a result of renal congestion, including orthostatic proteinuria (BULL 1948, 1949) and acute hypertensive renal vascular lesions may cause profuse excretion of blood and granular casts. The essential diagnostic point is that the presence of granular casts in the urine indicates that haematuria derives from the renal glomeruli and not from the lower urinary tract.

II. The nephrotic syndrome

In his reports on medical cases, published in 1827, RICHARD BRIGHT described 24 cases of "Anasarca with coagulable urine in patients with diseased kidneys". Most of the cases he described are typical of the disorder now generally referred to as the nephrotic syndrome. The outstanding feature is severe, persistent generalised oedema which may present as a manifestation of many forms of renal disease.

The common factor to all is heavy proteinuria, sufficiently long continued to produce marked reduction of plasma proteins. The blood cholesterol is usually elevated in such cases. Recent work has shown that the explanation of the oedema in this condition is one of extraordinary complexity — far removed from the simple Starling hypothesis of interstitial oedema resulting from reduced colloid osmotic pressure of the plasma proteins. In addition to hypoproteinaemia and hyperlipaemia a variety of metabolic disturbances are present, involving several homeostatic mechanisms. These include, increased production of antidiuretic hormone and aldosterone, reduction in plasma volume, hyponatraemia, increased protein catabolism, potassium depletion, and frequently urea retention. In seeking for the explanation of the persistent sequestration of fluid in the interstitial tissue there is often a tendency to think in terms of a single cause and to dismiss most of these metabolic changes as secondary in nature. There is good reason to believe however that the state of sustained oedema cannot be interpreted in terms of a disorder of any single variable, but that it represents a shift in equilibrium the maintenance of which depends on a combination of inter-related forces (LUETSCHER and JOHNSON 1954b).

The commonest cause of the nephrotic syndrome is Type II nephritis (ELLIS 1942) or so-called membranous nephritis (BELL 1950). It may also occur in the rapidly progressive course of Type I nephritis (subacute nephritis of VOLHARD), in diabetic glomerulosclerosis (KIMMELSTIEL and WILSON), particularly when severe generalised atherosclerosis leads to heart failure, and when the glomerular lesion is diffuse and associated with chronic ischaemic renal disease (SMITH, BOLTON and TURNBULL; GELLMAN et al.). More rarely the nephrotic syndrome is caused by amyloidosis of the kidney or collagen disease, and still more rarely by chronic renal venous congestion as in right heart failure, constrictive pericarditis (SQUIRE) 1953) or renal vein thrombosis. A number of chemical substances such as mercury and tridione have been incriminated in the development of the syndrome (WILSON, THOMSON and HOLZEL 1952; BARNETT, SIMONS and WELLS). It seems likely that they act antigenically in the production of Type II nephritis of varying severity since a number of vegetable antigens are known to act in this way (see reviews by EALES, and KARK et al. 1958). A group of cases with eosinophilia has been described (MCCALL; HARDWICKE et al.), suggesting a hypersensitivity reaction.

Relation of functional disorder to structural lesion. The basic functional disturbance of the nephrotic syndrome is increased permeability of the glomerular membrane to plasma proteins. There is a wide variation in the character and severity of structural glomerular changes in the conditions described above, but the degree of proteinuria is in no way related to the severity of glomerular damage. Gross proteinuria, hypoproteinaemia and oedema may be associated with minimal glomerular lesions — indeed occasionally no structural changes may be seen on light microscopy. Furthermore, patients with histologically severe and characteristic Type II nephritis may progress to terminal uraemia without the development of oedema at any time. Electronmicroscopic examination of renal biopsy tissue has revealed alterations in the glomerular epithelial cells leading to loss of the normal "foot processes", so that the cytoplasm appears continuous along the basement membrane (VERNIER 1961). Similar changes may occur however in the absence of the nephrotic syndrome, and their relation to abnormal glomerular permeability is uncertain. These considerations, together with the prompt and often unexpected reversibility of proteinuria in the nephrotic syndrome, suggest that the essential abnormality of glomerular permeability is functional and reversible rather than due to structural damage to the basement membrane.

Undoubtedly in the presence of severe glomerular damage a structural component of the proteinuria will be present and is likely to persist when the nephrotic syndrome resolves spontaneously or is reversed by treatment. There is some evidence that this structural component is associated with an increase in the proportion of larger protein molecules in the urine (HARDWICK and SQUIRE 1955). There is no evidence that reduced tubular reabsorption of filtered protein contributes to the proteinuira, indeed there is more probably an increase to a tubular maximum (RATHER 1952; HARDWICKE and SQUIRE 1955); reabsorption of the various protein fractions by the tubules appears to be non-preferential (HARDWICKE and SOOTHILL 1961). The renal tubular cells may be shown histologically to be filled with reabsorbed protein and lipid, and the presence of the latter in the epithelium and interstitial tissue explains the origin of the term "lipoid nephrosis". Secondary disorders of tubular reabsorption may lead to glycosuria and amino-aciduria (STANBURY and MACAULAY).

The biochemical lesion. Since the proteinuria is largely albumin and may amount to more than 30 G daily, reduction in plasma proteins chiefly affects the albumin fraction. A concentration of 2.0 G/100 ml. albumin is regarded as the "oedema level" but reduction to 1.0 G/100 ml. is not infrequent. The level of plasma globulins, especially the α_2 and β globulin fractions, increases (SQUIRE) whilst the smaller α_1 molecule is lost in the urine in considerable amounts. The high blood lipid concentration remains unexplained (SMITH 1951).

Whilst lowering of plasma colloid osmotic pressure must be a significant factor in the production and maintenance of oedema (LOEB et al. 1932; EPSTEIN 1917) there are many characteristics of the syndrome which it leaves unexplained. The plasma protein concentration may rise without any reduction of oedema, and on the other hand, wide fluctuations in the latter, including its complete disappearance, may take place while the plasma protein level remains unchanged (ROSCOE 1956). SQUIRE and his colleagues (SQUIRE, BLAINEY and HARDWICKE 1957) have attempted an explanation of these discrepancies on the basis of interstitial ground substance swelling pressure. There is obviously however a complex alteration in the homeostatic control of body water which cannot be explained by alteration of any single variable (Fig. 1). Hypovolaemia is a characteristic feature of the nephrotic syndrome and this gives rise to secondary changes which may help to perpetuate the disorder. There is marked increase in aldosterone production (FOX and SLOBODY; LUETSCHER and JOHNSON 1954 b) which on the one hand presumably increases sodium retention and on the other will aggravate the potassium depletion produced by increased protein catabolism (SQUIRE). The latter will contribute to nitrogen retention which is however chiefly due to lowering of glomerular filtration rate when hypovolaemia is severe. Increased secretion of antidiuretic hormone has been demonstrated (WILSON and MUIRHEAD) and this, together with other factors, such as passage of sodium into the cells, is in part responsible for the hyponatraemia and oliguria (RYTAND). Evidence has been produced for deficient synthesis of albumin by the liver (GITLIN, JANEWAY and FARR) even when protein intake is adequate. This multiplicity of biochemical disturbances explains the irregular and unpredictable response of the nephrotic syndrome to treatment. The homeostatic disturbance is obviously a very unstable one since a variety of circumstances may trigger off a sudden diuresis which may be accompanied by great reduction in protein excretion. This phenomenon was first described by BLACKALL in 1813[1]. Changes in water and electrolyte status

---

[1] BLACKALL distinguished between dropsy with and without coagulable urine. He observed that in one woman with dropsy "who had been scarified with relief, the urine became in a few days entirely devoid of serum".

such as are produced by diuretics, paracentesis, subcutaneous drainage and
steroids, may provide the necessary stimulus, but in other cases sudden and
massive diuresis may occur spontaneously or after an acute infection such as
measles. In other cases the condition is refractory to any form of treatment for
months or years. Yet even in these, oedema and proteinuria may eventually
resolve; this is most likely to occur in patients who have never exhibited hypertension or signs of active nephritis (e.g. haematuria with granular casts and
leucocytes in the urine deposit). Histologically, as demonstrated by renal biopsy,
such cases have minimal evidence of structural damage in the glomeruli. Rapid
removal of oedema by drainage, or prolonged use of diuretics, especially where
sodium depletion has been produced by a salt free diet, may cause serious collapse
with hypotension, vomiting and uraemia which may be fatal. Such severe sodium
depletion may take place even whilst oedema persists (LUETSCHER 1955). Of

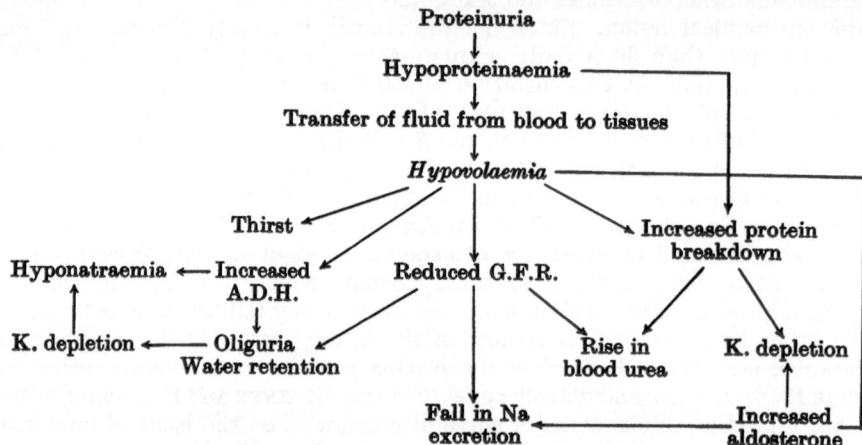

Fig. 1. Biochemical disturbances in the nephrotic syndrome

the many forms of treatment directed towards correcting the biochemical lesion
in the nephrotic syndrome successes have been obtained with ion exchange resins
(ROSENHEIM and SPENCER), adrenal steroids and ACTH (LUETSCHER, DEMING
and JOHNSON 1951; BARNETT et al. 1951; LAUSON et al. 1954; ROSS and SMITH
1963 and BLAINEY et al. 1960). Infusion of human salt free albumin may produce
a reduction in oedema, but this is usually temporary (THORN et al. 1945; LUET-
SCHER, HALL and KREMER 1950). We still do not understand the combination
of circumstances which is necessary to ensure a successful response to any of these
forms of treatment.

III. Pyelonephritis

Pyelonephritis in its various forms is one of the commonest causes of renal
disease and it presents many individual facets of disordered renal function which
have only recently been appreciated. It may arise as a primary infection of the
urinary tract or be superimposed on pre-existing renal damage. In the majority
of cases of acute pyelitis there is probably associated pyelonephritis. Even when
the acute attack has escaped recognition, pyelonephritis may progress insidiously
and this is perhaps the commonest cause of uraemia in patients who give no
previous history of renal disease. Diagnosis is difficult in the late stages since
evidence of urinary infection is often absent, hence the differentiation from

chronic glomerulonephritis may be difficult. A further reason for the high incidence of pyelonephritis, both acute and chronic, is the frequency with which it occurs as a complication of other forms of renal disease, particularly those associated with urinary tract obstruction. For this reason the kidneys may be unequally involved and not infrequently the condition may be unilateral. An important though inconstant feature of unilateral pyelonephritis is severe hypertension, and this has aroused great interest partly owing to the parallel with hypertension produced experimentally in animals by unilateral renal damage, but especially from the clinical similarity with essential hypertension owing to the absence of impaired renal function. It has therefore become a matter of paramount importance to search for evidence of unilateral renal disease in patients with unexplained hypertension. In recent years the concept of chronic pyelonephritis, already somewhat uncertain because of the obscure natural history of the disease, has become even less secure by the discovery that a similar histological picture may develop in chronic potassium depletion and as a result of chemotoxic renal damage, especially from long continued addiction to phenacetin (SPÜHLER and ZOLLINGER 1950; MOESCHLIN 1957; LINDENEG et al. 1959). Finally renal failure due to chronic pyelonephritis is occasionally characterised by very individual forms of tubular dysfunction, producing severe sodium depletion or hypokalaemia or renal diabetes insipidus. Some of these features have been referred to in previous sections, (see also under urinary tract obstruction).

Acute pyelonephritis as a concomitant of acute pyelitis and in the absence of other renal tract abnormalities rarely produces significant impairment of renal function. Occasionally however a massive ascending infection may produce acute necrotising papillitis. This is most often seen in elderly patients with diabetes but has in recent years been reported as a sequel of phenacetin addiction; the urine may contain blood and microscopic fragments of the renal medulla; intense toxaemia may confuse the diagnosis with diabetic coma, and acute uraemia may occur due to suppression of urine. If recovery occurs, deficiencies in the calyceal pattern may be revealed by pyelography (HULTENGRUN 1961). Acute pyelonephritis complicating obstructive lesions of the urinary tract, including neurogenic retention, is of especial importance in that its treatment is ineffective unless the underlying anatomical lesion is discovered and corrected.

Chronic pyelonephritis leads to progressive impairment in renal function closely resembling that described under chronic Type I nephritis, but with special characteristics which are helpful in diagnosis (BROD 1956). An important point is that albuminuria is less marked than in glomerulonephritis and may indeed be absent. This is presumably related to the fact that damage to the kidney is primarily interstitial leading secondarily to tubular atrophy and only later to ischaemic glomerular atrophy. Tubular dysfunction therefore appears earlier and is more marked than glomerular failure (KLEEMAN, HEWITT and GUZE 1960). Reduction in GFR is small compared with loss of urine concentrating power, and the urine is often hypotonic with fixation of specific gravity below 1010. Furthermore there may be considerable difference between the concentration of urine from the two kidneys. A further consequence of tubular damage is defective ammonia formation resulting in impaired acidification of the urine and excessive sodium loss (WRONG and DAVIES 1959). For these reasons polyuria may be more severe and chronic than in glomerulonephritis. Diminished tubular reabsorption of sodium may produce the picture which THORN, KOEPF and CLINTON (1944) termed "salt losing nephritis". Since then similar cases have been described in various types of chronic renal diseases but most commonly in chronic pyelonephritis. The condition may present with severe weakness, salt depletion, hypotension and pigmentation, a picture closely resembling Addison's disease, but differing in the lack of therapeutic response to cortisone in spite of a good response to sodium administration. Excessive potassium loss may be present in salt losing nephritis (EARLE et al. 1951 b) or may occur independently. The differential diagnosis between hypokalaemia due to chronic pyelonephritis and other forms of potassium depletion is a difficult one, since, as stated above, potassium depletion has been found to lead to a condition histologically resembling chronic pyelonephritis. This problem is discussed by MAHLER and STANBURY (1956). The explanation of hypokalaemic nephropathy is obscure; the early lesion is hydropic degeneration of the tubular epithelium (FOLLIS, ORENT-KEILES and McCOLLUM 1942); in rats renal sclerosis and tubular dilation develop (FOURMAN, McCANCE and PARKER 1956) and in man a picture resembling chronic pyelonephritis has been observed in aldosteronism and after intestinal potassium depletion (MILNE, MUEHRCKE and HEARD 1957). Hypertension is a common finding in chronic pyelonephritis and the frequency with which the malignant phase occurs is almost as great as in chronic nephritis (WEISS and PARKER 1939; BROD 1959). The association of hypertension with unilateral pyelonephritis which is discussed in the following section.

IV. Unilateral renal disease

Unilateral renal disease is of particular importance in surgical practice since it is one of the few disorders in which hypertension can be cured by removal of the cause. It presents special diagnostic problems since proteinuria may be absent and renal function is unimpaired, so that unless specific tests are carried out the condition may be misdiagnosed as essential hypertension. The recognition of this remediable form of high blood pressure has led therefore to the introduction of screening tests in cases of "hypertension without apparent cause", the most important of which is intravenous pyelography. As a result many causes of unilateral renal disease associated with hypertension have been recognised. These include unilateral pyelonephritis (BUTLER 1937; WEISS and PARKER 1939; PICKE-RING and HEPTINSTALL 1953), tuberculosis of the kidney (VAN GUIDSENHOVEN and VAN DEN BROUCKE 1946) renal injury, renal tumour (HOWARD et al. 1953) and the operation of tying an aberrant renal artery (BOEMINGHAUS and GOTZEN 1952). In all these conditions hypertension has been reported to improve or disappear following excision of the diseased kidney. Widely differing views have been expressed on the success of this operation however and SMITH (1956) reporting a cure rate of only 26% doubted the wisdom of nephrectomy in such cases. New light was thrown on the problem by the discovery that renal artery stenosis was one of the commoner forms of unilateral renal disease producing hypertension, and that hypertension was generally abolished when the lesion could be corrected surgically. In the recognition of this disorder aortography will indicate the anatomical lesion, but the functional significance of the stenosis in relation to the hypertension, and to the surgical prognosis, can only be decided by differential renal function tests. The value of such tests in unilateral renal disease was first clearly established by HOWARD, CONNOR and THOMAS (1956). Complete collection of urine from each ureter was attempted during water diuresis. A reduction of urine volume by 50% and in sodium concentration by 15% on the affected side was regarded as diagnostic of renal artery stenosis and was accepted as a criterion for successful reversal of the hypertension by relief of the renal artery constriction. Several writers have published the results of this and similar tests (PAGE, DUSTAN and POUTASSE 1959; HULET et al. 1960; CONNOR et al. 1960; YENDT et al. 1960; BROWN et al. 1960). SPENCER (1960) in a critical review concluded that the above criteria were reliable in the majority of cases. RAPOPORT (1960) attempted to avoid the difficulty of complete urine collection by comparing the creatinine to sodium ratio in incomplete collections from each ureter and this appears to be as reliable as the HOWARD test (BIRCHALL, BATSON and BRANNAN 1962). A more precise test, and one which probably has a wider diagnostic value is that described by STAMEY et al. (1961). These authors have shown that the essential functional pattern of the kidney with renal artery stenosis is increased tubular reabsorption of water and sodium relative to the GFR. This pattern is recognised not only by reduced urine volume and sodium excretion, but also by increased concentration of substances not subject to tubular reabsorption such as creatinine, inulin and PAH. These changes are accentuated by osmotic diuresis with urea or mannitol. Complete urine collections are necessary and this prodecure is not without risk of trauma to the ureters. In the hands of these authors, reduction of urine volume by at least 70% with increase in unilin concentration by 100% indicates main renal artery stenosis; figures of 50 and 16% respectively are considered diagnostic of segmental ischaemia due to branch renal artery stenosis. It is obvious that if renal artery stenosis, as revealed by aortography, is bilateral, the above tests are invalid — although they may still indicate the relative severity of the stenosis on the two sides. In other forms of unilateral renal disease such as pyelonephritis the above pattern will not be seen unless an ischaemic lesion is also present. Differential tests may reveal reduced urine flow but creatinine concentration is likely to be lower on the affected side compared with the healthy kidney (HOWARD and CONNOR 1962). A recent communication suggests that divided renal function tests can be satisfactorily made avoiding the risk of trauma involved in complete ureteric collections, by calculations based on analysis of the separate ureteric specimens and of the bladder urine (ROBERTS and WALL 1963).

The pattern of renal dysfunction produced by renal artery stenosis explains the characteristic features of the intravenous pyelogram. Delayed appearance of the contrast medium on the affected side is due to reduced rate of clearance, while the greater concentration achieved is explained by the excessive water reabsorption relative to the rate of excretion. Many recent papers have appeared on differential renal blood flow estimation by radio-active isotope techniques using either diodrast (WINTER 1957; WINTER and TAPLIN 1958; WINTER et al. 1959; SERRATTO, GRAYHACK and EARLE 1959), hippuran (BURBANK et al. 1961; TAUXE 1961; SCHWARTZ and MADELOFF 1962) or rubidium (TORRANCE, DAVIES and CLARK 1961). The results of STAMEY et al. (1961) indicate that hypertension may be caused by renal artery stenosis producing a differential renal blood flow of a little as 25%. In general however isotope renography is not sufficiently sensitive to recognise such a small difference hence false negative results are likely. Furthermore since other forms of unilateral renal disease may reduce renal blood flow considerably, false positive results will be not uncommon. However, as a preliminary screening test, combined with intravenous pyelography, this form of investigation is of value in selecting cases for aortography and measurement of differential renal function.

V. Renal function in essential hypertension

The diagnostic separation of essential hypertension into benign and malignant is based on the absence of papilloedema in the former and its presence in the latter. Impairment of renal function is a constant feature of malignant hypertension and increases with the duration of the disease. It is attributable to progressive vascular necrosis, chiefly in glomeruli and arterioles, with secondary interstitial fibrosis and tubular degeneration. Thus the pattern of renal failure is similar to that of a rapidly progressive chronic nephritis. It differs in the intensity of hypertensive complications such as left ventricular failure and hypertensive encephalopathy which usually prove fatal before nitrogen retention is more than moderate in degree i.e. uraemia as such is rarely the immediate cause of death in malignant hypertension. In the very early stages however there is evidence of tubular impairment. The specific gravity of the urine becomes fixed long before the blood urea rises, and nocturia due to loss of diurnal rhythm of tubular concentration is one of the earliest symptoms. Albuminuria may be absent when papilloedema is first recognised (ELLIS 1938) and is not usually more than moderate in degree, so that hypoproteinaemia is rare. Haematuria is occasionally severe due to haemorrhage from necrotising glomerulitis, but it is unusual to find granular casts in the urine. Recent work (ASSCHER and ANSON 1963) suggests that a renal vascular permeability factor may play a role in the causation of fibrinoid arterial necrosis in malignant hypertension. It may also contribute to the papilloedema, increased intra-cranial pressure and cerebral oedema. The latter manifestations are however more probably related to excessive local arterial constriction which BYROM (1954, 1963) has demonstrated in experimental malignant hypertension both in the brain and in the retina.

In benign essential hypertension impairment of renal function is rarely of clinical significance. It is possible to distinguish between functional changes due to the hypertension, and irreversible renal failure which is limited to the minority of cases in which severe arterial and arteriolar sclerosis lead to extensive ischaemic atrophy. The early functional changes were well defined by GOLDRING et al. (1941) using clearance studies. In a series of patients with essential hypertension of varying grades of severity, determination of inulin and diodone clearance showed reduction of glomerular filtration and renal blood flow, and also of tubular excretory mass. These changes increased with the severity of the hypertension. Renal blood floow was relatively more impaired than glomerular filtration, i.e. the filtration fraction was increased. This relative ischaemia of the functioning tubules was interpreted as due to efferent arteriolar constriction and it was shown that this was reversible since it could be increased by the action of pyrogens as in the normal kidney. Similar results were obtained by CARGILL (1949) using PAH extraction in place of diodone. A detailed account of clearance studies in essential hypertension is given by SMITH (1951) and the interpretations are discussed critically by PICKERING (1955). These observations may be taken to indicate that even in the early stages of benign hypertension there is some impairment of glomerular and tubular function although this produces no clinical effects and is not detected by the usual, less sensitive renal function tests. As the hypertension becomes more severe, even in the benign stage, nocturia may develop and the limits of urine specific gravity are narrowed.

When severe ischaemic fibrosis occurs, tests of tubular concentration become impaired i.e. urine specific gravity becomes fixed and there may be a moderate rise in blood urea. This has been termed "decompensated benign nephrosclerosis" and the degree of impaired renal function can be correlated with the severity of renal arteriolo-sclerosis (KIMMELSTIEL and WILSON 1936). Albuminuria is present in such cases, even in the absence of heart failure.

Hypokalaemia due to excessive potassium loss has been described in severe hypertension with grade III or grade IV retinopathy (DE WESSELOW and THOMSON 1939; HILDEN and KROGSGAARD 1958). In malignant hypertension

WRONG (1961) observed hypokalaemia in 50% of cases. In cases of unilateral or bilateral renal ischemia GOWENLOCK and WRONG (1962) observed hypokalaemia which they attributed to secondary aldosteronism. Increased aldosterone secretion has been found in severe, usually malignant, essential hypertension by several authors (LARAGH et al. 1960b; GENEST et al. 1960), and in severe hypertension produced by renal artery stenosis in dogs (CARPENTER, DAVIS and AYERS 1961b) and also after angiotensin infusion (LARAGH et al. 1960a; GENEST et al. 1961a). It is possible therefore that in malignant essential hypertension acute vascular lesions lead to areas of ischaemia and increased renin production; this in turn stimulates aldosterone secretion and results in hypokalaemia.

VI. Acute oliguric uraemia

(acute tubular necrosis, lower nephron nephrosis, acute cortical ischaemia).

1. Pathogenesis

It has already been pointed out that severe oliguria, seldom amounting to complete anuria, may occur in a variety of conditions in which renal blood flow and glomerular filtration are acutely reduced. If the reduction in renal blood flow is not extreme, or is of short duration, renal tubular function may be preserved. In this case, the small volume of urine produced is well concentrated and early restoration of renal blood flow leads to normal urine output. This disturbance (pre-renal uraemia) is distinct from acute (intrinsic) renal failure which may occur in similar circumstances and is characterised by the secretion of poorly concentrated urine. In these cases renal functional impairment with mounting azotaemia may persist for days or weeks after the precipitating trauma or shock has been successfully treated.

BYWATERS and BEALL (1941) described a series of patients in whom death from oliguric renal failure followed crushing injuries of the limbs. They noted the presence of pigment casts of myoglobin and haematin in the lumen of the tubules and suggested that these might have caused oliguria by obstructing the tubules. Shock and hypotension had been a prominent feature in most but not all of their cases. DUNN, GILLESPIE and NIVEN (1941) described in greater detail the histological lesions in the "crush syndrome" and noted segments of complete tubular disruption mainly in the ascending limb of the loop of HENLE and in the distal convoluted tubule. They noted no lesions in the proximal convoluted tubule or glomerulus. LUCKE (1946) used the term "lower nephron nephrosis" to describe the condition, which he believed to be essentially similar to that seen after haemorrhage, other forms of trauma, obstetric complications, burns and poisons. OLIVER, MACDOWELL and TRACY (1951) reviewed the lesions found in 31 cases of acute renal failure following trauma, burns, transfusion reactions and obstetrical complications and 23 cases due to poisoning. They showed by individual nephron dissection that segments of tubular disruption (tubulorrhexis) with disappearance of the basement membrane, were to be found at all levels from the proximal convolution onwards. These lesions were focal and many nephrons escaped damage; moreover they were not related to the occurrence of pigment casts in the lumen. A different type of lesion (nephrotoxic necrosis) was seen in poisoning, with more diffuse damage confined to the proximal tubules without disruption, the basement membrane remaining intact. It was concluded that tubulorrhexis was due to an episode of renal ischaemia. The condition is now frequently termed acute tubular necrosis, but this term is not althogether satisfactory since tubular lesions may be very slight in patients who have died in oliguric renal failure following trauma (BRUN and MUNCK 1957), but conspicuous in patients who have has no clinical evidence of renal failure, (SEVITT 1959). Renal cortical necrosis may be found in patients with acute renal failure, the great majority of cases being associated with concealed accidental ante-partum haemorrhage (utero-placental apoplexy: abruptio placentae). In this condition, although clinical signs of "shock" are usual, the blood pressure is often normal or high. SHEEHAN and MOORE (1952) studied the kidneys of 67 fatal cases of utero-placental apoplexy; there were 34 cases of renal cortical necrosis ranging from minute foci to gross cases which involved the whole of both renal cortices. In addition, there were 26 cases of less severe renal lesions, including focal tubular necroses. SHEEHAN and MOORE (1952) concluded that these less severe lesions and the renal cortical necrosis were both due to renal vasoconstriction of varying distribution and duration. In summary, in acute renal failure following trauma etc., histological lesions are usually confined to the tubules, they are focal and may be inconspicuous or even absent. In a few cases extensive renal cortical necrosis occurs. All these lesions are generally attributed to severe ischaemia. Nevertheless the syndrome of acute cortical ischaemia is not an invariable result of hypotensive shock, nor is it acceptable purely as a quantitatively more severe lesion than pre-renal azotaemia. There appears to be a selectively abnormal reaction of the renal blood vessels which determines the specific characteristics of the disorder.

2. Changes in renal function

Detailed investigation of renal function is difficult in critically ill patients. In animals, shock severe enough to produce renal ischaemia is usually irreversible and the clinical syndrome of oliguric renal failure is not easily reproduced. For purposes of description the illness may be divided into a *stage of onset* lasting about 48 hours after the original trauma, an *oliguric stage* with urine volumes under 500 ml. per day, and a *diuretic stage* from the first day in which the urine volume is over 500 ml. per day until normal homeostasis is secured (normal serum urea, creatinine and electrolytes).

Stage of onset. LAUSON, BRADLEY and COURNAND (1944) studied renal blood flow in shock in man, and found that it was reduced to a greater extent than the cardiac output, i.e. renal vasoconstriction occurred. This has been confirmed in man and animals (reviewed by FRANKLIN and MERRILL 1960b). Renal vaso-constriction also occurs in response to adrenaline injections and sympathetic nerve stimulation, and is reduced or abolished in shock by the use of adrenergic blocking agents and renal denervation. (In clinical practice, however, MOYER, MORRIS and BEAZLEY [1955] have shown that in shock from myocardial infarction, renal function may be improved by noradrenaline infusions.) TRUETA and his associates (1947) demonstrated cortical ischaemia in the rabbit due to shunting of blood through juxta-medullary glomeruli during shock, sciatic nerve stimulation and adrenaline infusion, but there is no evidence that medullary shunting occurs in man or the dog. KRAMER, THURAU and DEETJEN (1960) showed that during haemorrhagic shock in the dog cortical and medullary blood flows are reduced to an equal extent, and cortical capillary oxygen saturation is not lower than medullary. Renal oxygen consumption is reduced pari passu with renal blood flow down to a level of 30% of normal, and with this reduction there is no increase in renal arteriovenous oxygen difference or hypoxia of renal tissue (KRAMER and DEETJEN 1960). This is not attributable to shunting of blood through the medulla but to the fact that the greater part of the renal oxygen requirement is needed to provide energy for sodium transport; the amount of work involved is therefore proportional to the GFR At a RBF of 30% of normal, GFR is reduced to 1—2% of normal or less. Reduction of RBF below this level is accompanied by an exponential fall in oxygen consumption, widening A-V oxygen saturation difference and tissue hypoxia. Such low levels of RBF have not been satisfactorily demonstrated in animals or man with survival.

GRABER and SEVITT (1959) studied renal function in burned patients with shock. Gross reduction in GFR and isosthenuria frequently occurred, in some cases lasting only a few hours, but in others a sustained fall was seen and when GFR remained below 50% of normal for over 24 hours azotaemia developed. Not all patients had oliguria however but all those with a fall in GFR had a fall in osmolarity and in U/P concentration ratios for urea and creatinine. In most cases U/P sodium concentration ratios were low in the early stages (as would be expected if the tubules were reacting normally to aldosterone secretion during oligaemic shock). U/P ratios of potassium concentration were high (indicating continued tubular secretion). These findings are consistent with preservation of renal tubular function in the onset stage, the predominant renal disturbance being reduced glomerular filtration. The same result might be seen if urine formation was entirely due to a few surviving nephrons, and this finding does not exclude tubular necrosis as the cause of the renal failure since any nephron with a segment of complete tubular disruption cannot be secreting urine. Whether oliguria or azotaemia with normal urine volume occurs, is determined partly by the extent to which water is reabsorbed by the tubules. If the urine volume remains at about one litre per day, the functional disturbance resembles qualitatively that of the diuretic stage which follows the oliguric stage in the majority of cases.

Once glomerular filtration has reached a very low level (1%) sodium transport has usually ceased, and it will be impossible for the normal hyperosmolarity of the medullary interstium to be maintained. BOYLAN and ASSHAUER (quoted by KRAMER 1962) determined the osmotic pressure of slices of kidney from a shocked dog and found the normal gradient was abolished. This fits in with SELKURT'S (1962) findings that during the phase of shock renal venous blood contains more sodium than arterial blood. At a RBF of 30% of normal, with nil GFR. the small blood flow through the medulla is washing out the sodium from the interstium. Only as GFR recovers can the gradient be re-established, hence the U/P osmolality ratio rises with GFR as recovery takes place (KRAMER and DEETJEN 1960).

Stage of established oliguria. BULL, JOEKES and LOWE (1950) found the average duration of this stage to be 10—12 days, in rare cases it may last over three weeks. Large series of cases have been described from many centres (SWANN and MERRILL 1953; FRANKLIN and MERRILL 1960b; KILEY, POWER and BEEBE 1960; BLUEMLE, WEBSTER and ELKINTON 1951; PARSONS and McCRACHEN 1959; SHACKMAN, MILNE and STRUTHERS 1960; LOUGHRIDGE et al. 1960). BULL and his colleagues (1950) measured renal blood flow at this stage with PAH and found levels of 10% of normal or less. They concluded that the oliguria was associated with persistent renal ischaemia. MUNCK (1958) using radioactive Krypton however has found RBF 30—50% of normal in both the oliguric stage and the early diuretic stage. Hence it is difficult to attribute the oliguria to persistent ischaemia. All observers are agreed that the inulin and endogenous creatinine clearance are very low (about 1% of normal) at this stage and recover slowly in the diuretic stage. BULL, JOEKES and LOWE (1950) and earlier workers suggested that the creatinine or inulin clearance could not be relied upon to measure GFR since filtered creatinine or inulin might diffuse back passively through necrosed tubules. Nephrons in which this happened could not however be contributing to urine flow, and these clearances may be taken as indicating effective glomerular filtration. At the same time urine concentration is grossly reduced with U/P concentrations of creatinine and urea below 5:1, and often little more than 1:1, indicating reduced reabsorption of water. Urine sodium concentrations are variable. BULL, JOEKES and LOWE (1950) emphasised the relatively high concentrations sometimes found, but their results, and those of SWANN and MERRILL (1953), were variable, especially in the first few days, and in many cases sodium P/U concentration ratios of 5:1 or more may be seen. Urine potassium concentration is usually higher than in plasma. These electrolyte concentrations are similar to those expected in the response to injury (sodium conservation and potassium loss) and indicate some preservation of tubular function. Glycosuria occurs to a slight and variable extent and BULL, JOEKES and LOWE (1950) found tubular reabsorption of glucose to be impaired. Aminoaciduria is seen in a few patients (EMSLIE-SMITH et al. 1956). The p_H of the urine in the oliguric stage is often 5.5 or lower (FRANKLIN and MERRILL 1960b), a further indication of preservation of tubular function.

Diuretic stage. Once urine flow starts, the volume tends to rise in rapid steps, so that in a few days moderate to gross polyuria is established, but urinary concentrating power lags behind. BULL, JOEKES and LOWE (1950) found that it took an average of 10—12 days for U/P concentrations of creatinine to reach 20:1, or urea 10:1; at the same time higher P/U ratios sodium developed and excessive renal losses of water, sodium and potassium declined. Some impairment of renal function persisted for months, and even after 2—3 years, glomerular filtration and PAH clearances were seldom above the lower limits of normal (LOWE 1952) although complete *clinical* recovery was the rule.

3. Changes in body composition in oliguric renal failure

Expansion of the extracellular fluid volume, hyponatraemia and hypochloraemia occur in oliguric renal failure due to overloading with water on a daily intake of 1 litre (MERRILL 1955). HAMBURGER and MATHÉ, MERRILL (1955), and BLUEMLE, POTTER and ELKINTON (1956) pointed out that large amounts of fat and lesser amounts of other body solids are consumed during the oliguric period. The latter workers, measuring complete metabolic balances on eight cases, found a calorie soncumption of 2,500/day; 200 gm. of fat and 42 gm. of protein being consumed daily from the body stores in addition to 110 gm. carbohydrate, most of which was given as food. The water of oxidation produced was 303 ml./day and endogenous preformed water 124 ml./day. The insensible loss was 981 ml./day so that water required in excess of sensible loss was 550 ml./day. Loss of 0.2 to 0.5 kg./day in body weight would therefore occur if the patients were in exact water balance. Twice as much weight loss was to be expected in severe post-traumatic cases (FRANKLIN and MERRILL 1960b). During the diuretic phase there was a diminution of extracellular fluid and total body water with negative sodium and chloride balance. Some of this change was accounted for by elimination of water and electrolyte accumulated in the oliguric phase, but there was probably also some migration of sodium into the cells during the oliguric phase which was reversed in the diuretic phase. There was also a negative potassium balance in both oliguric and early diuretic phases, but serum potassium rose in the oliguric phase due to migration of potassium from the cells.

4. Relationship of clinical state to functional disturbance

The rate at which protein catabolism proceeds and azotaemia, acidosis and hyperkalaemia occur depends on the precipitating cause of the renal failure. In nephrotoxic poisoning, transfusion reactions and obstetric oliguria, the course is relatively favourable, the blood urea rising at from 10—30 mgm./100 ml. per day, and in the first week of oliguria few symptoms may occur. In post-traumatic cases on the other hand urea accumulation is much more sudden e.g. blood urea rises 30—120 mgm./100 ml. per day, hyperkalaemia and acidosis develop, and clinical deterioration is correspondingly rapid. *Hyperkalaemia* causes bradycardia, cardiac arrhythmia and death in ventricular systole at levels of potassium over 8.0 mEq/l.; muscle weakness and depressed tendon reflexes are also found. These serious effects are preceded by electrocardiographic signs at serum potassium levels of 6.5 to 8.0 mEq/l. The severity of the cardiac changes is greater when hyperkalaemia is accompanied by hypocalcaemia and acidosis, as is generally the case in the anuric state. *Expansion of extracellular fluid volume* (accumulation of sodium and water) causes oedema, raised venous pressure, tachycardia, sometimes raised arterial blood pressure and convulsions, and pulmonary oedema. It may be avoided in most cases by careful maintenance of fluid balance. *Acidosis* gives rise to rapid deep respiration (KUSSMAUL breathing). In advanced cases periodic breathing occurs (CHEYNE-STOKES respiration). Lethargy and mental confusion may be the result of several different disturbances, including raised serum urea (GROLLMAN and GROLLMAN 1959) and acidosis. Convulsions may be produced by hypertension but also occur in its absence. Tetany is rare. Exaggerated tendon reflexes with knee and ankle clonus are common. Asymmetry of muscle power and reflexes is not uncommon and may simulate cerebral vascular disease. These neurological disturbances have not been correlated with any particular pattern of electrolyte or acid base disturbance (LOCKE, MERRILL and TYLER 1961); they are sometimes temporarily made worse by haemodialysis (KENNEDY, LINTON and EATON 1962) probably because urea is removed from the extracellular fluid more rapidly than from the brain. A haemorrhagic state is seen in about half the cases with advanced uraemia; no abnormality of the clotting mechanism occurs specifically in uraemic states but various anomalies are seen from time to time (BLUEMLE, WEBSTER and ELKINTON 1951; FRANKLIN and MERRILL 1960b). Poor resistance to infection and failure of wound healing, commonly seen in these patients, may be mitigated by adequate dialysis (PARSONS and McCRACKEN 1959; TESCHAN et al. 1960). Intense thirst is usual in the oliguric subject who is given no more than his exact fluid requirements.

In the diuretic phase either sodium or potassium depletion may occur, and electrolyte loss has been observed for as long as 44 days (HUNTER and MUIRHEAD 1952). In the first few days of the diuresis the signs of uraemia may worsen and the blood urea may continue to rise, but when the urine volume exceeds 1500—2000 ml. a sustained fall in blood urea and rapid clinical improvement is generally seen. Within a few weeks the blood urea returns to normal and the patient goes into positive potassium and nitrogen balance during convalescence.

VII. Renal failure of extra-renal origin

The main extra-renal causes of disturbances of renal function are endocrine dieases, electrolyte imbalance, and circulatory disorders which impair renal blood flow. Reference has been made in other sections to the effects of endocrine disease and electrolyte imbalance. In addition, obstructive lesions of the urinary tract may produce disorders of renal function under a variety of circumstances.

These, together with certain extra-renal conditions of particular surgical interest will be described. Circulatory disorders will be included under postoperative renal failure.

1. Urinary tract obstruction

Renal function may be disordered in renal tract obstruction in a variety of ways. There may be chronic obstruction with hydronephrosis, or complete obstruction leading to acute retention of urine. Progressive or sudden obstruction may produce anuria. An entirely different situation is produced after the relief of obstructive retention. Finally infection, acute or chronic, may complicate the picture.

Investigation of chronic obstruction, usually due to prostatic enlargement, has been carried out by a number of workers (WILSON, REISMAN and MOYER 1951; PARSONS 1954; ROUSSAK and OLEESKY 1954; BRICKER et al. 1957; EDVALL 1959; BERLYNE 1961) and in hydronephrosis in infants and children by ZETTERSTROM, ERICSSON and WINBERG (1958) and WINBERG (1959). Chronic hydronephrosis interferes with both glomerular and tubular function. There is reduction in GFR to varying degree with rise in blood urea in most cases. Fluid retention may occur and plasma levels of sodium, potassium and chloride may be elevated even when nitrogen retention is slight or absent (PARSONS 1954). Tubular dysfunction is however most prominent and particularly affects distal tubular function (BERLYNE 1961). Incomplete acidification of the urine after an ammonium chloride load is characteristic and is associated with both defective excretion of ammonia and titratable acid. Maximal urinary concentration after pitressin is defective (BERLYNE 1961; ROUSSAK and OLEESKY 1954) and urinary hypotonicity and polyuria may be sufficient to warrant the term "nephrogenic diabetes insipidus". These findings can in part be explained on the basis of osmotic diuresis due to simple reduction in effective number of nephrons, but it seems likely there is also distal tubular damage with failure to respond to antidiuretic hormone. These results of tubular dysfunction are usually only observed in patients with nitrogen retention and it is obvious at this stage that severe dehydration and electrolyte depletion may be present. After relief of urinary tract obstruction these forms of distal nephron dysfunction may be reversible. When obstruction is suddenly relieved however massive diuresis with sodium, chloride and potassium loss may occur (WILSON, REISMAN and MOYER 1951; PARSONS 1954; BRICKER et al. 1957) and lead to severe clinical deterioration if replacement therapy is not promptly carried out.

2. Post-operative renal failure

All grades of severity of renal failure may occur after surgical operations, varying from moderate elevation of the blood urea to acute oliguric renal failure. There are numerous causative factors and the appropriate treatment depends on their early recognition.

Heart failure may occur, particularly in elderly patients with reduced cardiac reserve due to ischaemic heart disease. It may be precipitated by overloading of the circulation by intravenous infusions of blood, plasma or saline, by acute anaemia due to haemorrhage, or by infection. The blood urea is usually moderately elevated, rarely over 150 mgm.-%. The urine is reduced in amount and concentrated; a moderate degree of proteinuria may be found, with hyaline casts and occasionally granular casts in the deposit. This form of congestive uraemia rapidly improves on appropriate treatment of the heart failure. Occasionally cardiac infarction, which may be silent, during or immediately after operation, leads to acute hypotension and oliguria with severe nitrogen retention.

Hypotension may occur for a variety of reasons including traumatic shock, haemorrhage, dehydration and sodium depletion, adrenal failure, and as mentioned above, cardiac infarction. Oliguria or in severe cases anuria may follow, with progressive elevation of blood urea and failure of concentrating power. The condition is usually reversible if the blood pressure is elevated by correcting dehydration and, if necessary, intravenous infusion of vasoconstrictor drugs. If anuria persists, acute tubular necrosis must be suspected and treated by strict regulation of fluid and electrolyte balance or by haemodialysis.

Electrolyte disturbance. Sodium or potassium depletion may occur particularly in intestinal obstruction or ileus, with the consequences on renal function which have already been described. The electrocardiogram is a good indicator of potassium depletion. Alkalosis may be caused by excessive gastric drainage or vomiting or by overbreathing induced by anaesthesia or artifical respiration. Uraemia in such cases is largely due to the associated electrolyte disturbance.

Acute oliguric uraemia may occur as a complication of operations on the urinary tract or on the gall bladder, in cases of extensive muscle trauma, or the prolonged use of a limb tourniquet or following aortography, and occasionally intravenous pyelography. The disturbance of renal function is fully described on p. 451. Any form of prolonged hypotension may cause this form of renal failure with varying degrees of renal structural damage.

Increased protein catabolism may cause nitrogen retention by presenting an excessive metabolic load to a kidney already embarassed by one or more of the above factors. This occurs as a result of tissue trauma, infection, haemorrhage and dehydration, and may be aggravated by steroid administration.

3. Uretero-colic anastomosis

Renal Damage. Although patients may remain in excellent health for many years after uretero-colic anastomosis, the majority die eventually from renal failure. The cause of this appears to be hydronephrosis and pyelonephritis. During the last decade there have been many papers describing patients who have been observed for long periods after this operation. Unfortunately follow-up is often incomplete and adequate studies on renal function have not been performed. STEVENS (1940) collected 40 cases following uretero-colic anastomosis for ectopic bladder, with survival for at least ten years. There was evidence of renal damage in over half. GREY TURNER (1943) reported nine cases who had survived for at least 16 years. All patients were said to be in reasonable health although the excretion pyelogram showed abnormalities in each instance. HAR-VAD and THOMPSON (1951) reported 144 patients in whom the operation had been performed for bladder extrophy. Sixty-five per cent of deaths which occurred after discharge from hospital were due to renal complications and of 69 Patients surviving, more than two third showed evidence of renal damage. CORDONNIER and LAGE (1951) found evidence of pyelitis in 21 out of 48 patients examined by intravenous pyelography up to two years after operation. JACOBS and STIR-LING (1952) analysed case records of 1,673 patients from many centres. There was evidence of pyelonephritis in nearly half and 40% of all deaths (except those in which the operation was performed in cases of inoperable carcinoma) where due to renal causes. GARRETT and MERTZ (1954) found evidence of renal damage in six out of eleven patients followed for up to five years.

Electrolyte imbalance. BOYD (1931) first drew attention to a chronic state of acidosis which followed uretero-colic anastomosis. ALLISON (1933) described a patient who, following this operation, suffered from weakness, malaise and anorexia, which could be relieved by rectal darinage. FERRIS and ODEL (1950) were the first to make detailed studies of the serum electrolytes. In 141 patients operated on at the Mayo clinic about 80% were found to have hyperchloraemic acidosis; in the majority this developed during the first year after operation. Most patients were said to be well in spite of this disorder although some complained of weight loss, thirst, fatigue and of a salty taste in the mouth. LAPIDES (1951); CORDONNIER and LAGE (1951); BERGLIN and MATHISEN (1952); JACOBS and STIRLING (1952); CREEVY and REISSER (1952) and GARRETT and MERTZ (1954) described the same condition in between 40 and 100% of all cases subjected to uretero-colic anastomosis. In addition, low but fluctuating levels of serum potassium have been reported by LAPIDES (1951); JACOBS and STIRLING (1952); CREEVY and REISSER (1952) and WILKINSON (1952, 1954). The latter author considers that hypokalaemia is responsible for the majority of the symptoms although other workers disagree.

There has been considerable controversy whether these changes are due to selective reabsorption of chloride from the lumen of the bowel or to impairment of renal function. ANNIS and ALEXANDER (1952) found that if urine or normal saline is instilled into the bowel in patients with colostomy openings, chloride is absorbed more than sodium. ROSENBERG (1953) studied the absorption of isotopes from the colon, but was unable to demonstrate any selective absorption of chloride. In experiments on dogs, however, he found that the venous blood from the colon contained more chloride and ammonia and was of lower p_H when the colon contained urine. He concluded that absorption of urine constituents from the colon was the major factor in the development of hyperchloraemic acidosis. BOYD (1931) showed that dogs in which the ureters had been implanted into the caecum died in uraemia without severe renal damage, but that after ureteric implantation into the sigmoid colon the animal survived with slightly raised urea and chloride levels. Colostomy proximal to the ureteric openings restored urea and chloride level to normal. He concluded that the degree of absorption of urea and chloride from the colon is proportional to the area of bowel mucous membrane exposed to the urine.

KEKWICK et al. (1952) instilled urine into the colon in two patients who had had ileostomy or caecostomy. They found little evidence of absorption of urinary constituents. In addition, they reported four patients in whom one ureter had been implanted into the caecum and the other into the sigmoid colon. In three patients there was post-mortem evidence of pyelonephritis, but in the fourth, who had died with evidence of hyperchloraemic acidosis, there was some damage to the renal tubular cells but no pyelonephritis. They concluded that the syndrome was due to impairment of renal function rather than to reabsorption from the bowel and suggested that there might be tubular dysfunction in the absence of structural renal damage. LAPIDES (1951) demonstrated that the serum electrolytes remained normal in patients with no history of renal infection and normal pyelogram. This only occured in five out of 22 patients; in the remaining 15, in whom there was a history of renal infection or evidence of abnormalities in the pyelograms, there was hyperchloraemic acidosis. He gave urine enemata to patients with good renal function and found that this produced no change in serum electrolytes; in patients with renal impairment, hyperchloraemic acidosis could be demonstrated. He concluded that with good renal function reabsorption of chloride from the bowel produces no electrolyte change. JACOBS and STIRLING (1954) also found that electrolyte changes occurred mainly in patients in whom the kidney had been shown to be abnormal by pyelography.

BERGLIN and MATHISEN (1952) attributed the electrolyte changes to renal tubular dysfunction produced by increased back pressure on the kidney. WILKINSON (1952, 1954) considered that the urine acts as a colonic irritant and results in loss of excessive fluid and base, especially of potassium from the rectum. He ascribes all the electrolyte changes and symptoms to this. IRVINE, ALAN and WEBSTER (1956) studied groups of dogs with 1. uretero-colic anastomosis, 2. the same operation with proximal colostomy so that the urine drained into the isolated rectum and sigmoid colon, and 3. with ureteric impantation into a bladder made from an isolated loop of ileum. In the second and third groups in which the urine did not come into contact with the faecal stream there was little evidence of renal infection or damage, which was common in animals from the first group. Hyperchloraemic acidosis developed within several days of operation in the first, occurred occasionally in the second, but was never seen in the third group. Hypokalaemia occurred occasionally in animals from the first group but was not seen in the other two. In addition, they investigated the carbonic anhydrase activity of the kidney in all animals but found no abnormality. No other tests of glomerular or tubular function were performed. They concluded that reabsorption of constituents from the bowel is the probable cause of electrolyte imbalance following uretero-colic anastomosis.

The problem requires further study. No adequate tests of glomerular or tubular function have been performed either in patients or in experiments upon animals. The evidence suggests that both impairment of renal function and increased absorption of urinary constituents from the colon play a part in the development of this form of hyperchloraemic acidosis. It is obviously necessary to investigate glomerular and tubular function following uretero-colic anastomosis before serous renal damage has occurred from ascending pyelonephritis.

4. Renal impairment in cerebral states

Cerebral damage, arising from neoplasm, operative or accidental trauma, and other causes may be accompanied by a variety of disturbances of body water and electrolytes which may boht produce and result from impairment of renal function. The mechanisms underlying many of these disturbances are complex, involving centres in the brain for osmoregulation (VERNEY 1954), thirst (ANDERSSON and McCANN 1955) and possibly other centres which possess regulatory functions in electrolyte homeostasis. The disturbances which have been reported can be broadly classified and their pathogenesis will be briefly discussed. The subject has been surveyed in cases of head injury by HIGGINS et al (1951). The minor and transient disturbances of proteinuria and glycosuria, the latter due either to hyperglycaemia or to a lowered renal threshold, must be mentioned but require no further comment.

Water depletion. This is a very common occurrence and arises from a combination of inadequate fluid intake in the comatose patient and excessive water loss through fever, sweating and hyperpnoea which may occur in cerebral damage. The initial renal response to this is the excretion of a concentrated urine of high specific gravity and raised urea and sodium content. In severe cases the serum sodium level may be raised.

Hypernatraemia with hyponatriuria. In this state the serum sodium level may rise to 180 mEq/l. or more, whereas the urinary sodium concentration falls to 10 ml./l. of less. The blood urea level is raised and there is a high urinary output of potassium. Injuries to the frontal lobes are particularly associated with this condition (HIGGINS et al. 1951, GORDON and GOLDNER 1957) but the pathogenesis is far from clear. Dehydration may be a factor for reasons given above and the observed changes could occur through severe water depletion resulting in the „reaction of dehydration" (ELKINTON and TAFFEL 1942). There is frequently excessive protein catabolism and urea production in cerebral injuries which will tend to promote osmotic diuresis and further water loss. A possible explanation of this "reaction of dehydration" may be activation of the extracellular volume regulating mechanism leading to increased secretion of aldosterone, sodium retention and raised potassium excretion. In addition a diabetes insipidus state or impairment of the normal thirst mechanism, secondary to the cerebral injury, may be a major factor in the genesis of the dehydration (ALLOTT 1957; ENGSTROM and LIEBMAN 1953). However, not all cases show dehydration, and some show a raised rather than lowered urinary specific gravity, so that in these some other explanation must be sought (HIGGINS et al. 1951; NATELSON and ALEXANDER 1955; LEVITT, BELSKY and POLIMEROS 1959; METZ and COOPER 1958). The suggestion has been made that the set of the osmoregulatory centre has been altered by the cerebral damage, and it is interesting to note that attempts to reduce the serum sodium level by sodium restriction may result in symptoms of sodium depletion before the normal blood level has been reached.

Hyponatraemia with hypernatriuria. Attention was first drawn to this complication of cerebral injury by WELT et al. (1952) and later by HIGGINS et al. (1954) and CORT (1954), and to it the term "cerebral-salt-wasting" has been applied. The condition comes on insidiously, is rather chronic and not infrequently fatal. The serum sodium level is depressed below 130 mEq/l. whereas the urinary sodium is greater than 20 mEq/l. and may even exceed 100 mEq/l. The blood urea level is normal and there is a high urinary output of potassium. The patients reported earlier were dehydrated and resembled Addison's disease in some respects, but the serum potassium was normal or reduced, and the blood sugar level not depressed. The dehydration could be overcome by a high sodium chloride intake, but the hyponatraemia persistend even though sodium repletion was forced to the extent of oedema formation. Deoxycortone and cortisone were either ineffective or produced sodium retention without any change in the hyponatraemia. The mechanism of this disturbance is unknown although it has been suggested (WELT et al. 1952) that there may be impairment of proximal tubular reabsorption of sodium with consequent osmotic diuresis in the distal tubule and the excretion of a dilute urine containing sodium. This may be related to the salt losing state produced in dehydrated dogs after renal denervation (KAPLAN and RAPOPORT 1947), and it is interesting that in the case reported by CORT (1954) the lesion was restricted to the posterior part of the thalamus where it would interrupt the descending fibres of both the anterior and posterior parts of the hypothalamus. Cort suggested that there might be a nervous connection between the hypothalamus and the proximal tubules of the kidney influencing electrolyte reabsorption. The pathogenesis of "cerebral salt-wasting" is complicated by the fact that a number of patients have now been described in whom hyponatraemia and hypernatriuria was unaccompanied by dehydration. These patients suffered from diverse conditions including cerebral injuries, cerebrovascular lesions with infarction, subarachnoid haemorrhage and pituitary tumours (CARTER, RECTOR and SELDIN 1959; EPSTEIN and LEVITIN 1959; ROBERTS 1959; GOLDBERG and HANDLER 1960; VAN'T HOFF and ZILVA 1961). This disorder strikingly resembles the hyponatraemia reported in patients with bronchogenic carcinoma (SCHWARTZ et al. 1957; SCHWARTZ, TASSAL and BARTTER 1960). The symptoms in both are mainly those of water intoxication. Dehydration does not occur and consequently symptoms from hypovolaemia are absent. The disturbance has been attributed to inappropriate hypersecretion of anti-diuretic hormone, but verification of this is still lacking.

Respiratory alkalosis. When there is brain-stem damage with periodic breathing in which hyperpnoea exceeds hypopnoea, a respiratory alkalosis results with lowered plasma bicarbonate and raised chloride. Urinary chloride excretion is decreased and the urine is alkaline in reaction.

Acute anuria. Acute anuria, presumably arising from acute renal ischaemia, may complicate cerebral as well as any other form of trauma. Under these circumstances the rate of rise of blood urea through excess protein catabolism is particularly severe, and conservative treatment with protein sparing diets is relatively ineffective (TAYLOR 1957).

Reversal of diurnal urinary excretory rhythm. Reversal of the normal diurnal rhythm of urine excretion, resulting in nocturnal diuresis of water and sodium, has been reported following a head injury (PAYNE and DE WARDENER 1958). This condition may possibly be a manifestation of delayed water diuresis such as may be observed in patients with suprasellar tumours despite replacement doses of adrenal steroids (MARKS and HORNABROOK 1960).

References

ADDIS, T.: Glomerular nephritis — diagnosis and treatment. New York: Macmillan Co. 1949.
— E. BARRETT, L. J. POO, H. J. UREEN and R. W. LIPPMAN The relation between protein consumption and diurnal variations of endogenous creatinine clearance in normal individuals. J. clin. Invest. **30**, 206 (1951).
— — — and D. W. YUEN: The relation between the serum urea concentration and the protein consumption of normal individuals. J. clin. Invest. **26**, 869 (1947).
ALBRIGHT, F., W. BAUER, M. ROPES and J. C. AUB: Studies of calcium and phosphorus metabolism. IV. The effect of parathyroid hormone. J. clin. Invest. **7**, 139 (1929).
— C. H. BURNETT, W. PARSON, E. C. REIFENSTEIN jr. and A. ROOS: Osteomalacia and late rickets. The various etiologies met in the United States with emphasis on that resulting from a specific form of renal acidosis, the therapeutic indications for each etiological subgroup and the relationship between osteomalacia and Milkman's syndrome. Medicine (Baltimore) **25**, 399 (1946).
—, and E. C. REIFENSTEIN: The parathyroid glands and metabolic bone disease. Baltimore, Md.: Williams & Wilkins Company 1948.
ALEXANDER, H. B., J. DE J. PEMBERTON, E. J. KEPLER and A. C. BRODERS: Functional parathyroid tumours and hyperparathyroidism. Amer. J. Surg. **65**, 157 (1944).
ALEXANDER, J. D., E. D. PELLEGRINO, S. J. FARBER and D. P. EARLE: Observations on the relation of renal function changes to the electrolyte and glycosuric effects of A.C.T.H. in man. Endocrinology **49**, 136 (1951).
ALLBUTT, T. C.: Senile plethora or high arterial pressure in elderly persons. Abstracts Trans. Hunter. Soc. **77**, 38 (1895/96).
ALLISON, P. R.: Results of transplantation of ureters more than a quarter of a century after operation. Brit. J. Surg. **20**, 529 (1933).
ALLOTT, E. N.: Hypernatraemia and hyperchloraemia in bulbar poliomyelitis. Lancet **1957 I**, 246.
ANDERSON, I. A., A. MILLER and A. P. KENNY: Osteomalacia and renal glycosuria in adults. Quart. J. Med. **21**, 33 (1952).
ANDERSON, W. A. D., and W. R. BETHEA: Renal lesions following administration of hypertonic solutions of sucrose. J. Amer. med. Ass. **114**, 1983 (1940).
ANDERSSON, B., and S. M. MCCANN: Drinking, antidiuresis and milk ejection from electrical stimulation within the hypothalamus of the goat. Acta physiol. scand. **35**, 191 (1955).
ANNIS, D., and M. K. ALEXANDER: Differential absorption of electrolytes from the large bowel in relation to uretero-sigmoid anastomosis. Lancet **1952 II**, 603.
ASSCHER, A. W., and S. G. ANSON: A vascular permeability factor of renal origin. Nature (Lond.) **98**, 1097 (1963).
AUGUST, J. T., D. H. NELSON and G. W. THORN: Response of normal subjects to large amounts of aldosterone. J. clin. Invest. **37**, 1549 (1958).

BAINES, G. H., J. P. BARCLAY and W. T. COOKE: Nephrocalcinosis associated with hyper-
    chloraemia and low plasma bicarbonate. Quart. J. Med. 14, 113 (1945).
BARKER, E. S., R. B. SINGER, J. R. ELKINTON and J. K. CASH: The renal response in man
    to acute experimental respiratory alkalosis and acidosis. J. clin. Invest. 36, 515 (1957).
BARLOW, E. D., and H. E. DE WARDENER: Compulsive water drinking. Quart. J. Med. 28,
    235 (1959).
BARNES, B. A., O. COPE and T. HARRISON: Magnesium conservation in the human being on a
    low magnesium diet. J. clin. Invest. 37, 430 (1958).
BARNETT, H. L., C. W. FORMAN, H. MCNAMARA, W. W. MCCRORY, M. RAPOPORT, A. J.
    MICHIE and G. BARBERO: The effect of adrenocorticotrophic hormone in children with the
    nephrotic syndrome. J. clin. Invest. 30, 227 (1951).
— D. J. SIMONS and R. E. WELLS jr.: Nephrotic syndrome occurring during tridion therapy.
    Amer. J. Med. 4, 760 (1948).
BARTTER, F. C.: The rôle of aldosterone in normal homeostasis and in certain disease states.
    Metabolism 5, 369 (1956).
— and E. G. BIGLIERI: Primary aldosteronism. Ann. intern. Med. 48, 647 (1958).
— I. H. MILLS and D. S. GANN: Increase in aldosterone secretion by carotid artery constric-
    tion in the dog and its prevention by thyrocarotid arterial junction denervation. J. clin.
    Invest. 39, 1330 (1960).
BEARN, A. G.: Genetic and biochemical aspects of Wilson's disease. Amer. J. Med. 15, 442
    (1953).
— Renal function in Wilson's disease. Amer. J. Med. 22, 747 (1957).
BELL, E. T.: Renal diseases, 2nd edit. Philadelphia: Lea & Febiger 1950.
BERGLIN, T., and W. MATHISEN: Electrolyte imbalance following ureterocolic anastomosis.
    Acta chir. scand. 104, 130 (1952).
BERLINER, R. W.: Renal secretion of potassium and hydrogen ions. Fed. Proc. 11, 695 (1952).
— T. J. KENNEDY jr., and J. ORLOFF: Relationship between acidification of the urine and
    potassium metabolism. Amer. J. Med. 11, 274 (1951).
BERLYNE, G. M.: Distal tubular function in chronic hydronephrosis. Quart. J. Med. 30, 339
    (1961).
BERNER, A.: Les osteodystrophies d'origine renale. Étude systematique du squelette dans
    138 cas de maladies renales. Helv. med. Acta 11, 751 (1944).
BERNSTEIN, L. M., E. F. FOLEY and W. HOFFMAN: Renal function during and after diabetic
    coma. J. clin. Invest. 31, 711 (1952).
BICKEL, H.: Die Entwicklung der biochemischen Liaison bei der Lignac-Fanconischen Krank-
    heit. Helv. paediat. Acta 10, 259 (1955).
— H. S. BAAR, R. ASKEY, A. A. DOUGLAS, E. FINCH, H. HARRIS, G. G. C. HARVEY, E. M.
    HICKMANS, M. G. PHILPOT, W. C. SMALLWOOD, J. M. SMELLIE and C. E. TULL: Cystine
    storage disease with aminoaciduria and dwarfism (Lignac-Fanconi disease). Acta paediat.
    (Supp. 90), 42, 1 (1952).
—, and E. M. HICKMANS: Paper chromatographic investigation on the urine of patients. Arch.
    Dis. Childh. 27, 348 (1952).
—, and J. M. SMELLIE: Cystine storage disease with amino-aciduria: preliminary communica-
    tion. Lancet 1952 I, 1093.
—, and D. C. THURSBY-PELHAM: Hyperaminoaciduria in Lignac Fonconi disease, in galactos-
    aemia and in an obscure syndrome. Arch. Dis. Childh. 29, 224 (1954).
BING, J.: Studies on proteinuria. Acta med. scand., Suppl. 1, 76, 1 (1936).
BIRCHALL, R., H. M. BATSON and W. BRANNAN: Contribution of differential renal studies to
    the diagnosis of renal arterial hypertension with emphasis on the value of U sodium/
    U creatinine. Amer. J. Med. 32, 164 (1962).
BLACK, D. A. K.: Azotaemia in gastro-duodenal haemorrhage. Quart. J. Med., N.S. 11, 77
    (1942).
—, and E. W. EMERY: Tubular secretion of potassium. Brit. med. Bull. 13, 7 (1957).
—, and M. D. MILNE: Experimental potassium depletion in man. Lancet 1952 I, 244.
— R. PLATT, E. N. ROWLANDS and H. VARLEY: Renal haemodynamics in acute nephritis.
    Clin. Sci. 6, 295 (1948).
—, and R. T. WILLIAMS: The use of hypertonic saline in patients with renal failure. Quart.
    J. Med. 31, 57 (1962).
BLACKALL, J.: Observations on the nature and cure of dropsies, p. 121. London: Longman
    1813.
BLAINEY, J. D.: High protein diets in the treatment of the nephrotic syndrome. Clin. Sci.
    13, 567 (1954).
BLAINEY, J., D. BREWER, J. HARDWICKE and J. SOOTHILL: The nephrotic syndrome: diag-
    nosis by renal biopsy and biochemical and immunological analyses related to the response
    to steroid therapy. Quart. J. Med., N.S. 29, 249 (1960).

BLAKE, W. D., R. WEGRIA, H. P. WARD and C. W. FRANK: Effect of renal artery constriction on excretion of sodium and water. Amer. J. Physiol. 163, 422 (1950).

BLALOCK, A., and S. E. LEVY: Studies on the aetiology of renal hypertension. Ann. Surg. 106, 826 (1937).

BLUEMLE jr., L. W., H. P. POTTER and J. R. ELKINGTON: Changes in body composition in acute renal failure. J. clin. Invest. 35, 1094 (1956).

— G. D. WEBSTER and J. R. ELKINGTON: Acute tubular necrosis. Arch. intern. Med. 104, 180 (1951).

BOEMINGHAUS, H., and F. J. GOTZEN: Partieller Niereninfarkt und Hochdruck als Folge der Unterbindung akressorischer Gefäße. Medizinische 1952, 681.

BOLOMEY, A. A., A. J. MICHIE, C. MICHIE, E. S. BREED, G. E. SCHREINER and H. D. LAWSON: Simultaneous measurement of effective renal blood flow and cardiac output in resting normal subjects and patients with essential hypertension. J. clin. Invest. 28, 10 (1949).

BOLTE, E., M. VERDY, J. MARCAURELE, J. BROUILLET, P. BEAUREGARD and J. GENEST: Studies on new diuretic compounds: spirolactone and chlorothiazide. Canad. med. Ass. J. 79, 881 (1958).

BORST, J. R.: Disturbances in water and salt metabolism in the final stage of chronic renal insufficiency. Acta med. scand. 136, 1 (1950).

BOYCE, W. H., F. K. GARVEY and C. M. NORFLEET: Proteins and other biocolloids of urine in health and in calculous disease. J. clin. Invest. 33, 1287 (1954).

BOYD, J. D.: Chronic acidosis secondary to ureteral transplantation. Amer. J. Dis. Child. 42, 366 (1931).

BOYLAN, J. W., and E. ASSHAUER: Quoted by Kramer in „shock", p. 143 (1962).

BRADLEY, S. E.: The pathologic physiology of uraemia in chronic Bright's disease. Springfield, Illinois: Ch. C. Thomas 1948a.

— Physiology of essential hypertension. Amer. J. Med. 4, 398 (1948b).

— Acute diffuse glomerulonephritis. Amer. J. Med. 7, 382 (1949).

— G. P. BRADLEY, C. J. TYSON, J. J. CURRY and W. D. BLAKE: Renal function in renal diseases. Amer. J. Med. 9, 766 (1950).

BRAUN-MENENDEZ, E., J. L. FASCIOLO, C. F. LELOIR and J. M. MUNOZ: The substance causing renal hypertension. J. Physiol. (Lond.) 98, 283 (1940).

—, and I. H. PAGE: Suggested revision of nomenclature-angiotensin. Science 127, 242 (1958).

BRICKER, N. S., D. R. DEWEY, H. LUBOWITZ, J. STOKES and T. KIRKENSGAARD: Observations on the concentrating and diluting mechanisms of the diseased kidneys. J. clin. Invest. 38, 516 (1959).

— P. A. MORRIN and S. W. KIME jr.: The pathologic physiology of chronic Bright's disease. An exposition of the "intact nephron hypothesis". Amer. J. Med. 28, 77 (1960).

— E. I. SHWAYRI, J. B. REARDAN, D. KELLOG, J. P. MERRILL and J. H. HOLMES: An abnormality in renal function resulting from urinary tract obstruction. Amer. J. Med. 23, 554 (1957).

BRIGHT, R.: Reports of medical cases selected with a view of illustrating the symptoms and cure of disease by a reference to morbid anatomy. London: Longmans 1827.

— Tabular view of the morbid appearances in 100 cases connected with albuminous urine: with observations. Guy's Hosp. Rep. 1, 396 (1836).

BROD, J.: Chronic pyelonephritis. Lancet 1956 I, 973.

— Klinicky obraz, diferencialni diagnoza a terapie chronicke pyelonefritidy. Čas. Lék. čes. 98, 449 (1959). Quoted in: Renal disease by D. A. K. BLACK, p. 294. Oxford: Blackwell 1962.

— In: The pathogenesis of essential hypertension. Proceedings of Prague Symposiom 1961 (State Medical Publishing House).

— V. FENCL, L. HEJL, J. JIRKA and M. ULRYCH: General and regional haemodynamic pattern underlying essential hypertension. Clin. Sci. 23, 339 (1962).

BROOKS, R. V., R. R. MCSWINEY, F. T. G. PRUNTY and F. J. Y. WOOD: Potassium deficiency of renal and adrenal origin. Amer. J. Med. 23, 391 (1957).

BROWN, J. J., K. OWEN, W. S. PEART, J. I. S. ROBERTSON and D. SUTTON: The diagnosis and treatment of renal artery stenosis. Brit. med. J. 1960 II, 327.

BRUN, C., and O. MUNCK: Lesions of the kidney in acute renal failure following shock. Lancet 1957 I, 603.

BUCHEM, F. S. P. VAN, H. DOORENBOS and H. S. ELINGS: Primary aldosteronism due to adrenocortical hyperplasia. Lancet 1956 II, 335.

BULL, G. M.: Postural proteinuria. Clin. Sci. 7, 77 (1948/49).

— Uraemias. Lancet 1955 I, 731, 777.

— A. B. CARTER and K. J. LOWE: Hyperpotassaemic paralysis. Lancet 1953 II, 60.

— A. M. JOEKES and K. J. LOWE: Renal function studies in acute tubular necrosis. Clin. Sci. 9, 379 (1950).

BURBANK, M. K., J. C. HUNT, W. N. TAUXE and F. T. MAHER: Radioisotopic renography in evaluating hypertensive patients for renal arterial disease. Circulation **24**, 898 (1961).

BURNETT, C. H.: Actions of A.C.T.H. and cortisone on renal function in man. Trans. Conf. on renal function, p. 106. New York: Josiah Macey jr., Foundation 1950.

— B. A. BURROWS and R. R. COMMONS: Studies of alkalosis, renal function during and following alkalosis resulting from pyloric obstruction. J. clin. Invest. **29**, 169 (1950).

BURPUS, F. M., H. SCHWARZ and I. H. PAGE: Partial separation of the oxytocic principle from preparation of angiotensin. Circulat. Res. **4**, 488 (1956).

BUTLER, A. M.: Chronic pyelonephritis and arterial hypertension. J. clin. Invest. **16**, 889 (1937).

— L. L. WILSON and S. FARBER: Dehydration and acidosis with calcification of renal tubules. J. Pediat. **8**, 489 (1936).

BUTLER, E. A., and F. V. FLYNN: The proteinuria of renal tubular disorders. Lancet **1958 II**, 978.

BYROM, F. B.: The pathology of hypertensive encephalopathy and its relation to the malignant phase of hypertension. Lancet **1954 II**, 201.

— The nature of malignancy in hypertensive disease. Lancet **1963 I**, 516.

—, and L. F. DODSON: The mechanism of the vicious circle in chronic hypertension. Clin. Sci. **8**, 1 (1949).

BYWATERS, E. G. L., and D. BEALL: Crush injuries with impairment of renal function. Brit. med. J. **1941 I**, 427.

CAFFEY, J.: Lead poisoning associated with active rickets; report of a case with absence of lead lines in the skeleton. Amer. J. Dis. Child. **55**, 798 (1938).

CARGILL, W. H.: The measurement of glomerular and tubular plasma flow in the normal and diseased human kidney. J. clin. Invest. **28**, 533 (1949).

CARPENTER, C. C. J., J. O. DAVIS and C. R. AYERS: Concerning the rôle of arterial baroreceptors in the control of aldosterone secretion. J. clin. Invest. **40**, 1160 (1961a).

— — — Relation of renin, angiotensin II and experimental renal hypertension to aldosterone secretion. J. clin. Invest. **40**, 2026 (1961b).

CARTER, C., and M. SIMPKISS: The "carrier" state in nephrogenic diabtes insipidus. Lancet **1956 II**, 1069.

CARTER, N. W., F. C. RECTOR jr., and D. W. SELDIN: Pathogenesis of persistent hyponatraemia with water retention in cerebral disease. Clin. Res. **7**, 273 (1959).

CHANUTIN, A., and E. B. FERRIS: Experimental renal insufficiency produced by partial nephrectomy. Arch. intern. Med. **49**, 767 (1932).

CHAPLIN, H., and P. L. MOLLISON: Red sell life-span in nephritis and in hepatic cirrhosis. Clin. Sci. **12**, 351 (1953).

CHEYNE, A. I., and T. P. WHITEHEAD: Thorn's syndrome following excessive ingestion of alkalis. Lancet **1954 I**, 550.

CLARKE, E., B. M. EVANS, I. MACINTYRE and M. D. MILNE: Acidosis in experimental electrolyte depletion. Clin. Sci. **14**, 421 (1955).

CLARKSON, T. A., and J. E. KENCH: Urinary excretion of aminoacids by men absorbing heavy metals. Biochem. J. **62**, 361 (1956).

CLAY, R. D., E. M. DARMADY and M. HAWKINS: The nature of the renal lesion in the Fanconi syndrome. J. Path. Bact. **65**, 551 (1953).

CLAYTON, B. E., and A. D. PATRICK: Use of dimercaprol or penicillamine in the treatment of cystinosis. Lancet **1961 II**, 909.

COCKAYNE, E., and F. P. LEE LANDER: Rickets following an attack of acute nephritis. Arch. Dis. Childh. **7**, 321 (1932).

COHEN, S. I., M. G. FITZGERALD, P. FOURMAN, W. J. GRIFFITHS and H. E. DE WARDENER: Polyuria in hyperparathyroidism. Quart. J. Med., N.S. **26**, 423 (1957).

CONN, J. W.: Presidential address: painting background; primary aldosteronism, new clinical syndrome. J. Lab. clin. Med. **45**, 3 (1955a).

— Primary aldosteronism; a new clinical syndrome. J. Lab. clin. Med. **45**, 661 (1955b).

— Aldosterone in clinical medicine — past, present and future. Arch. intern. Med. **97**, 135 (1956).

— Aldosteronism and hypertension. Arch. intern. Med. **107**, 813 (1961).

CONNOR, T. B., W. C. THOMAS, L. HADDOCK and J. E. HOWARD: Unilateral renal disease as a cause of hypertension: its detection by uretheral catheterization studies. Ann. intern. Med. **52**, 544 (1960).

COOK, W. F., and G. W. PICKERING: The location of renin within the kidney. J. Physiol. (Lond.) **143**, 78P (1958).

COOPER, A. M., R. D. ECKHARDT, W. W. FALOON and C. S. DAVIDSON: Investigation of the aminoaciduria of Wilson's disease (hepato-lenticular degeneration). Demonstration of a defect in renal function. J. clin. Invest. **29**, 265 (1950).

CORDONNIER, J. J., and W. J. LAGE: An evaluation of ureterosigmoid anastomosis by mucosa to mucosa method after two and a half years experience. J. Urol. (Baltimore) 66, 565 (1951).

CORT, J. H.: Cerebral salt wasting. Lancet 1954 I, 752.

COUNIHAN, T. B., B. M. EVANS and M. D. MILNE: Observations on the pharmacology of the carbonic anhydrase inhibitor Diamox. Clin. Sci. 13, 583 (1954).

CRAIG, J. M., and R. SCHWARTZ: Histochemical study of the kidney of rats fed with diet deficient in potassium. Arch. Path. 64, 245 (1957).

CRAWFORD, T., C. E. DENT, P. LUCAS, N. H. MARTIN and J. M. NASSIM: Osteosclerosis associated with chronic renal failure. Lancet 1954 II, 981.

CREEVY, C. P., and M. P. RIESSER: Observations on reabsorption of urinary constituents after ureterosigmoidostomy; the importance of renal damage. Surg. Gynec. Obstet. 95, 589 (1952).

CROFTON, J., and L. TRUELOVE: Apparent acute glomerulonephritis without albuminuria. Lancet 1948 II, 54.

CUSHNY, A. K.: The secretion of the urine, 2nd edn., p. 243. London: Longmans 1926.

CUSHWORTH, D. C., C. E. DENT and F. V. FLYNN: The aminoaciduria in galactosaemia. Arch. Dis. Childh. 30, 150 (1955).

DAHL, L. K.: Possible rôle of salt intake in the development of essential hypertension. In: Essential Hypertension. Berlin-Göttingen-Heidelberg: Springer 1960.

DAMESHEK, W.: Biopsy of sternal bone marrow: its value in study of diseases of blood-forming organs. Amer. J. med. Sci. 190, 617 (1935).

DAMON, A., D. A. HOLUB, M. M. MELICOW and A. C. USON: Polycythaemia and renal carcinoma. Amer. J. Med. 25, 182 (1958).

DAVIES, D. F., and N. W. SHOCK: Age changes in glomerular filtration rate, effective renal plasma flow and tubular excretory capacity in adult males. J. clin. Invest. 29, 496 (1950).

DAVIES, H. E. F., B. EVANS, H. M. N. REES and P. FOURMAN: The defective absorption of phosphorus and calcium and the effect of Vitamin D in the Fanconi syndrome. Guy's Hosp. Rep. 107, 486 (1958).

DAVIS, J. O., C. R. AYERS and C. C. J. CARPENTER: Renal origin of an aldosterone-stimulating hormone in dogs with thoracic caval constriction and in sodium depleted dogs. J. clin. Invest. 40, 1466 (1961).

— C. C. J. CARPENTER, C. R. AYERS, J. E. HOLMAN and R. C. BAHN: Evidence for secretion of an aldosterone-stimulating hormone by the kidney. J. clin. Invest. 40, 684 (1961).

DAVSON, H., and J. F. DANIELLI: The permeabilty of natural membranes, p. 118. Cambridge 1952.

DEANE, H. W., and G. M. C. MASSON Adrenal cortical changes in rats with various types of experimental hypertension. J. clin. Endocr. 11, 193 (1951).

DEDMON, R. E., and O. WRONG: Excretion of citrate in patients with renal tubular acidosis and nephrocalcinosis. J. Lab. clin. Med. 56, 802 (1960).

DEFAZIO, V., R. C. CHRISTENSEN, T. J. REGAN, L. J. BAER, Y. MORITA and H. K. HELLEMS: Circulatory changes in acute glomerulonephritis. Circulation 20, 190 (1959).

DENT, C. E.: Rickets and osteomalacia from renal tubular defects. J. Bone Jt Surg. 34 B, 266 (1952).

— In: Recent advances in renal failure, p. 197 (Ed. M. D. Milne). London: Pitman 1960.

— C. M. HARPER and G. R. PHILPOT: Treatment of renal-glomerular osteodystrophy. Quart. J. Med. 30, 1 (1961).

—, and H. HARRIS: Hereditary forms of rickets and osteomalacia. J. Bone Jt Surg. 38 B, 204 (1956).

—, and C. J. HODSON: Radiological changes associated with certain metabolic bone diseases. Brit. J. Radiol. 27, 605 (1954).

—, and G. A. ROSE: Aminoacid metabolism in cystinuria. Quart. J. Med. 20, 205 (1951).

—, and B. SENIOR: Studies on the treatment of cystinuria. Brit. J. Urol. 27, 317 (1955).

— — and J. M. WALSHE: The pathogenesis of cystinuria. Polarographic studies on the metabolism of sulphur containing amino acids. J. clin. Invest. 33, 1216 (1954).

DE WESSELOW, O. L. V. S., and W. A. R. THOMSON: Study of some serum electrolytes in hypertension. Quart. J. Med., N.S. 8, 361 (1939).

DEXTER, L., and F. W. HAYNES: Relation of renin to human hypertension with particular reference to eclampsia, pre-eclampsia and acute glomerulonephritis. Proc. Soc. exp. Biol. (N.Y.) 55, 288 (1944).

DONIACH, I.: Uraemic edema of lungs. Amer. J. Roentgenol. 58, 620 (1947).

DUNN, J. S., M. GILLESPIE and J. S. F. NIVEN: Renal lesions in two cases of the crush syndrome. Lancet 1941 II, 549.

DUSTAN, H. P., A. C. CORCORAN and I. H. PAGE: Renal function in primary aldosteronism. J. clin. Invest. 35, 1357 (1956).

EALES, L.: Nephrotic syndrome: aetiological considerations. S. Afr. J. Lab. clin. Med. 1, 135 (1955).

EARL, C. J., M. J. MOULTON and B. SELVERSTONE: Metabolism of copper in Wilson's disease in normal subjects; studies with Cu-64. Amer. J. Med. 17, 205 (1954).

EARLE, D. P., S. J. FARBER and J. D. ALEXANDER: Renal function and oedema in acute nephritis. J. clin. Invest. 29, 810 (1950).

— — — and E. D. PELLEGRINO: Renal function and electrolyte metabolism in acute glomerulonephritis. J. clin. Invest. 30, 421 (1951a).

— S. SHERRY, L. W. EICHNA and N. J. CONAM: Low potassium syndrome due to defective renal tubular mechanisms for handling potassium. Amer. J. Med. 11, 283 (1951b).

EARLE jr., D. P., J. V. TAGGART and J. A. SHANNON: Glomerulonephritis: A survey of functional organisation of the kidney in various stages of diffuse glomerulonephritis. J. clin. Invest. 23, 119 (1944).

EDELMAN, C. M., H. L. BARNETT and V. TROUPKOU: Renal concentrating mechanisms in newborn infants. Effects of dietary protein and water content, rôle of urea, and responsiveness to antidiuretic hormone. J. clin. Invest. 39, 1062 (1960).

EDMONDS, C. J.: An aldosterone antagonist and diuretics in the treatment of chronic oedema and ascites. Lancet 1960 I, 509.

— and G. M. WILSON: The action of hydroflumethazide in relation to adrenal steroids and potassium loss. Lancet 1960 I, 505.

EDVALL, C. A.: Influence of ureteral obstruction (hydronephrosis) on renal function in man. J. appl. Physiol. 14, 855 (1959).

ELKINTON, J. R., E. J. HUTH, G. D. WEBSTER and R. A. McCANCE: The renal excretion of hydrogen ion, in renal tubular acidosis. Amer. J. Med. 29, 554 (1960).

—, and M. TAFFEL: Prolonged water deprivation in the dog. J. clin. Invest. 21, 787 (1942).

ELLIOT, D. F., and W. S. PEART: The aminoacid sequence in hypertension. Biochem. J. 65, 246 (1957).

ELLIS, A.: Malignant hypertension. Lancet 1938 I, 977.

— Natural history of Bright's disease: clinical, histological and experimental observations. Lancet 1942 I, 1, 34 and 72.

ELLIS, L. B., and S. WEISS: The measurement of capillary pressure under natural conditions and after arteriolar dilatation in normal subjects and in subjects with aterial hypertension and arteriosclerosis. J. clin. Invest. 8, 47 (1929).

EMSLIE-SMITH, D., J. H. JOHNSTONE, M. B. THOMPSON and K. G. LOWE: Aminoaciduria in acute tubular necrosis. Clin. Sci. 15, 171 (1956).

ENGLE, R. L., and L. M. WALLIS: Multiple myeloma and the adult Fanconi syndrome. Report of a case with cyst like deposits in the tumour cells and in the epithelial cells of the kidney. Amer. J. Med. 22, 5 (1957).

ENGSTROM, W. W., and A. LIEBMAN: Chronic hyperosmolarity of body fluids with cerebral lesion causing diabetes insipidus and anterior pituitary insufficiency. Amer. J. Med. 15, 180 (1953).

ENTICKNAP, J. B.: Condition of kidneys in salt-losing nephritis. Lancet 1952 II, 458.

EPSTEIN, A. A.: Concerning the causation of edema in chronic parenchymatous nephritis: method for its alleviation. Amer. J. med. Sci. 154, 638 (1917).

EPSTEIN, F. H., and H. LEVITIN: "Cerebral salt-wasting": an example of sustained inappropriate release of antidiuretic hormone. J. clin. Invest. 38, 1001 (1959).

EVANS, B. M., N. C. HUGHES-JONES, M. D. MILNE and S. STEINER: Electrolyte excretion during experimental potassium depletion in man. Clin. Sci. 13, 305 (1954).

—, and M. D. MILNE: Potassium-losing nephritis presenting as a case of periodic paralysis. Brit. med. J. 1954 II, 1067.

FANCONI, A., and G. A. ROSE: Ionised, complexed and protein-bound fractions of calcium in plasma. Quart. J. Med., N.S. 27, 463 (1958).

FANCONI, G.: Die nicht diabetischen Glykosurien und hyperglykämien des älteren Kindes. Jb. Kinderheilk. 133, 257 (1931).

— Der nephrotisch-glykosurische Zwergwuchs mit hypophosphatämischer Rachtitis. Dtsch. med. Wschr. 62, 1169 (1936a).

— Der frühinfantile nephrotisch-glykosurische Zwergwuchs mit hypophosphatämischer Rachitis. Jb. Kinderheilk. 147, 259 (1936b).

FERRIS, D. V., and H. M. ODEL: The electrolyte pattern of the blood after bilateral ureterosigmoidoscopy. J. Amer. med. Ass. 142, 634 (1950).

FISHBERG, A. M.: Hypertension and nephritis. London: Bailliere, Tindall & Cox 1954.

FLAX, L. J., and I. GERSH: Congenital renal tubular dysfunction (nephrogenic diabetes insipidus). Amer. J. Dis. Child. 89, 602 (1955).

FLETCHER, R. F., A. A. HENLY, H. G. SAMMONS and J. R. SQUIRE: A case of magnesium deficiency following massive intestinal resection. Lancet 1960 I, 522.

FLOYER, M. A.: The effect of nephrectomy and adrenalectomy upon the blood pressure of hypertensive and normotensive rats. Clin. Sci. 10, 405 (1951).
— Further studies on the mechanism of experimental hypertension in the rat. Clin. Sci. 14, 163 (1955).
— Rôle of the kidney in experimental hypertension. Brit. med. Bull. 13, 29 (1957).
FOLLIS jr., R. H.: Renal rickets and osteitis fibrosa in children and adolescents. Bull. Johns Hopk. Hosp. 87, 593 (1950).
—, and D. A. JACKSON: Renal osteomalacia and osteitis fibrosa in adults. Bull. Johns Hopk. Hosp. 72, 232 (1943).
— E. ORENT-KEILES and E. V. McCOLLUM: Production of cardiac failure and renal lesions in rats by diet extremely deficient in potassium. Amer. J. Path. 18, 28 (1942).
FOSS, G. L., C. B. PERRY and F. J. Y. WOOD: Renal tubular acidosis. Quart. J. Med. 25, 185 (1956).
FOURMAN, P.: Depletion of potassium induced in man with ion-exchange resin. Clin. Sci. 13, 93 (1954).
— Calcium metabolism and the bone, p. 79. Oxford; Blackwell 1960.
—, and G. R. HERVEY: An experimental study of oedema and potassium deficiency. Clin. Sci. 14, 75 (1955).
— R. A. McCANCE and R. A. PARKER: Renal disease in rats following a temporary deficiency of potassium. Brit. J. exp. Path. 37, 40 (1956).
— B. McCONKEY and J. W. G. SMITH: Defects of water reabsorption and of hydrogen-ion excretion by the renal tubules in hyperparathyroidism. Lancet 1960 I, 619.
FOWLER, D. I., H. HARRIS and F. L. WARREN: Plasma-cystine levels in cystinuria. Lancet 1952 I, 544.
FOX jr., C. L., and L. B. SLOBODY: Tissue changes in the nephrotic syndrome. Demonstration of potassium depletion. Paediatrics 7, 186 (1951).
FOYE jr., L. V., and T. V. FEICHTMEIR: Adrenal cortical carcinoma producing solely mineralocorticoid effect. Amer. J. Med. 29, 966 (1955).
FRANKLIN, S. S., and J. P. MERRILL: The kidney in health; the nephron in disease. Amer. J. Med. 28, 1 (1960a).
— — Acute renal failure. New Engl. J. Med. 262, 711, 761 (1960b).
— J. F. NIALL and J. P. MERRILL: The influence of solute load on the isosthenuria of renal disease. J. clin. Invest. 38, 1005 (1959).
FREIS, E. D.: Haemodynamics of hypertension. Phys. Rev. 40, 27 (1960).
FRICK, P. G., M. E. RUBINI and W. H. MERONEY: Recurrent nephrolithiasis associated with unusual tubular defect and hyperchloraemic acidosis. Amer. J. Med. 25, 590 (1958).
GARRETT, R. A., and J. H. MERTZ: Follow up studies of bladder extrophy with ureterosigmoidoscopy. J. Urol. (Baltimore) 71, 299 (1954).
GATZIMOS, C. D., D. M. SCHULZ and R. L. NEWNUM: Cystinosis (Lignac-Fanconi disease). Amer. J. Path. 31, 791 (1955).
GAUDINO, M., and M. F. LEVITT: Influence of the adrenal cortex on body water distribution and renal function. J. clin. Invest. 28, 1487 (1949).
GAUNT, R., A. A. RENZI and J. J. CHART: Aldosterone; a review. J. clin. Endocr. 15, 621 (1955).
GELLMAN, D. D., C. L. PIRANI, J. F. SOOTHILL, R. C. MUEHRCKE and R. M. KARK: Diabetic nephropathy; clinical and pathologic study based on renal biopsies. Medicine (Baltimore) 38, 321 (1959).
GENEST, J., P. BIRON, E. KOIW, W. NOWACZYNSKI, R. BOUCHER and M. CHRETIEN: Studies of the pathogenesis of human hypertension. The adrenal cortex and renal pressor mechanism. Ann. intern. Med. 55, 12 (1961a).
— — — — M. CHRETIEN and R. BOUCHER: Adrenocortical hormones in human hypertension and their relationship to angiotensin. Circulat. Res. 9, 775 (1961b).
— E. KOIW, P. BEAUREGARD, W. NOWACZYNSKI, T. SANDOR, J. BROUILLET, E. BOLTE, M. VERDY and J. MARC-AURELE: Electrolyte and corticosteroid studies in a 15 years old girl with primary aldosteronism and malignant hypertension. Metabolism 9, 624 (1960).
GILMOUR, J. R.: The parathyroid glands and skeleton in renal disease. London: Oxford Med. Pubs. 1947.
GITLIN, D., C. A. JANEWAY and L. E. FARR: Studies on the metabolism of plasma proteins in the nephrotic syndrome. J. clin. Invest. 35, 44 (1956).
GOIDSENHOVEN, I. VAN, and J. VANDENBROUCKE: Formes curables de l'hypertension renale chirurgicale ou urilogique (dix cas personnels). Presse méd. 54, 52 (1946).
GOLDBERG, M., and J. S. HANDLER: Hyponatraemia and renal wasting of sodium in patients with malformation of the central nervous system. New Engl. J. Med. 263, 1037 (1960).
GOLDBLATT, H.: Studies in experimental hypertension: production of persistent hypertension in monkeys by renal ischaemia. J. exp. Med. 65, 671 (1937a).

GOLDBLATT, H.: Studies in experimental hypertension: pathogenesis of hypertension due to renal ischaemia. Ann. intern. Med. 11, 69 (1937b).
— Studies in experimental hypertension. VII. The production of the malignant phase of hypertension. J. exp. Med. 67, 809 (1938).
— Renal origin of hypertension. Phys. Rev. 27, 120 (1947).
— J. R. KAHN and H. A. LEWIS: Studies in experimental hypertension; production of hypertension in sheep and goats. J. exp. Med. 77, 297 (1943).
— J. LYNCH, R. F. HANZAL and W. W. SUMMERVILLE: Studies in experimental hypertension; production of persistent elevation of systolic blood pressure by means of renal ischaemia. J. exp. Med. 59, 347 (1934).
GOLDMAN, R., and S. H. BASSETT: Phosphorus excretion in renal failure. J. clin. Invest. 33, 1623 (1954).
GOLDRING, W., and H. CHASIS: Hypertension and hypertensive diseases. New York: The Commonwealth Fund 1944.
— — H. A. RANGES and H. W. SMITH: Effective renal blood flow in subjects with essential hypertension. J. clin. Invest. 20, 637 (1941).
GOLDWASSER, E., and W. F. WHITE: Purification of sheep erythropoietin. Fed. Proc. 18, 236 (1959).
GOODWIN, J. F.: Mercurial diuretics and nephrosis. Brit. med. J. 1958 I, 1413.
GOORMAGHTIGH, N.: Existence of an endocrine gland in the media of the renal arterioles. Proc. Soc. exp. Biol. (N.Y.) 42, 688 (1939).
GORDON, G. L., and F. GOLDNER: Hypernatraemia, azotaemia and acidosis after cerebral injury. Amer. J. Med. 23, 543 (1957).
GOWENLOCK, A. H., and O. WRONG: Hyperaldosteronism secondary to renal ischaemia. Quart. J. M., N.S. 31, 323 (1962).
GRABER, I. G., and S. SEVITT: Renal function in burned patients. J. clin. Path. 12, 25 (1959).
—, and R. SHACKMAN: Divided renal function studies in hypertension. Brit. med. J. 1956 I, 1321.
GREY TURNER, G.: Transplantation of the ureter into the large bowel. Brit. med. J. 1943 I, 535.
GROLLMAN, A.: A simplified procedure for inducing chronic renal hypertension in the mammal. Proc. Soc. exp. Biol. (N.Y.) 57, 102 (1944).
— E. E. MUIRHEAD and J. VANATTA: Rôle of the kidney in the pathogenesis of hypertension as determined by study of bilateral nephrectomy and other procedures in the blood pressure of the dog. Amer. J. Physiol. 157, 21 (1949).
—, and C. RULE: Experimentally induced hypertension in parabiotic rats. Amer. J. Physiol. 138, 587 (1943).
GROLLMAN, E. F., and A. GROLLMAN: Toxicity of urea and its rôle in the pathogenesis of ureamia. J. clin. Invest. 38, 749 (1959).
GROSS, F.: Adrenocortical function and renal pressor mechanisms in experimental hypertension. In: Essential Hypertension, p. 92. Berlin-Göttingen-Heidelberg: Springer1960.
—, and W. D. DETTBARN: Water and salt loading in adrenalectomized dogs treated with cortexone, aldosterone and 9a-fluorocortisol: Acta endocr. (Kbh.) 22, 335 (1956).
— P. LOUSTALOT and R. MEIER: Production of experimental hypertension by aldosterone. Acta. endocr. (Kbh.) 26, 417 (1957).
GUTMAN, A. B., P. C. SWENSON and W. B. PARSONS: Differential diagnosis of hyperparathyroidism. J. Amer. med. Ass. 103, 87 (1934).
HAMBURGER, J., and G. MATHÉ: Fluid balance in anuria. Ciba Symposium on the kidney. London: Churchill 1954.
HANNA, S., and I. McINTYRE: The influence of aldosterone on magnesium metabolism. Lancet 1960 II, 348.
— K. A. K. NORTH, I. McINTYRE and R. FRASER: Magnesium metabolism in parathyroid disease. Brit. med. J. 1961 II, 1253.
HARDWICKE, J., and J. F. SOOTHILL: Glomerular damage and pore size. Ciba Symposium on Renal Biopsy. London: Churchill 1961.
— — J. R. SQUIRE and G. HOTT: The nephrotic syndrome with pollen hypersensitivity. Lancet 1959 I, 500.
—, and J. R. SQUIRE: The relationship between plasma albumin concentration and protein excretion in patients with proteinuria. Clin. Sci. 14, 509 (1955).
HARE, K., H. GOLDSTEIN, H. L. BARNETT, H. McNAMARA and R. S. HARE: Renal excretion of creatinine in man. Fed. Proc. 8, 67 (1949).
HARRIS, H.: Renal aminoaciduria. Brit. med. Bull. 13, 26 (1957).
— U. MITTWOCH, E. B. ROBSON and F. L. WARREN: The pattern of amino-acid excretion in cystinuria. Ann. hum. Genet. 19, 196 (1955a).
— — — — Phenotypes and genotypes in cystinuria. Ann. hum. Genet. 20, 57 (1955b).

HARRIS, H., and F. L. WARREN: Qualitative studies on the urinary cystine in patients with cystine stone formation and in their relatives. Ann. Eugen. (Lond.) 18, 125 (1953).

HARRISON, T. R., and M. F. MASON: Pathogenesis of the uraemic syndrome. Medicine (Baltimore) 16, 1 (1937).

HARTMANN, A. K.: Clinical studies in acidosis and alkalosis. Arch. intern. Med. 13, 940 (1939).

HARTROFT, P. M., and R. EDELMAN Renal juxtaglomerular cells in sodium deficiency. Hahnemann Symposium on oedema (Philadelphia) 1959, p. 63.

HARVARD, B. M., and G. J. THOMPSON: Congenital exstrophy of the urinary bladder; late results of treatment by the Coffey-Mayo method of ureterointestinal anastomosis. J. Urol. (Baltimore) 65, 223 (1951).

HAVARD, C. W. H., and P. H. N. WOOD: The effect of diuretics on renal water excretion in diabetes insipidus. Clin. Sci. 21, 321 (1961).

HAYNES, F. W., and L. DEXTER: Renin, hypertensinogen and hypertensinase concentration of the blood of dogs during the development of hypertension by constriction of the renal artery. Amer. J. Physiol. 150, 190 (1947).

HELMER, O. M.: Pressor substances in hypertension. In "Hypertension: Recent Advances". Philadelphia: Lea & Febiger 1961.

HERVEY, G. R., R. A. McCANCE and R. Q. C. TAYLOR: Forced diuresis during hydropenia. Nature (Lond.) 157, 1338 (1946).

HEWLETT, J. S., G. C. HOFFMAN, D. A. SENHAUSER and J. D. BATTLE jr.: Hypernephroma with erythrocythemia. Report of a case and assay of the tumour for an erythropoietic-stimulating substance. New Engl. J. Med. 262, 1058 (1960).

HIGGINS, G., W. LEWIN, J. R. P. O'BRIEN and W. H. TAYLOR: Metabolic disorders in head injury; hyperchloraemia and hypochloruria. Lancet 1951 I, 1295.

— — — — Metabolic disorders in head injury. Lancet 1954 I, 61.

HILDEN, P.: Diodrast clearance in acute nephritis. Acta med. scand. 116, 1 (1943).

HILDEN, T., and A. R. KROGSGAARD: Low serum potassium level in severe hypertension. Amer. J. med. Sci. 236, 487 (1958).

HILL, S. R., J. F. NICKERSON, S. B. CHENAULT, J. H. McNEIL, W. R. STARNES and B. S. GAUTNEY: Studies in man in hyper- and hypo-aldosteronism. Arch. intern. Med. 104, 982 (1959).

HODGKINSON, A.: Renal phosphate excretion indices in the diagnosis of hyperparathyroidism. Clin. Sci. 21, 125 (1961).

HOLZEL, A., G. M. KOMROWER and V. K. WILSON: Aminoaciduria in galactosaemia. Brit. med. J. 1952 I, 194.

HOWARD, J. E., M. BERTHRONG, R. D. SLOAN and E. R. YENDT: Relief of malignant hypertension by nephrectomy in four patients with unilateral renal disease. Trans. Ass. Amer. Phycns 66, 164 (1953).

—, and T. B. CONNOR: Hypertension produced by unilateral renal disease. Arch. intern. Med. 109, 8 (1962).

— — and W. C. THOMAS: A functional test for detection of hypertension produced by one kidney—preliminary studies. Trans. Ass. Amer. Phycns 69, 291 (1956).

HSIA, D. Y. Y., H. H. HSIA, S. GREEN, M. KAY and S. S. GELLIS: Aminoaciduria in galactosaemia. Amer. J. Dis. Child. 88, 458 (1954).

HUCHARD, H.: Traite clinique des maladies du cœur et de l'ororte. Paris 1899.

HUDSON, J. B., A. R. CHOBANIAN and A. S. RELMAN: Hypo-aldosteronism. A clinical study of a patient with an isolated adrenal mineralocorticoid deficiency, resulting in hyperkalaemia and Stokes-Adams attacks. New Engl. J. Med. 257, 529 (1957).

HULET, W. H., D. S. BALDWIN, A. W. BIGGS, E. A. GOMBOS and H. CHASIS: Renal function in the separate kidneys of man. J. clin. Invest. 39, 389 (1960).

HULTENGRUN, N.: Renal papillary necrosis. Acta chir. scand., Suppl 277 (1961).

HUNTER, R. B., and E. E. MUIRHEAD: Prolonged renal salt wasting. In: Lower nephron nephrosis. Ann. intern. Med. 36, 1297 (1952).

HUTH, E. J., G. D. WEBSTER and J. R. ELKINTON: The renal excretion of hydrogen ion in renal tubular acidosis. Amer. J. Med. 29, 586 (1960).

HUTT, M. S. R., J. L. PINNIGER and H. E. DE WARDENER: The relationship between the clinical and the histological features of acute glomerular nephritis. Quart. J. Med. 29, 265 (1958).

HYDE, R. D., R. Vaughan Jones, R. R. McSWINEY and F. T. G. PRUNTY: Investigation of hyperparathyroidism in the absence of bone disease (renal phosphorus threshold). Lancet 1960 I, 250.

IRVINE, W. T., C. M. ALLAN and D. R. WEBSTER: An experimental comparison of renal damage and electrolyte imbalance following various methods of urinary deviation. Surg. Forum 6, 593 (1956).

JACOBS, A., and W. B. STIRLING: Late results of ureterocolic anastomosis. Brit. J. Urol. 24, 259 (1952).

JACOBSON, L. O., E. GOLDWASSER, W. FRIED and L. PLZAK: Rôle of the kidney in erythropoiesis. Nature (Lond.) 179, 633 (1957).

JAENIKE, J. R., and C. WATERHOUSE: The renal response to sustained administration of vasopressin and water in man. J. clin. Endocr. 21, 231 (1961).

JAFFE, R. H., and H. STEINBERG: Über die vakuolare Nierendegeneration bei Chronische. Rhw. Virchows Arch. path. Anat. 227, 313 (1919).

JAMES, J., G. CORDILLO and J. METCOFF: Effects of infusion of hyperoncotic dextran in children with the nephrotic syndrome. J. clin. Invest. 33, 1346 (1954).

JENSEN, E. J., A. H. BAGGENSTOSS and J. A. BARGEN: Renal lesions associated with ulcerative colitis. Amer. J. med. Sci. 219, 281 (1950).

JEWELL, P. A., and E. B. VERNEY: An experimental attempt to determine the site of the neurohypophysial osmoreceptors in the dog. Phil. Trans. B 240, 197 (1957).

JOHNSON, B. B., A. H. LIEBERMAN and P. G. MULROW: Aldosterone excretion in normal subjects depleted of sodium and potassium. J. clin. Invest. 36, 757 (1957).

JOINER, C. L., and M. G. THORNE: Salt-losing nephritis. Lancet 1952 II, 454.

JONXIS, J. H. P.: Aminoaciduria and rickets. Helv. paediat. Acta 10, 245 (1955).

—, and T. H. J. HUISMAN: Aminoaciduria and ascorbic acid deficiency. Paediatrics 14, 238 (1954).

JOSKE, R. A., J. M. McALISTER and T. A. J. PRANKERD: Isotope investigations of red ceull production and destruction in chronic renal disease. Clin. Sci. 15, 511 (1956).

KAHN, J. R., L. T. SKEGGS, N. P. SHUMWAY and P. E. WISENBAUGH: Assay of hypertensin from the arterial blood of normotensive and hypertensive human beings. J. exp. Med. 195, 573 (1952).

KALCKAR, H. M., E. P. ANDERSON and K. J. ISSELBACHER: Galactosemia: a congenital defect in nucleotide transferase. Proc. nat. Acad. Sci. (Wash.) 42, 49 (1956).

KAPLAN, S. A., and S. RAPOPORT: Urinary excretion of sodium and chloride after splanchnicotomy; effect on the proximal tubule. Amer. J. Physiol. 164, 175 (1947).

KARK, R. M., C. L. PIRANI, V. E. POLLAK, R. C. MUEHRCKE and J. D. BLAINEY: The nephrotic syndrome in adults: A common disorder with many causes. Ann. intern. Med. 49, 751 (1958).

KEATING, R. E., T. E. WEICHSELBAIM, M. ALANIS, A. W. MARGRAF and R. ELMAN: The movement of potassium during experimental acidosis and alkalosis in the nephrectomised dog. Surg. Gynec. Obstet. 96, 323 (1953).

KEITH, N. M., and H. B. BURCHELL: Clinical intoxication with potassium, its occurrence in severe renal insufficiency. Amer. J. med. Sci. 217, 1 (1949).

KEKWICK, A., J. W. PAULLEY, E. W. RICHES and R. SEMPLE: Renal failure following ureterocaecostomy. Brit. J. Urol. 23, 112 (1951).

KENNEDY, A. C., A. C. LINTON and J. C. EATON: Urea levels in cerebro-spinal fluid after haemodialysis. Lancet 1962 I, 410.

KILEY, J. E., S. R. POWERS and R. T. BEEBE: Acute renal failure. New Engl. J. Med. 262, 481 (1960).

KIMMELSTIEL, P., and C. WILSON: Intercapillary lesions in the glomeruli of the kidney. Amer. J. Path. 12, 45 (1936).

KLEEMAN, C. R., W. L. HEWITT and L. B. GUZE: Pyelonephritis. Medicine (Baltimore) 39, 3 (1960).

KNOWLES jr., H. C., H. LEVITIN and H. BRIDGES: Salt losing nephritis with fixed urinary composition. Amer. J. Med. 22, 158 (1957).

KOHLSTAEDT, K. G., I. H. PAGE and O. M. HELMER: The activation of renin by blood. Amer. Heart J. 19, 92 (1948).

KOLFF, W. J.: Reduction of experimental renal hypertension by kidney perfusion. Circulation 17, 702 (1958).

—, and I. H. PAGE: Influence of protein and other factors on postnephrectomy hypertension in rats sustained with an improved method of peritoneal lavage. Amer. J. Physiol. 178, 69 (1954a).

— — Blood pressure reducing function of the kidney: reduction of renoprival hypertension by kidney perfusion. Amer. J. Physiol. 178, 75 (1954b).

— — Renoprival hypertension and antirenin. Amer. J. Physiol. 181, 575 (1955a).

— — Persistence of experimental renal hypertension after total nephrectomy in dog. Amer. J. Physiol. 182, 531 (1955b).

— — and A. C. CORCORAN: Pathogenesis of renoprival cardiovascular disease in dogs. Amer. J. Physiol. 178, 237 (1954).

KOMROWER, G. M.: L'amino-acidurie dans la galactosemie. Arch. f. Pediat. 10, 185 (1953).

KRAMER, K.: Renal failure in shock. In: Shock, ed. K. D. BOCK, p. 134. Berlin-Göttingen-Heidelberg: Springer 1962.
—, and P. DEETJEN: Beziehungen des O_2-Verbrauchs der Niere zu Durchblutung und Glomerulosfiltrat bei Änderung des arteriellen Druckes. Pflügers Arch. ges. Physiol. 271, 782 (1960).
— K. THURAU and P. DEETJEN: Hemodynamics of kidney medullary substance. Pflügers Arch. ges. Physiol. 270, 251 (1960).
LAMBREW, C. T., S. T. CARVER, R. T. PETERSON and M. MORWITH: Hypo-aldosteronism as a cause of hyperkalaemia and syncopal attacks in a patient with complete heart block. Amer. J. Med. 31, 81 (1961).
LAPIDES, J.: Mechanism of electrolyte imbalance following ureterosigmoid transplantation. Surg. Gynec. Obstet. 93, 691 (1951).
LARAGH, J. H.: Some effects of chlorothiazide on electrolyte metabolism and its use in edematous states. Ann. N.Y. Acad. Sci. 71, 419 (1958).
— The rôle of aldosterone in man. J. Amer. med. Ass. 174, 293 (1960).
— Relation of aldosterone secretion to hypertensive vascular disease. Circulat. Res. 9, 972 (1961).
— M. ANGERS, W. G. KELLY and S. LIEBERMAN: Hypotensive agents and pressor substances. The effect of epinephrine, norepinephrine, Angiotensin II and others on secretory rate of aldosterone in man. J. Amer. med. Ass. 174, 234 (1960a).
—, and H. C. STOERK: A study of the mechanism of secretion of the sodium-retaining hormone (aldosterone). J. clin. Invest. 36, 383 (1957).
— S. ULICK, V. JANUSZEWICZ, Q. B. DEMING, W. G. KELLY and S. LIEBERMAN: Aldosterone secretion and primary and malignant hypertension. J. clin. Invest. 39, 1091 (1960b).
LATNER, A. L., and E. B. BERNARD: Idiopathic hyperchloraemic renal acidosis of infants. Quart. J. Med. 19, 285 (1950).
LAUSON, H. D., S. E. BRADLEY and A. COURNAND: The renal circulation in shock. J. clin. Invest. 23, 381 (1944).
— C. W. FORMAN, H. MCNAMARA, G. MATTAR and H. L. BARNETT: The effect of corticotrophin (ACTH) on glomerular permeability to albumin in children with the nephrotic syndrome. J. clin. Invest. 33, 657 (1954).
LEAF, A., F. C. BARTTER, R. F. SANTOS and O. WRONG: Evidence in man that urinary electrolyte loss induced by pitressin is a function of water retention. J. clin. Invest. 32, 868 (1953).
—, and A. A. CAMARA: Renal tubular secretion of potassium in man. J. clin. Invest. 28, 1526 (1949).
—, and A. R. MAMBY: Antidiuretic mechanism not regulated by extracellular fluid tonicity. J. clin. Invest. 31, 60 (1952b).
LEAF, W., and A. R. MAMBY: Normal antidiuretic mechanism in man and dog: its regulation by extracellular fluid tonicity. J. clin. Invest. 31, 54 (1952a).
LEDINGHAM, J. M.: The nature of the hypertension occurring in the nephrectomised parabiotic rat. Clin. Sci. 10, 423 (1951).
— Tissue electrolytes in experimental hypertension. Ciba Foundation Symposium on Hypertension. London: Churchill 1954a.
— The influence of the adrenal on the water and electrolyte disturbances following nephrectomy and its relation to renoprival hypertension. Clin. Sci. 13, 535 (1954b).
LEVITT, M. F., M. BELSKY and D. POLIMEROS: Serum hypertonicity secondary to cerebral disease. Ann. intern. Med. 50, 788 (1959).
LEWIS, W. H., and A. S. ALVING: Changes with age in the renal function of adult man. I. Clearance of urea. II. Amount of urea nitrogen in the blood. III. Concentrating ability of the kidneys. Amer. J. Physiol. 123, 500 (1938).
LIDDLE, G. W.: Sodium diuresis induced by steroidal antagonists of aldosterone. Science 126, 1016 (1957).
— Aldosterone antagonists. Arch. intern. Med. 102, 998 (1958).
LIEBOW, A. A., W. MCFARLAND and R. TENNANT: The effects of potassium deficiency on tumour bearing mice. Yale J. Biol. Med. 13, 523 (1941).
LIGHTWOOD, R.: Calcium infarction of the kidneys in infants. Arch. Dis. Childh. 10, 205 (1935).
— Idiopathic hypocalcaemia with failure to thrive. Proc. roy. Soc. Med. 45, 397 (1952).
— W. W. PAYNE and J. A. BLACK: Infantile renal acidosis. Paediatrics 12, 628 (1953).
LIGNAC, G. O. E.: Über Störungen des Cystinstoffwechsels bei Kindern. Deutsch. Arch. klin. Med. 145, 139 (1924).
LINDENEG, O., S. FISCHER, J. PEDERSEN and N. J. NISSEN: Necrosis of the renal papillae and prolonged abuse of phenacetin. Acta med. scand. 165, 321 (1959).
LINDER, G. C., G. M. BULL and I. GRAYCE: Hypophosphataemic glycosuric rickets (Fanconi syndrome). Clin. Proc. 8, 1 (1949).

LIU, S. H., and H. I. CHU: Studies of calcium and phosphorus metabolism with special reference to pathogenesis and effect of dihydrotachysterol (AT 10) and iron. Medicine (Baltimore) 22, 103 (1943).

LOCKE, S., J. P. MERRILL, and R. H. TYLER: Neurologic complications of acute uraemia. Arch. intern. Med. 108, 519 (1961).

LOEB, R. F., D. W. ATCHLEY, E. M. BENEDICT and J. LELAND: Electrolyte balance studies in adrenalectomised dogs with particular reference to the excretion of sodium. J. exp. Med. 57, 775 (1933).

— — D. W. RICHARDS jr., E. M. BENEDICT and M. E. DRISCOLL: On the mechanism of nephrotic oedema. J. clin. Invest. 11 621 (1932).

LOUGHRIDGE, L. W., M. D. MILNE, R. SHACKMAN and I. D. P. WOOTON: The clinical course of uncomplicated tubular necrosis. Lancet 1960 II, 351.

LOWE, C. U., M. TERREY and E. A. MACLACHLAN: Organic aciduria, decreased renal ammonia production, hydrophthalma and mental retardation; clinical entity. Amer. J. dis. Child. 83, 164 (1952).

LOWE, K. G.: Late prognosis in acute tubular necrosis. Lancet 1952 I, 1086.

— G. MOODIE and M. B. THOMSON: Glycosuria in acute tubular necrosis. Clin. Sci. 13, 187 (1954).

LUCKE, B.: Lower nephron nephrosis. The renal lesion of the crush syndrome, of burns, transfusion and other conditions affecting the lower segments of the nephron. Milit. Surg. 99, 371 (1946).

LUETSCHER, J. A.: Problems of electrolyte and water balance in the nephrotic syndrome. Arch. intern. Med. 95, 380 (1955).

— Aldosterone. Adv. intern. Med. 8, 155 (1956).

— Q. B. DEMING and B. B. JOHNSON: The treatment of nephrosis with pituitary adrenocorticotropin. J. clin. Invest. 30, 1530 (1951).

— A. D. HALL and V. L. KREMER: Concentrated human serum albumin in nephrosis. II. J. clin. Invest. 29, 896 (1950).

—, and B. B. JOHNSON: Observations on the sodium-retaining corticoid (aldosterone) in the urine of children and adults in relation to sodium balance and oedema. J. clin. Invest. 33, 1441 (1954a).

— — Chromatographic separation of the sodium retaining corticoid from the urine of children with nephrosis. J. clin. Invest. 33, 276 (1954b).

MACDONALD, W. B.: Congenital pitressin resistant diabetes insipidus of renal origin. Paediatrics 15, 298 (1955).

MACLEAN, H., and O.L.V. DE WESSELOW: On the testing of renal efficiency, with observations on the 'urea coefficient'. Brit. J. exp. Path. 1, 53 (1920).

MACLEOD, M.: Systemic capillary pressure in acute glomerulonephritis estimated by direct micropuncture. Clin. Sci. 19, 27 (1960).

MADER, I. J., and L. T. ISERI: Spontaneous hypopotassemia, hypomagnesemia, alkalosis and tetany due to hypersecretion of corticosterone-like mineralocorticoid. Amer. J. Med. 19, 976 (1955).

MAHLER, R. F., and S. W. STANBURY: Potassium-losing renal disease. Quart. J. Med. 25, 21 (1956).

MAHONEY, J. P., A. A. SANDBERG, C. J. GUBLER, G. E. CARTWRIGHT and M. M. WINTROBE: Uric acid metabolism in hepatolenticular degeneration. Proc. Soc. exp. Biol. (N.Y.) 88, 427 (1955).

MARCHAND, J. F., and C. A. FINCH: Fatal spontaneous potassium intoxication in patients with uraemia. Arch. intern. Med. 73, 384 (1944).

MARKS, V., and R. W. HORNABROOK: Failure of cortisone to correct impaired water diuresis in patients with suprasellar tumours. Lancet 1960 II, 497.

MARRIOTT, H. L. L.: Some observations on the pathogenesis of cardiac oedema. Ann. intern. Med. 41, 377 (1954).

MARSHALL, D., and W. S. HOFFMAN: Nature of altered renal function in lower nephron nephrosis. J. Lab. clin. Med. 34, 31 (1949).

MASON, G. E.: Gastro-intestinal lesions occurring in uraemia. Ann. intern. Med. 37, 96 (1952).

MASTER, A. M., H. L. JAFFE and S. DACK: The heart in acute nephritis. Arch. intern. Med. 60, 1016 (1937).

McCALL, M. F.: Nephrotic syndrome in children treated with A.C.T.H. and cortisone. Arch. Dis. Childh. 27, 309 (1952).

McCANCE, R. A.: Osteomalacia with Looser's nodes (Milkman's syndrome) due to a raised resistance to vitamin D acquired about the age of 15 years. Quart J. Med. 16, 33 (1947).

— Renal physiology in infancy. Amer. J. Med. 9, 229 (1950).

—, and N. HATEMI: Control of acid-base stability in the newly born. Lancet 1961 I, 293.

McCANCE, R. A., and E. M. WIDDOWSON: Functional disorganisation of the kidney in disease. J. Physiol. (Lond.) 95, 36 (1939).
— — The correct physiological basis on which to compare infant and adult renal function. Lancet 1952 II, 860.
McGEOWN, M. G.: Normal standards of renal phosphate clearance and observations on calculus patients. Clin. Sci 16, 297 (1957).
—, and G. M. BULL: Pathogenesis of urinary calculus formation. Brit. med. Bull. 13, 53 (1957).
McINTOSH, J. F., R. MOLLER and D. D. VAN SLYKE: Studies of urea excretion. III. The influence of body size on urea output. J. clin. Invest. 6, 467 (1928).
McQUARRIE, I., W. H. THOMPSON and J. A. ANDERSON: Effects of excessive ingestion of sodium and potassium salts on carbohydrate metabolism and blood pressure in diabetic children. J. Nutr. 11, 77 (1936).
McQUEEN, E. G.: Quoted in Squire, J. R., J. HARDWICKE and J. F. SOOTHILL: "Proteinuria". In: Renal disease. Oxford: Ed. D. A. K. Black, Blackwell 1962.
MENDELSOHN, M. D., and O. H. PEARSON: Alterations in water and salt metabolism after bilateral adrenalectomy in man. J. clin. Endocr. 15, 409 (1955).
MENEELY, G. R., F. G. TUCKER, W. J. DARBY and S. H. AUERBACH: Chronic sodium chloride toxicity in albino rat; occurrence of hypertension and of syndrome of edema and renal failure. J. exp. Med. 98, 71 (1953).
MERRILL, A. J.: Edema and decreased renal blood flow in patients with chronic congestive heart failure: evidence of "forward failure" as primary cause of edema. J. clin. Invest. 25, 389 (1946).
—, and W. H. CARGILL: Effect of exercise on renal plasma flow and filtration rate of normal and cardiac subjects. J. clin. Invest. 27, 272 (1948).
MERRILL, J. P.: The treatment of renal failure. New York: Grune & Stratton 1955.
— C. GIORDANO and D. R. HEETDERKS: The rôle of the kidney in human hypertension. I. Failure of hypertension to develop in renoprival subjects. Amer. J. Med. 31, 931 (1961).
METZ, R. J. S., and W. COOPER: Salt retention and uraemia in brain injury. Lancet 1958 I, 435.
MILLER, J. H., and N. W. SHOCK: Age differences in the renal response to antidiuretic hormone. J. Gerontol. 8, 446 (1953).
MILLS, I. H., A. CASPER and F. C. BARTTER: On the rôle of the vagus in the control of aldosterone secretion. Science 128, 1140 (1958).
MILLS, J. N.: Aldosterone secretion in man. Brit. med. Bull. 18, 171 (1962).
MILNE, M. D.: Observations on the action of the parathyroid hormone. Clin. Sci. 10, 471 (1951).
— R. C. MUEHRCKE and I. AIRD: Primary aldosteronism: Quart. J. Med. 26, 317 (1957).
— — and B. E. HEARD: Potassium deficiency and the kidney. Brit. med. Bull. 13, 15 (1957).
— G. G. ROWE, K. SOMERS, R. C. MUEHRCKE and M. A. CRAWFORD: Observations on the pharmacology of mecamylamine. Clin. Sci. 16, 599 (1957).
— S. W. STANBURY and A. E. THOMSON: Observations on the Fanconi syndrome and renal hyperchloraemic acidosis in the adult. Quart. J. Med. 21, 61 (1952).
MITCHELL, A. G.: Nephrosclerosis (chronic interstitial nephritis) in childhood; with special reference to renal rickets. Amer. J. Dis. Child. 40, 101 and 345 (1930).
MOESCHLIN, S.: Phenacetinsucht und -schaden, Lungenkörperanämien und interstitielle Nephritis. Schweiz. med. Wschr. 87, 123 (1957).
MOVAT, H. L., J. W. STEINER and R. J. SLATER: Glomerular structure in Bright's disease. Ciba Symposium on Renal Biopsy. London: Churchill 1961.
MOYER, J. H., and L. C. MILLS: Hexamethonium — its effect on glomerular filtration rate, maximal tubular function and renal excretion of electrolytes. J. clin. Invest. 32, 172 (1953).
— G. C. MORRIS jr., and H. L. BEAZLEY: Renal haemodynamic response to vasopressor agents in the treatment of shock. Circulation 12, 96 (1955).
MUDGE, G. H.: Clinical patterns of tubular dysfunction. Amer. J. Med. 24, 785 (1958).
—, and I. M. WEINER: The mechanism of action of mercurial and xanthine diuretics. Ann. N.Y. Acad. Sci. 71, 344 (1958).
MUEHRCKE, R. C., R. M. KARK, C. I. PIRANI and V. E. POLLAK: Lupus nephritis: a clinical and pathologic study based on renal biopsies. Medicine (Baltimore) 36, 1 (1957).
MUELLER, C. B., A. SURTSHIN, M. R. CARLIN and H. L. WHITE: Glomerular and tubular influences on sodium and water excretion. Amer. J. Physiol. 165, 411 (1951).
MUIRHEAD, E. E., A. E. HALEY, S. HABERMAN and J. M. HILL: In: J. M. HILL and W. DAMESHEK, "Blood", special issue No 2. The Rh factor in the clinic and the laboratory, p. 101 (1948).
MUNCK, O.: Renal circulation in acute renal failure. Oxford: Blackwell 1958.
MURPHY, F. D., A. L. SETTIMI and N. J. KOZOKOFF: Renal disease with salt losing syndrome: report of 4 cases of so-called salt-losing nephritis. Ann. intern. Med. 38, 1160 (1953).

MURPHY, R. V., E. W. COFFMAN, B. H. PRINGLE and L. T. ISERI: Studies of sodium and potassium metabolism in salt-losing nephritis. Arch. intern. Med. **90**, 250 (1952).

MURRAY, J. E., J. P. MERRILL and J. H. HARRISON: Kidney transplantation between 7 pairs of identical twins. Ann. Surg. **148**, 343 (1958).

NATELSON, S., and M. O. ALEXANDER: Marked hypernatraemia and hyperchloraemia with damage to the central nervous system. Arch. intern. Med. **96**, 172 (1955).

NEWBURGH, L. H., and A. A. CAMARA: Lack of correlation between symptoms and degree of renal impairment. Ann. intern. Med. **35**, 39 (1951).

NICAUD, P., A. LAFITTE, A. GROSS and J. P. GAUTIER: Les lesions ossenses de l'intoxication chronique par le cadmium. Aspects radiologiques a type de syndrome de Milkman. Efficacite du traitement calcique et vitaminique (Vitamin D). Bull. Soc. méd. Hôp. Paris **58**, 204 (1942).

NICKEL, J. F., P. B. LAWRENCE, E. LEIFER and S. E. BRADLEY: Renal function, electrolyte excretion and body fluids in patients with chronic renal insufficiency before and after sodium deprivation. J. clin. Invest. **32**, 68 (1953).

NORDENSON, N. C.: The bone marrow in the anaemia of chronic nephritis. Folia haemat. (Lpz.) **59**, 1 (1938).

NORDIN, B. E. C., and R. FRASER: Assessment of urinary phosphate excretion. Lancet **1960 I**, 947.

NUSSBAUM, H. E., W. G. BERNHARD and V. D. MATTIE jr.: Chronic pyelonephritis simulating adrenocortical insufficiency. New Engl. J. Med. **246**, 289 (1952).

OGDEN, E.: The extra-renal sequence to experimental renal hypertension. Bull. N.Y. Acad. Med. **23**, 643 (1947).

OLIVER, J., M. MACDOWELL and A. TRACY: The pathogenesis of acute renal failure associated with traumatic and toxic injury. J. clin. Invest. **30**, 1307 (1951).

— — L. E. WELT, M. A. HOLLIDAY, W. HOLLANDER, R. W. WINTERS, T. F. WILLIAMS and W. R. SEGAN: The renal lesions of electrolyte imbalance. J. exp. Med. **106**, 563 (1957).

OLSEN, N. S., and J. W. BASSETT: Blood levels of urea nitrogen, phenol, guanidine and creatinine in uraemia. Amer. J. Med. **10**, 52 (1951).

OPPENHEIMER, E. T., and M. PRINZMETAL: Role of the arteries in the peripheral resistance of hypertension and related states. Arch. intern. Med. **60**, 772 (1937).

ORLOFF, J., and D. G. DAVIDSON: The mechanism of potassium excretion in the chicken. J. clin. Invest. **38**, 21 (1959).

— H. N. WAGNER and D. G. DAVIDSON: The effect of variations in solute excretion and vasopressin dosage on the excretion of water in the dog. J. clin. Invest. **37**, 458 (1958).

— L. G. WELT and L. STOWE: Effects of concentrated salt poor human albumin on the metabolism and excretion of water and electrolyte in nephrosis. J. clin. Invest. **29**, 1770 (1950).

OTTOLANDER, G. J. H. DEN, H. B. A. HELLENDOORA, H. DE JUGER and J. GERBRANDY: Acute hypercaliemie bij patienten met osteolytische metastasen van mamma carcinom. Ned. T. Geneesk. **101**, 2066 (1957).

PAGE, I. H.: The effect of bilateral adrenalectomy on arterial blood pressure of dogs with experimental hypertension. Amer. J. Physiol. **122**, 352 (1938).

— Method of producing persistent hypertension by cellophane. Science **89**, 273 (1939).

— H. P. DUSTAN and E. F. POUTASSE: Mechanisms, diagnosis and treatment of hypertension of renal vascular origin. Ann. intern. Med. **51**, 196 (1959).

PAPPENHEIMER, J.: Passage of molecules through capillary walls. Phys. Rev. **33**, 387 (1953).

PAPPER, E. M.: Renal function during general anaesthesia and operation. J. Amer. med. Ass. **152**, 1686 (1953).

PARSONS, F. M.: Chemical imbalance occurring in chronic prostatic obstruction; preliminary survey. Brit. J. Urol. **26**, 7 (1954).

—, and B. H. MCCRACHEN: The artificial kidney. Brit. med. J. **1959 I**, 740.

PAYNE, R. W., and H. E. DE WARDENER: Reversal of urinary diurnal rhythm following head injury. Lancet **1958 I**, 1098.

PEART, W. S.: Isolation of a hypertension. Biochem. J. **62**, 520 (1956).

— Hypertension and the kidney. Brit. med. J. **1959 II**, 1353, 1421.

PENINGTON, D. G.: Red cell regulators. Lancet **1960 I**, 975.

PERKINS, J. G., A. B. PETERSEN and J. A. RILEY: Renal and cardiac lesions in potassium deficiency due to chronic diarrhoea. Amer. J. Med. **8**, 115 (1950).

PETERS, J. P.: Edema of acute nephritis. Amer. J. Med. **14**, 448 (1953).

PHILLIPS, R. A., V. P. DOLE, P. B. HAMILTON, K. SMERSON, R. M. ARCHIBALD and D. O. VAN SLYKE: Effects of acute haemorrhagic and traumatic shock on renal function of dogs. Amer. J. Physiol. **145**, 314 (1945).

PICKERING, G. W.: The peripheral resistance in persistent arterial hypertension. Clin. Sci. **2**, 209 (1936).

PICKERING, G. W.: The role of the kidney in acute and chronic hypertension following renal artery constriction in the rabbit. Clin. Sci. 5, 229 (1945).
— High blood pressure. London: J. & A. Churchill 1955.
—, and R. H. HEPTINSTALL: Nephrectomy and other treatment for hypertension in pyelonephritis. Quart. J. Med. 16, 143 (1953).
—, and M. PRINZMETAL: Experimental hypertension of renal origin in the rabbit. Clin. Sci. 3, 357 (1938).
PINES, K. L., and G. H. MUDGE: Renal tubular acidosis with osteomalacia. Amer. J. Med. 11, 302 (1951).
PLATT, R.: Sodium and potassium excretion in chronic renal failure. Clin. Sci. 9, 367 (1950).
— Structural and functional adaptation in renal failure. Brit. med. J. 1952 I, 1313 and 1372.
— Some consequences of renal failure. Lancet 1959 I, 159.
— M. H. ROSCOE and F. W. SMITH: Experimental renal failure. Clin. Sci 11, 217 (1952).
POLONOVSKI, M., and M. F. JAYLE: Chimie biologique — sur la preparation d'une nouvelle fraction des proteins plasmatiques l'haptoglobine. C. R. Acad. Sci. (Paris) 211, 517 (1940).
PREEDY, J. R. K., and E. AITKEN: The effect of oestrogen on water and electrolyte metabolism. J. clin. Invest. 35, 423, 430, 443 (1956).
PRINZMETAL, M., and C. WILSON: The nature of the peripheral resistance in arterial hypertension with special reference to the vasomotor system. J. clin. Invest. 15, 63 (1936).
RAASCHOU, F.: Studies of chronic pyelonephritis with special reference to the kidney function. Copenhagen: Ejnar Munksgaard 1948.
RAMBACH, W. A., J. A. D. COOPER and H. L. ALT: Purification of erythropoietin by ion-exchange chromatography. Proc. Soc. exp. Biol. (N.Y.) 98, 602 (1958).
RAMEY, E. R., and M. S. GOLDSTEIN: The adrenal cortex and the sympathetic nervous system. Phys. Rev. 37, 155 (1957).
RAPOPORT, A.: Modification of the 'Howard test' for the detection of renal artery obstruction. New Engl. J. Med. 263, 1159 (1960).
RAPOPORT, S., W. A. BRODSKY, G. D. WEST and B. MACKLER: Urinary flow and excretion of solutes during osmotic diuresis in hydropenic man. Amer. J. Physiol. 156, 433 (1949).
— G. D. WEST and W. A. BRODSKY: Excretion of solutes and osmotic work during osmotic diuresis of hydropenic man. The ideal and the proximal and distal tubular work; the biological maximum of work. Amer. J. Physiol. 157, 363 (1949).
RATHER, L. J.: Filtration, reabsorption and excretion of protein by the kidney. Medicine (Baltimore) 131, 357 (1952).
RELMAN, A. S., and W. B. SCHWARTZ: The nephropathy of potassium deficiency. New Engl. J. Med. 255, 195 (1956).
— — The kidney and potassium depletion. Amer. J. Med. 24, 764 (1958).
REYNOLDS, T. B.: Observations on the pathogenesis of renal tubular acidosis. Amer. J. Med. 25, 503 (1958).
ROBERTS, H. J.: The syndrome of hyponatraemia and renal sodium loss probably resulting from inappropriate secretion of antidiuretic hormone. Ann. intern. Med. 51, 1420 (1959).
ROBERTS, K. E., and C. A. WALL: A new technique for differential renal function. J. clin. Invest. 42, 971 (1963).
ROBERTSON, B. R., R. C. HARRIS and D. J. McCUNE: Refractory rickets. Amer. J. Dis. Child. 64, 948 (1942).
ROBSON, E. B., and G. A. ROSE: The effects of intravenous lysine on the renal clearances of cystine, argenine and ornithine in normal subjects, in patients with cystinuria and in their relatives. Clin. Sci. 16, 75 (1957).
ROEMMELT, J. C., O. W. SARTORIUS and R. F. PITTS: Excretion and reabsorption of sodium and water in the adrenalectomised dog. Amer. J. Physiol. 159, 124 (1949).
ROSCOE, M. H.: Biochemical and haematological changes in type I and type II nephritis. Quart. J. Med. 19, 161 (1950).
— The nephrotic syndrome. Quart. J. Med. 25, 353 (1956).
ROSENBERG, M. L.: The physiology of hyperchloraemic acidosis following ureterosigmoidostomy: a study of urinary adsorption with isotopes. J. Urol. (Baltimore) 70, 569 (1953).
ROSENHEIM, M. L.: Sodium. Lancet 1951 II, 505.
—, and A. G. SPENCER: The treatment of the nephrotic syndrome with cation exchange resins and a high protein, low sodium diet. Lancet 1956 II, 313.
ROSS, E. J., and J. F. SMITH: The use of steroids in the treatment of the nephrotic syndrome in adults. Quart. J. Med. 32, 65 (1963).
ROUSSAK, N. J., and S. OLEESKY: Water losing nephritis. Quart. J. Med. 23, 147 (1954).
ROWNTREE, L. G., and A. M. SNELL: A clinical study of Addison's disease. Philadelphia: W.B. Saunders Company 1931.
RUBIN, M. I., E. BRUCK and M. RAPOPORT: Maturation of renal function in childhood clearance studies. J. clin. Invest. 28, 1144 (1949).

RUSBY, N. L., and C. WILSON: Lung purpura with nephritis. Quart. J. Med. **29**, 501 (1960).

RUYTER, J. H. C.: Über einen merkwürdigen Abschnitt der Vasa afferentia in der Mauseniere. Z. Zellforsch. **2**, 242 (1925).

RYTAND, D. A.- Chronologic separation of water and chloride diuresis in the nephrotic syndrome. Amer. J. Med. **4**, 624 (1948).

SARTORIUS, O. W., J. C. ROEMMELT and R. F. PITTS: The renal regulations of acid base balance in man. Nature of the renal compensations in ammonium chloride acidosis. J. clin. Invest. **28**, 423 (1949).

SAVILLE, P. D., J. R. NASSIM, F. H. STEVENSON and L. MULLIGAN: The Fanconi syndrome: metabolic studies on treatment. J. Bone Jt Surg. **37**B, 529 (1955).

SAWYER, W. H., and C. SOLEZ: Salt-losing nephritis simulating adrenocortical insufficiency; report of case. New Engl. J. Med. **240**, 210 (1949).

SCHOLZ, D. A.: Effects of steroid therapy on hypercalcaemia and renal insufficiency in sarcoidosis. J. Amer. med. Ass. **169**, 682 (1959).

SCHWARTZ, F. D., and M. S. MADELOFF: Use of radiohippuran in diagnosis of unilateral renal disease. J. Urol. (Baltimore) **87**, 249 (1962).

SCHWARTZ, V., L. GOLDBERG, G. M. KOMROWER and A. HOLZEL: Some disturbances of erythrocyte metabolism in galactosaemia. J. Biochem. **62**, 34 (1955).

SCHWARTZ, W. B., W. BENNETT, S. CURELOP and F. C. BARTTER: A syndrome of renal sodium loss and hyponatraemia probably resulting from inappropriate secretion of antidiuretic hormone. Amer. J. Med. **23**, 529 (1957).

— P. W. HALL, R. M. HAYS and A. S. RELMAN On the mechanism of acidosis in chronic renal disease. J. clin. Invest. **38**, 39 (1959).

—, and A. S. RELMAN: Metabolic and renal studies in chronic potassium depletion resulting from over-use of laxatives. J. clin. Invest. **32**, 258 (1953).

— D. TASSEL and F. C. BARTTER: Further observations on hyponatraemia and renal sodium loss probably resulting from inappropriate secretion of antidiuretic hormone. New Engl. J. Med. **262**, 743, 1037 (1960).

SCHWYZE, R., and P. SIEBER: New synthesis in the peptide field. Chimia **10**, 265 (1956).

SELKURT, E. E.: Nierendurchblutung und renale Clearances bei Blutverlust und im hämorrhagischen Schock. Ciba Schock-Symposion. Berlin-Göttingen-Heidelberg: Springer 1962.

— P. W. HALL and M. P. SPENCER: Influence of graded arterial pressure decrement on renal clearance of creatinine, p-aminohippurate and sodium. Amer. J. Physiol. **159**, 369 (1949).

SERRATTO, M., J. T. GRAYHACK and D. P. EARLE: A clinical evaluation of the iodopyracet (Diodrast) renogram. Arch. intern. Med. **103**, 851 (1959).

SEYMOUR, W. B., W. H. PRITCHARD, L. P. LONGLEY, J. M. HAYMAN jr.: Cardiac output, blood and interstitial fluid volumes, total circulating serum protein and kidney function during cardiac failure and after improvement. J. clin. Invest. **21**, 229 (1942).

SEVITT, S.: The pathogenesis of traumatic uraemia. Lancet **1959** II, 135.

SHACKMAN, R., G. D. CHISHOLM, A. J. HOLDEN and R. W. PIGOTT: Urea distribution in the body after haemodialysis. Brit. med. J. **1962** II, 355.

— M. D. MILNE and N. W. STRUTHERS: Oliguric renal failure of surgical origin. Brit. med. J. **1960** II, 1473.

SHARPEY-SCHAFER, E. P.: The response of the heart in acute nephritis. Lancet **1955** II, 841.

SHAW, C. C.: Enhancement of penicillin blood levels in man by means of new compound caronamide. Amer. J. Med. **3**, 206 (1947).

SHEEHAN, H. L., and H. C. MOORE: Renal cortical necrosis and the kidney of concealed accidental haemorrhage. Oxford: Blackwell 1952.

SHIPLEY, R. E.: Cited by I. H. PAGE, The mosaic theory of hypertension. Ciba Symposium on essential hypertension. Berlin-Göttingen-Heidelberg: Springer 1960.

SIMMONS, D. H., R. B. HARVEY and T. HOSHIKO: Effect of sodium intake on sodium loss due to osmotic diuresis: an empirical test for renal sodium-retaining activity. Amer. J. Physiol. **178**, 182 (1954).

SIMPSON, S. A., J. F. TAIT and I. E. BUSH: Secretion of salt-retaining hormone by mammalian adrenal cortex. Lancet **1952** II, 226.

— — A. WETTSTEIN, R. NEHER, J. v. EUW, O. SCHINDLER and T. REICHSTEIN: Aldosteron, Isolierung und Eigenschaften. Helv. chim. Acta **37**, 1163 (1954).

SIROTA, J. H.: Carbon tetrachloride poisoning in man. I. The mechanisms of renal failure and recovery. J. clin. Invest. **28**, 1412 (1949).

SKANSE, B., and B. HOKFELT: Hypo-aldosteronism with otherwise intact adrenocortical function, resulting in a characteristic clinical entity. Acta endocr. (Kbh.) **28**, 29 (1958).

SKEGGS, L. T., J. H. KAHN and N. P. SHUMWAY: Preparation and function of hypertensin-converting enzyme. J. exp. Med. **103**, 295 (1956a).

— — — Purification of hypertension. II. J. exp. Med. **103**, 301 (1956b).

SLATER, J. D. H., A. MOXHAM, R. HURTER and J. D. N. NABARRO: Clinical and metabolic effects of aldosterone antagonists. Lancet **1959 II**, 931.

SLYKE, D. D. VAN: Effects of shock on the kidney. Ann. intern. Med. **28**, 701 (1948).

SMITH, H. W.: William Henry Welch Lecture: Application of saturation methods to study of glomerular and tubular function in human kidney. J. Mt Sinai Hosp. **10**, 59 (1943).

— The kidney; structure and function in health and disease. New York: Oxford University Press 1951.

— Unilateral nephrectomy in hypertensive disease. J. Urol. (Baltimore) **76**, 685 (1956).

— W. GOLDRING and H. CHASIS: Measurement of tubular excretory mass, effective blood flow and filtration rate in the normal human kidney. J. clin. Invest. **17**, 263 (1938).

SMITH, J. F., J. R. BOLTON and A. L. TURNBULL: The renal complications of diabetes mellitus. J. Path. Bact. **70**, 475 (1955).

SMITH, W. V., and J. F. HAMMARSTEN: Serum magnesium in renal disease. Arch. intern. Med. **102**, 5 (1958).

SNAPPER, I.: Rare manifestations of metabolic bone disease. Springfield, Illinois 1952.

SPENCER, A. G.: Clearance studies in unilateral renal disease. In: Recent Advances in Renal Disease. London: Ed. M. D. Milne 1960.

—, and G. T. FRANGLEN: Gross aminoaciduria following a lysol burn. Lancet **1952 I**, 190.

SPUHLER, O., and H. V. ZOLLINGER: Die chronische interstitielle Nephritis. Helv. med. Acta **17**, 564 (1950).

SQUIRE, J. R.: The nephrotic syndrome. Brit. med. J. **1953 II**, 1389.

— J. D. BLAINEY and J. HARDWICKE: Physiology and pathology of the kidney, the nephrotic syndrome. Brit. med. Bull. **13**, No 1 (1957).

STAMEY, T. A., I. J. NUDELMAN, P. H. GOOD, F. N. SCHWENTKER and F. HENDRICKS: Functional characteristics of renovascular hypertension. Medicine (Baltimore) **40**, 347 (1961).

STANBURY, S. W.: Azotaemic renal osteodystrophy. Brit. med. Bull. **13**, 57 (1957).

— Some aspects of disordered tubular function. Advanc. intern. Med. **9**, 231 (1958).

— Renal osteodystrophy. In: Recent advances in renal disease. London: Ed. M. D. Milne Pitman 1960.

—, and G. A. LUMB: Metabolic studies of renal osteodystrophy. I. Calcium phosphorus and nitrogen metabolism in rickets, osteomalacia and hyperparathyroidism complicating chronic uraemia and in the osteomalacia of the adult Fanconi syndrome. Medicine (Baltimore) **41**, 1 (1962).

—, and D. MACAULAY: Renal tubular function in the nephrotic syndrome. Quart J. Med. **26**, 7 (1957).

—, and A. E. THOMSON: Diurnal variations in electrolyte excretion. Clin. Sci. **10**, 267 (1951).

STAPLETON, T.: Idiopathic renal acidosis in an infant with excessive loss of bicarbonate in the urine. Lancet **1949 I**, 683.

STEIN, W. H.: Excretion of amino acids in cystinuria. Proc. Soc. exp. Biol. (N.Y.) **78**, 705 (1951).

— A. G. BEARN and S. MOORE: The amino acid content of the blood and urine in Wilson's disease. J. clin. Invest. **33**, 410 (1954).

STEVENS, A. R.: Longevity following uretero-colic anastomosis with a report of cases. J. Urol. (Baltimore) **46**, 57 (1941).

STOWERS, J. M., and C. E. DENT: Studies on the mechanism of the Fanconi syndrome. Quart. J. Med. **16**, 275 (1947).

SURTSHIN, A., D. ROLF and H. L. WHITE: Constancy of sodium excretion in the presence of chronically altered filtration rate. Amer. J. Physiol. **165**, 429 (1951).

SWANN, G. F.: General softening of bone due to metabolic causes; pathogenesis of bone lesions in neurofibromatosis. Brit. J. Radiol. **27**, 623 (1954).

SWANN, R. C., and J. P. MERRILL: The clinical course of acute renal failure. Medicine (Baltimore) **32**, 215 (1953).

TAGGART, J. V.: Disorders of renal tubular function. Amer. J. Med. **20**, 448 (1956).

TALBOT, J. H., L. J. PECORA, R. S. MELVILLE and W. V. CONSOLAZIO: Renal function in patients with Addison's disease and in patients with adrenal insufficiency secondary to pituitary panhypofunction. J. clin. Invest. **21**, 107 (1942).

TAQUINI, A. C., and J. C. FASCIOLO: Renin in essential hypertension. Amer. Heart J. **32**, 357 (1946).

— — El papel de la renina circulante en la hipertension arterial. Rev. argent. Cardiol. **14**, 1 (1947).

TAUXE, W. N.: The radioisotope renogram in renal artery disease. Proc. Mayo Clin. **36**, 684 (1961).

— K. G. WAKIM and A. H. BAGGENSTOSS: The renal lesions in experimental deficiency of potassium. Amer. J. clin. Path. **28**, 221 (1957).

TAYLOR, W. H.: Management of acute renal failure following surgical operation and head injury. Lancet 1957 II, 703.

TEGELAERS, W. H. H., and H. W. TIDDENS: Nephrotic-glucosuric-aminoaciduric dwarfism and electrolyte metabolism. Helv. paediat. Acta 10, 269 (1955).

TESCHAN, P. E., C. R. BAXTER, J. F. O'BRIEN, J. N. FREYHOF and W. H. HALL: Prophylactic haemodialysis in the treatment of acute renal failure. Ann. intern. Med. 53, 992 (1960).

THORN, G. W., S. H. ARMSTRONG, N. D. DAVENPORT, L. M. WOODRUFF and F. H. TYLER: The use of salt-poor concentrated human albumin in the treatment of chronic Bright's disease. J. clin. Invest. 24, 802 (1945).

— G. F. KOEPF and M. CLINTON jr.: Renal failure simulating adrenocortical insufficiency. New Engl. J. Med. 231, 76 (1944).

TIGERSTEDT, R., and P. G. BERGMAN: „Niere und Kreislauf". Skand. Arch. Physiol. 8, 223 (1898).

TOBIAN, L.: Inter-relationship of electrolytes, juxtaglomerular cells and hypertension. Phys. Rev. 40, 280 (1960).

— J. JANECEK and A. TOMBOULIAN: Correlation between granulation of juxtaglomerular cells and extractable renin in rats with experimental hypertension. Proc. Soc. exp. Biol. (N.Y.) 100, 94 (1959).

— J. THOMPSON, R. TWEDT and J. JANECEK: The granulation of juxtaglomerular cells in renal hypertension, desoxycorticosterone and post desoxycorticosterone hypertension, adrenal regeneration hypertension and adrenal insufficiency. J. clin. Invest. 37, 660 (1958).

— B. WINN and J. JANECEK: Influence of arterial pressure on antihypertension action of a normal kidney: a biological servo-mechanism. J. clin. Invest. 40, 1085 (1961).

TONI, G. DE: Remarks on the relations between renal rickets (renal dwarfism) and renal diabetes. Acta paediat. 16, 479 (1933).

TORRANCE, H. B., R. P. DAVIES and P. CLARK: Detection of renal arterial stenosis in hypertension by the differential renal uptake of radioactive rubidium. Lancet 1961 II, 633.

TRUETA, J., A. E. BARCLAY, P. M. DANIEL, K. J. FRANKLIN and M. M. L. PRITCHARD: Studies of the renal circulation. Oxford: Blackwell 1947.

TWEEDY, W. R., and W. W. CAMPBELL: Effect of parathyroid extract upon distribution, retention and excretion of labelled phosphorus. J. biol. Chem. 154, 339 (1944).

UZMAN, L. L., and D. DENNY-BROWN: Aminoaciduria in hepato-lenticular degeneration Wilson's disease). Amer. J. med. Sci. 215, 599 (1948).

—, and B. HOOD: Familial nature of amino-aciduria of Wilson's disease (hepatolenticular degneration). Amer. J. med. Sci. 223, 392 (1952).

VANDER, A. J., R. L. MALVIN, W. S. WILDE, J. LAPIDES, L. P. SULLIVAN and V. M. McMURRAY: Effects of adrenalectomy and aldosterone on proximal and distal tubular sodium reabsorption. Proc. Soc. exp. Biol. (N.Y.) 99, 323 (1958).

VAN'T HOFF, W., and J. F. ZILVA: Chromophobe adenoma and hyponatraemia. Clin. Sci. 21, 345 (1961).

VEREL, D., A. TURNBULL, G. R. TUDHOPE and J. H. ROSS: Anaemia in Bright's disease. Quart. J. Med. 28, 491 (1959).

VERNEY, E. B.: Antidiuretic hormone and the factors which determine its release. Proc. roy. Soc. B 135, 25 (1947).

— Water diuresis (John Malet Purser lecture). Irish J. med. Sci. 6th series 377 (1954).

VERNIER, R. L.: The ultrastructure of the glomerulus. Ciba symposium on Renal Biopsy. London: J. & A. Churchill 1961.

VOLHARD, F.: MOHR und STACHELINs Handbuch der inneren Medizin. Berlin 1918.

—, and T. FAHR: Die Brightsche Nierenkrankheit, Klinik, Pathologie und Atlas. Berlin 1914.

VRIES, A. DE, S. KOCHWA, J. LAZEBNIK, M. FRANK and M. DJALDETTI: Glycinuria, a hereditary disorder associated with nephrolithiasis. Amer. J. Med. 23, 408 (1957).

WAKERLIN, G. E., R. B. BIRD, B. B. BRENNAN, M. H. FRANK, S. KREMEN, I. KUPERMAN and J. H. SKOM: Treatment and prophylaxis of experimental renal hypertension with "Renin". J. Lab. clin. Med. 41, 788 (1953).

— J. MARSHALL and H. MINATOVA: Renin concentration in the kidney in experimental renal hypertension. 2nd Conference Josiah Macey Foundation 1948, p. 61.

WALLIS, L. A., and R. L. ENGLE: The adult Fanconi syndrome. Amer. J. Med. 22, 13 (1957).

WARDENER, H. E. DE: Vasopressin tannate in oil and the urine concentration test. Lancet 1956 I, 1037.

—, and A. W. HERXHEIMER: The effect of a high water intake on the kidney's ability to concentrate the urine. J. Physiol. (Lond.) 139, 42 (1957).

WARREN, J. V., E. S. BRANNAN and A. J. MERRILL: Method of obtaining renal venous blood in unanaesthetized persons, with observations on extraction of oxygen and sodium para-amino hippurate. Science 100, 108 (1944).

WATERHOUSE, C., and E. H. KEUTMANN: Kidney function in adrenal insufficiency. J. clin. Invest. 27, 372 (1948).

WEBSTER, G. D., E. J. HUTH, J. R. ELKINTON and R. A. McCANCE: The renal excretion of hydrogen ion in renal tubular acidosis. Amer. J. Med. 29, 576 (1960).

WEISS, S., and F. PARKER: Pyelonephritis; its relation to vascular lesions and to arterial hypertension. Medicine (Baltimore) 18, 221 (1939).

WELT, L. G., D. W. SELDIN, W. P. NELSON, W. J. GERMAN and J. P. PETERS: Role of the central nervous system in metabolism of electrolytes and water. Arch. intern. Med. 90, 355 (1952).

WERKO, G., and H. LAGERLOF: Studies on the circulation in man. Iv. Cardiac output and blood pressure in the right auricle, right ventricle and pulmonary arteries in a patient with hypertensive cardiovascular disease. Acta med. scand. 133, 427 (1949).

WHITE, H. L., P. HEINBECKER and D. ROLF: Effects of the removal of the anterior lobe of the hypophysis on some renal function. Amer. J. Physiol. 136, 584 (1942).

— — — Some endocrine influences on renal function and cardiac output. Amer. J. Physiol. 149, 404 (1947).

WIDIMSKY, J., M. H. FEJFAROUA and Z. FEJFAR: Changes of cardiac output in hypertensive disease. Cardiologia (Basel) 31, 331 (1957).

WILKINSON, A. W.: Biochemical changes after uretero-colic anastomosis. Brit. J. Urol. 24, 46 (1952).

— Biochemical changes after transplantation of the ureters. Postgrad. med. J. 30, 405 (1954).

WILLIAMS, R. H., and C. HENRY: Nephrogenic diabetes insipidus: transmitted by females and appearing during infancy in males. Ann. intern. Med. 27, 84 (1947).

WILSON, B., D. D. REISMAN and C. A. MOYER: Fluid balance in the urological patient: disturbances in the renal regulation of the excretion of water and sodium salts following decompression of urinary bladder. J. Urol. (Baltimore) 66, 805 (1951).

WILSON, C.: Renal factors in the production of hypertension. Lancet 1958 II, 579, 632.

—, and F. B. BYROM: Renal changes in malignant hypertension. Lancet 1939 I, 136.

— — The vicious circle in chronic Bright's disease. Experimental evidence from the hypertensive rat. Quart. J. Med. 10, 65 (1941).

—, and G. W. PICKERING: Acute arterial lesions in rabbits with experimental renal hypertension. Clin. Sci. 3, 343 (1938).

WILSON, H. E. C., and H. MUIRHEAD: Evidence for the presence of a pitressin like substance in the tissue fluids in nephrosis. Acta paediat. 45, 77 (1956).

WILSON, V. K., M. L. THOMSON and C. E. DENT: Aminoaciduria in lead poisoning; a case in childhood. Lancet 1933 II, 66.

— — and A. HOLZEL: Mercury nephrosis in young children with special reference to teething powders containing mercury. Brit. med. J. 1952 I, 358.

WINBERG, J.: Renal function in water-losing syndrome due to lower urinary tract obstruction before and after treatment. Acta paediat. 48, 149 (1959).

WINER, N. J.: Renal function in diabetes insipidus. Arch. intern. Med. 70, 61 (1942).

WINKLER, A. W., P. K. SMITH and H. E. HOLT: Spontaneous potassium poisoning in the adrenalectomised animal. Fed. Proc. 1, 94 (1942).

WINTER, C. C.: Unilateral renal disease and hypertension: use of the radioactive diodrast renogram as a screening test. J. Urol. (Baltimore) 78, 107 (1957).

— M. H. MAXWELL, R. E. ROCKNEY and C. R. KLEEMAN: Results of the radioisotope renogram and comparison with other kidney tests among hypertensive persons. J. Urol. (Baltimore) 82, 674 (1959).

—, and G. V. TAPLIN: A clinical comparison and analysis of radioactive diodrast, hypaque, miokon and urokon renograms as tests of kidney function. J. Urol. (Baltimore) 79, 573 (1958).

WINTERS, R. W., J. B. GRAHAM, T. F. WILLIAMS and V. W. McFALLS: A genetic study of familial hypophosphataemia and vitamin D resistant rickets. Trans. Ass. Amer. Phycns 70, 234 (1957).

WOOD, J. E., and C. ETHRIDGE: Hypertension with arteriolar and glomerular changes in the albino rat following subtotal nephrectomy. Proc. Soc. exp. Biol. (N.Y.) 30, 1039 (1933).

WRONG, O.: Incidence of hypokalaemia in severe hypertension. Brit. med. J. 1961 II, 419.

—, and H. E. F. DAVIES: The excretion of acid in renal disease. Quart. J. Med. 28, 259 (1959).

WYNN, V., and O. GARROD: Spontaneous and induced water intoxication in two cases of hypopituitarism. Brit. med. J. 1955 I, 505.

YEH, H. L., W. FRANKL, M. S. DUNN, P. PARKER, B. HUGHES and P. GYORGY: The urinary excretion of aminoacids by a cystinuric subject. Amer. J. med. Sci. 214, 507 (1947).

YENDT, E. R., W. K. KERR, D. R. WILSON and Z. F. JAWORSKI: The diagnosis and treatment of renal hypertension. Ann. intern. Med. 28, 169 (1960).

ZETTERSTROM, R., N. O. ERICSSON and J. WINBERG: Separate renal function studies in predominantly unilateral hydronephrosis. Acta paediat. 47, 540 (1958).

Physiologie normale et pathologique des voies urinaires supérieures

Bernard Fey et Louis Quénu

Avec la collaboration de

W. v. Niederhäusern et de J. Auvigne et R. Lebatard-Sartre

Avec 6 figures

A. Physiologie normale des voies urinaires supérieures

L'urine secrétée par le rein ne coule pas dans les voies excrétrices suivant les lois de la pesanteur et de d'hydraulique. Elle est *propulsée* par la contraction du système musculaire des calices, du bassinet et de l'uretère. Le fonctionnement correct de cet appareil musculaire assure la vidange des voies excrétrices. Son fonctionnement défectueux est à la base de toute la pathologie du haut appareil urinaire.

Tout cela est connu depuis longtemps. On savait que l'urine est excrétée aussi bien chez le quadrupède que chez le bipède et, chez ce dernier, aussi bien en position couchée que debout. Les anatomistes avaient décrit avec minutie les parois des voies excrétrices, insistant sur l'épaisseur de la couche musculaire: ils en avaient même systématisé certaines structures particulières (Henle 1868). Les physiologistes trouvaient l'uretère commode pour étudier les propriétés des muscles lisses: dès 1869, Engelmann avait noté les mouvements de l'uretère et l'irritabilité automatique du muscle uretéral. En 1881, Sokoloff et Luchsinger perfusant l'uretère de chiens ou de lapins obtenaient des contractions régulières dont le nombre dépendait de la pression du liquide perfusé. Les chirurgiens au cours des opérations gynécologiques savaient reconnaitre l'uretère à ses mouvements de reptation. Ils avaient aussi remarqué qu'au cours des interventions en position de Trendelenburg, la vessie, évacuée par sondage au début, se retrouvait remplie à la fin. Enfin, les Urologues, au cours des cystoscopies, voyaient les orifices uretéraux se contracter et chasser l'urine dans la vessie par des éjaculations rythmiques et discontinues. Mais toutes ces notions isolées n'avaient pas abouti à une étude d'ensemble.

C'est en 1910 que Voelcker et v. Lichtenberg, en mettant au point la pyélographie, ont pu explorer directement les voies excrétrices. Malheureusement, la pyélographie donne un moulage purement morphologique: elle est incapable de distinguer une déformation physiologique d'une déformation pathologique et une dilatation temporaire d'une dilatation permanente. «Figure d'immobilité» (Leguéu), elle est mal adaptée à l'étude d'organes aussi mobiles que le bassinet et l'uretère.

Vers 1925, sous l'égide de Leguéu, nous avons controlé la pyélographie sous écran radioscopique et créé la pyéloscopie. Malgré ses difficultés et ses causes d'erreur, la pyéloscopie mettait en évidence la motricité pyélo-urétérale, ses variations pathologiques et les conséquences de ces variations sur l'appareil excréteur (hydronéphrose). La physiologie normale et pathologique de l'appareil excréteur sortait du domaine des laboratoires pour entrer dans la clinique journalière.

Dès lors, toutes les autres méthodes d'exploration, apparues depuis, se sont appliquées à l'étude de cette fonction motrice; d'abord l'Urographie (v. LICHTENBERG et SWICK, 1929) qui, exempte de toute cause d'erreur, a permis de vérifier et de contrôler les données de la pyéloscopie, ensuite la Kymographie, la Manométrie, etc, etc; ... pour aboutir à la plus récente et la plus complète, la Radiocinématographie.

I. L'appareil Pyélo-urétéral: L'outil

1. Anatomie

a) Le muscle pyélo-urétéral

L'anatomie des voies excrétrices a été étudiée ailleurs. Envisagée au point de vue physiologique, elle se résume à un tube musculaire étendu des papilles rénales à la vessie, formé de fibres lisses disposées schématiquement en deux couches, une interne longitudinale et une externe circulaire. Cette épaisse couche musculaire est limitée en dedans par la muqueuse, en dehors par l'adventice, le tout au milieu d'une atmosphère cellulaire lâche favorable à la motilité.

Couche circulaire et couche longitudinale sont plus ou moins distinctes et individualisées, selon les niveaux:

α) A la jonction papillo-calicielle

HENLE (1868) puis EBERTH, JARDET, HARRY HARRIS et NARATH distinguent une formation circulaire (sphincter papillaire de HENLE, sphincter fornicis de NARATH) et une formation longitudinale (le levator fornicis de NARATH).

β) Au collet des calices

— Au collet des calices, on retrouve une formation circulaire (sphincter calycis de NARATH); les fibres longitudinales sont plus problématiques.

L'ensemble des formations calicielles isole une cavité péripapillaire entre deux sphincters, celui de la papille en haut, celui du collet caliciel en bas, réalisant le dispositif schématique de «sas» que nous retrouverons d'étage en étage.

γ) Le bassinet

— Le bassinet a une paroi plus épaisse formée par un entrecroisement inextricable de fibres longitudinales obliques et circulaires, le tout entremêlé de fibres élastiques.

δ) L'uretère

— L'uretère est classiquement décrit avec deux couches, longitudinale interne et circulaire externe: en réalité les deux couches sont étroitement intriquées avec prédominance des fibres circulaires, et SCHLICHT a pu isoler des fibres en spirale qui unifient les deux variétés.

ε) L'uretère inférieur

— Au niveau de l'uretère inférieur, des modifications se produisent. Une couche longitudinale externe apparait, la couche de WALDEYER qui appartient en propre à la musculature vésicale dont elle partage l'innervation (KUNTZ).

Enfin, dans la portion intra-murale, les fibres circulaires s'espacent: elles existent cependant jusqu'au niveau de l'orifice vésical et NARATH souligne leur action sur le méat. Mais à ce niveau l'uretère est solidement engainé par le très épais détrusor vésical.

Toute cette jonction uretéro-vésicale et son dispositif anti-reflux intrigue les anatomistes depuis AMBROISE PARÉ. Elle est formée à la fois par la musculature de l'uretère et celle de la vessie et son fonctionnement dépend des deux organes.

b) L'innervation du muscle pyélo-urétéral

Nous passerons rapidement sur l'innervation de ce tube musculaire. On a vu la multiplicité des *nerfs extrinsèques* provenant des plexus rénaux, spermatiques et hypogastriques. *L'innervation intrinsèque* est constituée par un riche réseau nerveux dans l'adventice (plexus fondamental d'ENGELMANN) d'où partent des filets pénétrant la musculeuse et la sous-muqueuse. Ces filets sont en très petit nombre par rapport à celui des fibres musculaires (1 pour 50). REUNES, HAEBLER, ZANNE, ont vu des filets se terminer dans les fibres musculaires des calices et du bassinet. En revanche, HIRT, HAUFFMANN et GOTTLIEB affirment qu'au niveau de l'uretère les filets nerveux traversent la musculeuse pour se rendre à la sous-muqueuse sans donner de rameau musculaire.

Tout aussi problématique est la question des *ganglions nerveux* ou *cellules ganglionnaires*.

Certains (MAIER, PROTOPOPOW, ALSKNE, DISSE, SATANI, BOEMINGHAUS, CRACIUN) en trouvent sur toute la longueur de l'uretère. CRACIUN décrit même un centre supérieur au collet de l'uretère responsable du péristaltisme et un centre inférieur, dans l'uretère intra-mural, qui commande l'antipéristaltisme. ENGELMANN, HRYNTSCHACK, ne trouvent de cellules ganglionnaires que dans l'adventice du tiers inférieur de l'uretère — aucun ganglion dans la musculeuse ni la muqueuse. Même résultat chez le chien, quelques ganglions dans la musculeuse du tiers inférieur chez le chat; pas de ganglion ni de cellule nerveuse chez le porc.

Il y a donc peu à tirer des données anatomiques.

Nous enregistrons avec satisfaction les descriptions (HENLE, NARATH) de la musculature calicielle qui nous fournit (nous l'avons vu) un excellent exemple de «sas», des plus intéressant au point de vue de la physiologie.

En revanche, nous avons le regret de constater que les anatomistes ne trouvent ni modification musculaire, ni formation sphinctérienne, ni changement de vascularisation ou d'innervation, ni système ganglionnaire pour expliquer la segmentation de la rame urinaire au niveau de zones telles que la jonction pyélo-urétérale, ou les collets des cystoïdes, où toutes les explorations vont nous démontrer que cette segmentation existe, au moins, dans certaines circonstances. A la partie inférieure enfin, retenons l'intrication des formations musculaires urétérale et vésicale, ce qui nous explique bien la complexité de l'appareil anti-reflux.

Si l'anatomie nous déçoit, tournons nous vers le matériau dont est formé l'appareil excréteur, c'est-à-dire entreprenons l'étude du muscle lisse.

2. Physiologie du muscle lisse

Il est le même que dans tous les autres organes mais ici tellement prédominant qu'il nous parait indispensable de revoir rapidement ses propriétés.

Le muscle lisse a deux propriétés tissulaires qui caractérisent sa texture; l'extensibilité et l'élasticité, et deux propriétés vitales ou actives: la contractilité et la tonicité.

a) L'extensibilité

L'extensibilité permet au muscle de s'allonger sous l'action d'une traction. L'allongement n'est pas directement proportionnel à l'intensité de la traction; elle diminue au fur et à mesure que celle-ci augmente.

b) L'élasticité

L'élasticité permet au muscle de revenir à sa longueur primitive quand la traction cesse. L'élasticité du muscle lisse est parfaite tant que la fibre garde son intégrité.

Extensibilité et élasticité, propriétés tissulaires, résument les seuls modes de réaction du muscle. Toute excitation, quelles que soient sa nature et son intensité, ne peut provoquer qu'un allongement ou un raccourcissement s'il s'agit d'un muscle rectiligne, un changement de volume et de pression sur le contenu s'il s'agit d'un muscle creux. Les fonctions vitales, tonicité et contractilité ne peuvent se manifester qu'en déterminant des changements dans ce couple extensibilité-élasticité.

Tant que la fibre musculaire est saine, extensibilité et élasticité s'équilibrent harmonieusement: la fibre lisse est beaucoup plus résistante à ce point de vue que la fibre striée; il est classique de remarquer que la fibre lisse supporte les allongements considérables de la grossesse ou de la rétention vésicale sans perdre son élasticité.

Toutefois, cette résistance a des limites. Quand la fibre musculaire est abimée, l'extensibilité augmente et l'élasticité diminue; qnand elle est «cassée» on dit que le muscle est «distendu»; l'extensibilité et l'élasticité disparaissent.

c) La tonicité

La tonicité est une propriété vitale, active, beaucoup plus difficile à concevoir et à définir.

Les études de pathologie nerveuse du muscle strié (ROYLE et HUNTER, PIERON, FOIX et CHAVANY, etc.) ont abouti à des conceptions très savantes mais inapplicables au muscle lisse. Nous tacherons de simplifier et de nous cantonner à la conception suivante qui a au moins le mérite de la simplicité.

La tonicité est la faculté que possède le muscle de régler son extensibilité-élasticité pour l'adapter à un travail donné.

Un muscle à tonicité basse est mou, se laisse facilement allonger et revient sur lui-même avec une force élastique faible.

Un muscle à tonicité élevée est dur, résiste à l'extension et revient sur lui-même avec une force élastique puissante. Cette force élastique peut se mesurer au myographe isométrique.

La tonicité est indépendante de la longueur du muscle et celui-ci peut, avec des longueurs différentes exercer une force élastique équivalente.

S'il s'agit d'un *muscle creux*, la pression élastique exercée sur le contenu diminue avec une tonicité basse, augmente avec une tonicité élevée. Cette pression élastique se mesure au manomètre. La tonicité est, dans une certaine mesure, indépendante du volume du muscle creux et celui-ci peut avec des volumes différents exercer une pression élastique équivalente sur son contenu.

Mais cette indépendance ne joue que dans une certaine limite: lorsqu'elle est atteinte, et elle l'est assez rapidement pour les cavités pyélo-urétérale, si le contenu continue à augmenter, la pression augmente.

La tonicité est un état relativement stable et *statique* qui ne nécessite pas une grande dépense énergétique: nous aurons à revenir sur ce point. Il en résulte qu'un muscle au repos peut, selon les circonstances, augmenter ou diminuer la longueur de ses fibres d'une part et leur tension élastique d'autre part. S'il s'agit d'un muscle creux, il peut modifier son volume et adapter la pression qu'il exerce sur son contenu.

d) La contractilité

C'est la propriété active, efficiente du muscle. Elle est beaucoup plus facile à étudier d'autant que l'uretère s'est montré un matériel de choix pour l'étude de la contraction du muscle lisse.

α) La contraction en général

La contraction d'un muscle est caractérisée par un raccourcissement rapide, suivi à temps plus ou moins prolongé d'un allongement qui le ramène au point de départ.

L'élément de la contraction est la *secousse musculaire* dont la courbe nous est fournie par les myographes isotoniques ou isométriques. On sait que cette courbe comprend plusieurs temps: 1. temps perdu initial, 2. ascension rapide, 3. sommet, 4. descente progressive et prolongée (décontraction).

La secousse musculaire du muscle lisse est analogue à celle du muscle strié mais *considérablement allongée dans tous ses éléments*.

La secousse musculaire est obtenue par une excitation unique et instantanée: des excitations successives déterminent des secousses plus ou moins fusionnées en tétanos imparfait ou total.

Il semble aujourd'hui admis que la décontraction n'est pas seulement passive et due à la cessation de la contraction, mais nécessite l'intervention d'un second mécanisme actif et indépendant.

β) La contractilité du muscle pyélo-urétéral

1. *Qualité de l'excitation.* Pour qu'une excitation détermine une secousse musculaire, c'est-à-dire pour qu'elle soit efficace, *il faut qu'elle ait une certaine durée.* Les expériences d'ENGELMANN sur l'uretère de lapin ont montré l'importance de ce «temps physiologique». La mesure pratique du facteur temps est la chronaxie (LAPICQUE). Alors que la chronaxie des muscles striés est de l'ordre de quelques dixièmes de millième de seconde, la chronaxie de l'uretère de lapin est de 180 millièmes de seconde, celle de l'uretère de chat de 50 millièmes de seconde.

Une excitation très brève (par exemple l'onde d'ouverture de la bobine d'induction qui est de l'ordre du millième de seconde), efficace sur le muscle strié, est inopérante sur l'uretère; mais ces mêmes ondes répétées deviennent très efficaces: *pouvoir de sommation de la musculature lisse* (ENGELMANN), *addition latente* (CH. RICHET).

2. *Transmission des excitations.* ENGELMANN et plus récemment BOZLER admettent que le système nerveux intrinsèque ne joue qu'un rôle secondaire. Le muscle pyélo-urétéral, comme le muscle cardiaque, est un syncytium et l'excitation se transmet directement de cellule à cellule.

3. *Vitesse de transmission des excitations*. Elle est, dans l'uretère de lapin, de 20 mms. (par seconde), dans l'uretère de chat de 50 mms. (par seconde) (la vitesse de l'influx nerveux est d'environ 30 mètres par seconde).

Le muscle pyélo-urétéral présente une phase réfractaire très longue: 3 secondes pour l'uretère de lapin, 1,5 seconde pour l'uretère de chat (la phase réfractaire pour les nerfs est de quelques millièmes de seconde). *Aussi, est-il impossible de tétaniser un uretère* (BOZLER).

4. *Puissance de la contraction*. Elle dépend de l'état de la fibre musculaire et en particulier de sa longueur. La contraction est maxima pour une longueur moyenne. STARLING l'a établi pour le coeur et cette loi de STARLING «pourrait aussi bien être appelée la loi des tissus contractiles» (BINET).

Si la fibre musculaire est allongée ou raccourcie, la puissance de sa contraction diminue. Le fait a été vérifié au myographe isotonique sur des muscles soumis à une tension constante dont on fait varier la longueur.

5. *Les relations entre la tonicité et la contractilité*. On a voulu *confondre* la tonicité et la contractilité comme étant toutes deux une réaction de la fibre musculaire répondant à une excitation d'étirement par un raccourcissement.

De fait, toutes deux se manifestent par une modification dans le couple extensibilité-élasticité et il ne saurait en être autrement puisque ce couple résume les propriétés tissulaires du muscle donc ses seules possibilités de réaction. A ce point de vue, on peut dire avec EVANS: «qu'il n'y a aucun inconvénient à considérer la tonicité comme une contraction prolongée ou une décontraction inhibée».

Mais, le fait même que la contraction se prolonge ou que la décontraction s'inhibe montre qu'il s'agit d'une chose différente de la contraction et de la décontraction normales.

En réalité, tonicité et contractilité *sont choses différentes* car la *contraction* est un état *passager* qui, même prolongé en tétanos, n'est que temporaire, qui produit un *acte* dont le résultat tangible est la progression de l'urine qui entraine une dépense métabolique et qui, s'il est répété ou prolongé, aboutit à la fatigue.

La tonicité est un état *stable*, variant d'intensité mais lentement, qui ne produit pas d'acte mais reste statique (l'hypertonie augmente la pression mais ne fait pas progresser la bouchée urétérale), qui se maintient sans dépense énergétique et n'engendre pas de fatigue.

Tonicité et contractilité, quoique de natures différentes, ont cependant des rapports assez étroits. La loi de STARLING montre, en effet, que la puissance de la contraction dépend de la longueur de la fibre musculaire. Or, cette longueur est précisément réglée par la tonicité qui contrôle non seulement la longueur mais encore les capacités d'extensibilité et d'élasticité de la fibre musculaire.

TRENDELENBURG va plus loin et considère la tonicité comme le point de départ obligatoire, comme une «phase préparatoire» de la contraction.

On conçoit donc l'influence considérable de la tonicité sur la contraction. Un muscle de tonicité basse est allongé — le chemin à parcourir pour arriver à la contraction efficace est plus considérable mais sa fibre offre moins de résistance. Un muscle de forte tonicité est court et le chemin à parcourir est moins grand mais il offre plus de résistance.

La tonicité intervient donc dans la qualité de la contraction et il faudra tenir compte de ce fait dans les circonstances pathologiques.

e) Innervation

Au système intrinsèque du muscle excréteur aboutit un système nerveux extrinsèque provenant du sympathique et du para-sympathique entremêlés.

Ces nerfs extrinsèques ne commandent pas les contractions; le muscle excréteur constitue au même titre que le coeur, un système autonome. Ils modifient tout au plus les contractions en accélérant ou en ralentissant le rythme, en augmentant ou diminuant la puissance.

L'étude détaillée des sections et des excitations de ces *nerfs extrinsèques* à été faite par de nombreux auteurs (PROTOPOPOW, LOEWEN et MENWIRK, FREUDE, BRANDWSKY, LINA STERN, VALENTIN, SATANI etc., etc....). Tous leurs résultats sont incertains et souvent contradictoires et il n'y a rien à en retenir. Résumons les avec HORTOLOMEI dans le propos suivant : le parasympathique règle la motricité de l'uretère et le sympathique sa tonicité.

Pour *résumer ce chapitre*, il faut retenir que, pour que le muscle excréteur fonctionne correctement, il faut que soient réunies un certain nombre de conditions :

1. que le muscle ait une extensibilité-élasticité normale, son extensibilité étant considérable et son élasticité parfaite.

2. que la tonicité règle le couple extensibilité-élasticité à un niveau adéquat aux circonstances.

3. que la contractilité soit bonne, c'est-à-dire que la contraction et la dé-contraction se succèdent librement.

4. que le système nerveux extrinsèque et intrinsèque assure le réglage de ce système autonome.

f) Le mouvement péristaltique

Pour en terminer avec les généralités et avant d'étudier en détail le fonctionnement de l'excrétion urinaire, il faut rappeler en quelques mots ce qu'est un mouvement péristaltique en général.

Le mouvement péristaltique n'est pas spécial à l'appareil urinaire et son mécanisme encore fort obscur a surtout été étudié au niveau du tube digestif. Pourtant il est certainement plus pur au niveau de l'appareil urinaire, à cause de sa longueur limitée et surtout à cause de l'homogénéité de son contenu qui est et ne peut être que de l'urine, sans addition de gaz ni grande différence de densité.

Il ne nous appartient pas de discuter ici tous les travaux de BAYLISS et STARLING, d'UEXKULL, de TRENDELENBURG, d'ALVARES, HENDERSON, MORIN, etc.... concernant le péristaltisme en général.

Pour ce qui concerne plus spécialement le péristaltisme urétéral, on a le choix entre les conclusions suivantes :

— celle d'ENGELMANN qui n'accorde aucun rôle au système nerveux,

— celle de PROTOPOPOW pour qui l'intégrité du système ganglionnaire est indispensable au péristaltisme,

— celle de ZANNE qui distingue un centre nerveux supérieur d'où dépend l'isopéristaltisme et un centre inférieur qui commande l'antipéristaltisme.

Le péristaltisme dépend-il du système nerveux intrinsèque, est-il déclenché par la mise en tension du tube creux par son contenu ? est-ce la contraction qui est primitive et qui modèle son contenu ? le mouvement se propage-t-il de cellule à cellule ou sous l'action d'un clavier nerveux ? Toutes ces hypothèses ont été soulevées, aucune n'est démontrée. On constate l'existence du mouvement péristaltique, mais on ignore son mécanisme intime.

C'est lui cependant qui véhicule l'urine et l'entraine activement de la papille à la vessie. C'est lui que nous allons maintenant étudier dans ses variations physiologiques et pathologiques.

II. Moyens d'étude

Il faut distinguer:
1. L'expérimentation physiologique.
2. Les constatations cliniques.
3. Les constatations radiologiques.
4. Les méthodes spéciales.

1. Expérimentation physiologique

Inaugurées en 1869 par ENGELMANN, ces méthodes portent sur l'uretère, soit en place, soit plus souvent excisé et examiné en dehors de l'organisme. Le bassinet des animaux d'expérience étant intra-rénal n'a jamais été spécialement considéré.

L'intérêt de ces expériences est de pouvoir modifier les conditions de l'examen et d'apprécier les modifications qu'elles déterminent.

Ces études expérimentales sont déjà anciennes et bien connues. Nous les résumerons rapidement:

a) Mouvements spontanés

Un uretère, in situ, sectionné à sa partie supérieure, donc qui n'est plus traversé par de l'urine, présente, après une phase d'inhibition, des mouvements spontanés.

Un uretère, retiré de l'organisme, conservé à la glacière dans une solution physiologique, conserve une motricité virtuelle pendant plusieurs jours; si on le suspend, dans une solution de RINGER-LOCKE, bien oxygénée et maintenue à 38°, les contractions spontanées plus ou moins régulières reprennent après un certain temps.

b) Influence de la pression intra-urétérale

Si l'uretère se contracte, même sans qu'aucun liquide y circule, il n'en reste pas moins que le péristaltisme est normalement déclenché par la pression que détermine le débit urinaire (LAPIDES): l'urine met le muscle en tension et détermine une contraction locale qui se propage de proche en proche sans intervention du système nerveux.

En faisant varier la pression, on obtient les réactions suivantes (SOKOLOFF et LUCHSINGER — BINET et STOICESCO):

α) *Pression inférieure à 5 cm H_2O.* L'uretère peut rester sans réponse. En général, après une période latente de quelques secondes, il présente une contraction ou une série de contractions subintrantes, suivie après 50 à 150 secondes, d'autres groupes de contractions.

β) *Pression de 10 à 20 cm d'eau.* On obtient des contractions régulières qui peuvent se maintenir pendant 1 heure 1/2. Quelques minutes après le déclenchement de ces contractions, on peut supprimer la pression: les contractions deviennent moins fréquentes mais restent régulières et persistent pendant deux à trois heures.

γ) *Pression de 30 à 40 cm d'eau et plus.* Le rythme augmente de fréquence et l'amplitude diminue: la régularité est moins parfaite, l'uretère se fatigue rapidement.

δ) si on lie l'uretère et qu'on introduit dans sa cavité une certaine quantité de liquide, sous une pression donnée, on constate que:
— pression nulle: le rythme et l'amplitude ne se modifient pas
— pression de 5 cm. H_2O: les contractions sont plus fortes et la période de repos intermédiaire se raccourcit.
— pression de 10 à 15 cm. H_2O: même action, d'autant plus marquée que la pression est plus grande.

L'obstacle qui s'oppose à l'échappement du liquide contenu dans la cavité urétérale entraine une augmentation de la période de contraction et une diminution de la période de repos.

c) Influence de la composition du liquide urétéral

α) *Urine*. Binet et Stoicesco remplacent dans l'uretère le liquide de Ringer par l'*urine* du chien qui a fourni l'organe: ils observent, à pression égale, une augmentation de l'amplitude des contractions.

L'*acidification* et surtout l'*alcalinisation* de l'urine augmentent les contractions.

β) *Glucose*. L'addition de glucose à l'urine (ce qui modifie peu sa réaction mais change sa viscosité) augmente l'amplitude et diminue la fréquence des contractions.

γ) *Les solutions hypertoniques*. Les solutions hypertoniques modifient la contractilité (Trattner). Une solution de Locke hypertonique provoque une *augmentation* (parfois mais moins souvent un abaissement) de la *tonicité*, une *diminution* de l'*amplitude* et une *accélération du rythme des contractions*.

Une solution d'*iodure de sodium à 12%* diminue l'amplitude et accélère le rythme jusqu'au spasme; l'action est surtout nette dans le tiers supérieur de l'uretère.

Une solution de *Ténébryl à 35%* provoque une augmentation du tonus et une accélération du rythme, moins accusées que celles de l'Iodure de Sodium (Mingers).

d) Influence des variations du milieu dans lequel est placé l'uretère

α) *Variations de température*. Leur influence est nette.

Le passage rapide de 38° à 40° produit une augmentation de l'amplitude et de la fréquence puis, à la longue, une diminution de l'amplitude.

Le refroidissement brusque à 34° amène une diminution progressive du rythme puis un arrêt des contractions.

Le refroidissement lent produit une phase d'excitation qui précède l'arrêt.

Si on abaisse la température de l'extrémité vésicale d'un uretère, le péristaltisme continue mais l'amplitude est moindre dans la zône refroidie. Si la température est abaissée à l'extrémité rénale, le péristaltisme s'inverse en antipéristaltisme (Gruber).

β) *L'oxygénation*. L'oxygénation du bain augmente les contractions: l'arrêt du courant d'oxygène est suivi d'une diminution brutale des contractions.

γ) *Le chloroforme*. Le chloroforme paralyse l'uretère isolé. Administré par inhalation, il n'aurait, pour Lina Stern, aucun effet sur les contractions urétérales. D'autres auteurs, examinant des animaux avec exstrophie vésicale artificielle n'ont vu, pendant l'anesthésie, aucune éjaculation urétérale: celles-ci reprennent au réveil.

δ) L'éther. L'ether abolirait les contractions péristaltiques.

e) Influence des substances pharmaco-dynamiques

Elle est particulièrement importante depuis qu'à la notion de nerfs sympathiques et parasympathiques s'est substituée celle de nerfs adrénergiques et cholinergiques (DALE).

Les résultats obtenus par les divers auteurs ne concordent pas toujours: les conditions d'expérience et les doses employées expliquent ces variations. Nous nous attacherons surtout aux observations de BINET:

— *Adrénaline* (type des substances adrénergiques, libérées par excitation des fibres post ganglionnaires du sympathique). — Elle excite toutes les fonctions des nerfs sympathiques.
        Tonicité +
        Amplitude des contractions —
        Fréquence des contractions —
— *Ergotamine* (inhibiteur des fonctions excitatrices du sympathique):
        Contractilité amplitude —
        L'adrénaline ajoutée après action de l'ergotamine n'a plus d'action.
— *Yohimbine* (qui paralyse les effects des nerfs adrénergiques):
        seule: n'a pas d'action
        associée à l'adrénaline: inhibition totale des contractions.
— *Histamine* (le plus puissant excitant des contractions urétérales):
        fréquence des contractions ++
        amplitude des contractions —
— *Acétyl-choline* (type des substances libérées par les nerfs para-sympathiques):
        à faible dose: fréquence des contractions ++
        à forte dose: arrêt des contractions.
— *Pilocarpine* (excitant des fonctions parasympathiques):
        fréquence des contractions +
        Amplitudes des contractions au début + puis —
L'adrénaline ajoutée à la *pilocarpine:*
        fréquence des contractions —
        amplitude des contractions +
— *Esérine* (sensibilisateur des nerfs cholinergiques):
        fréquence des contractions +
        amplitude des contractions —
        Même action que la pilocarpine mais à dose beaucoup plus faible.
— *Atropine* (paralyse les effets des nerfs cholinergiques non pas en empêchant la libération d'acétylcholine, mais en rendant les tissus insensibles à son action). Schlicht déclare n'avoir obtenu aucun effet, ni de la phisiostigmine ni de la pilocarpine, ni de l'atropine ni de la nicotine.
        fréquence des contractions: non modifiées
        amplitude des contractions: légèrement +
Binet résume ainsi l'action des substances pharmaco-dynamiques:
— Les excitants des fonctions *sympathiques* augmentent *l'amplitude* des contractions.
— Les excitants des fonctions *parasympathiques* augmentant leur *fréquence.*

f) Influence de l'innervation

Elle a été étudiée p. 485 et nous avons vu qu'il est impossible d'en tirer des données nettes sur le rôle respectif du sympathique et du para-sympathique étroitement intriqués dans les plexus dont dépend l'innervation de cet appareil.

g) Influence de la vascularisation

La ligature de l'aorte ou de l'artère rénale qui provoque une anémie brusque de l'appareil pyélo-uretéral, amène un ralentissement puis un arrêt des contractions.

h) Motricité relative des différents segments de l'uretère

Pour l'étudier, on sectionne l'uretère en trois portions égales dont on étudie la motricité.

Placées dans des conditions analogues:
— c'est le tiers moyen qui est le moins actif,
— le tiers inférieur à des contractions plus amples,
— le tiers supérier les contractions les plus rapides.

Si on sectionne l'uretère à sa partie moyenne, le bout rénal continue à présenter des contractions normales. Sur le bout vésical, les contractions sont d'abord supprimées, puis elles reprennent plus lentes et plus fortes avec un rythme indépendant des contractions du bout supérieur. Sur le bout inférieur se produisent parfois des contractions antipéristaltiques.

Si on sectionne l'uretère en 3 segments, les segments supérieur et inférieur se comportent comme il vient d'être dit. Le segment intermédiaire ne présente pas de contractions spontanées.

Sur l'animal vivant, si l'on pratique une section portant haut et laissant attenant à l'uretère un segment de bassinet, l'uretère se contracte normalement (SETCHAVOW-ZANNE).

Si la section porte en plein uretère, au-dessous de la jonction pyélo-urétérale, les contractions sont moins fréquentes et parfois antipéristaltiques (ZANNE).

2. Constatations cliniques

a) Examen direct

Chez l'homme, au cours d'une intervention lombaire ou abdominale (interventions gynécologiques — opération de WERTHEIM) —

Chez les animaux de Laboratoire.

On a décrit deux variétés de mouvements:

1. des mouvements *pendulaires:* contractions rythmiques se produisant sur place, déplaçant l'uretère latéralement (BOEMINGHAUS); ils ne propulsent pas l'urine et ne sont peut être que des ébauches du mouvement péristaltique.

2. des mouvements *péristaltiques*, les seuls importants.

Rythmiques, plus ou moins espacés, se déplaçant de haut en bas. Le cordon de l'uretère aplati et rosé au repos, devient cylindrique, blanchâtre et se contracte. On distingue une contraction longitudinale qui raccourcit l'uretère et une contraction circulaire qui forme un anneau oblitérant la lumière. Ces deux contractions sont presque simultanées à l'extrémité supérieure, mais la contraction longitudinale s'étend plus rapidement et l'anneau contractile circulaire parcourt un uretère qui semble remonter à sa rencontre. En amont de la contraction, l'uretère est complètement relâché.

La fréquence des contractions varie de 2 à 8 par minute. Le rythme est irrégulier: tantôt elles restent isolées, tantôt elles se groupent et se succèdent à un rythme rapide, puis survient un temps d'arrêt plus ou moins prolongé.

Leur puissance est en raison inverse de leur fréquence: plus elles sont espacées, plus leur amplitude est grande. Leur vitesse de propagation varie selon l'espèce: (20 à 30 mm/s. chez le lapin).

L'excitation de l'uretère par contact ou pincement provoque l'apparition du péristaltisme et parfois celle d'antipéristaltisme; mais il semble que le résultat varie avec le segment d'uretère considéré.

Tout ceci ne concerne que l'uretère: le bassinet et les calices, intra-parenchy-mateux, échappent à l'examen direct. Seule la jonction pyélo-urétérale est visible; son excitation par contact détermine une contraction péristaltique qui survient après un temps perdu appréciable.

b) Cystoscopie

Elle permet de voir l'aboutissement vésical du péristaltisme sous forme d'*éjaculations urétérales*.

1er temps: l'orifice urétéral bombe et fait saillie dans la vessie.

2ème temps: forte rétraction de l'orifice qui fuit devant le cystoscope, efface la valvule muqueuse qui l'obture au repos.

3ème temps: l'orifice urétéral s'ouvre et l'éjaculation se produit, injectant avec force dans la vessie une certaine quantité d'urine, ce qui provoque un remous classiquement comparé à celui d'une goutte de glycérine tombant dans de l'eau. Cette éjaculation est surtout visible avec une urine colorée, soit par du sang, soit par de l'indigo carmin préalablement injecté.

4ème temps: le méat se referme et l'uretère reprend sa position de repos.

La méatoscopie permet d'étudier le rythme du péristaltisme et ses variations.

c) Examen des reins néphrectomisés

Cette méthode ne concerne, en principe, jamais des reins sains mais des reins enlevés pour lésion parenchymateuse qui peuvent avoir des voies excrétrices saines, susceptibles d'être étudiées. Cette étude est particulièrement passionnante sur les reins d'hydronéphrose (LEGUEU, FEY, PALAZZOLI).

Aussitôt après la néphrectomie, le rein et l'uretère prélevés sont plongés dans du serum à 37⁰.

On peut perfuser les voies excrétrices en introduisant une aiguille à travers le parenchyme avec une solution de serum coloré à l'éosine. On peut aussi introduire dans le bassinet une sonde urétérale coiffée d'un ballonnet de baudruche, la mettre en communication avec un tambour de MAREY et obtenir une courbe des contractions pyéliques.

Dans quelques cas, on voit se produire des contractions spontanées du bassinet qui se propagent à l'uretère; plus souvent il faut provoquer ces contractions par contact, pincement ou électrisation de la paroi pyélique ou par remplissage progressif du bassinet. L'excitation est particulièrement efficace dans le sinus du rein, c'est-à-dire à la partie supérieure du bassinet et au niveau de la jonction pyélo-urétérale. Une excitation portant sur l'uretère détermine une double contraction, péristaltique et anti-péristaltique, partant en sens inverse du point excité.

Il va de soi que les contractions obtenues au début de l'expérience sont plus nettes et plus énergiques et qu'elles vont s'atténuer progressivement. Le liquide perfusé, d'abord franchement éjaculé à l'extrémité du moignon urétéral, s'écoule en bavant: ce stade précède de peu la mort définitive de l'appareil neuro-musculaire.

Dans le cas particulier de l'hydronéphrose, il est curieux de noter qu'après néphrectomie, des bassinets trouvés atones d'après les explorations précédentes, retrouvent des contractions très nettes, très rapprochées et qui peuvent se prolonger spontanément plusieurs heures.

A noter, dans tous les cas, que toute contraction est suivie d'une phase réfractaire de plusieurs secondes, pendant lesquelles aucune réponse n'est obtenue, quelles que soient la qualité et l'intensité de l'excitation.

L'enregistrement graphique de la contraction permet de décomposer ses différents temps:

1. Au début, un temps perdu, court mais net, pendant lequel il ne se produit rien.

2. Une contraction systolique nette où le bassinet se contracte en masse, revient sur lui-même et se rétracte dans le hile du rein. Cette phase de contraction est rapide et énergique.

3. Une phase de diastole, beaucoup plus lente et plus longue pendant laquelle tout se détend et où le bassinet reprend son aspect initial.

4. Une phase d'inexcitabilité qui se prolonge plusieurs secondes.

La durée respective des différentes phases est de l'ordre de:
— temps perdu = 1 seconde,
— systole = $^1/_2$ seconde.
— diastole et phase réfractaire: = 10 à 15 secondes.

3. Constatations radiologiques

a) La pyélographie

«Figure d'immobilité» ne donne aucun renseignement.

b) La pyéloscopie

La pyéloscopie consiste à remplir le bassinet, préalablement cathétérisé, avec une substance opaque: l'injection du liquide opaque se fait sous écran radioscopique, en ayant soin de remplir les cavités rénales mais sans arriver à la distension (annoncée par la douleur). La sonde est alors retirée et l'on assiste sous écran à l'excrétion du liquide opaque.

Le bassinet et les calices sont d'abord seuls visibles: on y note des *mouvements de brassage* au cours desquels le bassinet est tantôt en systole (bassinet contracté, calices remplis) et en diastole (bassinet rempli et calices contractés).

Puis, au cours d'une systole plus prononcée, on voit le liquide opaque, non seulement refluer vers les calices, mais dessiner à la jonction pyélo-urétérale un prolongement conique plus ou moins allongé, que nous avons appelé le *bulbe uretéral* par analogie avec le bulbe duodénal qui apparait dans les mêmes conditions.

Nouvelle diastole, puis nouvelle systole pyélique au cours de laquelle le bulbe se détache de l'extrémité inférieure du bassinet qui reprend une forme arrondie. Le contenu du bulbe file dans l'uretère qu'il parcourt de haut en bas d'un mouvement uniforme pour aboutir à la vessie. C'est la *rame uretérale*.

Nouvelle systole, nouveau bulbe, nouvelle rame, plus ou moins précipités dans leur rythme. On assiste ainsi à l'excrétion progressive du liquide opaque intra-pyélique éliminé par bouchées intermittentes et rames urétérales progressant selon le mode péristaltique.

A noter que les bouchées pyéliques ne s'établissent qu'après une ou deux minutes de brassage inefficace, que les rames urétérales se succèdent à un rythme assez variable et à un intervalle d'environ 2 à 4 secondes, que le bassinet semble vidé après un temps qui est normalement d'environ une minute par centimètre cube de liquide opaque injecté.

A la pyéloscopie, le bassinet se comporte comme l'estomac (mouvements de brassage et évacuation par éclipses) et l'uretère comme l'intestin (péristaltisme).

Peut-on accepter ces données comme représentant exactement et avec certitude ce qui se passe en réalité ? La chose mérite d'être regardée de près.

Il y a dans la pyéloscopie trois causes d'erreur:

1. le cathétérisme préalable,

2. le remplissage du bassinet avec un liquide hypertonique,

3. son remplissage rapide avec une quantité de liquide probablement supérieure à celle qu'il contient normalement et qui ne doit se produire qu'en cas de polyurie exceptionnellement abondante.

Le cathétérisme préalable explique probablement la première phase de brassage inefficace; celle qui précède l'établissement des évacuations régulières.

L'hypertonie du milieu de contraste constitue une excitation anormale à laquelle le bassinet réagit par une réponse anormalement forte.

Enfin la quantité exagérée de liquide remplissant le bassinet peut modifier non seulement le rythme mais aussi la modalité de l'excrétion. C'est ce que pensent Hortolomei, Burghele et Stresa d'une part, Rubritius et Fuchs d'autre part. Pour eux, l'évacuation normale se ferait par mouvements péristaltiques continus. Ce n'est qu'en cas de polyurie, comme celle que réalise artificiellement l'injection de liquide opaque, que l'évacuation se ferait par «cystoïdes», le bassinet agissant à la façon d'une vessie pour retenir le liquide en excès et préserver le mince calibre de l'uretère contre un afflux trop brusque.

Nous aurons à revenir sur ce point, évidemment très important.

Malgré ces objections, les données de la pyéloscopie sont capitales. C'est la première exploration qui ait permis de suivre l'excrétion de bout en bout, des calices à la vessie et d'établir la succession de ses différents temps. Même si les mouvements vus à l'écran sont amplifiés ou troublés dans leur rythme, on est sûr qu'ils existent réellement et que ce sont eux, à l'exclusion de toute autre cause, qui assurent l'excrétion pyélo-urétérale.

Le plus gros inconvénient de la méthode est qu'il est long de s'adapter, que la protection contre le rayonnement est difficile à réaliser et qu'elle ne fournit que des renseignements subjectifs. Rares sont les Urologues qui l'ont pratiquée de façon suivie mais ceux là en ont tiré grands profits (Borgard).

c) L'urographie intra-veineuse

Elle montre l'aspect des voies excrétrices surpris aux différents temps et ceci dans leur réalité physiologique sans cause d'erreur d'ordre instrumental.

1. On retrouve, en Urographie, les différents temps de l'évacuation (Legueu, Fey, Truchot). Ces images sont plus vraies mais ne sont que des aspects successifs et transitoires. Pour les interpréter correctement il faut les multiplier et les replacer dans le cycle de l'évacuation établi par la pyéloscopie (Narath). Les sériographies (de Beaufond et Porcher) ont été faites dans ce but; elles ne sont qu'un timide acheminement vers la radiocinématographie.

2. Boeminghaus, Fuchs, ont utilisé l'Urographie dans l'étude des rapports de l'excrétion avec la secrétion rénale.

Pour une diurèse de 1 cc. par minute (1.500 cc. par 24 heures) ou pour une diurèse moindre, les voies excrétrices ont une même tonicité sur toute leur longueur; l'évacuation se fait par ondes péristaltiques continues, se propageant sans interruption le long du bassinet et de l'uretère.

Pour une diurèse de 2 cc. par minute (3.000 cc. par 24 heures), les voies excrétrices se mettent en état de *«segmentation fonctionnelle»* avec succession de segments hypotoniques ayant le caractère de détrusors, séparés par des segments hypertoniques ayant le caractère de sphincters. Chaque couple détrusor-sphincter constituant un «cystoïde». Il existerait un épicystoïde au niveau des calices, fermé par le sphincter calico-pyélique, un cystoïde pyélique fermé par le sphincter pyélo-uretéral, deux ou trois cystoïdes uretéraux dont l'inférieur est fermé par le sphincter uretéro-vésical. Le nombre de ces cystoïdes varie selon les sujets.

Chez un sujet néphrectomisé, le rein unique se comporte exactement de la même façon: évacuation continue pour une diurèse de 1.500 cc., évacuation segmentaire pour une diurèse de 3.000 cc. Le réglage excrétion-secrétion ne serait donc pas commandé par le rein ou le système nerveux rénal, mais bien par un centre nerveux que les auteurs pensent devoir exister dans le mésencéphale sur le plancher du IIIème ventricule. Les voies efférentes qui commandent ces changements de tonicité passeraient par les rami-communicantes de L2 pour l'uretère supérieur et de L3 pour l'uretère moyen et inférieur (BRANDESKY).

3. Un autre intérêt, primordial, de l'Urographie, est d'être la seule méthode qui permette d'explorer la *tonicité* des voies excrétrices. Pyélographie et pyéloscopie, qui comportent des causes d'erreur instrumentale, troublent certainement cette tonicité. Seule l'Urographie, parcequ'elle est physiologique, montre les voies excrétrices dans leur état réel et permet d'apprécier leur tonicité.

On apprécie la tonicité:

par le volume des différents éléments: dans l'ensemble, plus l'image est étalée, moins la tonicité est élevée, mais il existe des causes d'erreur:

— l'image opaque montre la surface mais non l'épaisseur, donc un seul des éléments du volume de la cavité,

— il y a des bassinets larges et d'autres étroits et ramifiés,

— la tonicité n'est pas toujours en relation directe avec le volume et certains bassinets dilatés et même très dilatés peuvent avoir une tonicité normale.

l'aspect des contours mous et arrondis pour les muscles de tonicité faible, rectilignes et angulés pour ceux de tonicité élevée.

par la réaction des voies excrétrices aux épreuves de compression et de décompression réalisées au cours de l'examen urographique.

La compression provoque une rétention et une augmentation de la pression interne. La décompression libère cette pression. A l'Urographie, on assiste, après 15 minutes de compression, à une certaine *expansion* des cavité pyélocalicielles en amont du point comprimé. Lors de la décompression, cette expansion disparait dans une plus ou moins grande proportion. Ces réactions mesurent très explicitement la réaction de la paroi musculaire à la pression qu'exerce son contenu. Une grande expansion à la compression suivie de faible retrait à la décompression, indique une tonicité basse; une expansion modérée, suivie d'un retrait net à la décompression, témoigne d'une tonicité élevée.

Dans l'ensemble, les pyélogrammes obtenus par pyélographie sont plus toniques et plus petits que ceux de l'Urographie parce que le bassinet réagit à l'injection de substance opaque en élevant sa tonicité.

A l'Urographie, la tonicité est en général moyenne ou basse et il faut se garder de considérer comme dilatés et pathologiques des bassinets hypotoniques mais parfaitement normaux.

L'étude de la tonicité normale des voies excrétrices est à peine ébauchée: on sait qu'elle dépend de multiples facteurs (nerveux, endocriniens, équilibre vago-sympathique, etc....) et aussi de la diurèse à laquelle elle doit adapter le travail de ses muscles.

A une augmentation de diurèse, correspondent des voies excrétrices mieux remplies, plus larges, à fibres musculaires plus allongées, c'est-à-dire de tonus diminué. La souplesse de ce mécanisme est une caractéristique des voies urinaires normales.

d) Radiocinématographie

Méthode récente rendue possible par les amplificateurs de brillance (1955): c'est le mode d'exploration du proche avenir dont il est, dès maintenant, possible de prévoir l'utilisation journalière en clinique.

Comme toutes les explorations nouvelles, elle a besoin d'une longue mise au point. Au début, les films ont été médiocres: leur qualité s'améliore mais il faut apprendre à les interpréter. Leur rapidité rend difficile la perception exacte de ce qui se passe en différents points et d'établir la coordination des différents éléments. Il faut recourir à des appareils de projection permettant le ralenti, le numérotage des vues dans le temps, l'arrêt et au besoin le retour en arrière. Nul doute que l'étude attentive de ces films n'arrive à résoudre toutes les questions qui se posent. Mais c'est là un travail de longue haleine qui n'est qu'à peine esquissé.

Il existe deux modalités de radiocinématographie:

1. *La pyélocinématographie*, qui utilise l'injection de produit d'opacité connue, donne d'excellents films mais est entachée des causes d'erreur des injections à contre-courant.

2. *L'Urocinématographie* après injection intra-veineuse du produit iodé: la concentration est beaucoup plus faible, les films moins nets, mais on se trouve placé dans les circonstances physio-pathologiques normales.

De même que la Pyélographie et l'Urographie, la Pyélocinématographie et l'Urocinématographie, loin de s'opposer, se recoupent et complètent leurs résultats respectifs.

Dans l'ensemble, la radiocinématographie est une pyéloscopie qui laisse un document qu'on peut lire et discuter à loisir.

Nous ne détaillerons pas ici les résultats parce qu'ils serviront de base, dans le chapitre suivant, à l'étude synthétique de l'excrétion.

Disons seulement que si son importance est primordiale en physiologie normale, elle sera surtout capitale en pathologie en permettant de distinguer les sténoses et les spasmes, les lésions passagères et les définitives, les retentissements étagés des différentes lésions, etc....

e) L'urokymographie

La Kymographie a été découverte par STUMPF en 1928. Ce procédé rend compte, sur un cliché, des mouvements divers survenus chez l'objet à photographier pendant le temps d'exposition.

Il a été appliqué à divers organes creux et contractiles et particulièrement à l'uretère.

A GREGOIR revient le mérite d'avoir utilisé de façon suivie, en pratique urologique, ce procédé qui n'était guère employé que dans un but de recherches.

α) Principes de la méthode

Devant la surface sensible se trouve placée une grille. Cette grille est perforée de fentes horizontales, aussi larges que le film, hautes de 0,5 mm. et disposées à un intervalle vertical de 12 mm.

Pendant le temps où passent les rayons, soit 20 secondes dans la technique de GREGOIR, la grille se déplace de 12 mm., selon un mouvement uniforme et dirigé verticalement de haut en bas. Il s'ensuit que les rayons parallèles issus de chaque fente vont balayer le film de haut en bas et y imprimer le contour des organes qu'ils ont traversés.

Le film obtenu est formé de bandes horizontales où figurent les organes photographiés, séparées les unes des autres par une ligne blanche. Chacune de ces bandes correspond au balayage d'une seule fente sur 12 mm. et pendant 20 secondes, nommée «secteur» par Gregoir.

— *Dans un secteur donné*, l'image de l'uretère normal, opacifié soit par pyélographie, soit par Urographie, apparait, soit discontinue, soit marquée d'incisures profondes.

Ceci nécessite une explication:

— Chaque secteur n'est pas un cliché instantané,

— Chaque secteur n'est pas non plus une suite de clichés horizontaux intéressant une seule et même tranche,

— Chaque secteur est constitué par une succession de clichés horizontaux, pris de haut en bas à des temps régulièrement successifs.

Ceci est assez complexe et les clichés ne peuvent être interprétés qu'en fonction de la technique utilisée, c'est-à-dire du temps de pose (20 secondes) et du déplacement de la grille. Ceci nécessite quelques calculs que Gregoir explique:

— la rame urétérale se déplace de haut en bas, à la vitesse de 2 à 6 cm. par seconde. En 20 secondes, temps d'exposition, elle se déplace de 40 à 120 cm. Elle croise donc nécessairement tous les secteurs.

— dans un secteur donné, systole et diastole urétérales sont nettement marquées.

On voit, par exemple, en haut du secteur, soit dans les premières secondes d'exposition, la systole. L'uretère est diminué de calibre, ou même invisible.

Plus tard, donc plus bas, apparait la diastole. L'uretère est élargi, opaque, bien visible.

Si le mouvement péristaltique est rapide, on peut voir encore en-dessous, toujours dans le même secteur, une nouvelle systole et même une nouvelle diastole.

En somme, chaque secteur offre une trace de l'activité péristaltique générale pendant 20 secondes.

De l'examen d'un seul secteur, on peut tirer d'abord le rythme.

Le rythme R. peut se calculer en divisant le temps de descente de la grille T par le nombre n de contractions enregistrées dans un secteur. Le chiffre obtenu a peu de valeur en raison de la petitesse de T.

De l'examen d'un seul secteur, on peut encore tirer des conclusions sur l'amplitude et l'énergie de la contraction uretérale.

— Le film est formé de secteurs étagés de haut en bas, tous balayés au même moment. Mais ces secteurs ne sont pas traversés par l'onde urétérale au même moment.

Il résulte de ceci un décalage entre les secteurs. Ce décalage permet d'apprécier l'isopéristaltisme.

Enfin l'examen de un ou deux secteurs permet de calculer la vitesse de propagation de l'onde:

$$V = \frac{AB \times E}{X \times T}$$

T = 20 secondes (Gregoir)

X = AB — E —

AB = distance séparant deux systoles

E = 12 mm.

β) Résultats

1. *Uretère* — En exposant les principes de la méthode et ses déductions mathématiques, nous avons pris l'uretère comme exemple.

C'est en effet au niveau de l'uretère que l'uretérokymographie offre le plus d'intérêt.

a) Elle donne des renseignements d'ordre général portant sur la totalité de l'uretère.

Elle permet de juger de la contractilité de l'uretère et de voir en particulier si un uretère qui apparait comme dilaté sur une Urographie, est inerte, acinétique, ou contractile.

C'est le plus grand mérite de la méthode. GRÉGOIR a étudié en détail le complexe systolo-diastolique et certains mouvements péristaltiques altérés. Dans ces cas, le cinéma est bien supérieur.

b) Elle donne des renseignements d'ordre local.

Elle met en évidence les zones uretérales totalement inertes dans un uretère contractile en d'autres points.

2. *Bassinet et calices.* Là, la kymographie montre encore si le muscle excréteur est inerte ou non.

Mais c'est à peu près tout ce qu'elle peut montrer car les données que l'on peut utiliser au niveau de l'uretère, conduit simple et traversé par des ondes régulières, ne valent plus rien au niveau du bassinet où les mouvements, le cinéma l'a montré, sont extrêmement complexes.

En conclusion, l'Urokymographie est une méthode fort intéressante, en ce sens qu'elle fait apparaitre sur les clichés le péristaltisme, ce que ne peuvent faire les clichés simples.

La méthode permet, au niveau de l'uretère, des déductions fort poussées sur le sens, le rythme, l'amplitude du mouvement péristaltique en général et sur les altérations éventuelles de ce mouvement. Elle permet aussi de déceler des altérations locales du muscle urétéral.

Au niveau du bassinet et des calices, l'Urokymographie traduit sur le cliché le péristaltisme mais aucune déduction ne peut en être tirée quant au fonctionnement des voies supérieures.

Certes, il est possible d'allonger le temps d'observation. GRÉGOIR peut renouveler la prise des clichées à intervalles de 30 secondes. Mais la kymographie, de par sa technique, ne peut rendre compte que de mouvements simples et est absolument impuissante à expliquer le fonctionnement des calices et du bassinet.

Elle a peut-être maintenant un intérêt pratique en pathologie. Elle n'en a plus aucun en physiologie car elle est détronée par la cinématographie d'étude.

4. Manométrie

Elle est destinée à mesurer les pressions au niveau des différentes cavités: bassinet, uretère et vessie.

a) Instrumentation

Schématiquement, on introduit une sonde dans la cavité à examiner et on la met en communication avec un manomètre enregistreur. Plusieurs difficultés se présentent:

— la sonde doit être de calibre suffisant pour que la pression se transmette librement.

— les mesures ne doivent être enregistrées qu'après les dix ou quinze minutes nécessaires pour que la secrétion compense la fuite de liquide vers le manomètre (Auvert).

— l'extrémité de la sonde doit être en bonne place; pour le bassinet, cette mise en place est facile si le rein est abordé chirurgicalement; elle est plus aléatoire si l'on recourt au cathétérisme et la vérification radiologique est nécessaire. Pour l'uretère, il faut également vérifier le niveau où la sonde s'arrête ou utiliser des sondes à orifices latéraux d'espacement connu (sonde de Bors et Blinn).

— le manomètre doit être de type isotonique. Le plus simple est le manomètre de Claude utilisé dans les ponctions lombaires. Mais les résultats sont plus exacts avec des manomètres électroniques: Electromanomètre de Baudoin utilisé par Rouffilange et Chaillet, Auvert, ou manomètre électronique de Knipper.

— les courbes de pression peuvent être enregistrées ce qui nécessite des montages complexes.

b) Résultats

Auvert a établi un excellent schéma des pressions successives auxquelles est soumise une goutte d'urine parcourant le rein et les voies excrétrices.

La pression artérielle moyenne est de 75 mm. Hg = 100 cm. H_2O.

La pression de filtration glomérulaire tombe à 40 mm. Hg = 52 cm. H_2O.

Elle diminue dans la traversée du tube contourné et la goutte d'urine perle à la papille et tombe dans le calice sous une pression d'environ 10 mm. Hg = 13 cm. H_2O: cette pression se maintient égale dans la traversée du calice et du bassinet; elle est sensiblement équivalente à la pression de la veine rénale.

Au niveau de l'uretère la pression augmente progressivement de haut en bas: 20 cm. H_2O dans le tiers supérieur, 30 cm. H_2O dans l'uretère moyen pour arriver à 50 à 70 cm. H_2O dans l'uretère terminal.

Notons qu'au niveau de la vessie, la pression très basse, 12 à 18 cm. H_2O au repos, monte au maximum à 100 cm. H_2O au moment de la miction.

Tel est le schéma au cours d'une excrétion libre dans un appareil excréteur normal. Si l'excrétion est bloquée (sonde bouchon introduite dans le méat), les pressions s'élèvent progressivement et un équilibre s'établit du glomérule à l'extrémité inférieure de l'uretère aux environs de 50 cm. H_2O qui correspond à la pression de filtration glomérulaire (pression urinaire maxima — (Auvert)).

Cette pression de base, en dehors de toute contraction varie avec les individus et les circonstances ce qui explique les chiffres variables obtenus par différents auteurs.

Au niveau du bassinet, les chiffres extrêmes sont de 3 à 5 cm. H_2O (Pisani) à 20 à 30 cm. H_2O (Pilcher, Bollmann et Mann).

Au niveau de l'uretère, mêmes variations amplifiées par celles qui dépendent du niveau envisagé.

La pression augmente, bien entendu, *au moment des contractions musculaires*, c'est-à-dire au moment du passage de l'onde péristaltique.

Au niveau du bassinet, la pression de contraction est difficile à mesurer à cause des petites dimensions de l'extrémité de la sonde. Auvert estime approximativement qu'au cours de la systole la pression passe de 10 à 20 cm. H_2O.

L'élévation de pression est beaucoup plus sensible au niveau de l'uretère où elle est en moyenne de 35 à 40 cm. H_2O (Swenson et Fischer); elle croit de haut en bas: 25 à 30 cm. H_2O pour l'uretère lombaire, 35 à 40 cm. H_2O pour l'uretère iliaque, 50 à 80 et même 100 et 120 cm. H_2O pour l'uretère pelvien

(Bors. Rattner). C'est donc sous une pression voisine de la pression vésicale de miction (100 cm. H_2O) que le contenu urétéral est éjaculé dans la vessie (Lapidès, Merenyi, Banchieri).

Bors et Blinn ont obtenu des courbes manométriques différentes selon les segments. Onde simple pour l'uretère lombaire, onde bifide pour l'uretère iliaque, onde triple ou quadruple pour l'uretère terminal.

La Manométrie est une méthode intéressante et pleine de promesse. Elle a permis à Knipper de noter que les analgésiques agissent sur le rythme des contractions et que les spasmolytiques influencent le tonus. Elle a fourni à Rouffilange et à Auvert des données pronostiques importantes dans des cas d'anurie et d'hydronéphrose. Malheureusement, elle est peu précise, difficile à appliquer au bassinet et passible de multiples causes d'erreur d'origine instrumentale. Finkentscher et Semm obtiennent des courbes totalement différentes selon la nature du liquide avec lequel ils perfusent l'uretère.

5. L'électro-urétérographie*

Cette méthode d'exploration, basée sur l'enregistrement de l'activité électrique de la musculature lisse de l'uretère in situ, c'est à dire dans des conditions se rapprochant autant que possible de celles du fonctionnement physiologique, s'adresse surtout à l'étude de la contraction péristaltique et en apprécie les différents caractères.

On conçoit donc son intérêt dans l'étude des perturbations pathologiques de la motricité urétérale.

α) Historique

L'idée d'enregistrer l'activité électrique des fibres lisses du muscle urétéral est venue tout d'abord à Orbeli et Brucke qui en 1910, réalisèrent le 1er tracé à partir d'un uretère isolé de lapin. Leur tentative chez l'homme, après exposition chirurgicale, échoua faute d'un appareillage électriquement satisfaisant.

En 1928, nouvelle tentative infructueuse de Trattner qui voulait contrôler les résultats de son hydrophorographe.

Ce n'est qu'en 1932 que Fasiani et Luisada réussirent le premier enregistrement pratiqué sur un uretère humain in situ. L'école italienne, en 1934, avec Ravasini, Chiatellino, et Paladini apporta sa contribution à cette étude.

De son côté Mingers en Belgique en 1936, construisait un appareil extrêmement complexe qui lui donna d'excellents résultats; c'était le polygraphe cathodique.

Puis, après 14 ans d'oubli, Hanley reprenait, avec des succès encourageants, l'étude de cette méthode et la rapportait au Congrès International de la Société d'Urologie en 1950.

Depuis, la littérature s'enrichit lentement de documents obtenus soit expérimentalement chez le chien, soit en clinique humaine, les enregistrements sur uretère pathologique étant encore fort peu nombreux. Parmi les auteurs ayant contribué à cet apport il faut citer les italiens Calafatti, Galli et Agnoletto; les anglais Hanley, Milton et Robb; et les américains Butcher et Sleator, Baker, Corey, Fite et Vest.

β) Appareillage

L'appareillage se compose essentiellement d'électrodes exploratrices reliées à un appareil enregistreur. Les caractéristiques de cet appareillage variant

* Ce chapitre est rédigé par J. Auvigne et R. Lebatard-Sartre.

suivant les experimentateurs c'est le matériel utilisé dans le Service de Clinique Urologique de la Faculté de Nantes qui sera décrit ici.

Les électrodes sont montées sur des sondes urétérales banales. Constituées par de petites bagues d'argent de 6 à 7 mm. de haut, elles sont au nombre de 2 ou 3, espacées de 35 à 40 mm., la première à 40 mm. de l'extrémité supérieure de la sonde. Elles sont reliées par des fils émaillés à des bagues identiques situées à l'autre extrémité de la sonde, les connexions avec l'appareil enregistreur s'effec-

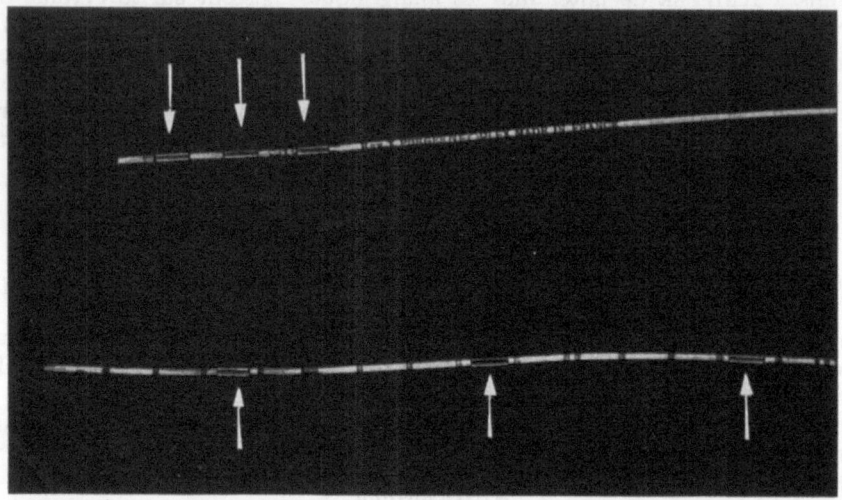

Fig. 1. Sonde urétérographique dont on ne voit que les extrémités. On remarque à l'extrémité supérieure les trois électrodes exploratrices et sur l'extrémité inférieure les trois contacts annulaires destinés à recevoir les «clips» assurant les connexions avec l'appareil enregistreur

tuant à l'aide de «Clips» (Fig. 1). La lumière de la sonde doit être en partie conservée pour permettre l'écoulement de l'urine.

L'appareil enregistreur le plus précis et le plus commode est, sans conteste, l'électro-encéphalographe standard, qui a l'avantage d'enregistrer plusieurs dérivations simultanément. Mais un électro-cardiographe banal à enregistrement direct peut être utilisé à la condition de n'employer que son circuit D.1.

Le tracé électrique sera obtenu, comme dans tous les enregistrements électrographiques, en utilisant plusieurs dérivations. On utilise à la fois des dérivations

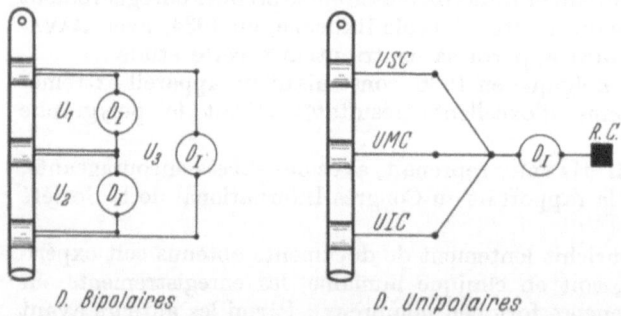

Fig. 2. Les dérivations utilisées en électro-urétérographie. *DI* appareil enregistreur. *R.C.* Référence commune (électrode cutanée)

bipolaires explorant simultanément 2 électrodes intra-urétérales et des dérivations unipolaires explorant une électrode intra-urétérale par rapport à un point électriquement neutre que l'on nomme la référence commune. L'expérience à fait adopter comme point optimum de référence commune, la peau de la partie moyenne de la cuisse du même côté que l'uretère exploré. Avec une sonde à 3 électrodes, c'est donc 6 dérivations qui seront étudiées successivement avec un électro-cardiographe ou mieux simultanément avec un électro-encéphalographe. La Fig. 2 représente ces différentes dérivations.

γ) Technique

Elle doit être standardisée pour obtenir des résultats comparables et pour écarter, dans la mesure du possible, les artéfacts.

Le malade qui a reçu une légère prémédication (Phénergan généralement) est installé aussi confortablement que possible sur la table d'examen de façon à obtenir une résolution musculaire complète. Après cathétérisme uni ou bilatéral des uretères on note l'heure et l'on peut prendre un cliché radiographique de contrôle (Fig. 3). Avant de commencer l'enregistrement *il faut attendre environ 20 minutes* pour permettre le retour au calme de la musculature lisse de l'uretère, excitée par le passage de la sonde. Cette attente doit être scrupuleusement observée, sous peine d'obtenir un tracé ininterprétable.

Pendant l'enregistrement qui sera pratiqué avec la vitesse lente de déroulement du papier on notera la fréquence du pouls et de la respiration ainsi que tous les mouvements ayant un retentissement sur le tracé.

La durée de l'enregistrement doit être longue et varie suivant l'aspect du tracé. Elle sera en moyenne de 5 minutes.

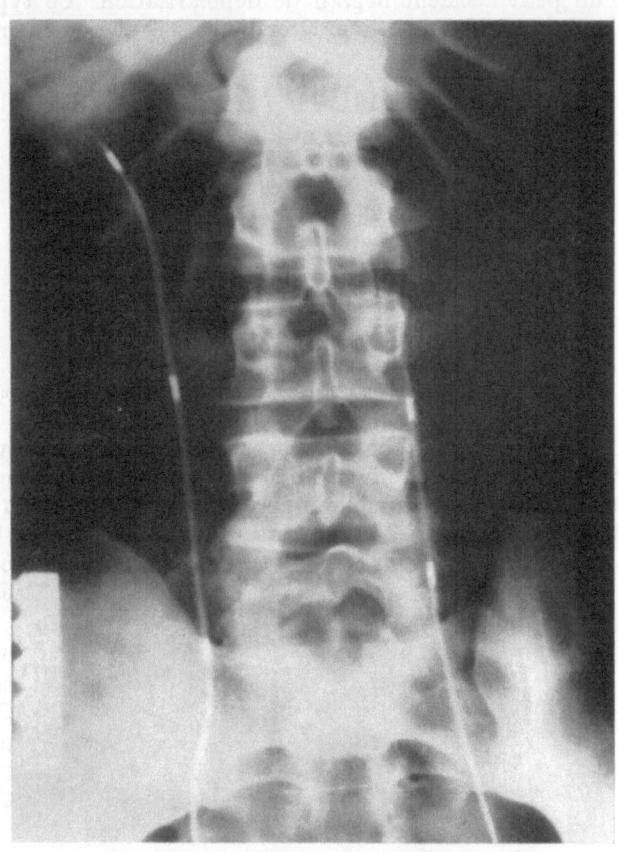

Fig. 3. Radiographie de contrôle montrant la position des sondes

Les suites sont celles de tout cathétérisme urétéral; il est prudent de donner systématiquement un sulfamide.

δ) Résultats

L'expérimentation humaine est encore assez réduite et le manque de standardisation de la technique de cet examen a entraîné des divergences dans les résultats obtenus par les différents auteurs.

Examen d'un uretère humain normal: Le tracé montre l'existence de 2 composantes principales.

1. La première composante de faible amplitude, est formée d'oscillations très plates donnant au tracé l'allure d'une sinusoïde très longue; elle représente l'activité tonique de la musculature urétérale (Fig. 4).

2. La deuxième est l'expression graphique de l'onde de contraction urétérale. Elle est plus intéressante à étudier.

— Aspect: Il est variable dans certaines limites; suivant le moment ou l'onde naît par rapport à l'activité électrique permanente de l'uretère, suivant le niveau de l'électrode exploratrice et enfin suivant la nature de l'appareil enregistreur (électro-cardiographe ou électro-encéphalographe). L'onde de contraction revêt essentiellement 3 types (Fig. 5).

— Type I: Monophasique, c'est une déflection positive précédée et suivie d'un petit accident négatif de dépolarisation. Ce type se voit surtout lorsque l'onde coïncide avec une ascendance marquée de l'onde de tonicité.

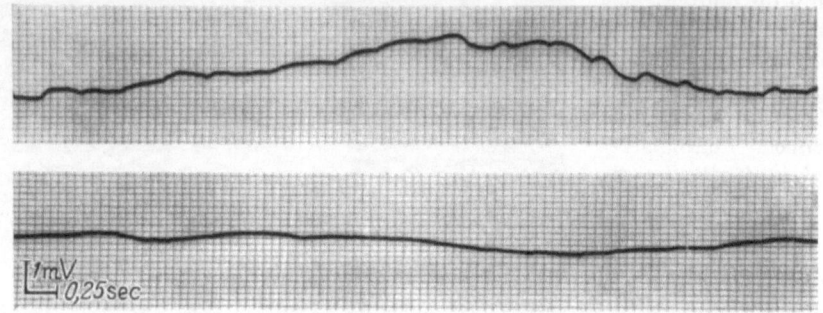

Fig. 4. Ondulations toniques de l'uretère enregistrées avec un électrocardiographe

— Type II: Diphasique, c'est l'aspect le plus typique constitué par une déflection positive suivie d'une négative, les deux accidents étant séparés par un ressaut plus ou moins important. Ce type est souvent précédé d'une petite déflection négative de dépolarisation. C'est l'aspect le plus fréquemment rencontré lorsqu'on utilise un électro-cardiographe.

—Type III: triphasique, c'est une déflection négative encadrée de 2 positives. C'est, avec le type I, l'aspect le plus fréquent sur les tracés obtenus avec un électro-encéphalographe.

Cette variabilité est un argument de plus en faveur de l'emploi de l'électro-encéphalographe où le tracé obtenu est beaucoup plus «parlant» et permet des recoupements faciles.

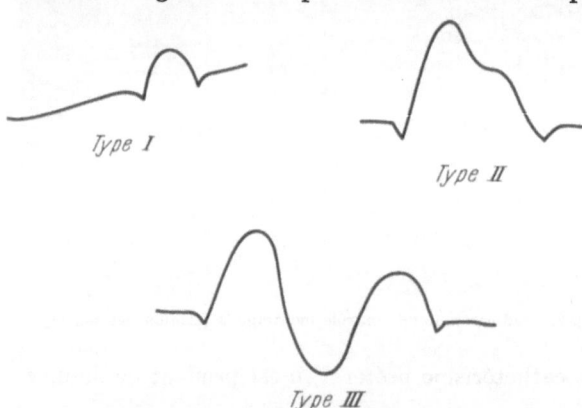

Fig. 5. Les trois types d'ondes de contraction péristaltique

— Voltage: Il est variable suivant les dérivations; le chiffre moyen est en bipolaire de 0,8 mV. et en unipolaire de 4 mV. lorsqu'on utilise l'électro-cardiographe. Si l'on emploie un électro-encéphalographe le voltage moyen est légèrement supérieur (environ 1,1 mV.) du fait de la plus grande sensibilité de l'appareil. Mais, fait remarquable, le voltage croit à mesure que l'électrode exploratrice se rapproche de l'extrémité inférieure de l'uretère.

— Durée: Elle varie évidemment suivant le type de l'onde péristaltique; les limites moyennes sont de 0,7 à 2,5 secondes.

— Fréquence: Elle est variable suivant l'activité que l'uretère doit fournir. Elle est en moyenne de 4 contractions par minute.

— Vitesse de propagation: Notion très importante et qui semble facile à calculer connaissant l'espacement des électrodes exploratrices, elle est en moyenne de 20 mm./sec. Elle est plus facile à déterminer si on utilise un électro-encéphalographe qui permet un enregistrement simultané des dérivations (Fig. 6).

— Direction: De haut en bas c'est à dire isopéristaltique. Il semble qu'il existe parfois, même sur des uretères sains, quelques rares contractions antipéristaltiques de même aspect que les isopéristaltiques, mais inversées. Leur voltage est sensiblement le même mais leur durée semble plus réduite.

La variabilité des caractéristiques de l'onde de contraction péristaltique est à souligner; elle rend difficile encore l'interprétation correcte des tracés.

Applications: Les applications de l'électro-urétérographie sont encore, sur bien des points, du domaine de l'avenir, car les expérimentations pratiquées jusqu'à ce jour sont encore en nombre insuffisant pour permettre d'en tirer des conclusions absolues.

I. Dans le domaine de la physiologie et de la physiopathogénie, cette méthode permet d'étudier le comportement urétéral à l'état normal ou après stimulation physique ou chimique; elle rend possible aussi l'étude des réactions urétérales consécutives à la mobilisation chirurgicale, à la ligature ou à la suture d'un uretère.

Il n'est pas permis pour l'instant de tirer des conclusions fermes mais il semble que les points les plus importants sont les modifications portant sur le voltage et surtout sur la vitesse de propagation de l'onde.

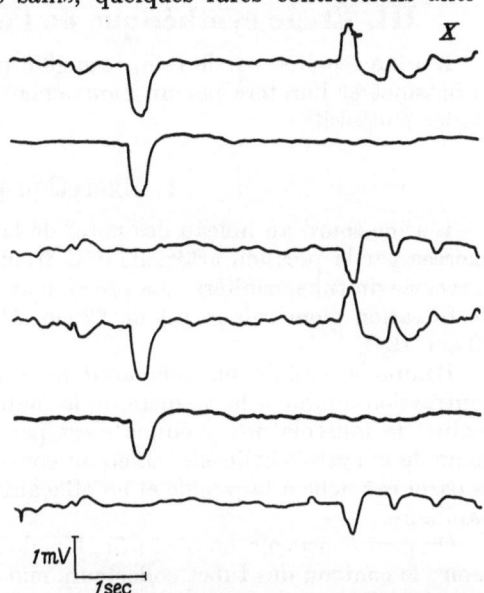

Fig. 6. Tracé simultané (obtenu avec un électro-encéphalographe) permettant de calculer la vitesse de propagation de l'onde de contraction. — Le tracé supérieur représente la dérivation bipolaire mettant en jeu les électrodes supérieure et inférieure; les deux tracés suivants représentent successivement les unipolaires obtenues avec l'électrode supérieure et l'électrode inférieure (les trois tracés inférieurs ne sont que la répétition des trois précédents pour des raisons de contrôle de l'appareil enregistreur). — La contraction, passée sous l'électrode supérieure, est enregistrée par la dérivation unipolaire correspondante (ligne 2) et par la dérivation bipolaire (ligne 1). — Puis lorsqu'elle passe au niveau de l'électrode inférieure, elle s'enregistre sur l'unipolaire correspondante (ligne 3) et sur la même bipolaire mais, là, en sens inverse, du fait de la différencialité de l'appareil. — Connaissant la distance entre les deux électrodes, la vitesse de déroulement du papier et la distance entre deux points précis et identiques des ondes, une simple règle de trois donne la vitesse de propagation

II. En pathologie il n'y a que très peu d'observations et les seuls tracés pratiqués concernent quelques cas de méga-uretères congénitaux (4 cas), de bifidité urétérale (1 cas), d'urétéro-hydronéphroses (7 cas), d'urétérites dites «spastiques» (HANLEY) et de troubles péristaltiques urétéraux chez les traumatisés de la moelle épinière (14 cas).

Il semble donc prématuré d'envisager des résultats précis. Cependant l'électro-urétérographie est appelée à prendre place à côté des autres moyens d'exploration, qu'elle complètera.

En particulier, elle permettra de mieux approcher le problème très difficile de la récupération fonctionnelle d'un uretère dilaté et atone. Car, là où la radio-cinématographie et la manométrie ne montrent qu'un conduit immobile, le

tracé électro-urétérographique pourra peut-être du fait de la persistance d'une
activité électrique, faire prévoir une récupération fonctionnelle et orienter les
décisions thérapeutiques.

Par ailleurs, cette méthode pourrait éclaircir les problèmes pathogéniques
posés par les méga-uretères en montrant s'ils sont dus à une maladie primitive
de la fibre lisse ou à un trouble fonctionnel.

III. Étude synthétique de l'excrétion pyélo-urétérale

L'urine secrétée par le rein, recueillie par les calices, est propulsée à travers
le bassinet et l'uretère par un mouvement péristaltique dont il faut étudier les
stades successifs.

1. Excrétion papillaire

L'urine sourd au niveau des pores de la papille sous l'action de la vis a tergo,
exercée par la pression artérielle déjà freinée par la filtration glomérulaire et la
traversée du tube urinifère. La pression artérielle est de 100 cm. H_2O, la pression
de filtration glomérulaire est de 52 cm. H_2O, la pression dans le calice de 8 à
10 cm. H_2O.

HENLE accordait un rôle actif au muscle annulaire de la papille dont la
contraction agirait à la manière de la main du vacher trayant le mamelon. En
réalité, la musculature pyélique n'est pas adaptée à cette action (NARATH) au
cours de la systole calicielle. Bien au contraire, il est probable qu'en appliquant
la paroi calicielle à la papille et en effaçant le fornix, la systole arrête l'excrétion
papillaire.

On peut concevoir, en revanche, lors de la diastole, que la cavité qui se forme,
aspire le contenu des tubes collecteurs mais la radiocinématographie montre que
c'est le reflux du contenu pyélique qui remplit cette cavité.

Le calice n'intervient donc pas activement dans l'excrétion papillaire et
AUVERT a vu, à bassinet ouvert, en l'absence de toute contraction calicielle,
l'urine colorée par l'indigo carmin, sourdre des pores papillaires et remplir le
fornix.

2. Au niveau des calices

On distingue à l'Urographie deux aspects des calices: *la diastole* avec cavité
largement béante et pied fermé et *la systole* avec cavité effacée, la paroi calicielle étant étroitement appliquée à la saillie papillaire et pied largement ouvert.

Le cinéma montre un aspect intermédiaire de *position indifférente* où la
cavité est moyennement remplie et où le pied entrouvert laisse communiquer
le calice avec le bassinet.

Comment se succèdent ces trois temps sur un même calice?

Partons de la position indifférente, la plus longue: *la diastole* se produit
brusquement au moment de la systole pyélique qui surprend le calice en position
indifférente et y injecte une certaine quantité de son contenu — le calice s'étale
largement et ferme son pied, limitant ainsi le reflux. Cette diastole dont l'apparition est instantanée, brutale, persiste un temps appréciable pendant lequel sa
paroi se met en tension et *la systole* apparait. La cavité s'efface, la paroi se moule
sur la papille, le pied s'ouvre et donne issue au contenu caliciel dans le bassinet
relâché, jusqu'à ce que les pressions calicielle et pyélique s'égalisent; le calice
ne s'efface donc pas complètement; il revient à sa position indifférente.

La succession des trois temps est de l'ordre de 2 à 3 secondes pour la diastole, 1 seconde pour la systole, 7 à 9 secondes pour la période indifférente; ces chiffres ne doivent être considérés que dans leur relativité, car ils dépendent de plusieurs facteurs:

— de la capacité du calice: les petits calices isolés se contractent plus souvent et plus vite que les grand calices bifurqués ou trifurqués de capacité plus grande.

— de la tonicité des différents calices qui peut être différente au moins dans les cas pathologiques.

— de la quantité d'urine secrétée par le territoire de parenchyme correspondant.

Considérons maintenant l'ensemble du système pyélo-caliciel et les rapports qui existent dans le fonctionnement des différents calices d'une part et du bassinet d'autre part.

Une chose est constante: tous les calices entrent en diastole en même temps: cette diastole est provoquée par la systole du bassinet.

Ensuite, chaque calice reprend son individualité, chacun se remplit à son rythme et fait sa systole quand il est mis en tension: il n'existe ni alternance, ni synergie entre les différents calices.

Il peut arriver que deux calices fassent coïncider leur systole; leurs systoles suivantes seront séparées. Ces systoles successives remplissent le bassinet le mettent en tension et la systole pyélique se déclenche.

Dans l'intervalle de 10 à 15″ environ qui sépare deux systoles pyéliques successives, le nombre des systoles calicielles est variable: en général, tous les calices ont le temps de se contracter une fois mais il arrive que certains ne se contractent pas du tout, alors que d'autres effectueront deux systoles. On peut aussi voir une diastole caliciélle avorter lors d'une systole pyélique parceque à ce moment le calice était en systole et non en période indifférente.

Il peut arriver que la systole d'un des calices soit suivie d'une systole pyélique, puis urétérale. Il semble que le mouvement péristaltique ait pris naissance à l'extrémité d'un calice et se soit propagé sans interruption tout au long du bassinet et de l'uretére. Il ne s'agit que d'une coïncidence fortuite: Il suffit pour s'en convaincre de compter pendant un temps donné le nombre total des systoles calicielles et celui des systoles pyéliques: ces dernières sont beaucoup moins nombreuses (nous avons pu compter 26 systoles calicielles pour 5 systoles pyéliques).

PFEIFER spécifie que la succession systole diastole des calices dépend de celle du bassinet; mais il précise aussi que les calices possèdent en outre un rythme de contraction propre et indépendant du bassinet. C'est du bassinet lui-même que nous verrons partir la véritable onde péristaltique efficace. FUCHS a raison de distinguer les épicystoïdes des calices des véritables cystoïdes pyéliques et uretéraux: les calices fonctionnent bien à la manière d'un cystoïde, c'est-à-dire d'un système détrusor-sphincter. Chacun d'eux dépend du cystoïde principal pyélique, mais ils ne font pas partie du mouvement principal qui commence au bassinet.

MAINTZ, MEESE et WUELLENWEBER ont constaté à la kymographie que si le mouvement péristaltique se poursuit sans arrêt du bassinet à l'uretère, toutes les combinaisons de phases sont possibles entre les calices et le bassinet.

3. Au niveau du bassinet

Toutes les 8 à 15″ environ, le bassinet, progressivement rempli par les systoles calicielles, met son détrusor en tension et entre *en systole.*

Cette systole est nette et brusque: les bords se contractent, le volume diminue sans disparaitre complètement et l'ensemble du bassinet se rétracte vers le hile du rein (Pfeifer).

Les calices, surpris en position indifférente se remplissent par reflux et ferment leur pied avant la fin de la systole: à ce moment, le pyélogramme montre un petit bassinet contracté et tous les calices, en diastole, remplis.

En même temps, la jonction pyélo-urétérale s'ouvre et le contenu pyélique passe dans l'uretère; ce passage, beaucoup plus prolongé que le reflux caliciel, va durer pendant toute la systole. Lorsque celle-ci-cesse, la jonction pyélo-urétérale se referme et le bassinet reprend un contour régulièrement arrondi à son pôle inférieur.

L'écart entre deux systoles pyéliques est d'environ 10 secondes mais il varie dans de larges limites selon la diurèse, l'état de tonicité, la réplétion vésicale et aussi selon les mouvements respiratoires, la position du corps et les facteurs pathologiques.

La systole pyélique dure environ $1^1/_2$ à 2 secondes; la diastole serait pour Pfeifer de 2 à 3 secondes mais il distingue une troisième phase «phase de repos» analogue à la période indifférente. Pour cet auteur, en cas d'*oligurie* avec systoles espacées à un intervalle de 20 secondes, la durée de la systole et de la diastole restent les mêmes; la période de repos s'allonge à 17 secondes.

En *polyurie* (3 systoles en 20 secondes), systole et diastole gardent leur rythme: c'est la période de repos qui diminue.

Le bassinet est l'organe principal de l'excrétion urinaire. D'un côte il déclenche la diastole des calices, de l'autre il donne naissance au mouvement péristaltique uretéral. C'est lui enfin qui, en réglant le rythme alternatif des systoles et des diastoles, fragmente l'évacuation grâce au mécanisme de la jonction pyélo-urétérale que nous allons maintenant étudier.

4. Au niveau de la jonction pyélo-urétérale

On sait, qu'au point de vue anatomique, rien ne distingue cette jonction: ni sphincter, ni disposition spéciale des fibres musculaires, des nerfs, ou des ganglions nerveux. Tout au plus, note-t-on une ligne sinueuse séparant la muqueuse pyélique plus blanche de la muqueuse urétérale plus vascularisée et plus mince.

Au point de vue physiologique, en revanche, Pannet a démontré l'excitabilité spéciale de la région; il prélève un anneau pyélique au-dessus de la jonction et un anneau urétéral au-dessous d'elle: l'anneau pyélique a des mouvements spontanés augmentés par l'action de l'adrénaline, l'anneau uretéral n'a pas de mouvements spontanés mais l'adrénaline y provoque des contractions deux fois plus fortes et plus rapides que celles de l'anneau pyélique.

Pannet également injecte sous pression faible et continue un liquide dans l'uretère: celui-ci se dilate, son péristaltisme diminue puis s'arrête: la dilatation s'arrête à la jonction.

Inversement, il injecte le liquide dans le bassinet par une canule introduite dans le bord convexe du rein: le bassinet se dilate seul. Si on insiste, la dilatation s'étend à l'uretère, mais bassinet et uretère restent séparés par une contraction localisée à leur jonction.

Setchavow, Zanne, sectionnent chez l'animal vivant le bassinet en laissant attenant à l'uretère le segment inférieur du bassinet: l'uretère se contracte normalement. Si la section porte au-dessous de la jonction, les contractions sont rares et quelquefois antipéristaltiques.

Tout segment urétéral soustrait par section à l'influence de la jonction pyélo-urétérale, continue à se contracter mais de façon anarchique et avec une efficacité douteuse.

La jonction commande la régularité du péristaltisme. C'est le «pace maker» des auteurs anglo-saxons.

Cette importance devient évidente en pathologie si on tient compte des hydronéphroses par trouble de cette jonction.

La pyéloscopie nous avait amenés à décrire le fonctionnement au niveau de la jonction d'un «bulbe urétéral» analogue au bulbe duodénal. Il s'agissait d'une courte évagination du bassinet vers l'uretère en forme d'entonnoir : elle restait visible pendant un certain temps puis se séparait du bassinet qui reprenait sa limite convexe.

En réalité, quand, au lieu de scopie, on employait la sériographie ou l'urographie, ce bulbe apparaissait beaucoup plus long que ne le laissait voir la scopie.

La cinématographie nous a fourni l'explication et nous a démontré que le bulbe n'existe pas. Ce que nous avons pris pour un bulbe, c'est l'entonnoir pyélo-urétéral visible à cause de sa relative épaisseur alors que le trop mince uretère lombaire n'est pas perceptible à l'oeil. Tout le temps où le bulbe est visible correspond au passage continu de liquide qui dure tout le temps de la systole et mesure sa durée.

Or cette durée de la systole pyélique est relativement longue : quand on voit en pyéloscopie le bulbe se former, c'est que le passage commence ; tant qu'il reste visible, c'est que le passage continue, quand on voit le bulbe se détacher, c'est que le passage cesse, que le bassinet ferme la communication et se remet en diastole.

Pour résumer le rôle de la jonction pyélo-urétérale :

1. région de haute différenciation qui commande la fonction de tout l'uretère.

2. région à valeur sphinctérienne, car c'est elle qui interrompt la vidange pyélique, la rend intermittente par rames uretérales. Le passage est ouvert pendant toute la systole du bassinet. Il se ferme hermétiquement pendant la diastole.

3. Pendant toute la systole, le liquide passe dans l'uretère. Il n'y a pas de système bulbaire analogue au bulbe duodénal, au moins dans les circonstances normales.

5. Au niveau de l'uretère

La systole pyélique injecte dans l'uretère une certaine quantité de liquide : celle-ci parcourt le mince canal urétéral de haut en bas, véhiculée par une onde péristaltique qui la chasse devant elle.

Cette «rame urétérale» remplit une certaine longueur du conduit, mais ne le remplit jamais de bout en bout.

A la scopie, on voit le liquide opaque effectuer une reptation qui dessine de haut en bas les sinuosités du conduit, montant sur le psoas, contournant le détroit supérieur, plongeant dans le petit bassin et revenant vers la ligne médiane pour s'évanouir en arrivant à la vessie.

Ce ruban opaque n'a pas un calibre uniforme : il s'étale dans les trois fuseaux lombaire, iliaque et pelvien, se ramasse dans les rétrécissements intermédiaires, tout relatifs d'ailleurs. Son calibre est plus grand à sa partie moyenne, effilé à ses deux extrémités. La vite de propagation de la rame est de 2 à 3 centimètres par seconde. CHAILLET a déterminé au manomètre qu'elle parcourt 10 centimètres en 2 à 3 secondes. La durée totale du parcours urétéral est donc d'environ 7 à 8 secondes. Le rythme des rames successives est celui des systoles pyéliques, donc de 10 à 15 secondes; ce rythme s'accélère en polyurie, se ralentit en oligurie (MORALIS) et lors de la réplétion vésicale (NARATH).

Tous ces temps très relatifs varient avec la tonicité, la dilatation, la force de propulsion pyélique etc., etc....

La rame uretérale est-elle continue? Le mouvement péristaltique parcourt-il l'uretère régulièrement de bout en bout, ou se fait-il une segmentation, l'uretère étant formé de 2 ou 3 systèmes cystoïdes surperposés? Les opinions varient.

Certains auteurs (NARATH, BEGG, AUVERT) considèrent l'évacuation par cystoïdes comme normale en toutes circonstances. Chaque cystoïde se remplit isolément: une fois plein il se contracte et injecte le cystoïde sous jacent et ainsi de suite. Il y aurait un arrêt normal au niveau des trois sphincters inter-cystoïdiques.

BOEMINGHAUS, FUCHS, MURNAGHAN pensent que:

— pour un débit normal (1 cc. minute) et une basse pression (de 2 à 10 cm. H$_2$O) la progression est continue.

— en polyurie (> 2000) et avec une forte pression, la contraction est discontinue et se fait par cystoïdes.

MURNAGHAN distingue pour chacun des 3 cystoïdes des modes de contraction différents liés à leurs différences de structure.

Le cystoïde lombaire, en continuité avec le bassinet, et formé en majorité de fibres spirales, est un segment de transmission et supporte difficilement la dilatation.

Le cystoïde moyen à prédominance de fibres circulaires, se laisse, au contraire, facilement dilater par la moindre hyperpression: il s'y accumule beaucoup d'urine et quand la contraction se produit, il s'aplatit en masse: c'est le plus cystoïdique des trois segments.

Le cystoïde inférieur est de calibre plus mince, les fibres longitudinales prédominent. Il ne se laisse pas dilater et réagit fortement par une contraction qui consiste surtout en un accourcissement.

Pour notre part, nous n'avons jamais vu dans des voies excrétrices normales, ni au cours d'un millier de pyéloscopies, ni dans nos films radiocinématographiques, le moindre arrêt se produire dans la progression de la rame uretérale: or, l'injection de liquide opaque dans le bassinet place dans les conditions d'une forte polyurie.

Dans les voies excrétrices normales, nous pensons donc que l'évacuation se fait de manière continue sans trace d'arrêt cystoïdique.

Il n'en est pas toujours ainsi: dans les voies excrétrices pathologiques ou soumises à un obstacle, leur existence devient évidente: l'onde péristaltique s'arrête à la zône inférieure sphinctérienne des trois cystoïdes. Il existe à ce niveau des points particulièrement sensibles capables de déterminer une stase dans la zône qu'ils contrôlent.

La question est de savoir si cette segmentation existe dans des circonstances normales ou si elle ne se produit qu'en présence d'une excitation physio pathologique anormale, ce que, pour notre part, nous pensons.

6. Au niveau de l'abouchement urétéro-vésical

Deux points sont à considérer à ce niveau:

1. L'aboutissement de la rame uretérale et son passage dans la vessie: c'est *l'éjaculation uretérale.*

2. Le mécanisme d'occlusion de l'orifice urétéro-vésical qui s'oppose au retour du contenu vésical vers les voies excrétrices supérieures: c'est le *système anti-reflux* dont l'importance physio pathologique est considérable.

a) Ejaculation urétérale

Elle est préparée par la contraction de l'uretère inférieur. On sait que ce segment inférieur, le cystoïde pelvien, réagit avec énergie à la réplétion, qu'à son niveau les fibres longitudinales prédominent et que leur contraction raccourcit et redresse l'obliquité selon laquelle l'uretère aborde et traverse la vessie.

L'uretère garde son individualité anatomique et physiologique dans cette traversée de la paroi vésicale. Dans l'intervalle des mictions, où le detrusor est relâché, rien ne s'oppose au libre passage de l'urine.

On sait aussi que la pression dans l'uretère inférieur est maxima, 70 à 80 cm. H_2O, alors que la pression vésicale, dans l'intervalle des mictions, est aux environs de 20 cm. H_2O. Morat et Doyen remarquent qu'étant donné le faible calibre de l'uretère comparé à celui de la vessie, le muscle urétéral a un avantage considérable sur le muscle vésical: exactement comme le petit cylindre de la presse hydraulique à l'égard du grand.

Tout est préparé pour que le contenu urétéral soit projeté dans la vessie avec une grande force: c'est l'éjaculation urétérale que la cystoscopie rend visible dans ses moindres détails.

b) Système anti-reflux

Normalement, la vessie et l'uretère collaborent pour former un systéme anti-reflux parfait. Même pendant la rétention vésicale aiguë, il n'y a pas de reflux (Guyon et Albarran).

Ce système doit être envisagé, d'abord *dans l'intervalle des mictions*, puis *au cours des mictions vésicales*. Dans les deux cas il réunit plusieurs facteurs vésicaux et uretéraux.

α) Dans l'intervalle des mictions

Rôle de la valvule uretérale. Son rôle est évident sur le cadavre où tous les autres facteurs s'éliminent. On peut alors injecter de l'air ou de l'eau jusqu'à faire éclater la vessie, rien ne ressort par l'uretère.

Si on écarte la valvule par cathétérisme, si on sectionne le méat sur I cm. $^1/_2$ (Draer et Braasch), si on l'excise totalement ou partiellement (Robert Gayet), le reflux se produit dans un certain nombre de cas (I sur 10 environ).

Auer et Seager obtiennent une proportion beaucoup plus grande de reflux en infiltrant l'uretère intra mural avec du serum physiologique, l'oedème ainsi créé s'opposant à l'occlusion de la valvule (33% de reflux chez le cobaye, 81% chez le lapin, 82% chez le chien). Quand l'oedème est résorbé, le reflux cesse.

A noter les constatations contradictoires des opérations endoscopiques: les sections longitudinales du méat (lèvre supérieure) pour extraction de calcul, ne sont pas suivies de reflux. En revanche, certaines électrocoagulations pour tumeur ou papillome juxta-méatiques donnent quelquefois un reflux.

D'où l'intérêt dans l'urétéro-cysto-néostomie de rétablir un abouchement oblique pour reconstituer une valvule (Marion, Darget).

Rôle de la musculature vésicale. Ce rôle est primordial et justifie l'aphorisme de Guyon qui déclare que c'est «la vessie qui est la gardienne de l'uretère».

Courtade et J. F. Guyon, Lepoutre, en sectionnant chez le chien ou le chat la sangle musculaire péri-urétérale, obtiennent un reflux constant. Si la section est unilatérale, le reflux ne se produit que du côté sectionné.

Avec une musculature vésicale saine, le reflux ne doit donc pas être possible. Pourtant il se produit tout de même dans un certain nombre de cas expérimentaux ou d'exploration cystographiques et les circonstances de ces «*reflux surprise*» méritent d'être précisées.

Expérimentalement, ce reflux s'observe facilement chez le lapin, difficilement chez le chat, rarement chez le chien et le porc.

Au cours des cystographies, le reflux se produit pour de petites quantités de liquide injecté; pour provoquer le reflux, la meilleure méthode est d'injecter doucement une dizaine de centimètres cubes, puis très brutalement trente centimètres cubes — une fois la vessie remplie, on ne provoque plus de reflux surprise.

Courtade et J. F. Guyon, Lervier, Goldschmidt, Wislocki et O'Connor, Henningsen, Graves et Davidoff, obtiennent du reflux dans les vessies à réponse isotonique courte, jamais dans les vessies passives qui se laissent distendre sans contraction.

Tous s'accordent à déclarer que tout ce qui provoque et augmente le tonus vésical aide au reflux. Pavone insiste sur le rôle du déclenchement brusque d'une miction impérieuse, surtout chez les rétentionnistes aigus ou chroniques. Il a vu des reflux se produire au cours des manoeuvres d'aspiration vésicale avec l'appareil de Duchastelet, alors que les orifices uretéraux paraissaient normaux.

Tout ceci montre que si le reflux ne se produit pas dans une vessie saine, le reflux surprise devient possible avec une musculature vésicale rendue hypertonique par des causes pathologiques ou par hyperpression brutale.

Dans un autre ordre d'idée, Oberniedermayer a établi expérimentalement que la narcose favorise le reflux:

— sur 15 essais sans narcose il obtient 2 reflux,
— sur 5 anesthésies vésicales   —   3 reflux,
— sur 11 narcoses profondes   —   11 reflux.

Rôle du péristaltisme uretéral. Il s'oppose très efficacement au reflux: rappelons encore la sensibilité du cystoïde inférieur à la distension et l'efficacité de ses contractions.

Encore faut-il que ce péristaltisme ne soit pas inhibé.

De nombreux auteurs (Seres, Pfanner, Graves et Davidoff, Sampson, Krutzmann), ont établi l'influence de la réplétion vésicale sur le péristaltisme uretéral. Le remplissage modéré de la vessie augmente le péristaltisme. Le remplissage total provoque des contractions plus lentes et vigoureuses.

La distension vésicale est suivie de dilatation de l'uretère dont les mouvements deviennent rapides et mous puis cessent complètement. Stern, Farrel pensent qu'il s'agit d'un reflexe dont la partie afférente passe par les splanchniques.

β) Au cours de la miction

Les conditions changent du tout au tout. Les pressions s'inversent, la pression de miction de 100 à 120 cm. H_2O devient égale ou supérieure à celle de l'uretère inférieur.

Rôle de la valvule muqueuse. Il devient très efficace: la pression intra-vésicale favorisant et assurant l'occlusion passive de l'orifice méatique à condition que la contraction urétérale, si elle se produit au même instant, ne vienne pas l'effacer en redressant l'uretère.

Rôle de la contraction vésicale. Lorsque le détrusor se contracte, il redresse mais, en même temps, aplatit l'uretère et assure son obstruction (Sampson).

Rôle du péristaltisme urétéral. Tant que dure la miction, il y a arrêt du péristaltisme urétéral. Boeminghaus ne voit à la cystoscopie aucune éjaculation lorsque le patient fait un effort de miction. Farrel constate l'absence de toute contraction pendant la miction: dès que la contraction active de la vessie cesse, l'élimination urétérale reprend.

La synergie fonctionnelle entre la vessie et l'uretère assure donc normalement l'absence d'éjaculation urétérale pendant la miction.

Mais cette synergie peut être troublée. GRAVES et DAVIDOFF, WISLOCKI et O'CONNOR, voient le reflux se produire après injection intra-veineuse de chlorure de baryum qui déclenche des contractions urétérales subintrantes et désordonnées.

Le système anti-reflux est donc adapté pour agir efficacement, non seulement en phase de repos mais spécialement au moment de la miction vésicale.

De tout ce qui précède, il résulte:

1. Que dans un appareil urétéro-vésical normal, le reflux ne peut pas se produire. «Comme la femme de CÉSAR, dit BRANSFORT-LEWIS, la continence de l'orifice urétéro-vésical ne doit pas être suspectée».

2. Cette occlusion est particulièrement efficace au moment de la miction pour s'opposer au renversement de pression entre vessie et uretère.

3. Le système anti-reflux comprend un facteur anatomique, la valvule ostiale, et des facteurs musculaires vésical et uretéral. C'est la synergie de ces deux facteurs musculaires qui assure son efficacité.

4. Il arrive cependant que cette synergie soit troublée (hypertonie vésicale, hyperkinésie urétérale, etc....). Le reflux surprise se produit alors mais il est sous la dépendance de causes pathologiques, expérimentales ou d'exploration.

5. Le reflux peut notamment se produire au cours des anesthésies générales (BLUM, LINNER, OBERNIEDERMAYER) ou de la rachi-anesthésie (LEPOUTRE), et au cours du cathétérisme de l'uretère (BOEMINGHAUS).

B. Physiologie pathologique des voies urinaires supérieures

I. Étude expérimentale des obstructions urétérales

La première idée des expérimentateurs devait être de réaliser une *obstruction complète de l'appareil excréteur par ligature de l'uretère*.

Mais il y avait loin de cette ligature totale aux conditions réalisées par les lésions pathologiques et on a cherché à se rapprocher de celles-ci en pratiquant *des ligatures partielles ou temporaires*.

Dans le même esprit, on a tenté de créer des lésions de plus en plus légères susceptibles de provoquer des *troubles fonctionnels sans diminution anatomique de la lumière uretérale*.

Ces deux dernières séries d'expériences ne sont exemptes ni de difficultés ni de causes d'erreur et il ne faut en attendre ni constance ni unanimité des résultats.

Toute l'expérimentation a porté sur l'uretère moyen: elle laisse dans l'ombre les variations segmentaires.

1. Obstruction totale des voies excrétrices par ligature complète et définitive de l'uretère

L'obstruction de l'uretère est réalisée par simple ligature, par section entre deux ligatures, ou par un noeud fait avec le bout supérieur de l'uretère sectionné.

a) Modifications de la motricité

α) *Aussitôt après la ligature* le péristaltisme s'arrête du fait du traumatisme opératoire.

Bientôt, les contractions reparaissent mais elle ne sont plus synchrones ni de même amplitude dans les deux bouts:

— dans le bout supérieur, elles sont exagérées de force et de fréquence,

— dans le bout inférieur, elles sont plus rares et amples.

Si on fait une double ligature, le segment intermédiaire est inerte mais réagit aux excitations.

β) Puis la musculature se fatigue et les contractions spontanées disparaissent, mais *dans les trois premières semaines qui suivent la ligature,* l'uretère réagit encore aux agents pharmaco-dynamiques (acétyl-choline, adrénaline, histamine — Binet et Seringe): il ne s'agit plus d'un péristaltisme vrai; seules les fibres circulaires se contractent et leurs contractions sont plus espacées, plus prolongées et surtout plus amples que normalement.

γ) Cette excitabilité persiste *jusqu'à 3 mois* chez le chien (Wislocki et O. Connor), plus longtemps dans le segment inférieur que dans la partie supérieure.

Pendant tout ce temps, il est possible de voir réapparaitre des contractions spontanées en vidant partiellement la poche hydronéphrotique; elles cessent dès qu'on remplit à nouveau la poche.

δ) Au delà de 3 mois, le bassinet et l'uretère sont totalement inertes.

b) Modifications de l'appareil excréteur

α) Dilatation pyélo-urétérale

— *En amont de la ligature* se produit une dilatation qui croit progressivement et proportionnellement à la durée de la ligature: la dilatation se fait de bas en haut, d'abord sur l'*uretère supérieur* qui, en même temps qu'il se dilate, s'allonge et devient flexueux, puis sur le *bassinet,* enfin sur les *calices.*

— *En aval de la ligature* Camossa et Verliac, Fey et Ferrier, ont remarqué que si la ligature porte sur la partie moyenne de l'uretère, la dilatation ne se fait qu'en amont; si la ligature porte sur l'extrémité toute supérieure de l'uretère, on voit une fois sur deux une dilatation de l'uretère sous jacent.

— Très exceptionnellement, la dilatation sus-stricturale ne se produit pas. La ligature détermine une atrophie rénale, un arrêt brusque et total de la secrétion sans dilatation pyélique.

Dans un cas de de Berne Lagarde, cette atrophie s'explique par une ligature accidentelle de l'artère rénale. Hinman et Hepler, sur plusieurs centaines de ligatures urétérales n'ont observé que trois atrophies primitives; dans les trois cas il y avait de l'infection.

L'atrophie primitive est donc exceptionnelle, due, soit à un arrêt de la circulation, soit au développement brutal de l'infection.

β) Altérations de la paroi pyélo-urétérale

La *muqueuse,* d'abord hyperhémiée, peut être le siège d'hémorragies sous-épithéliales. Très rapidement la muqueuse comprimée s'anémie et desquame: elle peut subir une évolution mucoïde aboutissant à une véritable dégénérescence microkystique de l'endothélium (Gouygou).

Dans la *sous-muqueuse* un tissu conjonctif abondant prolifère d'où épaississement de la paroi et rigidité du bassinet et des calices.

La tunique musculaire présente d'abord une hypertrophie marquée. L. Loeffler, étudiant des bassinets et des uretères d'hydronéphrose, trouve la musculature constamment hypertrophiée. Dans le bassinet, où les fibres circulaires prédominent normalement, ce sont les fibres longitudinales qui se développent le plus. Dans l'uretère, c'est l'inverse. Les faisceaux musculaires néoformés suivent le trajet des vaisseaux.

Plus tard, on assiste à la dissociation et à l'atrophie des fibres musculaires qui se réduisent à quelques éléments disséminés dans du tissu fibreux.

γ) Contenu de la poche sus-stricturale

La poche contient une urine, mais une urine modifiée.

D'une part, il y a une baisse de concentration qui porte sur tous les éléments de l'urine, notamment sur l'urée. Cette baisse est due à l'altération de la fonction rénale et est d'autant plus accusée que la ligature est plus ancienne.

D'autre part, le contenu de la poche est soumis à des phénomènes de résorption; les colorants injectés dans sa cavité s'atténuent puis disparaissent. Cette résorption sera étudiée plus loin (voir p. 522).

Un équilibre s'établit entre la secrétion qui continue et la résorption et cet équilibre se stabilise à un niveau variable. On est souvent surpris de trouver dans les hydronéphroses des taux de concentration encore valables.

δ) Mise en tension du bassinet — Pression pyélique

La pression pyélique, normalement de 10 à 15 cm. H_2O, monte rapidement jusqu'à un certain niveau qu'on appelle la *pression de secrétion.*

Celle-ci atteint le niveau de la pression de filtration glomérulaire mais, comme elle, reste toujours inférieure à la pression artérielle. Grâce à cette marge différentielle, la filtration glomérulaire continue. Cette marge différentielle n'existe que pour les reins glomérulés: chez les animaux à reins aglomérulés, on ne l'observe pas plus que dans les autres glandes de l'économie.

La pression de secrétion se stabilise sous la double action de la dilatation sus-stricturale et de la baisse de la fonction rénale. Puis elle diminue lentement.

Deux éléments interviennent dans son évolution: d'une part la fatigue et l'atrophie musculaire, d'autre part les phénomènes de résorption sur lesquels nous reviendrons (voir p. 522).

Voici les chiffres de pression de secrétion obtenus pas différents auteurs:

	au bout de:						
	20 minutes	une heure	4 heures	26 jours	60 jours	72 jours	au delà
GUYON-ALBARRAN et CHABRIER	40 mms. Hg	65 à 70	45	11		3	
HUBER		60 à 65					
STARLING		70 à 95					
OBNISKY		62 à 105					
HINMAN et LEE-BROWN .		70 à 90			15		0

Seuls McDONALD, MANN et PRIESTLEY obtiennent des chiffres plus élevés parce qu'ils opèrent chez des chiens non anesthésiés: ils obtiennent en moyenne 101 cm. d'urine (= 78 mm. Hg) avec, comme extrêmes, 93 cm. d'urine (= 72 mm. Hg) et 125 cc. d'urine (= 96 mms. Hg).

L'anesthésie diminuerait donc la pression d'environ 30%.

L'énervation préalable du pédicule rénal n'a qu'une faible influence.

En déclenchant une polyurie par injection intra-veineuse de sulfate de soude et de glucose, ils obtiennent une hausse rapide de la pression qui atteint son maximum en une heure et sa valeur devient de 30% supérieure à la normale.

La pression de secrétion est donc influencée par la diurèse.

c) Conséquences de la rétention pyélique sur le parenchyme rénal

La rétention et la pression pyélo-rénale entrainent: *un refoulement du parenchyme rénal, la dilatation des tubes du rein et des troubles circulatoires:* l'ensemble aboutit à *l'atrophie du parenchyme rénal.*

Les expériences faites à ce sujet sont innombrables et leurs résultats varient avec le choix de l'animal et les techniques employées. L'atrophie du rein est d'autant plus rapide qu'on opère sur un rein plus petit; Les chiffres de Hinman et Hepler, Hosford, le prouvent:

Rat: poids du rein: 20 gr. atrophie réalisée en   2 mois.
Lapin: —   40 —   —   8 mois.
Chien: —   70 —   —   16 mois.

Mais un même observateur opérant sur des animaux de même espèce, avec une même technique, n'obtient pas toujours des résultats identiques: il y a des variations individuelles, tenant à l'état des tissus, l'âge, l'état de nutrition etc....

En outre, les lésions ne frappent pas le parenchyme dans sa totalité: elles sont d'abord parcellaires, en ilôts séparés par du tissu sain; ces résultats varient selon le point examiné et sur une même coupe on trouve côte à côte des stades successifs.

Aussi n'envisagerons nous que les grandes lignes de ces divers processus.

α) Refoulement du parenchyme

Dès les premiers jours, la papille s'aplatit. A la 3ème semaine, elle est atrophiée et ne fait plus saillie dans le calice. En même temps la médullaire s'amincit, refoule la corticale contre la capsule inextensible.

β) Dilatation tubulaire

Dès les 24 premières heures, la dilatation tubulaire se manifeste par une distension des branches ascendantes des anses de Henle et des segments intermédiaires.

Elle s'étend ensuite aux tubes contournés, puis à l'espace glomérulaire. Cependant, Camossa et Verliac n'ont pas observé cette ectasie des tubes contournés qui seraient d'emblée aplatis par la pression des parties saines, étranglées dans la capsule rénale inextensible.

Les tubes collecteurs résistent mieux et se dilatent les derniers.

A la troisième semaine, le tube rénal est totalement dilaté du glomérule à la papille.

γ) Troubles circulatoires

La pression interne est équivalente dans toute l'étendue du tube urinifère, du glomérule à l'uretère. Elle comprime les vaisseaux rénaux aussi bien dans le parenchyme qu'au niveau du bassinet (Lee-Brown).

— La compression agit d'*abord* sur les capillaires veineux: la circulation artérielle est encore normale, d'où engorgement des capillaires et hyperémie.

— *A la fin de la première semaine,* les capillaires artériels et les artères glomérulaires sont comprimés, d'où arrêt de la circulation glomérulaire et atrophie.

L'arrêt de la circulation glomérulaire par hyperpression tubulaire a été observé directement par Hayman sur le rein de grenouille: comprimant un tube rénal et mesurant la pression intra-capsulaire avec un manomètre, il voit, au fur et à mesure que la pression monte:

— la capsule se distendre, puis le peloton vasculaire diminuer de volume,

— le courant sanguin devenir pulsatile par ralentissement puis arrêt diastolique.

— enfin l'arrêt total de la circulation.

A cette compression mécanique, s'ajoute vraisemblablement une constriction vasomotrice par spasme reflexe.

— Après 14 jours, les glomérules périphériques sont plus ou moins atrophiés: les glomérules plus profonds de la zône cortico-médullaire s'hypertrophient; cette hypertrophie compensatrice est rendue possible parce que leurs vaisseaux afférents viennent de troncs artériels plus volumineux, donc à pression sanguine supérieure et parce que leurs vaisseaux efférents descendent directement dans les gros vaisseaux droits de la médullaire. Notons que cette constatation annonce le phénomène décrit par Trueta.

— Plus tard, ces vaisseaux droits eux-mêmes sont comprimés et coudés par la distension pyélique: ils deviennent tortueux et la circulation s'y ralentit. D'où atrophie totale et définitive de tous les glomérules.

δ) Atrophie rénale

L'atrophie glomérulo-tubulaire est rapide. C. M. Johnson, utilisant la méthode de macération tissulaire décrite par Huber, a disséqué des tubes rénaux de lapin à des stades successifs d'hydronéphrose provoquée.

— à la fin du premier mois, l'atrophie porte sur les glomérules, les tubes de Henle et les segments intermédiaires: les tubes collecteurs se dilatent encore.

— à la fin du 3ème mois, les glomérules semblent s'implanter directement sur des tubes collecteurs énormes.

— à partir du 5ème mois, les tubes collecteurs diminuent de volume.

— au 8ème mois, l'atrophie est pratiquement totale.

Strauss et Germont, Verliac, de Berne Lagarde, etc.... sont arrivés à des résultats analogues.

Le rein est alors transformé en un sac volumineux, bosselé, presque translucide. L'intérieur de la poche est divisé par des cloisons falciformes, formées de tissu conjonctif et de quelques vaisseaux, vestiges des colonnes de Bertin. Ce n'est qu'à la base d'implantation de ces colonnes qu'on retrouve quelques traces de parenchyme.

L'atrophie du parenchyme rénal ne provient donc pas uniquement du refoulement mécanique: celui-ci serait bien vite arrêté du fait de la chute progressive de la pression de secrétion. Elle est due aux *troubles circulatoires et à l'ischémie* progressive à laquelle échappent seuls quelques territoires de parenchyme irrigués par de gros vaisseaux encore perméables.

Le rôle de l'ischémie sur l'atrophie rénale a été prouvé par les *expériences de* Hinman *et* Hepler.

Ils opèrent sur des animaux dont un uretère a été sectionné entre deux ligatures et obstruent, soit partiellement l'artère rénale (par compression), soit totalement la branche rétro pyélique (par section).

Obstruction partielle de l'artère rénale: dilatation pyélique et atrophie parenchymateuse se développent beaucoup plus rapidement (2 fois environ) que sur les animaux témoins dont l'uretère seul a été lié.

Les altérations histologiques sont beaucoup plus marquées: après 21 jours le tissu conjonctif et fibreux prédomine dans le parenchyme; on ne trouve plus que quelques glomérules atrophiés: cet aspect ne se produit que beaucoup plus tard dans l'hydronéphrose simple.

Ligature de la rétro-pyélique: 7 fois sur 12 Hinman et Hepler voient à partir du 14ème jour, une volumineuse poche se développer en arrière du bassinet dilaté: il s'agit d'un véritable diverticule pyélique développé aux dépens du parenchyme

33*

postérieur ischémié. La pression pyélique s'est exercée dans toutes les directions, mais a trouvé dans la zône ischémiée un point de moindre résistance.

Dans un cas, la ligature portait, non sur la rétro-pyélique, mais sur une branche polaire inférieure; au 28ème jour, un énorme diverticule inférieur était appendu au bassinet dilaté.

Hosford, de son côté, provoque l'ischémie par obstruction partielle de la veine rénale. Il obtient d'abord une accélération du développement de la dilatation du fait de l'accroissement de la pression secrétrice; puis le rythme devient identique à celui d'une hydronéphrose simple: la circulation collatérale est très augmentée.

Si on détruit alors cette circulation collatérale péri-rénale, on détermine une atrophie rapide par insuffisance circulatoire.

ε) État du rein opposé après ligature de l'uretère

On a décrit, dans le rein opposé, des lésions assez vagues de néphrite qui seraient dues aux produits de désintégration des cellules épithéliales du rein opéré en voie d'atrophie, le rein dilaté produirait des *néphrotoxines* agissant sur le rein opposé (Castaigne et Rathery).

La majorité des auteurs n'ont observé que des modifications d'hypertrophie compensatrice, identiques à celles qui se développent après néphrectomie. Les lésions dégénératives n'existent qu'en cas d'infection (de Berne-Lagarde, Camossa et Verliac).

2. Obstruction des voies excrétrices par ligature temporaire. Recupération anatomique et fonctionnelle après levée de la ligature

L'expérimentation est ici particulièrement délicate. Ces ligatures temporaires laissent après leur levée des lésions définitives qui aboutissent à l'obstruction totale ou au moins partielle de l'uretère.

a) Appareil excréteur

Ce point a été peu étudié. Cependant, Pflaumer a vu, après une ligature complète au catgut qui se résorbe en moins de 3 semaines, l'uretère se contracter normalement 12 semaines plus tard.

b) Secrétion

Après quelques heures, la levée de l'obstacle est suivie d'une polyurie importante avec diminution de concentration de l'urée et des chlorures (Guyon, Hermann, Pfaundler):

— après 24 heures: le rein récupère une fonction normale (Corbett).

— après 2 à 4 jours, la secrétion de l'indigocarmin est bonne (Kawasoye). Au point de vue anatomique, Camossa et Verliac trouvent deux fois un rein normal, deux fois des lésions de sclérose, vraisemblablement antérieures à l'expérience, mais nettement plus accentuées qu'au niveau du rein opposé.

— à la 2ème semaine, l'élimination de l'indigocarmin devient médiocre (Kawasoye). Cependant le rein (lapin) récupère un fonctionnement suffisant pour permettre la néphrectomie du rein opposé (Johnson); cette récupération est lente: un mois pour une ligature maintenue 7 jours, 5 mois pour une ligature de 14 jours.

— après 30 à 60 jours, Hinman pratique une urétéro-cysto-néostomie: il observe toujours une phase temporaire de réparation anatomique, importante après 30 jours, insignifiante après 60 jours. Dans les deux cas, un an plus tard, le parenchyme est totalement atrophié bien que l'anastomose soit restée perméable.

— après 42 jours (chien) HINMAN injecte les artères d'une hydronéphrose; seuls les gros vaisseaux et quelques capillaires sont perméables: dans une hydronéphrose de même durée, dont on a levé l'obstruction depuis 3 jours, il trouve des capillaires injectés mais en faible proportion.

Les altérations vasculaires secondaires à l'hydronéphrose sont donc partiellement reversibles et ceci explique les récupérations fonctionnelles observées après néphrostomie pour hydronéphrose.

Dans l'ensemble, les lésions produites par obstruction totale de l'uretère sont *rapidement définitives*. Une semaine après la ligature les lésions peuvent être considérées comme irréversibles.

3. Obstruction anatomique partielle des voies excrétrices par ligature incomplète de l'uretère

L'obstruction partielle a été réalisée:

— *par compression indirecte* plus ou moins prolongée à travers la paroi abdominale.

— *en opposant à l'élimination urétérale une certaine pression*

— *par ligature peu serrée de l'uretère.*

— *par coudure aiguë et fixée de l'uretère.*

— *en déterminant une péri-urétérite.*

Toutes ces techniques sont approximatives et leur effet ne peut en être ni mesuré ni apprécié avec rigueur. Les résultats ne peuvent donc être qu'imprécis: il convient surtout de noter leurs différences avec les résultats de ligature complète.

a) Modifications de la motricité

1. *Obstruction légère:* le muscle urétéral renforce ses contractions et peut vaincre l'obstacle: la musculeuse s'hypertrophie, il ne se fait pas de dilatation (GRAVES et DAVIDOFF).

2. *Obstruction plus marquée:* la motricité est longtemps conservée (PENFIELD, WISLOCKI, O'CONNOR). Il y a dissociation de rythme et d'intensité entre les contractions des deux bouts uretéraux.

— *En amont de l'obstacle*, les ondulations péristaltiques sont plus fortes et moins nombreuses: on peut voir des ondulations antipéristaltiques remonter de l'obstacle vers le bassinet.

Si on vide par aspiration le contenu de la poche, les contractions deviennent plus fréquentes et plus vigoureuses.

L'excitation de l'uretère supérieur par pincement ou contact d'un cristal de chlorure de baryum forme un anneau de constriction d'où partent des ondulations vers le haut et vers le bas: cet anneau de constriction bloque les contractions péristaltiques venues du bassinet.

— *En aval de l'obstacle* on observe des contractions indépendantes des contractions du segment supérieur.

— GOUVERNEUR et H. MARION obtiennent des résultats identiques en plaçant la ligature sans serrer l'uretère «comme une bague autour d'un doigt».

— KREUTZMANN réalise l'obstruction partielle chez l'homme en introduisant dans l'uretère une sonde uretérale No 12 montée jusqu'à 10 cms. du méat et reliée à un manomètre, donc imperméable à l'urine, mais celle-ci peut continuer à filtrer autour de la sonde.

La pression augmente rapidement avec des contractions péristaltiques normales; bientôt celles-ci deviennent plus fréquentes et plus violentes et la pression monte à 15, à 25 mms. Hg. Puis les contractions faiblissent et deviennent irrégulières. Après 15 ou 20 minutes, on débouche la sonde et on laisse l'urine s'écouler librement pendant 10 minutes; puis on la relie de nouveau au manomètre: malgré ce temps de repos, les contractions restent faibles.

Cette expérience indique combien les modifications de la contractilité sont rapides pour une faible obstruction urétérale.

— Winsbury White provoque l'obstruction partielle en provoquant une péri-uretérite (lapin) par injection péri-urétérale d'iode à 10%. Neuf à douze mois plus tard, il trouve une masse de tissu sclérosé au contact de l'uretère, mais celui-ci ne présente ni sténose, ni dilatation sus-jacente. Il est probable que l'uretère, protégé par son adhérence au péritoine, n'est pas totalement entouré de sclérose.

b) Modifications anatomiques

Toute compression de l'uretère, même temporaire (comme celle qu'on réalise au cour de l'Urographie), entraine une dilatation pyélo-urétérale en amont, mais cette dilatation est facilement étalée par le jeu de la tonicité.

Une obstruction incomplète et permanente de l'uretère provoque des lésions anatomiques analogues à celles d'une ligature complète, mais elles se constituent plus lentement parce que la pression pyélique est moindre et augmente plus lentement (Tuffier, Mangeais, Albarran et Legueu).

Dans les obstructions basses, tant que la pression intra-urétérale n'atteint pas, chez le chien, 30 cm. d'eau, l'uretère peut, en renforçant ses contractions, vaincre la résistance, sans qu'il se fasse de dilatation pyélique (Lucas)... au moins pendant un certain temps.

En général, la dilatation est plus lente à s'établir mais elle devient plus considérable qu'après ligature complète parce que la secrétion rénale persiste.

L'uretère augmente de diamètre et s'allonge, se coude et devient flexueux.

La poche pyélique est globuleuse et dissocie les éléments du pédicule rénal; certains vaisseaux deviennent aberrants et croisent l'uretère.

La muqueuse est amincie. La musculeuse, d'abord *hypertrophiée*, *s'atrophie à la longue.*

c) Conséquences de l'obstruction partielle sur le parenchyme rénal

Le refoulement du parenchyme et les lésions vasculaires sont analogues à celles des ligatures complètes, mais elles s'établissent beaucoup moins rapidement parce que la pression de secrétion est limitée, dans une certaine mesure, par la perméabilité que conserve l'uretère.

C'est de cet équilibre entre la pression pyélique et la contre-pression due à l'obstacle, et aussi à la permanence ou à l'intermittence de cet obstacle, qu'est due la plus ou moins grande rapidité avec laquelle se produisent les lésions.

Plusieurs expérimentateurs ont étudié le fonctionnement d'un rein à l'excrétion duquel on oppose une contre-pression variable.

— Avec une contre-pression faible (10 cm. d'eau), on observe une diurèse augmentée, avec hyperconcentration des chlorures et diminution de l'acidité (Schwarz, Brodie et Miss Cullis). La polyurie serait due, pour Cushny, à un reflexe vaso-dilatateur à point de départ urétéral.

— Avec une contre-pression inférieure à 30 cm. d'eau, Pilcher, Bollmann et Mann, n'observent aucune différence qualitative ou quantitative: l'uretère étant capable de vaincre la résistance par renforcement de ses contractions.

Avec une contre-pression de 40 à 60 cm d'eau, HERMANN, LINDEMANN, LEPINE et ses collaborateurs, CUSHNY, ALLARD observent:
— une grosse diminution de la diurèse,
— une diminution importante du débit des chlorures sans modification de la concentration,
— une diminution légère du débit avec concentration augmentée de l'urée, des sulfates, des phosphates et de l'indigo-carmin,

WINTON, PILCHER, BOLLMANN et MANN ont des résultats à peu près identiques.

d) Récupération fonctionnelle

Disparition ou atténuation des lésions dépendent de leur intensité et de leur ancienneté, mais on peut dire, qu'après un certain temps d'obstruction partielle, les lésions ne disparaissent jamais complètement.

KEITH et PULFORD ont vu la fonction rénale se rétablir quand la ligature était levée dans la semaine: au delà s'installent des lésions chroniques et définitives.

CAMOSSA et VERLIAC, après ligature incomplète de 2 jours, trouvent le rein prélevé de 13 à 19 jours après l'intervention, absolument sain.

Après ligature incomplète de 4 à 11 jours, ils trouvent, après 2 à 4 semaines, une légère dilatation des cavités glomérulaires.

Après ligature incomplète de 15 jours, ils trouvent après 35 à 40 jours, la dilatation d'un certain nombre de tubes excréteurs et d'anses de HENLE.

4. Perturbations fonctionnelles provoquées sans diminution anatomique de la lumière urétérale

On les a obtenues:
a) Par excitation localisée de l'uretère.
b) Par contre-pression.
c) Par section de l'uretère suivie du rétablissement de sa continuité.
d) Par dénudation et énervation extrinsèque de l'uretère.
e) Par injection de toxines et par infection.

a) Excitations localisées de l'uretère

Toute excitation (électrique, pincement, piqûre, attouchement avec un cristal de chlorure de Baryum, etc....) pratiquée en un point quelconque de l'uretère, provoque un anneau de constriction d'où partent vers le bassinet une ou plusieurs ondulations anti-péristaltiques, et vers la vessie une ou plusieurs ondulations péristaltiques.

Si l'anneau de constriction persiste assez longtemps pour que les contractions normales de l'uretère sus-jacent aient le temps de se produire, on voit ces ondulations s'arrêter à son niveau, sans jamais les franchir; le segment sous jacent présente des contractions indépendantes de rythme et d'intensité.

Une excitation localisée de l'uretère équivaut donc à une véritable section physiologique temporaire du canal.

Mais, pour être efficace, il faut que l'excitation porte sur la musculeuse: si elle est limitée à la muqueuse ou à l'adventice, l'anneau de constriction ne se produit pas (ENGELMANN).

Pour SAMPSON, une excitation interne provoque bien des contractions péristaltiques plus fortes, mais jamais l'antipéristaltisme. WISLOCKI et O'CONNOR poussent, chez le chien, une sonde urétérale à 8 cms.: les contractions péristaltiques s'arrêtent à l'extrémité de la sonde, sans antipéristaltisme. Si on injecte du serum, les vagues péristaltiques sont renforcées et luttent contre l'ascension du liquide; si on augmente la pression de l'injection, les contractions faiblissent et s'arrêtent.

Ces données sont confirmées par Boeminghaus: il est facile de les vérifier au cours de la pyéloscopie lorsqu'on procède au remplissage du bassinet sous écran.

Seule l'excitation de l'extrémité inférieure de l'uretère, telle que la réalise l'injection au cours de l'uretéro-pyélographie rétrograde, provoquerait des mouvements antipéristaltiques (Chevassu).

b) Contre-pressions exercées sur l'uretère

On réalise cette contre-pression en obstruant partiellement l'uretère inférieur par introduction d'une sonde à olive (sonde de Gudin).

On note d'abord une augmentation de fréquence et d'amplitude des contractions uretérales, celles-ci deviennent subintrantes mais s'affaiblissent et deviennent inefficaces: c'est le rythme pendulaire (Chaillet) comparable à la fibrillation cardiaque.

La pression s'élève en amont: la lutte entre la pression d'origine rénale et la contre-pression de l'obstacle aboutit à un équilibre entre la pression de secrétion et d'excrétion. C'est la pression urinaire maxima (Auvert) qui est de l'ordre de 50 cm. H_2O.

Murnaghan, en faisant varier la valeur de la contre-pression a fait les constatations suivantes:

— Avec une contre-pression de 6 cm. H_2O on voit le fuseau inférieur refouler son contenu dans le fuseau moyen: le bassinet et l'uretère supérieur continuent à se contracter normalement, le cystoïde moyen se distend et ses contractions deviennent faibles.

— Avec une contre-pression de 11 cm. H_2O, les trois fuseaux uretéraux se distendent: leurs contractions restent puissantes à condition que l'urine puisse s'écouler malgré la contre-pression. Il se produit un reflux vers le bassinet. Si on obstrue complètement l'uretère, les contractions cessent: c'est toujours le fuseau inférieur qui persiste le dernier à se contracter.

— Avec une contre-pression de 20 cm. H_2O, les contractions ne sont plus visibles que dans le fuseau inférieur mais ces contractions se traduisent pas un simple accourcissement sans qu'aucune onde efficace parvienne à la vessie.

c) Section de l'uretère suivie de rétablissement de sa continuité

(Alskne, Gouverneur, Iselin, Gouverneur et Henri Marion, Zanne etc....)

Que la continuité soit rétablie par un tube de verre (Alskne, Beach) ou par suture bout à bout, le résultat immédiat est le même.

L'extrémité pyélique se contracte et réagit fortement aux excitations: les contractions, spontanées ou provoquées, s'arrêtent toujours au niveau de la solution de continuité: il y a un «obstacle invincible à la propagation de l'onde» (Gouverneur). L'urine s'accumule à ce niveau puis filtre dans l'uretère inférieur qui l'évacue dans la vessie.

Il se produit cependant un arrêt suffisant pour entrainer une *dilatation sus-jacente* qui est constante pendant les premières semaines.

Ultérieurement, une sténose cicatricielle peut se produire au niveau de la suture et on rentre dans le cas précédemment étudié d'obstruction partielle de l'uretère.

Mais si la suture est parfaite et ne provoque aucun rétrécissement de la lumière du conduit, que deviennent alors la fonction et le calibre du conduit ? Il y a divergence dans les constatations des différents expérimentateurs.

Pour ISELIN, après une phase d'akinésie, l'uretère reprend une motricité et une morphologie parfaites : les ondes péristaltiques franchissent à nouveau la ligne de suture.

BEACH sectionne chez le chien la couche musculaire jusqu'à ce que les ondulations péristaltiques ne franchissent plus la zône opérée : 50 jours après, il n'y a pas de dilatation et le péristaltisme normal a repris.

GOUVERNEUR et HENRI MARION, ZANNE voient, au contraire, l'arrêt des contractions persister au niveau de la suture : le péristaltisme normal ne se rétablit pas et il en résulte une dilatation progressive de l'uretère et du bassinet en amont.

Résultats contradictoires en apparence, mais expériences trop peu nombreuses et trop peu suivies.

Cette expérimentation a actuellement perdu son intérêt parce qu'elle est dépassée par l'expérience chirurgicale. Les sutures bout à bout de l'uretère, faites avec une bonne technique, donnent après un certain délai, des récupérations anatomiques et fonctionnelles parfaites (RENÉ KÜSS).

d) Dénudation et énervation extrinséque pyélo-urétérales

La dénudation ou l'énervation d'un segment plus ou moins étendu des voies excrétrices provoquent des troubles de la motricité. Les techniques employées par les auteurs sont assez variées : pourtant leurs résultats sont identiques, bien qu'ils aient généralement ignoré les travaux de leurs prédécesseurs.

STEWART et BARBER dépouillent l'uretère d'un chien sur une certaine longueur. Ils obtiennent une dilatation urétéro-pyélique et une diminution de la contractilité. Alors que, avant l'intervention, les contractions se produisaient toutes les 9 secondes, elles s'espacent à 16 secondes, puis, après dépouillement plus étendu, à 25 secondes ; après dépouillement total, l'uretère ne présente plus que quelques contractions fibrillaires espacées de 69 secondes. L'examen histologique des pièces a montré des lésions identiques à celles des obstructions mécaniques.

Dossot a repris ces expériences sur le lapin en 1925 : les résultats sont identiques.

ANDLER : l'énervation (sans dénudation) de l'uretère et de la partie voisine du bassinet ne provoque aucun trouble morphologique ni dynamique.

Mais en combinant la dénudation à l'énervation du pédicule rénal, il observe une augmentation des contractions pyélique et urétérales, suivie d'une paralysie complète avec dilatation. La sympathectomie bilatérale faite dans la même séance, peut même être suivie de mort par urémie. Si l'énervation est faite d'un côté, puis. après un certain intervalle, de l'autre, les animaux vivent : l'excrétion s'améliore même dans une certaine mesure jusque vers le 14ème jour, mais le péristaltisme n'est plus normal, l'élimination urinaire reste insuffisante et une urétéro-hydronéphrose se constitue.

CAPORALE réalise une sympathectomie péri-urétérale par destruction de l'adventice sur 1 à 3 cms. avec ou sans badigeonnage à l'isophénol. Il observe immédiatement un anneau de constriction au niveau de la zône énervée. Plus tard, il constate :

— à la pyéloscopie, une dilatation notable de la zône énervée et des voies excrétrices en amont : les ondes péristaltiques existent mais elles sont moins énergiques et plus rares que du côté opposé et s'arrêtent à la région opérée,

— à la cystoscopie, l'élimination de l'indigo-carmin se fait par éjaculations retardées, faibles et arythmiques,

— à l'autopsie: uretéro-hydronéphrose typique.

Blatt dénude, chez le lapin, au bistouri et à l'iso-phénol, le tiers supérieur, puis le tiers moyen et enfin le tiers inférieur de l'uretère. Dans les 3 mois qui suivent, il constate à la pyélographie et à l'autopsie une dilatation sus-jacente à l'énervation, toute possibilité d'erreur d'origine mécanique ayant été éliminée.

Gouverneur et Henri Marion dénudent au bistouri un segment d'uretère de chien: le segment sus-jacent est inerte mais réagit à l'excitation, l'onde provoquée ne franchit pas la zône dénudée.

De 10 à 30 jours plus tard, le segment supérieur est dilaté: il reste excitable mais la contraction ne franchit pas la zône dénudée: le segment inférieur conserve des contractions aboutissant à une éjaculation urétérale rythmée; l'excitation de ce segment inférieur provoque une onde vers le bas et une onde antipéristaltique qui remonte au point dénudé sans le franchir.

Beach badigeonne 2 à 3 cms. d'uretère moyen à la nicotine; quelques minutes après, la zône touchée est dilatée. Plus tard, les ondes péristaltiques s'arrêtent à la zône traumatisée: les contractions du segment inférieur sont normales. Les excitations en amont et en aval provoquent des contractions qui ne franchissent pas le point badigeonné.

L'uretère est fortement dilaté en amont, avec d'abord hypertrophie puis atrophie de la musculeuse. Le bassinet et les calices sont également dilatés.

L'uretère sous jacent est légèrement dilaté avec légère atrophie musculaire. Cette dilatation est temporaire.

Plus récemment, Ragnotti, Zanne et Henry Duvergey ont repris ces expériences et en ont confirmé les résultats.

e) Injection de toxines et infection

Primbs a étudié les effets des toxines colibacillaires et staphylococciques sur la motricité de l'uretère prélevé et examiné in vitro. Les bouillons de culture filtrés sont mis au contact de la muqueuse: une toxine très diluée augmente les contractions et provoque des spasmes, une toxine concentrée arrête les contractions.

Lütjens confirme l'action des toxines microbiennes et obtient des effets identiques des toxines de désintégration tissulaire.

Zanne obtient:

— avec du pus stérile et exempt de toxine, un renforcement de la contractilité uretérale,

— avec des cultures microbiennes (staphylocoque, streptocoque, colibacille) une longue période d'excitation suivie de parésie,

— avec du pus de pyonéphrose, une courte période d'excitation suivie de paralysie définitive. Si la toxine est mise au contact de l'adventice, la paralysie est plus durable et la dilatation plus importante que si elle est mise au contact de la muqueuse.

II. Résorption pyélo-rénale

En 1894, Tuffier injecte de la strychnine dans le bassinet d'un chien sans provoquer de troubles. Il lie alors l'uretère, réinjecte de la strychnine: le chien meurt rapidement en opisthotonos.

Cette expérience établit que le bassinet qui n'absorbe rien dans les circonstances normales, résorbe les poisons lorsque se produisent à son niveau une stase et une hyperpression.

Huber (1895) reprend l'expérience en injectant de l'iodure et du ferrocyanure de potassium qu'il retrouve dans la salive: il baptise le phénomène: *résorption pyélo-rénale.*

Depuis lors la question a été reprise, précisée dans:
1. son existence,
2. ses variétés,
3. son mécanisme,
4. ses conséquences pathologiques.

Une phrase d'HINMAN suffit à en montrer l'importance: «Le contenu d'une poche pyélique au-dessus d'un obstacle, dit-il, est, non pas une mare stagnante, mais bien un lac aux eaux courantes».

1. Expériences démontrant l'existence de la résorption pyélo-rénale

Nous passerons rapidement. Après TUFFIER et HUBER:

MACHT vérifie la résorption d'autres toxiques: aconitine, apomorphine, etc....

MARCUS, BASTLER, LEWIN, celle de particules colorantes d'indigo ou de vert d'outre-mer.

VERRIÈRE celle de collargol ou d'encre de chine,

WELD injecte de l'iodure de potassium, HINMAN et VICKI, MAGOUN, BURNS et SCHWARTZ de la sulfone phénol phtaléine qu'ils retrouvent dans la secrétion du rein opposé.

V. SAUER, BOEMINGHAUS utilisent les opacifiants radiologiques et obtiennent des urographies du rein opposé.

BOEMINGHAUS remplit de liquide opaque le bassinet isolé d'une part, un segment d'uretère d'autre part: il constate par des radiographies en série que la résorption est beaucoup plus rapide au niveau du bassinet que dans l'uretère.

HINMAN et REDWILL perfusent un rein avec une solution de citrate de fer ammoniacal et recueillent le liquide sortant de la veine dans un récipient contenant de l'acide chlorhydrique. Ils injectent alors dans l'uretère une solution de ferrocyanure de potassium et voient se produire, dans l'acide chlorhydrique, un précipité de bleu de Prusse.

Ces mêmes auteurs établissent que la résorption est plus forte pour l'urine alcaline que pour l'urine acide: un lot de rats est soumis à un régime alcalin; un autre au régime acide pendant 15 jours; on lie l'uretère: 48 heures après, les rats acides ont un bassinet dilaté, les rats alcalins ne présentent pas de dilatation.

2. Les différentes variétés de résorption pyélo-rénale

La résorption pyélique se fait selon 4 mécanismes qui ont été précisés par les travaux de VERRIÈRE (1932), de NARATH (1938) et par la remarquable mise au point d'AUVERT (1957): nous le suivrons de très près dans sa nomenclature et son texte.

a) Reflux pyélo-canaliculaire ou pyélo-tubulaire

Dans certaines conditions, qu'il faudra préciser, l'urine contenue dans les calices peut refluer dans les tubes collecteurs de la papille et même remonter dans le tube contourné et y être résorbée.

Il s'agit là d'un *véritable reflux* à contre-courant.

VERRIÈRE injectant du collargol ou de l'encre de chine dans le bassinet, retrouve des grains dans les tubes collecteurs et jusque dans les tubes contournés.

BIRD et MOISE, employant le citrate de fer ammoniacal et le ferrocyanure de potassium, retrouvent des cristaux de bleu de Prusse dans les tubes collecteurs, dans les deux branches de l'anse de HENLÉ et jusque dans la capsule glomérulaire. Ils reprennent les mêmes expériences sur des rein hydronéphrotiques et constatent que les glomérules de la corticale, les premiers atrophiés par l'hydro-néphrose, sont envahis bien avant les glomérules profonds, que l'absorption est d'autant plus importante qu'on a affaire à un segment plus élevé du tube urinaire.

BIETER confirme cette dernière notion en injectant une solution de sulfone phénol phtaléine par l'uretère. Si le colorant n'atteint que les tubes collecteurs, il n'y a pas d'absorption, s'il arrive aux tubes contournés, il y a élimination rapide par le rein opposé.

Enfin, *la pyélographie* donne de temps en temps une preuve tangible de ce reflux sous forme de pinceaux en brosse débordant le fond d'un ou plusieurs calices.

b) Diffusion pyélo-interstitielle

L'existence de cette diffusion repose sur quelques rares pyélographies où l'on voit, soit le prolongement en corne d'un angle caliciel, soit une série d'images dentelées en couronne partant du fond du calice. Cette diffusion pourrait devenir «très abondante et même monstrueuse». Une fois résorbé dans le tissu inter-stitiel, le contenu pyélique diffuse dans l'espace cellulaire en se dirigeant, soit le long des pyramides jusque sous la capsule, soit vers la graisse intra-sinusale.

Elle n'a jamais été reproduite expérimentalement, mais il est probable qu'elle est responsable de certains épanchements sous capsulaires rencontrés au cours d'interventions (CIBERT).

Cette diffusion peut se faire par rupture du fornix (voir plus loin) mais NARATH pense qu'il s'agit souvent d'une simple diffusion dans le tissu interstitiel qui entoure le fond du calice. L'épithélium du fornix, particulièrement mince, pour-rait, sous l'action de la distension, devenir perméable à l'urine. De fait, si, après avoir constaté la fuite au cours d'une pyélographie, on vide le bassinet et qu'on refasse immédiatement une seconde pyélographie, la fuite ne se reproduit pas.

c) Réabsorption pyélo-lymphatique

Le contenu pyélique résorbé peut envahir les lymphatiques.

LEWIN et GOLDSCHMIDT ont retrouvé des traces de produit injecté dans les ganglions lymphatiques du hile et dans ceux de la paroi lombaire. Mais c'est encore la *pyélographie* qui met le fait en évidence en montrant l'injection, soit des collecteurs lymphatiques du sinus rénal, soit des trajets aberrants, le long de l'uretère et jusque dans l'atmosphère périrénale après traversée de la capsule.

Trois hypothèses peuvent expliquer ce phénomène:

— celle de l'effraction au niveau du fornix établissant une communication directe entre le calice et les lymphatiques et veines qui l'entourent,

— celle du passage à travers la paroi pyélique elle-même (RENIY-VAMOS, BALOGH et SZENDROÏ),

— celle de la réabsorption simple du liquide épanché dans le tissu inter-stitiel, dans les conditions étudiées ci-dessus: la réabsorption pyélolymphatique serait alors la conséquence obligatoire et «révélatrice» de la résorption pyélo-interstitielle à laquelle elle succède obligatoirement.

d) Effraction pyélo-veineuse

Il s'agit d'une *lésion traumatique* due à la rupture du calice d'une part, des lacs veineux péricaliciels d'autre part.

Cette lésion a été maintes fois réalisée expérimentalement. On la retrouve sur certaines pyélographies sous forme d'images courbes en arceau, en pinces de homard, objectivant le trajet des veines interlobaires, d'où partent des stries rayonnantes correspondant aux veines intra lobulaires. Sur de telles pyélographies, on constate souvent des diffusions mixtes, pyélo-interstitielles, pyélolymphatiques et pyélo-veineuses, difficiles à interpréter.

La rupture calicielle se produit toujours à l'angle calico-papillaire. Depuis GIGON (1856) tous les auteurs l'ont vérifié. Il y a là une zone de moindre résistance à la jonction du versant papillaire inextensible et du versant externe mince et entouré de graisse. De plus, ce versant externe (LEE, BROWN et LAIDLEY, TRANT) fait corps avec les vaisseaux qui traversent le sinus dont l'adventice renforce le tissu sous-muqueux; au niveau de l'angle calico-papillaire, les vaisseaux abandonnent la paroi calicielle pour pénétrer dans la colonne de BERTIN et la sous-muqueuse se réduit à quelques fibres élastiques.

La rupture veineuse intéresse l'anneau veineux qui entoure le calice et forme un véritable lac veineux anastomosant les veines interlobaires. Le contenu du calice dilaté passe directement dans les grosses veines pédiculaires, la veine cave, etc.... on l'a suivi jusqué dans le coeur, le foie, la rate. Il remonte d'autre part dans les veines rénales interlobaires et interlobulaires dilatées elles-mêmes par la distension du bassinet.

3. Mécanisme de production de la résorption
a) Hyperpression pyélique

La condition nécessaire et constante de tout phénomène de résorption est l'*hyperpression du contenu pyélique.*

TUFFIER a du lier l'uretère, HUBER provoquer une hyperpression de 55 cm. H$_2$O, HINMAN et REDWILL voient le précipité de bleu de Prusse se produire à 35 mm. Hg et MAGOUN a retrouvé la phénol sulfone phtaléine dans le rein opposé en faisant monter la pression pyélique de 20 à 45 puis 55 cm. H$_2$O etc....

Cette hyperpression est obtenue par différents procédés:

a) Injection du bassinet par l'uretère sous pression controlée: C'est le cas des pyélographies.

b) Injection dans un bassinet dont on lie l'uretère: on injecte directement sous pression, ou bien on remplit seulement le bassinet et on attend que la secrétion rénale provoque l'hyperpression.

c) Injection dans un bassinet déjà hydronéphrosé par ligature antérieure de l'uretère (HINMAN, VERRIÈRE).

d) Hyperpression provoquée par reflux vésico-pyélique (LEWIN et GOLDSCHMIDT, GRAVES et DAVIDOFF, VERRIÈRE).

Quelques expériences fournissent des données plus précises:

HINMAN et LEE-BROWN injectent dans un bassinet de lapin du bromure de sodium à 50%. Sous une pression de 10 à 20 mm. Hg le pyélogramme est normal. A 30 mm. Hg le passage dans les veines est visible. A 40 mm. Hg le liquide opaque apparait dans les grosses veines.

Les mêmes auteurs, chez un chien dont la pression secrétoire est de 63 mm. Hg, injectent de la phénolsulfone phtaléine à la pression de 50 mm. Hg et laissent la pression monter sous l'action de la secrétion. En dix minutes, la pression est de 60 mm. Hg et le colorant passe dans l'urine du rein opposé. Ils lavent alors le bassinet au serum pour enlever toute trace de colorant: dans les vingt minutes suivantes, les deux reins secrètent la phénol sulfone phtaléine.

Pour ces auteurs, l'effraction pyélo-veineuse se produit à 60 mm. Hg = 80 cm. H$_2$O. Une fois la rupture produite, la résorption continue sous une pression très inférieure (20 mm. Hg = 27 cm. H$_2$O) mais maintenue un assez long temps.

Verrière qui injecte par l'uretère du collargol ou de l'encre de Chine, fixe à 70 mm. Hg = 95 cm. H_2O la pression nécessaire pour obtenir le reflux pyélo-veineux.

Rolnick et Singer ont étudié la gamme de lésions déterminées par des pressions allant de 20 à 150 mm. Hg (30 à 200 cm. H_2O). Les faibles pressions donnent des diffusions limitées avec lymphographie. Les fortes pressions seules déterminent l'effraction pyélo-veineuse.

Auvert a repris les expériences pyélographiques de Narath en les complétant par un contrôle manométrique. Les conclusions sont les suivantes:

— les types de diffusion sont variés et *imprévisibles*.

— la lymphographie est obtenue par injection rapide de 4 à 6 cm³. sous une pression de 120 cm. H_2O.

— la phlébographie nécessite une injection plus abondante (10 cm³.) et une pression plus élevée (150 cm. H_2O).

— la mise en tension préalable du bassinet facilite les diffusions ascendantes.

Aucun des animaux soumis à des agressions pyéliques répétées n'a présenté de phénomène de pyonéphrose, d'insuffisance rénale ou d'hématurie persistante.

En résumé: on peut, avec Verrière, distinguer: les *agressions à minima* qui se limitent aux trois premières variétés de résorption, c'est-à-dire au reflux pyélo-tubulaire et à l'absorption pyélo-interstitielle suivie de l'élimination pyélo-lymphatique, et l'*agression a maxima* qui comporte l'effraction anatomique pyélo-veineuse.

Cette dernière, parce qu'elle a un substratum anatomique est la seule qu'on puisse reproduire expérimentalement. On l'obtient pour une hyperpression qui varie selon les auteurs de 60 à 80 mm. Hg = 80 à 100 cm. H_2O.

Les autres variétés ont été découvertes par la pyélographie: elles sont imprévisibles (Auvert) et leur mode de production reste imprécis. Ce sont pourtant les plus importantes parce qu'elles se produisent aux hyperpressions modérées observées dans les circonstances pathologiques courantes.

b) Autres conditions

1. *Les contractions du bassinet.* Elles augmentent évidemment la pression mais cette augmentation est relativement faible (10 à 20 cm. H_2O) et intermittente.

2. *L'état de la muqueuse pyélique.* Son inflammation détermine une hyper-vascularisation et des modifications du tonus en plus ou en moins. Dans l'ensemble, la résorption semble se produire plus difficilement sur des bassinets atteints de pyélite que sur des bassinets sains.

Lee Brown et Laidley pensent que la muqueuse s'épaissit au niveau de la jonction papillo-calicielle dont l'angle est en partie comblé par du tissu scléreux. Le reflux est difficile ou même impossible à provoquer, malgré une pression élevée (120 mm. Hg).

Verrière a également constaté que dans les cas où il n'a pas obtenu de reflux, il s'agissait de reins malades atteints de lésions infectieuses chroniques, de sclérose, ou appartenant à des animaux âgés.

3. *La colique néphrétique* favorise incontestablement les résorptions en créant une hyperpression quelquefois considérable (50 à 90 cm. H_2O). Auvert insiste sur la fréquence des images de résorption obtenues sur des urographies pratiquées au cours de la colique néphrétique. Les aspects d'extravasation assez déroutants évoqueraient des lésions variées telles que tuberculose, tumeur ou pyonéphrose s'ils n'étaient passagers, c'est-à-dire s'ils ne disparaissaient pas aux urographies pratiquées après la crise.

4. *Le reflux vésico-uretéro-pyélique* peut être à l'origine de résorption pyélique et ceci se conçoit puisque dans le reflux, tant actif que passif, la pression de miction qui est d'environ 100 cm. H_2O est transmise aux cavités pyélo-calicielles.

4. Conséquences physio-pathologiques de la résorption

1. D'abord quelques conclusions d'ordre pratique: toute hyperpression provoquée, au cours d'un cathétérisme, d'un lavage du bassinet, d'une pyélographie et même d'une compression abdominale au cours d'une urographie, peut causer des accidents de résorption.

2. Parmi les résorptions, la plus grave est l'effraction pyélo-veineuse (agression a maxima) qui est une lésion anatomique: elle est responsable des hématuries au cours de l'hydronéphrose et des septicémies brutales survenant après pyélographie ou cathétérisme de certaines poches hydronéphrotiques.

Les autres variétés et plus spécialement le reflux pyélo-tubulaire sont probablement d'ordre physiologique et AUVERT fait remarquer l'extraordinaire tolérance de l'organisme à la plupart des diffusions observées au cours des pyélographies: elles ne provoquent aucun symptôme et ne laissent après elle ni séquelle ni trouble de la secrétion rénale.

FUCHS voit dans cette résorption un agent de coordination entre la secrétion rénale et l'excrétion pyélo-urétérale. Il peut arriver, en cas de polyurie excessive, que le pouvoir d'évacuation de l'uretère soit dépassé: la résorption entre alors en jeu. Ceci expliquerait les poussées fébriles parfois observées à la fin de l'épreuve de VOLHARD chez les malades atteints de pyélonéphrite.

3. C'est grâce à cette résorption que le contenu de la poche d'hydronéphrose se stabilise au point de vue chimique et au point de vue de la pression. L'hyperpression qui suit la ligature (>80 cm. H_2O) ne se maintient guère plus de 12 à 24 heures (OBNISKI) et décroit ensuite: 40 cm. H_2O au cinquième jour (PAVONE), 20 cm. H_2O après le quinzième jour (GRÉHANT) 4 cm. H_2O après soixante jours (GUYON).

4. C'est grâce à cette résorption que le rein (seul de toutes les glandes) continue à secréter après ligature de son canal excréteur et peut, de ce fait, récupérer une certaine valeur fonctionnelle après levée de l'obstacle.

5. C'est elle qui explique en partie les variations inattendues et même paradoxales du volume des poches d'hydronéphrose: un obstacle très accentué ne donnant qu'une rétention modérée alors que des poches monstrueuses correspondent à des lésions assez minimes pour n'être pas décelables.

6. Il ne faudrait pas conclure de tout ceci que la résorption n'a que des conséquences favorables. Il est probable qu'elle est notamment à la base du processus de pyélonéphrite ascendante. Tout ce qui précède ne concerne que les rétentions strictement aseptiques. Tout change dès que l'infection se met de la partie. Mais ceci concerne la pathologie.

III. Le reflux vésico-urétéral

A côté des «obstacles» très variés qui intéressent la voie excrétrice elle-même, il est une cause d'hyperpression qui, bien qu'indépendante d'elle, n'en retentit pas moins sur son fonctionnement: c'est le *reflux vésico-uretéro-pyélique*.

Son origine est dans l'appareil urinaire inférieur (urètre-prostate-vessie); son résultat est de gêner l'excrétion du haut appareil et de retentir sur le rein. Par lui, les lésions de l'appareil urinaire inférieur aboutissent finalement à l'insuffisance rénale.

1. *Avant même que le reflux ne se produise*, les dysfonctionnements de l'appareil urinaire inférieur peuvent retentir sur l'excrétion pyélo-urétérale.

GUYON et ALBARRAN lient l'urètre d'un chien. Après 24 heures, les contractions des uretères sont abolies; après 48 heures, l'uretère et le bassinet sont dilatés et atones. Il suffit à ce moment de ponctionner la vessie pour voir l'uretère se vider et reprendre ses contractions. Plus tard, la dilatation est irréversible. Jamais, au cours de ces expériences, on n'observe de reflux.

SAMPSON et KREUTZMANN enregistrant les pressions de la vessie et de l'uretère inférieur dans diverses circonstances, montrent que la pression de l'uretère inférieur, normalement toujours supérieure à la pression vésicale, devient nettement inférieure sur la vessie distendue.

On conçoit que l'uretère s'épuise à injecter sous pression l'urine dans une vessie contenant 500 à 1000 ou 1500 cm³, que ses contractions d'abord plus fortes et plus rares, finissent par s'affaiblir et s'arrêter.

Ceci explique déjà le fait bien connu en clinique jornalière, de la déficience de la fonction rénale chez les rétentionnistes vésicaux, surtout chez les distendus.

2. Plus grave encore est le *reflux* et de ces *reflux-pyélo-urétéraux*, on distingue plusieurs variétés.

a) *Le reflux surprise* que nous avons vu (voir p. 511) se produire rarement et de manière intermittente et artificielle avec une vessie et un uretère sains.

Ce reflux disparait dès que la pression vésicale accidentelle cesse: elle n'a pas de conséquences pathologiques.

b) Plus grave est le *reflux* dit *actif*, c'est-à-dire celui qui se produit au moment où la miction détermine une hyperpression vésicale importante.

Ce reflux est décrit par LEPOUTRE dans les termes suivants: «l'urine remonte de la vessie dans l'uretère sous forme d'une colonne ininterrompue. Elle rencontre l'onde péristaltique, la repousse et tout remonte vers le haut. Si la pression vésicale se relâche, le péristaltisme urétéral reprend et évacue l'urine refoulée par ondes et bouchées régulières». Ce reflux peut être suivi facilement par cystographie sous contrôle radioscopique.

La lutte entre l'injection vésicale à contre-courant et les ondes péristaltiques urétérales régulières a pu faire croire à des ondes antipéristaltiques (LEWIN et GOLDSCHMIDT). Cette interprétation est erronée (WISLOCKI et O'CONNOR) car l'ascension se fait beaucoup plus rapidement que les ondes antipéristaltiques qui ne se déplacent jamais à plus de 40 cms. par seconde.

Ce reflux actif correspond à un *uretère forcé*; il ne devrait jamais se produire avec une vessie et un uretère sains. Mais la lésion est légère et, à la cystoscopie, le méat urétéral apparait normal.

Il ne nous appartient pas d'énumérer les causes pathologiques de l'uretère forcé: il s'agit en général d'une lésion de cystite ou de sclérose vésicale localisée à une ou aux deux zones méatiques. L'inflammation, l'oedème ou la sclérose gênent le fonctionnement et détruisent la synergie fonctionnelle qui existe normalement entre la vessie et l'uretère inférieur.

Le retentissement du reflux actif sur les voies excrétrices et le rein sont très variables:

— si le reflux actif est épisodique et intermittent, l'uretère lutte efficacement, son péristaltisme refoule le liquide reflué.

— si le reflux devient habituel, les voies excrétrices se fatiguent et se dilatent; AUVERT fait remarquer que cette uretéro-hydronéphrose est un moyen de défense du parenchyme rénal à condition de rester aseptique. Si les urines s'infectent, il se produit une pyélonéphrite ascendante plus néfaste encore que l'atrophie hydronéphrotique par compression.

— si le reflux actif s'installe, le sphincter méatique se laisse forcer et on voit s'installer successivement:

c) *Un reflux mixte* avec renforcement mictionnel, et enfin:

d) *Le reflux passif pur* (GRUBER). La vessie et l'uretère communiquent librement et toute modification de la pression vésicale est immédiatement transmise à la cavité urétéro-pyélique. Celle-ci, étant moins résistante que la cavité vésicale, se dilate, s'amincit, s'atrophie et les mouvements péristaltiques disparaissent. Ce n'est pas un reflux à proprement parler, c'est une cavité diverticulaire de la cavité vésicale, qui se remplit avec elle et se vide passivement.

Le retentissement sur le rein est extrêmement variable et dépend de la pression développée par la vessie dans l'intervalle et au moment des mictions, mais cette hyperpression est continuelle et lèse le rein. Il faut remarquer que cette hyperpression est plus élevée donc plus dangereuse avec une vessie de faible capacité et surtout à sensibilité atténuée. La sauvegarde du rein est dans la pollakiurie et celle-ci n'est pas toujours suffisante pour protéger le haut appareil (CIBERT).

Données cliniques et radiologiques au point de vue physio-pathologique

L'expérimentation crée un obstacle et constate ses conséquences. La pathologie constate des symptômes et en cherche l'origine. Leur point de vue est différent, mais chaque observation clinique, chaque cliché radiologique est une expérience in vivo dont les résultats doivent être interprétés en fonction des données physio-pathologiques.

Sans empiéter sur le territoire de la pathologie, nous étudierons dans ce chapitre qui manquera d'homogénéité:

1. Les deux grands symptômes de la maladie excrétrice: la *dilatation* et la *rétention*, en les envisageant sous l'angle physio-pathologique car tous deux ont une valeur et une signification bien différentes selon les cas.

2. *Les réactions segmentaires* des voies excrétrices, dont l'expérimentation soupçonne l'existence mais que la pathologie affirme avec beaucoup plus de netteté.

3. Certains *aspects radiologiques* de *pratique courante* envisagés, eux aussi, sous l'angle de la physiologie pathologique.

1. La dilatation et la rétention envisagées sous l'angle physio-pathologique
a) La dilatation

C'est la première et principale réaction à l'«obstacle». Les cavités pyélo-urétérales sont agrandies dans leurs trois dimensions par l'allongement de leurs fibres musculaires circulaires, longitudinales ou obliques.

Dans quelle mesure cet allongement est-il compatible avec l'intégrité de la fibre musculaire, dans quelle mesure compromet-il les fonctions musculaires (extensibilité, élasticité, tonicité et contractilité)?

Il est indispensable, à ce point de vue, de préciser la définition de certains termes. On emploie souvent à côté du terme «dilatation» celui de «distension», on a même tendance à les confondre. Cette confusion a peut être peu d'inconvénient en clinique, elle en a de très grands en physiologie pathologique.

Le terme *dilatation* doit être réservé à l'allongement d'une fibre musculaire saine: cet allongement est physiologique et reversible.

A son moindre degré, la dilatation n'est qu'une adaptation des voies excrétrices aux variations de la polyurie.

Mais elle peut être beaucoup plus considérable et la clinique en fournit des exemples fréquents : par exemple, ces énormes dilatations provoquées par un calcul de l'uretère qui disparaissent totalement après levée de l'obstacle.

La fibre musculaire lisse possède, on le sait, une extensibilité considérable : l'utérus gravide et la vessie de rétention aiguë en fournissent des exemples évidents. Son élasticité parfaite la ramène ensuite à une longueur normale.

Seule, la tonicité qui adapte cette extensibilité-élasticité aux circonstances physiologiques et physio-pathologiques, intervient. La dilatation est donc un phénomène physiologique et totalement reversible : on peut même la considérer comme un moyen de défense. *On ne saurait trop s'élever contre la facilité avec laquelle certains baptisent hydronéphrotiques des bassinets qui ne sont qu'atones.*

Il en va tout autrement de la *distension*. La distension est «le résultat d'une extension *trop* considérable» (LITTRÉ). C'est dire que l'extension de la fibre musculaire a dépassé les facultés, grandes mais non illimitées, de son extensibilité. D'où élongation, microtraumatisme et même déchirure, bref, *lésion anatomique* qui compromet l'architecture et les propriétés tissulaires. L'extensibilité normale diminue, mais surtout, l'élasticité n'étant plus parfaite, la fibre musculaire ne revient pas à sa longueur d'origine. Les cavités pyélo-uretérales ne reviennent pas à leur volume primitif : elles sont *distendues* et cette distension n'est plus que partiellement reversible ou même totalement irréversible.

Autre conséquence : la tonicité ne peut plus adapter l'extensibilité-élasticité aux circonstances pathologiques. Son adaptation n'est plus possible que dans des limites plus ou moins étroites et le rôle de protection assuré par la tonicité se trouve compromis.

Dilatation et distension doivent donc être nettement distinguées au point de vue physio-pathologique dans leurs conséquences et leur pronostic.

b) La rétention

La rétention est la stase de l'urine au-dessus d'un «obstacle». L'urine peut encore couler mais n'est plus propulsée par le mouvement péristaltique qui, selon les degrés, est inefficace, ou interrompu, ou supprimé. Il s'agit d'un *trouble de la contractilité*.

Celle-ci peut être exagérée : c'est l'*hyperkinésie*, presque toujours temporaire et sans grande conséquence pathologique. Mais l'hyperkinésie peut aboutir au pasme ou à la contracture spasmodique qui peut se prolonger des jours et même des semaines, puisque, par le jeu de la tonicité, elle s'établit sans dépense énergétique donc sans provoquer de fatique musculaire (voir p. 483).

La contractilité peut aussi être affaiblie dans sa puissance ou ralentie dans son rythme : c'est l'*hypokinésie*, ou même totalement supprimée : c'est l'*akinésie*.

Ajoutons, pour être complets, des *mouvements antipéristaltiques* qui n'existent pas en physiologie normale, mais se produisent à la suite de certaines excitations pathologiques, notamment celles qui s'adressent à l'uretère inférieur.

Spasme d'une part, hypo et akinésie d'autre part, reproduisent au niveau du bassinet toutes les variétés de rétention bien connues au niveau de la vessie.

La pyeloscopie a permis d'individualiser notamment :

— *La rétention complète aiguë*: celle de la colique néphrétique,
— *La rétention incomplète sans dilatation*: avec résidu pyélique,
— *La rétention intermittente*: spéciale au rein mobile,
— *La rétention incomplète avec distension* et hypokinésic,
— *La rétention chronique complète*.

Ces deux dernières variétés constituant l'hydronéphrose.

En quoi consistent ces troubles de la contractilité?

Pour que le muscle se contracte, il faut qu'il soit sain au point de vue anatomique et physiologique.

— *au point de vue anatomique:* c'est-à-dire que toutes les lésions traumatiques, inflammatoires ou infectieuses, congénitales, etc.... troublent sa fonction.

— *au point de vue physiologique:* c'est-à-dire que les propriétés musculaires doivent être intactes.

En premier lieu, ses propriétés tissulaires: il faut que son extensibilité-élasticité soit suffisante; un muscle distendu ne peut plus se contracter qu'autant qu'une proportion notable de ses fibres ont conservé leur extensibilité-élasticité.

Mais cela ne suffit pas et il faut encore qu'il ait conservé sa tonicité. On sait les rapports étroits de la tonicité et de la contractilité (voir p. 483). La loi de STARLING établit que la puissance de la contraction dépend de la longueur de la fibre musculaire et cette longueur est réglée par la tonicité.

En cas d'hypertonie, les contractions sont moins amples et plus fréquentes; en poussant à l'extrême, c'est-à-dire à la contraction spasmodique, elles deviennent impossibles.

En cas d'hypotonie, les contractions sont plus amples et plus espacées: en poussant à l'extrême, c'est-à-dire à la grande dilatation (sans même faire intervenir la distension) les contractions s'arrêtent. Ce dernier fait a été maintes fois observé de façon quasi-expérimentale: on opère pour une grande hydronéphrose, on constate que la poche est inerte, on retire par ponction 20 ou 30 cc. et on voit reprendre des contractions efficaces qui vident complètement la poche.

Dans l'ensemble, dilatation et rétention sont parallèles et marchent de pair. Toute dilatation importante s'accompagne d'une rétention plus ou moins marquée et toute rétention provoque en amont une dilatation.

On note cependant des dissociations: certaines poches d'hydronéphrose, même volumineuses, se vident avec retard mais se vident: leur contractilité persiste alors que la tonicité est effondrée. Cela se produit dans certaines hydronéphroses opérées où la dilatation persiste alors que la motricité a repris une certaine valeur.

Tant que le tissu musculaire possède ses propriétés tissulaires et vitales, il s'adapte, et se défend: lorsqu'une de ces propriétés disparait, son absence retentit sur les autres et un véritable cercle vicieux s'établit qui aboutit, après une phase de lutte, à la fatigue du muscle, à sa distension et à sa destruction physiologique puis anatomique.

2. Les réactions segmentaires de l'appareil excréteur

On sait que l'appareil excréteur est formé par la succession de plusieurs systèmes détrusor-sphincter successifs appelés *cystoïdes*.

On distingue:

— les épicystoïdes caliciels,

— le cystoïde pyélique,

— les trois cystoïdes de l'uretère lombaire iliaque et pelvien.

Il existe à l'extrémité inférieure de chacun de ces cystoïdes une zone douée d'un pouvoir sphinctérien, capable de freiner ou d'arrêter l'onde péristaltique dans certaines circonstances.

Il est logique de penser que ces zones que rien ne différencie anatomiquement, sont physiologiquement douées d'un tonus plus élevé que celui des fuseaux intermédiaires.

Cela explique les dilatations et rétrécissements décrits pas les anatomistes sur des moulages d'uretère, alors qu'ils sont invisibles sur l'uretère vivant. De même certaines urographies reproduisent la topographie cystoïdique en dessinant des fuseaux séparés par des défilés.

34*

En physiologie normale, dans l'excrétion normale, un seul de ces cystoïdes se manifeste: le cystoïde pyélique, le «pace maker» du mouvement péristaltique qui assure la segmentation du flux urinaire et l'évacuation rythmée des rames uretérales. Au delà, la traversée des trois cystoïdes ureteraux se fait de façon continue (voir p. 508).

En cas de polyurie, l'évacuation pourrait prendre l'allure cystoïdique, chacun des cystoïdes ureteraux présentant des caractères anatomiques et fonctionnels bien étudiés par MURNAGHAN (voir p. 508).

Dans certains cas pathologiques le rôle des sphincters successifs devient évident et indiscutable. Toute excitation portant au niveau de ces zones de tonus élevé détermine l'arrêt de l'onde péristaltique, quelquefois même la production d'ondes antipéristaltiques.

Ici encore c'est la jonction pyélo-uretérale qui est la plus sensible: la fréquence prédominante des hydronéphroses de la jonction en est une preuve manifeste. Mais tous les sphincters cystoïdiens peuvent être touchés.

La radiocinématographie nous a fourni récemment deux observations de valeur expérimentale.

Dans la première, il s'agit d'un calcul de la jonction pyélo-uretérale: les épicystoïdes des calices sont distendus, le bassinet, d'abord invisible, ne se dessine que progressivement et lentement: il ne reçoit des épicystoïdes caliciels que la quantité réduite de liquide dont le calcul permet l'élimination.

Dans la seconde, il existe un rétrécissement de l'uretère inférieur; le film montre au niveau de l'articulation sacro-iliaque l'aspect d'un second rétrécissement aussi serré. Les contractions du bassinet et de l'uretère supérieur se produisent avec force; mais quand l'onde arrive au niveau de la sacro-iliaque, une petite partie s'engage lentement dans le cystoïde pelvien et franchit le rétrécissement. La plus grosse partie de la rame uretérale est brutalement refoulée jusque dans le bassinet par des mouvements antipéristaltiques violents.

Des examens ultérieurs ont prouvé que la zône incriminée était de calibre normal: l'aspect de pseudo rétrécissement était du à la contracture de la zône intermédiaire aux cystoïdes iliaque et pelvien.

Les cas de ce genre sont trop peu nombreux pour en tirer des déductions valables mais, dans les deux cas que nous venons de rapporter, tout se passe comme si le cystoïde situé au-dessus de l'obstacle ne laissait strictement passer que la quantité susceptible de se faufiler au niveau de la zône sténosée.

Cette protection d'un segment uretéral par le segment sus-jacent est-il la règle? dans quelle mesure et pour combien de temps cette protection est-elle efficace? Il est impossible de le dire actuellement. Tout ce qu'on peut affirmer c'est qu'il existe des réactions segmentaires et étagées des voies excrétrices.

3. Aspects radiologiques envisagées en physiopathologie

a) Rein muet

Plusieurs éventualités sont à envisager:

a) Le rein n'existe pas.

b) Le rein est insuffisant, son pouvoir de concentration est trop faible pour donner une opacité décelable aux rayons. A noter que certains reins, et notamment les reins hydronéphrotiques, ont une secrétion retardée: leur opacification demande plusieurs heures et la répétition de l'injection intra-veineuse.

c) La secrétion est bloquée par l'hyperpression pyélique aiguë et reversible: c'est le cas des coliques néphrétiques de toutes origines (calcul, crise d'hydronéphrose, etc....). Auvert, mesurant les pressions au cours des coliques néphrétiques et des anuries par obstruction, a trouvé des chiffres variant de 20 à 90 cm. H_2O. Cette pression en excrétion bloquée est d'autant plus basse que le rein est plus altéré. Une pression supérieure à 50 cm. H_2O laisse prévoir une récupération valable. Une pression inférieure à 40 cm. H_2O correspond à une insuffisance rénale.

b) Néphrographie

Il existe plusieurs variétés d'opacification du parenchyme rénal, avec ou sans opacification des voies excrétrices:

α) *La néphrographie physiologique* qui correspond au stade capillaire du passage de la substance opaque. On peut la surprendre au cours de l'artériographie suivant immédiatement le stade artériel et précédant le stade veineux et l'opacification des calices. Cette néphrographie physiologique, très courte, peut être observée par hasard sur des urographies sériées à court intervalle. L'injection intra-veineuse doit être abondante, très rapidement poussée: la néphrographie survient environ quarante secondes après le début de l'injection. Elle est suivie d'un pyélogramme normal.

β) *Les néphrographies* s'observent fréquemment *au cours des coliques néphrétiques* (Fey et Jacques Michon). Néphrographie ou rein muet ont la même origine: l'hyperpression pyélique, et la même signification, mais le rein muet correspond à une faible concentration alors que la néphrographie prouve une excellente fonction rénale.

Cette néphrographie est relativement tardive (cinq à dix minutes après l'injection), sans pyélogramme avant la fin de la crise. Si la colique néphrétique vient à céder au cours de l'examen, le pyélogramme apparait aussitôt.

Le stockage de la substance opaque se fait dans les tubes urinifères (Narath).

Hickel a proposé de provoquer cette néphrographie par l'hyperpression à 80 cm. H_2O pour mettre en évidence le volume et les contours du rein.

γ) La néphrographie peut également se produire dans des rétentions chroniques (hydronéphrose de la jonction, rétrécissements de l'uretère). Il s'agit d'une hyperpression chronique mais équilibrée avec conservation d'une secrétion valable. Si on libère cette rétention par cathétérisme ou ponction, la néphrographie disparait et le pyélogramme se dessine.

Le stockage iodé se fait dans les tubes (Narath, Puigvert) et dans les espaces interstitiels péritubulaires (H. Smith).

c) Dilatation élective des calices
(Fey, Dossot et Truchot)

C'est l'aspect des calices, seuls dessinés et de forme régulièrement circulaire, en «boules», à l'exclusion de toute opacification pyélique. Les calices apparaissent tardivement, d'abord très pales: le liquide opaque s'y accumule lentement, on peut y constater un niveau liquide; ce n'est qu'après plusieurs heures que le liquide opaque s'écoule et dessine un bassinet toujours dilaté.

Cet aspect est du à la dilatation des calices dans lesquels la papille refoulée n'imprime plus son empreinte convexe et surtout à l'atonie et à l'acinésie de leur musculature. Le contenu de ces calices n'est plus brassé par la systole pyélique et ne s'écoule que par simple pesanteur. Il s'agit donc d'une paralysie à la fois pyélique et calicielle coïncidant avec une secrétion parenchymateuse encore valable.

Conclusion

L'expérimentation est destinée à expliquer la pathologie: elle ne l'explique qu'en partie.

L'expérimentateur, quelle que soit son ingéniosité, n'oppose et ne peut opposer à l'excrétion que des obstacles mécaniques: ce sont peut être les principaux, ce ne sont surement pas les seuls. En pathologie, le choix est plus riche: obstacles congénitaux par malformation ou aplasie, traumatiques et micro-traumatiques, tumoraux, inflammatoires, cicatriciels, par sténose, compression ou obstruction, etc., etc.... Sans compter les cas assez nombreux où l'exploration la plus complète, avec nos moyens d'investigation actuels, ne révèle aucun obstacle et laisse un doute sur son existence elle-même. On peut alors se demander s'il ne s'agit pas d'un trouble purement fonctionnel sans base anatomique: ici, comme ailleurs, un tel trouble peut, s'il se prolonge, créer des lésions anatomiques secondaires. Toutes ces questions, l'expérimentation est incapable de les résoudre.

Ce que l'expérimentation nous apprend, c'est la succession, l'évolution et les conséquences des troubles de l'excrétion, quel que soit l'obstacle à l'excrétion, qu'il s'agisse de ligature complète ou incomplète, temporaire ou définitive, d'excitation prolongée ou de dénudation, les troubles déclenchés évoluent toujours selon le même cycle:

a) *stade d'adaptation physiologique:* la motricité s'arrête, la tonicité se relache, une certaine dilatation se produit: aucune lésion n'existe et tout reprend.

b) *stade de lutte et d'hypertrophie musculaire:* le muscle allongé se contracte avec son maximum de puissance tente de forcer l'obstacle et s'hypertrophie: sa tonicité lutte contre la dilatation.

c) *stade de fatigue musculaire.* Cette fatigue n'atteint pas les propriétés tissulaires: l'extensibilité et l'élasticité sont intactes, mais la tonicité faiblit et la dilatation augmente, les contractions sont plus fréquentes mais perdent leur ampleur et leur efficacité.

Plus tard, toute motricité apparente cesse: pourtant, longtemps encore, elle peut reprendre: la simple ponction de la poche suffit à la faire réapparaitre et les fibres musculaires restent excitables.

Si l'obstacle est levé à ce stade, ces lésions sont totalement reversibles.

d) *stade de distension et de dégénérescence musculaire.* Les fibres musculaires sont anatomiquement lésées et progressivement détruites: non seulement la motricité et la tonicité ont disparu mais l'extensibilité et l'élasticité sont également touchées. Les lésions ne sont plus que partiellement reversibles selon l'importance des lésions anatomiques.

e) *stade de sclérose.* Le muscle n'est plus du muscle. Les fibres musculaires et élastiques sont remplacées par un tissu de sclérose rigide et inextensible. La lésion est totalement irréversible.

L'expérimentation démontre aussi les conséquences physiologiques et anatomiques des troubles excréteurs sur la glande rénale: compression du parenchyme par hyperpression, déficience secrétoire, troubles circulatoires, ischémie, etc.... aboutissant à l'insuffisance rénale d'une part, à la destruction anatomique du parenchyme par le processus hydronéphrotique.

Ce cycle est constant et son déroulement inéluctable et c'est l'expérimentation qui a permis de l'établir.

En revanche, elle est incapable de dire en combien de temps ce cycle évoluera parceque cela dépend de la nature et du degré de l'obstacle, de sa constance ou de son intermittence: selon les cas, la durée d'évolution sera, ici de quelques jours et là de plusieurs années.

Il reste à la pathologie, non seulement à découvrir l'obstacle pour le supprimer, mais aussi à déterminer à quel stade du cycle on est parvenu, pour évaluer les possibilités pronostiques de la thérapeutique.

La divergence capitale qui oppose l'expérimentation à la clinique réside dans l'intervention de l'*infection*.

Pour l'expérimentateur, l'infection est l'ennemi. Elle fausse ses expériences, trouble leurs résultats, rend leur interprétation impossible. Les problèmes qu'elle introduit nécessiteraient de nouvelles séries d'expériences d'une complexité insurmontable.

Pour le clinicien, l'infection est le pain quotidien. Le vieil adage urologique «stase égale infection» reste intangible. Il y a sans doute des stases stériles, l'hydronéphrose est là pour le démontrer. Mais, toute poche stasique est un lieu de moindre résistance à n'importe quelle infection d'ordre général ou local et, une fois infectée, une poche de stase ne se désinfecte pratiquement jamais.

L'infection elle-même est génératrice de stase par parésie, oedème, infiltration et sclérose. Ainsi s'établit le cercle vicieux qui complique tout. Ici il attaque sournoisement la valeur fonctionnelle par le mécanisme de la pyélonéphrite ascendante; là il infiltre et détruit la couche musculaire avant même que la dilatation se soit produite; là enfin, il transforme le processus hydronéphrotique en celui, beaucoup plus grave et compliqué de la pyonéphrose.

On se trouve bien loin des règles schématiques que l'expérimentation avait tenté d'établir.

Bibliographie

A. Physiologie normale des voies urinaires supérieures

II. Moyens d'étude. Expérimentation physiologique

ALVAREZ and H. ZIMMERMANN: The absence of inhibition ahead of peristaltic rushes. Amer. J. Physiol. 83, 52—59 (1927). — BINET, L., et P. SERINGE: L'uretère isolé provenant de chiens atteints de néphrite ou d'hydronéphrose expérimentales. Presse méd. 1936, Nr 103, 2086—2087. — BINET, L., et S. STOICESCO: Recherches sur la motricité de l'uretère isolé. Arch. urol. de la Clin. Necker 7, 1—15 (1931). — BOEMINGHAUS, H.: Experimentelle Untersuchungen über den nervösen Zusammenhang zwischen Nieren- und Blasentätigkeit. Verh. Dtsch. Ges. Urol., 8. Kongr., S. 538—540, Berlin (1928). — BOZLER, E.: Electric stimulation and conduction of excitation in smooth muscle. Amer. J. Physiol. 122, 614—623 (1938). — The response of smooth muscle to stretch. Amer. J. Physiol. 149, 299—301 (1947). — EVANS, N.: The physiology of plain muscle. Physiol. Rev. 6, 358—398 (1926). — GRUBER, C. M.: The peristaltic and antiperistaltic movements in excised ureters as affected by drugs. J. Urol. (Baltimore) 20, 27—60 (1928). — The autonomic innervation of the genito-urinary system. Physiol. Rev. 13, 497—609 (1933). — HAEBLER, H.: Zur Anatomie und Physiologie des Nierenbeckens. Z. Urol. 19, 332 (1925). — HENDERSON, V. E.: The mecanism of intestinal peristaltism. Amer. J. Physiol. (Lond.) 86 (I), 82—98 (1928). — HIRT: Über den Faserverlauf der Nierennerven. Z. Anat. Entwickl.-Gesch. 78, 260—276 (1926). — HORTOLOMEI, N., T. BURGELE and M. STRESA: Considérations sur la physiologie des voies urinaires supérieures. J. Urol. méd. chir. 43, 399—424 (1937). — HRYNTSCHACK, T.: Beiträge zur Physiologie des Ureters. Pflügers Arch. ges. Physiol. 209, 542 (1925). — KUNTZ, A.: The autonomic nervous system, 3. édit., p. 284—295. Philadelphia: Lea and Febiger 1947. — LAPICQUE, L.: La motricité nerveuse. Paris: Flammarion 1943. — LAPIDES, J.: The physiology of the human intact ureter. J. Urol. (Baltimore) 59, 501—537 (1948). — LEGUEU, F., B. FEY et P. TRUCHOT: La pyéloscopie. Paris: Maloine 1927. — LEGUEU, F., B. FEY et M. PALAZZOLI: La motricité du bassinet étudiée sur le rein fraîchement néphrectomisé. J. Urol. méd. chir. 24, 61—67 (1927). — MINGERS, P.: Contribution à l'étude physiologique de l'uretère. Thèse Bruxelles 1937. — Mise en évidence de l'action de l'uroselectan et de l'uropan sur les contractions de l'uretère au moyen du polygramme cathodique de l'uretère. VIème Congr. de l' Assoc. Internat. d'Urologie, Wien 1936, p. 277—280. Paris: Doin. — MORIN: La motricité gastro-intestinale chez les mammifères. Rapp. à la 12ème Sess. de l'Assoc. des Physiologistes, Louvain 1938. C. R. Ass. Physiol. et Physico-chim. biol. 14, 321—327 (1938). — NARATH, P. A.: Renal pelvis and ureter. New

536   BERNARD FEY et LOUIS QUÉNU:

York: Grune & Stratton 1951. — RUBRITIUS, H., et F. FUCHS: Physiologie und Pathologie der Nierenexkretion. VIème Congr. de l'Assoc. Internat. d'Urologie, Wien 1936. C. R. L., 499—561 (1936). — SCHLICHT, L.: Le transport des fluides dans l'uretère. Z. Urol. 47, 517 à 526 (1954). — TRATTNER, H. R.: Graphic registration of the function of the human physiology and pathologic physiology of the ureter. J. Urol. (Baltimore) 28 (I), 1—33 (1932). — ZANNE, D. A.: Experime elle Studien zur Dynamik der oberen Harnwege. Z. Urol. 31, 171—200 (1937). — Die Dynamik der oberen Harnwege. Z. Urol. 31, 464—472 (1937). — ZANNE, D. A., G. GEORGESCU et CRACIUN: Dynamisme des voies urinaires supérieures, étude expérimentale 5ème Congr. de la Soc. Roumaine d'Urologie, 1935.

Constatations radiologiques

BEAUFOND, H. DE, et P. PORCHER: L'exploration fonctionnelle du canal excréteur du rein. Arch. Mal. Reins 3, 27—56 (1927). — BORGARD, W.: Roentgennachweis flüchtiger Nierenbeckenentleerungsstörungen. Med. Klin. 42, 359—369 (1947). — FUCHS, F.: Die Hydromechanik der Niere. Z. urol. Chir. 33, 1 (1931). — Theorie der Harnwegfunktionen. Z. urol. Chir. 37, 154 (1933). — GREGOIR, W.: L'urokymographie et la radiomanométrie urinaire. Paris: Masson et Cie. 1953. — HORTOLOMEI, N., T. BURGHELE et M. STRESA: Considérations sur la physiologie des voies urinaires supérieures. J. Urol. méd. chir. 43, 399—429 (1937). — LEGUEU, F., B. FEY et P. TRUCHOT: La pyéloscopie. Paris: Maloine 1927. — RUBRITIUS, H., et F. FUCHS: Die Physiologie der ableitenden Harnwege. VI. Congr. de la Soc. Internat. d'Urologie, Wien 1936. C. R., p. 499—574. Paris: Doin 1936. — STUMPF, P.: Das röntgenographische Bewegungsbild und seine Anwendung. Leipzig: Georg Thieme 1931.

Manométrie

AUVERT, J.: Les reflux à partir du bassinet. Rapp. à la 51ème Session de l'Assoc. Franç. d'Urologie 1957. Secrétariat de l'Assoc. Paris 1957. — BORS, E., and K.A. BLINN: A new method of recording ureteral peristalsis «ureteral kymography». J. Urol. (Baltimore) 74, 322—330 (1955). — CHAILLET, B.: Electromanomètrie urinaire, contribution à l'étude de la dynamique urinaire. Thèse Paris 1957. — FINKLE, A.L., and D.R. SMITH: Concepts of ureteral physiology. J. Urol. (Baltimore) 74, 312—321 (1955). — LAPIDES, J.: The physiology of the intact human ureter. J. Urol. (Baltimore) 59, 501—533 (1948). — MERENYI, I.: Recent investigations on human ureter. Mag. Sebész. 5, 121—126 (1952). — PILCHER, F., J.C. BOLLMANN et F.C. MANN: Effet d'une hausse de la pression intra-uretérale sur la fonction rénale. J. Urol. (Baltimore) 38, 202 (1937). — PISANI, G.: Patologia della escrezione renale. VIème Congr. de la Soc. Internat. d'Urologie, p. 380—498. Paris: Doin. — RATTNER, H.: Hydrodynamics of the intact human ureter and renal pelvis. 42. Clinical Congr. Acs, San Francisco and Philadelphie 1956. — ROUFFILANGE, F.: Discussion du Rapp. au 51ème Congr. Français d'Urologie, p. 381—389. Paris: Doin 1957. — SWENSON, O., et J.H. FISCHER: A new concept of étiology in megalo ureters. New Engl. J. Med. 246, 41—46 (1952). — New techniques in the diagnosis and treatment of megalo-ureter. Pediatrics 18, 304—313 (1956). — SWENSON, O., et D. MARCHANT: Uretero pelvic obstruction in infants and childhood. J. Urol. (Baltimore) 73, 945 (1955).

L'Electro-urétérographie

BAKER, R.: — Ureteral electromyography in congenital megalo-ureter. Amer. J. Dis. Child. 87, 7—15 (1954). — BAKER, R., and J. HUFFER: Ureteral electromyography. J. Urol. (Baltimore) 70, 874—883 (1953). — Electromyography in the normal, dilated, transsectend and transplanted ureter. Amer. J. Physiol. 180, 261—276 (1955). — BUTCHER, H. R., et W. SLEATOR: A study of the electical activity of intact an partially mobilized human ureters. J. Urol. (Baltimore) 73, 970—986 (1955). — The effect of ureteral anastomosis upon conduction of peristaltic waves: an electroureterographic study. J. Urol. (Baltimore) 75, 650—658 (1956). — BUTCHER, H.R., W. SLEATOR and W. P. SCHMANDT: A study of the peristaltic conduction mechanism in the canine ureter. J. Urol. (Baltimore) 78, 221—231 (1957). — COREY, E. L., E. H. FITE and S. A. VEST: Electropotential changes in the normal human ureter. J. Urol. (Baltimore) 75, 244—249 (1956). — FASIANI, G. M., e A. LUISADA: L'elletrogramma del uretere umano. Minerva med. (Torino) 23, 1 (1932). — HANLEY, H. G.: VII. Congr. Internat. Soc. d'Urol. Barcelone 2, 56 (1950). — The electro-ureterogram. Brit. J. Urol. 25, 358 (1953). — LEBATARD-SARTRE, R.: L'électro-urétérographie. Mémoire de Médaille d'Or de l'internat des Hôpitaux de Nantes 1958. — MILTON, G. W., and W. A. T. ROBB: Electrical studies in hydroureterer: Report of two. cases. Brit. J. Urol. 26, 274 (1954). — MINGERS, P.: Le polygramme cathodique de l'uretère. C. R. Soc. Biol. (Paris) 1936, 123, 107. — ORBELI, L., et T. E. BRUCKE: Beiträge zur Physiologie der autonom innervierten Muskulatur. Pflügers Arch. ges. Physiol. 133, 341—364 (1910).

III. Étude synthétique de l'excrétion pyélo-uretérale

AUVERT, J.: Les reflux à partir du bassinet. Rapp. à la 51ème Session de l'Assoc. Française d'Urologie. Paris: Au secrétariat de l'Association 1957. — BEGG, R. C.: Physiological variations in pyelograms commonly interpreted as pathological. Brit. J. Urol. 18, 176 (1946). — CHAILLET, B.: Electromanométrie urinaire. Contribution à l'étude de la dynamique urinaire. Thèse Paris 1957. — FUCHS, F.: Die Hydromechanik der Niere. Z. urol. Chir. 33, 1 (1931). — Theorie der Harnwegfunktionen. Z. urol. Chir. 37, 154 (1933). — MAINTZ, M., J. MEESE u. G. WÜLLENWEBER: Röntgenkymographische Untersuchungen über normale und krankhafte Bewegungsvorgänge an den abführenden Harnwegen. Z. Urol. 32, 682 (1938). — MORALES, P. A., CH. H. CROWDER, A. P. FISHMAN and M. H. MAXWELL: The response of the ureter and pelvis to changing urine flows. J. Urol. (Baltimore) 67, 484 bis 491 (1952). — MURNAGHAN, G. F.: Experimental investigation of the dynamics of the normal an dilated ureter. Brit. J. Urol. 29, 403—409 (1957). — NARATH, P. A.: Renal pelvis and ureter. New York: Grune & Stratton 1951. — PFEIFER, W.: Grundlagen der funktionellen urologischen Röntgendiagnostik. Stuttgart: Georg Thieme 1949. — ZANNE, D.: Experimentelle Studien zur Dynamik der oberen Harnwege. Z. urol. Chir. 31, 171 (1937).

Abouchement uretéro-vésical

AUER, J., and L. D. SEAGER: Experimental local bladder edema causing urine reflux into ureters and kidneys. Proc. Soc. exp. Biol. (N.Y.) 35, 361 (1936). — J. exp. Med. 66, 741 (1957). — BLUM, V.: Physiologie und Pathologie des Harnleiters. Z. Urol. 19, 161 (1925). — BOEMINGHAUS, H.: Über funktionelle Zusammenhänge zwischen Harnblase und Niere (vesicorenaler Reflux). Langenbecks Arch. klin. Chir. 154, 114 (1929). — DARGET, R.: Les anomalies pyélo-uretérales congénitales et leurs conséquences chirurgicales. (Partie expérimentale p. 127 à 136.) Rapp. à la 36ème Session de l'Assoc. Française d'Urologie. Paris: Doin 1936. — FARREL, J. I.: A study of vesicorenal reflexes and of the possibility of renorenal reflex. J. Urol. (Baltimore) 25, 487—496 (1931). — GAYET, R.: L'uretère intra-mural. Étude anatomophysiologique. Troubles fonctionnels et leur traitement. Thèse Lyon 1937. — GRAVES, R. C., et L. M. DAVIDOFF: Studies on the ureter and bladder with special reference to regurgitation of the vesical contents. J. Urol. 10, 185—231 (1923); 12, 93—103 (1924). — Studies on the ureter and bladder with special reference to regurgitation of the vesical contents; regurgitation as observed in cats an dogs. J. Urol. (Baltimore) 14, 1—17 (1925). — HENNINGSEN, O.: Klinisch- experimentelle Untersuchungen über die Möglichkeiten eines Blasen-Harnleiterrückflusses. Z. Urol. 31, 505 (1937). — KREUTZMANN, H. A. R.: Studies on normal ureter and vesical pressure. J. Urol. (Baltimore) 19, 517—524 (1928). — LEPOUTRE, M.: Le reflux vésico-uretéral. Rapp. à la 26ème Session de l'Assoc. Française d'Urologie. Paris: Doin 1926. — OBERNIEDERMAYER, A.: Experimenteller Beitrag zur Frage des Harnblasen-Harnleiter refluxes. Z. Urol. 30, 295 (1936). — PAVONE, M.: Influenza dell'anestesia locale, generale, rachidiane e regionale sus reflosso vesico-ureterale. Arch. ital. Urol. 4 (6) (1928).

B. Physiologie pathologique des voies urinaires supérieures

I. Étude expérimentale des obstructions uretérales

ALKSNIS, A.: Ein Beitrag zur Wiederherstellung des durchschnittenen Harnleiters. Chirurg 20, 35 (1949). — ANDLER, J.: Über Ureteratonie. Z. urol. Chir. 17, 298—357. — AUVERT, J.: Les reflux à partir du bassinet. Rapp. à la 51ème Session de l'Assoc. Française d'Urologie. Paris: Secrétariat de l'Association 1957. — CAPORALE, L.: Au sujet de l'énervation de l'uretère. J. Urol. méd. chir. 28, 28—29 (1929). — The dynamic hydronephrosis and sympathectomy of the ureter. J. Urol. (Baltimore) 33, 83—89 (1935). — CHAILLET, B.: Electromanométrie urinaire — Contribution à l'étude de la dynamique urinaire. Thèse Paris 1947. — CUSHNY, A. R.: The secretion of the urine. London: Longmann Green & Cie. 1928. — DOSSOT, R.: Physiologie et traitement de l'hydronéphrose. Rapp. au 8ème Congr. de la Société Internat. d'Urologie, p. 79—152. Paris: Doin 1949. — DUVERGEY, H.: Dilatations pyélo-uretérales d'origine dynamique. Thèse Bordeaux 1937. — GOUYGOU, C.: Étude systématique de l'appareil musculaire lisse excrétourinaire supérieur. J. Urol. méd. chir. 55, 296 (1949). — GOUVERNEUR, R., et H. MARION: La suture de l'uretère. Étude expérimentale. J. Urol. méd. chir. 27, 155—161 (1929). — HEPLER, J.: Intra renal changes in hydronephrosis. J. Urol. (Baltimore) 38, 593—604 (1937). — HINMAN, F.: Hydronephrosis. I. The structural changes. J. Surg. 17, 816 (1945). — HINMAN, F., and J. HEPLER: Experimental hydronephrosis, the effect of changes in blood messure and blood flow on its sate of development. Arch. Surg. (Chicago) 11, 578—585, 649—659, 917—932 (1925); 12, 830—853 (1926). — ISELIN, M.: Recherches experimentales sur la réparation de l'uretère. J. Urol. méd. chir. 27, 529—536 (1929). — Recherches expérimentales sur la suture de l'uretère. Bull. Soc. Chir. (Paris) 54, 650—655 (1928). — KREUTZMANN, H. A. R.: Studies on normal ureter an vesical pressure. J. Urol. (Baltimore) 19, 517—524 (1928). — KÜSS, R.: A propos de 2 cas de suture de l'uretère. J. Urol. méd. chir. 57, 427—431 (1951). — LÖFFLER, L.: Muskelveränderungen am Nierenbecken und Ureter bei Stauung in den harnableitenden Wegen. Z. urol. Chir. 36, 384 (1933). — LÜTJENS, W.: Über die Automatie des Harnleiters und den Einfluß von Bakterientoxinen auf die Bewegungen des Harnleiters. Z. Urol. 27, 587 (1933). — MCDONALD, J. R, F. C. MANN and J. T. PRIESTLEY: The maximal intra pelvis pressure (secretion pressure) of the kidney of the dog. J. Urol. (Baltimore) 37, 326—332 (1937). — MURNAGHAN, G. F.: Experimental investigation of the dynamics of the normal and dilated ureter. Brit. J. Urol. 29, 403—409 (1957). — PILCHER, F., J. L. BOLLMANN and F. C. MANN: The effect of increased intra ureteral pressure on renal function. J. Urol. (Baltimore) 38, 202—211 (1937). — RAGNOTTI: Considerazioni e ricerche sul significato patologico et sulla produzione sperimentale delle idronefrosi dinamica. Arch. ital. Chir. 4 (1934). — WINSBURY WHITE, H. P.: The pathology of hydronephrosis. Brit. J. Surg. 13, 50, 247—281 (1926). — The influence of infection of the lower urinary tract and reproductive organs on the kidneys with special reference to lithiasis an hydronephrosis. J. Urol. (Baltimore) 36, 469 (1936). — WINTON, F. R.: Physical factors involved in the activities of the mammation kidney. Physiol. Rev. 17, 408 (1937). — ZANNE, D.: Dinamica cailor urinare superiorare studiu experimental. 5ème Congr. de la Société Roumaine d'Urol. 1935. — Experimentelle Studien zur Dynamik der oberen Harnwege. Z. urol. Chir. 31, 171 (1937). — ZANNE, D., et G. GEORGESCU: Étude experimentale et clinique de la physiologie normale et pathologique de l'uretère. Revista Romania de Urol. Avril 1935.

II. Résorption pyélo-rénale

AUVERT, J.: Les reflux à partir du bassinet. Rapp. à la 51ème Session de l'Assoc. Française d'Urologie. Paris: Secrétariat de l'Association 1957. — BIETER, R. N.: The reabsorptive function of the tubule in the frog's kidney. Amer. J. Physiol. 93, 574—577 (1930). — BIRD, C. E., et T. S. MOISE: Pyelovenous back flow. J. Amer. med. Ass. 86, 661—663 (1926). — BOEMINGHAUS, H.: Röntgenologische Untersuchungen über die Resorption schattengebender Lösungen in verschiedenen Hohlorganen, insbesondere in Nieren, Nierenbecken und Ureter bei akuten Stauungszuständen. Langenbecks Arch. klin. Chir. 155, 451—468 (1929). — FUCHS, F.: Pyelovenous back flow in the human kidney. J. Urol. (Baltimore) 23, 685—692 (1930). — Pyelovenöser Reflux und Hydronephrose. Dtsch. Z. Chir. 224, 353—382 (1930). — Zur Frage der pyelographisch sichtbaren Nierenbeckenextravasate. Mitteil. Urol. Chir. 30, 392 à 403 (1930). — GREHANT, C.: Recherches physiologiques sur l'excrétion de l'urée. Thèse Paris 1930. — HINMAN, F.: Pyélovenous back flow at time of pyelography. S. G. O. 44, 592 (1927). — HINMAN, F., and F. H. REDWILL: Pyelovenous back flow. J. Amer. med. Ass. 87, 1287—1293 (1926). — HINMAN, F., et M, VICKI: Pyelovenous backflow. J. Urol. (Baltimore) 15, 267—271 (1926). — LEE-BROWN, R. K. and J. W. S. LAIDLEY: Some observations on the microscopical anatomy of the kidney. J. Urol. (Baltimore) 21, 259—274 (1929). — MAGOUN, J. A. H.: The absorption of phenolsulfone phtalein from the human pelvie. J. Urol. (Baltimore) 22, 127—131 (1929). — PAVONE, M.: Il riassorbimento del liquido del bacinetto nelle idronefrosi sperimentali. Cultura méd. mod. 3 (1936). — RÉNYI-VÁMOS F., F. BALOGH u. Z. SZENDROŸ: Über einige Probleme des Pyelonverschlusses. Schweiz. med. Wschr. 82, 1084 (1952). — ROLNICK, H. C., and P. L. SINGER: Effects of overdistension of the renal pelvis and ureter: a study of pyelovenous backflow. J. Urol. (Baltimore) 57, 834 (1947). — SAUER, v. H.: Über Ureteratonie. Langenbecks Arch. klin. Chir. 166, 659 (1931). — VERRIERE, P.: Reflux pyélo-veineux — Absorption intra-rénale. Thèse Lyon 1932.

Données cliniques et radiologiques au point de vue physio-pathologique

AUVERT, J.: Les reflux à partir du bassinet. Rapp. à la 51ème Session de l'Assoc. Française d'Urologie. Paris: Secrétariat de l'Association 1957. — FEY, B., R. DOSSOT et P. TRUCHOT: La dilatation élective des calices. J. Urol. méd. chir. 52, 161—175 (1944). — FEY, B., et J. MICHON: Les réactions fonctionnelles et morphologiques de l'appareil urinaire au cours et au décours de la colique néphrétique. J. Urol. méd. chir. 53, 201—227 (1947). — HICKEL, R.: Figures urographiques particulières: les ombres péripapillaires (ou images dites en boule) et la néphrographie. J. Radiol. Électrol. 27, 509—515 (1946). — MURNAGHAN, G. F.: Experimental investigation of the dynamics of the normal and dilated ureter. Brit. J. Urol. 29, 403—409 (1957). — PUIGVERT, A.: Rotura calicilar y reflujo pielo-canalicular. Med. clin. (Barcelone) 1, 1—8 (1942). — SMITH, H. W.: The kidney. New York: Oxford University Press 1951).

Cette bibliographie est arrêtée à 1958, année où futzemis le manuscrit.

Physiology of urinary bladder and urethra, normal and pathological

By

ALBERT KUNTZ †

With 3 figures

A. Anatomical relationships and structure

Urinary bladder. The urinary bladder is a musculo-membranous hollow organ that acts as a reservoir for the urine. In the newborn it is ovoid and lies chiefly in the abdomen, adjacent to the ventral abdominal wall. Its base is located behind the symphysis pubis. With growth and development it assumes a lower position. In the adult, when empty, it lies wholly within the pelvis; when distended it extends above the symphysis pubis and becomes in part an abdominal organ. Its form and relationships, consequently, vary according to the volume of liquid it contains. When empty, it has the form of a flattened tetrahedron, with its vertex directed toward the upper border of the symphysis pubis. From the vertex the middle umbilical ligament extends upward to the umbilicus. This ligament is covered by a fold of peritoneum, the middle umbilical fold. The fundus is directed downward and backward. It is triangular in shape and separated from the rectum by the rectovesical fascia, the seminal vesicles and the terminal portions of the ductus deferentes. The triangular superior surface is bounded on either side by a lateral border which separates it from the inferior surface. Posteriorly the superior surface is separated from the fundus by a line joining the two ureters. From the lateral borders, which extend from the ureters to the vertex, the peritoneum is reflected to the walls of the pelvis. A depression of the peritoneum on either side of the bladder is called the paravesical fossa. When the bladder is moderately full it assumes an oval form, the long diameter of which measures about 12 cm. and is directed upward and forward. In this condition it exhibits a ventro-caudal, a dorso-rostral, and two lateral surfaces, a summit and a fundus. The fundus is more or less fixed; consequently, it is only slightly depressed, as the viscus fills, but the rostral surface gradually rises into the abdominal cavity carrying with it the peritoneal covering.

In the female, the relationships of the bladder to the symphysis pubis and the anterior body wall are essentially the same as in the male, but dorsally it lies in relation to the uterus and the rostral portion of the vagina. It is separated from the body of the uterus by the vesicouterine excavation, but it is connected with the cervix of the uterus and the upper part of the anterior vaginal wall by areolar tissue.

Structure. The bladder wall is made up of four layers: adventitia, muscularis, submucosa and mucosa.

The adventitia consists in part of loose areolar connective tissue that blends with the connective tissue of the peritoneum which covers the rostral and lateral surfaces of the bladder and forms a serous layer. The remaining portion of the bladder wall is not covered with peritoneum, but is attached to the pelvic fascia by the adventitial connective tissue.

The muscularis is a relatively thick layer. It consists of three strata of smooth muscle. In the outer and the inner layers the muscle fibers in general are arranged in longitudinal bundles. In the middle stratum the fiber bundles in general are arranged circularly. Dorsally fibers of the outer stratum blend with the deep layer of the retrovesical fascia. This stratum is thickest on the dorsal and ventral surfaces and very thin or absent on the lateral surfaces. The middle stratum is thickest and the circular fibers are densely interlaced. The internal urethral sphincter is made up of fibers derived from the outer and middle strata. The inner stratum is thin and its fiber fascicles show a reticular arrangement. It includes two bands of oblique fibers, the muscles of the ureters, that extend from behind the orifices of the ureters to the middle lobe of the prostate. They serve to maintain the oblique direction of the ureters in the bladder wall and to prevent the reflux of urine from the bladder.

The trigonal muscle is made up of fibers derived from the longitudinal layers of the ureters. After intermingling in the trigone, the fibers of these muscles extend caudad and insert in the posterior urethra.

The submucosa is a thin layer of highly vascular areolar connective tissue that intervenes between the muscularis and the mucosa. The mucosa consists of a layer of transitional epithelium and a subepithelial layer of connective tissue containing numerous lymphocytes. The mucosa of the bladder is continuous rostrally with that of the ureters and caudally with that of the urethra. A definite basement membrane beneath the epithelium is not apparent. When the bladder is empty the mucosa is thrown into folds or rugae except in the area of the trigone where it is closely attached to the muscularis. In this condition the epithelium appears to be several cell layers thick. When the bladder is distended folds of the mucosa are not apparent and the epithelium is thin and appears to be made up of only two or three layers of flattened cells.

The orifices of the ureters are located at the dorsolateral angles of the trigone. The internal urethral orifice is located at the apex of the trigone in the most dependent part of the bladder. In the contracted bladder the ureteral orifices are approximately 2.5 cm. apart and each is approximately the same distance from the internal urethral orifice. In the distended bladder these measurements may be increased to approximately 5 cm. Immediately behind the internal urethral orifice is a slight elevation of the mucosa, the uvula vesicae, caused by the middle lobe of the prostate.

Urethra. The male urethra is divisible into a prostatic, a membranous and a cavernous portion. The prostatic portion, approximately 3—4 cm. in length, is surrounded by the prostate gland. Extending into its lumen from the dorsal wall of this portion is a conical elevation, the seminal colliculus, on either side of which are the slit-like openings of the ejaculatory ducts. This portion of the urethra also receives the ducts of the prostate gland through numerous small openings. The membranous portion, approximately 1 cm. in length, is the shortest and also the narrowest portion. The cavernous portion extends through the penis and opens at the tip of the glans. It is surrounded by the corpus cavernosum urethrae, or corpus spongiosum. In its first part the lumen is enlarged to form the bulb of the urethra. In the glans there is a dorso-ventral enlargement of the lumen known as the fossa navicularis. The mucous membrane varies in structure in the different portions. In the prostatic portion the epithelium is transitional like that of the bladder. The membranous and cavernous portions are lined with stratified columnar or pseudostratified epithelium to the fossa navicularis. The remaining portion is lined with stratified squamous epithelium which at the external urethral orifice becomes continuous with the epidermis. More or less extensive areas of stratified squamous epithelium frequently occur throughout the entire length of the urethra. The urethral epithelium rests on a thin basement membrane beneath which is a loose connective tissue stroma that is rich in elastic fibers. In its deeper portion lies a plexus of capillaries and thin-walled veins. A definite submucosa is not apparent.

Many deep crypts or lacunae due to longitudinal foldings of the mucosa occur in the lumen of the urethra. The ducts of branched tubular glands, the glands of Littré, which lie chiefly in the stroma but penetrate into the corpus spongiosum, lead into these lacunae. They are most numerous in the cavernous portion. Mucous cells, either isolated or in groups, also occur scattered in the epithelium of the mucosa.

The female urethra is a narrow membranous canal that extends from the internal to the external urethral orifice. It usually does not exceed 4 or 5 cm. in length. The epithelium lining its proximal portion is usually transitional like that of the bladder. The remaining portion is lined chiefly with stratified squamous epithelium, but patches of statified columnar or pseudostratified epithelium also occur. The mucosa is commonly folded longitudinally. Opening into the lacunae between the folds are glands of Littré, which are fewer than in the male. The stroma which is abundant includes many elastic fibers and contains a rich plexus of thin-walled veins. External to the stroma is an indefinite muscularis that contains both longitudinal and circular muscle fibers, many of which extend into the stroma between the veins. The urethral sphincter is formed by an outer layer of striated muscle.

The distal two-thirds of the female urethra, as described by KRANTZ (1951), is imbedded in the ventral vaginal wall and is inseparable from it. The circular muscle of the distal one-third of the vagina encircles the urethra. The longitudinal smooth muscle of the urethra lies close to the lumen and is continuous with the longitudinal muscle of the bladder. It is encircled in a spiral fashion throughout the length of the urethra by smooth muscle that is continuous with the circular muscle of the bladder. The middle one-third of the urethra is encircled by striated muscle derived from the decussating ischiocavernous and bulbocavernous muscles to form a striated muscle sphincter. A localized smooth muscle sphincter does not exist; consequently, the urethra and the bladder constitute an anatomical and functional unit.

Blood and lymph vessels. The bladder is supplied chiefly through the superior, middle and inferior vesical arteries, derived from the anterior trunk of the hypogastric artery. Small branches of the obturator and inferior gluteal arteries also reach the bladder. In the female the uterine and vaginal arteries supply additional branches to the bladder. In most cases, according to KRANTZ (1951), a small artery courses along either side of the umbilical ligament that sends branches medially into the rostral surface of the bladder. The superior vesical artery usually divides into three branches of which the two rostral ones supply the dome of the bladder. The caudal one, the middle vesical artery, penetrates the bladder wall on the dorso-lateral surface in the region of the trigone. Branches of the inferior vesical artery frequently penetrate the base of the bladder. The veins conform to no specific pattern, but form part of a large plexuses that drains into the hypogastric vein. Blood vessels enter the bladder mainly along the lateral margins.

The urethral bulb is supplied by a short artery of large caliber, the artery of the urethral bulb, that arises from the internal pudendal artery, pierces the inferior fascia of the urogenital diaphragm, and gives off branches to the urethral bulb and the proximal portion of the corpus cavernosum urethrae. The more distal parts of the urethra and the corpus cavernosum urethrae are supplied through the urethral artery that arises a short distance in front of the artery of the urethral bulb.

The veins of the prostatic and membranous portions of the urethra drain into the prostatic venous plexus which communicates with the pudendal and vesical plexuses and with tributaries of the vertebral veins. Those of the cavernous portion of the urethra drain mainly into the deep dorsal vein of the penis.

The efferent lymph vessels of the bladder arise in an intra- and an extramuscular plexus. They are arranged in two groups, one from the ventral and the other from the dorsal surface of the bladder. Those from the ventral surface lead into the external iliac nodes. Those from the dorsal surface lead into the hypogastric, external and common iliac nodes. In the female anastomoses of the lymphatics of the bladder and the cervix uteri are common.

B. Development

The urinary bladder is a derivative of the cloaca which in the higher mammals is subdivided into a dorsal rectum and a ventral bladder, urethra and urogenital sinus. The cloacal subdivision also gives rise to the perineum, separating the urogenital vent from the rectal orifice. Before complete division is attained, the human cloaca recapitulates several developmental stages that remain permanent in lower mammals.

In human embryos that exhibit six somites the future cloaca is represented by a blind, caudal expansion of the hindgut which already lies in contact ventrally with the ectoderm. The cloacal membrane arises in this area of union. This membrane at first extends from the tail bud to the body stalk, but later its extent is relatively decreased by the ingrowth of mesoderm to form the infra-umbilical body wall. Rostrally the cloaca gives off the allantoic stalk. Laterally it receives the mesonephritic ducts and caudally it is prolonged into the transitory tail-gut. The interval between the hind-gut and the allantoic stalk gradually becomes invaded by mesoderm that forms the cloacal, or urorectal, septum. This mesodermal structure gradually extends caudad until the division of the cloaca into a dorsal rectum and a ventral bladder and urogenital sinus is completed during the seventh week (AREY 1954). Certain future regions can be recognized in the ventral portion even before the cloacal division is completed. The continuity of the bladder with the allantois is recognizable at the end of the sixth week. At its caudal end the bladder receives the common stems of the paired mesonephritic ducts and the ureters. The orifices of these ducts mark the approximate rostral border of the primitive urogenital sinus, in which the pelvic portion, nearest the bladder, and the more distal phallic portion, that extends into the genital tubercle, are clearly outlined.

When the bladder first appears as a separate entity, it still receives on either side the common stem of the mesonephritic duct and the ureter. As growth advances, these common stems soon become absorbed and the four ducts acquire separate openings (AREY 1954). The mesonephritic ducts are displaced caudad for a short distance and open close together in an elevation in the future urethra known as MÜLLER's tubercle. The two ureters enter the bladder well apart from each other. The triangular area on the dorsal walls of the bladder and the urethra, as outlined by the ureteral orifices and MÜLLER's tubercle, represents the trigone of the adult bladder. Temporarily, this area is lined with mesodermal epithelium, but this is gradually replaced, as growth advances, by entodermal epithelium.

The bladder gradually expands into a sac-like epithelial organ the apex of which tapers into an elongate tube, the urachus, which is continuous at the umbilicus with the remnant of the allantoic stalk. As the infraumbilical body wall develops progressively, the bladder and urachus elongate proportionately. The splanchnic mesoderm of the bladder wall begins to be differentiated into interlacing bands of smooth muscle and an outer covering of connective tissue during the third month. The layers characteristic of the adult bladder wall are clearly recognizable by the fourth month. During the latter part of fetal life the urachal lumen usually is obliterated, leaving an epithelioid cord surrounded by fibrous tissue that extends from the apex of the bladder to the umbilicus. It increases in length with the growth of the body and the descent of the fundus of the bladder, and is then known as the middle umbilical ligament. The paired lateral umbilical ligaments are formed from the postnatally closed portions of the umbilical, or allantoic, arteries.

In the female the urethra is derived from the originally short neck between the bladder and the urogenital sinus. The slit-like vestibule into which the urinary and the genital ducts open separately is formed by fusion of the pelvic and phallic portions of the sinus. The counterpart in the male of the entire female urethra is the portion extending from the bladder to MÜLLER's tubercle which becomes the permanent seminal colliculus. It comprises the major portion of the prostatic urethra. The pelvic portion of the urogenital sinus in the male gives rise to the remaining portion of the prostatic and all of the membranous urethra. The cavernous portion of the urethra, which extends through the penis, is derived from the phallic portion of the sinus.

1. Bladder anomalies

Vesical agenesis. Absence of the bladder occurs only rarely. It is of anatomical rather than clinical interest since the infant devoid of a bladder exhibits other urogenital anomalies and usually dies of pyelonephritis. In a child that lives, the dilated ureters opening into the urethra act as reservoirs for the urine and the musculofibrous tissue at the constricted orifices exerts a sphincteric action (HUBER 1936).

Hypoplasia. Underdevelopment of the bladder resulting in an organ of minute size is extremely rare and is usually associated with other urogenital anomalies that are incompatible with prolonged life. CAMPBELL (1937) reported a hypoplastic bladder measuring 2 by 0.8 cm. in a stillborn male with hypospadias and horseshoe kidney.

Reduplication. Reduplication of the bladder may be complete or incomplete, but complete doubling is most common. A classification of congenital bladder divisions in three categories has been proposed by SENGER and SANTARE (1951). The first category includes complete and incomplete reduplication of the bladder and incomplete sagittal septum. The second category includes complete and incomplete frontal or transverse division and hourglass bladder. The third category includes multilocular bladder.

In sagittal bladder reduplication, the ureter from each kidney drains into the segment on the same side. The urethra may or may not be reduplicated. In multilocular bladder there usually are as many ureters as loculi (WEHRBEIN 1940; SENGER and SANTARE 1951).

Bladder reduplication is usually accompanied by other urogenital anomalies. In some instances it resembles bladder diverticulum so closely that clinical differentiation of the one from the other is difficult.

Congenital bladder diverticulum. True congenital bladder diverticulum is extremely rare. It usually is associated with some form of intravesical obstruction. Bladder diverticulum in the adult is nearly always acquired due to some pathological condition such as some form of prostatism in the male and contracture of the neck of the bladder in the female.

Exstrophy of the bladder. Eversion of the dorsal bladder wall usually is associated with absence of the lower abdominal and ventral bladder walls. The incidence of bladder exstrophy is relatively low. It is always accompanied by genital anomalies such as wide open epispadiac urethra. The exstrophy usually is complete, but in rare cases in which the defect in the abdominal wall is relatively slight it may be incomplete.

Urachal cysts. Partial persistence of the lumen of the allantoic stalk may result in a small epithelial lined cavity that tends to become filled with liquid and becomes a nonmalignant cyst surrounded by a thick-walled connective tissue capsule. A cyst of this type may develop without internal connection with the bladder or external opening at the umbilicus, or it may occur as a dilated cavity in the course of a narrow lumen throughout the entire length of the urachus. A persistent allantoic lumen of this kind permits leakage of urine from the umbilicus and is known as an umbilico-urinary fistula, or patent urachus.

Trigonal folds. Redundancy of the trigonal mucosa may result in a valve-like leaflet that, with urination, flaps over and obstructs the vesical outlet. The incidence of this condition is relatively low.

2. Urethral anomalies

Complete absence or atresia of the urethra is an unusual condition that usually kills the fetus in utero. Distension of the bladder caused by the secreted urine causes pressure upon the umbilical arteries with marked embarassment of the fetal circulation. Secondary rupture of the bladder into the rectum or a persistent patent urachus has made possible the birth of a viable child in a few instances.

Congenital urethral stricture causing stenosis of the external meatus of the pin-point variety occurs frequently and usually remains unnoticed until urinary or urethral infection or dysuria develops or an attempt is made at instrumentation. The incidence of this condition is only slightly lower in female than in male infants.

Accessory urethral canals occur in wide variety. The term, double urethra, implies complete reduplication, but unfortunately it is frequently applied to channels that represent only incomplete reduplication. Accessory urethral channels may be located either dorsal or ventral to the urethra, but the dorsal location is less frequent than the ventral. Histologically the accessory urethra resembles the normal one.

Epispadias is the absence of the upper wall of the urethra. Complete epispadias occurs in both sexes. In this condition the urethra is entirely open from the neck of the bladder outward. Sphincters are poorly developed and control of urine is faulty or absent. In incomplete penile epispadias the urethral opening may be anywhere from the suspensary ligament to the postglandular sulcus, but it is most often at the base of the penis. In the female the degrees of epispadias may be designated as complete, subsymphyseal and clitoric.

Hypospadias is a congenital defect in which the urethral canal opens ventral and proximal to the normal site of the meatus. The opening may occur at any point from the normal site to the perineum. The post proximal portion of the urethra is never involved; consequently, the sphincters develop and function normally. Hypospadias is one of the most common of urogenital anomalies and occurs in both sexes.

In the male, balanitic hypospadias is the most common type. The urethral orifice occurs near the normal site. It seldom produces symptoms other than those due to a tight meatus. In penile hypospadias the urethra opens ventrally at some point between the glandular sulcus and the penoscrotal junction. In penoscrotal hypospadias the urethral orifice is situated at the penoscrotal junction and is commonly stenosed. It is usually associated with extreme penile deformity. Perineal hypospadias is characterized by a wide open funnel-shaped urethral orifice in the perineal area and thoroughly anomalous development of the genitalia, with rudimentary penis often covered by a preputial hood, or engulfed in an overlying bifid scrotum.

In the female, the hypospadiac urethra opens obliquely on the ventral vaginal wall proximal to the normal site of the meatus. The orifice is frequently stenosed. Urinary leakage may occur in all except the mildest degrees of hypospadias in the female.

Congenital diverticulum of the urethra may be single or multiple. The diverticulum is most instances probably is secondary to peripheral obstruction, notably stenosis of the external urethral meatus, but in some instances it may represent a modified form of an accessory urethral canal (CAMPBELL 1933; KRETSCHMER 1936). It occurs predominantly in the male. The site of congenital diverticulum formation, according to incidence, is 1. the pendulous urethra, 2. the penoscrotal junction, 3. the region of the frenum and 4. the bulbous urethra (CAMPBELL 1954).

Congenital urethral cyst occurs only rarely, but may be located at any point from the external meatus to the neck of the bladder. It usually obstructs ducts of structures such as COWPER's gland, the utricle or anterior urethral glands. The usual clinical manifestation is urethral obstruction.

3. Innervation

Extrinsic nerves. The urinary bladder and the urethra are innervated chiefly through the pelvic and the hypogastric plexuses. The pelvic plexuses are located along the lateral aspects of the pelvic viscera. They are continuous with the hypogastric plexus rostrally. The pelvic plexus on either side comprises an extensive meshwork of nerve fiber bundles that spread out between the viscera and the body wall. It receives parasympathetic preganglionic and visceral afferent fibers through the visceral rami of the 2nd, 3rd and 4th sacral nerves which unite to form the pelvic nerve. The preganglionic fibers in these rami constitute the sacral parasympathetic outflow. The sympathetic preganglionic fibers that reach the pelvic plexuses traverse the hypogastric plexus. They are splanchnic nerve components some of which have their origin as far rostrad as the 10th thoracic segment (Fig. 1).

The hypogastric plexus also conveys postganglionic sympathetic fibers into the pelvic plexus. Of these, some arise in lumbar sympathetic trunk ganglia, some in the inferior mesenteric ganglia and ganglia associated with the intermesenteric nerves. Some also arise in ganglia in the hypogastric plexus. Slender rami that arise from the sacral segments of the sympathetic trunks also join the pelvic plexuses. They probably are made up predominantly of postganglionic fibers.

Each pelvic plexus includes numerous ganglia made up of both parasympathetic and sympathetic ganglion cells. In an experimental anatomical study of the pelvic plexuses in the cat, KUNTZ and MOSELEY (1936) demonstrated that some of the ganglia receive preganglionic fibers exclusively through the sacral parasympathetic outflow, some exclusively though the thoracolumbar sympathetic outflow and some through both the sacral and the thoraco-lumbar outflows. The pelvic ganglion cells that are synaptically connected with parasympathetic preganglionic fibers are more numerous than those that are synaptically connected with sympathetic preganglionic fibers.

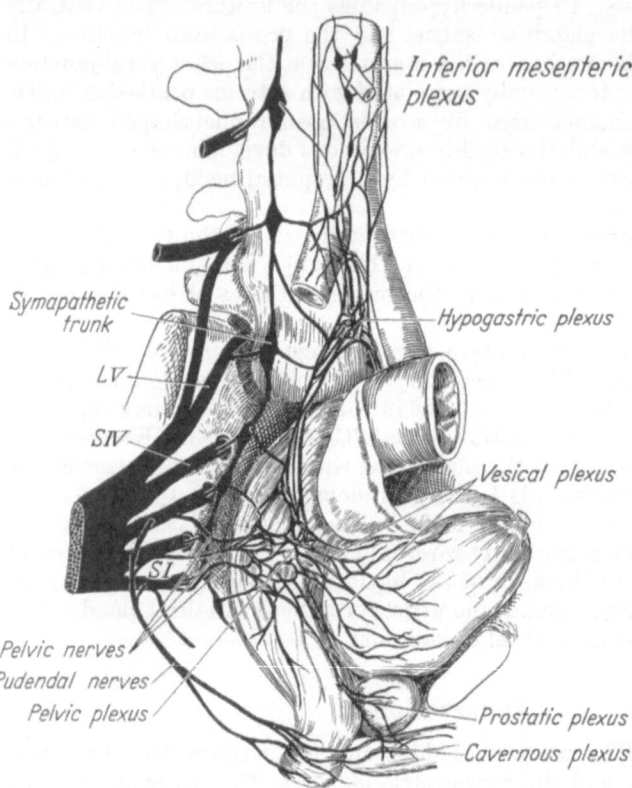

The regional subdivisions of each pelvic plexus are named according to the organs to which they are anatomically and functionally related. The paired subdivisions through which the urinary bladder is innervated, consequently, are called the vesical plexuses. The one on either side extends from the region of the trigone along the lateral aspect of the bladder. It receives preganglionic and visceral afferent fibers through both the pelvic and the hypogastric nerves. The parasympathetic preganglionic fibers that are concerned with the innervation of the bladder are derived chiefly through the 2nd and 3rd sacral nerves

Fig. 1. Autonomic nerves and ganglia in the pelvis

(KUHN 1949). The external vesical sphincter is innervated through the pudendal nerves. These nerves also convey afferent fibers to the internal vesical sphinter and adjacent parts of the bladder.

The sympathetic preganglionic fibers concerned with the innervation of the bladder terminate predominantly in ganglia in the vesical plexus. Some probably terminate in lumbar sympathetic trunk ganglia and ganglia in the hypogastric plexus. Like other ganglia in the pelvic plexus, those in the vesical plexus are neither exclusively parasympathetic nor exclusively sympathetic, but preganglionic fibers of both the sacral parasympathetic and the thoraco-lumbar sympathetic outflows make synaptic connections in them.

The male urethra is innervated through the prostatic and cavernous subdivisions of the pelvic plexus. Like the vesical plexus, they include both parasympathetic and sympathetic components. The prostatic plexus is continuous with the vesical plexus. It lies in intimate contact with the prostate gland and supplies fibers to the neck of the bladder, the prostate gland and the prostatic urethra. The cavernous plexus is continuous with the prostatic plexus and extends along the urethra. Nerves derived from it are distributed to the corpora cavernosa penis, and, in association with branches of the pudendal nerves, to the corpus cavernosum urethrae and the penile portion of the urethra (Fig. 2).

The female urethra is innervated through the vaginal plexus. It is composed chiefly of parasympathetic fibers derived from the pelvic plexus, but it includes some sympathetic fibers derived through the pelvic plexus and some that enter it directly from sacral segments of the sympathetic trunk. The external vesical sphincter and the compressor urethrae muscles are innervated through the pudendal nerves (Fig. 3).

Both the parasympathetic and the sympathetic nerves of the bladder and the urethra are accompanied by afferent nerve fibers. Those that accompany the parasympathetic nerves are sacral nerve components. Those that accompany the sympathetic nerves are components of the splanchnic nerves. The vesical sphincters and adjacent areas are also supplied with afferent fibers through the pudendal nerves. The afferent fibers make reflex connections in the spinal cord, but they also make synaptic connections with neurons in the spinal cord through which impulses are conducted cephalad.

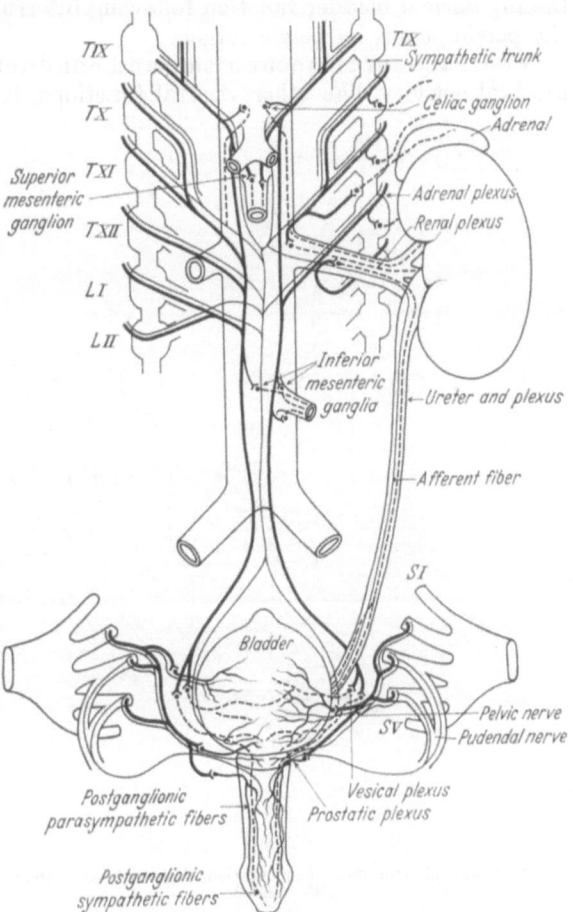

Fig. 2. Autonomic and visceral afferent innervation of the urinary system in the male

In addition to the nerves of the bladder outlined above, some nerves reach this organ through a perivascular route along the blood vessels in the endopelvic fascia within the lateral walls of the pelvis. As described by McCREA and KIMMEL (1952), most of the fibers of this system are derived from the 2nd, 3rd and 4th sacral nerve roots, but some arise directly from the sympathetic trunk. Small ganglia have also been demonstrated along these nerves. Their course to the bladder is independent of that of fibers derived through the pelvic and the hypogastric plexuses, except that near the bladder wall there is some intermingling of fibers of the two systems. The nerves that reach the bladder along the blood vessels enter it at the level of the orifices of the ureters. Within the bladder wall their distribution completely overlaps that of the nerves derived through the pelvic and hypogastric plexuses.

In view of the sources of the fibers that circumvent the usual pathways through the pelvic plexus to the bladder and the presence of ganglia in their courses, it may be assumed that these nerves include both parasympathetic and sympathetic and afferent fibers. On the basis of clinical data, McCREA and KIMMEL (1954) have advanced the opinion that these nerves are capable of maintaining normal bladder function following interruption of the pathways through the pelvic plexus by pelvic surgery.

Central neural mechanisms and conduction pathways. Bladder and urethral activity, like other visceral functions, is influenced through reflex and correlation centers in the brain stem and by impulses that emanate from the cerebral cortex. Ascending conduction pathways, consequently, must convey impulses from these organs to centers in the brain stem and the cerebral cortex and descending pathways must conduct impulses from the cortex and from centers in the brain stem to the preganglionic neurons through which the bladder and the urethra are innervated. Both the ascending and the descending conduction required for bladder and urethral regulation appears to be mediated in part through pathways made up of short neurons with frequent synaptic relays and in part through pathways made up of long neurons.

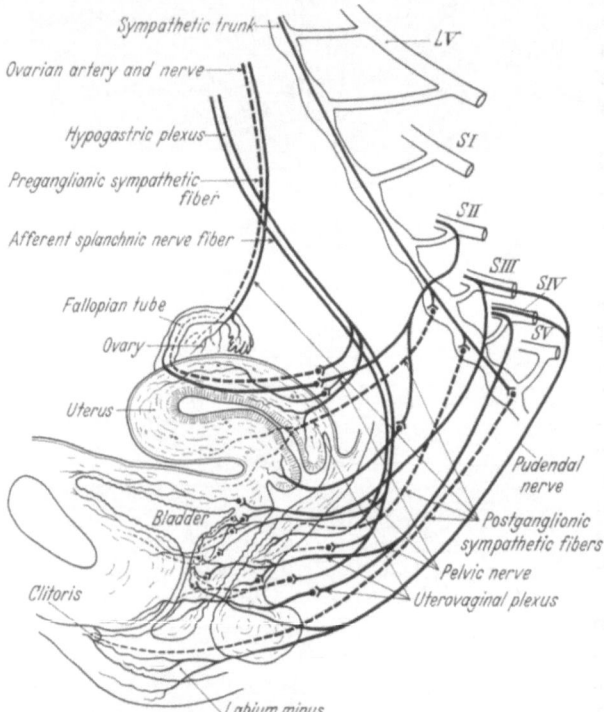

Fig. 3. Autonomic and visceral innervation of the urinary system in the female

On the basis of clinical data and histological examination of sections of spinal cords following cordotomies for the relief of pain of bladder origin, NATHAN and SMITH (1951) advanced the conclusions (a) that the afferent pathway subserving the sensation that bladder is full, and giving rise to the desire to micturate; and the one subserving the sensation of pain from the bladder, urethra and lower ends of the ureters, and sensations of temperature from the urethra are located in the lateral spinothalamic tract, and that (b) the pathways that subserve sensations of touch or pressure or tension from the urethra are located within the dorsal columns.

Data relative to the descending central conduction pathways concerned in the regulation of bladder and urethral activity indicate that in the caudal region of the diencephalon the fibers that conduct impulses from the hypothalamic centers lie widely scattered. Most of them traverse the tegmental portions of the mesencephalon and the pons. Experimental lesions in some hypothalamic areas result in descending degeneration into the spinal cord. Some of the fibers in question appear to terminate in the reticular formation in the brain stem. Others extend into the intermediolateral cell column in the spinal cord where they probably make synaptic connections either directly or through intercalated neurons with preganglionic neurons. According to ALLEN (1932), the reticulospinal tracts are in part visceral. Since many of the short fibers that descend from the hypothalamus terminate in the reticular formation in relation to neurons that descend in the reticulospinal tracts, the latter play a role in the conduction of impulses to visceral organs from the hypothalamus as well as from the reticular formation of the mesencephalon and the pons.

Data relative to the pathways through which autonomic impulses are conducted caudad in the brain stem and the spinal cord, as summarized by MAGOUN (1940), support the conclusion that they include some long fibers and an extensive system of short ones arranged in relays. In the medulla oblongata these pathways lie chiefly in the lateral portion of the reticular formation. In the spinal cord they lie chiefly in the ventral portion of the lateral funiculus. Most of the fibers in question are limited to one side, but some cross the median plane in the brain stem or at more caudal levels in the spinal cord. Pathways through which impulses emanating from the hypothalamus are conducted to the urinary bladder, according to WANG and CLARK (1940), include decussations in the brain stem and in the lower lumbar segments of the spinal cord, but none in the intervening portions of their courses.

Centers. A neural mechanism at the level of the pontine midbrain junction that is concerned with the regulation of bladder activity has long been known. According to BARRINGTON (1925), this area includes a reflex center for micturition. This conclusion has been confirmed by LANGWORTHY and KOLB (1933, 1935) and TANG and RUCH (1955). Bladder activity is also influenced by impulses emanating from the rostral portion of the midbrain and the caudal and rostral portions of the hypothalamus (KABAT, MAGOUN and RANSON 1936); the septum pellucidum and the preoptic area (KABAT, MAGOUN and RANSON 1936; HESS and BRUEGGER 1943), the putamen and the globus pallidum (STROM and UVNAS 1950) and the walls of the cruciate sulcus (LANGWORTHY and KOLB 1935).

Conduction from the midbrain and more rostral centers into the reticular formation probably is mediated through short neurons. As has been suggested by KABAT et al. (1936), there may be many synaptic relays between the preoptic area and the level of the inferior colliculus, but data advanced by GROSSMAN and WANG (1955) seem to indicate that few if any neurones in the preoptic area that are concerned in bladder function synapse before reaching the micturition center at the junction of the midbrain and the pons. Impulses emanating from the hypothalamus reach the bladder through both sympathetic and parasympathetic nerves. According to ROTHFELD and RABINER (1954), impulses emanating from the cerebral cortex reach the sacral spinal micturition center through fibers that arise in the cortex and traverse the corticospinal tracts. The lower motor neurons in question have bilateral cortical representation, as is indicated by the persistence of sphincter control in patients with pathology in only one hemisphere. Data advanced by ROTHFELD and RABINER also indicate that the fibers through which cerebral control of micturition is mediated are older phylogenetically than the younger pyramidal tract fibers and become involved late, if at all, in the course of disease.

Intramural vesical nerves. The nerves in the bladder wall form a plexiform structure that includes numerous ganglia. This structure is abundantly connected with the vesical plexus through nerves that penetrate the bladder wall. Intramural ganglia are most abundant in the trigone and gradually decrease in abundance as the distance from the trigone increases. An extensive area of the dome of the bladder is devoid of ganglia. The larger intramural ganglia and some of the smaller ones lie just beneath the fibrosa. Other small ganglia are located between muscle bundles, but relatively few are deeply imbedded in the muscle. Like the ganglia in the vesical plexus, the intramural ganglia receive preganglionic fibers through both the sacral parasympathetic and the thoracolumbar sympathetic outflows. On the basis of data obtained in an experimental study carried out on cats, MOSELEY (1936) concluded that approximately 40 per cent of the intramural ganglia receive only parasympathetic, approximately 40 per cent receive only sympathetic and approximately 20 per cent receive both parasympathetic and sympathetic preganglionic fibers. This does not mean that parasympathetic and sympathetic ganglion cells occur in approximately equal numbers. In general, the parasympathetic ganglia in the bladder wall are larger than the sympathetic ones. Most of the ganglia that receive both parasympathetic and sympathetic preganglionic fibers also are relatively small. The parasympathetic ganglion cells, consequently, greatly exceed the sympathetic in numbers. A similar relationship of parasympathetic and sympathetic ganglion cells probably obtains throughout the pelvic plexuses.

A preponderance of parasympathetic ganglion cells in the pelvic plexuses is also indicated by data relative to the histogenesis of the pelvic ganglia. As observed by KUNTZ (1952), the primordia of the pelvic plexuses arise somewhat later than those of the sympathetic trunks, due to the relatively late differentiation of the pelvic region of the embryo. The visceral rami of the sacral nerves play a role in the early development of the pelvic plexuses comparable to that of the thoracic and rostral lumbar nerves in the development of the sympathetic trunks and the abdominal prevertebral plexuses. The cells of neural origin that appear earliest in the primordia of the pelvic plexus are displaced from the central nervous system along the sacral nerves and their visceral rami. Cells displaced from the primordia of the abdominal prevertebral plexuses and from the sympathetic trunks along the lumbar splanchnic nerves enter the primordia of the pelvic plexuses somewhat later along the nerve fiber bundles in the hypogastric plexus, but those derived from the sacral segments of the central nervous system via the sacral nerves greatly exceed in number those derived from the thoracolumbar segments via the hypogastric nerves. In general, the cells that become differentiated into autonomic ganglion cells become synaptically connected with preganglionic fibers in the nerves along the paths of their displacement from the central nervous system. Since most of these cells are displaced into the pelvic plexus along the visceral rami of the sacral nerves the embryological data are consistent with the demonstration of both parasympathetic and sympathetic ganglion cells in the pelvic ganglia and with the assumption that the pelvic organs are innervated more abundantly through parasympathetic than through sympathetic nerves.

The nerve fibers within the bladder wall are predominantly unmyelinated and of small caliber. Most of the myelinated ones penetrate deeply into the bladder wall and undoubtedly are afferent. Nerve fiber terminations, presumably afferent, in the mucosa have been described by various investigators. Receptive end organs appear to be widely distributed in the mucosa and the submucosa. According to LANGWORTHY and MURPHY (1939), most of those in the trigone and adjacent areas are connected with afferent fibers that traverse the hypogastric nerves and most of those farther removed from the base of the bladder are connected with afferent components of the pelvic nerves. Complex terminal arborizations of relatively large afferent fibers in the bladder musculature have been demonstrated by KLEYNTJENS and LANGWORTHY (1937) which they have interpreted as stretch receptors since, in their experiments, the bladder did not respond in a normal manner following section of the dorsal sacral nerve roots.

The data obtained by LANGWORTHY and MURPHY (1939) relative to the distribution of sympathetic and parasympathetic nerve fibers in the bladder musculature led them to conclude that the efferent innervation of the detrusor muscle is exclusively parasympathetic and that the sympathetic fibers in the bladder wall are distributed to the blood vessels, BELL's muscle and the crista of the urethra. VAN DUZEN and DUNCAN (1953) concur in the opinion that the efferent innervation of the detrusor muscle is solely parasympathetic, and that the muscle of the trigone is innervated through sympathetic nerves. In sections of the urinary bladder and adjacent tissues in newborn kittens prepared by the silver technic that, according to NONIDEZ (1939), differentially impregnate sympathetic and parasympathetic nerve fibers in young animals, KUNTZ and SACCOMANO (1944) obtained data that support the assumption that the detrusor muscle is innervated through both parasympathetic and sympathetic fibers. In these sections, the heavily impregnated fibers, presumably parasympathetic, appeared to be distributed exclusively to the muscle tissue, whereas the less heavily impregnated ones, presumably sympathetic, appeared to be distributed both to the bladder musculature and to the blood vessels throughout the bladder wall. The point of view that the detrusor muscle is innervated through both parasympathetic and sympathetic nerves is also supported by experimental data (KUNTZ and SACCOMANO 1944; INGERSOLL et al. 1954).

The intramural nerves of the bladder are related primarily to the blood vessels, the musculature and the mucosa. Many of the larger fiber bundles are closely associated with blood vessels. They give rise to branches that ramify throughout the bladder wall and frequently inosculate to form coarse meshworks from which fibers in small bundles or individually course among the tissue elements. The neuroeffector relationships in the bladder are similar to those in other muscular hollow organs, such as the gastro-intestinal tract, the respiratory tract and the bile ducts, but intramural ganglion cells are relatively few.

SCHABADASCH (1934) described three intramural neural plexuses in the bladder of mammalian species, including man: an intramuscular, a subepithelial and an intraepithelial plexus. The intramuscular and the subepithelial plexus are predominantly autonomic, but they also include afferent fibers. The intraepithelial plexus is predominantly afferent.

The intramuscular plexus, as described by SCHABADASCH in methylene blue preparations stained intravitally, includes a relatively coarse fundamental meshwork of frequently inosculating nerve fiber bundles and a terminal syncytial network that lies in intimate relation to the bundles of muscle fibers and individual muscle cells. The fibers in the syncytial neural structure are derived directly from the larger bundles and nodes of the fundamental meshwork. The branching of the nerve fiber bundles and their topographic relationships are related to the pattern of the muscle bundles. Most of the cells in the syncytial structure appear to be neurilemma cells, but some are regarded as interstitial cells of CAJAL. Periterminal autonomic neuroeffector formations that are devoid of neurilemma cells and lie in intimate contact with the effector cells are also described.

The subepithelial plexus is intimately connected with the intramuscular plexus. It is located in the tunica propria of the mucosa and is made up predominantly of unmyelinated fibers imbedded in a syncytium of neurilemma cells.

The intraepithelial plexus is located in the transitional epithelium. It is less abundant than the subepithelial plexus and is made up predominantly of fine, varicose unmyelinated fibers that anastomose freely. A large part of this plexus extends beyond the limits of the syncytial plasmodium and is devoid of neurilemma cells. Terminal arborizations of myelinated afferent fibers occur particularly in the region of the trigone.

Since the publication of SCHABADASCH account of the intramural nerves of the urinary bladder, autonomic neuroeffector formations have been studied extensively in various organs, including the urinary bladder. On the basis of observations on intravital methylene blue preparations of the rat's bladder, studied in whole mounts, MEYLING (1953) concluded that every smooth muscle cell in the muscularis is surrounded by processes of interstitial cells of CAJAL. According to his point of view, the cells that make up the syncytial plasmodium in contact with the muscle fibers are interstitial cells which he regards as primitive neurons. This point of view has been controverted, but the fibrous processes in question undoubtedly represent the final links in the autonomic neural pathways and serve to transmit the nerve impulses to the muscle cells. The nerve fibers in contact with the smooth muscle are essentially varicose. The varicosities, according to LEEUWE (1937), are not artifacts, but are the structures through which the transmission of nerve impulses to the smooth muscle cells is mediated. On the basis of studies of both methylene blue and silver preparations, he concluded that the neurofibrillar structure in the varicosities extends into the protoplasm of the muscle cells and that the functional connections of the nerve fibers with the muscle cells occur at these points. According to his findings, the varicosities remain in the same positions on the smooth muscle cells both during contraction and relaxation; consequently, the part of the nerve fiber between two connections with muscle cells appears wavy during contraction and straight during relaxation. The findings of LEEUWE have been corroborated by MEYLING (1953) in intravitally stained methylene blue preparations of the urinary bladder of the rat. According to his account, based on favorable preparations, a connection between the nerve fiber and the smooth muscle exists at every varicosity. A single smooth muscle cell may be innervated in this manner at more than one point.

Our observations on preparations of the rat's bladder stained intravitally with methylene blue in general corroborate those of MEYLING with respect to the existence of a syncytial plasmodium in relation to the bladder musculature in which the anastomosing varicose nerve fibers are imbedded that make anatomical and functional contacts with the smooth muscle cells. We do not, however, concur in MEYLING'S concept of the peripheral syncytial structure as a third link in the autonomic efferent pathway. Various other investigators also differ with MEYLING in their concepts of the anatomical nature of the autonomic conduction pathways.

According to one point of view, the postganglionic nerve fibers retain their individuality as they approach the effector tissues and end in separate terminal structures. Such endings in the bladder musculature have been described by KLEYNTJENS and LANGWORTHY (1937). In the light of the findings of SCHABADASCH (1934) and MEYLING (1953) it seems probable that the preparations studied by KLEYNTJENS and LANGWORTHY did not reveal the complete picture of the neuroeffector formations.

According to another point of view that has been supported by the results of numerous investigations, the postganglionic nerve fibers lose their individuality at the periphery and become incorporated in the common terminal neural network that consists of anastomosing protoplasmic strands which include neurilemma nuclei and a network of neurofibrils, but reveals no discrete nerve endings. The absence of discrete nerve endings in autonomic neuroeffector formations has been emphasized by STÖHR (1935, 1950) and others. Neurofibrillar enlargements in the course of the terminal neural network that extend into the protoplasm of the effector cells similar to the varicosities described by LEEUWE (1937) and MEYLING (1953) have also been described by BOEKE (1942, 1949).

According to a third point of view, the postganglionic fibers do not lose their individuality in the neurilemmal plasmodium, but make functional connections with the terminal syncytial formation that is composed of interstitial cells of CAJAL. This point of view has been supported particularly by JABONERO (1952), JABONERO et al. (1953) and MEYLING (1953). Participation of interstitial cells in autonomic neuroeffector formations have also been described by NELEMANS (1948), SPOERRI (1949) and others. According to BOEKE (1949), neuroeffector formations are made up in part of anastomosing neurilemma cells and in part of interstitial cells of CAJAL. According to his concept, the protoplasm of the interstitial cells is continuous with that of the neurilemma cells, but the functional contact with the effector tissue is made by the interstitial cells. JABONERO and MEYLING do not admit that neurilemma cells take part in the formation of the distal neural syncytium, but maintain that it is made up solely of interstitial cells and is interposed between the postganglionic nerve fibers and the effector tissue. According to MEYLING, the interstitial cells are synaptically related to postganglionic fibers.

Our observations on preparations of the rat's urinary bladder stained intra-vitally with methylene blue and similar preparations of other smooth muscle and blood vessels (KUNTZ and NAPOLITANO 1956) support the assumption that auto-nomic neuroeffector formations include closed plexiform networks. The nuclei in the plasmodial structure in which the conducting elements are imbedded resemble neurilemma nuclei. Those located within strands of axons anastomos-ing neurofibrils usually are oval in outline. Those located at nodal points in the plexiform structure usually are spheroidal or triangular. If any of the cells in-corporated in the plasmodial structure of the atutonomic neuroeffector formations are interstitial cells of CAJAL, they cannot be differentiated from neurilemma cells on the basis of nuclear morphology alone or by the neurofibrillar structure im-bedded in the plasmodium.

If the autonomic neuroeffector formation consists of a syncytial network of interstitial cells with which postganglionic nerve fibers make synaptic connections, this network ought to remain intact following degeneration of the postganglionic nerve fibers. Data bearing on this point are not unequivocal. Our observations on preparations of blood vessels of the rat's hind limb following degeneration due to interruption of all the nerves that enter the limb indicate complete degeneration of the plexiform neural network in the vessel walls.

C. Physiology

1. Regulation of normal bladder function

Spontaneous activity of the bladder musculature. Spontaneous contractions of the urinary bladder in the intact animal have been reported frequently. STEWART (1900) described both simple and compound rhythmic contractions. According to his account, the simple rhythms are sometimes irregular and the compound rhythms may consist of two or more regular or irregular ones, due to contractions at different rates in two or more different areas of the viscus.

Although the smooth muscle of the bladder in common with all smooth muscle, has the inherent capacity to contract, spontaneous contractions of the bladder appear to be neurogenic. According to INGERSOLL and HEGRE (1951), all regions of the bladder exhibit spontaneous activity. In experiments on anesthetized cats, they observed that when the bladder is but slightly distended the detrusor muscle exhibits unsynchronized writhing movements. According to DENNY-BROWN and ROBERTSON, this unorganized activity is due to a continual bombardment of the muscle by nerve impulses. Certain other investigators have supported the assumption that detrusor activity of this kind is myogenic (GRUBER 1933). Such waves of contraction in the slightly distended bladder appear to be inadequate to initiate the micturition reflex (LANGWORTHY et al. 1940).

In bladders that are moderately to well distended, as observed by INGERSOLL and HEGRE, a given wave of contraction usually is initiated at the base of the bladder and advances along its long axis toward the apex. This finding seems to support the assumption that there exists a pace maker or a nodal point at the base of the viscus. The assumption that in micturition a peristaltic wave of contraction passes from the base of the bladder to the apex is supported by both clinical and experimental data. According to MUELLNER (1950), the first step in micturition is a downward pull in the region of the internal sphincter followed by a wave of contraction that starts from the internal sphincter and spreads over the base to the sides and dome of the bladder.

Specific responses to sympathetic and parasympathetic stimulation. According to current concepts the musculature of the bladder is innervated through sympathetic and parasympathetic nerves, but there is no general agreement relative to the distribution of sympathetic and parasympathetic nerve fibers in the bladder wall. The reported data relative to the effects on the bladder of sympathetic and parasympathetic nerve stimulation are not unequivocal. Stimulation of the parasympathetic nerves of the bladder commonly results in functional activity. The effects of stimulation of the sympathetic nerves of the bladder are less certain. Some of the data reported, furthermore, have led to conflicting conclusions. Some investigators have supported the assumption that sympathetic stimulation generally results in inhibition of bladder function and contraction of the internal vesical sphincter. Others have supported the assumption that the internal vesical sphincter does not respond to sympathetic stimulation. In the Rhesus monkey, as reported by VAN DUZEN (1932), stimulation of the hypogastric nerves had little effect, if any, on the internal vesical sphincter. Clinical observations also support this point of view. CLOAKE, LEARMONTH and BARRINGTON (1932), on the contrary, reported that stimulation of the hypogastric nerves resulted in contraction of the internal vesical sphincter and section of these nerves caused its relaxation.

In a study of the action potentials of the nerves supplying the bladder in the cat, EVANS (1936) obtained no conclusive evidence that the sympathetic nerves play any part in vesical function. In experiments on cats reported by LANGWORTHY, KOLB and LEWIS (1940), sympathetic stimulation caused an initial rise in intravesical pressure followed by a fall below the normal resting level, when the volume was held constant, and an initial diminution in the vesical volume followed by an increase, when the intravesical pressure was held constant. Stimulation of the hypogastric nerves also resulted in closure of the ureteral orifices and a decrease in the distance between them. BELL's muscle also contracted, resulting in caudad displacement of the base of the bladder. Following section of the hypogastric nerves the bladder accommodated a smaller volume of urine before micturition occurred, than before sympathetic denervation. On the basis of these results they advanced the opinion that the detrusor muscle is devoid of functional sympathetic innervation.

In experiments carried out on male human subjects under spinal anesthesia, reported by LEARMONTH (1931), stimulation of the entire sympathetic supply to the bladder resulted in powerful contraction of the ureteric orifices, increased tonus in the trigone and contraction of the internal vesical sphincter, but no observable effect on the detrusor muscle except that it was inhibited. Stimulation of either hypogastric nerve resulted in contraction of the ureteric orifice on the same side, increased tonus of the trigone and contraction of the internal sphincter. Reflex responses in the bladder could not be elicited by stimulation of the proximal portion of one hypogastric nerve after its section alone or after section of the entire sympathetic supply to the bladder. The immediate results of section of the sympathetic nerves were relaxation of the ureteric orifices, the entire trigone and the internal sphincter, but no observable change in the detrusor muscle. After an interval of approximately 21 days the ureteric orifices close in the intervals between jets of urine, the relaxation of the trigone is less marked than immediately after sympathetic nerve section and the internal sphincter may close completely, but it offers less resistance than the normally innervated sphincter to the advancing beak of the cystoscope. In LEARMONTH'S experiments, intravenous injection of adrenin in appropriate dosage resulted in immediate active dilatation of the bladder that lasted approximately five minutes. These findings support the assumption that the sympathetic innervation of the detrusor muscle in man includes inhibitory fibers.

In experiments on cats and dogs reported by KUNTZ and SACCOMANNO (1944), stimulation of the hypogastric nerves while the intravesical pressure was kept constant resulted in an initial decrease in the vesical volume followed by a moderate increase. The same stimulation under conditions of constant vesical volume resulted in an initial rise in intravesical pressure followed by a fall below the normal resting level. These findings corroborate those of LANGWORTHY, KOLB and LEWIS cited above.

In order to determine the response of the detrusor muscle alone to sympathetic stimulation, experiments were carried out in which the responses of this muscle were recorded under conditions designed to eliminate any effect on the record of responses elicited by the same stimulation in the musculature at the base of the bladder. In these experiments, mild faradic stimulation of the hypogastric nerves elicited a slight contraction of the muscle followed by moderate inhibition. Stronger stimulation elicited a more marked initial contraction followed by marked, prolonged inhibition. Similar responses of the detrusor muscle to hypogastric nerve stimulation were also obtained following section of the sacral parasympathetic outflow. The results of these experiments also support the assumption that the sympathetic nerves of the bladder play a role in the activity of the detrusor muscle.

In an experimental study reported by HEGRE and INGERSOLL (1949) in which the responses of the detrusor muscle in the cat to electrical stimulation of the hypogastric nerves were analyzed it was found that all parts of the detrusor muscle participate in a diphasic response to sympathetic stimulation. The magnitude of each phase of the response appears to be conditioned by the physiological state of the bladder at the time of the stimulation. Under given experimental conditions the responses elicited in various regions of the bladder also show characteristic differences.

It has been assumed quite generally that each lateral half of the bladder receives hypogastric nerve fibers only from the hypogastric nerve on the same side. On the basis of an extensive review of the pertinent literature, Gruber (1933) concluded that the bladder responses elicited by stimulation of the distal portion of a divided hypograstric nerve are limited to the corresponding half of the viscus, but affects equally all parts of the detrusor muscle on that side. In a further study of the effects of hypogastric nerve stimulation on the bladder musculature in cats and dogs, Ingersoll, Jones and Hegre (1954) found that unilateral hypogastric nerve stimulation invariably elicited on the corresponding side prompt contraction of all parts of the detrusor muscle followed immediately by relaxation. The response, however, was not limited to the ipsolateral half of the bladder. In over 50 per cent of the trials unilateral stimulation elicited a response in the contralateral half of the bladder that was similar to the one on the side of the stimulation. In some instances there was a latent period of 1 to 4 seconds before the onset of contraction on the contralateral side. When the distal portion of a divided hypogastric nerve was stimulated, the latent period before the onset of contraction on the contralateral side was somewhat increased. In some instances the initial response on the contralateral side was one of relaxation. In some of these instances relaxation was the only response; in others the initial relaxation was followed in some regions by contraction and subsequent relaxation. The amplitude of the contraction on the side of the stimulation was always greater than that of the contraction on the contralateral side. The least responsive areas in any single trial were on the contralateral side, usually along the lateral margin of the bladder and within or adjacent to the fundus. These findings support the assumption that all parts of the bladder musculature are supplied with fibers from each hypogastric nerve, but the abundance of this supply is highly variable, particularly on the contralateral side, along the lateral margin of the bladder.

In experiments carried out on dogs, Henderson and Roepke (1934) observed that tonic stimulation of the bladder resulted in liberation of an acetylcholine-like substance. The tonic response, furthermore, was abolished by atropine. Contractile stimulation, on the other hand, did not result in the liberation of an acetylcholine-like substance and the response was not abolished by atropine. On the basis of these findings, they advanced the hypothesis that the functional activity of the bladder involves both a tonic and a contractile mechanism.

Mellanby and Pratt (1940) reported the results of experiments on cats in which instantaneous change from a condition of constant intravesical pressure to one of constant volume caused either an isometric contraction or a state of quiescence at zero pressure, depending on the phase of isotonic rhythm at which the change was made. The isometric contraction was followed by a quiescent state at zero pressure of indefinite duration or by a series of rhythmic contractions. Section of the pelvic nerve abolished the isometric contractions, but stimulation of its distal portion elicited maximal isometric contractions. Prompt responses similar to isometric contractions were elicited by acetylcholine. Similar responses after a long latent period were also elicited by adrenin. The isometric contractions were abolished more readily than the isotonic rhythmic contractions by atropine.

It has been assumed that stimulation of either pelvic nerve elicits contraction of the corresponding lateral half of the detrusor muscle without appreciably affecting the contralateral half. Some of the data at present available do not support this assumption. It has long been known that stimulation of the intact pelvic nerve several weeks after section of the one on the opposite side results in contraction of the entire bladder musculature. Section of both pelvic nerves results in marked atony of the detrusor muscle and closure of the internal vesical sphincter. The liquid content of the bladder is held at a higher pressure than in the normally innervated viscus and for the first few days the capacity of the bladder is increased, but when automatic micturition begins it drops somewhat below the normal level. The emptying reflex is then initiated earlier than in the bladder with intact nerve supply.

In experiments on cats, INGERSOLL, JONES and HEGRE (1955) found that unilateral stimulation of the intact pelvic nerves usually elicited an immediate, vigorous and sustained contraction of the detrusor muscle on the side of the stimulation and a slightly weaker and often somewhat delayed contraction on the opposite side. Occasionally the contraction on the contralateral side was preceded by relaxation. In some instances the relaxation continued throughout the period of stimulation. Stimulation of the distal portion of a severed pelvic nerve elicited a bladder response similar to that elicited by stimulation of the intact nerve. The bladder response to stimulation of the distal portion of one pelvic nerve after bilateral pelvic nerve section was essentially similar in most respects to that elicited by the same stimulation with both pelvic nerves intact. In some instances the shortening of the muscle per unit length was actually greater on the contralateral side following bilateral pelvic nerve section than in the bladder with intact innervation. The general pattern of the bladder response to stimulation of either the intact or sectioned pelvic nerves was not altered by section of the hypogastric nerves.

Stimulation of the central end of a severed pelvic nerve while the one on the opposite side was intact elicited a well marked contraction of the entire bladder after a latent period of several seconds. This response was abolished by section of the contralateral pelvic nerve even though the hypogastric nerves were intact.

Responses to stimulation of central neural mechanisms. Electrical stimulation of the brain stem at the level of the inferior colliculus in the cat evokes contraction of the bladder, whereas bilateral chronic lesions in this area result in inability to completely empty the bladder (BARRINGTON 1925; LANGWORTHY and KOLB 1933; TANG and RUCH 1955). Contractions of the bladder have also been evoked by stimulation of the rostral portion of the midbrain and the posterior and anterior portions of the hypothalamus (KABAT, MAGOUN and RANSON 1936), the medial preoptic area and the septum pellucidum (KABAT et al. 1936; HESS and BRUEGGER 1943), the putamen and globus pallidum and adjacent areas (STROM and UVNAS 1950).

As observed by GROSSMAN and WANG (1955), the typical bladder responses elicited by diencephalic stimulation in the cat are either a series of small contractions or a smooth contraction sustained throughout the duration of the electrical excitation, depending on the frequency and the intensity of the stimulus. These responses are mediated through the parasympathetic nerves. Unsustained contractions of the bladder evoked by hypothalamic stimulation after section or atropinization of the sacral nerve roots have also been reported (WANG and HARRISON 1939). They resemble the unsustained contractions of the bladder that can be evoked by stimulation of the hypogastric nerves (LANGWORTHY and REEVES 1934). They obviously are mediated through sympathetic nerves. This is also suggested by their association with pressor reactions. Stimulation of the posterior portion of the hypothalamus, as reported by BEATTIE and KERR (1936), resulted in diminution of intravesicular pressure. This response probably is also mediated through sympathetic nerves. Inconsistancies in the responses in the bladder to hypothalamic stimulation can probably be explained most satisfactorily on the basis of the initial bladder tonus and the frequency of the stimulus.

The significance of brain stem mechanism in the functional regulation of the bladder is not fully understood. Preoptic and hypothalamic mechanisms may play a role in integrating the influences on the bladder exerted through the sympathetic and parasympathetic nerves. The center in the caudal region of the midbrain through which the bladder is influenced appears to be the only known brain stem mechanism that gives any indication of being a center for micturition in the sense that it has the capacity to coordinate autonomic and somatic reactions concerned in the act of micturition (GROSSMAN and WANG 1956).

Bladder activity is strongly influenced by emotional stimulation that eminates predominantly from the hypothalamus. Strong emotional excitation, such as anxiety or fright, frequently gives rise to an urge to micturate and under certain conditions, actually results in involuntary micturition. Milder emotional stimulation also plays a role in the regulation of bladder function.

The assumption that impulses emanating from the cerebral cortex play a role in the regulation of bladder activity is supported by both experimental and clinical data. Bilateral lesions in the motor and the premotor cortex, particularly on the medial surfaces of the cerebral hemispheres may result in defective voluntary control of micturition and urinary incontinence. Hyperexcitability of the bladder musculature in some cases and hypotonicity in others associated with brain tumors and cortical lesions have been reported. Attempts to elicit purely sympathetic and purely parasympathetic responses in the bladder by electrical stimulation of selected cortical areas in the cat, as reported by INGERSOLL et al. (1951), yielded only negative results.

Micturition. Normal micturition is carried out through coordinated reflex activity, but it is in part a voluntary act. The voluntary neural mechanisms concerned have engaged the attention of many investigators. The voluntary impulses emanating from the cerebral cortex probably are not conducted to the bladder musculature, but to the external sphincter which is a voluntary muscle. The peripheral fibers through which these impulses reach the external sphincter traverse the pudendal nerves. The direct response to these impulses is relaxation of the external sphincter. Afferent impulses initiated by this response are conducted back to the spinal cord through afferent pudendal nerve fibers that make reflex connections with visceral efferent components of the pelvic nerves through which impulses are conducted to the bladder musculature. Thus the micturition reflex initiated by voluntary inhibition of a striated muscle is carried out as a spinal reflex through the appropriate visceral efferent conduction pathways, like the spinal reflexes concerned in the functional regulation of other visceral organs.

The modes of action of the vesical muscles and the sphincters in the act of micturition have been studied extensively. YOUNG (1915) advanced the hypothesis that the muscle of the trigone assists in the opening of the internal sphincter by its contraction. According to this point of view, the opening of the internal vesical orifice is not an inhibitory reaction, but the result of contraction of the trigone.

On the basis of data advanced by YOUNG and WESSON (1921) and YOUNG and MACHT (1923) and his own observations, VAN DUZEN (1935) described the act of micturition in three phases. During the first phase contraction of the trigone depresses the posterior portion of the internal sphincter orifice. In the second phase a wave of contraction of the detrusor muscle is initiated in the region of the internal sphincter orifice and extends toward the dome of the bladder. This results in a lateral pull on the internal orifice that tends to open it further. If the trigone is paralyzed by drug action or sympathetic nerve section, the first phase, i.e., the depression of the posterior lip of the internal vesical orifice, is omitted. The internal vesical orifice must then be opened by lateral pull on the circular fibers around the orifice due to contraction of the detrusor muscle and increasing intravesical pressure. This is less effective than the normal mechanism. Paralysis of the detrusor muscle results in atonicity of the bladder and absence of expulsive force and, consequently, complete retention of urine. The third phase of micturition consists of contraction of the abdominal muscles, resulting in increased intra-abdominal pressure that augments the expulsive force exerted by contraction of the bladder.

YOUNG (1937) emphasized the importance of VAN DUZEN's demonstration of the role of the lateral detrusor muscles in holding open the internal vesical orifice. It seems to confirm the view that the act of micturition is an active process throughout, being initiated by the trigone which, with the assistance of the lateral muscles, holds the internal urethral orifice open. The lateral muscles, with the other detrusors, exert the expulsive power.

LEARMONTH (1931) explained the act of micturition as a modified autonomic reflex, that may be initiated and completed by a stimulus applied either to the vesical musculature, for which the adequate stimulus is the degree of distention of the viscus, or the internal vesical sphincter. When the adequate stimulus is applied to the bladder musculature, the opening of the internal spincter orifice comes about automatically. This is the mechanism of micturition evoked by the urge to urinate. When the internal sphincter is relaxed voluntary contraction of the detrusor muscle follows automatically. This is the mechanism of voluntary micturition.

LEARMONTH recognized that there may be reasonable objection to the application of the term "reflex" to a process that may be interrupted voluntarily at any point in the cycle by voluntary closure of the external vesical sphincter. Such sudden interruption of urination is not necessarily followed by an automatic effort of the bladder musculature to overcome an obstruction at the outlet, but as the internal sphincter is closed, following closure of the external sphincter, the contraction of the detrusor muscle is arrested and assumes a degree of tonus, commensurate with the vesical content at the moment. Surgical experience also indicates that the flow of urine can be interrupted without discomfort to the patient after prostatectomy, when, due to surgical destruction of the internal sphincter, the external sphincter alone is available to close the orifice. The change in the behavior of the detrusor muscle is the result either of a reflex initiated in the internal sphincter, in which case the reflex may be purely autonomic, or a reflex initiated in the external sphincter, in which case the afferent limb of reflex arc is somatic or the impulses that result in closure of the sphincter are integrated at a higher level from which impulses are conducted simultaneously to the sphincter and the detrusor muscle. The concept of micturition as a pure reflex, according to this point of view, must be limited to infancy. The gradual development of voluntary control of micturition involves more and more complete subjugation of an originally primitive spinal reflex function to influences emanating from the cerebral cortex. In the female the external vesical sphincter is relatively poorly developed and plays a less important role in the control of bladder function than in the male.

On the basis of data obtained in experiments carried out on decerebrate cats, BARRINGTON (1921) described a series of six mixturition reflexes: (1) A hindbrain reflex initiated by distention of the bladder that results in contraction of the detrusor muscle. The peripheral links of both the afferent and the efferent limbs of the reflex arcs employed in this reflex are components of the pelvic nerves. (2) A hindbrain reflex through which stimulation of the urethra by running water through it elicits contraction of the detrusor muscle. The afferent limbs of the reflex arcs employed in this reflex traverse the pudendal nerves and the efferent limbs traverse the pelvic nerves. (3) A spinal reflex through which distention of the proximal portion of the urethra elicits a slight transitory contraction of the bladder. Both the afferent and the efferent limbs of the reflex arcs employed in this reflex traverse the hypogastric nerves. (4) A spinal reflex through which stimulation of the urethra by running water through it elicits its relaxation. Both the afferent and the efferent limbs of the reflex arcs employed in this reflex traverse the pudendal nerves. (5) A spinal reflex through which distention of the bladder elicits relaxation of the urethra. The afferent limbs of the reflex arcs employed in this reflex traverse the pelvic nerves; the efferent limbs traverse the pudendal nerves. (6) A spinal reflex through which distention of the bladder elicits relaxation of the smooth muscle of the urethra particularly in its proximal one-third. Both the afferent and the efferent limbs of the reflex arcs employed in this reflex traverse the pelvic nerves.

In decerebrate animals, according to BARRINGTON, reflex contraction of the detrusor muscle is elicited by distention of the bladder through filling. This in turn elicits reflex relaxation of the urethra. This relaxation of the urethra elicits further reflex contraction of the detrusor muscle, resulting in complete emptying of the bladder. These reflexes are carried out in part through centers in the spinal cord and in part through centers in the brain stem. On the basis of all the pertinent data, BARRINGTON (1942) advanced the hypothesis that stimulation of the urethra by passing liquid through it elicits contraction of the detrusor muscle through a hind brain reflex that is mediated through afferent components of the pudendal and efferent components of the pelvic nerves or through a spinal reflex mediated through afferent and efferent components of the pelvic nerves. The hind brain reflex is elicited more easily than the spinal reflex and results in stronger contraction. This spinal reflex has been referred to as the seventh micturation reflex of BARRINGTON (NATHAN 1952).

In NATHAN'S (1952) clinical experience movements of the catheter or the cystoscope in and out of the urethra in man caused no obvious change in intravesical pressure and no contraction of the detrusor muscle. Since this seemed to contradict the findings of BARRINGTON in the cat, a further detailed investigation in human subjects was undertaken. In some experiments a cystoscope was passed and connected with a water manometer. In others a catheter was passed into the bladder and connected with a manometer. The bladder was then filled until the subject felt the urge to micturate. At this point contraction of the detrusor muscle occurred spontaneously or could be easily evoked by adding a little more liquid or by increasing intraabdominal pressure. During cystoscopy the bladder was examined for detrusor activity and during catheterization the intravesical pressure was recorded. When the detrusor activity elicited by the filling of the bladder had subsided, movement of the cystoscope or the catheter in and out along the urethra caused neither a rise in intravesical pressure nor detrusor contraction. Neither did moderate dilatation or stimulation of the urethra by liquid flowing through it elicit contraction of the bladder. The data obtained by NATHAN, therefore, afford no evidence that reflex contraction of the bladder elicited by moving a smooth foreign body along the urethra or by irrigating the urethra with liquid, as reported by BARRINGTON in decerebrate cats, occurs in man. The question why in man the bladder usually continues to expel its contents after its pressure has fallen to a level too low to evoke contraction seems to remain unanswered.

In experiments carried out on dogs by DENNING (1924), irrigation of the distal portion of the urethra failed to elicit contraction of the bladder. He, therefore, concluded that opening of the external sphincter constitutes the adequate stimulus for reflex micturition. He also demonstrated experimentally that voluntary micturition can be carried out following interruption of the pudendal nerves. Closure of the sphincters is less perfect following bilateral interruption of the pudendal nerves than before, but dogs that had been previously trained to micturate at a designated place persisted in this habit, following the operation, and expelled urine voluntarily whenever they were brought to the place in question. No other somatic efferent nerve fibers reach the bladder or the urethra. The ease with which the flow of urine was brought about also seems to rule out any direct stimulating effect on the bladder of increased intra-abdominal pressure. DENNING, therefore, concluded that voluntary nerve impulses may exert a direct influence on the bladder through the autonomic nerves. The autonomic nerves concerned, furthermore, appear to be parasympathetic, since, section of the hypogastric nerves, following section of the pudendal nerves, did not abolish voluntary micturition, but it was abolished by section of the pelvic nerves, leaving the hypogastric nerves intact, until the bladder became adjusted so that it would contract in response to intra-abdominal pressure due to contraction of the abdominal muscles.

The results of DENNING's experiments also shed some light on the specific functional defects of the bladder that result from elimination of any one of the several components of its nerve supply. Interruption of the pudendal nerves results in imperfect closure of the sphincter and loss of sensibility in the urethra, but it does not otherwise cause marked disturbance of the normal functioning of the bladder. Hypogastric nerve section either alone or in conjunction with section of the pudendal nerves results in no marked alteration in bladder function. Interruption of the pelvic nerves results in profound functional and trophic disturbances of the bladder. Section of all the extrinsic nerves of the bladder is followed by a more or less constant flow of urine in small quantities and by periodic discharges of larger quantities brought about by mechanical stimulation to which the bladder is now hypersensitive. Under these conditions incomplete emptying and cystitis are common.

The observation of DENNING that voluntary micturition can be carried out after section of the pudendal nerves led certain other investigators to assume that autonomic neural mechanisms that are concerned in micturition are subject to direct voluntary influences. This obviously is true of some of them, but conclusive evidence that contraction of the detrusor muscle can be initiated or continued by direct voluntary effort is wanting. Voluntary micturition cannot be adequately explained, however, on the assumption that the proximal portion of the urethra and the external vesical sphincter constitute the only "trigger zone" for initiation of the act. As has been pointed out by LEARMONTH (1931) on the basis of all the available data, including clinical and experimental observations on human subjects, the internal sphincter and the bladder musculature also constitute a "trigger zone" for the initiation of voluntary micturition.

Reflex micturition is mediated through reflex centers located in the sacral segments of the spinal cord. Reflex inhibition of the detrusor muscle and contraction of the internal vesical sphincter are mediated through centers located in the first and second lumbar segments of the spinal cord. Afferent impulses are conducted to these centers not only from the urinary bladder and its outlet, including the internal and external vesical sphincters, but also from other parts of the body; consequently, micturition may be facilitated or inhibited by stimuli that are effective in widely separated areas. Reflex bladder responses, however, are elicited with greater facility by stimulation in certain parts of the body than in others. In patients with extensive spinal cord lesions, automatic emptying of the bladder can be evoked by stimulation of the lower extremities or other parts of the body below the level of the lesion. This has generally been regarded as part of a "mass reflex", but it could be interpreted otherwise. HOLMES (1933) has pointed out that the involuntary micturition that frequently is associated with spasms of the lower extremities, in patients with spinal cord lesions, may be, not the direct result of stimulation of the lower extremities, but of associated spastic contraction of the abdominal muscles, which, by increasing the intra-abdominal pressure, suddenly increases the tension on the bladder musculature. In patients with complete transverse spinal cord lesions, contractions of the bladder do not occur simultaneously with the contractions of the abdominal muscles, but after an interval. This seems to indicate that the overflow of impulses into the micturition reflex center does not take place immediately. The more powerful contraction of the bladder that expels the urine usually is preceded by a short series of oscillations of pressure. In patients with spinal cord lesions too low to permit the reflexes elicited by stimulation of the lower extremities to spread to the abdominal muscles, spasm of the extremities is not accompanied by bladder evacuation. The effectiveness of stimulating the abdominal wall by rubbing or by percussion in order to elicit reflex mixturition in patients without spinal cord lesions in whom evacuation of the bladder is difficult has been emphasized by SCHLESINGER (1933). If the first reflex response does not result in complete emptying of the bladder, the reflex may be elicited repeatedly after short intervening intervals.

Bladder sensitivity. Normal sensation from the bladder, according to DENNY-BROWN and ROBERTSON (1933), is derived in part from the tension due to the vesical content. During progressive increase in the volume of liquid in the bladder a series of sensations are evoked with the vague reference that characterizes all visceral sensations and culminates in actual pain. These sensations are not directly related to the internal vesical pressure, since they are not evoked by strong passive pressure upon the bladder when the volume is low. In their experiments a pressure of 18 cm. of water was not found to be necessary to evoke the desire to micturate. Extreme discomfort was sometimes experienced at much lower pressures. Spontaneous vesical contraction does not necessarily evoke sensation, but if the volume is sufficient to evoke some sensation, it is intensified by contraction of the bladder. If the active vesical contraction be sufficiently powerful the entire series of sensations culminating in acute pain may be experienced as the tension of the muscle is increased although the volume remains so small that it would cause no sensation in the resting bladder. It is apparent, therefore, that the receptors concerned may be adequately stimulated both by passive stretching of the muscle and increased tension due to active contraction. The effects of these stimuli can be simulated, and, if the resultant sensation is moderately constant, it can be suppressed from consciousness. Fluctuations in the perception of sensations associated with the desire to micturate do not necessarily reflect equivalent fluctuations in the degree of distention of the bladder or active contraction of its musculature, but presumably they have a psychological basis.

The bladder, like other viscera, is relatively insensitive to mechanical stimulation and probably wholly insensitive to thermal stimulation. On the basis of experimental data, LANGWORTHY, KOLB and LEWIS (1940) concluded that the bladder mucosa is slightly responsive to heat, cold and touch. Sensations due to tactile stimulation of the mucosa are essentially vague and not definitely localizable. Data relative to thermal sensitivity of the bladder are not unequivocal. The urethra undoubtedly is sensitive to thermal stimulation. Thermal sensations that have been regarded as arising in the bladder probably arose from thermal stimulation of the urethra. Using a double walled glass urethral catheter to avoid thermal stimulation of the urethra, WALTZ (1922) obtained no evidence that the bladder is sensitive to thermal stimulation. In experiments reported by NATHAN (1952), carried out on 15 patients, the bladder was emptied and then gradually filled with liquid of known temperature introduced through a suprapubic tube. This was done repeatedly with liquids at temperatures near 45°C or 15° C. The patients was encouraged to compare the sensations associated with each irrigation with those produced by the previous one. No satisfactory report that the bladder possesses thermal receptors was obtained from any of the patients. It seems highly probable, therefore, that the disagreement concerning the data obtained in experiments carried out to determine whether the bladder possesses thermal sensitivity by passing liquids at various temperatures into the bladder through the urethra is due to the neglect in some instances to exclude thermal stimulation of the urethra.

DENNING (1924) reported experiments on animals in which marked distention of the bladder by the introduction of liquid through a urethral catheter resulted in uneasiness on the part of the animal. If reflex contraction of the bladder was elicited by the distention, the animal exhibited increased uneasiness until the liquid began to flow out around the catheter and the internal pressure was reduced. The uneasiness of the animal caused by artifical distention of the bladder was not relieved by section of the pudendal nerves, but it was much less marked after section of both the hypogastric and the pelvic nerves, although the pudendal nerves remained intact. After section of all the nerves to the bladder, artificial distention of the bladder to any degree no longer caused uneasiness of the animal. It may be assumed, therefore, that the impulses resulting from distention of the bladder are conducted through either the hypogastric or the pelvic nerves. Since afferent impulses from the bladder that result in the desire to micturate and that initiate reflex micturition are conducted through the pelvic nerves it may be assumed that the pelvic nerves play the major role in the conduction of impulses caused by artificial distention of the bladder, but clinical data indicate that afferent impulses from the bladder are also conducted through the hypogastric nerves. The impulses that give rise to the sensation of emptying of the bladder probably are mediated through the pudendal nerves.

Electrical stimulation of the fundus of the bladder, according to FRÖHLICH and MEYER (1922), gives rise to afferent impulses conducted through the pelvic nerves that result in painful sensations. The same stimulation in the region of the sphincter gives rise to afferent impulses that are conducted through the pudendal nerves which also evoke painful sensations. These results afford definite information relative to afferent pathways for impulses that arise in circumscribed areas of the bladder, but they afford no unmistakable information relative to the pathways of afferent impulses that evoke the desire to micturate.

The assumption that both contraction of the detrusor muscle and opening of the internal sphincter play a part in the urge to micturate is supported by both experimental and clinical data. The sensations associated with this phenomenon are not all of the same quality. Indefinite sensations localized in the region of the bladder probably are evoked by impulses that arise in the bladder musculature.

36*

More acute sensations that are more or less definitely localizable at the neck of the bladder probably are evoked by afferent impulses that arise in that region. Since contraction of the detrusor muscle assists in opening of the internal vesical sphincter, emptying of the bladder can only be prevented by voluntary contraction of the external sphincter. If the external sphincter holds, a short period of rest usually ensues during which the detrusor muscle relaxes in some degree and relieves the internal vesical pressure. If the bladder content is not reduced, stronger contractions of the detrusor muscle set in and, if a few drops of urine are pressed into the urethra, the impulse to micturate becomes irrestible and reflex micturition takes place. If the external sphincter keeps the urethral orifice closed during repeated contractions of the detrusor muscle, this muscle may become inactive, so that soon after the urge to micturate reaches its maximum strength spontaneous micturition becomes impossible. The afferent impulses concerned in these phenomena that arise within the bladder are conducted predominantly through the pelvic nerves. Those that arise in the external sphincter and in part those that arise in the internal vesical sphincter are conducted through the pudendal nerves.

Certain experimental data reported by TALAAT (1937) support the assumption that some receptors in the bladder wall are stimulated by rapid changes in the volume of the bladder contents and contraction of the detrusor muscle and others are stimulated by a rise in intravesical pressure. The former adapt rapidly. The latter adapt slowly and vary within a wide range in threshold of excitation. Receptors located outside the bladder wall are stimulated by changes in the position of the viscus. Impulses that arise within and without the bladder wall are conducted through both the hypogastric and the pelvic nerves. Those immediately concerned with micturition are conducted predominantly through the pelvic nerves. Impulses that evoke sensations of pain in the bladder, particularly pain due to distention of the viscus, probably arise in receptors that adapt slowly and are conducted predominantly through the hypogastric nerves, but the pelvic nerves also play a part in the mediation of bladder pain.

Regulation of the urethra. The smooth muscle in the wall of the urethra, like the internal vesical sphincter, relaxes during active contraction of the detrusor muscle. It also undergoes tonic contraction simultaneously with contraction of the internal sphincter. Relaxation of the smooth musculature of the urethra is brought about by parasympathetic nerve stimulation and contraction of the musculature is brought about by sympathetic nerve stimulation. The response of the urethral musculature, like that of the internal sphincter, is the opposite to that of the detrusor muscle. This is generally regarded as a functional adaptation to facilitate the flow of urine during micturition and to support the sphincter mechanism during relaxation of the detrusor muscle and filling of the bladder. Voluntary contraction of the external vesical sphincter and the compressor urethrae muscles also plays a part in the reflex regulation of the smooth muscle of the urethra.

2. Pathological physiology

Enuresis. Enuresis is the unintentional and unconscious voiding of urine, usually in a full steady stream. It occurs predominantly during sleep, and less frequently during the waking state. Involuntary voiding of urine is a normal condition of infancy. Essential enuresis, as defined by CROSBY (1950), is the involuntary and unconscious voiding of urine after an arbitrary age limit of three years, in the absence of congenital or acquired defects of the urogenital and nervous systems, and in the absence of significant psychological abnormality. Persistence of enuresis after the age of ten years in boys and after the onset of menstruation in girls is uncommon and ususally indicates organic defect or a marked psychological problem (JOHNSON and MARSHALL 1954). The occurrence of involuntary voiding of urine that is associated with organic disease, whether in children or in adults, is more accurately designated as incontinence of urine.

On the basis of incidence alone, enuresis must be regarded as the most important functional urological disorder of childhood and, in view of its social consequences, its importance as a potential deterrent to normal development during childhood can hardly be exaggerated. The failure to attain control of the bladder before the third or fourth year presents the child with a physical situation to which it has to make some mental adjustment. If the condition persists longer, as it frequently does, anxiety regarding the future is added to the depression caused by the present state.

Etiology. Enuresis may be classified in two categories: true enuresis, which is functional or psychogenic in origin, and enuresis caused by organic defect. According to CAMPBELL (1954), 90 to 95 per cent of all cases fall into the first category. True enuresis may be regarded as a personality disorder due to a single one or a combination of psychological conditions in the child. As chief among these JOHNSON and MARSHALL (1954) mentioned a subconscious resentment toward the parents, a subconscious desire to remain in, or return to the irresponsible and protected state of infancy, and the lack of maturity with respect to bladder control. Defective habit training must also be regarded as an important etiological factor. Failure of many children to attain urinary continence until the age of eight or ten years undoubtedly can be explained on this basis. Organic enuresis is commonly associated with uropathology, chiefly in the lower urinary tract. Involuntary micturition or frequency caused by infection is not true organic enuresis. Neuromuscular dysfunction of the bladder, urethral diverticulum, ectopic ureteral orifices and certain other organic defects with which involuntary micturition is associated do not fall within the category of enuresis, but rather into that of incontinence or pseudoincontinence.

Descriptive classification. For descriptive purposes enuresis may be classified as follows: (1) Nocturnal. — In this form, which is the most common, involuntary voiding occurs during sleep or immediately on awakening. (2) Diurnal. — In this form, which is relatively uncommon, involuntary voiding usually occurs only during the day without concomitant nocturnal enuresis. (3) Continuous from infancy. (4) Regular, i.e., bed-wetting usually occurs every night unless precautions are taken. (5) Reappearing after a period during which bed-wetting has not occurred. (6) Sporadic, in which there is a succession of periods of bed-wetting with intervening periods of continence. (7) Facititious, i.e., voluntary micturition occurs due to cold, fear of the dark or other reasons. This is not true enuresis.

Urinary continence. Under physiological conditions intravesical pressure constitutes the normal stimulus for micturation. Pressure of about 16 cm. of water may evoke spontaneous micturition. In adults the first desire to micturate is generally experienced at about half the volume of bladder content required to cause imperative urination (BEST and TAYLOR 1945). This is approximately half the anatomical capacity of the bladder. The physiological effects of intravesical tension vary with the rate of filling, the emotional state of the individual, environmental temperature and other factors. For example, in cold weather the volume of urine required to cause urgency may be no more than half the volume required to produce the same degree of urgency in hot weather. CROSBY (1950) has expressed the opinion that an understanding of continence cannot be gained from studies of micturition alone. He has pointed out that to insure nocturnal continence both detrusor activity and micturition must be inhibited so that urination does not occur too early in response to increasing bladder volume. Such inhibition in conjunction with the increasing anatomical capacity of the bladder as the child grows older may insure continence during the night if the volume of urine in the bladder remains below the threshold value required to initiate micturition. Secondly, this inhibition must predominate over visceral afferent stimuli that tend to initiate micturition until sleep is dispersed by the discomfort of the filling bladder, and the waking state allows voluntary micturition.

In both continent and enuritic children the bladder contents eventually reach the physiological limit. When this occurs the continent child awakens, but the enuritic child does not. CROSBY's experimental findings suggest that in enuritic children involuntary micturition commonly occurs before filling of the bladder has reached the physiological limit.

The threshold intravesical pressure required to disperse sleep or to initiate micturition varies in both normal and enuritic children and adults, as is indicated by the variation in the volume of urine voided by continent individuals on being awakened by the urge to urinate. This indicates an essential difference between the continent and the enuritic child, and illustrates the reserve of inhibition that is available in the normal child during deep sleep due to fatigue. After continence is well established the discomfort due to filling of the bladder may amount to severe pain on awakening from deep sleep.

Conversion from enuresis to continence. In most enuritic children the defect is basically physiological and is not associated with a primary anatomical defect, a pathological condition or a psychological aberration. Conversion to continence, therefore, can usually be accomplished by physiological responses, regardless of whether it occurs spontaneously or is acquired by artificial means such as toilet training, suggestion, volitional attempts to extend control during sleep, etc.

According to CROSBY (1950), the discomfort of a wet bed, which he calls "somatic discomfort", acts as an inhibitory stimulus at the onset of involuntary micturition that elicits an unconditioned response tending to terminate the flow of urine by inhibition of the detrusor muscle and contraction of the internal vesical sphincter. Reinforcement of this response by its repeated elicitation by the stimuli of repeated somatic discomfort to wetting should be expected to result in a gradual increase in the strength of the inhibition produced so that a larger volume of urine would be required to initiate micturition. Then as the bladder fills the prepotency of its inhibition over the increasing current of impulses conducted by the afferent limb of the reflex arc employed in the micturition reflex diminishes. Increasing bladder distension concurrently gives rise to an increasing volume of impulses that are conducted to the brain and tend to awaken the child. The afferent impulses that arise in the filling bladder of the sleeping child are active both at the bladder reflex centers in the spinal cord and at the center responsible for the waking state. The resultant effect is determined by three coexisting factors: the afferent stimulation excited by filling of the bladder, the degree of inhibition of the bladder and the depth of sleep. If the inhibition of the bladder is sufficiently prepotent, the child will be awakened by the discomfort of the filled bladder before reflex micturation is initiated. The natural process of conversion may be reinforced by appropriate training methods if such methods are applied wisely. Inappropriate attempts at training may interfere with the natural process in enuritic children and aggravate the condition.

BOSTOCK and SHACKLETON (1951) have pointed out that toilet training of enuretic children can be beneficial only if it is carried out wisely and with patience and affection. It must be performed so kindly and smoothly that no tension is produced in the child. Rigid toilet training frequently results in frustration. Habits acquired under a rigid toilet training regime frequently break down. Habits acquired under frustration are unstable and tend to disintegrate with further frustration because the conditioning is linked with discomfort and sometimes with fear. Regression tends to occur when frustration and fear are again experienced. In the experience of BOSTOCK and SHACKLETON with enuretic children, the secondary frustrations produced by rigid training regimes introduce new characteristics. The child is less susceptible to punishment and reward, and any change in his behavior is apt to be hostile or regressive. The removal of frustrating factors must be regarded as highly desirable in the management of enuretic children.

A certain percentage of enuritic children that do not respond to judicious toilet training or routine medical or psychiatric treatment will, on examination, exhibit organic changes in the urinary tract. A complete urological examination of children with refractory enuresis, therefore, is indicated particularly, those that show additional symptoms of urinary tract instability. Many enuritic children that exhibit pathological alterations in the urinary tract may actually be functional enurities, but correction of the urinary tract abnormalities may be essential to prevent later recurrence or later irreparable damage (JOHNSON and MARSHALL 1954).

In some instances enuresis continues into adult life. The problem of enuresis in adults is essentially the same as that of chronic enuresis in children. In all adults with functional urinary incontinence the disorder has persisted since childhood (HUBBLE 1950). Obviously, the longer the habit has persisted the more difficult its correction becomes. Enuresis in adults is more common in males than in females. Involuntary micturition occurs not only during sleep but frequently diurnal precipitate micturition occurs which amounts almost to incontinence and which can be held back voluntarily only with difficulty. When in severe cases the condition gradually improves — as rule with sporadic recurrences — the bladder remains weak with a tendency to diurnal precipitate action throughout life (MARSHALL 1954).

3. Nocturia in the aged

Nocturnal frequency of micturition may occur in the aged with or without excessive production of urine. Its chief causes, as outlined by RUBIN and NAGEL (1951), are (1) physiological, (2) psychological, (3) cardiac, (4) renal and (5) obstructive or urological.

The physiological cause is most evident after excessive liquid intake. The psychological cause is not clearly definable. The aged usually sleep less soundly than younger persons. When the aged person awakens in the night and cannot readily return to sleep, he may find it convenient to urinate, although he may experience no real urgency. The habit of getting up at night may be acquired in this way. Frequently, such a habit acquired during a period of illness persists. This is illustrated particularly by older men who have sufferend long from obstruction of the proximal portion of the urethra and have delayed adequate therapy for years. Nocturia usually is more severe and persistent in older men who have had a long history of urinary frequency prior to prostatectomy, whereas, men who have had prostatectomy soon after the onset of symptoms usually have little or no residual urinary frequency. In long standing cases of chronic prostatitis nocturia may persist after prostatectomy due to chronic cystitis with hypertrophy and fibrosis of the bladder wall.

The cardiac cause of nocturia is frequently manifested in incipient or frank edema. In a healthy person more urine per hour is secreted during activity than during sleep. When the heart is functioning normally liquid retention in the tissues is not apparent. Slight lowering of blood pressure during sleep also lowers the filtration pressure in the kidneys. In cardiac disease nocturia may be the earliest sign of decompensation. The elimination of retained liquid, furthermore, is facilitated by the recumbent position. It has long been assumed that kidney function is facilitated by the recumbent posture either because of better venous return or other factors.

In renal disease in which the urine is not concentrated abnormally large amounts of urine of low specific gravity are produced and larger volumes are voided during both day and night. This results in both diurnal and nocturnal frequency.

Urological causes of nocturia are the most important. They have been classified by RUBEN and NAGEL as (1) infective, (2) reflex, (3) diminished bladder capacity, and (4) obstructive. Obstructive lesions are the most serious causes. They include constriction of the neck of the bladder, bladder calculi, diverticulum, and cystocele. In the male prostatic hyperplasia either benign or malignant and conditions following prostatectomy probably are the most common causes of nocturia in the aged.

4. Stress incontinence of urine

Stress incontinence of urine may be defined as the leakage of small quantities of urine on strain, coughing, sneezing or increasing intra-abdominal pressure. It varies within wide limits. The amount of urine discharged may be only a few drops or a considerable quantity. Leakage may occur frequently or only at infrequent intervals.

This defect is much more common in females than in males. It has been investigated most extensively in gynecological patients. Among the common causes are obstetric trauma, surgical trauma or unsatisfactory wound healing following plastic surgery involving the urethra and the anterior vaginal wall. Other predisposing conditions are congenital underdevelopment of the urethra and its supporting structures and involutional tissue changes incidental to the menopause.

Since the control of micturition depends on normal functional balance between the urethral sphincter mechanism and the expulsive force of the bladder, leakage of urine may occur through a normal urethra if intravesical pressure becomes excessive. Abnormally high intravesical pressure may arise at times due to external pressure on the bladder, uterine prolapse, abnormalities of the motor innervation of the bladder musculature or reflex instability of the bladder due to inflammation of the urinary tract, but leakage of urine through a normal urethra caused by excessive intravesical pressure is not true stress incontinence.

Stress incontinence is commonly associated with gross anatomical changes involving the bladder and the urethra and their supporting structures. The urethra and the neck of the bladder usually are displaced downward and ventrad from their normal positions beneath the pubic arch. The lumen of the urethra is increased in caliber due to relaxation of the urethral musculature and damage to supporting structures. In the presence of marked relaxation, the proximal one-third to one-half of the urethral lumen may remain open and become an extension of the bladder cavity, thus reducing the length of the urethral canal. Such alterations are probably invariably accompanied by some degree of relaxation, destruction and perhaps distortion of the urethral sphincter muscles, resulting in functional defects (ALDRIDGE 1952). In most instances, according to MOORE (1953), the region of the urethrovesical junction occupies the bottom of a funnel-shaped area of relaxation at the base of the bladder while the patient is standing or straining or there is a significant increase in the tonus of the detrusor muscle. He also pointed out that injury to the tissue in the region of the neck of the bladder, without gross changes in the structure supporting the bladder, may be sufficient to cause exertional incontinence.

Data obtained by the use of cystourethrography in which either ventro-dorsal or oblique exposure of the bladder and urethra was employed (SCHUBERT 1929; MIKULICZ-RADECKI 1931; BALL 1950, and BALL et al. 1950) seem to support the assumption that the anatomical changes characteristic of stress incontinence are (1) funneling of the internal urethral meatus, (2) undue descent of the neck of the bladder on straining and (3) sometimes dilatation of the urethra. These alterations, according to ROBERTS (1952) and JEFFCOATE and ROBERTS (1952) are not the most constant features. The most characteristic anatomical changes, according to their point of view, become apparent only when the pelvic organs are X-rayed from the side. As described by JEFFCOATE and ROBERTS (1952), the base of the full normal bladder, when viewed laterally, lies just above and parallel to a line extending from the lower border of the symphysis pubis to the fifth sacral vertebra. The junction of the urethra with the bladder is T-shaped and the angles on the ventral and dorsal aspects of the junction are clearly defined. The urethra is essentially straight. The anatomical relationships of the bladder and urethra are not significantly altered by strong bearing down effort. During micturition the bladder becomes more ovoid in shape, the dorsal urethrovesical angle is obliterated and the proximal portion of the urethra comes into line with the trigone of the bladder. The entire urethra becomes somewhat dilated and the funneling of the internal meatus is associated with the obliteration of the dorsal urethrovesical angle.

In the presence of uterovaginal prolapse without incontinence of urine the urethrovesical junction descends on straining. The proximal portion of the urethra is also displaced dorsad and caudad. Since these alterations are not accompanied by leakage of urine, it is apparent that displacement of the bladder and urethra does not in itself cause incontinence. In this condition the bladder and urethra descend together without alteration of their anatomical relationships to each other, and the ventral and dorsal urethrovesical angles remain clearly defined. The normal anatomical relationships of the bladder and urethra to each other are also maintained during micturition. The only anomalous relationship is that the proximal portion of the urethra may be so low that the stream of urine is directed upward in the first part of its course.

In cases of stress incontinence with or without uterovaginal prolapse there is frequently some descent of the base of the bladder and the urethrovesical junction on straining. This is more accurately a measure of the degree of prolapse than of the severity of the incontinence. The most characteristic anatomical alteration appears to be obliteration of the dorsal urethrovesical angle so that the urethra and the trigone lie in the same plane, i.e., the relationships of the bladder and the urethra to each other are essentially similar to those that exist during micturition in normal subjects. It has also been demonstrated radiologically that when stress incontinence is controlled temporarily by finger pressure in the region of the urethrovesical junction, or by a pessary, the dorsal urethrovesical angle is restored. This appears to be more important in stopping the leakage than upward or ventrad displacement of either the bladder or the urethra.

Although there exists no definitive internal vesical sphincter in the female, the muscles adjacent to the internal urethral orifice subserve the function of a sphincter in some degree. In both the male and the female the muscle layers at the urethrovesical junction tend to form two U-shaped slings, one ventral and the other dorsal. A sphincter mechanism is thus provided that normally holds the urine at this level. These slings function reciprocally with the detrusor muscle, contracting when the rest of the bladder is relaxed and vice versa. The relaxation of the musculature around the internal urethral orifice simultaneously with the contraction of the detrusor muscle during micturition allows funneling of the proximal portion of the urethra. The downward movement of the base of the bladder and the proximal portion of the urethra, however, results from relaxation of the floor of the pelvis, the urethra moving with the vagina.

The voluntary muscles around the urethra probably serve to empty it at the end of micturition. They also subserve voluntary interruption of the act of micturition. They probably also provide a second line of defense against incontinence. Urine that has passed into the urethra might be arrested by the contraction of these muscles and returned to the bladder when the crisis is passed. A major factor in urinary control, according to JEFFCOATE and ROBERTS (1952), is the maintenance of the angle between the proximal portion of the urethra and the bladder. The mechanism by which this angle is maintained as yet is unknown. It is known, as they have pointed out, that it is maintained in many instances in the presence of gross uterovaginal prolapse with distortion of all supporting structures of the pelvic organs. This suggests that its maintenance is a function of the intrinsic musculature of the bladder and the urethra rather than of the accessory muscles.

5. Urinary retention

Urinary retention in children. Pronounced urinary retention in children is usually related to congenital lesions of the urogenital tract. In many instances neurological factors play a significant role, although neurological defects may not be demonstrable.

Etiology. The etiological factors are chiefly mechanical and neuromuscular. Mechanical obstruction may be due to a pinpoint meatus, urethral stricture, contracture of the vesical neck, giant verumontanum or true valves without infection (POWELL 1953). Infection in conjunction with any of the obstructions mentioned above may result in atony of the bladder. Neuromuscular causes of urinary retention include both upper and lower motor neuron lesions and lesions of the bladder musculature. The neural defects may be associated with cerebral palsy, spinal cord lesions, spina bifida with meningocele, arachnoiditis, anomalies of the spine and sacrum, poliomyelitis, etc. Lesions of the bladder musculature are in some instances associated with congenital megalocolon (HIRSCHSPRUNG'S disease). In such cases the bladder may exhibit a deficiency in intrinsic ganglion cells comparable to the deficiency in the myenteric plexus in the colon (SWENSON 1952). Clinical observations on patients with urinary retention associated with congenital megalocolon also indicate neuromuscular dysfunction of the bladder. Urinary retention in adults is commonly associated with urethral obstruction or spinal cord lesions, including multiple sclerosis.

Dynamics of urinary retention. Significant data relative to the dynamics of urinary retention have been obtained in experiments carried out on dogs by Lawson and Tomlinson (1951). The animals under pentothal sodium anesthesia were given constant intravenous infusion of 2.5 per cent glucose, in distilled water at a constant rate sufficient to give them 1500 to 200 cc. in 36 hours. An appropriate catheter was inserted and attached to a water manometer.

During acute urinary retention, in these experiments, the intravesical pressure increased to a peak and then progressively decreased, although the bladder was constantly increasing in volume. Exogenous filling of the bladder at a slow constant rate resulted in abnormally high intravesical pressure with extravasation of liquid into the peritoneal cavity without apparent rupture of the bladder wall. The intravesical pressure then decreased as it does in the normal bladder. When the intravesical pressure was sufficient to cause increased intranephric pressure, during acute urinary retention, the output of urine decreased. The low peak of bladder pressure that normally occurs during acute urinary retention probably can be explained on this basis. Reflex inhibition probably is also a factor in the decreased production of urine. Bilateral stasis of urine in the ureter and the pelvis of the kidney occurred within 24 to 36 hours in every instance of induced acute urinary retention, but no evidence of incompetence at the urethrovesical junction was obtained in any instance.

6. Urethral stenosis

Congenital stenosis is the most common developmental anomaly of the urethra. Its frequency in males is approximately six times the frequency in females (Herbut 1952). It is usually discovered during the first year of life because of difficulty and frequently pain associated with urination. In some instances it does not become apparent until the second or third year and occasionally not until adulthood is attained.

Congenital urethral stenosis represents an abnormally tight closure, during fetal life, of the urethral furrow or arrest of the canalization of the urethral epithelium. In both males and females the stenosus usually occurs at the external meatus. The narrowing exists as a ring or a fold along the inferior margin of the urethra at or near the external meatus. In the male narrowing of the lumen may also occur just proximal to the fossa navicularis or at the junction of the bulbar and the membranous portions of the urethra. Because of incomplete emptying of the urethra, dribbling of urine frequently occurs. Emptying of the bladder is incomplete, and incontinence may result due to overflow from the over-distended bladder.

Acquired urethral stenosis may be due to various forms of injury. Roen and Stept (1946) have emphasized urethral stricture as a cause of urethritis with the development of periurethral fibrosis which in turn results in further stricture.

7. Neurogenic vesical dysfunction

General considerations. Neurgenic vesical dysfunction is a highly controversial subject and not fully understood. All types of vesical dysfunction that result from lesions of the central nervous system and peripheral nerves are commonly included in this category. In cases of complete transverse interruption of the spinal cord, particularly in a young adult, the physiological aspects of the bladder dysfunction are relatively clear and well defined. In cases of incomplete interruption of the spinal cord, particularly in older patients, the urological manifestation due to the neural lesion may not be clearly recognizable. In certain cases clear differentiation of the neurogenic vesical dysfunction from urethral obstruction or simple prostatism may be impossible. Obviously many patients that exhibit neurogenic bladder dysfunction also exhibit bladder dysfunction of non-neurogenic origin.

Animal experimental data. Much of our early knowledge of neurogenic vesical dysfunction has been derived from experimentation on animals, particularly dogs. A complete review of this work cannot be included in the present chapter. The significant data have been summarized by DENNY-BROWN and ROBERTSON (1933).

In the dog complete destruction of the lumbo-sacral segments of the spinal cord results in atony of the bladder with contracted sphincter and resultant retention of urine. In the course of a few days this phase passes and intermittent discharge from a small bladder takes place. The subsequent state is one of intermittent automatic micturition and hypertrophy of the detrusor muscle (GOLTZ and EWALD 1896).

In the dog and other animals complete transverse section of the spinal cord rostral to the lumbar segments results in a period of depression of bladder function followed by the gradual development of "automatic micturition". Large quantities of urine that nearly completely empty the bladder are discharged periodically each in a steady stream (GOLTZ 1874, SHERRINGTON 1892). This action is facilitated by light momentary intermittent abdominal pressure or perineal stimulation, and abolished by strong reflex activity of the limbs (SHERRINGTON 1900). In cats, according to BARRINGTON (1915), the external vesical sphincter is highly tonic during the period of depression and becomes less tonic during the development of automatic micturition, but this part of the urethra still resists the outflow even after section of the pudendal nerves (BARRINGTON 1928). Stimulation of the intact sciatic nerve in the spinal animal causes micturition (STEWART 1899, ELLIOT 1907) with relaxation of the internal sphincter. The micturition reflexes described by BARRINGTON in anesthetized and spinal animals are outlined in an earlier section of the present chapter. As indicated by certain clinical data (NATHAN 1952), certain of these reflexes are not duplicated in man. On the basis of animal experimentation it appears to be well established, as reported by JACOBSON (1945), that bladder function is altered following transection of the spinal cord, the specific alteration depending on the level of the transection. If the sacral segments of the cord are destroyed or both pelvic nerves are interrupted, in the dog, the bladder wall becomes thickened, hypertrophied and trabeculated. Unilateral section of the pelvic nerve results in unilateral hypertrophy involving only half of the bladder. Transverse section of the spinal cord rostral to sacral segments results in less hypertrophy of the bladder musculature than destruction of the sacral segments.

8. Cord bladder in man

Acute and chronic stages. Immediately following a complete transverse spinal cord lesion, regardless of its level, reflex activity is abolished below the level of the lesion. The bladder is flaccid and there is no sensory awareness of its distention or desire to micturate. If not drained by artificial means, overflow dribbling occurs. The older concept of the complete loss of detrusor tonus during this stage is no longer tenable, since NESBIT et al. (1941) have shown that vesical tonus is not lost. The acute stage during which artificial drainage of the bladder is required lasts for a variable period, from several weeks or months to a year or longer, when the bladder enters the chronic or recovery stage.

The chronic stage is characterized by (1) impaired urinary control, (2) incontinence and (3) relatively large amounts of residual urine frequently associated with urinary infection. The ability of the bladder to accomodate readily to increase in volume of its contents is greatly reduced. All of these factors vary with the site and severity of the lesion, its degree of completeness and the extent to which recovery has taken place.

Classification. Cord bladders are commonly classified as (1) atonic neurogenic bladder, (2) automatic or reflex bladder, (3) autonomous bladder, (4) voluntary neurogenic bladder and (5) unihibited bladder.

Atonic neurogenic bladder. This is essentially the acute phase of neurogenic bladder dysfunction. As the patient gradually recovers from the spinal shock, the bladder becomes either automatic or autonomous depending on the level of the neural lesion. MUNRO (1952) has described two intermediate phases in the process of conversion. The first intermediate phase is characterized by ineffective and abortive emptying contractions. The capacity of the bladder gradually diminishes and its basic tonus is increased, but the internal sphincter remains contracted. Frequent voiding of small quantities of urine commonly occurs. This phase may be of short duration and in some instances it may escape recognition. The second intermediate phase is characterized by hypertrophy of the bladder wall. The detrusor muscle is overactive and may exhibit an almost constant state of spasm. Its basic tonus, consequently, is high. The internal sphincter exhibits physiological relaxation. The external sphincter relaxes reflexly. Beyond this point the bladder either relapses to atonicity or progresses toward automaticity (Ross 1956).

The automatic neurogenic bladder functions essentially reflexly. It requires the integrity of the sacral spinal micturition reflex center, consequently, it can develop only when the neural lesion is located at a higher level and the sacral portion of the cord remains intact. The patient with an automatic bladder has no control of micturition. It usually occurs at intervals up to three or four hours, but it may occur more frequently. The urine is forcibly evacuated, usually several ounces at a time. The amount of residual urine usually is large, but varies from patient to patient. Although in the absence of vesical sensations the desire to urinate is not experienced, the patient may experience some vague sensations of fullness in the suprapubic or perineal areas due to impulses conducted through the hypogastric and splanchnic nerves. This can occur only if the afferent splanchnic nerve fibers in question enter the spinal cord rostral to the lesion.

The capacity of the automatic or reflex bladder is highly variable. It may be greater or less than normal. The variations in capacity have given rise to terms such as hypotonic, hypertonic, spastic and irritable reflex bladder. If the capacity is large the tonus of the bladder musculature usually is relatively low. An automatic bladder of small capacity on the other hand, may be expected to exhibit hypertonus. The smaller the capacity, the shorter will be the intervals between voidings. In some instances the bladder capacity becomes so small and the intervals between voidings so short that the intermittent spurts of the autonomous or nonreflex bladder are simulated. The increased irritability of the automatic bladder of small capacity may be caused by various factors among which may be mentioned infection, extravesical mass reflexes of the lower extremities and abdominal muscles, irritation in the region of the neck of the bladder due to obstruction or other causes.

The autonomous neurogenic bladder is commonly the result of destruction of the sacral micturition reflex center or interruption of the micturition reflex arcs. Interruption of these arcs may result from injury to the cauda equina. Normal vesical sensation is abolished, although the afferent splanchnic nerve fibers that traverse the hypogastric nerves are intact. Vague sensations due to sensory stimuli that may arise in the bladder or adjacent tissues and are mediated through afferent splanchnic nerve fibers are felt, but they play no part in the functioning of the bladder. Voluntary control is completely abolished and the bladder exhibits little or no reflex activity. Evacuation of urine occurs irregularily in intermittent jets or spurts. If the abdominal muscles are intact some urine may be expressed by voluntary contraction of the abdominal wall or manual compression of the abdomen.

The capacity of the autonomous bladder is variable, but the volume of residual urine usually is large. The capacity of the bladder to accomodate to increasing volume of urine is limited. The cystoscopic appearance of the bladder varies with the duration of the lesion. The bladder wall, including the neck, appears thick and hypertrophied. Trabeculation of the bladder is usually well marked (EMMETT 1954).

The autonomous bladder is commonly regarded as non-reflex. According to current concepts, if the sacral spinal cord lesion is complete, subsequent reflex activity of the bladder should not return. Varying degrees of apparent reflex bladder activity after complete destruction of the sacral micturition reflex center, however, have been reported. Two possible explanations of this phenomenon have been advanced: (1) Some sacral micturition reflex arcs may have remained intact, and (2) the observed bladder contractions may represent the contractile capacity inherent in smooth muscle or activity initiated in the intramural ganglia of the bladder. The possibility of reflex bladder activity mediated through intrinsic reflex arcs is not precluded, but data in support of this hypothesis are wanting. The feeble contractions observed in the autonomous bladder, furthermore, are inadequate to expel urine.

With regard to persistence of intact micturition reflex arcs, BORS (1952) has advanced the opinion that the damage to the sacral micturition center and the reflex arcs can be quite accurately assessed by means of the bulbocavernous anal reflexes and the anal tonus. If the reflex arcs are intact squeezing of the glans penis should elicit brisk contraction of the sphincter ani. A similar reflex response of the sphincter ani should be elicited by appropriate stimulation of the perianal skin. These reflexes may not be elicited if the anal sphincter is in a state of high tonus, but, as BORS has pointed out, spasticity of the anal sphincter would itself indicate intact reflex arcs through the sacral spinal cord centers. SEMBA et al. (1956) have also demonstrated reflex inhibition of the external anal sphincter and the bulvocavernous muscle in response to rapidly increasing internal vesical pressure in unanesthetized spinal dogs. How much reliance can be placed on these reflexes as indicators of the functional state of the reflex micturition mechanisms remain to be demonstrated.

Voluntary Neurogenic Bladder is commonly associated with an incomplete transverse spinal cord lesion. Immediately after the injury both bladder sensitivity and voluntary control of bladder function may be completely abolished, but with the lapse of time, bladder sensitivity and voluntary control of micturition may be restored in some degree. The degree of possible recovery is dependent on the extent and the level of spinal cord injury. The level of the lesion has been emphasized by various investigators, since the final type of vesical dysfunction is determined in a large measure by the amount of damage suffered by the sacral cord and the micturition reflex arcs. In the absence of injury to the sacral spinal cord, the patient with voluntary neurogenic bladder may hope to achieve voluntary micturition, although control is imperfect.

The Uninhibited Neurogenic Bladder exhibits only minimal functional deviation from the normal. Its most characteristic symptom is imperative micturition. According to McLELLAN (1939), it occurs chiefly in patients who exhibit lack or loss of cerebral inhibition due to failure of development, unilateral cortical disease or subtotal destruction of spinal cord pathways. The sensory conduction pathways need not be impaired.

The classification of cord bladders outlined above is significant and useful for purposes of description, but of limited practical value. A working classification has been devised by BORS (1951) that is based on the following significant factors: (1) the level of the lesion, (2) the completeness of the lesion, and (3) the functional efficiency of the bladder as determined by the amount of residual urine in proportion to the capacity of the bladder. Bladder efficiency, therefore, is expressed in terms of balance. THOMPSON (1953) also emphasized the importance of classifying cord bladders according to their functional state as efficient or inefficient. If the patient can empty or nearly empty the bladder it is efficient, although urination may take place at relatively long intervals, Pyuria is absent or minimal, the bladder and upper parts of the urinary tract are free from calculi and febrile attacks occur only rarely or not at all. If the bladder does not empty it is inefficient. It usually contains 5 fluid ounces or more urine which frequently is infected. An extreme urgency type of incontinence occurs commonly. Vesical calculi are sometimes present and febrile attacks occur frequently. An inefficient cord bladder can in some instances be converted into an efficient one by transurethral resection of the vesical neck.

Basic factors in neurogenic vesical disfunction: During the acute stage the bladder fills and becomes distended, due to loss of tonus and reflex activity, and overflow dribbling occurs. The major problems during this stage are drainage to prevent overdistention of the bladder and the control of infection. During the chronic stage the major problems are related to (1) incontinence, (2) residual urine, and (3) shortness of the time between ejections of urine. Problems of lesser importance include (1) inability to recognize imminence of voiding, (2) inability to inhibit, and (3) inability to initiate micturition.

Incontinence in the chronic stage is usually associated with normal or increased tonicity of the vesical sphincters. The underlying mechanical cause is the repeated irregular and unsuccessful attempts of the bladder to expel its contents. The incontinence, consequently, is not a passive but an active process. Remedial measures should, therefore, be directed toward improvement in the efficiency of detrusor activity and the promotion of reciprocal relaxation of the sphincters to permit evacuation of the bladder contents.

Residual urine constitutes the basic underlying factor in most of the problems associated with neurogenic vesical dysfunction. The amount of urine that cannot be evacuated, which is the chief factor in determining the efficiency of a cord bladder, varies within wide limits. In an automatic bladder due to a spinal cord lesion above the sacral segments, the reflex arcs for micturition are intact. Vesical tonus usually is within normal limits or slightly higher, and the reflex contractions of the bladder may be equal in power or more powerful than those of the normal bladder, but the urine is not completely evacuated, probably because reciprocal relaxation of the vesical sphincter does not take place or the detrusor contractions are not sufficiently sustained. According to one point of view, sufficiently well-sustained contractions to insure complete evacuation of the bladder cannot be achieved without impulses that emanate from the brain stem.

The basis for residual urine in an autonomous or nonreflex bladder is more readily understood. Because the reflex arcs for micturition are destroyed, what-

ever detrusor activity there is depends on the inherent capacity of the muscle
to contract or on local reflex mechanism in the bladder wall. The contractions
that take place are usually small and exert little expulsive power. In rare instances they may become sufficiently powerful to resemble the contractions of
the reflex bladder. On the other hand, the autonomous bladder has the advantage
of hypertrophy of the detrusor muscle, high intravesical pressure and the ability
to respond to abdominal training. The hypertrophy and hypertonicity, however,
extend into the vesical neck where they act as an obstruction.

In the normal person micturition is not initiated by contraction of the abdominal muscles or manual expression regardless of the height to which the intravesical pressure is raised. While micturition is in progress, however, the force of
the urinary stream can be increased by these measures. This also applies to the
true automatic or reflex bladder, but in some cases the hyperirritable bladder
may be stimulated to contract by contraction of the abdominal muscles. In
autonomous bladders, micturition may be initiated and maintained by increasing
abdominal pressure either manually or by abdominal contraction. It is possible
by contraction of the intact abdominal muscles to raise the intravesical pressure
to 50 to 70 cm. of water (EMMETT 1954) which is higher than the pressure required
for normal micturition and would suffice to evacuate the bladder in the absence
of obstruction at the outlet. Hypertrophy of the muscles and failure of the
vesical neck and the sphincters to relax undoubtedly are significant factors in
incomplete emptying of the bladder in the presence of spinal cord lesions. The
assumption that the vesical sphincters constitute an important cause of residual
urine is also supported by consideration of all spinal cord injuries rostral to the
sacral segments as upper motor neuron lesions, since such lesions result in spasticity of the muscles affected. Data advanced by DARST et al. (1951) strongly
suggest that this is a significant factor in relation to residual urine. The two
major factors responsible for residual urine obviously are (1) the resistance to the
outflow from the bladder and (2) inefficient and inadequate expulsion of urine.
It may be impossible in most instances to determine which of these factors is the
more important. It is significant, however, as has been pointed out by EMMETT
(1954), to note that the most significant advances that have been made in the
treatment of neurogenic vesical dysfunction have been directed toward weakening
of the sphincter mechanisms.

9. Bladder dysfunction caused by neural lesions other than partial or complete transection of the spinal cord

Interruption of afferent limbs of reflex arcs. Section of the dorsal
sacral nerve roots in cats (BARRINGTON 1915; DEES and LANGWORTHY 1935) and
dogs (BURNS 1917, 1931) results in inability to carry out normal micturition. The
bladder becomes flaccid with progressive enlargement and dilatation, resulting
in overflow incontinence. Intravesical pressure is low and cystometric records
show no waves of contraction. The flaccid condition of the bladder appears to
be due to interruption of the sacral reflex arcs. The bladder becomes overdistended
due to abolition of the desire to micturate that results from interruption of the
sacral afferent pathways from the bladder (LANGWORTHY et al. 1940). The overdistention results in further damage to the bladder musculature.

Tabes dorsalis. Neurogenic vesical dysfunction associated with tabes dorsalis appears to be due to destruction of the afferent limbs of the sacral reflex
arcs and degeneration of afferent conduction pathways in the spinal cord. The
bladder manifestations of this disease are similar to those produced in experi-

mental animals by section of the dorsal sacral nerve roots. The patient gradually experiences difficulty in voiding and large amounts of residual urine remain in the bladder. Nocturnal incontinence develops gradually, and, as the disease progresses, diurnal incontinence. The bladder becomes large and atonic and may or may not show evidence of trabeculation. Intravesical pressure is low. In the absence of bladder sensations mediated through the sacral nerves the urge to urinate may be completely abolished. If any urge is experienced it occurs only after a very large volume of urine has accumulated in the bladder. The lack of desire to micturate, according to EMMETT (1954), is a significant factor in the accumulation of residual urine. As the bladder becomes increasingly distended it becomes atonic and flaccid and an imbalance between the detrusor muscle and the vesical sphincters develops, which in turn results in residual urine and retention. Under these conditions the vesical neck may obstruct the outflow of urine. Most male patients suffering from tabes dorsalis, furthermore, have reached the age of prostatism, and exhibit some degree of prostatic hyperplasia.

The urinary incontinence associated with tabes dorsalis is of two types: (1) overflow from a greatly distended bladder which occurs as a more or less constant dribble of urine, and (2) involuntary micturition caused by reflex contraction of the bladder. Such involuntary micturition cannot be voluntarily inhibited or postponed. Impulses arising in the bladder and the urethral sphincters are not conducted to the higher neural centers from which the efferent impulses emanate that normally inhibit bladder emptying contractions.

Diabetic neuritis. This is a disease that involves chiefly the sensory nerves. It is characterized by pain, paresthesia and areflexia without corresponding motor impairment. It is frequently accompanied by vesical dysfunction resembling that associated with tabes dorsalis. The vesical dysfunction is characterized by urinary retention in a distended atonic bladder. Its onset and development are usually insidious, so that it may not be recognized until the bladder is markedly enlarged and nocturnal incontinence due to overflow from a distended bladder has set in. The intervals between voiding gradually increase until micturition may be necessary only once or twice daily, but diurnal incontinence may also occur. As in tabes dorsalis, the chief neural factor in the bladder dysfunction is the damage to the afferent limbs of the micturition reflex arcs and the failure of impulses arising in the bladder to be conducted to the appropriate center in the brain stem and the cerebral cortex.

Spina bifida (myelodysplasia). Spina bifida is a congenital defect characterized by failure of fusion of the walls of the neural canal, usually in the sacral segments. The degree of disability associated with it is determined by the extent of the damage to the spinal cord and the nerve roots. Among the functional defects associated with frank spinal bifida may be mentioned flaccid paralysis of the lower extremities, absence of reflexes in the areas affected, impairment or absence of sensation in the perineal region, loss of rectal tonus and urinary incontinence.

The urinary dysfunction associated with spina bifida usually is manifested in varying degrees of incontinence and varying degrees of retention. In some instances, in which the neural defect is very limited, bladder function may be adequate until late in life or until some additional factor causes strain on the bladder musculature (LANGWORTHY, KOLB and LEWIS 1940). In typical cases the intravesical pressure is low and rhythmic contractions are absent or minimal. This suggests involvement predominantly of the afferent nerves. If both the afferent and the efferent nerves were involved the intravesical pressure ought to be higher and the rhythmic contractions stronger and better sustained. The lack of sensory innervation of the perineum undoubtedly is a factor in the incompetence of the external vesical sphincter and possibly the vesical neck. This, in EMMETT's (1954) opinion, sets off the vesical dysfunction associated with spina bifida from that usually associated with transverse spinal cord lesions.

Lesions of the cerebral cortex and projection fibers. Bladder activity, like other visceral functions, is subject to regulatory influences emanating from the cerebral cortex. Patients with vesical dysfunction associated with bilateral lesions of the motor cortex or its projection fibers, as reported by LANGWORTHY et al. (1940), commonly exhibit loss of the ability to initiate micturition easily and to interrupt it voluntarily when once started. The inability to initiate micturition is due to failure of impulses emanating from the cortex to reach the micturition center in the spinal cord. The inability to inhibit micturition voluntarily is due to loss of voluntary control of the external vesical sphincter. Urgency and frequency of urination and consequently incontinence are experienced by these patients even more frequently than the loss of voluntary control. These reactions are due to disordered activity of the sacral micturition center released from cortical control.

Since the activity of the detrusor muscle is built upon the basis of the stretch reflex, it becomes hyperactive in the absence of inhibitory impulses from the cortex. As the bladder fills, therefore, strong contractions of the muscle take place even though the volume of the bladder contents is relatively small. Similar slight responses to stretch take place under normal conditions, but the magnitude of the contractions is not sufficient to expel the urine until filling is completed. The extent of the vesical dysfunction is dependent on the degree of loss of cortical influence on the micturition reflex mechanisms and loss of voluntary control of the external sphincter.

Multiple sclerosis. The most common types of vesical dysfunction associated with multiple sclerosis are (1) urgency and urgency incontinence and (2) obstructive symptoms simulating those of simple obstruction of the vesical neck. Since the sclerotic lesions may involve almost any part of the central nervous system in almost any degree, the vesical dysfunction will vary with the pathways involved. The specific character of the dysfunction is depentent on whether the neural damage involves predominantly afferent or efferent or both afferent and efferent conduction pathways.

PARKINSON's disease. Vesical dysfunction associated with PARKINSON's disease has been reported, but it is not a significant factor in this disease. Only a small percentage of Parkinsonian patients complain of frequency of micturition or urgency and when residual urine becomes a problem it is due to causes other than the neural lesion responsible for the Parkinsonian syndrome. The intravesical pressure is generally high in these patients (WALSHE 1929) and the capacity of the bladder is well below normal. The increased tonus of the bladder musculature prevents normal adaptation to increasing volume (LANGWORTHY et al. 1940), but since the stretch reflex is not hyperactive, urgency is not commonly experienced. Frequency of micturition may result from decreased vesical capacity.

Cerebrovascular accidents. Complete urinary retention is a common immediate result of cerebrovascular accidents. The subsequent state of bladder function is dependent on the degree of recovery. Urgency and urgency incontinence are common, due to the loss of inhibitory impulses emanating from the cortex. Difficulty in the initiation of micturition also occurs frequently. If the lesion is severe and there is little recovery, the continuance of artificial drainage is imperative.

Poliomyelitis. Lesions of poliomyelitis in the sacral spinal cord segments affect primarily the motor neurons, but do not necessarily involve the parasympathetic preganglionic neurons. In many cases, however, the parasympathetic preganglionic neurons are damaged and vesical dysfunction becomes a manifestation of the disease. TOOMEY (1933) observed vesical dysfunction, usually complete vesical paralysis, in 60 of 386 patients during the acute stage of the disease. Urine accumulated even though both the detrusor muscle and the sphincters were paralyzed, and the urethra offered no resistance to the passage of a catheter. In some cases, paralysis of the bladder may be recognized earlier than that of the extremities. In TOOMEY's experience the ability to urinate was usually restored within one week after the onset of the paralysis. WRIGHT (1936) also pointed out that in some instances acute urinary retention is the first indication of the disease. In his experience, disturbed urinary function varied from slowness in starting micturition to complete urinary retention. Urinary disorders occured more frequently in the older than in the younger children.

Of 211 adult patients with poliomyelitis, as reported by WRIGHT, 135 exhibited vesical dysfunction varying from slight, transient dysuria to complete bladder paralysis. In some of these patients urinary incontinence and failure to recognize fullness of the bladder were the earliest indications of the disease.

In most instances the immediate urinary disorder appears to be due to the peripheral neuritis involving the nerves of the bladder. In certain patients, according to WRIGHT, the cause appears to be central. He explained the painful irritable bladders, the spasmodic sphincters and acute retention on this basis, and attributed the remote urinary complications to (a) stretching and overactivity of the bladder musculature during the acute stage of the neuritis when these muscles should have been at rest, (b) the chronic retention due to hypotonia and atony and long periods of supine position, and (c) infection resulting from frequent catherization.

In a man 26 years of age who was completely paralyzed below the level of the umbilicus and showed urinary incontinence with overflow eight weeks after the onset of poliomyelitis, LANGWORTHY et al. (1940) found marked pain on vesical distention, probably related to tenderness of other paralyzed muscles. Intravesical pressure was low and the bladder showed no waves of contraction during or at the end of filling. Some degree of bladder function returned after a few weeks. Two years after the onset of the disease he still had difficulty in initiating the flow of urine. The recovery of bladder function in this patient was much better than that of the skeletal muscle since there had been almost no return of muscle function below the umbilicus.

10. Postoperative urinary retention

Acute urinary retention may occur after surgery in any area, but it occurs frequently after pelvic surgery. The incidence of retention appears to increase with the nearness of the site of operation to the bladder. It is a common complication of inguinal herniorrhaphy and surgery involving the sigmoid colon and the rectum. The vesical dysfunction may vary from moderate difficulty in micturition with varying amounts of residual urine to complete urinary retention. After drainage of the bladder for a week or longer by means of an indwelling catheter, some patients experience difficulty in micturition after the catheter is removed and require intermittent catherization for some time longer. In a small percentage of patients this annoying complication is persistent. In general the urinary retention is transitory and can be relieved by catherization or cholinergic stimulation of the bladder.

The causes of urinary dysfunction associated with surgery are not fully understood. Among those that have been suggested are depression of reflex activity of the bladder due to anesthesia, pain, psychic influences and injury to the pelvic nerves. In many instances vesical dysfunction associated with surgery undoubtedly is neurogenic, due to surgical trauma or actual damage to the pelvic nerves (McCREA 1947). If, however, the pelvic nerves have suffered sufficient damage to account for the complete urinary retention, explanation of the degree of recovery that many of these patients show within a few weeks offers some difficulty. In this connection it is of interest to recall that McCREA and KIMMEL (1952) described a system of nerves that reach the bladder by coursing along blood vessels in the pelvic fascia. Since they do not traverse the pelvic plexus they would be less apt to be damaged by pelvic surgery than the nerves that reach the bladder through the pelvic plexus. McCREA and KIMMEL (1954), on the basis of clinical data, advanced the opinion that normal bladder function can be mediated through these nerves following interruption of the neural pathways that traverse the pelvic plexus.

In corroboration of the neurogenic hypothesis it has been pointed out that cystometrograms frequently show that the bladder is atonic and intravesical pressure is low. The patient, furthermore, has no desire to micturate. The cystometrograms resemble those of tabetic bladders or of bladers with long-standing obstruction at the vesical neck associated with bladder decompensation. In criticism of evidence of this kind, EMMETT (1954) has called attention to the difficulty of understanding how only the sensory nerves become traumatized by surgery.

In many cases the primary cause of vesical dysfunction associated with surgery undoubtedly is obstruction at the neck of the bladder caused by edema, prostatic hyperplasia and injury to supporting structures adjacent to the bladder and the urethra that cause sagging of the bladder (ENGEL 1939; COLLER and EASTMAN 1943). EMMETT and CRISTOL (1944) and EMMETT and BISQUERTT (1947) have supported the hypothesis that the urinary difficulty is due, in most instances, to obstruction at the neck of the bladder and bladder decompensation that have been precipitated by the operative trauma to the bladder, prostate and urethra. A high percentage of the patients in question are males many of whom exhibit prostatism in some degree and have experienced some difficulty in micturition before operation.

References

ALDRIDGE, A. H.: Stress incontinence of urine. J. Obst. Gynaec. Brit. Emp. 59, 681—720 (1952). — ALLEN, W. F.: Formatio reticularis and reticulospinal tracts, their visceral functions and possible relationships to tonicity and clonic contractions. J. Wash. Acad. Sci. 22, 16—17 (1932). — AREY, L. B.: Developmental anatomy, 6th edit. Chapt. VI, The urinary system. Philadelphia: W. B. Saunders Company 1954. — BALL, T. L.: Topographic urethrography. Amer. J. Obstet. Gynec. 59, 1243—1251 (1950). — BALL, T. L., R. G. DOUGLAS and L. L. FULKERSON: Topographic urethrography. Amer. J. Obstet. Gynec. 59, 1252—1259 (1950). — BARRINGTON, F. J. F.: The effect of division of the hypogastric nerves on frequency of micturition. Quart. J. exp. Physiol. 9, 261—264 (1915). — Relations of hindbrain to micturition. Brain 44, 23—53 (1921). — The effect of lesions of the hindbrain and midbrain on micturition in the cat. Quart. J. exp. Physiol. 15, 81—102 (1925). — Affections of micurition resulting from lesions of nervous system. Proc. roy. Soc. Med., see Urol. 20, 22—27) (1927). — Central nervous control of micturition. Brain 51, 209—220 (1928). — The component reflexes of micturition in cat. Brain 64, 239—243 (1942). — BEATTIE, J., and A. S. KERR: Effects of diencephalic stimulation of urinary bladder tonus. Brain 59,

302—314 (1936). — Best, C. H., and N. B. Taylor: The physiological basis of medical practice, 4th edit. Baltimore: Williams & Wilkins Company 1945. — Boeke, J.: The problem of interstitial cells in the nervous endformation. Proc. kon. med. Akad. Wet. 14, 1—8 (1942). — The sympathetic end-formation, its synaptology, the interstitial cells, the periterminal network and its bearing on the neuron theory. Discussion and critique. Acta anat. (Basel) 8, 18—161 (1949). — Bors, E.: Neurogenic bladder. In G. M. Piersol, The encyclopedia of medicine, surgery, vol. 9, p. 603—614. Specialties, F. A. Davis Co. 1951. — Effect of eletric stimulation of the pudenal nerves in the vesical neck; its significance for function of cord bladder: preliminary report. J. Urol. (Baltimore) 67, 925—935 (1952). — Bostock, J., and M. G. Shackleton: Enuresis and toilet training. Med. J. Aust. 2, 100—113 (1951). — Burns, J. E.: The bladder changes due to lesions of the central nervous system. Surg. Gynec. Obstet. 24, 659—668 (1917). — Burns, J. E., and F. C. Helwig: Bladder disturbances in relation to abnormalities of lumbosacral spine. Trans. Amer. Ass. gen.-urin. Surg. 24, 323—339 (1931). — Campbell, M. F.: Diverticula of urethra. J. Urol. (Baltimore) 30, 113—121 (1933). — Dwarf bladder. Pediatric urology, vol. 1, p. 294. New York: Macmillan & Co. 1937. — Anomalies of the urethra. In Urology, vol. 1, sec. IV, p. 408—452. Philadelphia: W. B. Saunders Company 1954. — Cloake, P. C., J. R. Learmonth and F. J. F. Barrington: Discussion on innervation of bladder. Proc. roy. Soc. Med. 25, 547—561 (1932). — Coller, F. A., and P. F. Eastman: Urinary retention following combined abdominoperineal resection. Surgery 14, 223—228 (1943). — Crosby, N. D.: Essential enuresis: successful treatment based on physiological concepts. Med. J. Aust. 2, 533—543 (1950). — Dees, J. E., and O. R. Langworthy: Experimental study of bladder disturbances analogous to those of tabes dorsalis. J. Urol. (Baltimore) 34, 359—371 (1935). — Denning, H.: Untersuchungen über die Innervation der Harnblase und des Mastdarmes. Z. Biol. 80, 239—254 (1924). — Denny-Brown, D., and E. G. Robertson: On physiology of micturition. Brain 56, 149—190 (1933). — Duzen, R. E. van: Effect of resection of presacral nerve on vesical function. Sth. med. J. (Bgham, Ala.) 25, 964—967 (1932). — Anatomy of the prostate and vesical neck. Sth. med. J. (Bgham, Ala.) 28, 785—791 (1935). — Duzen, R. E. van, and C. G. Duncan: Anatomy and nerve supply of urinary bladder. J. Amer. med. Ass. 153, 1345—1347 (1953). — Elliott, T. R.: The innervation of the bladder and urethra. J. Physiol. (Lond.) 35, 367—445 (1907). — Emmett, J. L.: Urology. Sect. XI, chapt. 1, Physiology of normal bladder: neurophysiology of micturition; chapt. 2, neurogenic vesical dysfunction (cord bladder) and neuromuscular ureteral dysfunction. Edited by F. Meredith Campbell: Philadelphia: W. B. Saunders Company 1954. — Emmett, J. L., and J. E. Bisquertt: Transurethral resection in treatment of vesical dysfunction secondary to inflammatory degenerative and traumatic lesions of spinal cord. S. Clin. N. Amer. 27, 950—977 (1947). — Emmett, J. L., and D. S. Cristol: Urinary retention following surgical operation on rectum and sigmoid; treatment by transurethral resection. J. Amer. med. Ass. 126, 1077—1079 (1944). — Evans, J. P.: Observations on the nerves of supply to the bladder and urethra of the cat, with a study their action potentials. J. Physiol. (Lond.) 86, 396—414 (1936). — Frohlich, A., and H. H. Meyer: Visceral sensibility. Klin. Wschr. 1, 1368—1369 (1922). — Goltz, F.: Über den Einfluß des Nervensystems auf die Vorgänge während der Schwangerschaft und des Gebärakts. Pflügers Arch. ges. Physiol. 60, 552—565 (1874). — Goltz, F., u. J. R. Ewald: Der Hund mit verkürzten Rückenmark. Pflügers Arch. ges. Physiol. 68, 362—400 (1896). — Grossman, R. G., S. C. Wang: Diencephalic mechanism of control of the urinary bladder of cat. Yale J. Biol. Med. 28, 285—297 (1956). — Gruber, C. M.: The autonomic innervation of the genito-urinary organs. Physiol. Rev. 13, 497—609 (1933). — Hegre, E. S., and E. H. Ingersoll: Analysis of regional variations in response of detrusor muscle to electrical stimulations of hypogastric nerves. J. Urol. (Baltimore) 61, 1037—1047 (1949). — Henderson, V. E., and M. H. Roepke: Role of acetylcholine in bladder contractile mechanisms and in parasympathetic ganglia. J. Pharmacol. exp. Ther. 51, 97—111 (1934). — Herbut, P. A.: Urological pathology. Vol. 1, chapt. II, Urethra. Philadelphia: Lea and Febiger 1952. — Hess, W. R., u. M. Brugger: Der Miktions- und der Defäkationsakt als Erfolg zentraler Reizung. Helv. physiol. pharmacol. Acta 1, 511 (1943). — Holmes, G.: Observations on the paralyzed bladder. Brain 56, 383—396 (1953). — Hubble, D.: Enuresis. Brit. med. J. 1950, 1108—1111. — Huber, H. G.: Nabelkoliken bei Doppelbildung mit Verengung des Ureters. Kinderärztl. Prax. 7, 254 (1936). — Ingersoll, E. H., and E. S. Hegre: Spontaneous activity of detrusor muscle in cat. J. Urol. (Baltimore) 66, 758—764 (1951). — Ingersoll, E. H., L. L. Jones and E. S. Hegre: Urinary bladder response to unilateral stimulation of hypogastric nerves. J. Urol. (Baltimore) 72, 178—190 (1954). — Urinary bladder response to unilateral stimulation of pelvic nerves. Proc. Soc. exp. Biol. (N.Y.) 88, 46—49 (1955). — Jabonero, V.: Die interstitiellen Zellen des vegetativen Nervensystems mit ihrer vermutlichen Analogie zu anderen Elementen. I und II. Acta neurovegetativa 5, 1—24, 266—280 (1952). — Jabonero, V., P. Gomez-Bosque, F. Bordallo u.

J. PEREZ CASIS: Der anatomische Aufbau des peripheren vegetativen Systems. Acta neuroveg. (Wien) Suppl. 4, 1—159 (1953). — JACOBSON jr., C. E.: Neurogenic vesical dysfunction;
experimental study. J. Urol. (Baltimore) 53, 670—695 (1945). — JEFFCOATE, T. N. A., and
H. ROBERTS: Observations on stress incontinence of urine. Amer. J. Obstet. Gynec. 64,
721—738 (1952). — Stress incontinence of urine. J. Obstet. Gynaec. Brit. Emp. 59, 685—697
(1952). — JOHNSON, S. H., III and M. MARSHALL jr.: Enuresis. J. Urol. (Baltimore) 71,
554—559 (1954). — KABAT, H., H. W. MAGOUN and S. W. RANSON: Reaction of bladder
to stimulation of points in forebrain and mid-brain. J. comp. Neurol. 63, 211—239 (1936). —
KLEYNTJENS, F., and O. R. LANGWORTHY: Sensory nerve endings on smooth muscle of
urinary bladder. J. comp. Neurol. 67, 367—380 (1937). — KRANTZ, K. E.: The anatomy of
the urethra and anterior vaginal wall. Amer. J. Obstet. Gynec. 62, 374—386 (1951). —
KRETSCHMER, H. L.: Diverticula of the anterior urethra in male children. Surg. Gynec.
Obstet. 62, 634 (1936). — KUHN, R. A.: Note on the identification of motor supply to detrusor
during anterior dorsolumbar rhizotomy. J. Neurosurg. 6, 320—323 (1949). — KUNTZ, A.:
Visceral functions of nervous system. Ann. Rev. Physiol. 14, 409—432 (1949). — Origin
and early development of pelvic neural plexuses. J. comp. Neurol. 96, 345—357 (1952). —
KUNTZ, A., and R. L. MOSELEY: Experimental analysis of pelvec autonomic ganglia in cat.
J. comp. Neurol. 64, 63—75 (1936). — KUNTZ, A., and L. M. NAPOLITANO: Autonomic
neuroeffector formations. J. comp. Neurol. 104, 17—31 (1956). — KUNTZ, A., and G. SACCO-
MANNO: Reflex inhibition of intestinal motility mediated through decentralized prevertebral
ganglia. J. Neurophysiol. 7, 163—170 (1944). — LANGWORTHY, O. R., and L. C. KOLB:
Encephalic control of tone in musculature of urinary bladder. Brain 56, 371—382 (1933). —
Demonstration of encephalic control of micturition by electrical stimulation. Bull. Johns
Hopk. Hosp. 56, 37 (1935). — LANGWORTHY, O. R., L. C. KOLB and L. G. LEWIS: Physio-
logy of micturition. Baltimore: Williams & Wilkins Company 1940. — LANGWORTHY, O. R.,
and E. L. MURPHY: Nerve endings in urinary bladder. J. comp. Neurol. 71, 487—509 (1939). —
LANGWORTHY, O. R., D. L. REEVES and E. S. TAUBER: Autonomic control of urinary bladder.
Brain 57, 266—290 (1934). — LAWSON, J. D., and W. B. TOMLINSON: Observations on
dynamics of acute urinary retention in dog. J. Urol. (Baltimore) 66, 678—685 (1951). —
LEARMONTH, J. R.: Contribution to neurophysiology of urinary bladder in man. Brain 54,
147—176 (1931). — Neurosurgery in treatment of diseases of urinary bladder; anatomic
and surgical considerations. J. Urol. (Baltimore) 25, 531—549 (1931). — Neurosurgery in
treatment of diseases of urinary bladder; treatment of vesical pain. J. Urol. (Baltimore)
26, 13—24 (1931). — Neurosurgery in treatment of diseases of urinary bladder; treatment
of certain types of vesical paralysis. J. Urol. (Baltimore) 26, 229—232 (1931). — LEEUWE, H.:
Over de interstitielle cel (Cajal). Diss. Utrecht 1937. — MAGOUN, H. W.: Descending connections from hypothalamus. A. Research. Nerv. & Ment. Dis., Proc. 1939 20, 270—285
(1940). — MARSHALL, C. J.: Peristent adult bed-wetting treated by sacral neurotomy.
Brit. med. J. 1954 I, 308—311. — MCCREA, L. E.: Vesical dysfunction following recto-
sigmoid resection. Urol. cutan. Rev. 50, 710—712 (1946). — Management of vesical dysfunction following operation on lower bowel. Med. Rec. (Houston) 41, 312—315 (1947). —
MCCREA, L. E., and D. L. KIMMELL: A new concept of vesical innervation and its relationship
to bladder management following abdominoperineal proctosigmoidectomy. Amer. J. Surg.
84, 518—523 (1952). — MCLELLAN, F. C.: The neurogenic bladder. Springfield, Ill.: Ch. C.
Thomas 1939. — MELLANBY, J., and C. L. G. PRATT: Reactions of urinary bladder of cat
under conditions of constant volume. Proc. roy. Soc. B 128, 186—201 (1940). — MEYLING,
H. A.: Structure and significance of peripheral extension of autonomic nervous system.
J. comp. Neurol. 99, 495—543 (1953). — MIKULICZ-RADECKI, F.: Röntgenologische Studien
zur Ätiologie der urethralen Inkontinenz. Zbl. Gynäk. 55, 795—810 (1931). — MOORE,
J. G.: Stress incontinence of urine; considerations of etiologic factors in women. Calif.
Med. 78, 227—231 (1953). — MOORE, T.: Bladder neck obstruction in women. Proc. roy.
Soc. Med. 46, 558—563 (1953). — MOSELEY, R. L.: Preganglionic connections of intramural
ganglia of urinary bladder. Proc. Soc. exp. Biol. (N.Y.) 34, 728—730 (1936). — MUELLNER,
S. R.: The physiology of micturition. Its clinical application. Bull. New Engl. Med. Cent.
12, 93 (1950). — MUNRO, D.: Anterior-rootlet rhizotomy; method of controlling spasm with
retention of voluntary motion. NEW ENGL. J. Med. 246, 161—166 (1952). — NATHAN, P. W.:
Micturition reflexes in man. J. Neurol. Neurosurg. Psychiat. 15, 148—149 (1952). — Thermal
sensation in the bladder. J. Neurol. Neurosurg. Psychiat. 15, 150—151 (1952). — NATHAN,
P. W., and M. C. SMITH: The centripetal pathway from the bladder and urethra within the
spinal cord. J. Neurol. Neurosurg. Psychiat. 14, 262—280 (1951). — Spinal pathways subserving defecation and sensation from the lower bowel. J. Neurol., Neurosurg. Psychiat.
16, 245—256 (1953). — NELEMANS, F. A.: The innervation of the smallest blood vessels.
Amer. J. Anat. 83, 43—66 (1948). — NESBIT, R. M., and W. G. GORDON: Management of
urinary bladder in traumatic lesions of spinal cord and cauda equina. Surg. Gynec. Obstet.
72, 328—331 (1941). — NONIDEZ, J. F.: Studies on innervation of heart; distribution of

cardiac nerves with special reference to identification of sympathetic and parasympathetic postganglionics. Amer. J. Anat. 65, 361—413 (1939). — POWELL, T. A.: Clinical management of urinary retention in children. J. Amer. med. Ass. 153, 1341—1345 (1953). — ROBERTS, H.: Cystourethrography in women. Brit. J. Radiol. 25, 253—259 (1952). — ROEN, P. R., and R. R. STEPT: Urethritis in girls. Amer. J. Dis. Child. 72, 529—535 (1946). — ROSS, J. C.: Treatment of the bladder in paraplegia. Brit. J. Urol. 28, 14—23 (1956). — ROTHFELD, S. H., and A. M. RABINER: Vesical sphincter and nervous system; note on pathways conducting cerebral control of micturition. N.Y. J. Med. 54, 368—371 (1954). — RUBIN, S. W., and H. NAGEL: Nocturia in aged. J. Amer. med. Ass. 147, 840—841 (1951). — SCHABA-DASCH, A.: Studien über Architektonik des vegetativen Nervensystems und intramurale Nervengeflechte der Harnblase und des Harnleiters. Z. Zellforsch. 21, 657—732 (1934). — SCHER, S.: Some observations on anatomy of bladder neck and posterior urethra with reference to prostatic observation. Brit. J. Urol. 22, 116—124 (1950). — SCHLESINGER, H.: Der Bauchdecken-Austreibungsreflex der Harnblase. Ein bisher unbekannter therapeutisch verwertbarer Reflex. Med. Klin. 29, 538—539 (1933). — SCHUBERT, E.: Topographie der Harnblase in Schwangerschaft, Geburt und Wochenbett. Zbl. Gynäk. 53, 2541—2550 (1929). — Topographie des Uterus und der Harnblase im Röntgenprofilbild. Zbl. Gynäk. 53, 1182—1193 (1929). — SEMBA, T., H. MISHIMA and T. DATE: Studies on a vesico-anal inhibitory reflex. Jap. J. Physiol. 6, 108—111 (1956). — SEMBA, T., H. MISHIMA and T. HIRAOKA: A motor reflex from the urinary bladder to the colon. Jap. J. Physiol. 6, 112—117 (1956). — SENGER, F. L., and V. J. SANTARE: Congenital multilocular bladder. Trans. Amer. Ass. gen.-urin. Surg. 43, 114 (1951). — SHERRINGTON, C. S.: Experiments in examination of peripheral distribution of the fibers of the posterior roots of some spinal nerves. Proc. roy. Soc. 52, 333—337 (1892). — The spinal cord. Chapter in E. A. SCHAFER's Textbook of physiology, p. 783—883. New York: Macmillan & Co. 1900. (See sections on visceral reflexes and urinary bladder.) — SPOERRI, R.: Histological studies on nerve elements and their endings at the epithelial cells of the gastric mucosa. J. comp. Neurol. 90, 151—171 (1949). — STEWART, C. C.: The relaxation of the bladder muscles of cat. Amer. J. Physiol. 8, 8 (1899). — Mammalian smooth muscle; the cat's bladder. Amer. J. Physiol. 8, 185—208 (1900). — STOHR jr., P.: Beobachtungen und Bemerkungen über die Endausbreitung des vegetativen Nervensystems. Z. Anat. Entwickl.-Gesch. 104, 133—158 (1935). — Bemerkungen über die Endigungsweise des vegetativen Nervensystems und über den Aufbau des Organismus. Acta neuroveg. (Wien) 1, 74—86 (1950). — STROM, G., and B. UVNAS: Motor responses of gastrointestinal tract and bladder to topical stimulation of frontal lobe, basal ganglia and hypothalamus in cat. Acta physiol. scand. 21, 90—104 (1950). — SWENSON, O.: New concept of pathology of megaloureters. Surgery 32, 367—371 (1952). — TALAAT, M.: Afferent impulses in nerves supplying urinary bladder. J. Physiol. (Lond.) 89, 1—13 (1937). — TANG, P. C., and T. C. RUCH: Non-neurogenic basis of bladder tonus. Amer. J. Physiol. 181, 249—257 (1955). — THOMPSON, G. J.: Practical points in management of cord bladder. J. Amer. med. Ass. 153, 1337—1341 (1953). — TOOMEY, J. A.: Intestine and urinary bladder in poliomyelitis. Amer. J. Dis. Child. 45, 1211—1215 (1933). — WALSHE, F. M. R.: Oliver-Sharpey lectures on physiological analysis of some clincially observed disorders of movement; tremor-rigidity, symptom complex. Lancet 1929 I, 1024—1029. — WALTZ, W.: Über die Blasensensibilität. Dtsch. Z. Nervenheilk. 74, 278—284 (1922). — WANG, S. C., and G. CLARK: Descussation of sacral autonomic pathways of bladder from hypothalamus. Amer. J. Physiol. 130, 74—80 (1940). — WANG, S. C., and F. HARRISON: Nature of bladder responses following stimulation of anterior hypothalamus. Amer. J. Physiol. 125, 301—309 (1939). — WANG, S. C., and S. C. RANSON: Descending pathways from the hypothalamus to the medulla and spinal cord: observation on blood pressure and bladder responses. J. comp. Neurol. 71, 457 (1939). — WEHRBEIN, H. L.: Double kidney, double ureter and bilocular bladder in child. J. Urol. (Baltimore) 43, 804—810 (1940). — WRIGHT, B. W.: Urinary complications in epidemic of poliomyelitis. J. Urol. (Baltimore) 35, 618—629 (1936). — YOUNG, H. H.: Changes in the trigone due to tuberculosis. Surg. Gynec. Obstet. 26, 603—615 (1918). — Prostatic surgery. Sth. med. J. (Bgham, Ala.) 30, 1157—1162 (1937). — Diagnosis and therapeutic indications of various diseases of prostate. Med. Clin. N. Amer. 21, 1417—1447 (1937). — YOUNG, H. H., and D. I. MACHT: The physiology of micturition. J. Pharmacol. 12, 329—354 (1923). — YOUNG, H. H., and M. B. WESSON: The Anatomy and surgery of the trigon. Arch. Surg. (Chicago) 3, 1—37 (1921).

The physiology and physiopathology of the male sexual glands

By

D. F. McDONALD

With 17 figures

A. Testis

I. Anatomy, growth, function and development

1. Fetal testis

During the formation of the embryo, the first sexual structures to develop are the fetal testes. This is followed by differentiation of the genital tracts and accessory organs from a dual set of sex ducts and from common primordia. The testis is probably important in the differentiation of the genital tract in the male by the elaboration of hormonal factors, JOST. The hormonal theory of differentiation is supported by the fact that ablation of the genital ridge in placental animals results in a feminine differentiation in the fetus whether the removed tissue was ovary or testis. If the testis is removed after sex differentiation has begun, however, it proceeds in the development of male genitalia. From these observations, it is concluded that the fetal testicular hormone has a stimulative effect on the Wolffian duct and common primordia and an inhibitory action on the Müllerian structures. Presence of testicular hormone has not been detected in the very young embryo during the critical period of sex differentiation but androgens have been extracted from sex differentiated bovine fetal testis and fetal rats. The fetal testicular hormone produced during sexual differentiation resembles adult androgenic hormone in its ability to stimulate the development of male organs (Wolffian duct, urogenital sinus and external genitalia). However, the adult androgenic hormone lacks the ability to suppress the development of the Müllerian duct system. It may be that more than one hormone is elaborated by the fetal testis. The cellular origin of testicular hormone is not known. Large numbers of interstitial cells appear in the testis late in embryogenesis that are similar to Leydig cells. These are apparently stimulated to develop by maternal gonadotropins. Their presence in the fetal testis suggests that androgenic hormone may be secreted. This may be similar to adult testicular androgenic hormone and may participate in the final sexual development and descent of the testis into the scrotum.

The elaboration of a fetal testicular hormone may be controlled by the hypophysis. Decapitation in the rabbit prior to the stage of sex differentiation produces sexual modification. This is not so in the mouse and rat. Human anencephalic monsters are females in the great majority, PERRIN. However, there is no evidence in man that hypophyseal control is present.

The germinal epithelium begins to develop during the fifth and sixth weeks of embryonic life. At first a superficial layer of cells separates from a thickening of the peritoneum near the urogenital ridge to form the germinal epithelium. These ridges of germinal epithelium contain primordial germ cells which are isosexual. The germ cells lie within a mass of proliferating epithelium. They then separate and begin to branch into cords. By the seventh week, the differentiation has progressed sufficiently to distinguish testicular from ovarian tissue.

The testis cords converge in a radial fashion to form the mesorchium which soon becomes attached to the gonadal mesentery, the rete testis. The seminiferous tubules are soon recognizable. Two groups of tubules are distinguishable. Those adjacent to the rete testis are known as tubuli recti. The distal tubules are the tubuli contorti. The seminiferous tubules have two cell types, the spermatogonia and undifferentiated cells. The latter at puberty mature as Sertoli cells. The seminiferous tubules are separated by connective tissue radials which connect to the tunica albuginea on the surface and contain the large, pale staining Leydig cells in the intratesticular portion. The Leydig cells appear late in the prenatal period presumably as a result of a maternal chorionic gonadotropic hormone influence.

2. Pre-puberal testis

Until the onset of puberty, there is little change from the neonatal testis in size and weight. The cells in the seminiferous tubulus are enclosed by a thin basement membrane. The tubules are solidly packed with undifferentiated cells and spermatogonia. The abundant undifferentiated cells have large sharply defined nuclei that are either oval or round with coarse chromatin granules. The cytoplasm is pale staining and poorly outlined. A few spermatogonia are distinguished by larger round nuclei with large clumps of chromatin, lying on a clearly defined basement membrane. Sertoli cells are not yet recognizable. The connective tissue between the tubules contains large numbers of fibroblasts. In the first few months of neonatal life, Leydig interstitial cells are present. They then disappear to reappear with the onset of adolescence. The Leydig cells are large, often polygonal in shape with a central or eccentric nucleus and a nucleolus. Coarse clumps of chromatin are often condensed along a distinct nuclear membrane. The cytoplasm is abundant, well outlined and contains granules. In the pre-puberal testis, ROOSEN-RUNGE and BARLOW found cells which have nuclei similar to the Leydig cell but the cytoplasm was sparse. They did not appear to be hormonally active.

3. Puberal testis

During puberty, DeROBERTS and coauthors report that the seminiferous tubules enlarged from a pre-puberal diameter of 40—80 μ to 150—250 μ. They grew longer, became tortuous, and tubular lumens appeared. The spermatogonia began to show more mature forms as spermatogenesis began. Spermatogonia, primary and secondary spermatocytes, spermatids and finally spermatozoa were seen. Sertoli cells appeared in the seminiferous tubules from the undifferentiated cells as larger with a nucleolus. The basement membrane lining the tubules thickened and acquired elastic fibers. In the interstitium, Leydig cells made their reappearance in small groups around blood vessels. The interstitial tissue was compressed by the enlarging tubular elements.

At the time of puberty, the testis and the adenohypophysis engage in a permanent reciprocal relationship. The pituitary gonadotrophins stimulate and regulate testicular function. In turn, the testis exerts hormonal control of the production of stimulating hormones from the pituitary.

Gonadotrophins, secreted by the anterior lobe of the pituitary, are similar in males and females, Witschi. The human male pituitary has been shown to contain three gonadotrophins. FSH (follicle stimulating hormone) acts on the epithelium of the seminiferous tubules to stimulate spermatogenesis. Luteinizing hormone (LH) or interstitial cell stimulating hormone (ICSH) stimulates the Leydig cells to elaborate testosterone. Luteotrophic hormone, which is present in males and females, maintains the corpus luteum. FSH and LH are produced by the basophilic cells of the pituitary. Luteinizing hormone is also known as the lactogenic principle.

The pituitary gonadotrophic function is regulated, in part, by environmental factors in some species (Cowie). They have no effect in man in normal physiologic terms. The hypothalamus may have an important role in the secretion of gonadotrophins by the pituitary. Very little of the mechanism is known in man, but some conclusions may be drawn from animal experimentation. Destruction of the anterior portion of the hypothalamus produces a decrease in the secretion of hormones from the anterior pituitary. Stimulation appears to increase secretions. Two pathways are hypothesized. One is the hypothalamo-hypophyseal nerve tract which ends in the posterior pituitary (Green and Harris). The other is a vascular connection, the hypophyseal portal system (Green). This conducts blood from the median eminence of the hypothalamus into the pituitary. This appears to be particularly important in gonadotrophin secretion because destruction of this area leads to gonadal atrophy without the other signs of hypopituitism in rat. In the ferret this is not so; pituitary gonadotrophic activity is uninterrupted.

Inanition produces gonadal hypofunction and atrophy in the experimental animal (Werner). Pituitary gonadotrophic activity declines early in the course of starvation. There is evidence that this is due to deficiencies of the B vitamins (Meites). Direct influence of the pituitary gonadotrophins is best demonstrated by the administration of adequate amounts of FSH and ICSH to immature animals. Gonadal maturation and pubescent changes occur. In the hypophysectomized animals, seminiferous tubules degenerate, interstitial cells disappear and the testes become soft and atrophic. None of the pituitary hormones can completely replace the others in gonadotrophic activity. Their effects on the testis are synergistic. Administration of FSH to the hypophysectomized animal maintains spermatogenesis, but at an immature level. Leydig cell atrophy occurs. ICSH alone will produce Leydig cell hyperplasia and tend to restore some of the seminiferous tubule activity. Combination of ICSH and FSH will produce histologic growth and development of the testis as well as development of secondary sex characteristics. The addition of luteotrophic hormone and growth hormone further restores the testis to normal, however, no specific histologic defect can be seen in the absence of these.

The administration of androgenic compounds to the newly hypophysectomized animal can prevent spermatogenic involution (Nelson). If this is attempted too late, tubular atrophy and sclerosis occurs. In hypogonadotrophic eunuchoid males, the administration of chorionic gonadotrophin results in Leydig cell hyperplasia and increase in size of the seminiferous tubules. Chorionic gonadotrophin has an ICSH like activity which increases urinary 17 ketosteroid excretion. There is no spermatogenic activity. However, when FSH is added to the regimen, all stages of spermatogenesis are seen.

Under varying physiological conditions, the pituitary responds to changes in the hormonal secretion of the testis by altering the secretion of gonadotrophins. Histologic changes in the pituitary occur after castration in man

(BIGGART) and rat (LEHMAN). These consist of the appearance of large vacuolated basophilic cells, the "castration cell" in the anterior lobe. The increased gonadotrophic activity consists of secretion of FSH and ICSH, FSH being secreted in larger quantities than ICSH. Similar changes are seen after irradiation, sterilization, and surgically induced cryptorchidism. These artificial situations produce mainly seminiferous tubular degeneration and do not greatly disturb physiology or histology of the interstitial cells. In the normal state, then, there appears to be a substance that has the ability to inhibit the secretion of FSH and prevents the "castration cells" from appearing in the pituitary. This substance has been termed "inhibin or X hormone". Its existence has not been conclusively proven. After castration, hypersecretion of gonadotrophins can be prevented by the administration of testosterone. It has also been found that androgen administration decreased FSH secretion in both sexes (HELLER and NELSON). In the adult male, castration produces increased gonadotrophin excretion as does removal of the ovaries in the adult female. In cryptorchidism and certain types of seminiferous tubular atrophy and sclerosis, increased gonadotrophin secretion occurs. These conditions generally show little change in Leydig cell formation.

The administration of large doses of androgens and estrogens lowers gonadotrophin secretion in the human much as it does in lower animals. FSH is primarily affected. Estrogen and androgen suppress adenohypophyseal activity. Estrogen is more potent.

4. Adult testis

a) Spermatogenesis

The adult seminiferous tubule measures 150—250 μ. Its epithelium consists of two cell types, the spermatogenic cells (in all stages of maturation), and the Sertoli cells. The seminiferous tubules occupy about two-third the total volume of the testis. ROOSE-RUNGE calculated that of the volume of the seminiferous tubule, about one-half is accounted for by the spermatogenic series of cells and one-third by the Sertoli cells. The process of spermatogenesis is not uniform in the human seminiferous tubule. Varying stages of development will be found in adjacent areas of a tubule. Nevertheless, in any given area of a tubule, most of the cells will be near the same developmental stage.

The peripheral layer of cells in the active seminiferous tubule has two cell types: the Sertoli cell and the spermatogonium. They are derived from the primitive seminiferous cords of the coelomic epithelium. The spermatogonia are precursors of gametes while the Sertoli cells appear to serve as supportive and nutritive elements. Spermatogenesis consists of the proliferation of large numbers of spermatogonia and a succession of morphologic and chromosomal changes resulting in the production of spermatozoa. The morphologic transformation of the precursor cells involved in spermatogenesis (spermatids) into the mature spermatozoa is calles spermiogenesis. The precursors of the spermatogenic cells are the spermatogonia. They are in contact with the basement membrane at the periphery of the seminiferous tubule and constitute the outermost of 4—8 layers of spermatogenic cells. They are round or cuboidal with a diameter of 4—12 μ. The nucleus is round and highly chromatic. The structure of the spermatogonia is similar to that seen in the fetal and prepuberal testes. The spermatogonia undergo marked proliferation by ordinary mitotic division, each cell having 48 chromosomes. This is known as the preliminary period of proliferation and produces several generations of spermatogonia which become slightly smaller as they are pushed to the center of the tubule. Some spermatogonia remain at the periphery to serve as a future source of spermatozoa. The centrally located spermatogonia undergo active proliferation and enlargement to produce primary spermatocytes which are located still more centrally and have a diameter of 18 μ. The nucleus shows considerable mitotic activity. After attaining full development, the primary spermatocyte divides to produce two centrally located secondary spermatocytes with a diameter of 12 μ. These then rapidly divide again to form two spermatids. They have a diameter of 9 μ and lie in the lumen of the tubule. The two maturation divisions result in four spermatids which are haploid (24 chromosomes). The cell division resulting in decreasing the chromosome number is called meiosis. Since the sex chromosomes of the male are X and Y, half of the spermatids contain an X chromosome and half contain a Y chromosome. The two mitotic divisions differ from each other. The first includes a reduction in chromosome number and results in a separation of pairs of chromosomes. Each chromosome divides longitudinally to form two chromatids. Genetic material is interchanged in the division. The daughter cell is composed of 12 pairs of chromosomes as compared to 24 in the mother cell. The cells contain genes from either parent. The second division is mitotic but haploid in nature. Each spermatid thus contains 12 pairs of chromosomes and all of the chromosomes are identical. A single chromosome in the parent cell may undergo a reductional or an equational division in either the first or the second miotic division. Thus the process of spermatogenic maturation serves two functions. First, it is essential that the spermatozoon (gamete) contain a haploid number of chromosomes. Second, the reduction division results in a random distribution of paternal genes. The daughter germ cell may contain a distinctly unique collection of genes providing for a diversity in the offspring. Spermiogenesis is the transformation of spermatids into mature spermatozoa. The spermatids are attached to the Sertoli cells from which they apparently derive their nourishment.

b) Sperm morphology

The head of the spermatozoon is derived from the nucleus and part of the cytoplasm. The Golgi, mitochondria, and cytoplasmic material contribute to the formation of the tail and sheath. The human spermatozoon is 55—65 μ long. With the light microscope and ordinary magnification, only a head and tail can be distinguished. SCHULTZ-LARSEN with use of higher magnification or electron-microscopy, discerned a short neck and two parts to the tail. Proximally it has a long whipping tail with a distal terminal filament. In the formation of the head of the spermatozoon, the principle changes involve the centrioles and acroblast. The anterior part of the head becomes covered by the acroblast. This surface membrane is derived from part of the Golgi apparatus. The head is oval or elliptic when viewed from its flattened aspect and pear shaped when seen laterally. It measures 4—5 μ in length and 3 μ in width. About one-third of the head was observed by SCHNALL to be occupied by the acrosome and two-thirds by the nucleus. The acrosome usually contains 1—3 vacuoles. It is covered by a thin clear cup-like structure. The mechanism of formation of the neck piece is not conclusive. It may be formed as described by AREY and MAXIMOW and BLOOM from the distal and proximal centrioles together or it may be comprised of just the proximal centriole with the distal centriole situated at the caudal end of the neck. The neck is a fragile structure, the weakest part of the cell. It is approximately 5 μ long. Two thickened areas are noted proximally and distally, the anterior and posterior knobs. Through the neck run long fibrils grouped into two fasicles. Posterior to the short neck WILLIAMS described a body that is thicker than the neck and cylindrical or spindle shaped when viewed in the light microscope. Under the electron microscope, SCHNALL showed it to be narrower than the neck. Its central core contains the axial filament that begins in the foremost part of the neck in the anterior end knob. The axial filament is a continuation of the fasicles described in the neck. An axial sheath covers the axial filament. This in turn is surrounded by JENSEN's spiral body, a sheath of mitochondrial origin that wraps around the axial filament in 6—15 turns (CULP and BEST). Enclosing the entire middle piece, SCHULTZ-LARSEN described a cytoplasmic sheath containing microsomes. At the distal limit of the middle piece is a disc, JENSEN's ring, through which the axial filament courses. It is apparently derived from the distal centriole. The tail is about 40—50 μ long with a terminal filament of 5—10 μ in length. The terminal filament is comprised of 9—11 fibrils and is surrounded by a translucent sheath which is absent distally leaving the end piece exposed. Tightly wound around the axis and its sheath is an extremely fine cortical helix. These fibrils begin at JENSEN's ring and continue the entire length of the tail. The presence of the end piece in man is not conclusive.

The Sertoli cells as described by SNIFFEN are arranged radially, extending from the basement membrane to the lumen. The eosinophilic cytoplasm is reticulated and contains waxy fibrils, fine granules staining with iron hematoxylin, mitochondria, lipid droplets and a crystalloid body.

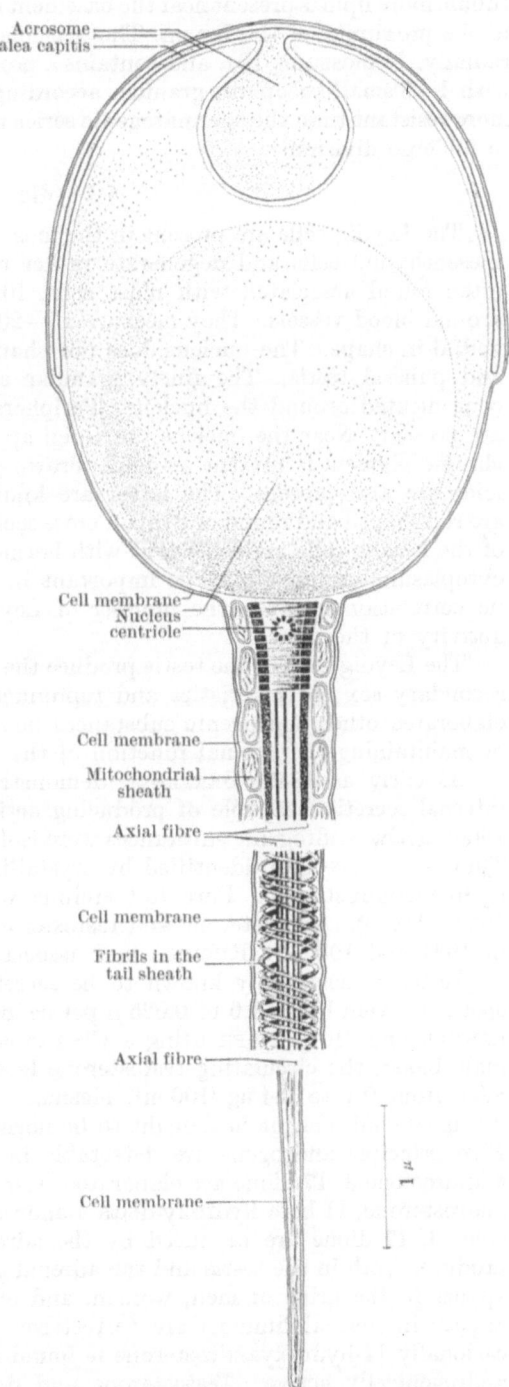

Fig. 1. Sperm morphology as learned through electron microscopy (after SCHULTZ-LARSEN 1958). "Frontal" section

There is a variation in the amount of lipid content of the Sertoli cells. In the normal tubule more lipid is present near the basement membrane and in larger droplets than in the proximity of the lumen. The vesicular nucleus has its long axis directed radially. It measures $10\,\mu$ and contains a prominent nucleolus that is eosinophilic with 1—3 small basophilic granules according to Maximow and Bloom. They are more resistant than the spermatogenic series to noxious stimuli and do not appear to undergo division.

c) Leydig cells

The Leydig cells are present in the loose interstitial stroma. They arise from mesenchymal cells and degenerate rather than revert to fibroblasts. They are often found associated with mast cells, fibroblasts and histiocytes in clusters around blood vessels. They measure 15—$20\,\mu$ in diameter and are oval or polyhedral in shape. The nucleus does not change from that seen in the prepuberal and puberal testis. The finely granular eosinophilic cytoplasm is apt to be concentrated around the nucleus. Peripherally fat droplets and small vacuoles are present. Near the nucleus the Golgi apparatus encircles a clear zone. Lipochrome pigment is present as goldenbrown granules. Mitochondria and crystalloids are also present. The latter are known as "Reinke crystalloids". They are rod shaped and round or oval on cross section. The histological characteristics of the Leydig cells are consistent with hormone production. The presence of the cytoplasmic granules may be important in this function. There appears to be no correlation between the number of Leydig cells present and the hormonal activity of the gonad.

The Leydig cells of the testis produce the hormone that is responsible for male secondary sex characteristics and reproductive structures. The adrenal cortex elaborates other androgenic substances but only testicular androgen is capable of maintaining the normal function of the male sex organs.

As early as 1849, Berthold demonstrated that the testis elaborated an internal secretion capable of producing active androgenic effects. In the early 1900's active androgenic substances were isolated from the urine of normal males. They have since been identified by crystallization as pure androsterone and dehydroepiandrosterone. Pure testosterone was isolated from the bull testis in 1935 (David). Androsterone and testosterone were synthesized from cholesterol in 1934 and 1935 by Ruzicka and associates.

Testosterone is only known to be secreted by the adult testis. In human spermatic vein blood 1.6 to $0.025\,\mu$ per cc. of plasma has been detected by Hollander and Hollander using a C^{14} testosterone dilution method. In human male blood, the circulating testosterone level has been measured in normals to vary from 0.1 to 0.4 ug./100 ml. plasma. In adult normal females a level of 0.1 ug./100 ml. plasma is thought to be normal by Finkelstein and co-workers. Five principle androgens are detectable in the blood. Testosterone and delta 4-androstene-3, 17-dione are elaborated from the testis. Dehydroepiandrosterone, androsterone, 11 beta-hydroxy-delta 4-androstene-3, 17 dione, and delta 4-androstene-3, 17 dione are produced by the adrenal cortex. The latter hormone is produced both in the testis and the adrenal gland. Biologically active androgens appear in the urine of men, women, and children of both sexes. Those which appear in normal humans are testosterone and dehydroepiandrosterone. Occasionally 11-hydroxyandrosterone is found in the urine of normal males and is androgenically active. Testosterone and delta 4-androsterone-3, 17 dione are both biologically active androgens.

The biological activity of androgens can be measured by various bio-assay tests. These depend upon the growth response of the comb of a capon or baby chick. They are also measured by the weight response of the ventral prostate and seminal vesicles of the castrate rat, the myotropic effect on the levator ani and the estimation of fructose and citric acid in the prostate of the same animal

The normal androgen content of human urine is approximately 63—68 international units for 24 hours in males and 42—56 in females as measured by comb growth (GALLAGHER). There is tremendous variation between the values seen clinically in normal individuals, however. Castration reduces excretion to one-sixth normal in men and one-half normal in women. Castrates will often have levels which fall into the range seen in normal men (DORFMAN).

The determination of 17 ketosteroids is more practical than bio-assay methods (DORFMAN). These substances are urinary degradation compounds of androgens produced by the adrenal cortex and the testis. Two-thirds are produced in the adrenal gland and one-third in the testis. The total quantity roughly parallels the androgen content of the blood. Testosterone is not measured but 3 alpha-hydroxyetiocholane-17-one will be, which is biologically inert. The 24 hour urinary 17 ketosteroid level is a good rough method for determining the androgenic level of the organism. Normal adult men excrete 10—18 mgm. of 17 keto-steroids per 24 hours and normal adult women 7—15 mgm. The difference in the amount excreted is attributed to the testis. Children 0—6 years excrete up to 1.0 mg., 6—12 years 5.0 mg. and 12—20 years 5—12 mg. per 24 hours.

d) Histochemistry of the testis

Histochemical techniques visualize, identify and localize the chemical structure and biological activity of cells. The study of lipid metabolism by such techniques is important in testicular physiology because testis hormones are steroidal in nature. Glycogen and enzymatic activity are also helpful in elucidating the metabolic functions. Much of the recorded data is incomplete, conflicting, and is derived from study of lower animals. Interpretation insofar as human physiologic mechanisms are concerned is speculative.

Numerous water insoluble, fat-like substances have been studied by their solubility in benzene, chloroform, ether and acetone. The major lipids studied, are the total lipids, neutral lipids, and unsaturated steroids (cholesterol, cholesterol esters and ketosteroids). Various histochemical methods are available for differentiating these compounds: The total lipids can be stained with the sudan stains; the neutral lipids with Nile blue sulfate; unsaturated steroids with the Schultz modification of the Lieberman-Burchardt reaction; ketosteroids with dinitrophenylhydrazine reaction or naphthoic acid hydrazide (Ashbel-Seligman procedure); and free cholesterol can be demonstrated with digitonide refringence methods. These methods have varying specificities depending on the physical state of the substance being studied (amorphous or crystalline). The presence of lipids has been demonstrated in all of the cells of the seminiferous tubules and the Leydig cells. Sudanophilic granules have also been noted in most cells and fibroblast-like cells in the interstitium (MONTAGNA). The seminiferous tubules contain a prominent band of sudanophilic lipid just inside the tubular wall in the spermatocytes and basal Sertoli cells. Finer particles are found in the more centrally located primary and secondary spermatocytes and Sertoli cells. In the mature spermatozoa, found in the ejaculate, lipid material is concentrated in the sheath surrounding the middle piece (MANN). In general, increasing age is associated with an increase in Sertoli cell lipid and a decrease in Leydig cell lipid (SCOTT and LYNCH). The presence of lipid material in a cell does not necessarily reflect metabolic activity. The cell may elaborate or utilize steroidal compounds and hence be actively engaged in hormonal processes, without storage of the compound in the cell itself. The Sertoli cell lipid may be essential for spermatogenesis and is found stored in the cell in the aging individual as activity declines. The accumulation of lipid in the Sertoli cells that have attached or adjacent sperm heads gives further importance to its probable role in spermatozoa maturation.

Glycogen, as demonstrated by the Schiff acid fuchsin procedure is absent in the interstitial cells. The Sertoli cells, spermatogonia and primary spermatocytes contain large amounts. The remainder of the germinal epithelial cells contain no glycogen. The glycogen content, then, is probably related to active spermatogenic activity (LONG and ENGLE). Alkaline phosphatase activity is found in the fibroblast-like cells and endothelial cells of the interstitial tissue. Sertoli cells contain minute amounts while centrally located germinal cells contain abundant quantities (MONTAGNA). Lipase, indicative of active lipid metabolism, has not been studied extensively but is found in Leydig cells and other interstitial cells (LONG and ENGEL).

5. Senile testis

No abrupt change is noted in the testes of aging males. Spermatogenesis has been noted in the ninth decade. Generally there is a decrease in the spermatogenic activity with age. The decrease in activity is noted histologically as an enlargement of the lumen of the tubule. The most constant feature associated with aging is fibrosis and thickening of the basement membrane. This is also noted in pathological situations. The Leydig cells show only an increase in pigment. They do not appear to decrease in number in the human but may do so in animals.

II. Descent of the testis

The scrotum begins development during the second month of gestation (AREY). It is first recognized as genital folds which first enlarge, then grow medially and posteriorly to meet in the midline to form the scrotum externally. A scrotal septum is formed internally. The scrotal sac forms by an evagination of the peritoneal cavity into the scrotum to form the processus vaginalis. The gubernaculum testis is formed from rudimentary layers of the abdominal wall and consists of a band of fibromuscular tissue which anchors the testis to the connective tissue of the scrotal sac.

The testis is suspended from the posterior abdominal wall by the ligaments of the regressing mesonephros. The cranial ligament or suspensory ligament is transitory and disappears. The caudal ligament develops into the gubernaculum testis. By the tenth week, the testis is suspended by the mesorchium and is found in the lateral part of the greater pelvis, i.e. the iliac fossa. It is devoid of ligaments other than the gubernaculum testis and maintains its original blood supply. The testis carries its original blood supply and the vas deferens with it during its descent. At the seventh month it moves into the scrotal sac. It slides beneath the peritoneum of the posterior abdominal wall into the scrotal sac where the processes vaginalis invests it to form the visceral layer of the tunica vaginalis (WELLS, WYNDHAM). Obliteration of the processes vaginalis takes place from the abdominal wall to the terminal portion of the part covering the testis.

The role of the gubernaculum in testicular descent is not clear. AREY believes it is possible that it actively brings the testis into the scrotum but it may merely guide the testis. In the experimental animal, BURROWS observed that absence of the gubernaculum may cause the testis to descend into the wrong compartment.

Hormones play an important role in the descent of the testis. In hypophysectomized immature male animals, descent does not take place. In mice and rats, the testes do not descend until puberty and rodent testes descend only during the rutting season. The frequently observed effectiveness of chorionic gonadotrophin in enlarging and causing descent of the inguinal testis in adolescent males lends further support to the importance of hormonal factors in testicular descent. Maternal chorionic gonadotrophin may play an important part in fetal descent according to ENGLE.

III. Cryptorchidism

1. Testis temperature and function

Maldescended testes generally do not exhibit normal function. The higher temperature of their extrascrotal location is deleterious. The seminiferous tubules sustain most of the injury. MOORE and QUICK have established that the temperature gradient between the intraabdominal and inguinal areas and scrotum is essential for normal spermatogenesis. This is true in man as well as in lower animals. With increased temperatures, the seminiferous tubules show varying degrees of degenerative changes depending upon the degree of temperature elevation and the length of the period over which it takes place. In the undescended testis, SHOVAL found complete tubular degeneration with atrophy and fibrosis in some cases. The tubular changes resulted from increased body temperature. Oligospermia has been observed by MACLEOD and HOTCHKISS following hyperpyrexia with illness. The effect was temporary. Sperm counts returned to normal in 30—60 days. The normal temperature differential between the abdomen and the scrotum is 2.2° C.

Experimentally induced elevation of scrotal temperature 2° C for two weeks has resulted in absence of spermatozoa in the seminiferous tubules. GLOVER found that scrotal insulation for only five days produces seminal degeneration and elevation of scrotal temperature of 5° C for only 24 hours produces similar changes. Varicoceles in YOUNG's experience may produce a rise in intrascrotal temperature of as much as 2.8° C with resultant tubular degeneration. In rabbits a reduction in fertility is induced by high environmental temperature directly and indirectly by changes in thyroid metabolism.

Data on the effect of low temperatures on spermatogenesis is sparse. In the rat, MACDONALD and HARRISON observed that spermatogenisis is markedly impaired. Spermatozoa can survive very low temperatures. The scrotum protects the testis against low temperatures. A greater degree of destructive change is noted if the testis is exposed directly to the cold.

2. Clinical features of cryptorchidism

Testes which are not in the normal scrotal location can best be divided into three categories. The retractile testis is found in the superficial tissues of the inguinal canal and can be pulled into the scrotum. The histologic structure is generally normal and the location is secondary to a hyperactive cremasteric muscle. This condition is frequently seen in children. The parent will often note that the testis was seen in the scrotum at one time or another. With the onset of puberty, these testes may or may not descend into the scrotum. The ectopic testis lies in the inguinal canal. It can usually be palpated by having the patient relax the abdominal muscles and pressing laterally and downward over the canal. Pressing it medially generally makes it disappear. It does not descend at puberty. Failure of normal formation of the inguinal canal occurs usually because of fusion of Scarpa's fascia to the symphysis pubis. The truly un-descended or cryptorchid testis lies within the abdominal cavity and cannot be palpated.

Undescended testes occur in the adult population with a frequency of 1:200. In the premature infant, 33% have one or both testes undescended. In the full-term child, 4% have undescended testis. The incidence at one year approximates that seen in the adult. Scorer believes that very few testes that are un-descended at one year of age will descend at puberty.

The histo-pathology seen in the cryptorchid testis is variable. Early it appears to be an immature gonad that does not differ from normal. With the onset of adolescence pathologic changes become apparent. The seminiferous tubules become atrophic. The basement membrane thickens and shows hyalinization. Leydig cells show variable changes. They may be either decreased or increased in number. A few tubules show spermatogenic activity. Mack and associates found that only 3.9% of all the tubules of undescended testes demonstrated some spermatogenesis. In the ectopic testis, about 7.4% and in the normal or retractile testes 26.5% of the tubules were fertile. He concluded that both the ectopic and true undescended testis were defective with a decreased number of germ cells. In 10% of the patients he biopsied with ectopic testes, normal spermatogenesis was seen in the fertile tubules. In the cryptorchid testis, the vast majority of the tubules were pathologic. Androgen production by the cryptorchid testis was depressed. Engberg and associates found androgen pro-duction to be about 50% of normal in adult males with bilaterally cryptorchid testis. There was also associated decrease in acid phosphatase content of the semen in the patients studied by Raboch and Homolka. In the lower animals, Moore found surgical cryptorchidism decreased androgen secretion. Clegg saw a decrease in the clear areas in the epithelial cells of the prostate with a decrease in the weight of secondary sex glands.

Treatment of the patient with undescended testes with chorionic gonado-trophin was often successful in Gordon and Field's study. Testosterone also induced descent (Zelson and Steinitz), but caused degeneration of seminiferous tubules (Hamilton and Lenard). Thyroid extract, when used with chorionic gonadotrophin also promoted descent of the testis into the scrotum (Gordon, Gordon, and Fields). Surgical treatment of bilateral undescended testes preserved fertile seminiferous tubules from further degeneration. Gross and Jewett reported fertility in 79% of patients surgically treated for bilateral undescended testes between ages of 10 and 14 years. Hinman Jr. described histological changes in the undescended testis which led him to conclude that orchiopexy at earlier ages might be worthwhile.

IV. Hypogonadism

Hypogonadism is present when the adult male testis is incapable of pro-ducing fertile spermatozoa or elaborating adequate amounts of the male sex hormone. The state may be due to testicular maldevelopment (Primary hypo-gonadism) or to extratesticular factors (Secondary hypogonadism).

1. Cytogenetic types of primary hypogonadism

Primary congenital hypogonadal states in the male are: true hermaphroditism, male pseudohermaphroditism, Klinefelter's syndrome, Turner's syndrome and a variety of other chromosomal anomalies. Rapid advancement in the study of chromosomal analysis in recent years has led to clarification of some of these interesting clinical entities. In 1956, TIJO and LEVAN demonstrated that the normal human chromosome number is forty-six rather than forty-eight. In the same period, BARR and associates discovered the existence of a distinctive chromocenter, the sex chromatin, in the intermitotic nuclei of females and its absence in the nuclei of males. The application of methods of nuclear sexing in clinical states of hypogonadism has led to the discovery of discrepancies between the genetic sex and nuclear sex in the above syndromes. True hermaphrodites may be either sex chromatin negative or sex chromatin positive. MILLER'S

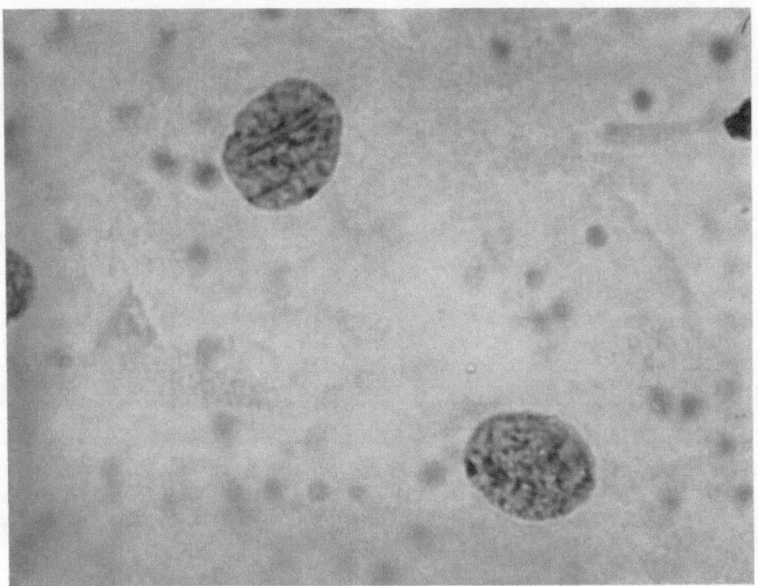

Fig. 2. Sex chromatin body of leucocyte characteristic of female nuclei. Buccal smear. (Courtesy Dr. H. A. THIEDE)

techniques for the study of cytogenetics involves: 1. the use of tissue culture techniques to obtain large number of cells from any part of the body, most commonly from the skin, bone marrow and blood, 2. colchicine treatment of tissue culture cells to increase the number of cells in mitosis at the metaphase, 3. treatment of tissue culture cells with hypotonic solutions prior to fixation in order to swell the cells and disperse nuclear elements throughout the cytoplasm and to destroy the nuclear membrane, 4. flattening of the cytoplasm of the cells in metaphase so that chromosomes are more widely dispersed and in a single plane, 5. photographing the cells and matching of their chromosomes for karyotype analysis for comparison with other cells from the same individual or cells from other individuals with the same abnormality.

a) Normal

In normal females and males chromosome analyses have borne out the XY—XX sex determining mechanism in man. Normal females (XX), Fig. 2, are found to be sex chromatin positive. The sex chromatin material is a FEULGEN positive body or chromocenter lying opposed to the nuclear membrane in the interphase nucleus. The number of sex chromatin bodies present is always the number of X chromosomes minus one (n-1). Thus, the normal male XY has no chromocenter and is chromatin negative. The study of sex chromatin bodies revealed them to be present in many but not all tissues. The first ones found were in skin biopsy sections, but they are also present in the buccal mucosa and the availability of these cells makes them preferable for use. The mode of action by which the Y chromosomes brings about male sex differentiation is not known. Probably one or more genes on the Y chromosome are responsible. Complete sex

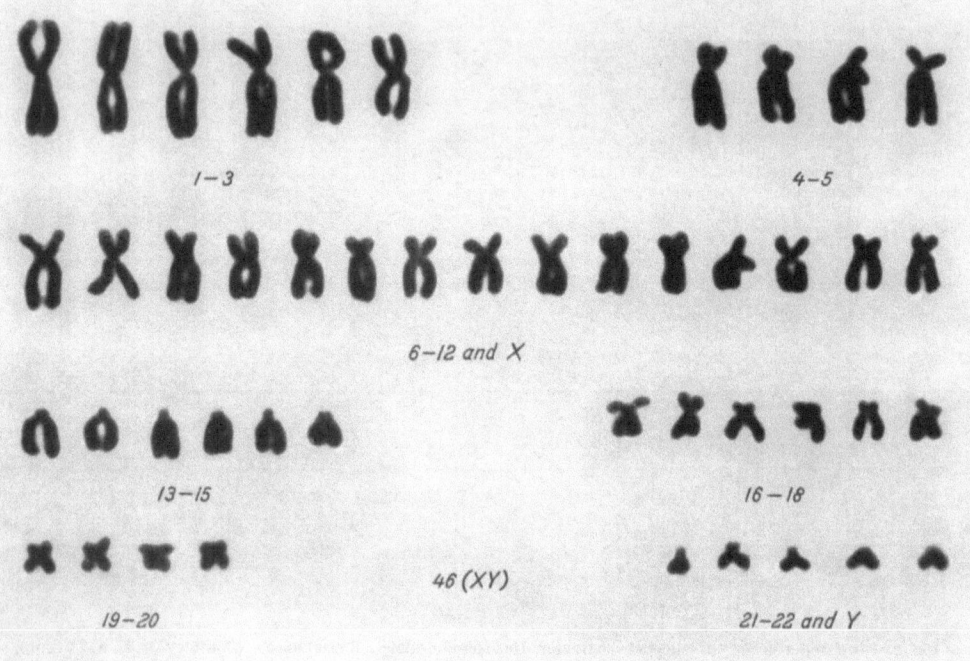

Fig. 3. Karyotype of normal. (Courtesy of Dr. HENRY A. THIEDE)

reversal has been reported in a female, with ovaries, with XY chromosome complement. They may be due to a mutation of a gene on the Y chromosome.

b) Male pseudohermaphroditism

Male pseudohermaphroditism may take two clinical forms. In one, elements of abnormal sexual development are present in the form of abnormal genitalia. The nuclear sex chromatin and the sex chromosome complement corresponds to the gonads present. The modal chromosome pattern is the normal forty-six and in the male pseudohermaphrodite the XY complex is present. A variety of this condition is the testicular feminization syndrome. The individuals are phenotypic females and go unnoticed until adult life. They have undescended testes and primary amenorrhea but they have normal external genitalia, normal breast development and a feminine habitus. Familial cases have been reported that are transmitted through the maternal line. JACOBS and coworkers suggest that the syndrome is sex linked recessive recessive or sex linked autosomal dominant. True hermaphrodites possess male and female elements not only in the genital tract but in the gonadal tissue as well. Both testes and ovaries or ovotestes with or without a testis or an ovary is present. They may be either sex chromatin positive or negative.

c) KLINEFELTER's syndrome

Patients with KLINEFELTER's syndrome are phenotypic males with positive sex chromatin. They have anatomic derangement (sclerosing tubular fibrosis,

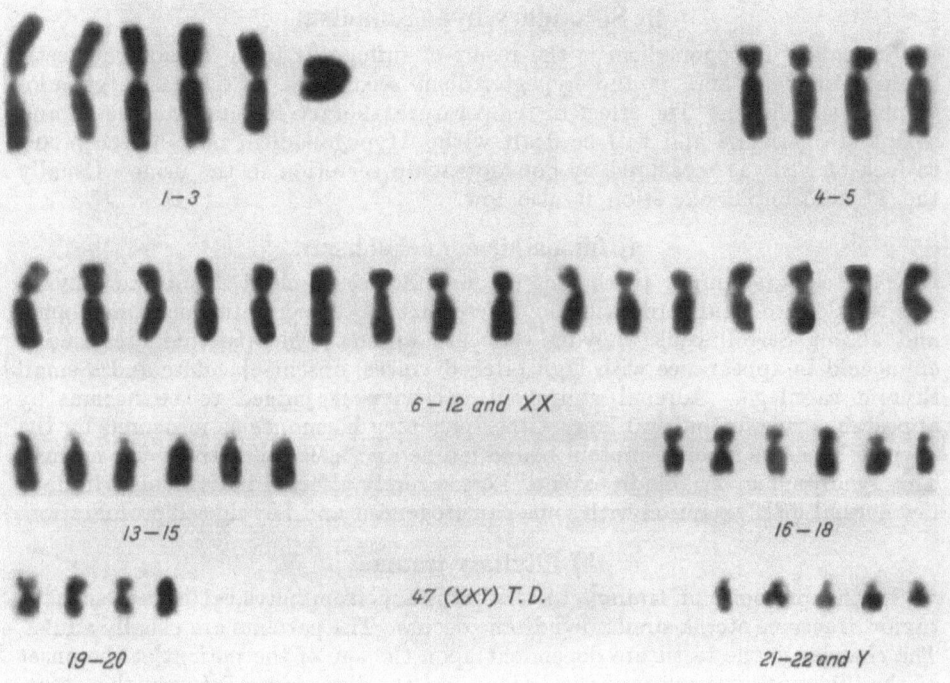

Fig. 4. Karyoptype KLINEFELTER's syndrome, usual XXY type. (Courtesy Dr. HENRY A. THIEDE)

seminiferous tubular dysgenesis and microorchism) and functional impairment (sterility and androgen deficiency) of the testis. Clinically there is associated, but not invariable, gynecomastia, eunuchoid habitus, raised urinary gonadotrophin excretion and mental defects. 17 ketosteroid excretion may be normal or low. The chromosome constitution in the majority of the chromatin positive patients is (47) XXY. There may be a mosaic of chromosomes XX/XXY in some patients. A variety of karyotype patterns have been encountered in a small number of patients with KLINEFELTER's syndrome that makes it appear that the entity is not a homogeneous one and that its features may be simulated by a variety of conditions. The most common karyotype in KLINEFELTER's is XXY (Fig. 4), and is apparently the result of a non-dysjunction of the sex chromosome during gametogenesis of either parent.

d) TURNER's syndrome

Individuals with TURNER's syndrome are phenotypic females with normal but underdeveloped female genitalia and absence of secondary sexual characteristics at puberty. They usually have increased gonadotrophins and usually exhibit a variety of associated anomalies (short stature, webbing of the neck, broad shield-like chest and cubitus valgus). The gonads arc replaced by fibrous streaks. About 80 percent of the patients arc chromatin negative. The karyotype is forty-five chromosomes with an XO sex chromosome complement. Mosaicism is frequently present. The condition appears to be due to non-dysjunction during gametogenesis account for the XO karyotype. Either the sperm or the ovum lacks a sex chromosome producing the XO zygote.

2. Secondary hypogonadism

Secondary hypogonadism is the result of influences from outside the testis itself. Pertinent here is the hypogonadism secondary to decreased gonado-trophic stimulation. The effect of temperature, dietary factors, irradiation and toxins are germane and will be dealt with. Hypogonadism may be secondary to lack of FSH as measured by gonadotrophin secretion in the urine. Usually the 17 ketosteroid excretion is also low.

a) Idiopathic eunuchoidism

The testis is similar to that of the pre-adolescent child (TIJO and LEVAN) The tubules are solid cords with no differentiation of spermatogenic components and absent Sertoli cells. Leydig cells are absent. The patients are usually eunuchoid in appearance with high pitched voices, absent ejaculate and a small thyroid cartilage. Adrenal androgenic activity is judged to be normal by appearance time of puberal hair. Other pituitary hormones as measured by the thyroid hormone level as protein bound iodine and islet cell activity are normal. This syndrome is variable in extent. Less severely affected individuals will have low normal FSH excretion with some gametogenesis and Leydig cell proliferation.

b) Pituitary trauma

In the presence of trauma to the pituitary from physical causes such as tumor, fractures etc., a similar syndrome occurs. The patients are usually adults. The changes in the testis are dependent upon the age of the patient at the onset of the illness, the severity of the lesion, and the time lapse between the occurrence of the lesion and the testis biopsy. There is great variability. Generally, there tends to be progressive hypospermatogenesis, excessive desquamation of germinal epithelium, accumulation of lipid droplets in the Sertoli cell cytoplasm, decrease in tubular diameter and thickening and fibrosis of the basement membrane. Leydig cells tend to disappear. Eventually, the histologic picture may be that of sclerotic cords separated by interstitial tissue.

c) Estrogen treatment

For the most part, the changes are the result of abnormal estrogen-androgen ratio and depression of the gonadotrophin levels from adenohypophysis. The histologic changes noted in the testes are similar to those seen in patients with organic lesions of the pituitary. There is depression of spermatogenesis, desquamation of germinal epithelium, accumulation of Sertoli cell lipid, decrease in the size of the tubules, basement membrane thickening and reduction in the number of Leydig cells. The end result is characterized by fibrotic tubules separated by thick collagenous tissue.

The estrogen effect is reversible if the drug is administered only over a short period. After 30 days of estrogen treatment, CHARNEY saw complete regeneration of the seminiferous tubules in 6 to 8 weeks. Tubular regeneration may follow after up to 96 days of estrogen therapy. However, most observers feel that irrepairable damage may take place with long term estrogen therapy.

d) Dietary deficiencies

Little is known about the effects of dietary deficiency states on human testicular physiology. There is little information in the literature that enables one to make any conclusive statements. With caloric restriction, in animals, atrophy of the testis and degeneration of the spermatogenic series of cells takes place. However, this may be secondary to decreased gonadotrophin secretion by the pituitary secondary to inanition. Decreased spermatogenesis may also be due to the deficiency of one or more essential dietary elements and not only due to caloric restriction. The lack of a specific vitamin in the diet has not been demonstrated to produce testicular lesions in the human. Various investigations have reported conflicting findings in laboratory animals on diets deficient in vitamins A, B, C, and E. Deficiencies of the trace elements generally do not produce obvious histopathological changes. Tubular atrophy has been reported to follow manganese deficiency.

Diets low in protein or specific amino acids are not known to have any specific effect in the human. Deficiencies of typtophane, lysine or arginine produces severe cytological degeneration in the rat testis (SHETTLES).

V. Irradiation effects on testis

The germinal epithelium is particularly sensitive to radioactive agents. The spermatogenic series of cells suffers the majority of the damage. The Sertoli and Leydig cells are relatively resistant. The histopathology in suitably irradiated testes shows almost complete disappearance of the germinal epithelium. Spermatogonia and spermatozoa are present. Intermediate cell forms are absent. There appears to be an inhibition of division at the level of the spermatogonium. The main effect according to FRIEDMAN and DRUTZ is in the chromatin material. The mature spermatozoa in the ejaculate following irradiation show little cytological change. However, these cells are usually infertile or incapable of inducing normal fertilization.

The changes produced by irradiation may be permanent if the dosage is sufficiently intensive or prolonged. In the rat, 300—400 r. applied directly to the testis is necessary to cause suppression of spermatogenesis while 950—1500 r. are required for permanent arrest (CALLAWAY, MOSELEY and BAREFOOT). In individuals exposed to the atom bomb, the ionizing radiation appears to be the most important factor. VORDER BRUEGGE observed that the damage appears in the first few days and progresses to atrophic tubules with replacement of the germinal epithelium by Sertoli cells. Total body dose of 40—50% of the lethal dose of atomic irradiation has no permanent effect on human fertility, Committee on Pathologic Effects of Atomic Radiation, report of.

B. Epididymis. vas deferens and ejaculatory ducts
I. Epididymis

The spermatozoa leave the seminiferous tubules through the efferent ductules. Ligation of the vasa efferentia caused atrophy of the seminiferous tubular epithelium whereas SMITH observed no such change after vasoligation. The epididymis appears to be able to cushion the effect of vasoligation possibly by absorbing the secretions of the testis. The epididymis receives the spermatozoa as produced and holds them for variable periods of time. The epididymis has been calculated to be 20 feet long by BELFIELD and ROLNICK. They believe that the epididymis stores spermatozoa providing them at time of mating. OSLUND has observed that spermatozoa transport in the epididymis is related to the pressure of formation of new spermatozoa and fluid in the seminiferous tubules. During copulation the rate of transport is augmented by rhythmic contraction of epididymis and vas deferens. VON LANZ and coauthors believe they have established that the tail of the epididymis is a reservoir for spermatozoa. In dogs, spermatozoa were not found in the tail of the epididymis until 48 hours after ejaculation. TOOTHILL and YOUNG have measured the transit time of India ink through the epididymis of guinea pigs. Whereas the normal time is 14—18 days, after ligation of the head of the epididymis 25—28 days are required. This evidence supports the view of the role of the secretory pressure of the seminiferous tubules in epididymal sperm transport. SHAVE found ink particles removed from the lumen of the epididymis by the stereocilia and hence into the columnar cells lining the epididymis. This he suggests may be physiologic means of removing cellular debris and secretion. The contribution of the epididymis to maturation is incompletely established. Whether the epididymis contributes a maturation principle to the spermatozoa or whether the spermatozoa are given a period of time during transport to accomplish this unaided is not known. Fertility of spermatozoa held in the epididymis has been observed by KNAUS after 40 days. Glycogen granules were demonstrated by NICANDER in the epididymal columnar epithelium and secretion. Whereas in some species including man, cells resembling Leydig cells have been observed in the epididymis and spermatic cord tissues in the rat Lawless could not demonstrate physiologic evidence of androgen production by the epididymis in castrate rats.

II. Vas deferens

The vas deferens is about 20 inches long. Spermatozoa are actively transported by peristaltic contractions of the vas deferens during copulation. Spermatozoa removed from the vas deferens were found by BISHOP to be non-motile. He speculates that low oxygen tension and carbohydrate levels may explain lack of sperm motility. The vas deferens motility appears to be subject to hormonal control. MARTINS and VALLE found that androgen decreased contractility and excitability of the deferens whereas estrogen had the opposite effect in vitro. MOORE (1931) and LYNN and NESBET have reported experimental and clinical data that vasoligation does not appreciably alter spermatogenesis. These observations in the absence of dilatation of the vas deferens suggest that the epididymis must dispose of the spermatozoa when the vas is occluded.

III. Ejaculatory ducts

The ejaculatory ducts course obliquely through the posterior prostate. They allow emptying of the spermatozoa and seminal vesicle secretion into the proximal urethra during ejaculation. The average length of the ejaculatory duct was found by IVANIZKY to be 23 mm. No specific function or secretion is attributed to the ejaculatory duct.

IV. Colliculus seminalis-verumontanum

The colliculus seminalis is a $9 \times 3 \times 3$ mm. eminence which is the termination of the ejaculatory ducts. It is located at the apex of the prostate about 4 mm.

from the external urinary sphincter. The colliculus seminalis is a remnant of the Müllerian duct, as such it is exceedingly responsive to estrogenic hormone.

V. Cowper's (bulbo-urethral) glands

Cowper's glands are pea size compound racemose mucus secreting glands whose main structures lie in the urogenital diaphragm. The 2.5 cm. long ducts empty into the membranous urethra. To these glands and to the multiple small urethral glands of Littré no special function is attributed. The secretions of these glands are supposed to serve a lubricative purpose at time of coitus.

C. The prostate gland
I. The growth, development and involution of the prostate

The human prostate is first in evidence in the 12 week old fetus. Five groups of epithelial buds originate from the proximal urethra. These groups form anterior, posterior (post-spermatic), middle and lateral portions of the prostate. At 16 weeks, the epithelial buds have branched into tubules lined with low cuboidal cells. Lowsley described an average of 63 excretory prostatic ducts emptying into the urethra.

From three weeks before birth to three weeks after birth the neonatal prostate displays squamous metaplasia. Originally described by Aschoff in 1894, its relationship to maternal hormones was correctly suggested by Schlacta. By three weeks of age, the prostate re-

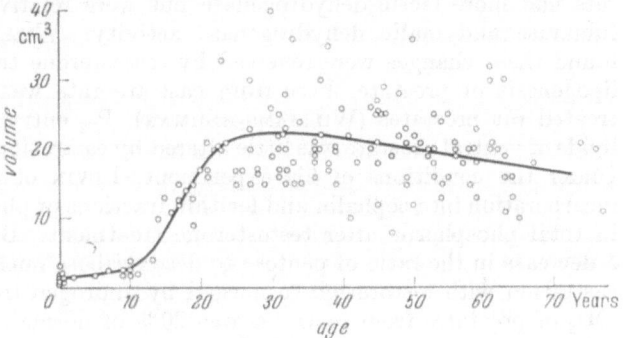

Fig. 5. Prostate volume. (Redrawn from Swyer 1944)

verts to low cuboidal epithelium until onset of puberty. At puberty, in response to hormonal stimulation, the prostate grows to its adult volume considered to be 10—13 cc. by Moore or 16—22 cc. by Swyer (Fig. 5). From age 13—45 years, the adult size and histologic appearance prevails. Moore describes onset of histologic atrophic changes at age 45—50 years, with decreased secretory activity 50—60 years, and sclerotic atrophy from age 60—65. In prostates not involved by benign or malignant hypertrophy, smooth muscle atrophy with a relative increase in connective tissue is seen after 60 years. The normal prostate size and histologic appearance depend upon numerous known factors many of which have been experimentally confirmed. The most important consideration appears to be an adequate supply of the male sex hormone.

Moore, Hughes and Gallagher described the histologic changes in rat prostate following castration and replacement treatment with testis extracts. Within five days of castration, the typical secretion vacuoles disappeared. In 20 days, the prostatic epithelium became cuboidal. Administration of testis extracts prevented castration changes or restored the previously atrophic epithelium to normal. The seminal vesicle was found to be even more rapidly responsive to castration than the prostate. Recognizable decrease in epithelial height and cytoplasmic vacuolization appeared in 24 hours. Moore and Gallagher reported functional evidence of impaired secretion of prostate and seminal vesicles following castration. In the guinea pig ejaculation of progressively smaller volumes of secretion of altered character may persist for 2—3 months. After 2—3 weeks of treatment of the castrate with testis extract, the volume and appearance of the ejaculate returned to normal.

Although starvation leads to complete cessation of prostatic function in dogs, Pazos and Huggins maintained prostatic secretory responses to pilocarpine by administration of gonadotrophin or testosterone during starvation. Hence, the effect of starvation must be the result of pseudohypophysectomy. These observations were confirmed in irradiated and starved rats by Lutwak-Mann and Mann and in vitamin B_1 deficiency by Moore and Samuels. In groups of castrate rats on deficient diets, Grayhack and Scott found a diminished prostate growth response to testosterone proprionate as compared with controls on normal diets. Where castrate rats are treated with suboptimal quantities of testosterone, Moore and Price found the prostate more responsive than the seminal vesicle.

With few exceptions, the chemical, enzyme content and metabolism of the prostate decreased after castration and returned to or toward normal soon after adequate replacement treatment with androgen. The prostatic tissues of castrate rats had more lactic dehydrogenase but were relatively deficient in aconitase, fumarase and malic dehydrogenase activity. Williams-Ashman and Banks found these changes were reversed by testosterone treatment. Respiration and lipogenesis of prostate slices from castrate rats was lower than in normal or treated rat prostates (Williams-Ashman). P_{32} entry into proteins or phospholipids of ventral prostate was little altered by castration or testosterone treatment. Under the conditions of his experiment, Levin et al. reported increased P_{32} incorporation into cephalin and lecithin fractions of phospholipids and an increase in total phosphorus after testosterone treatment. Butler and Schade found a decrease in the ratio of pentose to desoxyribose nucleic acids of 2.4 to 0.9 after castration with restoration to normal by androgen treatment. They also found QO_2 of prostates from castrates was 20% of normal. R.Q. was decreased from 0.9 to 0.4 and zymohexase decreased to 5—10% of normal. Alpha glycerophosphate dehydrogenase activity was doubled after castration. Acid phosphatase activity was not found to be affected by castration, estrogen or testosterone.

Marvin and Awapara found the decrease in number and quantity of free amino acids associated with post-castration prostatic atrophy reversible by replacement therapy. The mechanism of action of testosterone in producing these striking changes is incompletely known. However, the effect of testosterone can be a direct one since Grayhack (1958), was able to induce localized growth of the prostate by means of intraprostatic administration of androgen. Testosterone C_{14} is avidly retained by the prostate especially when previously given estrogen treatment (McDonald).

II. Hormonal interrelationships in prostatic growth

The pituitary exercises indirect and apparently a direct synergistic action on prostatic growth. Scott's sketch (Fig. 6), illustrates the interrelationships of testosterone and luteotrophin (prolactin) in prostatic growth. Grayhack, Bunce, Kearns and Scott showed that prostate growth in response to testosterone in hypophysectomized castrates was much inferior to that observed in nonhypophysectomized castrates or in castrates treated with luteotrophin. Radioactive luteotrophin has been found to localize in prostate by SONENBERG. HUGGINS and RUSSELL observed more profound prostatic atrophy after hypophysectomy than after castration in dogs. Histologically, the prostate returned to the prepuberal appearance which was easily distinguishable from post-castration atrophy. Acid phosphatase content was much reduced below castrate level. GOODWIN. RASMUSSEN, TAXDAL, FERREIRA and SCOTT have found that in hypophysectomized dogs the volume of prostatic secretion can be restored to normal by testosterone apparently without the need for luteotrophin. In humans, the

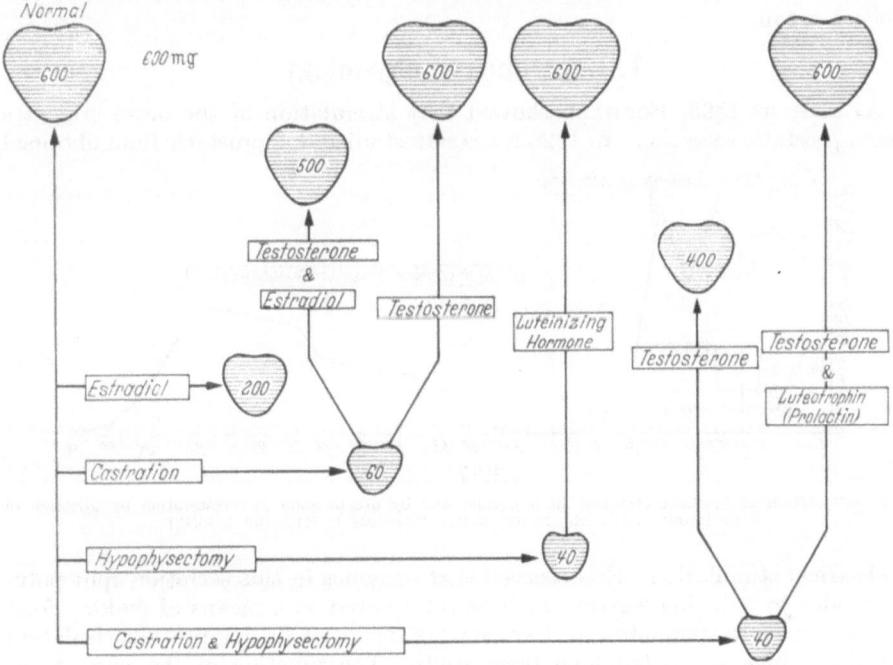

Fig. 6. Total prostate weights (milligrams) of young adult rats subjected to several endocrine manipulations.
(Courtesy W. W. SCOTT)

effect of hypophysectomy is most marked if it takes place before development of secondary sex characters which then fail to develop. SCOTT (1954) reported that the older the individual the less marked the decrease in secondary sex characters.

The adrenal contributes little or nothing to normal prostate growth. In the absence of the testis at an early age, the adrenal can apparently produce sufficient androgenic steroid to permit rather normal growth and development of the rodent prostate until 30—40 days of age after which atrophy takes place (PRICE). These observations are supported by those of HOWARD (1941) in castrate rats of 21 days of age. Simultaneous adrenalectomy resulted in a further decrease in prostate weight. In mice, HOWARD (1946), did not find adrenal androgens contributed to prostate and seminal vesicle growth.

Although SMELSER (1939) reported decrease in the weight of the prostate and seminal vesicles following thyroidectomy (SCOTT 1956), found the magnitude of the effect much less striking than the effect of other hormones. At least in vitro, insulin 5—10 mg-% stimulates growth of mouse prostate (FRANKS 1961).

III. The physiology of the prostate

The prostate gland because of its strategic periurethral location is the frequent cause of clinically symptomatic disease. For 30 years, prostatic function has been extensively studied. However, its contribution to the well being of the total organism even solely to its reproductive function has not been established. Various methods have been applied to the investigation of the prostate. In the present compilation of the relevant literature of the past 30 years an attempt was made to select only those studies subsequently confirmed which elucidate the unique chemical, metabolic and physiologic characteristics of this unusual organ.

1. Experimental physiology

As early as 1863, Eckhard showed that stimulation of the nervi erigentes caused prostatic secretion. In 1926 Karassik studied dog prostatic fluid obtained

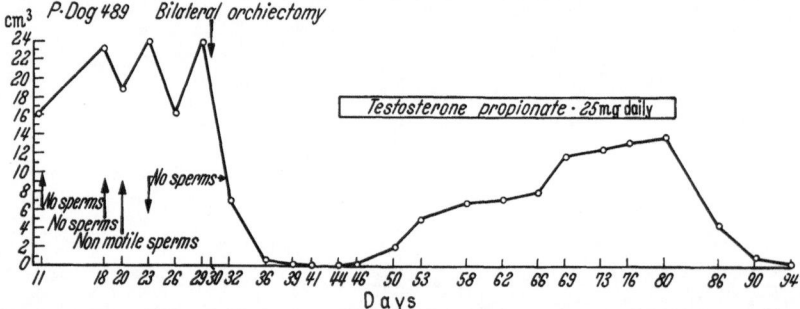

Fig. 7. Elimination of prostatic secretion in a normal dog by orchiectomy and restoration by injection of testosterone propionate, 25 mg. daily. (Courtesy C. Huggins 1946/47)

by electrical stimulation. He observed that enzymes in this secretion split polysaccharides to reducing sugars which he interpreted as a means of making food stuffs available to spermatozoa. Farrell (1931) devised a dog prostatic isolation operation which permitted long term study. The function of the prostate in response to intravenously administered pilocarpine and the secretion was made available for analysis. He made the observation (Farrell 1938), that alcohol was secreted by the prostate in concentrations similar to those in blood and urine. He also discovered that dog prostatic fluid had bacteriocidal properties. Youmans, Liebling and Lyman confirmed this observation and determined that the activity was stable in the cold but was heat labile. No complement or lysozyme activity was demonstrated.

Huggins (1945, 1946) summarized his research on the physiology and biochemistry of the prostate and its secretion. His many references to the literature will not be duplicated. Whereas, the resting secretion in the dog varied from 0.1 to 2 cc./hour, after pilocarpine injection, the prostate secreted 2—4 times its weight of prostatic fluid. The prostatic secretory response varied with the quantity of pilocarpine given. Tripling the dose increased the volume 25 times. Not only was the volume of secretion increased, but it contained more solids and enzymes (Rosenkrantz and Mason). Administration of testosterone propionate 5 mg. i.m. daily to immature prostatic fistula dogs initiated secretory responses to pilocarpine in as little as four days. Maturation of the prostate and increasing secretory ability continued over a 40 day period in adult normal dogs. The quantity of prostatic fluid secreted in response to pilocarpine was relatively constant within accepted biological limits. If the animal became ill, the prostate failed to respond normally presumably due to the secondary effects of pseudo-hypophysectomy. After castration (Fig. 7), the prostate lost its secretory capacity in one to three weeks. Replacement treatment with testosterone proprionate injections restored the prostatic function in two weeks.

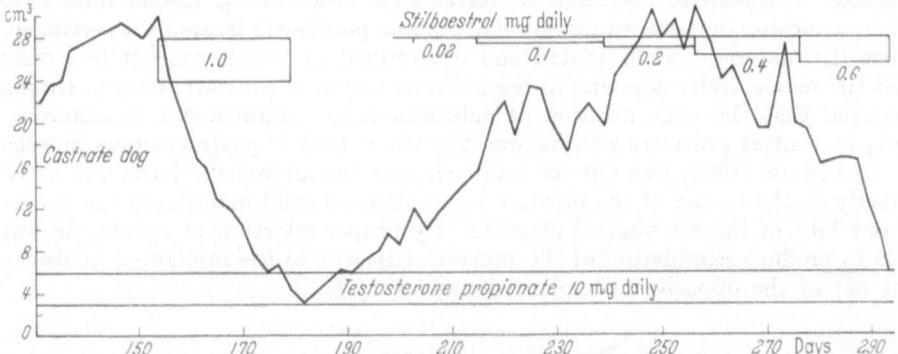

Fig. 8. Castrate immature dog has been injected daily with testosterone propionate, 10 mg. for 160 days, during which time secretion had risen from 0.1 to 30.2 cc. This androgen was continued at same rate throughout experiment and, in addition, stilbestrol injections were begun. Daily amounts of stilbestrol, 1.0 mg. and 0.6 mg., caused great decrease of secretion, while dosages of 0.02, 0.1 and 0.2 mg. did not affect the output: stilbestrol 0.4 mg. caused leveling of rate of secretion (dog 5—10). [Courtesy C. HUGGINS, J. Exp. Med. 72, 747 (1940)]

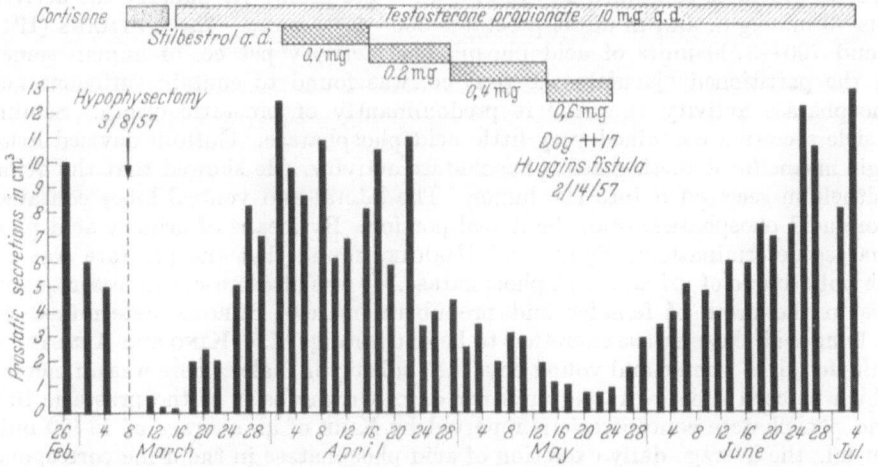

Fig. 9. Hypophysectomy in adult dog in which prostatic fistula has been prepared previously leads to marked reduction in volume of prostatic secretion within one week. Daily injections of testosterone propionate restore prostatic secretion to pre-hypophysectomy levels and, as in castrate dog stilbestrol in sufficient dosage inhibits testosterone-maintained secretion. (Courtesy GOODWIN et al. 1961)

In intact prostatic fistula dogs, prostatic secretion was markedly depressed in seven days by daily intra-muscular injections of 0.1 mg. stilbestrol. Secretion was restored by simultaneous treatment with 400 i.u. gonadotrophin daily. In the castrate prostatic fistula dog maintained on daily 10 mgm. injections of testosterone proprionate, the simultaneous injection of progressively larger quantities of stilbestrol permitted determination of the androgen to estrogen equivalent for the prostate. As seen in Fig. 8, this ratio is 1:25, i.e. 0.4 mg. stilbestrol inhibits the effect of 10 mg. testosterone proprionate. In hypophysectomized testosterone treated prostatic fistula dogs, GOODWIN et al. (Fig. 9) found a ratio of 1:50. The only data concerning the sensitivity of human prostatic tissues to minimal doses of stilbestrol are those of BAKER relating to prostatic carcinoma. These data indicate that as little as 0.25 mg. daily will reduce the level of serum acid phosphatase and give symptomatic improvement.

McDONALD reported evidence that testosterone is avidly taken up by the prostate. Intra-aortic injections of physiologic doses of C_{14} testosterone were found to localize in the prostate especially in rats previously treated with estrogen. Since the material was extracted and determined as testosterone, it is certain that the radioactivity was due to testosterone bound in prostatic tissue. GREER observed that the concentration of subcutaneously administered testosterone-4-C_{14} in ventral prostates of rats was $2^1/_2$ times that of gastrocnemius muscle.

GRAYHACK (1958) was able to establish that the androgenic hormones acted directly on the tissues of the prostate by implanting solid material in the tissues of one lobe of the rat ventral prostate. By proper selection of agents, he was able to produce stimulation of the prostate adjacent to the implanted androgen but not of the opposite unimplanted prostatic lobe.

2. Prostatic acid phosphatase

The GUTMANS (1932 and 1939) found high concentrations of phosphatase activity at pH 5.0 in extracts of human and animal prostates. The enzyme was inhibited by sodium fluoride and propyl alcohol. The acid phosphatase of pre-puberal prostates contained less than 5 units per gram. At puberty the activity was 73 units/gm. and in adult prostates 500—2000 units. The GUTMANS (1941) found 700—3700 units of acid phosphatase activity per cc. of human semen. In the partitioned ejaculate the first cc. was found to contain sufficient acid phosphatase activity to make it predominantly of prostatic origin. Seminal vesicle secretion contained very little acid phosphatase. GOMORI devised histo-logic means for detecting acid phosphatase activity. He showed that the acinar epithelium secreted it into the lumen. The lateral and ventral lobes contained more acid phosphatase than the dorsal portion. By means of urinary acid phos-phatase determinations, SCOTT and HUGGINS found that the prostate was not the only source of urinary acid phosphatase. It was also present in lesser quanti-ties in the urine of females and prepuberal males. BURGEN determined the 24 hour acid phosphatase excretion to be in the range of 50 KING and ARMSTRONG units for girls, women and young boys. At puberty in males, there was an increase which reached a peak of 350 units per day. On the basis of the prostatic fluid acid phosphatase concentrations reported by KIRK of an average of 14400 units per ml., the average daily excretion of acid phosphatase in the urine corresponds to 0.02 ml. of prostatic fluid. KIRK also observed that average prostatic fluid acid phosphatase activity decreased with age. Hence, it was presumably related to declining androgen stimulation of the aging prostate. These observations were experimentally confirmed by STAFFORD, RUBINSTEIN and MEYER who found decreased prostatic acid phosphatase in castrate rats could be restored by testo-sterone treatment. Despite contentions that certain phosphatase activity may be of specific origin in the prostate, DELORY and HETHERINGTON found that acid phosphatases of urine from females was similar to prostatic acid phosphatase in response to additions of tartrate and formalin. GOETSCH histochemically showed that acid phosphatase was formed in the cytoplasm of the prostatic cell, secreted into the acinar lumen and excreted in the semen. Little is known of its function. Seminal acid phosphatase can split phosphoryl choline, HUDSON, SCOTT, and BUTLER, which may be its natural substrate (LUNDQUIST). Prostatic phosphatase extracts can be inactivated by calcium ions. The inhibition can be reversed by phosphate compounds such as ATP or monosodium phosphate. Although the acid phosphatase content of prostate is one of its most characteristic features, it also contains unusual quantities of citric acid and zinc. HUGGINS and BARRON found a concentration of 645 mg.-% of citrate in prostatic adenoma. Aconitase, also present in high concentration, may be responsible for high citrate level. Citrate is apparently produced in greater quantities than can be metabolized. Citric acid is secreted by the prostate into the semen of many species (MANN). Its usefulness to the spermatozoa is unknown.

3. Zinc

Zinc is present in the posterior prostate in rats in concentrations 5—10 times that of other soft tissues. MAWSON and FISCHER also found considerable amounts of zinc in human prostate. FISCHER, TIKKALA and MAWSON observed that the

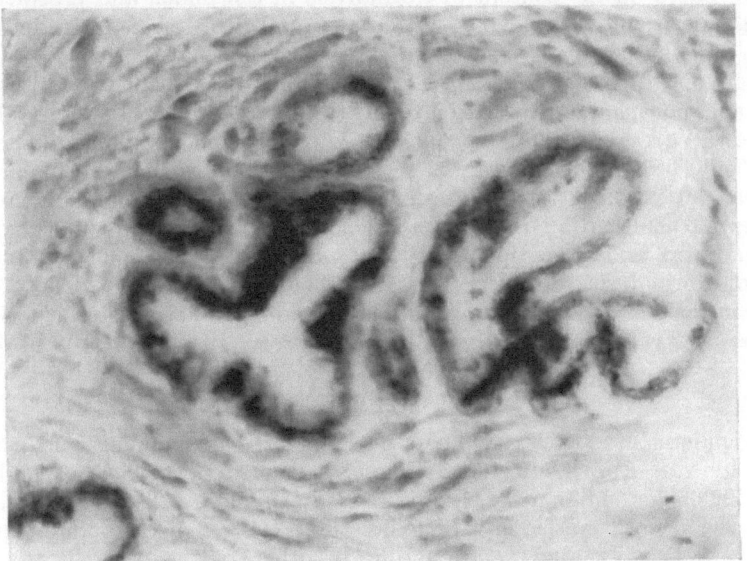

Fig. 10. Zn^{65} radioautography of human prostate. (Courtesy W. WHITMORE)

zinc content of prostate increased with maturation to 300 micrograms per gram. DANIEL, HADDAD, PROUT, and WHITMORE injected Zn 65 intravenously and found it localized in the prostatic epithelium. Fig. 10 is an autoradiograph of Zn 65 in the human prostate. GUNN and GOULD studied the localization of Zn 65 in rat prostate after castration and estrogen treatment. Following castration, the zinc concentration of the prostate decreased. Testosterone treatment of castrates restored the zinc levels. Although estrogen treatment decreased the size of the prostate, Zn 65 uptake was increased. The zinc content of prostate is not proportional to the quantity of epithelium. This is particularly true of carcinoma of the prostate which is low in zinc (HOARE, DELORY and PENNER). MILLAR, ELCOATE and MAWSON established that zinc concentration and Zn 65 uptake in the rat prostate is normally controlled by testosterone. These observations were confirmed and extended to the dog prostate by PROUT, DANIEL, and WHITMORE and PROUT, SIERP and WHITMORE. McDONALD (1960) has shown that administration of a zinc chelator, dithizone, to animals and humans causes regression and in some instances extensive necrosis of the prostate. Lo has found testosterone pre-treatment may improve the degree of destruction of prostatic carcinoma induced by dithizone injection.

4. Fibrinolysin

Enzymes participating in coagulation and fibrinolysis are to be found in the prostate and its secretion. In the monkey, van Wagener reported coagulation of seminal vesicle secretion by extracts of the cranial lobe but not by caudal lobe secretions. Human prostatic fluid contains an enzyme which liquefies coagulated blood and fibrin (Huggins and Neal). Although Huggins and Vail found that the prostatic fibrinolysis resembled trypsin in many respects, Huggins and Neal found prostatic fibrinolysin differed from trypsin in that it failed to digest hemoglobin. Huggins and McDonald (1944) found more rapid fibrinolysis with cell free prostatic fluid from patients with increased numbers of leucocytes in the secretion. Based on the content of fibrinolysis in the semen and prostatic fluid in the same patient, Ying, Day, Whitmore and Tagnon estimated that the prostate contributed about 50 percent of the volume of the semen. Whereas, it had been long appreciated that prostatic malignancy frequently led to increases in serum acid phosphatase it was first reported in 1952 and later amply established by Tagnon, Whitmore, Schulman, and Kravitz that increased blood fibrinolytic activity could be demonstrated in 12 percent of patients with extensive prostatic carcinoma. McNicol, Fletcher, Alkjaersig, and Sherry found that epsilon amino caproic acid had a specific anti-fibrinolytic action which could be demonstrated in vitro and in patients. A concentration of 10^{-3} moles (13 mg.-%) prevented fibrinolysis. Rasmussen and Albrechtsen identified prostatic fibrinolysins as heat stable and heat labile plasminogen activators. No plasmin, lipokinase or trypsin inhibitor were found.

5. Prostaglandin

Prostaglandin in extracts of prostate glands of many animals and man was reported by von Euler (1934), to exercise a pressor action corresponding to 0.001 to 0.005 mg. adrenaline per gram of fresh organ. These extracts also inhibited the smooth muscle of rabbit intestine. He was of the opinion that the observed effects were due to adrenalin. In other extracts, v. Euler (1926), reported vasodilator and smooth muscle stimulating principles. Eliason further characterized this latter principle as a carboxylic acid in ester linkage. Hawkins and Labrum quantitated the prostaglandin titer in semen. They found an average of 6.1 microgram per ml.

6. Antibacterial action

Another interesting attribute of prostatic fluid is its antibacterial action. Taylor and Morgan found a heat stable dializable substance which inhibited the growth of Staphylococcus aureus, Escherichia coli and Neisseria gonorrheae and meningitidis. The antibacterial agent was present in a concentration whose effectiveness approached that of two micrograms of pencillin per ml.

7. Lipids and chemical composition

The normal human prostatic secretion is an opalescent milky homogeneous fluid. It does not usually contain spermatozoa. There are urethral and prostatic epithelial cells in small numbers. Numberous doubly refractile spherical secretion granules varying in size from barely visible up to almost the size of a red blood cell are present, the cephalin bodies. Three to five leucocytes per high power field are usually present. Provided they are not associated with clumps of leucocytes, they are not considered to be evidence of infection. The prostatic secretion is usually sterile.

The lipid bodies of the prostatic secretion constitute a well recognized and characteristic feature. SCOTT (1945) found 286 mg.-% total lipid content. Phospholipid constituted over 65% of the total lipid and cephalin composed 82% of the phospholipid. Lecithin was present in very small amounts. Hence, the

Table. *Chemical composition of human and canine prostatic fluids* (Courtesy C. HUGGINS 1945)

	Man resting fluid	Dog pilocarpine stimulation
pH	6.3—6.45 (67)	5.29—6.16 (64)
Values per liter of fluid		
Water, gram	927—936 (67)	981±3 (64)
Sodium, m.eq	149—158 (67)	159 ±2.6 (64)
Potassium, m.eq	28.7—61.4 (67)	5.1±0.2 (64)
Calcium, m.eq	28.7—32.7 (67)	0.3 (64)
Chloride, m.eq	34.8—46.1 (63)	160 ±2.7 (64)
Acid-soluble P, m.eq	0.65—1.77 (63)	Trace (64)
Carbon dioxide, m.M.	3.1—5.4 (67)	0.8—0.9 (64)
Values per 100 cc. of fluid		
Total nitrogen, mgm	295—511 (67)	154 (64)
Non-protein nitrogen, mgm	30—90 (67)	22 (64)
Total protein, gram	2.46—2.64 (67)	0.8 (64)
Glucose, mgm	Trace—16.4 (63)	0—30 (64)
Ascorbic acid, mgm	0.54 (3)	0.76 (3)
Citric acid, grams	0,48—2.68 (66); 7.0 (123)	0.0026 (66)
Acid phosphatase, King and Armstrong units (76)	255—1727	3—286 (3)
Alkaline phosphatase, King and Armstrong units (76)		0—106 (3)
Total lipids, mgm	286 (124)	
Cholestrol, mgm	62—105 (124)	
	86—618	130—210 (106)
Specific gravity	1.022 (106)	1.005—1.008 (3)

doubly refractile bodies found on microscopy of prostatic secretion should be identified as cephalin bodies not lecithin bodies.

The chemical composition, table, of human prostatic fluid is worthy of comment. An usually high concentration of calcium and citrate and low levels of chloride, bicarbonate and phosphate are found. The proteins of prostatic fluid are proteoses. Spermine is present in high concentration, 100 mg.-%.

8. Carbohydrate metabolism

The carbohydrate metabolism of human and animal prostates is similar. Respiration, 2 μl./mg./hr. and aerobic glycolysis, 2.2, are low and anerobic glycolysis, 5.4 μl./mg./hr. is relatively high. BARRON and HUGGINS described increased oxygen utilization by human prostate when succinate and pyruvate were added. Citrate, alpha ketoglutarate, glutamate and alanine were without effect. Synthesis of citrate and transamination were observed. The high citric acid level in prostate was probably due to non-utilization. Although the majority of enzyme activities were reduced by adverse endocrine manipulations, AWAPARA did not find a change in transaminases after castration. The mechanism of action of

the sex hormones on the prostate has been studied in vitro. BERN found a level
of 50 μg./ml. of testosterone decreased aerobic glycolysis of rat ventral prostate.
McDONALD and LATTA (1956) observed that concentrations of 2 to 500 micrograms
of testosterone per ml. inhibited anerobic glycolysis of human benign hypertrophy slices from 20 to 58% of control values. They found testosterone inhibition to be reversible by washing of the slices. WOTIZ and LEMON found that
human prostate actively metabolized testosterone under aerobic conditions.
There was no evidence of decreasing effectiveness of testosterone inhibition by
virtue of metabolic inactivation under anerobic conditions in the experiments
of McDONALD and LATTA (1954).

D. The seminal vesicle
I. Function

Comparatively little is known of the human seminal vesicles. They can
be presumed to undergo differentiation and maturation at puberty much as has
been found for prostate. The primary interest in the seminal vesicle, since it
is much less prone to important
disease, is its role in fertility.
MORRISSEY expressed the opinion that vesiculectomy was
invariably followed by sterility
and often by impotence. ROL-
NICK suggested from his studies
of seminal vesiculograms that
the seminal vesicles were reservoirs for the semen. BEAMS
and KING on examination of
many rat seminal vesicles never found spermatozoa. In
post-mortem human seminal
vesicles insufficient spermatozoa were found to consider the
seminal vesicles important in
sperm storage. MACLEOD and
HOTCHKISS observed in partitioned human ejaculates that
75% of the spermatozoa were
found in the first portion. The
second portion contained more
reducing sugar. They also noted

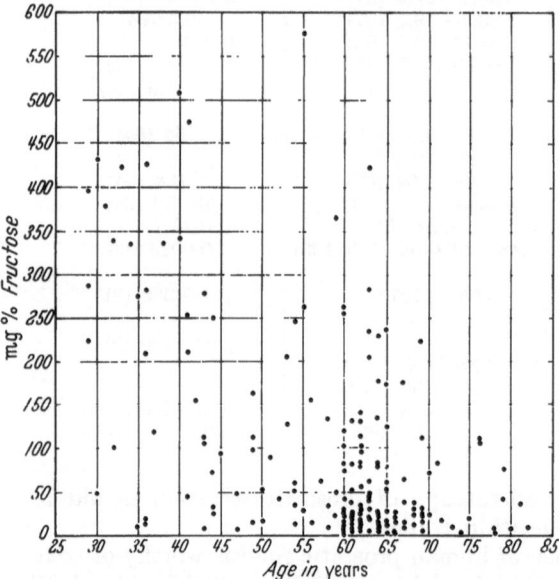

Fig. 11. Fructose concentration of seminal vesicle fluid obtained at
autopsy from men of varying ages. Each dot represents fructose
concentration in single specimen. (Courtesy J. T. GRAYHACK 1961)

that in azospermia the glucose content of semen was nearly doubled and the
lactate content halved. These changes they interpreted as metabolism of glucose
to lactate by the spermatozoa in normal semen and lack of same in aspermia.
MANN established that survival of sperm in semen depends upon the amount of
reducing sugar present in the semen. His studies conclusively established that
the reducing sugar present in semen is largely derived from the seminal vesicles
and that it is fructose not glucose. LENARD, PERLMAN and KURZROK added
seminal vesicle extract to testis homogenate. A greater quantity of hyaluronidase
activity was thereby achieved than was observed when other extracts including
that of prostate were added. They suggested that the seminal vesicles stimulated
the spermatozoa to produce hyaluronidase.

II. Aging

GRAYHACK observed in an autopsy series that the size of the seminal vesicles was relatively constant between 20 and 80 years. Only after 80 did they atrophy. Fructose content of the seminal vesicles was found to decrease with age. He interpreted these observations (Fig. 11) as indicating that androgen production even in the older age groups was sufficient to maintain size and histologic appearance but inadequate to preserve function. CHWALLA and ZANDANELL reported increased seminal vesicle weight in patients with benign prostatic hyperplasia.

III. Endocrine relationships

The seminal vesicle develops and is maintained only in the presence of adequate quantities and qualities of androgenic hormone. The seminal vesicle is reported to be more responsive to alterations in its endocrine environment than the prostate. This sensitivity has led DEANESLY and PARKES to suggest the use of the weight of the immature mouse seminal vesicles as an androgen bioassay method. LEVEY and SZEGO found both size and fructose content of the rat seminal vesicles increased by testosterone injections. In the very immature castrate mouse, HOWARD found adrenal androgens capable of maintaining the seminal vesicles for 100 days. By means of local pellet implants of testosterone, ROBSON was able to maintain the seminal vesicle in castrate rats. Androsterone was much less potent than testosterone and its ester. These studies suggested that the androgenic hormones acted directly as such without prior conjugation or chemical change in the body.

IV. Secretion

The typical seminal vesicle secretion appears as a gelatinous opalescent yellowish branched cast of the lumen of the gland. In semen it is found at the bottom of the specimen. In 15 minutes the majority of the secretion liquefies with the possible exception of a few translucent masses. Microscopic examination of the normal secretion before liquefaction shows parallel strands separated by clear or finely granular material. Rarely are spermatozoa seen in the interstices of these strands. Cells or leucocytes are absent or few in number. HUGGINS, SCOTT and HEINEN found seminal vesicle secretion much richer in protein, ascorbic acid and reducing sugar than prostatic fluid. The data of SCOTT (1945) on prostatic fluid and seminal plasma lipids can be interpreted as minimizing the lipid contribution of the seminal vesicle to the semen. This supposition is supported by the report of PORTER for the rat seminal vesicle secretion which contains no lipid. LUNDQUIST and SEEDORFF found pepsinogen activity in the semen in the same concentration as found in gastric juice. They attributed this seminal pepsinogen activity to the seminal vesicle. ELIASON asserts that prostaglandin in human semen is derived from seminal vesicle. It may induce emptying of the accessory sex organs and stimulate sperm motility. The metabolic activity of the seminal vesicle was assessed by PELC and GAHAN by means of H_3 thymidine uptake. They found an unsuspectedly high uptake of H_3 thymidine which is an indication of active metabolism.

V. Chronic hemospermia

When hemospermia persists longer than a month and is not associated with antecedent history of acute predisposing disease or trauma it is apt to become chronic for years. Among the demonstrable causes of chronic hemospermia, tuberculosis and bilharzial seminal vesiculities should be mentioned. Often complete study of the lower urinary tract fails to disclose abnormality. Chronic non-specific seminal vesiculitis has been cited as a cause of chronic hemospermia. Instillations of silver nitrate have been recommended. In idiopathic hemo-spermia, HUGGINS and McDONALD observed a characteristic syndrome. The majority of the patients noted a rusty brown rather than bright red color to the semen. When partitioned into three containers there was always more blood or rusty pigment in the third glass. Microscopically the third glass showed red blood cells singly and in clumps. There were many large macrophages filled with yellowish-brown coarse granular inclusions. Leucocytes and epithelial cells were few in number. Chemical analysis of the partitioned ejaculates substan-tiated the view that the bleeding came from the seminal vesicles. Temporary suppression of the seminal vesicle function by administration of estrogen orally for 1—2 months effected cessation of hemospermia without causing impotence or permanent oligospermia.

E. Estrogen and the accessory sex glands

Any of the potent synthetic or natural estrogenic hormones in suitable dose will induce characteristic changes in the accessory sex organs. Some of these changes relate to the reduction in androgenic function of the testis which follows pituitary suppression. Other effects are attributed to a direct action on the organs. With the aid of colchicine, TISLOWITZ was able to demonstrate that in addition to stratification and cornification of the epithelium of the prostatic acini there was increased mitotic acti-vity in stromal muscle and connec-tive tissue. Intraocular seminal ve-sicle implants in female rabbits were observed by MELCHIONNA and FLAN-DERS to show hypertrophy and hyper-plasia of smooth muscle. THORBORG observed that in all species of ani-mals studied estrogen administration caused germinal testicular atrophy. Interstitial cell atrophy as was seen after hypophysectomy was not seen

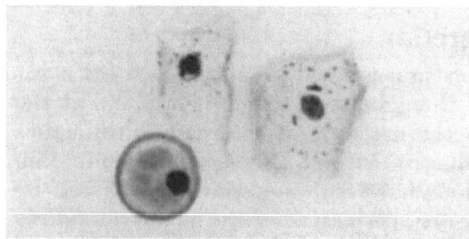

Fig. 12. Single "glycogenic" prostatic epithelial cell and two squamous epithelial cells in prostatic secretion after estrogen treatment. (Courtesy I. N. FRANK)

histologically. The indirect changes observed in the secondary sex organs resem-bled castration effects. But estrogens exerted a direct stimulatory effect on the smooth muscle of epididymis, vas deferens, prostate, most marked in the seminal vesicle. Metaplasia and edema were most intense at the level of the verumontanum which appeared to be the most estrogen sensitive of the male sex organs. HUGGINS and WEBSTER have commented on the difference in response of the anterior and posterior prostate to estrogen. In man, mouse, and rat, the anterior portion of the prostate underwent squamous metaplasia. The posterior or dorsal prostate was less responsive. In vitro studies by LASNITZKI later confirmed by FRANKS substantiated the direct inhibitory action of estrogen on prostatic epithelium. The desquamated cells of the prostatic epithelium which make their way into the prostatic secretion have a characteristic appearance in the sexually mature male. FRANK has observed that estrogen induced the prostatic epithelial cells to undergo a characteristic change in shape from columnar to spherical. The cytoplasm lost its usual staining properties and was filled with glycogen (Fig. 12). Squamous cells were more numerous in prostatic secretions from estrogen treated patients.

F. The penis
I. Growth and development

SCHONFELD has applied precise mensuration and statistical method to the determination of the median growth curve for the penis. Fig. 13 gives this growth curve. Slight increase in size of the penis during the first ten years of life culminates in a rapid growth phase during puberty. During the six year period starting at an average age of 11.5 years, puberty changes take place in the following sequence according to REYNOLDS and WINES: At age 11.5 years, enlargment of the scrotum is observed. Pubic hair first appears at age 12. Enlargment of the penis begins at 12.5 years. At 13.5 years, pubic hair becomes more abundant and curly. There is increased sculpturing of the penis. Pigmentation of the genitalia is more pronounced. Adult genital development is complete at 17.5 years. Puberty in the male also is accompanied by a spurt in longitudinal body growth. Temporary gynecomastia probably due to pituitary gonadotrophin reaches its peak in mid-puberty. Axillary and body hair and growth of the beard parallel genital development reaching maximum at the end of puberty. Laryngeal growth with deepening of the voice also reaches its adult stage at the end of puberty.

Experimental studies in growth of the penis have indicated that testosterone

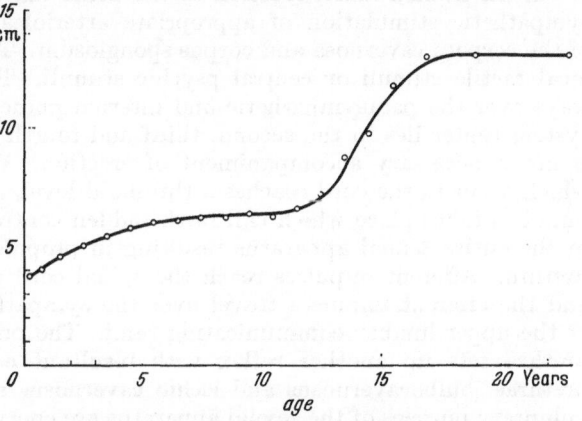

Fig. 13. Median curve for growth in length of penis. (Redrawn from SCHONFELD 1943)

alone is not complete replacement for the testis and pituitary function. THYBERG and LYONS treated hypophysectomized castrate male rats with testosterone. Although the weight of the penis was larger than that of control animals, the os penis was shorter.

LYONS, ABERNATHY, and GROPPER were unable to induce growth of the penis with pituitary somatotrophin in hypophysectomized castrate rats. Simultaneous treatment with testosterone and somatotrophin induced better growth of the os penis.

Pituitary gonadotrophin treatment of prepuberal patients with undescended testes may produce adult genital development in a few months. THOMPSON, HECKEL and BEVAN observed marked genital growth in one-third of patients treated with as little as 3000 units. The treatment of hypogenitalism in adult males who have had hypogonadism or are eunuchs can be best accomplished by injections of testosterone proprionate or long acting derivative of testosterone. VEST and HOWARD have reported that initial therapy with 25 mg. testosterone proprionate daily for two weeks can induce improved erections and ejaculations. Penis growth reached a maximum in six months. SMART and ESCAMILLA followed a castrate over a 10 year period during which time they found that fluoxymestrone and methyltestosterone linguettes did not provide satisfactory replacement therapy. Most satisfactory replacement was provided by injections of 200 mg. testosterone enanthate every 4 to 6 weeks and methyltestosterone 20 mg. daily sublingually.

II. Erection

Achievement of penile erection is the result of interrelationships between neuro-physiological, circulatory, pharmacological, anatomical and hormonal mechanisms. The neuro-physiological mechanism is the most widely investigated major influence upon erection. Eckhard first produced erections of the penis of the dog by stimulating branches of the sacral nerve which he called nervi erigenti in 1863. Semans and Langworthy noted stimulation of the second sacral nerve roots produced strong erections in the cat and stimulation of the sympathetic nerves caused emission of seminal fluid into the urethra. To cause ejaculation of the fluid, it was necessary to stimulate the internal pudendal nerves containing somatic, parasympathetic and sympathetic fibers. Excitation of a sympathetic pathway resulted in subsidence of erection.

In the human male, erection of the penis takes place as the result of parasympathetic stimulation of appropriate arterioles with resultant engorgement of the corpora cavernosa and corpus spongiosum. The reflex is initiated by either local tactile stimuli or central psychic stimuli. The nerve impulses pass both ways over the parasympathetic and internal pudic nerves. The central nervous system center lies in the second, third and fourth sacral segments. Ejaculation is not a necessary accompaniment of erection. When summation of impulses which occur in the cord reaches a threshold level, a sudden discharge of efferent impulses takes place which call forth sudden contraction of smooth musculature of the entire sexual apparatus resulting in propulsion of seminal fluid into the urethra. Afferent impulses reach the spinal cord over the internal pudic nerve and the efferent impulses travel over the sympathetic nervous system by way of the upper lumbar communicating rami. The presence of seminal fluid in the urethra sets up another reflex with resultant contraction of the constrictor urethrae, bulbocavernosus and ischio cavernosus muscles. All the striated and voluntary muscles of the sexual apparatus are enervated by the somatic neurones of the pudic nerves. The spinal cord segments that are involved in ejaculation are the second, third, and fourth sacral and upper lumbar segments.

Ejaculation also is basically a spinal-segmental reflex function. Monro, Horne, and Paull believe the integrity of the low thoracic and high lumbar sympathetic central connections is an important link in the neurologic chain. They found 28 patients with transections of the spinal cord between the sixth thoracic and third lumbar segment were incapable of ejaculation. They concluded that to prevent ejaculation cord damage must be within this area and also be extensive.

The second step of ejaculation, also reflex, is initiated by the presence of semen in the posterior urethra causing efferent impulses which travel over the internal pudic nerves by way of the second, third, and fourth sacral segments. Hence, transection of sacral segments and cauda equina can also prevent ejaculation in most individuals. The role of the autonomic nervous system in erection ejaculation is illustrated in a study of 84 patients with cord injuries at various levels by Monro, Horne, and Paull. They found 74% were capable of erections and 7% had ejaculations. They concluded erection takes place on a purely segmental-reflex basis and that afferent sensory impulses that initiate the action, travel to the second, third, and fourth sacral segments by way of the internal pudic nerves. Efferent impulses leave the same segment by way of the parasympathetic supply and cause dilatation of the arterioles of the penis. The efferent impulses travel the same segments over the internal pudic nerves to cause contraction of the peri-urethral muscles resulting in compression of venous drainage channels. MONRO concluded destruction of the sacral segments of the cord and transection and destruction of the cauda equina and pelvic parasympathetic plexus are the only neurologic-anatomic lesions preventing occurrence of erection. ZEITLIN, COTTRELL, and LLOYD corroborate MONRO's work by presenting 100 patients with spinal lesions of one year or more duration. They agree that reflex erections are mediated through the sacral portion of the spinal cord and can occur in face of any lesion above the sacral level. They conclude that the higher the spinal lesion the more probable is the occurrence of satisfactory erection. They noted 64% of the group had complete erections but only 26% had successful intercourse. 5% underwent orgasm and 3% had ejaculation while only one of them conceived. 33% of the men with cervical cord lesions were able to carry out successful intercourse while 28% of the upper thoracic group and 15% of the lower thoracic group succeeded.

Recent work by MacLEAN, PLOOG, and ROBINSON elucidates supra-segmental influence upon erection. They observed stimulation in the septum or medial preoptic region of the hypothalamus at rates of 20—30 per second caused erection in the squirrel monkey in 2—3 seconds. In subsequent work, they were able to determine the cerebral representation of penile erection. They found positive loci to involve parts of three cortico-subcortical subdivisions of the limbic system which coincide with the anatomical distribution of the hippo-campal projections to parts of the septum, anterior and midline thalamic nuclei, and hypothalamus. They noted other loci in respective parts of the anatomical system comprising the mammillary bodies, mammillothalamic tract, anterior thalamus cingulate gyrus, gyrus rectus, medial part of the medial dorsal nucleus of the thalamus, and inferior thalamic peduncle. The cortico-subcortical subdivisions of the limbic system although not directly associated with the motor function of erection does seem to reflect the role of olfactory and visual influence upon erection and does alter motor function according to these forms of sensory stimulation.

Although the nervous system has a considerable influence upon erection, the arteries and veins play a direct role in the production of erection. There is much contradictory evidence regarding the histological structures and anatomical relationships of blood vessels in the penis. DEYSACH demonstrated in his studies of the vascular anatomy of the penis two features of major importance concerning erection of the penis which does not contain a long os penis. One is the artery-like nature of the deep veins referred to as venae profundae in the corpus cavernosum. The other is the small peculiar side branches of the venae profundae referred to as sluice channels. He feels these two features together with the thick walls of the venae profundae form a complex or multiple sluice valve which he thinks is the most important part of the mechanism of erection in animals not possessing a long os penis. He classifies erections according to the predominant vascular component. The "arterial erection" is one in which the arteries of the penis dilate thus permitting a greater amount of blood to flow into the erectile bodies causing a mild state of erection. The "venous erection" is attained by compression of veins which conduct blood away from the organ also resulting in a mild state of erection. Both the forenamed types are inadequate for mammalian copulation. The third type of erection occurs only in mammals not possessing a long os penis and is referred to as a "sluice valve erection". This type achieves the greatest degree of turgescence. Conti in a long anatomical study of 20 zoo specimens presents the theory that musculo-epithelial cells selectively shunt blood into the corpora cavernosa thereby inducing turgescence.

The role of pharmacological agents in erection is questionable. HENDERSON and ROEPKE present evidence through dog experimentation that vasodilatation upon stimulating the dilator nerves to the penis is due to a local hormonal mechanism which possibly can be acetyl-choline-like in action. They were unable to present direct evidence that the local hormonal mechanism of dilatation is due to this action. However, physostigmine administration through the parietal branch of the hypogastric artery caused increase in stimulation effect, hence strongly suggested an acetylcholine mechanism. It is questionable how much influence androgens exert on erection. Sexual abilities have been described in castrate men by Rowe and Lawrence. The possibility of some degree of stimulation by androgens from extragonadal sources has remained largely an undetermined factor. Hamilton presented two cases of men castrated for 13 and 18 years who had marked capacity for penile erection in face of having low titers of urinary androgens and clinical and laboratory evidence of testicular insufficiency including supra-normal values for urinary gonadotrophins indicating no considerable extragonadal source of androgenic secretion. In view of these cases, they felt that a marked capacity for penile erection may continue for many years subsequent to castration and that this phenomenon is not the result of stimulation by extragonadal androgen sources because it occurs in individuals with definitely subnormal titers of androgens in body tissues and fluids. Their study suggests that prolonged erection ability is an exceptional phenomenon for castrates. Price and Penna attempted to determine the efficacy of estrogen in controlling post-circumcision erections through a study of 125 men given the drug. They found 10 mgm. of diethylstilbestrol per day for three days pre-operatively and for five postoperatively would reduce erection to 31% of the untreated control subjects.

The fourth influence upon erection-ejaculation is muscular in origin. Henderson and Roepke believed skeletal muscle participates in erection. They noted short spontaneous voluntary contractions of the ischio-cavernosus muscle occur followed by a gain in erection after each contraction through compression of the corpora lying between them. Monro, Horne, and Paull state that the bulbo-cavernosus and ischio-cavernosus muscles act in erection by compression of the efferent veins. Ejaculation takes place reflexly as a result of contraction of the musculature of the vasa deferentia, seminal vesicles and by voluntary contractions of the periurethral muscles.

III. Priapism

1. Definition

Priapism is persistent prolonged usually painful penile erection unaccompanied by sexual desire. It must be distinguished from transitory and nocturnal erections related to local disease usually inflammatory in character and susceptible to standard therapy. True priapism is resistant to therapy, subsides gradually, and rarely leaves its victim potent.

2. Etiology

In 1914, Hinman collected 170 cases. The majority occurred between the ages of 20 and 50 years. He classified the cases into neurogenic 20% and "mechanical" 80%. He believe thrombosis of the corpora cavernosa was the most prevalent mechanical cause of priapism. Abeshouse and Tankin in 1950, were able to collect 378 reported cases. Neurogenic causes included multiple sclerosis, paraplegia due to trauma, abscess and tabes dorsalis. Local mechanical causes included testosterone therapy in eunuchs, leukemia, sickle cell disease,

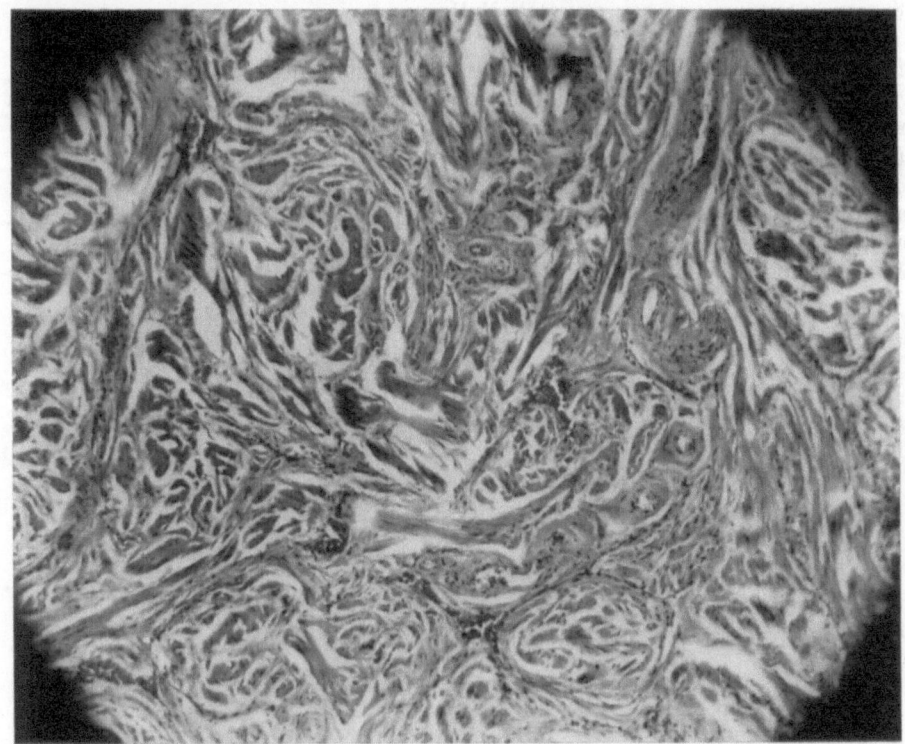

Fig. 14. Cross section of normal corpus cavernosum. (Courtesy F. HINMAN Jr.)

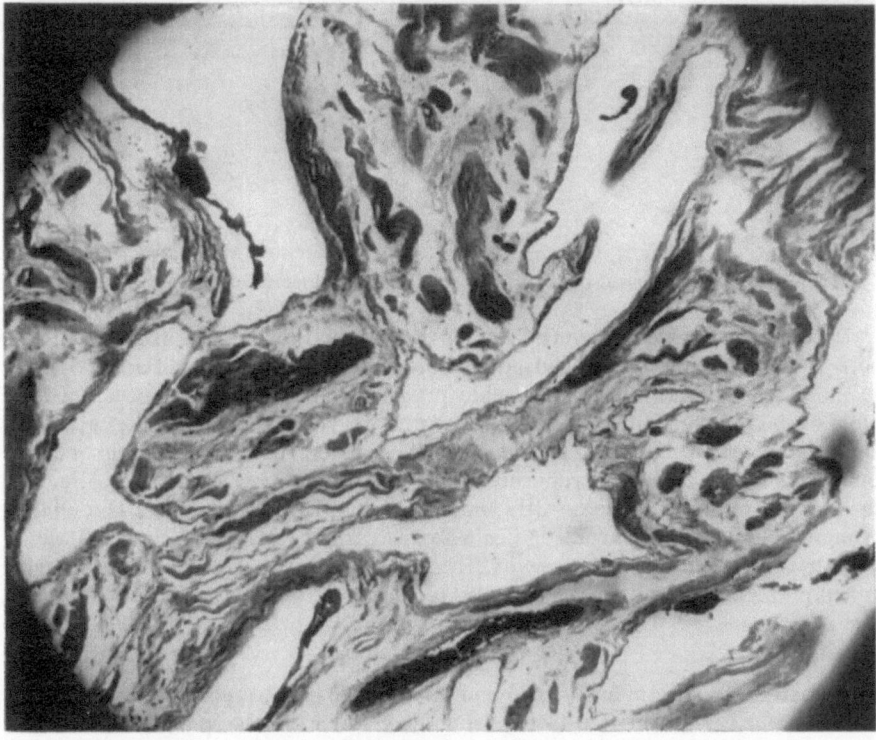

Fig. 15. Cross section of corpus cavernosum in priapism. (Courtesy F. HINMAN Jr.)

inflammatory disease, metastatic tumor from kidney, prostate, bladder, urethra, liver, rectum, trauma, impacted urethral calculus, tularemia, thrombophlebitis and pelvic abscess. Priapism has been attributed to lead poisoning and the ingestion of aphrodisiacs, notably cantharides.

HINMAN Jr. has observed characteristic histologic changes in biopsy material from the corpora cavernosa in idopathic priapism. Compared with the normal corpus cavernosum (Fig. 14), the septa of the priapic corpora (Fig. 15), are thickened and edematous. Thus failure to effect complete detumescence by

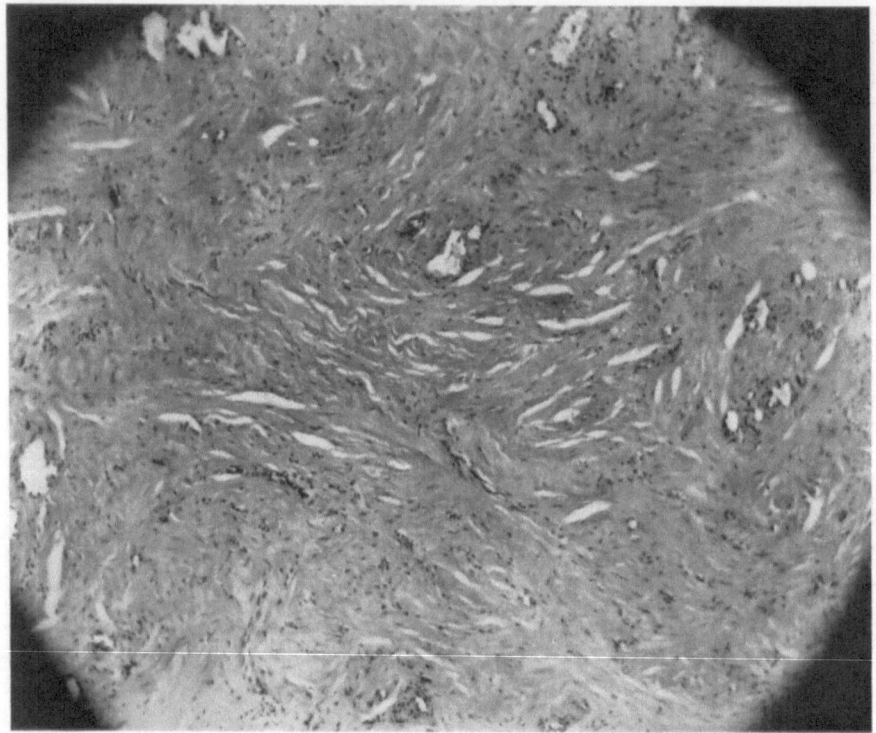

Fig 16. Cross section corpus cavernosum some time after priapism. (Courtesy F. HINMAN Jr.)

aspiration of the corpora cavernosa is explained. Subsequent fibrosis of the corpora (Fig. 16), explains the consequent erectile impotency which often follows priapism. His explanation of idiopathic priapism is, "Erection is prolonged by psychic or local excitatory factors, resulting in venous stasis. The viscosity of the blood rises from the increased carbon dioxide tension, producing relative venous occlusion at the site of juncture of the cavernous spaces with the collecting veins. Edema of the trabeculae fills the corpora and further reduces the chance for venous outflow. Eventually, occlusion of the arterioles occurs, allowing aspiration to reverse the processes. Fibrosis in the trabeculae combined with disruption of the arteriovenous supply mechanism makes adequate erections impossible."

3. Treatment

The usual early treatment of priapism of unknown cause consists of sedatives and narcotics. When these fail and the discomfort of the patient continues, regional anesthesia is induced. This also fails in most instances. Traditionally at this stage of the refractory condition, the patient is advised that incision and drainage or aspiration with massage is indicated. By this time the patient beset by pain and distraught with the enduring nature of his affliction accepts operative treatment. Multiple incision or puncture and massage reduces the degree of erection which, however, does not subside to normal for days or weeks. Once deturgescence is complete the corporal fibroplasia described by HINMAN, Jr. may be the cause of permanent impotency.

A growing number of case reports describe treatment which causes the priapism to subside without permanent impotency. EIMAN and BLOOMBERG report stilbestrol 25—50 mg. i.m. daily for a week effected gradual but complete cure of priapism associated with sickle cell anemia with preservation of potency. OLDFIELD reported success following anticoagulant treatment and massage under anesthesia. WILLIAMS reported streptokinase and streptodornase injections following aspiration of the corpora gave good results. ULM used Arfonad ® to produced hypotension and vasodilatation. Combined with aspirations, the treatment succeeded. BURT, SCHIRMER and SCOTT ligated one internal pudendal artery following which the priapism subsided. An unusual feature of this patient was the observation that the dorsal penile vein contained well-oxygenated apparently arterial blood. Potency was preserved in this patient. The successful treatment of priapism secondary to leukemic infiltrates with an alkylating agent was reported by HAAR, SHANBROM and MILLER. FINKLER found testosterone-induced priapism in a eunuch lasted seven days.

It is probable that improved methods of treatment will be forthcoming for idiopathic priapism. Some of the newer methods which may preserve potency would seem worthy of trial early in the course of the malady. Certainly, anti-coagulants, estrogens, and vasodilators would be relatively innocuous. Multiple puncture aspiration or incision and traumatic massage would best be reserved for refractory cases.

IV. Impotency

Impotence is the inability to perform normal sexual intercourse and encompasses many manifestation of sexual insufficiency such as lack of desire, desire with inability to have erection, faulty ejaculation, ejaculation without erection, painful erection or ejaculation, or physical defects precluding the technical possibility of satisfactory intercourse.

1. Etiology

HAHMAN and SCOTT classify impotence into four causes which led to interference with normal sex function: (1) the organic urologic disease, (2) physiological inferiority, (3) purely psychological disturbances, (4) a combination of organic urologic disease and psychologic disturbance. They believed organic etiology was more frequently the starting point of impotency. Psychological abberations were responsible for continuation of the problem. The latter cause was more frequently found in men in the prime of life. WOLBARST in a study of 300 cases found 44% gave a history of gonorrhea, 51% admitted long continued "withdrawal", excessively frequent coitus, frequent masturbation and ungratified sex desires. Urethroscopically, abnormality was observed in 89% with a gonorrheal history and in 77% of non-gonorrheal cases with a history of abnormal sex activity. He opined that seminal vesiculitis was the invariably common factor observed in all cases regardless of history and abnormality in the posterior urethra was not the cause of the impotence but reflected the primary

condition existing in the vesicles. Dahlen and Goodwin pointed out that men
who became impotent after open perineal prostatic biopsy were older than those
whose potency was retained post-operatively. They emphasized that a certain
number of aging men became impotent spontaneously unrelated to any surgical
procedure. They presented 24 cases of men who underwent open perineal
biopsies and no further treatment. Twenty-nine percent became totally impotent, 37% had diminution in sexual power and 33% claimed unchanged or
increased potency. Finkle and Moyers performed the same procedure on 54
patients and found 23% were impotent following the biopsy. They think problems
other than the prostatic operation per se are equally contributory or causative
of sexual impotency. Hvidt did 211 open prostatectomies and found 43%
became impotent in all age groups. Eleven percent of patients under 60 became
impotent and seminal emission stopped in 78% of those with preserved potency.
The role of age in impotency was presented in Newman and Nichol's series of
250 geriatric subjects aging from 60 to 90 years. They found 54% of those who
were married were still active. They found sexual interest and activity does
decline with advancing years but cessation of sexual activity in the oldest subjects was often found to be related to a decline in physical health of one or both
of the marital partners. Finkle et al. studied 101 men over 55 years of age and
found sexual potency in twice as many men under the age of 70 as over the
70 year age level. A prevalence of impotency was found in patients with diabetes
mellitus. Rubin found 25% of diabetic men ages 30 to 34 years were impotent.
Seventy percent of the men who had the disease less than one year were impotent
because of various uncontrolled states of the disease. He compared 168 diabetic
men with 168 healthy married men and concluded impotency is 2—5 times
higher in the diabetic male and reaches 53.6% for men 50 to 54 years of age.
Drugs with atropine-like and ganglionic blocking action were associated with
impotency. Robinson and Schwartz found impotency uniformly coincident
with methantheline bromide ingestion. Partial impotency may be the earliest
manifestation of impaired pelvic blood flow and may be present with minimal
occlusive disease of the aorta or iliac vessels according to O'Conor. He claimed
the mechanism was reflex vasospasm of the pelvic arteries. Leriche described
the foremost complaints of young adults with thrombotic obliteration of the
aortic bifurcation as impotency and lower extremity fatigue. Huhner proposed
that the organic cause for impotence was congestion of the prostatic urethra.
Wolbarst corroborated his findings and described congestion, erosion, granulations, polyps, cysts, excrescences, hypertrophy, swelling, and distortion of the
verumontanum associated with organic impotency. According to Tuthill
psychological impotency was primarily due to faulty development of sexual
reflexes due to restraints of society which in sensitive people inhibited them from
spontaneous response and action.

2. Diagnosis

The diagnosis of impotency is based on a thorough investigation. Keshin
and Pinck stated that a systematized and comprehensive evalution is essential.
It is necessary to delve into specific detail about the many features associated
with impotency. Drug addiction, alcoholism, marital incompatibility are important contributing factors. The past history is probed to disclose any antecedent
episodes of trauma, venereal disease, childhood illnesses which are sometimes
provocative of orchitis, and hereditary disposition to sexual weakness. During
the physical examination, special attention is devoted to distribution of fat

and hair as well as genital abnormalities. Examination of scrotal contents, perineum, and prostate deserve particular care. Microscopic study of prostate-vesicular secretion and sperm are performed as well as laboratory tests to procure leads concerning infections and metabolic or endocrine dysfunction. Cysto-scopy can divulge disease of the posterior urethra. In rare instances, seminal vesiculography may be considered important in diagnosis.

3. Physical findings

SCOTT and HAHMAN outlined criteria for physical abnormalities as causative agents in impotence. Inflammatory conditions of the prostatic urethra, veru-montanum, seminal vesicles, and ejaculatory ducts show swelling of the veru, congestion of the posterior urethral mucosa and abnormal granulations replacing the epithelium. Infectious inflammatory reactions from trauma secondary to calculi or foreign body introduction may show the same appearance. Surgical injury to the nerve supply of this area may at times disturb the mechanism of erection. New growths of the prostate and posterior urethra also may interfere with potency either as a primary cause or through secondary inflammation or ulceration. Prostatitis and vesiculitis give rise to verumontanum and posterior urethral reaction. Neurologic injury to the pudic nerves or lower cord result in impotency. WOLBARST supports HAHMAN and SCOTT'S findings in presenting 114 cases of impotent men without gonorrhea who were determined to have hypertrophy, swelling, and distortion of the verumontanum with trabeculation of the urethral floor. He believes these findings represent seminal vesiculitis in which the organs are palpably tender, the prostate atonic, soft, flat, sometimes enlarged with indistinct margins. The vasa deferentia may present with con-siderable thickening and occlusions with inflammatory detritus. Pus is fre-quently found in the urine. KESHIN and PINCK believe the inflammatory reac-tion of the posterior urethra produces an irritation to the nerve endings resulting in premature ejaculation which leads to impotence. Several factors may account for this: (1) the nerve endings which were originally over-stimulated are damaged and lose their conductive property, (2) the center of ejaculation and erection may become damaged as a result of excessive number of stimuli coming to them.

4. Treatment

The treatment of impotency is directed for the most part towards eradication of organic pathology followed by psychiatric intervention provided a basis for the latter is the prominent etiology. WOLBARST believes methods of treatment must deal with the man's entire complex of mental and physical equipment not merely his sex organs. Endocrine dysfunction must be corrected, obesity corrected, and occasionally organic replacement products administered. Under-lying inhibitions must be uncovered and treated by psychiatrist. Congenital pathology can be rectified along with other measures. Urethral pathology is treated with decongesting methods consisting of massage and local applications of silver nitrate solution. Urethral irrigations must not be given too frequently. WOLBARST considered in the vast majority of cases, vasotomy the most effective single therapeutic measure for vesiculitis associated with impotency. He claimed 77% cures for impotency provided all etiologic factors were accorded appropriate treatment. HUHNER stated that impotence is most often due to locally congested secondary sex organs. His treatment was directed to the prostatic urethra and verumontanum. He gave prostatic gentle massage followed by instillation of

weak silver nitrate solution into the urethra every week for seven weeks. He
believed the muscles of erection become weakened and atonic. Therefore, he
used sinusoidal-faradic current to invigorate them. KESHIN and PINCK in their
comprehensive work indicated that surgical therapy is rarely required but
various procedures have been devised to control erection such as deep dorsal
vein ligation, vasa deferentia ligation to increase the number of interstitial cells
with resultant increased hormonal secretion (STEINACH). Plication of the bulbo-
cavernosus and ischiocavernosus muscles allowed greater compressibility of the
veins leading from the penis. However, these procedures have met with limited
success. KOVACS believed physiotherapy played a most important role in relieving
congestion of the posterior urethra. He claimed faradic current, urethral instillations, hot and cold douches and showers and rectal diathermy relieved posterior
urethral congestion and acted as stimulants to the central nervous system.
TUTHILL treated erectile impotence with 100 to 200 mgm. testosterone implants
and found all those treated improved. CARMICHAEL stated that if the sex glands
are not impaired or deficient they would not respond to endocrine stimulation.
In general, testosterone was a substitution or supplement to the testis secretion
and aided to stimulate the secondary sex apparatus. ZUCHERMAN stated that
severe injury can result to the seminiferous tubules from excess administration
of the hormones. Testosterone seemed of little value in cases which had no
endocrine disturbance. Cases which were purely psychiatric in nature should
be handled by a physician trained in psychiatry. However, all organic diseases
must be ruled out or treated before referral is made.

V. Peyronie's disease or plastic induration of the penis

1. Introduction

PERONIE'S disease or plastic induration of the penis is an affliction characterized by fibrous infiltration which begins in the septum between the corpora
cavernosa in any part of the organ. It may extend laterally into BUCK'S fascia
on either side to form uneven plaques (Fig. 17). It rarely involves the cavernous
bodies. Although evidence of the disease is alluded to in early pre-christian
literature, the first accurate description of the disease is credited to LA PEYRONIE
in 1743. There has been a paucity of information about this malady because
of difficulty encountered in extracting adequate histories and follow-up information.

2. Incidence

Fully two-thirds of the reported cases of PEYRONIE'S disease have been in
men between the ages of 40 and 60 years. LOWSLEY reports the disease may
occur in younger men. A few cases have been reported in men in the third decade
of life and 12 cases in men under 25 years of age.

3. Etiology

The cause remains unknown. Attempts to etiologically associate induratio
penis plastica with venereal disease, gout, and arthritis have been unsuccessful.
CALLOMON states that the indurative tissue changes of gonorrhea and syphilis
have nothing to do with the nodules, streaks or shields characteristic of plastic
induration. The corpora cavernosa in PEYRONIE'S disease are almost never
involved. The indurations are devoid of inflammatory elements, and the skin is
freely movable over the lesion. Lymphogranuloma inguinale also has equally

distinct differences from induratio penis plastica. It is equally difficult to impli-
cate diabetes and gout. ZUR VERTH and SCHEELE found only 29 cases of diabetes
mellitus and gout in 203 cases of plastic induration. CALLOMON and BURFORD noted
only 15 cases of diabetes in 156 cases of plastic induration. Hence, it seems
likely that association of induratio penis plastica and gout or diabetes may be
coincidence. Likewise it is possible for gout and diabetes to have an occasional
association with DUPUYTREN's contracture. Because of its more frequent occurrence in the elderly and its pathologic similarity to PEYRONIE's disease, the
two conditions may be due to a degenerative process. The occasional case in

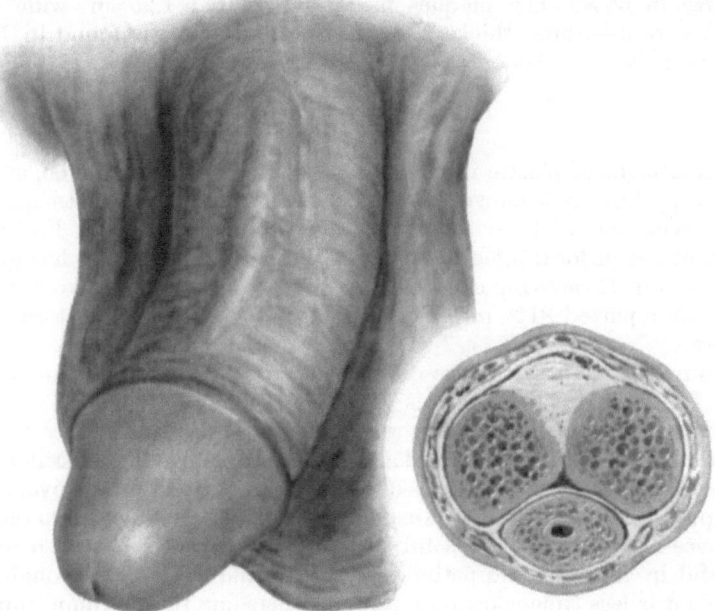

Fig. 17. PEYRONIE's disease

youth seems to refute this hypothesis. At present no degenerative process common to both diseases has been discovered. Trauma has a relationship to palmar
contracture and plastic induration. Many authors have observed that DUPUY-
TREN's contracture is more common in manual laborers although it has also
been found in professional men. WESSON advances the theory of internal trauma
produced by psychogenic "irritation" as a principle cause of induration. Regardless of the various methods of injury, it appears that trauma may favor fascial
disease development as a secondary factor where individual predispostion may
act as a primary force.

4. Pathology

The histological appearance is that of thick plaques oʃ partly hyalinized connective tissue poor in cells and elastic tissue. There are few if any inflammatory
changes. Some investigators have found pronounced vascular changes with
thickening of the intima. In about 10% of cases there are calcareous deposits
or irregular cartilage or bone formation within the hardened tissue. This latter
finding has led WHIRSCH to postulate the disease as atavistic reversion to the
os priapi found in some animals. However, this is unfounded because it is well-

known that bone formation often occurs in various parts of the body where it is not normally found. Bone formation in plastic induration of the penis is considered by Schaurup to be "simple" metaplasia.

5. Clinical appearance

The most common subjective findings are deformity, tender masses, unsatisfactory intercourse, and pain. Lowsley and Boyce presented 50 cases in which dorsal deformity was found in 66%, lateral deformity in 11%, and ventral in 12%. Pain on erection was found in 46%, impotency in 36%, and unsatisfactory intercourse in 64%. The plaques usually measured 1.25 cm. wide and 3 cm. long and were 3—7 mm. thick. Hyaline degeneration was found in 76%, calcification in 20%, and bone formation in 4% of cases.

6. Treatment

The treatment of plastic induration of the penis with medicine, surgery, and radio-therapy have not shown convincing results. Medical treatment consisting of lacto-vegetarian diet, iodine and thiosinamine have given limited results. More recent use of local injections of cortisone into the plaques has given 100% improvement in 24 cases reported by Teasley. Scardino and Scott and Waller and Preese reported 81% improvement in 33 patients on long-term tocopherol treatment.

Radium treatment of fibrous cavernositis also varies widely in its degree of success. Barford treated 18 cases with an average of 150 mg. r. claiming 84% improvement or cure and Fricke and Vormey treated 141 cases with heavily filtered radium over the entire shaft. They acquired only 10% excellent and 20% good results. 44% of those treated claimed no benefit at all over a six year follow-up. Soiland acquired 7 cures out of 18 cases using a 4 gram radium pack. He believes radium is "only useful". X-ray therapy also has been found to be only useful in checking the activity of plastic induration. Although this form of treatment is less time-consuming and cumbersome than radium, improvement ranges between 20 and 45%.

According to Lowsley the surgical treatment by which a number of good results have been obtained consists of total extirpation of the indurated tissue through a longitudinal incision on the dorsum of the penis. The excision may be complicated by hemorrhage if the induration extends wedge-shaped down between the two corpora cavernosa. Objection to surgical treatment is that it may leave a scar which is no improvement over the affliction. Besides, vessel and nerve injury may jeopardize complete erections especially if surgery involves the corpora cavernosa. He treated seven cases with surgical excision and acquired gratifying improvement in six of them. The failure was a result of wide incision because of extensive lateral wall induration which led to a new deformity. In a more recent series of 50 patients, Lowsley and Boyce claim 78% of them were cured or markedly improved through surgical treatment.

References

Testis

Arey, L. B.: Developmental anatomy, 6th edit., pp. 24, 28, 316. Philadelphia and London: W. B. Saunders Company 1954. — Ashbel, R., and A. M. Seligman: A new reagent for the histochemical demonstration of active carboxyl groups. A new method for staining ketonic steroids. Endocrinology 44, 565 (1949).

BAILEY's tectbook of histology, revised by P. E. SMITH and W. M. COPENHAVER, p 551. Baltimore, Maryland: Williams & Wilkins Company 1948. — BARR, M. L.: Sex chromatin and phenotype in man. Science 130, 679 (1959). — BERTHOLD, A. A.: Transplantation der Hoden. Arch. Anat., Physiol. u. wiss. Med. 1849, 42—26. — BIGGART, J. H.: Hypophysis of human castrate. Bull. Johns Hopk. Hosp. 54, 157 (1934). — BURROWS, A.: Influence of oestrogenic compounds in causing hernia and descent of testes in mice. Brit. J. Surg. 23, 658 (1936).

CALLAWAY, J. L., V. MOSELEY and S. W. BAREFOOT: Effects of roentgen ray irradiation on the testis of rabbits. Possible harmful effects on human testes from low voltage roentgen ray therapy. Arch. Derm. Syph. (Chic.) 56, 471 (1947). — CHARNEY, C. W.: Discussion. Fertil. and Steril. 3, 42 (1952). — CLEGG, E. J.: Some effects of artificial cryptorchidism on the accessory sexual organs of the rat. J. Endocr. 18, 27 (1959). — Committee on pathologic effects of atomic radiation, report of. Science 124, 60 (1956). — COWIE, A. T., and S. J. FOLLEY: Physiology of the gonadotropins and lactogenic hormone. Hormones 3, 309 (1955). — CULP, O. S., and J. W. BEST: Morphology of human spermatozoa: Observations with the electron microscope. J. Urol. (Baltimore) 61, 446 (1949).

DAVID, K., E. DINGEMANSE, J. FREUD and E. LAQUER: Über krystallinisches männliches Hormon aus Hoden (Testosteron), wirksamer als aus Harn oder aus Cholesterin bereitetes Androsteron. Hoppe-Seylers Z. physiol. Chem. 233, 281 (1935). — DE ROBERTS, E. D. P., W. W. NOWINSKI and F. A. SALZ: General cytology, 2nd edit. Philadelphia: W. B. Saunders Company 1954. — DORFMAN, R. I.: Biochemistry of androgens. Hormones 1, 467 (1948).

ENGBERG, H., E. ANDERSON, B. SURY and J. RAFT: Possibility of determining androgen production by measuring acid phosphatase in semen; Investigation in cryptorchid testes. J. Endocr. 5, 42 (1947). — ENGLE, E. T.: Experimentally induced descent of testis in macacus monkey by hormones from anterior pituitary and pregnancy urine. Endocrinology 16, 513 (1932).

FINKELSTEIN, M., E. FORCHIELI and R. I. DORFMAN: Estimation of testosterone in human plasma. J. clin. Endocr. 21, 98 (1961). — FORD, C. E., P. E. POLANI, J. H. BRIGGS and P. M. F. BISHOP: A presumptive human XXY/XX mosaic. Nature (Lond.) 183, 1030 (1959). — FRIEDMAN, N. B., and E. DRUTZ: Certain effects of irradiation, nitrogen mustard, urethane and colchicine on the testis. J. Urol. (Baltimore) 85, 609 (1961).

GALLAGHER, T. F., D. G. PETERSON, R. I. DORFMAN, A. T. KENYON and F. C. KOCH: Daily urinary excretion of estrogenic and androgenic substances by normal men and women. J. clin. Invest. 16, 695 (1937). — GLOVER, T. D.: The effect of a short period of scrotal insulation in the ram. Proc. physiol. Soc. 4, 31 (1958). — GORDON, M. B.: Endocrine study of hypogonadism and cryptorchidism. N.Y. J. Med. 36, 1313 (1936). — GORDON, M. B., and E. M. FIELDS: Comparative values of chorionic gonadotropic hormone and testosterone propionate in treatment of cryptorchidism and hypogenitalism. J. Endocr. 2, 531 (1942). — GREEN, J. D.: The comparative anatomy of the hypophysis with special reference to its blood supply and innervation. Amer. J. Anat. 88, 225 (1951). — GREEN, J. D., and G. W. HARRIS: The neurovascular link between the neurohypophysis and the adenohypophysis. J. Endocr. 5, 136 (1947). — GROSS, R. E., and T. C. JEWETT jr.: Surgical experience from 1222 operations for undescended testis. J. Amer. med. Ass. 160, 634 (1956).

HAMILTON, J. D., and S. L. LENARD: Effect of male hormone substance on testes and on spermatogenesis. Anat. Rec. 71, 105 (1938). — HANES, F. M., and C. W. HOOKER: Hormone production in undescended testes. Proc. Soc. exp. Biol. (N.Y.) 35, 549 (1937). — HELLER, C. G., and W. O. NELSON: Testis-pituitary relationship in man. Recent Progr. Hormone Res. 3, 229 (1948). — HINMAN Jr., F.: Optimum time for orchiopexy in cryptorchidism. Fertil. and Steril. 6, 206 (1955). — HOLLANDER, N., and V. P. HOLLANDER: Testosterone content of human spermatic vein blood, microdetermination. J. clin. Endocr. 18, 966 (1958).

JACOBS, P. A., A. G. BAIKIE, W. M. COURT, BROWN, H. FOREST, J. R. ROY, J. S. S. STEWART and B. LENNOX: Chromosomal sex in the syndrome of testicular feminization. Lancet 1959 II, 591. — JEFFRIES, M. E.: Production of experimental cryptorchid rat testes as indicated by seminal vesicles and prostate cytology tests. Anat. Rec. 48, 131 (1931). — JOST, A.: Problems of fetal endocrinology: The gonadal and hypophyseal hormones. Recent Progr. Hormone Res. 8, 379 (1953).

KLINEFELTER jr., H. F., E. C. REIFENSTEIN jr. and F. ALBRIGHT: Syndrome characterized by gynecomastia, aspermatogenesis without A-Leydigism and increased excretion of follicle stimulating hormone. J. clin. Endocr. 2, 615 (1942).

LEHMAN, J.: Zur Frage der Geschlechtsspezifizität der Keimdrüseninkrete. Inkretwirkung und Veränderung der Kastrationshypophyse der Ratte. Arch. des Physiol. 216, 729 (1927). — LONG, M. E., and E. T. ENGLE: Cytochemistry of the human testis. Ann. N.Y. Acad. Sci. 55, 619 (1952).

MACDONALD, J., and R. G. HARRISON: Effect of low temperatures on rat spermatogenesis. Fertil. and Steril. 5, 205 (1954). — MACLEOD, J., and R. S. HOTCHKISS: Effect of hyperpyrexia upon spermatozoa counts in men. Endocrinology **28**, 780 (1941). — MACK, W. S., L. S. SCOTT, M. A. FERGUSON-SMITH and B. LENNOX: Ectopic testis and true unde- scended testis: A histological comparison. J. Path. Bact. **82**, 439 (1961). — MANN, T.: The biochemistry of semen. New York: John Wiley & Sons 1954. — MAXIMOW, A. A., and W. BLOOM: A textbook of histology, 6th edit., p. 464. Philadelphia and London: W. B. Saunders Company 1952. — MEITES, J.: The relation of nutrition to endocrine and repro- ductive functions. Iowa St. Coll. J. Sci. **28**, 19 (1953). — MILLER, O. J.: Sex determination: The sex chromosomes and the sex chromatin pattern. Fertil. and Steril. **13**, 93 (1962). — MONTAGNA, W.: The distribution of lipids, glycogen and phosphatases in the human testis. Fertil and Steril. **3**, 27 (1952). — Cytochemical observations on human testes and epididymis. Ann. N.Y. Acad. Sci. **55**, 629 (1952). — MOORE, C. R.: Hormone secretion by experimental cryptorchid testes. Yale J. Biol. Med. **17**, 203 (1944). — MOORE, C. R., and W. J. QUICK: The scrotum as a temperature regulator for the testis. Amer. J. Physiol. **68**, 70 (1924).

NELSON, W. O.: Gametogenic and endocrine functions of testis. Cold Spr. Harb. Symp. quant. Biol. **5**, 123 (1937).

PERRIN, E. V., and K. BENIRSCHKE: Somatic sex of anencephalic infants. J. clin. Endocr. **18**, 327 (1958).

RABOCH, J., and J. HOMOLKA: Acid phosphatases in the ejaculate of men with distur- bances of somatosexual development. Fertil. and Steril. **12**, 368 (1961). — ROOSEN-RUNGE, E. C.: Quantitative investigations on human testicular biopsies. Fertil. and Steril. **7**, 251 (1956). — ROOSEN-RUNGE, E. C., and F. D. BARLOW: Quantitative studies on human sper- matogenesis: Spermatogonia. Amer. J. Anat. **93**, 143 (1953). — RUZICKA, L., M. W. GOLD- BERG, J. MEYER, H. BRÜNGGER u. E. EICHENBERGER: Zur Kenntnis der Sexualhormone. II. Über die Synthese des Testikelhormons (Androsteron) und Stereoisomerer desselben durch Abbau hydrierter Sterine. Helv. chim. Acta **17**, 1395 (1934).

SCHNALL, M. D.: Electronmicroscopic study of human spermatozoa. Fertil. and Steril. **3**, 62 (1952). — SCHULTZ-LARSEN, J.: Spermatozoa-electron microscopy of ultrastructure. Acta path. microbiol. scand., Suppl. **128**, 1 (1958). — SCORER, C. G.: Descent of the testicle in the first year of life. Brit. J. Urol. **27**, 374 (1955). — SCOTT, W. W., and K. M. LYNCH: The Sertoli cell in studies on testis ovary, eggs, and sperm. Edit. by E. T. ENGLE, p. 37. Springfield (Ill.): Ch. C. Thomas 1952. — SHETTLES, L. B.: Relation of dietary deficiencies to male fertility. Fertil. and Steril. **11**, 88 (1960). — SHOVAL, A. R.: Histopathology of cryptorchidism. A study based upon the comparative histology of retained and scrotal testes from birth to maturity. Amer. J. Med. **16**, 346 (1954). — SNIFFEN, R.: The testis: I. The normal testis. Arch. Path. **50**, 259 (1950). — STEINACH, E., and H. KUN: Hyperemia as a test of male sex hormone. Lancet **1940 I**, 688.

TJIO, J. H., and A. LEVAN: The chromosome number of man. Hereditas (Lund) **42**, 1 (1956). — TURNER, H. H.: A syndrome of infantilism, congenital webbed neck, and cubitus valgus. Endocrinology **23**, 566 (1938).

VELARDO, J. T.: The endocrinology of reproduction. New York: Oxford Univ. Press 1958. — VORDER BRUEGGE, C. F.: Radiation injury following an A-bomb explosion. Ann. intern. Med. **36**, 1444 (1952).

WELLS, A. J.: Descent of the testis. Surgery **14**, 436 (1942). — WERNER, S. C.: Failure of gonadotropic function of rat hypophysis during chronic inanition. Proc. Soc. exp. Biol. (N.Y.) **41**, 101 (1939). — WILLIAMS, W. W.: Cytology of the human spermatozoön. Fertil. and Steril. **1**, 199 (1950). — WITSCHI, E., and G. M. RILEY: Quantitative studies on the hormones of human pituitaries. Endocrinology **26**, 565 (1940). — WYNDHAM, N. R.: A morphological study of testicular descent. J. Anat. (Lond.) **77**, 179 (1943).

YOUNG, D.: The influence of varicocele on human spermatogenesis. Brit. J. Urol. **28**, 426 (1956).

ZELSON, C., and E. STEINITZ: Treatment of cryptorchidism with male sex hormone. J. Pediat. **15**, 522 (1939).

Epididymis, vas deferens, ejaculatory ducts, and penis

ABESHOUSE, B. S., and L. A. TANKIN: True priapism; Report of 4 cases and review of literature. Urol. cutan, Rev. **54**, 449 (1950).

BARFORD, E. H.: Fibrous cavernositis. J. Urol. (Baltimore) **43**, 208 (1946). — BELFIELD. W. T., and H. C. ROLNICK: Obervations on the physiology and therapy of the seminal duct. J. Amer. med. Ass. **89**, 2104 (1927). — BISHOP, D. W., and H. P. MATHEWS: Significance of intravas pH in relation to motility. Science **115**, 209 (1952). — BURT, F. B., H. K. SCHIRMER and W. W. SCOTT: A new concept in the management of priapism. J. Urol. (Baltimore) **83**, 60 (1960).

CALLOMON, F. T.: Induratio penis plastica. The problems of its etiology and patho- genesis. Urol. cutan. Rev. **49**, 742 (1945). — CARMICHAEL, H. T., W. J. NOONAN and A. L.

KENYON: The effects of testosterone propionate in impotence. Amer. J. Psychiat. 97, 919 (1941). — CONTI, A.: L'erection du penis humain et ses bases morphologico-vasculaires. Acta anat. (Basel) 14, 217 (1952).
DAHLEN, C. P., and W. E. GOODWIN: Sexual potency after perineal biopsy of prostate. J. Urol. (Baltimore) 77, 660 (1957). — DAHLEN, C. P., L. KAPLAN and W. E. GOODWIN: Priapism as complication of tularemia. J. Urol. (Baltimore) 72, 1192 (1954). — DEYSACH. L. J.: The comparative morphology of the erectile tissue of the penis with especial emphasis on the probable mechanism of erection. Amer. J. Anat. 64, 11 (1939).
ECKHARD, C.: Untersuchungen über die Erektion des Penis beim Hunde. Beitr. Anat. Physiol. 3, 123 (1863). — EIMAN, S., and H. H. BLOOMBERG: Priapism in sickle cell anemia: Treatment by estrogenic hormone. J. Urol. (Baltimore) 84, 345 (1960).
FINKLE, A. L., T. A. MOYERS, M. I. TOBENKIN and S. L. KARG: Sexual potency in aging males. J. Amer. med. Ass. 170, 1391 (1959). — FINKLER. R. S.:Initial priapism during therapy with testosterone propionate in eunuchoid man. J. Urol. (Baltimore) 43, 866 (1940). — FRICKE, R. H.. and J. A. VORMEY: PEYRONIE's disease and its treatment with radium. J. Urol. (Baltimore) 59, 627 (1948).
HAAR, H., E. SHANBROM and S. MILLER: The treatment of leukemic priapism with A-139. J. Urol. (Baltimore) 83, 429 (1960). — HAHMAN, L. B., and W. W. SCOTT: Combined psychiatric and urologic study of sexual impotency. J. Urol. (Baltimore) 29, 59 (1933). — HAMILTON, J. B.: Demonstrated ability of erection in castrate men with markedly low titers of urinary androgens. Proc. Soc. exp. Biol. (N.Y.) 54, 309 (1943). — HENDERSON. V. E., and M. H. ROEPKE: The mechanism of erection. Amer. J. Physiol. 106, 441 (1933). — HINMAN, F.: Priapism: Report of cases and a clinical study of the literature with reference to its pathogenesis and surgical treatment. Ann. Surg. 60. 689 (1914). — HINMAN jr., F.: Priapism: Reasons for failure of therapy. Trans. Amer. Ass. gen.-urin. Surg. 51, 82 (1959). — HUHNER. M.: Masturbation and impotence from urologic standpoint. J. Urol. (Baltimore) 36, 770 (1936). — HVIDT, V.: Patensforhold efter prostatectomie. Nord. Med. 62, 1684 (1959).
IVANIZKY, M.: Beiträge zur Anatomie des Ductus ejaculatorius. Z. Anat. Entwickl.-Gesch. 87, 11 (1923).
KESHIN, J. G., and B. D. PINCK: Impotencia. N. Y. J. Med. 49, 269 (1949). — KNAUS, H.: Zur Physiologie der Spermatozoen. Arch. Gynäk. 151, 302 (1932). — KOVACS, R.: Electrotherapy and light therapy. Philadelphia: Lea & Febiger 1945. — KUNTZ, A.: The autonomic nervous system, third edition. Philadelphia: Lea & Febiger 1945.
LANZ, T. v., T. WALLRAFF and U. HANDFEST u. K. WIMMER: Der Nebenhodenschweif des Menschen als Samenspeicher. Z. mikr.-anat. Forsch. 37, 259 (1935). — LAWLESS, J. J.: Castration in rat with and without removal of epididymides. Anat. Rec. 66, 455 (1936). — LERICHE, R.: De la resection du carrefour aorticoiliaque avec double sympathectomie lombaire pour thrombose arteritique de l'aorte le syndrome de l'obliteration terminoartique par arterete. Presse méd. 48, 601 (1940). — LOWSLEY, O. S.: Surgical treatment of plastic induration of the penis — PEYRONIE's disease. N.Y. J. Med. 43, 2273 (1943). — LOWSLEY. O. S., and W. H. BOYCE: Further experience with an operation for cure of PEYRONIE's disease. J. Urol. (Baltimore) 63, 888 (1950). — LYNN, J. M., and R. M. NESBIT: Influence of vasectomy upon incidence of epididymitis following TUR prostatectomy. J. Urol. (Baltimore) 59, 229 (1948). — LYONS, W. R., E. ABERNATHY and M. GROPPER: Effects of androgen and somatotrophin (growth hormone) on os penis of rat. Proc. Soc. exp. Biol. (N.Y.) 73, 193 (1950).
MACLEAN, P. D., D. W. PLOOG and B. W. ROBINSON: Circulatory effects of limbic stimulation with special reference to the male genital organ. Physiol. Rev. 40, 105 (1960). — MARTINS, T., and J. R. VALLE: Endocrine control of motility of male accessory genital glands. Endocrinology 25, 80 (1939). — MCCARTHY, J. F., J. S. RITTER and P. KLEMPERER: Anatomical and histological study of the verumontanum with special reference to the ejaculatory ducts. J. Urol. (Baltimore) 17, 1 (1927). — MONRO, D., H. W. HORNE and D. P. PAULL: The effects of injury to the spinal cord and cauda equina on the sexual potency of men. New Engl. J. Med. 239, 903 (1948). — MOORE, C. R.: Supplementary observations on mammalian testes activity; vas efferentia ligation; atypical scrota. Anat. Rec. 48, 105 (1931).
NEWMAN, G., and C. R. NICHOLS: Sexual activities and attitudes in older persons. J. Amer. med. Ass. 173, 117 (1960). — NICANDER, L.: Glycogen secretion in the epididymis. Nature (Lond.) 174, 700 (1954). — NOWSKY, D. O., and I. S. MELMAN: Plastic induration. Urol. cutan. Rev. 41, 185 (1937).
O'CONOR jr., V.: Impotence and Leriche syndrome. J. Urol. (Baltimore) 80, 195 (1958). — OLDFIELD, J.: Management of primary priapism. Brit. med. J. 1959 II, 1227. — OSLUND, R. M.: The physiology of the male reproductive system. J. Amer. med. Ass. 90, 829 (1928).
PRICE, R. A., and O. J. PENNA: Effectiveness of drugs in preventing postoperative penile erections. Surgery 24, 980 (1948).

Reynolds, E. L., and J. V. Wines: Physical changes associated with adolescence in boys. Amer. J. Dis. Child. 82, 529 (1951). — Robinson, B. D., and N. H. Schwartz: Impotence due to methantheline bromide. N.Y. J. Med. 52, 1530 (1952). — Rowe, A., and C. Lawrence: Studies of the endocrine glands. Endocrinology 12, 591 (1928). — Rubin, A.: Studies in human reproduction. II. The influence of diabetes mellitus in men upon reproduction. Amer. J. Obstet. Gynec. 76, 25 (1958). — Rubin, A., and D. Babbott: Impotence and diabetes mellitus, statistics. J. Amer. med. Ass. 168, 498 (1958).

Scardino, R. L., and W. W. Scott: Use of tocopherols in treatment of Peyronie's disease. Ann. N.Y. Acad. Sci. 52, 390 (1949). — Schaurup, K.: Plastic induration of the penis. Acta radiol. (Stockh.) 26, 313 (1945). — Schonfeld, W. A.: Primary and secondary sexual characteristics. Study of their development in males from birth thru maturity with biometric study of penis and testes. Amer. J. Dis. Child. 65, 535 (1943). — Schonfeld, W. A., and G. W. Beebe: Normal growth and variation from birth to maturity. J. Urol. (Baltimore) 48, 759 (1942). — Semans, J. H., and O. R. Langworthy: Neurophysiology of sexual function in the male cat. J. Urol. (Baltimore) 40, 836 (1938). — Shave, S. L.: Role of sterocilia in removing India ink particles from lumen of rat epididymis. Anat. Rec. 119, 177 (1954). — Smart, W. R., and R. F. Escamilla: Simultaneous bilateral testicular seminomas: Report of a case after a 10 year follow-up period with discussion of substitution androgen therapy. J. Urol. (Baltimore) 86, 614 (1961). — Smith, G.: The effects of ligation of the vasa efferentia and vasectomy on testicular function in the adult rat. J. Endocr. 23, 385 (1962). — Soiland, A.: Peyronie's disease or plastic induration. Radiology 42, 183 (1944). — Strandness, D. E., and M. Paulken: Priapism secondary to metastatic malignancy: Report of a case. Arch. Surg. 76, 644 (1958).

Teasley, G. H.: Peyronie's disease. A new approach. J. Urol. (Baltimore) 71, 611 (1954). — Thompson, W. O., N. J. Heckel and A. D. Bevan: Influence of anterior pituitary-like principle on external genitalia of young boys. J. Urol. (Baltimore) 40, 145 (1938). — Thyberg, W. G., and W. R. Lyons: Androgen induced growth of os penis of hypophysectomized-gonadectomized rats. Proc. Soc. exp. Biol. (N.Y.) 69, 158 (1948). — Toothill, M. C., and W. C. Young: Time consumed by spermatozoa in passing through ductus epididymis of guinea pig as determined by means of India ink injections. Anat. Rec. 50, 95 (1931). — Tuthill, J. F.: Impotence. Lancet 1955 I, 124.

Ulm, A. H.: The treatment of 1° priapism with Arfonad. J. Urol. (Baltimore) 81, 291 (1959).

Vest, S. A., and J. E. Howard: Clinical experiments with the use of male sex hormones. I. Use of testosterone proprionate in hypogonadism. J. Urol. (Baltimore) 40, 154 (1938).

Waller, J. I., and W. C. Preese: Peyronie's disease associated with Dupuytren's contractures. J. Urol. (Baltimore) 68, 623 (1952). — Wesson, M. B.: Peyronie's disease — cause and treatment. J. Urol. (Baltimore) 49, 350 (1943). — Whirsch, E.: Relation of os penis of mammals to bone formation in human penis. Urol. cutan. Rev. 34, 453 (1930). — Williams jr., D. C.: Treatment of priapism by tryptic enzymes. Trans. s.-east. Sect. Amer. urol. Ass. 21, 12 (1957). — Wolbarst, A. L.: Urologic aspects of sexual impotence. J. Urol. (Baltimore) 29, 77 (1933).

Zeitlin, A. B., T. L. Cottrell and F. A. Lloyd: Sexology of the paraplegic male. Fertil. and Steril. 8, 337 (1957).

The prostate gland, the seminal vesicle and estrogen and the accessory organs

Aschoff, L.: Ein Beitrag zur normalen und pathologischen Anatomie der Schleimhaut der Harnwege und ihrer drüsigen Anhänge. Virchows Arch. path. Anat. 138, 119 (1894). — Awapara, J.: The influence of sex hormones on the transaminases. Endocrinology 51, 75 (1952).

Baker, R., D. Govan, J. Huffer and J. Cason: Biologic titration of diethylstilbestrol against activity of cancer. Effect on serum aldolase. J. clin. Endocr. 13, 383 (1953). — Barron, E. S. G.: Citric acid and aconitase content of the prostate. Proc. Soc. exp. Biol. (N.Y.) 62, 195 (1946). — Barron, E. S. G., and C. Huggins: The metabolism of prostate, transamination and citric acid. J. Urol. (Baltimore) 55, 385 (1946). — Beams, H. W., and R. L. King: The sperm storage function of the seminal vesicles. J. Urol. (Baltimore) 29, 95 (1933). — Bern, H. A.: The effect of sex steroids on the respiration of the rat ventral prostate in vitro. J. Endocr. 9, 312 (1953). — Brandes, D., and D. P. Groth: The fine structure of the rat prostatic complex. Exp. Cell Res. 23, 159 (1961). — Burgen, A. S. V.: Urinary excretion of phosphatases in man. Lancet 1947 I, 329. — Burrows, H.: Pathological conditions induced by oestrogenic compounds in the coagulating gland in the prostate of the mouse. Amer. J. Cancer 23, 490 (1935). — Butler III, W. W. S., and A. I. Schade: The effects of castration and androgen replacement on the nucleic acid composition, metabolism, and enzymatic capacities of the rat ventral prostate. Endocrinology 63, 271 (1958).

CHWALLA, R., u. E. ZANDANELL: Untersuchungen über die Samenblasengröße bei Prostatikern, über die diffuse Prostatahyperplasie und die Samenblasenhyperplasie. Urol. int.
(Basel) 7, 199 (1958).
DANIEL, O., F. HADDAD, G. PROUT and W. F. WHITMORE: Some observations of the
distribution of radioactive zinc in prostatic and other human tissues. Brit. J. Urol. 28, 271
(1956). — DEANESLY, R., and A. PARKES: Size changes in seminal vesicles of the mouse
during development and after castration. J. Physiol. (Lond.) 78, 442 (1933). — DE LORY,
G. E., and M. HETHERINGTON: The determination of urinary acid phosphatase. Canad. J.
Med. Sci. 30. 1 (1952).
ECKHARD, C., quoted by C. HUGGINS: The prostatic secretion. Harvey Lect. 42, 148
(1946/47). — ELIASON, R.: Prostaglandin occurrence, form and biological properties. Acta
physiol. scand. 46, 1 (1959). — EULER, U. S. v.: Specific vasodilating and plain muscle
stimulating substances from accessory genital glands in man and certain animals. J. Physiol.
(Lond.) 88, 213 (1926). — An adrenaline-like action in extracts from prostatic and related
glands. J. Physiol. (Lond.) 81, 102 (1934).
FARRELL. J. I.: Studies on the secretion of the prostatic gland: Method for collecting
pure secretion in dogs; Factors influencing secretion of the prostatic fluid; Some properties
of prostatic secretions in dogs. Trans. Amer. Ass. gen.-urin. Surg. 24, 221 (1931). — The
newer physiology of the prostate gland. J. Urol. (Baltimore) 39, 171 (1938). — The secretion
of alcohol by the genital tract; experimental study. J. Urol. (Baltimore) 40, 62 (1938). —
FISCHER. M. I., A. O. TIKKALA and C. A. MAWSON: Zinc, carbonic anhydrase, and phosphatase in the rat. Canad. J. Biochem. 33, 181 (1955). — FRANK, I. N.: A cytologic evaluation of the prostatic smear in carcinoma of the prostate. J. Urol. (Baltimore) 73, 128 (1955). —
FRANKS, L. M.: The growth of mouse prostate during culture in vitro in chemically defined
and natural media, and after transplantation in vivo. The effects of insulin and normal
human serum. Exp. Cell Res. 22, 56 (1961). — Estrogen and testosterone on cultures of
prostate from mice of various ages. Brit. J. Cancer 13, 59 (1959).
GOETSCH. J. B.: A clinical and histochemical study of acid and alkaline phosphatase in
normal and abnormal prostatic tissue. J. Urol. (Baltimore) 84, 636 (1960). — GOMORI, G.:
Distribution of acid phosphatase in the tissues under normal and under pathologic conditions. Arch. Path. 32, 189 (1941). — GOODWIN, D. A., D. S. RASMUSSEN-TAXDAL, A. A. FER
REIRA and W. W. SCOTT: Estrogen inhibition of androgen maintained prostatic secretions
in the hypophysectomized dog. J. Urol. (Baltimore) 86, 134 (1961). — GRAYHACK, J. T.:
The effect of local testosterone administration on the prostate of the rat. Endocrinology 63,
399 (1958). — Changes with aging in human seminal vesicles. Fluid fructose concentration
and seminal vesicle weight. J. Urol. (Baltimore) 86, 142 (1961). — GRAYHACK, J. T., P. L.
BUNCE, J. W. KEARNS and W. W. SCOTT: The influence of pituitary on prostatic response to
androgen in the rat. Bull. Johns Hopk. Hosp. 96, 154 (1955). — GRAYHACK, J. T., and W. W.
SCOTT: The effect of general dietary deficiencies on the response of prostate of albino rat to
testosterone propionate. Endocrinology 50, 406 (1952). — GREER, D. S.: The distribution
of radioactivity in non-excretory organs of the male rat after injection of testosterone 4 C¹⁴.
Endocrinology 64, 898 (1959). — GUNN, S. A., and T. C. GOULD: Relative importance of
androgen and estrogen in the selective uptake of Zn 65 by dorsolateral prostate of the rat.
Endocrinology 58, 443 (1956). — GUTMAN, A. B., and E. G. GUTMAN: Acid phosphatase and
functional activity of prostate (man) and preputial glands (rat). Proc. Soc. exp. Biol. (N.Y.)
39, 529 (1932). — Adult phosphatase levels in the prepubertal rhesus prostate tissue after
testosterone propionate. Proc. Soc. exp. Biol. (N.Y.) 41, 277 (1939). — Quantitative relations
of a prostatic component (acid phosphatase) of human seminal fluid. Endocrinology 28,
115 (1941).
HAWKINS, D. F., and A. H. LABRUM: Semen prostaglandin levels in fifty patients attending a fertility clinic. J. Reprod. Fertil. 2, 1 (1961). — HOARE, R., G. E. DELORY and D. W.
PENNER: Zinc and acid phosphatase in human prostate. Cancer (Philad.) 9, 721 (1956). —
HOWARD, E.: Effects of adrenalectomy and desoxycorticosterone therapy on castrated rat
prostate; Evidence of andromimetic function of immature rat adrenal. Endrocrinology 29,
746 (1941). — The effect of adrenalectomy on accessory reproductive glands of mice castrated
for short periods. Endocrinology 38, 156 (1946). — Effects of castration on seminal vesicles
as influenced by age considered in relation to degree of development of adrenal X zone.
Amer. J. Anat. 65, 105 (1939). — HUDSON, P. B., and W. W. S. BUTLER III.: A study of the
enzyme acid phosphatase and its possible role in intermediary carbohydrate metabolism of
prostate gland and secretion in man and dog. J. Urol. (Baltimore) 63, 323 (1950). — HUG
GINS, C.: The physiology of the prostate gland. Physiol. Rev. 25, 281 (1945). — The prostatic
secretion. Harvey Lect. 42, 148 (1946/47). — HUGGINS, C., and E. S. BARRON: The metabolism of isolated prostatic tissue. J. Urol. (Baltimore) 51, 630 (1944). — HUGGINS, C., and
D. F. McDONALD: Proteolytic enzymes and acid phosphatase in the prostatic fluid in chronic
prostatitis. J. Urol. (Baltimore) 52, 472 (1944). — Chronic hemospermia; Its origin and

treatment with estrogen. J. clin. Endocr. 5, 226 (1945). — HUGGINS, C., and W. NEAL: Coagulation and liquefaction of semen; Proteolytic enzymes and citrate in prostatic fluid. J. exp. Med. 76, 527 (1942). — HUGGINS, C., and P. S. RUSSELL: Quantitative effects of hypophysectomy on testis and prostate of dogs. Endocrinology 39, 1 (1946). — HUGGINS, C., W. W. SCOTT and J. H. HEINEN: Chemical composition of human semen and of the secretion of the prostate and seminal vesicles. Amer. J. Physiol. 136, 467 (1942). — HUGGINS, C. and V. C. VAIL: Plasma coagulation and fibrinogenolysin by prostatic fluid and trypsin. Amer. J. Physiol. 139, 129 (1943). — HUGGINS, C., and W. O. WEBSTER: Duality of human prostate in response to estrogens. J. Urol. (Baltimore) 59, 258 (1948). — HUMPHREY, G. F., and T. MANN: Citric acid in semen. Nature (Lond.) 61, 353 (1948).

KARASSIK, W. M.: Über die fermentativen Eigenschaften des Prostatasekrets in Zusammenhang mit der Bedeutung der Prostata in der Spermatozoenbewegung. Z. ges. exp. Med. 53, 734 (1926). — KIRK, J. E., A. EISENSTEIN and C. M. MACBRYDE: The acid phosphatase concentration of the prostatic exprimate during normal puberty. J. clin. Endocr. 12, 338 (1952).

LASNITZKI, I.: The effect of estrogen alone and combined with 20 methylcholanthrene on mouse prostate glands grown in vitro. Cancer Res. 14, 632 (1954). — LEONARD, S. L., P. L. PERLMAN and R. KURZROK: The effect of the prostate and seminal vesicles on the production of hyaluronidase by rat testes homogenate. Endocrinology 40, 199 (1947). — LEVEY, H. A., and C. M. SZEGO: The effect of androgen on fructose production by the sex accessories of male guinea pigs and rats. Endocrinology 56, 404 (1955). — LEVIN, E., S. ALBERT and R. M. JOHNSON: Phospholipid metabolism during hypertrophy and hyperplasia in rat prostates and seminal vesicles (studies using P^{32}). Arch. Biochem. 56, 59 (1955). — LO, M. C.: Clinical application of diphenylthiocarbazone in carcinoma of the prostate. Canad. med. Ass. J. 82, 1203 (1960). — LOWSLEY, O. S.: The development of the human prostate gland with reference to development of other structures at the neck of the bladder. Amer. J. Anat. 13, 299 (1912). — LUNDQUIST, F.: Studies on biochemistry of human semen. I. The natural substrate of prostatic phosphatase. Acta physiol. scand. 13, 322 (1947). — LUNDQUIST, F., and H. H. SEEDORFF: Pepsinogen in human seminal fluid. Nature (Lond.) 170, 1115 (1952). — LUTWAK-MANN, C., and T. MANN: Restoration of secretory function in male accessory glands of vitamin B-deficient rats by means of chorionic gonadotrophin. Nature (Lond.) 165, 556 (1950).

MACLEOD, J., and R. S. HOTCHKISS: The distribution of spermatozoa and of certain chemical constituents in the human ejaculate. J. Urol. (Baltimore) 48, 225 (1942). — MANN, T.: Fructose and fructolysis in semen in relation to fertility. Lancet 1948 I, 446. — MARVIN, H. N., and J. AWAPARA: Effect of androgen on concentration of certain amino acids in the rat prostate. Proc. Soc. exp. Biol. (N.Y.) 72, 93 (1949). — MAWSON, C. A., and M. J. FISCHER: I. Carbonic anhydrase and zinc in prostate glands of the rat and rabbit. Arch. Biochem. 36, 485 (1952). — McDONALD, D. F.: Symposium on therapy for disseminated prostatic cancer. Proc. III. National Cancer Conference. Philadelphia: J. B. Lippincott Company 1956. — Effect of diphenylthiocarbazone on prostates of animals and in human prostatic cancer. J. Urol. (Baltimore) 83, 458 (1960). — McDONALD, D. F., and M. J. LATTA: Anerobic glycolysis of human benign prostatic hypertrophy slices: Inhibition by testosterone. J. appl. Physiol. 7, 325 (1954). — Anerobic glycolysis of human prostatic adenoma. II. In vitro inhibition by estrogen and by androgen and estrogen. Endocrinology 59, 159 (1956). — McNICOL, G. P., A. P. FLETCHER, H. ALKJÄERSIG and S. SHERRY: The absorption, distribution and excretion of E. aminocaproic acid following oral or intravenous administration to man. J. Lab. clin. Med. 59, 15 (1962). — MELCHIONNA, R. H., and S. FLANDERS: The physiological response of ocular transplants of the seminal vesicle in female rabbits. Endocrinology 23, 468 (1938). — MILLAR, M. J., P. V. ELCOATE and C. A. MAWSON: Sex hormone control of the zinc content of the prostate. Canad. J. Biochem. 35, 865 (1957). — MOORE, C. R., and T. F. GALLAGHER: Seminal vesicle and prostate function as a testis hormone indicator: The electric ejaculation test. Amer. J. Anat. 45, 39 (1930). — MOORE, C. R., W. HUGHES and T. F. GALLAGHER: Rat seminal vesicle cytology as testis hormone indication and prevention of castration changes by testis extract. Amer. J. Anat. 45, 109 (1930). — MOORE, C. R., and D. PRICE: Effects of testosterone and testosterone propionate in rat. Anat. Rec. 71, 59 (1938). — MOORE, C. R., and L. T. SAMUELS: The action of testis hormone in correcting changes induced in rat prostate and seminal vesicles by vitamin B deficiency or partial inanition. Amer. J. Physiol. 96, 278 (1931). — MOORE, R. A.: The evolution and involution of the prostate gland. Amer. J. Path. 12, 599 (1936). — MORRISSEY, J. H.: Surgical drainage of the seminal vesicles and prostate. Surg. Gynec. Obstet. 46, 341 (1928).

NYDEN, S. J., and H. G. WILLIAMS-ASHMAN: Influence of androgens on synthetic reactions in ventral prostate tissue. Amer. J. Physiol. 172, 588 (1953).

PAZOS jr., R., and C. HUGGINS: Effect of androgen on the prostate in starvation. Endocrinology 36, 416 (1945). — PELC, S. R., and P. B. GAHAN: Incorporation of labelled thymidine in the seminal vesicles of the mouse. Nature (Lond.) **183**, 335 (1959). — PORTER, J. C., and R. M. MELAMPY: Effects of testosterone propionate on the seminal vesicles of the rat. Endocrinology **51**, 412 (1952). — PRICE, D.: Normal development in rat with study of experimental post-natal modifications. Amer. J. Anat. **60**, 79 (1936). — PROUT, G. R., O. DANIEL and W. F. WHITMORE jr.: The occurrence of intravenously injected radio-active zinc in the prostate and prostatic fluid of dogs. J. Urol. (Baltimore) **78**, 471 (1957). — PROUT jr., G. R., M. SIERP and W. F. WHITMORE jr.: Radioactive zinc in the prostate. Some factors influencing concentration in dogs and men. J. Amer. med. Ass. **169**, 1703 (1959).

RASMUSSEN, J., and O. K. ALBRECHTSEN: Characterization of the fibrinolytic component in the human prostate. Scand. J. clin. Lab. Invest. **12**, 261 (1960). — ROBSON, J. M.: Local action of steroids on secondary sex organs of male rats. J. Physiol. (Lond.) **113**, 537 (1951). — ROLNICK, H. C.: Infections of the seminal ducts. Arch. phys. Ther. (Omaha) **8**, 163 (1927). — ROSEN-KRANTZ, H., and M. MASON: The influence of hormones and pilocarpine on biochemical constituents of canine prostatic fluid. Cancer Chemother. Reports **12**, 143 (1961).

SCHLACTA, J.: Beiträge zur mikroskopischen Anatomie der Prostate und Mamma des Neugeborenen. Arch. mikr. Anat. **64**, 405 (1904). — SCOTT, W. W.: The lipids of prostatic fluid seminal plasma and enlarged prostate gland of man. J. Urol. (Baltimore) **53**, 712 (1945).— Role of pituitary in normal and abnormal prostatic growth. Trans. Amer. Ass. gen.-urin. Surg. **46**, 33 (1954). — SCOTT, W. W., and C. HUGGINS: The acid phosphatase activity of human urine; An index of prostatic secretions. Endocrinology **30**, 107 (1942). — SELYE, H., and S. ALBERT: The pubertal increase in response of accessory sex organs to steroid hormones. Proc. Soc. exp. Biol. (N.Y.) **49**, 361 (1942). — SMELSER, G. K.: Effect of thyroidectomy on reproductive system and hypophysis of adult male rats. Anat. Rec. **74**, 7 (1939). — SONENBERG, M.: Studies with radioactively labelled anterior pituitary preparations. Ciba Found Coll. Endocrin. **4**, 229 (1951). — STAFFORD, R. O., I. N. RUBINSTEIN and R. K. MEYER: Effect of testosterone propionate on phosphatases in the seminal vesicle of the rat. Proc. Soc. exp. Biol. (N.Y.) **71**, 353 (1949). — SWYER, G. J. M.: Postnatal growth changes in human prostate. J. Anat. (Lond.) **78**, 130 (1944).

TAGNON, H. J., and A. STEEN-LIEVENS: Reversible inactivation of acid phosphatase in human prostatic extracts in vitro. Cancer (Philad.) **13**, 507 (1960). — TAGNON, H. J., W. F. WHITMORE jr., P. SCHULMAN and S. C. KRAVITZ: The significance of fibrinolysis occurring in patients with metastatic cancer. Cancer (Philad.) **6**, 63 (1953). — TAYLOR, P. W., and H. R. MORGAN: Antibacterial substances in human semen and prostatic fluid. Surg. Gynec. Obstet. **94**, 662 (1952). — TEEM, M. V.: Size and weight of normal and of pathologic prostatic gland. Arch. Path. **22**, 817 (1936). — THORBORG, J. V.: Influence of estrogenic hormones on male accessory genital system with special reference to prostate and etiology of senile hypertrophy of human prostate. Acta endocr. (Kbh.) **1**, 1 (1948). — TISLOWITZ, R.: The action of estrogens in inducing mitosis in muscle, connective tissue, and epithelium of the prostate and seminal vesicle of mice as determined by the colchicine technique. Anat. Rec. **75**, 265 (1939). — TURK, E.: The acid phosphatase of prostatic fluid in young, middle aged, and old individuals. J. Geront. **3**, 98 (1948).

WAGENER, G. VAN: The coagulating function of the cranial lobe of the prostate gland in the monkey. Anat. Rec. **66**, 411 (1936). — WILLIAMS-ASHMAN, H. G.: Changes in enzymatic constitution of ventral prostate gland induced by androgenic hormones. Endocrinology **54**, 121 (1954). — WILLIAMS-ASHMAN, H. G., and J. BANKS: The synthesis and degradation of citric acid by ventral prostate tissue. I. Enzymatic mechanisms. J. biol. Chem. **208**, 337 (1954). — WOTIZ, H. H., and H. M. LEMON: Studies in steroid metabolism; metabolism of testosterone by human prostatic tissue slices. J. biol. Chem. **206**, 525 (1954).

YING, S. H., E. DAY, W. F. WHITMORE jr. and J. H. TAGNON: Fibrinolytic activity in human prostatic fluid and semen. Fertil. and Steril. **7**, 80 (1956). — YOUMANS, G. P., J. LIERLING and R. Y. LYMAN: Bacterial action of prostatic fluid in dogs. J. infect. Dis. **63**, 117 (1938).

Endokrinologie

Von

F. Heni

Mit 66 Abbildungen

A. Entwicklung der Keimdrüsen und der Geschlechtsorgane

An der medialen Seite der Urnierenfalte beginnt bei Embryonen von 5 mm Länge das Cölomepithel und gleichzeitig das darunterliegende embryonale Bindegewebe zu wuchern, so daß sich eine neue Falte, die *Keimdrüsenleiste* (Genitalleiste, Plica genitalis) abhebt (etwa 4. Schwangerschaftswoche). Das Cölomepithel wird mehrschichtig und bildet das Keimdrüsenepithel, den Cortex. Gleichzeitig verdichtet sich das unter dem Epithel gelegene Mesenchym, hier treten die primären Keimstränge auf, die den Markanteil der Gonade darstellen. In diese Anlage wandern die bipotentiellen primitiven Keimzellen, die Gonien, die sich im Mark zu Spermatogonien, in der Rinde zu den Ovogonien entwickeln. Witschi (1957) schätzt ihre Zahl auf 2000.

Rinde und Mark sind heterogene Strukturen, ähnlich den Wolffschen und den Müllerschen Gängen, deren Entwicklung klar bestimmt ist. Die Rinde kann sich nur als Ovar und das Mark nur als Hoden entwickeln.

Bei beiden Geschlechtern überwiegt anfänglich der Markanteil und jede primitive Gonade beginnt sich zuerst in Richtung eines Hodens zu differenzieren, erst sekundär erfolgt die Umwandlung in weiblicher Richtung. Witschi nimmt an, daß Rinde und Mark eigene Induktoren besitzen (Cortexin bzw. Medullarin), die in Widerstreit stehen und die von einem gewissen Stadium ab die Leitung der Entwicklungsvorgänge übernehmen. Normalerweise entscheidet die genetische Konstitution, ob der Rinden- oder Markinduktor die Führung übernimmt. Schädigung des genetisch überlegenen Induktors gibt dem schwächeren Gelegenheit, die Führung zu übernehmen.

Die weitere Entwicklung beginnt beim männlichen Geschlecht früher als beim weiblichen. Bei 13 mm langen (männlichen) Embryonen zerfällt der Markanteil in eine Reihe von soliden Zellhaufen (Keim- oder Hodenstränge), die durch Bindegewebe voneinander getrennt werden und an den inneren Enden durch quere Verbindungen miteinander zusammenhängen (Rete testis). Die Keimstränge wachsen in die Länge und bilden Schlingen (Tubuli contorti s. seminiferi). Sie bestehen aus „indifferenten" Zellen und Geschlechtszellen (Spermiogonien), die sich aus den Urgeschlechtszellen ableiten. Aus den Keimstrangzellen werden die Stütz-(Sertoli)Zellen, im Bindegewebe treten bei 40 mm-Embryonen große Zellen auf, die Leydigschen Zwischenzellen. Im Bereich des Rete testis verdichtet sich das Bindegewebe zum Mediastinum testis. Durch die sog. Urogenitalverbindung finden die Hodenstränge im 4. Fetalmonat Anschluß an den Ductus epididymis. Der Rindenanteil bildet sich zurück.

Im 3. Schwangerschaftsmonat wachsen die fetalen Kanälchen als Folge der vermehrten Choriongonadotropinproduktion in die Länge und Dicke, das Zwischengewebe nimmt zu. Bis zum 10. Monat wachsen die Kanälchen langsam weiter, die Masse der Zwischenzellen, die im 4. Monat ihre höchste Ausbildung erreicht, nimmt vom 5. Monat an langsam ab; nach der Geburt bilden sie sich rasch zurück, verschwinden ganz und sind von Bindegewebszellen nicht mehr zu unterscheiden, der Kanälchendurchmesser schwindet auf 45—50 μ. Die lumenlosen Kanälchen enthalten undifferenzierte Zellen und einzelne Spermatogonien.

Die weibliche Keimdrüse entwickelt sich erst bei 18—20 mm langen Embryonen, indem der Markanteil zerfällt und sich im Rindenanteil kleine Zellnester ausbilden. Nur in der Nähe des späteren Mesovariums bleiben Markstränge erhalten und werden zum Rete ovarii. Durch weitere Bindegewebswucherung und Zerteilung der Zellnester entstehen in der Rinde bei einem Fet von 150 mm Länge die Primärfollikel, die eine mittelständig große Zelle, die Ovogonie und einen Kranz von Hüllzellen (Granulosazellen) aufweisen.

Die interstitiellen Zellen des Hoden zeigen bei einer Fetlänge von 31 mm die ersten Zeichen der Spezialisierung. Beim 50 mm-Fet nehmen die „großen Zellen" den größten Teil des Hodens ein, die größte Ausdehnung wird mit 160 bis 190 mm Länge (18.—21. Schwangerschaftswoche) erreicht. Die Entwicklung dieser embryonalen Leydigzellen folgt dem starken Anstieg der Choriongonadotropinausscheidung der 5.—6. Schwangerschaftswoche und fällt mit der Degeneration des weiblichen Gangsystems (10. Schwangerschaftswoche), der Ausbildung der Prostata, Samenblasen und des äußeren Genitale (12. Schwangerschaftswoche) und der Wanderung der Hoden in das Scrotum (16. Schwangerschaftswoche) zusammen, so daß man die Androgene des embryonalen Hoden mit Recht als Induktoren für die Ausbildung des männlichen Gangsystems ansieht.

Im indifferenten Stadium der Gonadendifferenzierung verfügt der Embryo über Anlagen der Genitalwege für das männliche und weibliche Geschlecht. OVERZIER nimmt an, daß die Anlage des Gangsystems durch die primitive Gonade induziert wird. Fehlt die Gonadenanlage, dann bleibt auch die Anlage des Gangsystems aus. Dieses besteht aus den beiden paarigen Geschlechtsgängen, Urnieren oder Wolffschen Gängen und den Müllerschen Gängen, sowie dem unpaarigen Urogenitalrohr und den Anlagen für das äußere Genitale. Aus dem Wolffschen Gang entsteht der Ductus epididymis, das Vas deferens, die Samenblase und der Ductus ejaculatorius. Prostata, Cowpersche Drüse und Littrésche Drüsen entwickeln sich aus dem Urogenitalsinus. Der Müllersche Gang bildet sich zurück, als Reste bleiben der Utriculus spermaticus und die Appendix testis.

Für die Entwicklung des Gangsystems und des äußeren Genitale in männlicher Richtung ist ein weiterer Induktor, nämlich funktionierendes Hodengewebe während des Differenzierungsstadiums notwendig. Dies geht aus den experimentellen Untersuchungen von JOST; RAYNAUD und FRILLEY 1947 hervor. Ein männlicher Kaninchenfet, der bis zum Alter von 19 Tagen kastriert wurde (operative Entfernung der Hodenanlage, Zerstörung durch Röntgenstrahlen, Ausschaltung der Hypophyse durch Dekapitation) entwickelt sich in weiblicher Richtung mit Tuben, Uterus, Vagina und normalem äußerem weiblichen Genitale. Wird die Kastration etwas später vorgenommen (19.—24. Tag), dann ist die Umwandlung im weiblichen Sinne unvollständig. Werden die Feten zwischen dem 21. und 22. Tag kastriert, dann bleiben verschiedene Abschnitte der Müllerschen Gänge und Überreste der Wolffschen erhalten, die Prostata ist kleiner, das äußere Genitale feminin oder hypospad. Bei Kastrationen nach dem 24. Tag entwickeln sich alle männlichen Gewebe vollständig, sie sind nur etwas kleiner angelegt. Diese Unterentwicklung betrifft besonders gerne die Prostata und die

Samenblasen. Der vom Hoden ausgehende Impuls, der die Genitalentwicklung in männlicher Richtung treibt, ist also nur während einer ganz kurzen Zeitspanne wirksam. Auf den Menschen bezogen liegt dieses Entwicklungsstadium zwischen der Fetlänge von 30 und 50 mm, also 50—60 Tage nach der Befruchtung des Eies. Bei Ausfall der embryonalen Hodenfunktion, die in die sich um dieselbe Zeit entwickelnden Zwischenzellen verlegt wird, kann ein Individuum genetisch und gonadal ein männliches, gonophor, was die Entwicklung des Gangsystems anlangt, aber ein weibliches Geschlecht haben (s. Tabelle 1).

Nicht nur der Zeitpunkt des Ausfalls der embryonalen internen Hodensekretion ist wichtig, sondern auch ihre Stärke. Bei teilweiser Zerstörung entwickeln sich die dem Hoden naheliegenden Gewebe normal — Ductus epididymis und Vas deferens, Rückbildung der Müllerschen Gänge. In den entfernter liegenden reicht die Potenz jedoch nicht aus, so daß ein weibliches äußeres Genitale oder ein Urogenitalsinus oder nur eine einfache Hypospadie als Zeichen

Tabelle 1. *Hauptsächlichste Abnormitäten des männlichen Kaninchenfeten durch Schädigung der Hodenanlage nach* JOST. (AUS JONES und SCOTT 1958)[1]

Gangsysteme	Prostata	Äußeres Genitale	Art des experimentellen Eingriffs
1. Weiblich	∅	♀	frühzeitige Kastration
2. Anteile der Müllerschen und Wolffschen Gänge	+ bis +÷	♀ oder Hypospadie	Kastration am 21. oder 22. Tag
3. Männlich mit kleineren Abnormitäten	+ bis ++	♀	Dekapitation vor dem 21. Tag
4. Männlich	÷+ bis +++	± Hypospadie	Dekapitation nach dem 21. Tag
5. Fehlender Ductus deferens	+++	♂	Kastration am 23. Tag
6. Eine Seite weiblich, andere männlich	−++	♂	frühzeitige einseitige Kastration

der unterwertigen Hodenfunktion während dieses kurzen Stadiums der embryonalen Entwicklung für immer bestehenbleibt. Man neigt heute dazu, diesen Mechanismus voll und ganz für die Deutung der häufigen Mißbildungen des äußeren und inneren Genitales des Menschen heranzuziehen.

Die Bedeutung der hypophysären Gonadotropine des Feten ist bei den einzelnen Arten verschieden. Ratten und Mäuse entwickeln sich auch nach Dekapitation normal, Kaninchen und Opossum jedoch nicht. Beim Menschen weiß man nichts Sicheres. Anencephale haben meist unterentwickelte Hoden und normale äußere und innere Genitalien, ebenso einige Fälle von kongenitalem Fehlen der Hypophyse.

B. Histologie des normalen Hodens

I. Vor der Pubertät

CHARNY unterscheidet bei der Entwicklung des Hodens nach der Geburt die Phase des Wachstums und die Phase der Reifung.

Beim Neugeborenen sind die lumenlosen Tubuli klein, haben einen Durchmesser von 45—50 μ und sind angefüllt mit undifferenzierten Zellen, randständig sieht man einige Samenmutterzellen (Spermatogonien). In den ersten 14 Tagen bilden sich die Leydigzellen, die beim Fet stark entwickelt sind, zurück, werden Bindegewebszellen ähnlich oder gehen zugrunde (Gewicht 0,2 g).

---

[1] Mit Erlaubnis des Verlages The Williams & Wilkins Company, Baltimore.

Die Wachstumsphase reicht von der Geburt bis etwa zum 10. Lebensjahr. In dieser Periode vollzieht sich eine geringe Volumenvergrößerung des Organs durch Wachstum der Tubuli seminiferi, die zum Körperwachstum in Beziehung steht. Die Wandung besteht aus undifferenzierten Zellen des späteren Sertolizellverbandes, die in mehreren Schichten liegen. Spermatogonien sind nur in geringer Zahl nachweisbar. Später entstehen durch zerfallende Zellen im Zentrum kleine Lichtungen. Das Kanälchenepithel ordnet sich in einer zweischichtigen Kernlage. Leydigzellen fehlen. Im 8.—10. Lebensjahr schreitet die Lumenbildung fort, der Durchmesser beträgt 65—70 μ. Das Epithel ist mehrschichtig, die Spermatogonien haben sich vermehrt. Die Zwischenräume sind noch schmal und ausgefüllt von einem feinfaserigen Bindegewebe mit Bindegewebszellen ohne Leydigzellen (Gewicht Ende des 1. Lebensjahres 0,7—1,0 g; 10.—13. Lebensjahr 1,3—1,6 g).

Die Reifungsphase beginnt ziemlich plötzlich, etwa im 10.—12. Lebensjahr. Der puberale Hoden ist gekennzeichnet durch das Auftreten von Mitosen der

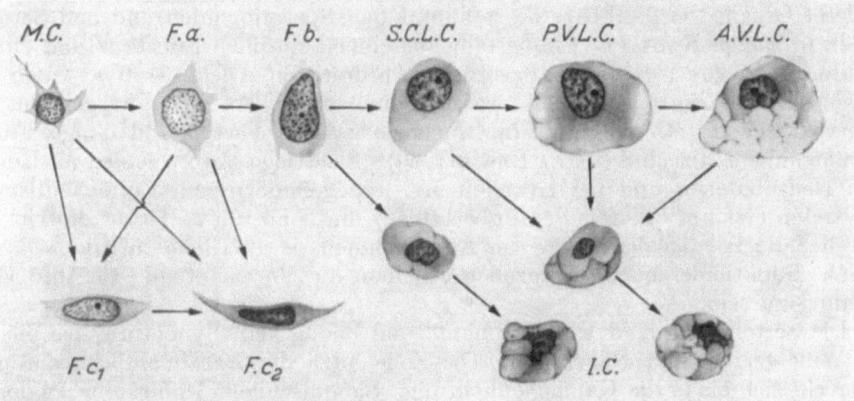

Abb. 1. Entwicklung der Leydig-Zellen nach DE LA BALZE u. Mitarb.[1] *M.C.* mesenchymähnliche Zellen; *F.a.* Fibroblasten-Typ a; *F.b.* Fibroblasten-Typ b; *F.C₁* und *F.C₂* Unterformen von Fibroblasten des Typs C; *S.C.L.C.* kleine kompakte Leydigzelle; *P.V.L.C.* spärlich vacuolisierte Leydigzelle; *R.V.L.C.* reichlich vacuolisierte Leydigzelle; *J.C.* Involutionsformen, links aus Fibroblasten des Typ b, rechts aus Leydigzellen

Spermatogonien und die Entwicklung von Spermatocyten I. Ordnung. Erst mit der Reifung der Samenzellen entwickeln sich aus den undifferenzierten Zellen die Sertolizellen. Ihr Kern nimmt seine charakteristische längsovale Form an, das feinverteilte Chromatin umschließt einen deutlichen Nucleolus. Der Differenzierungsgrad der Sertolizellen kann als Reifezeichen der Kanälchen gewertet werden (SNIFFEN). DE LA BALZE u. Mitarb. haben kürzlich den Reifungsvorgängen des Interstitiums eine eingehende Studie gewidmet. Sie unterscheiden vier Fibroblastenarten im Zwischengewebe. Aus dem Typ b, Zellen mit kleinen Kernen, dichtem Chromatin und einem Nucleolus entwickeln sich in der ersten Phase der Reifung Vorläufer der Leydigzellen mit positiver Reaktion für Lipoide, Ascorbinsäure und Nucleoproteiden (vgl. Abb. 1). In der zweiten Phase werden daraus Zellen mit größerem rundlich oder polygonal begrenztem granuliertem Cytoplasma und kleinen dichten Kernen mit dicker Membran und großem Nucleolus. In der dritten Phase sieht man neben kleinen, kompakten Leydigzellen zwei neue Typen, die sich vorwiegend im Ausmaß der Vacuolisierung unterscheiden. Außerdem erscheinen schon im Stadium 2 und 3 involvierte Leydigzellen mit pyknotischem Kern, reichlichem Cytoplasma und zahlreichen Vacuolen.

[1] J. clin. Endocr. and Metabol. **10**, 269 (1960). Courtesy of Charles C. Thomas, Publisher.

Die Ableitung der Leydigzellen aus mesenchymalen Zellen ist allgemein anerkannt (Hooker 1948, Williams, Albert, Sniffen 1950, 1952). Die früher vielfach verbreitete Ansicht, daß während der Reifung die Spermatozoen vor den Leydigzellen auftreten, wird von de la Balze (1960), Tonutti u.a. nicht geteilt. Kleine, kompakte Leydigzellen erkennt man gleichzeitig mit der Reifung des Samenkanälchens.

II. Nach der Pubertät

Beim *Erwachsenen* beträgt der Kanälchendurchmesser zwischen 170 und 260 μ. Schuchardt errechnet für den äußeren im Mittel 193 μ, für den inneren 173 μ. Auf die Wand entfallen also 20 μ. Der Anteil der Kanälchen beträgt 85,4%, der des Interstitiums 14,6%. Andere errechnen für die Kanälchen 66%, für das gesamte Interstitium 34%, für die Leydigzellen 12%.

Die Kanälchenwand (Gesamtdicke 7—20 μ) wird von der Basalmembran und der Tunica propria gebildet. Die Basalmembran (Glashaut) ist mit derjenigen anderer Organe vergleichbar, sie steht mit den Spermiogonien und den Sertolizellen in engem Kontakt. Sie besteht aus einer amorphen Substanz und einem dichten Netz von reticulären Fasern und Fibrocyten, Dicke 3—6 μ. Auch die Tunica propria wird aus einer intercellulären amorphen Substanz gebildet, in der vorwiegend reticuläre Fasern, wenige elastische Fasern und einige Fibroblasten eingebettet sind (de la Balze 1960). Elastische Fasern fehlen im Hoden von Neugeborenen und bei Kranken mit hypogonadotropem Eunuchoidismus. Sie treten erst um die Zeit der Pubertät auf und sind um so besser entwickelt, je reifer die Leydigzellen sind. Im Alter nehmen sie an Dicke zu (de la Balze 1954). Funktionierende Leydigzellen scheinen die Voraussetzung für ihre Entstehung zu sein.

Die Sertolizellen sind Einzelelemente und bilden kein Syncytium, sie dienen als reine Stütz- und Nährzellen. Die Zelle sitzt der Basalmembran auf und erstreckt sich bis in die Kanälchenlichtung. Sie umschließt Hohlräume, in denen die basalen Zellen des Samenepithels liegen. Ihr Kern ist oval, der Rand zeigt oft charakteristische Einkerbungen, im feinen Netzwerk liegt ein großer und dichter Nucleolus. Sie enthalten Lipoide, die Produktion von Oestrogenen ist nicht erwiesen.

Die *Keimzellen* liegen in einer Schicht von 4—8 Lagen. Die Spermatogonien entwickeln sich zu den großen primären Spermatocyten. Diese enthalten 44 Autosome und 2 XX- oder XY-Geschlechtschromosomen. Beim Menschen finden drei Teilungen statt, so daß aus einer Spermatocyte über zwei Präspermatiden I. Ordnung vier Präspermatiden II. Ordnung endlich acht Spermatiden entstehen, die dann zu den Spermatozoen ausreifen. Die Kanälchenweite ist ein Maß für die Stärke der Spermiogenese, je weiter um so mehr Spermien, die nur zum Teil im Lumen erhalten bleiben, werden produziert. Das *Zwischengewebe* enthält neben kollagenen Fasern, Blut- und Lymphgefäßen, Nerven, mehrere Fibroblastenarten, Wanderzellen, Mastzellen und embryonale perivasculäre Zellen. Die Gefäße verlaufen nur im Interstitium. Die Versorgung des Keimepithels muß also durch die Tunica propria erfolgen.

Im reifen Hoden liegen die Leydigzellen in Nestern, messen 15—20 μ im Durchmesser, sind oval oder polyedrisch. Der Kern ist groß und vesiculär und liegt oft exzentrisch. Er enthält eine oder mehrere Nucleolen, das Protoplasma ist fein granuliert und um den Kern herum etwas verdichtet. Es enthält zahlreiche Mitochondrien, lipochromes Pigment und Kristalloide (Reinke-Kristalloide). Diese Einschlüsse wurden bis jetzt in keiner anderen Zelle des Körpers beobachtet und scheinen spezifisch für den Menschen.

SNIFFEN (1952) teilt die Zwischenzellen in drei Formen ein:

1. Unreife mit spindelförmigen oder polygonalen Kernen, die von einem kleinen, fusiformen Protoplasmaleib mit acidophiler Körnelung umgeben sind.

2. Mittelgroße, polygonal begrenzte Zellen mit runden, meist exzentrisch liegenden Kernen, deren Protoplasma homogen granuliert ist und vereinzelte Vacuolen zeigt.

3. Große polygonale Zwischenzellen mit runden, exzentrisch gelegenen Kernen, die zentral von einem granulierten, peripher von einem wabigen Protoplasma umgeben sind, in dem sich zahlreiche Vacuolen finden. Diese Zellen enthalten vereinzelt grobe Granula und Pigmentkernchen. Nach der Pubertät zählt man auf ein Kanälchen etwa sechs Zellen (SNIFFEN 1952).

Bei der Involution bilden sie sich wieder zu fibroblastenähnlichen Zellen zurück oder aber es entstehen oxyphile vacuolisierte Zellen mit pyknischen Kernen oder Fettgewebszellen. Entwicklung und Involution zeigt ein Schema von DE LA BALZE (Abb. 1).

Die Beurteilung des Funktionszustandes ist schwierig. Die zur Verfügung stehenden histochemischen Methoden geben noch kein vollständiges Bild. NELSON und HELLER (1948) schließen aus Beobachtungen beim Hypogonadismus, daß Verlust der Granulation, Abnahme der Kern- und Zellgröße und abweichende Formen ein funktionelles Versagen anzeigen. Gleichzeitig vermehren sich die Fibrocyten, die Fettzellen und das intertubuläre Bindegewebe. Histochemische Untersuchungen ergeben einen hohen Gehalt an Ascorbinsäure und Lipoiden. Das Protoplasma enthält Alkohol und acetonlösliches Material, zeigt Doppelbrechung und färbt sich mit Phenylhydrazin. Die Lipoide färben sich auch mit Sudanschwarz, mit Nilblau, sie sind schiffpositiv und geben die für die Anwesenheit von Cholesterin charakteristische Schultzsche Reaktion. Die unreifen Zellen enthalten wohl Lipoide, aber keine „Steroide", während in den reifen alle Reaktionen positiv werden. Mit den gegenwärtig gebräuchlichen Methoden können die echten Steroide nicht sicher von ihren Vorstufen abgetrennt werden (MANCINI). Bei jugendlichen Ratten ist der Cholesteringehalt der interstitiellen Zellen gering im Vergleich zu dem hohen des Kanälchenepithels (PEARLMAN). Sertolizellen und Spermatogonien färben sich auch mit der Reaktion nach ASHBEL und SELIGMANN deutlich an.

C. Regulation der Hodenfunktion

I. Die hypophysären Gonadotropine

CROWE, CUSHING und HOMANS beobachteten als erste 1909 bei einem Menschen nach Entfernung der Hypophyse eine Atrophie der Hoden. ASHNER beschreibt 1912 nach Exstirpation der Hypophyse beim männlichen Hund ebenfalls einen Schwund der Keimdrüsen. Ihnen folgen HOUSSAY 1921, REICHERT 1922 u. a., aber erst SMITH gelang es 1926, die Pars distalis der Hypophyse allein zu entfernen. Er erbrachte damit den Beweis, daß der Vorderlappen der Hypophyse die Funktion der Keimdrüsen reguliert.

Bei jugendlichen Tieren bleibt die Entwicklung der Keimdrüsen nach der *Hypophysektomie* auf einer primitiven Stufe stehen, die Zwischenzellen bleiben unentwickelt, das Keimepithel besteht nur aus ein bis zwei Schichten von Spermatogonien. Beim ausgewachsenen Tier atrophiert der Hoden allmählich, der Schwund erreicht bei Ratten erst nach 3—4 Wochen die volle Schwere. Zuerst verschwinden die Spermatozoen, dann die Spermatiden, während die Spermatogonien und Spermatocyten in gewissem Umfang erhalten bleiben. Die Sertoli-

zellen zeigen keine nennenswerten Veränderungen, die Leydigschen Zwischenzellen, das innersekretorische Organ des Hodens, fällt ebenfalls einer Atrophie
anheim. Tonutti (1955) hat die früher am Hoden hypophysektomierter Ratten
erhobenen Befunde ergänzt. Er beschreibt seine Beobachtungen folgendermaßen:
An den *Leydigzellen* verschwindet der normal große epitheloide Plasmaleib so
weitgehend, daß es schwerfällt, noch einen feinen Saum um die Zellkerne zu
erkennen. Diese liegen daher dicht gepackt im Interstitium und scheinen vermehrt. Das fein verteilte Chromatin der bläschenförmigen, rundlichen Kerne
verschwindet. Diese werden plump und oval und zeigen im Hämatoxylinbild
eine charakteristische, dichte, fleckförmige Lagerung des Chromatins, die an ein
Schachbrettmuster erinnert. Das Volumen der Kerne vermindert sich von
$100—110 \mu^3$ bei Kontrolltieren, auf $50—55 \mu^3$ beim hypophysektomierten Tier.
Eine völlige Entdifferenzierung zu Bindegewebszellen findet nicht statt, zahlen-
mäßig tritt keine Verminderung ein. Als Folge einer fibrösen Entartung des
Zwischengewebes entwickelt sich eine Vermehrung der Bindegewebsfasern, so
daß die geschwundenen Leydigzellen in einem Maschenwerk von Bindegewebszügen liegen.

In den *Kanälchen* kommt die Spermatogenese zum Erliegen, die Tubuli
contorti sind nur noch von einer zwei- bis dreischichtigen Zellreihe ausgekleidet
(Albert 1956, Albright 1937, Bahn 1953, Tonutti). Außer Sertolizellen sieht
man noch Spermatogonien und Spermatocyten I. Ordnung. Die Teilungsfähigkeit der Spermatogonien bleibt erhalten, man sieht zahlreiche Teilungsstadien.
Spermatocyten sind seltener als normal, die weiteren Stadien der Spermiogenese
fehlen vollständig. Nicht selten finden sich abgestoßene Zellen im Lumen der
Kanälchen, im Volumen der Spermatogonien ergeben sich keine Unterschiede.

Bei anderen Arten ist die Kanälchenatrophie eine weitgehendere. Bei Affen
besteht der Tubulusinhalt nach 30 Tagen nur noch aus Sertolizellen und Spermatogonien, ebenso bei Kaninchen und Katzen (P. S. Smith 1944). Die Unterschiede hängen wahrscheinlich mit der bei den einzelnen Tierarten mehr oder
weniger vollständig durchführbaren Hypophysektomie zusammen. Beim *Menschen* ist die Atrophie bei Zerstörung der Hypophyse ebenfalls eine vollständige.
In den kleinen Kanälchen finden sich nur noch Sertolizellen und Spermatogonien bzw. undifferenzierte Formen.

Die *Sertolizellen* zeigen keine gröberen Abweichungen von der Norm. Die
Tunica propria der Tubuli verdickt sich beträchtlich, der Durchmesser der
Kanälchen schwindet stark. Da sich nach Zerstörung des Keimepithels durch
Röntgenstrahlen die Kanälchenwand trotz des Schwundes des Kanälchendurch-
messers nicht verdickt, nehmen de la Balze (1954) und Tonutti (1956) an,
daß für die Strukturierung der Tubuluswand hormonale Einflüsse maßgebend sind.

Die Verdickung der Tunica propria erlaubt ein Urteil über den Zeitpunkt
des Ausfalls der Gonadotropine. Sie fehlt beim Jugendlichen, aber auch beim
erwachsenen Menschen, wenn Leydigzellen und Kanälchen noch nie entwickelt
waren, wenn also schon immer ein hypogonadotroper Hypogonadismus bestanden
hat. In diesen Fällen fehlen auch die elastischen Fasern (de la Balze 1954).

Als Folge des Erlöschens der hormonalen Leistung atrophieren die Samenblasen und die Prostata rasch und ebenso stark wie bei kastrierten Tieren.

Zondek (1926) implantierte jungen Mäusen Vorderlappengewebe und beobachtete nach 4—5 Tagen eine Verhornung des Vaginalepithels wie im Oestrus,
eine Entwicklung der Follikel und die Bildung von Gelbkörpern. Aschheim
fand im Urin schwangerer Frauen eine Substanz, die in ihrer Wirkung Hypo-
physenimplantaten gleicht, indem sie auf Ovarien ausgesprochen luteinisierend
wirkt, ein Befund, der später oft bestätigt wurde. Im Urin von kastrierten

oder klimakterischen Frauen läßt sich dagegen eine Substanz anreichern, die vorwiegend das Follikelwachstum anregt. Prolan A und B wurden von ZONDEK abgetrennt.

Die weitere Forschung führte zur Abtrennung von zwei großen Gruppen von Gonadotropinen, die vom Hypophysenvorderlappen gebildeten, die aus der Hypophyse extrahierbar sind und sich in Blut und Urin nachweisen lassen, und die sog. Choriongonadotropine, die in den Körperflüssigkeiten nur festgestellt werden können, wenn der Organismus eine fetale Placenta oder ein Äquivalent davon in sich birgt.

Bei *männlichen Ratten* beobachtete E. P. SMITH (1927) nach Implantation von Vorderlappengewebe eine vorzeitige Entwicklung des Hodens. Nach Injektion von Hypophysenextrakten hypertrophieren bei jugendlichen Tieren die Leydigzellen, die Prostata und Samenblasen vergrößern sich (STEINACH und KUN 1928, VOSS und LOEWE 1928, ENGLE 1932 u. a.). E. P. SMITH (1927) konnte beim hypophysektomierten Tier mit Extrakten aus dem Hypophysenvorderlappen den Genitalapparat erhalten.

1. FSH und ICSH

Durch chemische Aufarbeitung von *Hypophysenextrakten* gelang es (FEVOLD, EVANS 1935, VAN DYKE 1950, LI 1949) zwei nicht ganz reine Prinzipien darzustellen, die als *follikelstimulierendes Hormon (FSH)* bzw. Follikelreifungshormon (FRH) und als *Luteinisierungshormon (LH)* bzw. die interstitiellen Zellen stimulierendes Hormon (ICSH) bezeichnet werden. Beide verhalten sich bei der Elektrophorese und in der Ultrazentrifuge wie einheitliche Eiweißkörper.

Verhältnismäßig reine FSH-Präparate wurden aus Hypophysen von Schafen und von Schweinen und des Menschen gewonnen. Das Verhältnis FSH:LH wechselt in Hypophysenextrakten je nach Tierart und Reinheitsgrad der Präparate. Extrakte aus Ochsenhypophysen wirken vorwiegend luteinisierend, aus menschlichen haben stärkere FSH-Eigenschaften (BAHN 1953). Die aus tierischen Hypophysen dargestellten reinen FSH-Präparate sind bis jetzt alle mit kleinen LH-Mengen verunreinigt, so daß man bei hypophysektomierten weiblichen Ratten mit den Präparaten von LI (1949), von VAN DYKE (1950), dem Armour Standard in höheren Dosen nicht nur eine Gewichtszunahme des Ovars, sondern auch des Uterus erhält. Auch das von SEGALOFF und STEEMAN (1959) aus menschlichen Hypophysen dargestellte FSH hat noch geringe LH-Eigenschaften. Die Gewinnung von reinem hypophysärem *ICSH* gelingt dagegen leichter (SEGALOFF 1959, SIMPSON 1944).

Wie das ACTH können auch die hypophysären Gonadotropine durch enzymatische Andauung in niedrigmolekulare Produkte mit höherer Wirkung als das bis jetzt reinste FSH-Präparat von LI (1949) gespalten werden. Man vermutet, daß die Gonadotropine selbst keine Proteine sind, sondern daß die Wirkung Polypeptiden zukommt, die an ein unwirksames Protein gebunden sind.

Die Prüfung dieser isolierten Extrakte muß an hypophysektomierten Tieren vorgenommen werden, da die eigene Hypophyse erwachsener und jugendlicher Tiere in nicht sicher vorausschaubarer Weise an der Reaktion teilnimmt. Die meisten Untersuchungen wurden an der Maus und Ratte durchgeführt. Meerschweinchen und Kaninchen verhalten sich etwas anders. Dabei besteht ein Unterschied, ob die einzelnen Hormone den Tieren direkt nach der Entfernung der Hypophyse oder erst 4—6 Wochen später gegeben werden. Im letzteren Fall ist die Reaktion bedeutend schwächer, während im ersteren die für das einzelne Hormon typische Reaktion nachweisbar ist. Die Erklärung sieht man darin, daß direkt nach der Hypophysektomie noch endogene Hormone des Vorderlappens zirkulieren bzw. im Gewebe der Gonaden haften (Li 1949). Die Gonaden müssen einen bestimmten Funktionsgrad aufweisen, damit künstlich zugeführte reine Hormone überhaupt wirksam werden können. Dieser scheint nur gewährleistet, wenn gewisse Mengen von *ICSH* und von *FSH* gleichzeitig vorhanden sind. Die zum Teil recht beträchtlichen Unterschiede der Ergebnisse der einzelnen Autoren sind auf die Beimengung anderer Wirkstoffe, auf die verschiedene Dosierung, auf den verschiedenen Zeitpunkt der Anwendung und auf die verwandte Tierart zurückzuführen. Es ist wahrscheinlich, daß auch andere Hormone wie das Wachstumshormon, Thyroxin und die Nebennierenrindenhormone für die Aufrechterhaltung der normalen Funktion der Keimdrüsen nötig sind. Wie bei weniger differenzierten Geweben, scheint auch bei den hochdifferenzierten das Erhaltensein der Homöostase eine der Voraussetzungen für den normalen Reaktionsablauf (Li 1949).

Bei der *weiblichen* hypophysektomierten Ratte löst die Gabe von gereinigtem *FSH* die Differenzierung und das Wachstum von zahlreichen Follikeln aus. Uterus und Vagina bleiben infantil, da die Graafschen Follikel unter der Wirkung des reinen FSH kein Oestrogen abgeben (Greep 1950). Erst nach der Zugabe von kleinsten Mengen von LH, die allein verabreicht keine Luteinisierung bewirken, werden reichlich Oestrogene sezerniert, es folgt der Oestrus.

Guten Aufschluß über die Verhältnisse gibt die *parabiotische* Vereinigung von zwei oder drei Tieren, denen Hypophyse bzw. Keimdrüsen entfernt sind. Wenn eine hypophysektomierte mit einer kastrierten *weiblichen* Ratte vereinigt wird, dann wachsen im Ovar des hypophysektomierten Tieres viele große Graafsche Follikel heran, die nicht springen und sich nicht in Corpora lutea umwandeln. Diese cystisch degenerierten Ovarien zeigen histologisch ein gut entwickeltes Zwischengewebe. Die Hypophyse des kastrierten weiblichen Tieres bildet also vorwiegend FSH und nur so kleine Mengen von ICSH, daß die Umwandlung in Corpora lutea nicht erfolgen kann. Bei parabiotischer Vereinigung von *männlichen* Tieren derselben Art bleiben sowohl tubuläres und interstitielles Gewebe und die akzessorischen Drüsen des hypophysektomierten Partners voll erhalten. Die für die Luteinisierung des Ovars nötige Menge von ICSH scheint größer als die für die Erhaltung des Zwischengewebes in Ovar und Hoden, vielleicht bildet das männliche Tier aber auch mehr ICSH als FSH (Turner 1948).

Bei jungen *männlichen* Ratten, deren Hypophyse entfernt ist, vergrößert gereinigtes FSH nur den Durchmesser der Kanälchen und regt die Spermiogenese etwas an, sie wird nicht normalisiert, die Leydigzellen werden nicht entfaltet, die atrophischen Adnexe bleiben klein. Man spricht auch vom *gametokinetischen Hormon*. Die meisten Autoren nehmen an, daß FSH-Extrakte des HVL, die die Spermiogenese der hypophysektomierten Ratte völlig normalisieren, auch kleine Mengen von LH enthalten (Heller u. Nelson 1948, Nelson 1956, Turner 1938). Die Umwandlung der Spermatiden in Spermatozoen erfolgt bei der Ratte nur bei Anwesenheit von Testosteron (Nelson 1956). *ICSH* regt die Zwischenzellen zur Androgenbildung an, erhöht das Gewicht des ventralen Anteils der Prostata der Ratte und der Samenblasen und stellt das Epithel dieser Organe wieder her. Mit langsam steigenden Dosen von ICSH konnten Simpson u. Mitarb., van Dyke und Chow bei hypophysektomierten Ratten und Mäusen nicht nur die Zwischenzellen aktivieren, sondern auch die Spermiogenese wieder in Gang bringen. Die Wiederherstellung der Kanälchen wird dabei den in den Leydigzellen gebildeten Androgenen zugeschrieben. Gleichzeitige Gabe von FSH und ICSH wirkt synergistisch, es genügen so kleine Hormonmengen zur völligen Wiederherstellung des Hodens, die allein gegeben, wirkungslos sind.

Beim *Menschen* gelten dieselben Beziehungen, wie HELLER und NELSON (1948) zeigen konnten. Sie behandelten hypophysäre Eunuchoide mit Choriongonadotropin (HCG), das wie ICSH wirkt. Darunter traten Leydigzellen auf, die vorher gänzlich gefehlt hatten, die Kanälchen vergrößerten sich, die Spermiogenese kam jedoch nicht in Gang. Erst nachdem zu dem HCG ein gereinigter, FSH enthaltender Hypophysenextrakt vom Tier gegeben wurde, enthielten die Kanälchen nach 6—30wöchiger Behandlung in einigen ausgewählten Fällen alle Stadien der Spermiogenese, auch reife Spermatozoen.

Aus Schweins- und Schafshypophysen gewonnene FSH-Präparate ergaben bei klinischer Prüfung sehr unterschiedliche Ergebnisse, ein Teil der Untersucher beschreibt eindeutige hormonale Wirkung, andere vermissen sie ganz. Die Ursache liegt im Artunterschied, es werden frühzeitig Antikörper gebildet, die nicht nur die exogen zugeführten, sondern auch die endogen gebildeten Hormone blockieren können (EVANS 1929).

Neuerdings wurden Extrakte aus menschlichen Hypophysen geprüft und mit HMG 20 verglichen (GEMZELL 1958). Die Ergebnisse beim Menschen sind schwer zu deuten, da die Ausgangssituation von Fall zu Fall verschieden ist. Amenorrhoische Frauen reagieren auf Hypophysenextrakte mit der Bildung großer, polycystischer Ovarien und mit starker Vermehrung der Oestrogensekretion. Wird FSH mit HCG kombiniert, dann kommt es in den meisten Fällen zur Ovulation und zur Corpus luteum-Bildung. FSH allein führt nicht zur Ovulation, auch nicht HCG allein, nur wenn beide zusammen gegeben werden, kann man den Follikelsprung erreichen. Neben der Oestrogenausscheidung steigt im Urin auch Pregnandiol etwas an, während die 17-Ketosteroide und die 17-Hydroxycorticoide unverändert bleiben.

Auch die seltenen Krankheitsbilder von isoliertem Fehlen eines gonadotropen Hormons, des FSH bzw. des ICSH, sprechen für den Dualismus der Gonadotropine.

Die Erforschung der hypophysären Gonadotropine ist keineswegs abgeschlossen. Manche Befunde lassen vermuten, daß das von männlichen Hypophysen gewonnene ICSH von dem aus weiblichen gewonnenen LH etwas abweicht. Bis vor kurzem waren alle Versuche fehlgeschlagen, die beiden Hormone im Urin voneinander zu trennen, so daß manche Forscher an der Existenz von zwei verschiedenen hypophysären Gonadotropinen zweifeln und nur von den hypophysären Harngonadotropinen (HGP) sprechen. So sind für ARON FSH und ICSH nur Artefakte, die bei der Aufarbeitung entstehen. ARON experimentierte nur mit Meerschweinchen und Kaninchen. Bei diesen Arten besteht in der Tat kein Unterschied in der biologischen Wirkung von Choriongonadotropin des Menschen und dem Serumgonadotropin von Pferden (PMS).

Testet man denselben Urinextrakt mit verschiedenen Methoden (Rattenovar, ventrale Prostata, Mäuseuterus), dann verhalten sich die von der Dosis abhängigen Gewichtskurven der Organe mit Urinextrakten von Männern, von menstruierenden Frauen, von klimakterischen Frauen und von kastrierten Frauen gleich, d.h. der Gehalt an FSH und LH-Aktivität des hypophysären Gonadotropins im Urin steht in allen Lebensaltern im gleichen Verhältnis zueinander, eine Feststellung, die ebenfalls für die Einheitlichkeit des hypophysären Gonadotropins spricht. Das Wirkungsverhältnis der verschiedenen Urinextrakte im Ovar- und Uterustest liegt immer zwischen 1,8—2,2. Grundsätzlich ist es also gleichgültig, welcher biologische Test für die Bestimmung der Uringonadotropine angewandt wird.

Kürzlich scheint es SEGALOFF und STEELMAN bei Aufarbeitung großer Urinmengen gelungen zu sein, aus Urin von Männern ein praktisch reines ICSH und aus Urin klimakterischer Frauen ein praktisch reines FSH darzustellen, ein Ergebnis, das noch der Bestätigung bedarf.

2. Prolactin

Als drittes Hypophysenhormon wird von ASTWOOD (1941) das *Prolactin* (Luteotropin) den hypophysären Gonadotropinen zugeordnet. Beim Säugetier erhält der Faktor die sekretorische Tätigkeit des Corpus luteum und regt die Bildung des Progesterons an, hat aber keinen Einfluß auf die Umwandlung der Theca- und Granulosazellen in die Luteinisierungszellen. Bei weiblichen Nagern ist er für die Entwicklung der Brustdrüse und für die Milchsekretion mitverantwortlich. Das Wachstum der Kropfdrüse von Tauben wird als spezifischer Test verwendet (Taubenkropftest). Prolactin enthält keine Hexose, es besitzt wie STH keinen hormonalen Gegenspieler — kein feed-back mechanismus —, seine Bildung wird in die eosinophilen Zellen verlegt. Hypophysen von Rindern und Schafen enthalten 30—40 TE/g Frischdrüse (BATES und RIDDLE 1930). Prolactin ist auch in menschlichen Hypophysen nachgewiesen. CURRIE u. Mitarb. (1961) fanden mit der qualitativen Methode an pseudograviden Kaninchen in allen Hypophysen von Männern und Frauen zwischen 50 und 80 Jahren Prolactin, mit zunehmendem Lebensalter steigt der Gehalt an, der höchste Wert wurde unter Cortisongabe festgestellt. Die Bedeutung des Hormons im männlichen Organismus ist nicht bekannt. FIORI u. Mitarb. berichten bei männlichen Ratten über eine Anregung der Leydigzellen zur Androgenbildung, PASQUALINI (1953) über eine direkte Wirkung auf die männlichen Adnexe, indem die Sekretion der Samenblasen kastrierter Ratten bei der kombinierten Gabe von Prolactin und Testosteron beträchtlich größer ist als bei Testosterongabe allein. Seine diabetogene Wirkung ist umstritten (vgl. RIDDLE und BATES 1935, PASQUALINI 1953). Die Prolactinausscheidung ist wenig untersucht. Beim gesunden Mann schwankt sie zwischen 0 und 305 E (Taubenkropftest), beim präpuberalen Jugendlichen ist nichts nachzuweisen, während die Ausscheidung im Alter hoch sein soll (LOPPEDGE). Im Blut von Frauen konnte es in der zweiten Cyclushälfte und in der Stillperiode festgestellt werden, nicht bei Kindern, jungen Männern und in der ersten Cyclushälfte.

3. Lokalisation der Hypophysenhormone

FSH und ICSH sind Glykoproteide, ebenso wie das thyreotrope Hormon. Die Anwendung neuer histochemischer Reaktionen, besonders der Perjodsäure-Leukofuchsin-Reaktion, erlaubte die Abtrennung mehrerer Arten von basophilen Zellen — PAS färbt Kohlenhydrate in fixiertem Gewebe. Die eine liegt mehr an der Oberfläche und gegen die Pars intermedia, es sind dies die „blassen" Basophilen oder Hypocyanophilen, auch δ-Zellen genannt, in sie wird die Bildung von FSH und ICSH bzw. LH verlegt. Die Intensität der Glykoproteidreaktion scheint dem Gonadotropingehalt parallel zu gehen. Die zweite Gruppe (β-Zellen) liegt mehr im Zentrum des HVL und wird als Bildungsstätte des thyreotropen Hormons (thyreotrophs) angesehen (PRUNTY 1953). Eine Bestätigung dieser Deutung brachte die Trennung der Granula von Hypophysenhomogenaten mit Hilfe der Ultrazentrifuge. McManus-positiv reagierende, also basophile Granula, ergaben bei infantilen Ratten, Meerschweinchen, Kaninchen ausgesprochen gonadotrope Effekte. Die Bildung von Prolactin, das wie Wachstumshormon (STH) ein einfacher Eiweißkörper ist, wird wie dieses in die acidophilen Zellen verlegt, und zwar in die Carminophilen (FRIEDGOOD), in die Orangeophilen von ROMEIS

(1940) bzw. in die α-Zellen, wobei die Identität dieser drei Zellarten noch nicht geklärt ist (TONUTTI 1955).

4. Gehalt der menschlichen Hypophyse

BAHN u. Mitarb. (1953) verarbeiteten Hypophysen von Frauen und Männern, die 3—4 Std nach Tod entfernt werden konnten. Ein Homogenat aus 3 mg feuchtem Gewebe von Mann und Frau enthält 1 RE FSH und 1 RE ICSH. Der gesamte Vorderlappen des Mannes enthält etwa 200 RE von beiden Hormonen. Da das Hypophysengewicht von Frauen größer ist als das der Männer, ist die Gesamthormonmenge bei Frauen etwas höher. Bei einem vierjährigen Kind fand sich ein Zehntel der Menge. Die Hypophyse von Frauen in der Menopause enthält pro 1 mg 3 E FSH und 1 E LH. Die Hypophyse von graviden Frauen enthält keine Gonadotropine. CURRIE u. Mitarb. extrahierten menschliche Hypophyse mit 2%iger Kochsalzlösung und bestimmten die gonadotropen Hormone mit Hilfe des Ovargewichtstestes jugendlicher Ratten im Vergleich zu HMG 20a als Standard. Die Hypophyse von Frauen zwischen 49 und 76 Jahren enthielt etwa 1000 HMG 20a E, die von Männern zwischen 52 und 86 Jahren etwa 1100 HMG 20a E. Nach Entfernung der Ovarien ist der Gehalt erhöht, nach Verabreichung von Cortison etwas vermindert. Das Verhältnis von FSH und ICSH in Hypophysen von Männern beträgt 1:1. Fällt man menschliche Hypophysenextrakte mit 55—75% Ammoniumsulfat, dann erhält man Präparate mit stärkerer FSH- als ICSH-Aktivität, ein durch 55% Ammoniumsulfatfällung gewonnenes Produkt regt dagegen vorwiegend die Leydigzellen an (GEMZELL 1958).

5. Ausscheidung im Urin

Die Erfassung der im Hypophysenvorderlappen gebildeten und mit dem Urin ausgeschiedenen Gonadotropine gibt Auskunft über die Aktivität einer Teilfunktion dieses Organs. Die quantitative Bestimmung erlaubt die Abgrenzung der primären und sekundären Keimdrüseninsuffizienz von Mann und Frau. Bei der primären, deren Ursache in den Keimdrüsen selbst zu suchen ist, werden die Gonadotropine, ebenso wie in der Menopause und beim Kastraten, in vermehrtem Maße ausgeschieden, bei Störungen des Hypophysen-Zwischenhirnsystems dagegen vermindert. Man hat errechnet, daß etwa 10—20% in unveränderter Form im Harn erscheinen.

Die Uringonadotropine können nach verschiedenen biologischen Methoden bestimmt werden. Die chemischen, die meist auf der Messung des Zuckerrestes im Gonadotropinmolekül basieren, sind noch zu unzuverlässig, als daß sie in der Klinik Anwendung finden könnten (BUTT 1956).

Biologische Methoden, die vorwiegend FSH erfassen, sind: die *Gewichtszunahme des Ovars* von hypophysektomierten Mäusen oder Ratten. Der Test ist hochspezifisch, erfordert aber sehr viel Aufwand. Obwohl Mäuse viel empfindlicher sind als Ratten, setzt sich wegen der geringeren Schwankungsbreite der Ovargewichte allmählich der Rattenovartest durch. Statt hypophysektomierter Tiere verwendet man im klinischen Betrieb infantile, die ein bestimmtes Gewicht nicht überschreiten dürfen. ALBERT hat den Rattenovartest standardisiert, er versteht unter einer Rattenovargewichtseinheit die Menge an HPG, die eine 100%ige Gewichtszunahme des Ovars über nicht injizierte Kontrollen auslöst. Die *Zunahme des Hodengewichtes* hypophysektomierter Ratten ist ebenfalls vorwiegend ein Maß der FSH-Aktivität. Demgegenüber stehen Methoden, die vorwiegend die ICSH-Eigenschaften erfassen. Die sicherste und empfindlichste ist

die Messung der Gewichtszunahme des *ventralen Teiles der Prostata* hypophysektomierter Ratten. Eine Prostata-Einheit (VPA) ist definiert als die HPG-
Menge, die eine 100%ige Gewichtszunahme der ventralen Prostata gegenüber
nicht injizierten hypophysektomierten Kontrollen auslöst.

Als *unspezifischer* Test hat die Verfolgung des *Gewichtes des Mäuse-Uterus*
(MUT) infantiler Tiere wegen seiner einfachen Durchführung die größte Verbreitung erfahren. Hierbei wird eine Mischung von FSH und ICSH gemessen.
Wenn das Ergebnis nicht auf ME, sondern auf ein Standard-Gonadotropin,
gewonnen aus Urin klimakterischer Frauen, z.B. HMG 20 A[1] oder HMG-J oder
von Männern, z.B. AMW (ALBERT 1956) bezogen wird, erhält man nicht nur
brauchbare, sondern auch vergleichbare Ergebnisse, die für klinische Bedürfnisse
ausreichen und ebensoviel aussagen, wie die komplizierten Teste an hypophysektomierten Tieren, da das Verhältnis von FSH und ICSH bzw. LH im Urin
bei allen Lebensaltern und Geschlechtern dasselbe ist (ALBERT, MCARTHUR u.a.).
Ausfällungs- und Konzentrierungsmethoden unterscheiden sich wohl erheblich
voneinander, alle Reinigungs- und Konzentrierungsverfahren ergeben aber End-
produkte mit denselben biologischen Eigenschaften, so daß die Unterschiede
der einzelnen Verfahren nur quantitativer und nicht qualitativer Art sind (AL-
BERT 1958).

Gonadotropine werden im allgemeinen erst um die Zeit der Pubertät nachweisbar. Im Urin von Mädchen erhält man etwa 1 Jahr vor Eintritt der Menses positive
Ergebnisse (NATHANSON 1942, 1943). Einzelne haben bei gesunden Kindern
4 ME (LLOYD 1949), 2 ME (CATCHPOLE 1938), 2—5 ME (JSELSTÖGER) bestimmt.

Bei gesunden Männern fallen Methoden, die mit der Alkoholpräcipitation
arbeiten, häufig negativ aus. Bei Verwendung des Mäuse-Uterusgewichtes als
Test fand PEDERSEN-BJERGAARD nach Erreichung der Höchstwerte mit der
Pubertät einen langsamen Abfall bis gegen das 60. Lebensjahr, danach einen
kräftigen Anstieg, andere finden im Greisenalter einen Abfall (HELLER u. SHIPLEY).
Beim gesunden Mann erfolgt im höheren Alter kein nennenswerter Anstieg. Normalwerte: HELLER und SHIPLEY für junge Männer 4—64 MUE bei 15% negativen,
ENGLE (1939, 1952) 5—30 MUE, KLINEFELTER (1943) 6,6—52,8 MUE, in den
meisten Fällen mehr als 13,2 und weniger als 52,8 MUE, MCCULLAGH u. Mitarb.
(1953) 13,2—105,6 MUE, TAUBERT und WELLER 10—40 MUE. Mit dem Hyper-
ämietest der Mäuseovars stellen LLOYD u. Mitarb. (1949) beim gesunden Mann
4—16 MOE, mit dem Mäuse-Uterustest 8—16 MUE fest. Ein Gipfel in der
Mitte des Cyclus ergibt sich nur bei Verwendung der Prostatamethode (MCARTHUR
1952). Nach der größten Untersuchungsserie von PEDERSEN-BJERGAARD
(360 Frauen) steigt bei der Frau die Ausscheidung vom 40. bis zum 60. Lebensjahr an, um nach dem 80. Lebensjahr wieder abzufallen. ALBERT findet zwischen
dem 20. und 40. Lebensjahr gleichbleibende Werte (4—14), dann präklimak-
terischer Anstieg auf 22, hohe klimakterische Werte zwischen 50 und 65 Jahren
(60—100 ROE), dann wieder langsamer Abfall. ROSEMBERG (1960) bestimmt
im MUT zwischen 14—43 Jahren 0,2—2,4 μg Oestronäquivalente bei 11% negativen bei Männern und 0,6—2,3 μg Oestronäquivalente bei Frauen. Frühere
Angaben über starke Schwankungen der Ausscheidung beim gleichen Menschen
von Tag zu Tag (5—10fache) (HELLER 1939) können bei Verwendung der stan-
dardisierten Methode nicht bestätigt werden. Extrakte aus Blättern von *Lithospermum officinale* heben die Wirkung der hypophysären Gonadotropine in vitro
und in vivo auf, auch die des Choriongonadotropins und des Serumgonadotropins
(LOESER).

---

[1] Eine HMG-Einheit entspricht der gonadotropen Wirkung von 1 mg HMG 20 A (human
menopausal gonadotropin charge 20 A) (Organon).

McArthur u. Mitarb. konnten bei 3 von 12 Kindern vor der Pubertät eine geringe Zunahme des Prostatagewichtes im Prostatatest feststellen, weibliche Erwachsene scheiden in der Mitte des Cyclus etwa 4 RE aus, erwachsene Männer mehr. Der Nachweis gelingt bei 16 von 17 Untersuchten, wobei ein deutlicher Unterschied zwischen gesunden Freiwilligen (4 und 24 RE) und hospitalisierten Patienten mit verschiedenen Allgemeinkrankheiten besteht. Bei letzteren liegt die Ausscheidung zwischen 2 und 8 RE. Die höchsten Werte finden sich bei klimakterischen Frauen mit 24—96 RE. Die gleichzeitige Bestimmung des Hodengewichtes erlaubt auch einen Rückschluß auf den Gehalt an FSH, dieses nimmt in derselben Urinkonzentration proportional dem Prostatagewicht zu, das Verhältnis von FSH und ICSH ist also bei allen untersuchten Gruppen etwa dasselbe, eine Beobachtung, die die Ergebnisse von ALBERT u. Mitarb. bestätigt (ALBERT 1960). Eine Ausnahme machen vielleicht Jugendliche vor der Pubertät, bei denen FSH-Aktivität häufiger nachweisbar war als ICSH-Aktivität, ein Befund, der die Beobachtung am menschlichen Hoden bestätigen würde, daß die Reifung der Kanälchen dem Auftreten von aktiven Leydigzellen vorausgeht.

Schon lange ist bekannt, daß Hunger, Unterernährung und chronische Krankheiten der verschiedensten Art die Gonadotropinausscheidung vermindern. Der Einfluß von ACTH bzw. von Cortison ist unsicher, in eigenen Untersuchungen konnten wir keinen Anstieg feststellen. Beim unbehandelten Myxödem ist die Ausscheidung vermindert, unter Thyroxingabe wird sie normal, die Unterschiede sind gering.

Im Plasma klimakterischer Frauen bestimmt APOSTOLAKIS den sehr hohen Wert von 32 (17—59) HMG E in 100 cm^3, der Konzentrationsunterschied zwischen Plasma und Urin beträgt 5,3, die Nierenclearance 0,04—0,43 ml/min.

II. Choriongonadotropin

ASCHHEIM und ZONDEK fanden im Blut und Urin von graviden Frauen eine gonadotrop wirkende Substanz, die bei infantilen Mäusen und Ratten die Follikel zur Reifung bringt, Oestrus, Ovulation und Luteinisierung des Ovars auslöst. Sie wird in den syncytialen und Langhans-Zellen des Trophoblasten der Placenta gebildet. In der 12. Schwangerschaftswoche ist der Gehalt in Blut und Urin am höchsten (O. W. SMITH 1952). Außerhalb der Schwangerschaft findet man HCG bei der Blasenmole, dem Chorionepitheliom und bei teratoiden Geschwülsten. Die höchsten Titer wurden bei Lebermetastasen solcher Tumoren festgestellt.

Der Aschheim-Zondek-Schwangerschaftstest beruht darauf, daß der Urin Schwangerer in den Ovarien von Mäusen und Ratten 96 Std nach der Injektion die Bildung von Blutpunkten oder von Corpora lutea auslöst. Dies beruht auf einer synergistischen Wirkung von HCG und dem eigenen FSH der Tiere. Teste an Amphibien sparen Zeit und sind wahrscheinlich zuverlässiger als die mit Säugern. Weibliche Frösche ovulieren 6—8 Std nach der Injektion von Schwangerenurin und schon 3 Std nach der Injektion können in der Kloake männlicher Tiere Spermatozoen nachgewiesen werden.

HCG hat ähnliche biologische Eigenschaften wie ICSH. Bei normalen Nagern führt es zur Luteinisierung des Ovars, Entwicklung der Follikel, Ovulation und Keratinisierung der Vagina. Die erreichbare Zunahme des Ovarialgewichtes und die Anregung des Wachstums nur weniger Follikel zeigt, daß ihm nur eine beschränkte FSH-Wirkung zukommt. Bei der hypophysektomierten Ratte stellt es nur das interstitielle Gewebe des Ovars wieder her (EVANS 1950), der Uterus wächst nicht und die Verhornung des Vaginalepithels bleibt aus, die Oestrogenbildung wird also nicht angeregt. Nur wenn man sehr hohe Dosen injiziert,

wachsen auch die Follikel (MAINZER). HCG unterscheidet sich im Uterus- und
Ovartest beträchtlich vom HPG. Im Uterustest, also in der Auslösung der
Oestrogensekretion des Ovars, ist HCG sechsmal so stark wirksam wie HPG
(ALBERT 1958).

Zwischen HCG und FSH besteht derselbe Synergismus wie zwischen LH
und FSH. Erst wenn etwa 14 Tage nach der Hypophysektomie FSH bei weiblichen Ratten ausgeschieden und das Ovar atrophisch geworden ist, sieht man
die reine LH-Wirkung auf das interstitielle Gewebe (LI 1953).

Bei der hypophysektomierten *männlichen* Ratte regt HCG die Tätigkeit der
Leydigzellen an, Prostata und Samenblasen entwickeln sich, während die Spermatozoenbildung nicht in Gang kommt (COLLIP, DICZFALUSY 1954). Mit sehr hohen
Dosen konnte jedoch nicht nur die Funktion der Leydigzellen, sondern auch
das Kanälchenepithel erhalten bleiben oder wiederhergestellt werden (SCHMIDT-
VOIGT). HCG besitzt also auch gewisse FSH-Eigenschaften, so daß man neuerdings annimmt, daß HCG zu einem kleinen Teil aus FSH besteht.

TONUTTI hat die unterschiedlichen Angaben der Literatur nochmals an hypophysektomierten *Ratten* geprüft. Seine Beobachtungen weichen von den früher
erhobenen ab, wahrscheinlich deshalb, weil das HCG erst 4 Wochen nach der
Entfernung der Hypophyse gegeben wurde, zu einem Zeitpunkt also, zu dem
nicht nur die Atrophie des Hodens vollständig war, sondern auch das endogene
FSH ausgeschieden war. An den *Leydigzellen* erfolgt eine Zunahme des Kern-
volumens auf über das Doppelte, so daß an der oberen Grenze der Norm liegende
Werte erreicht werden. Gleichzeitig entfaltet sich der Plasmaleib dieser Zellen.
Die vollständige Ausbildung der Prostata und der Samenblasen zeigt eine völlig
normalisierte Leistung dieser Gewebe an. Am *Keimepithel* sind die Änderungen
nur geringgradig. Die Zahl der Spermatocyten I. Ordnung wird etwas vermehrt,
es erfolgt aber keine weitere Reifung. Über die Spermatocyten I. Ordnung geht
die Spermiogenese ohne einen zweiten Faktor nicht hinaus.

HCG wirkt mit FSH gametokinetisch über die Androgenbildung in den
Leydigzellen. Die vermehrte Androgenbildung hat nur einen indirekten Einfluß
auf das Keimepithel, wie TONUTTI annimmt, über die Verbesserung der Permeabilität der Zellwand. Die Tubuluswand wird unter der Behandlung wieder
dünn und normal strukturiert. TONUTTI stellt diese Kontaktwirkung der Androgene deren Fernwirkung gegenüber. Die Sertolizellen bleiben unbeeinflußt.

Trotz der Ähnlichkeit der Wirkung bestehen zwischen ICSH und HCG chemische und biologische *Unterschiede*. Beim infantilen Tier wirkt ICSH nicht gonadotrop, obwohl es mit FSH zusammen ebenso wirksam ist wie HCG. HCG verhält
sich dagegen auch beim jugendlichen Tier wie ein volles Gonadotropin. Aus
diesem Unterschied schließt man, daß HCG die Hypophyse zur Bildung von
FSH anregt, während der Hypophysenvorderlappen durch ICSH nicht stimuliert wird. Injiziert man ICSH intraperitoneal, dann wird gleichzeitig subcutan
gegebenes Gonadotropin gehemmt, während HCG dessen Wirkung fördert.

Mit kristallisiertem HCG kann man bei Jugendlichen mit Oligo- bzw. Azoospermie und Hypogonadismus die sexuelle Entwicklung fördern und die Spermiogenese in Gang bringen. Man nimmt an, daß, wie im Tierexperiment, die eigene
Hypophyse durch das HCG zur Abgabe von FSH angeregt wird. HCG fördert
wie Testosteron die Reifung der Regulationszentren im Zwischenhirn. Bei funktionellen Störungen im Hypophysen-Zwischenhirnsystem — verzögerte Pubertät.
hypophysärer Infantilismus — kann man unter Umständen eine Ausheilung des
Hypogonadismus erreichen. Organische Defekte sind nicht ausgleichbar. Sehr
hohe Dosen schädigen das Keimepithel. MADDOCK und NELSON verabreichten
fünf gesunden Erwachsenen im Alter von 33—67 Jahren über mehrere Wochen

dreimal 5000 E HCG pro Woche. Die Aktivierung der Leydigzellen wurde in einem Anstieg der 17-Ketosteroide auf das Doppelte und der Oestrogene auf das Zehnfache im Urin sichtbar, auch das Plasmaandrosteron erhöht sich (EIK-NES 1959). Histologisch entwickelten sich bei allen Patienten regressive Veränderungen an den Kanälchen, bestehend in einer Verkleinerung des Durchmessers, in vermehrter Hyalinisierung der Basalmembran, in peritubulärer Fibrose und in Untergang von Keimzellen, die Sertolizellen bleiben normal. Wie unter der Verabreichung von Androgenen oder Oestrogenen wird die FSH-Abgabe im HVL gehemmt. Dadurch wird trotz der lokal in großer Menge vorhandenen Sexualhormone die Keimzellreifung gestört. Nach Absetzen des HCG erholen sich die Kanälchen wieder und es kann vorübergehend eine bessere Reifung der Spermatozoen nachweisbar sein (s. bei Rebound-Phänomen).

Es ist klar, daß dieser Mechanismus sehr von der individuellen Empfindlichkeit des einzelnen Menschen abhängig ist, so daß dieselbe Choriongonadotropindosis die hypophysäre Gonadotropinbildung einmal hemmt, das andere Mal eher anregt. Der immer wieder angenommene Einfluß des Choriongonadotropins auf die Nebennieren ist bis heute nicht bewiesen. Das Gewicht des Uterus kastrierter Rattenweibchen wird durch 100 E nicht geändert. Beim menschlichen Kastraten erhöhen Dosen bis 5000 E täglich die 17-Ketosteroidausscheidung nicht.

Antihormone werden nicht gebildet, da es sich um ein von Menschen selbst stammendes Hormon handelt. Umschriebene Rötung der Haut an der Injektionsstelle, kleine Infiltrate, Urticaria, leichte Übelkeit können in einzelnen Fällen auftreten.

III. Serumgonadotropin

Das Serumgonadotropin wurde 1930 von COLE und HART aus dem Serum von trächtigen Stuten isoliert. Aus 1 mg Endometrium erhält man bis zu 300 i.E. PMSG wird nicht im Urin ausgeschieden, nach parenteraler Injektion bleibt es mehrere Tage im Serum nachweisbar. Das Molekulargewicht beträgt etwa 30000, es ist ein Glykoproteid, das ziemlich viel Galaktose enthält.

Die biologische Wirkung von PMSG ist mit der eines hypophysären Extraktes mit vorwiegender FSH-Wirkung vergleichbar. Beim weiblichen Tier wird die Entwicklung der Follikel und des interstitiellen Gewebes angeregt, beim männlichen sowohl die Spermatogenese als auch die Leydigzellen (EVANS 1950). Bei hypophysektomierten Ratten und Mäusen erhält es die Spermiogenese.

Die Ergebnisse der Tierversuche sind je nach Tierart etwas verschieden, so daß noch keine einheitliche Auffassung über die biologische Wirkungsweise besteht.

IV. Antikörperbildung gegen artfremde Gonadotropine und ihre klinische Bedeutung

Die Entstehung von Antikörpern nach Verabreichung von artfremden *Gonadotropinen*, die die Wirkung des injizierten Hormons aufheben, verhindert bis heute die Anwendung hypophysärer Gonadotropine und des Serumgonadotropins von Tieren beim Menschen. Solche Antikörper werden im Serum von Kaninchen nachweisbar, wenn diese mit Hypophysenvorderlappenextrakten von Rindern oder von Schafen behandelt werden, sie sind auch beim Menschen nach Verabreichung von Serumgonadotropinen des Pferdes (JAILER 1940, LEATHEM 1948, ROWLANDS 1929), nach hypophysärem Gonadotropin von Pferden (LEATHEM 1947) und von Schafen festgestellt (LEATHEM 1948). Die eingehenden Untersuchungen von Maddock (1949) zeigen das ganze Risiko. Er verabreichte sieben Menschen täglich 50 E hypophysäres Gonadotropin, das aus Schafshypophysen gewonnen war und das vorwiegend FSH enthält. Nach 45—60 Tagen wurden Antikörper nachweisbar, 0,9 cm³ Plasma der Behandelten inaktivierte etwa 4 E Schafsgonadotropin, so daß im gesamten zirkulierenden Plasma etwa 3000 bis 10000 E vorhanden waren. Die Antikörper verschwanden erst 3—5¹/₂ Monate nach der letzten Injektion des tierischen FSH-Präparates, einmal waren sie noch nach 283 Tagen vorhanden. Bei einigen Kranken, bei denen das Ejaculat untersucht werden konnte, verminderte sich die Zahl der Spermatozoen 60 bis 140 Tage nach Behandlungsbeginn, bei zweien zeigte die Biopsie eine beträchtliche Abnahme des Kanälchendurchmessers, ein Stehenbleiben der Keimzellreifung auf der Stufe der primären Spermatocyten mit Abstoßung zahlreicher unreifer Formen in das Lumen, eine beträchtliche Verdickung der Kanälchenwand und ein Verschwinden der Leydigzellen im Interstitium, d.h. also, ähnliche Veränderungen wie nach Entfernung der Hypophyse (Jungck 1949).

Die besondere Bedeutung dieser Antikörper besteht darin, daß auch die aus dem Urin kastrierter Männer gewonnenen hypophysären Gonadotropine durch das Serum in vitro inaktiviert werden, auch menschliches Choriongonadotropin wird in vitro wirkungslos gemacht. Diese Antikörper sind also nicht hormonspezifisch. Die Produktion der eigenen hypophysären Gonadotropine wird dabei nicht gestört, die Vereinigung mit dem Antikörper findet erst im strömenden Blut statt, der Komplex scheint in der Niere wieder gespalten zu werden, denn im Urin der behandelten Menschen sind die hypophysären Gonadotropine nachweisbar, während die Antikörper nicht ausgeschieden werden (Maddock 1949).

Diese Beobachtungen sind für die Behandlung des Menschen mit artfremden Gonadotropinen von grundsätzlicher Bedeutung, sie können aber zur Entscheidung der Frage, ob der Antikörper gegen das Hormon oder gegen ein Begleiteiweiß gerichtet ist nicht herangezogen werden, da bei all diesen Untersuchungen nur wenig gereinigte Präparate verwendet wurden. Henry und van Dyke sensibilisierten neuerdings Kaninchen mit hochgereinigtem ICSH aus Schafshypophysen, auch mit einem Präparat von Dr. Li. Die entstehenden Antikörper trennen sich bei der Untersuchung mit der Ouchterlony-Technik in vier bis sechs Präcipitatsbanden. Nach Absorption mit verschiedenen Seren und Hypophysenextrakten bleibt eine Bande übrig, die die Autoren als Präcipitatlinie des reinen ICSH mit seinem spezifischen Antikörper deuten. Der Schafs-ICSH-Antikörper präcipitiert auch das ICSH von Ochsen, nicht dagegen von Schweinen und nicht das menschliche Choriongonadotropin. Wie zu erwarten, wird ICSH aus Schafs- und Ochsenhypophysen auch in vitro inaktiviert. Wird der Antikörper Ratten injiziert, dann bleibt die Wirkung der eigenen hypophysären Gonadotropine der Tiere erhalten. Wahrscheinlich bedeuten diese biologischen Unterschiede der Gonadotropine verschiedener Tierarten auch Unterschiede in der Struktur und im Molekulargewicht, wie sie neuerdings für das STH gefunden wurden (Hajashida). Ob es einmal gelingen wird, die Bildung der Antikörper durch Verwendung von noch biologisch wirksamen Bruchstücken der hypophysären Gonadotropine zu vermeiden, ist nicht bekannt. Vorläufig muß bei Anwendung von artfremden Gonadotropinen beim Menschen mit der Bildung von präcipitierenden, das Hormon inaktivierenden Antikörpern gerechnet werden, wobei die Inaktivierung um so weiter reicht, je unreiner das verwandte Gonadotropinpräparat ist. Eine Ausnahme macht nur das hypophysäre Gonadotropin von Affen. Bei der idiopathischen Pubertas praecox wären solche Antikörper therapeutisch wertvoll. Maddock u. Mitarb. (1949) berichten über ein sieben-jähriges menstruierendes Mädchen, das unter einem FSH enthaltenden Schweine-hypophysenextrakt vorübergehend die Menstruation verlor.

V. Das Selbstreglersystem (Feed-back mechanismus)

Nicht nur die Funktion der Keimdrüsen wird durch die glandotropen Hormone des Hypophysenvorderlappens reguliert, sondern dessen Leistung ist abhängig von der Menge der zirkulierenden peripheren Sexualhormone. Es besteht ein Selbstreglermechanismus zwischen den spezifischen Funktionen des HVL und den zugeordneten peripheren Hormondrüsen. Ein Absinken des Hormonspiegels im Blut führt zu einer erhöhten, ein Ansteigen zu einer verminderten Produktion des übergeordneten Vorderlappenhormons (Feed-back mechanismus).

Dieses Selbstreglersystem ist ein komplizierter und nur teilweise erforschter Mechanismus. In den letzten Jahren wurde die Zwischenschaltung des Hypothalamus immer breiter bestätigt. Man nimmt an, daß die Sexualhormone direkt die Sexualregion des Hypothalamus hemmen und den Vorderlappen nur indirekt beeinflussen. Verschiedene Beobachtungen weisen darauf hin, daß die *Empfindlichkeit der Sexualregion* gegenüber den Sexualhormonen variabel ist. Besonders HOHLWEG u. Mitarb. (1934, 1953) haben sich mit dieser Frage beschäftigt. Bei erwachsenen Rattenmännchen bewirkt z.B. die Zufuhr von wöchentlich 10 µg Oestradiolbenzoat eine Atrophie der Hoden, die nach 2 Monaten ihren Höhepunkt erreicht. Trotz gleichbleibender Hormonzufuhr erholen sich die Organe wieder und sind trotz fortgesetzter Behandlung nach 7 Monaten in Größe und Funktion nicht von den unbehandelten Kontrollen zu unterscheiden. Bei der Gabe von 100 µg Oestradiolbenzoat täglich ist die Erholung nach 7 Monaten nur noch gering, bei 1000 µg wöchentlich bleibt sie aus. Die Atrophie von Tieren, die 6 Wochen lang 20 µg pro Woche erhalten, ist viel stärker ausgeprägt als die von Tieren mit anfänglich hohen Dosen (1000 µg pro Woche) 6 Wochen lang und anschließend 100 µg pro Woche für 6 Wochen (HOHLWEG 1953). Gibt man Rattenweibchen zweimal wöchentlich 0,5 mg Testosteronpropionat, so wird der Sexualcyclus anfangs gehemmt. Nach der zweiten oder dritten Injektion tritt kein Oestrus mehr auf. Trotz gleichbleibender Hormonzufuhr setzt die Ovarialtätigkeit nach 8 Wochen wieder ein und nach 12 Wochen haben von 24 Tieren 19 wieder normale Cyclen. Bei der zehnfachen Dosis Testosteron trat keine Adaptation mehr ein.

HOHLWEG hat schon 1934 auf diese *Desensibilisierung* des Hypophysen-Zwischenhirnsystems aufmerksam gemacht. Er konnte bei geschlechtsreifen Rattenweibchen durch regelmäßige Follikelhormongabe den Oestruscyclus hemmen. Wurde die Behandlung nach 2 Monaten unterbrochen, so traten bald wieder Cyclen auf, deren Anzahl und Dauer auf eine erhöhte Ovarialtätigkeit hinwies. Diese Umstellung der Empfindlichkeit des Sexualzentrums gilt auch für den Menschen, wie die Beobachtungen von HECKEL, HELLER und NELSON (1943, 1950), HEINKE und TONUTTI u.a. zeigen. Wie im Tierexperiment, kann dieses Rebound-Phänomen nicht nur durch Testosteron, sondern auch durch Choriongonadotropin und durch Oestrogene ausgelöst werden (KARNS).

DÖRNER und HOHLWEG bestimmten den Gonadotropingehalt der Rattenhypophysen unter der Behandlung mit Testosteronpropionat. Während einer fünfwöchigen Gabe ist er deutlich vermindert, nach Absetzen des Androgens steigt er im Laufe von 8 Wochen über den Wert der Kontrollen an. Auch histologisch zeigt die Hypophyse eine starke Aktivität.

Gibt man statt Testosteron *Choriongonadotropin* (HCG), so tritt schon während der Hormongabe eine Überfunktion der Leydigzellen der Hoden ein. Die vermehrte Testosteron- und Oestrogenproduktion hemmen die Adenohypophyse. Nach Absetzen des HCG verstärkt die nachfolgende erhöhte Gonadotropinbildung der eigenen Hypophyse die Androgenbildung noch mehr, das Gewicht der Samenblasen steigt weiter an. Auch in diesen Versuchen ist der Gonadotropingehalt der Hypophyse erhöht. Hohlweg spricht vom „Überproduktionseffekt" (overproduction effect).

1. Desensibilisierungseffekt

Die Erklärung für dieses Verhalten kann nach Hohlweg (1951) nur über eine Änderung der Empfindlichkeit der Sexualregion im Zwischenhirn geschehen. Dieses adaptiert sich an den höheren Hormonspiegel im Blut, der fälschlicherweise als physiologisch genommen wird. Wird die künstliche Zufuhr von Keimdrüsenhormonen eingestellt, dann steigt die gonadotrope Funktion des Vorderlappens an, da die Receptoren ein Absinken des „physiologischen" Keimdrüsenhormonspiegels im Blut registrieren und eine vermehrte Abgabe des humoralen Wirkstoffes veranlassen. Bei einer Unterfunktion der Keimdrüsen, die auf einer Überempfindlichkeit des Zentrums beruht, kann durch eine länger dauernde Hormonbehandlung eine Desensibilisierung erfolgen, so daß nach Abbruch der Hormonbehandlung mehr Gonadotropine gebildet werden als vorher.

Schon das infantile Tier bildet eine gewisse Menge von Gonadotropinen. Hohlweg (1951) kastrierte infantile Rattenweibchen. Implantierte er solchen Tieren nicht sofort, sondern erst nach 3 Wochen Ovarien in die Nieren, dann trat ein Oestrus auf. Die implantierten Ovarien zeigten große Follikel und Corpora lutea. Hohlweg nimmt an, daß als Folge der Kastration eine vermehrte Produktion von gonadotropen Hormonen in der Hypophyse eingetreten ist. Dadurch entwickelt sich das infantile Ovar und nimmt seine Funktion auf. Der Oestrus erfolgt jedoch nur einmal, die vorzeitige Pubertät bleibt aus. Das implantierte und funktionierende Ovar hemmt offenbar das Sexualzentrum und damit die Gonadotropinbildung im Hypophysenvorderlappen wieder, so daß bis zur Zeit der normalen Pubertät wieder ein Ruhezustand eintritt. Dann erst beginnen die implantierten Ovarien rhythmisch zu funktionieren. Bei infantilen Rattenweibchen genügen 0,01 μg Oestradiolbenzoat pro Tag, um die gonadotrope Funktion des Hypophysenvorderlappens kastrierter Tiere zu hemmen, bei ausgewachsenen Tieren ist die 30fache Dosis notwendig (0,3 μg pro Tag). Das Sexualzentrum des infantilen Organismus ist offenbar viel empfindlicher als das des Erwachsenen. Hohlweg bezeichnet die Pubertät als „physiologische Desensibilisierung".

Besonders Nelson und Heller, Heinke und Tonutti u.a. heben hervor, daß bei der Behandlung der verspäteten Pubertät mit Choriongonadotropin, aber auch mit Androgenen, Dauererfolge zu erreichen sind. Die Hodenvergrößerung bleibt nach Absetzen der Therapie nicht nur bestehen, sondern schreitet weiter. Wahrscheinlich ist auch hier die Desensibilisierung der maßgebende Mechanismus.

Eine schöne experimentelle Bestätigung dieser Hohlwegschen Anschauung haben Bahner u. Mitarb. gegeben. Erhalten junge männliche Ratten vom 14.—33. Tag 20 Tage lang je 5 mg Testosteron, dann steigt das Gewicht der Hoden bis zum 34. Tag auf das Dreifache an und entspricht dem unbehandelter Tiere vom 50. Lebenstag. Histologisch sind die Kanälchen kleiner, aber die Differenzierung entspricht dem 50 Tage älteren Tiere. Die Pubertät wird also um $^1/_3$ der Lebenszeit vorverlegt. Frühere Testosterongabe ist ohne Wirkung. Auf den Menschen übertragen bedeutet dies, daß man in den Jahren vor der

Pubertät mit einer intensiveren und länger dauernden Testosteron- oder Gonadotropinbehandlung zurückhaltend sein muß. Therapeutisch macht man sich diesen Mechanismus bei der Behandlung des hypophysären Minderwuchses zunutze.

Beim Menschen hat man den begründeten Eindruck, daß die Reife des Sexualzentrums an die somatische Reife gekoppelt ist. Erst wenn diese einen gewissen Grad erreicht hat, beginnt die Pubertät. Wird die körperliche Reifung durch schwere Allgemeinerkrankungen verzögert (Sprue, hämolytische Anämie u.ä.), dann bleibt sie aus. Dem widerspricht nicht, daß die Gonadotropinbildung nach den Untersuchungen von JOST (1953) schon einmal in den ersten Embryonalmonaten aufgenommen war. Die somatische Reife kann durch Wachstumshormon enthaltende Extrakte menschlicher Hypophysen beschleunigt werden, nach klinischer Erfahrung aber auch durch Testosteron, Oestrogene und anabole Steroide. Wahrscheinlich sind es die anabolen Eigenschaften der Steroide, die die Reifung der Sexualregion bedingen, also die physiologische Desensibilisierung auslösen.

Für die Behandlung des Prostatacarcinoms mit Oestrogenen ist dieser Desensibilisierungseffekt wahrscheinlich von großer Bedeutung, da die Hypophyse nach Gewöhnung an die hohen Hormondosen die Gonadotropinbildung und damit wieder die Androgenproduktion im Hoden aufnehmen kann!

2. Einfluß der Kastration

Wie zahlreiche Untersucher immer wieder festgestellt haben, steigt nach Entfernung der Gonaden (Kastration) die Ausscheidung der gonadotropen Hormone im Urin stark an. Dies gilt für den Menschen und alle untersuchten Tiere in gleichem Maße. Die Hypophyse des Kastraten vergrößert sich und wandelt sich in ganz charakteristischer Weise um (BIGGART, BERBLINGER, ROMEIS). Bei der Ratte erhöht sich Zahl und Volumen der Basophilen. Kolloidartige Massen drängen den Zellkern zur Seite, so daß Siegelring- oder Kastrationszellen entstehen. Beim Menschen sind die Veränderungen unspezifisch und fehlen oft ganz. BERBLINGER findet eine auffallende Vermehrung und Vergrößerung der α-Zellen, BIGGART viele große chromophobe Zellen, die er als Übergänge zu den Basophilen ansieht, Siegelringzellen fehlen. Auch beim künstlichen Kryptorchismus der Ratte ohne Zeichen des Hypogonadismus wandelt sich die Hypophyse allmählich zur Kastrationshypophyse mit typischen Siegelringzellen um, ebenso nach Zerstörung des Keimepithels durch Röntgenstrahlen. Das Kanälchenepithel hemmt also die Gonadotropinbildung der Hypophyse.

Der Gehalt der Hypophysen kastrierter Tiere und des Menschen an gonadotropen Hormonen ist beträchtlich erhöht, auch die Jugendlicher (EVANS, McCULLAGH, FINERTY, SMITH). Diese Hypophysen enthalten vorwiegend FSH und weniger ICSH. Wichtig ist, daß schon die Hypophyse des infantilen Organismus unter der Bremswirkung der Gonaden steht. Kastriert man infantile männliche Ratten, dann enthält die Hypophyse, im Implantationsversuch geprüft, mehr gonadotropes Hormon als diejenige von nicht kastrierten erwachsenen Kontrollen (EVANS).

Endlich sei an die Versuche von HARRIS (1950) erinnert, der zeigen konnte, daß auch die Hypophysen neugeborener Tiere, wenn sie ihren hypophysektomierten Müttern in die Sella gelegt werden, eine normale Funktion aufnehmen können. Gibt man dem Kastraten oestrogene oder androgene Wirkstoffe, dann bildet sich die Kastrationshypophyse wieder zurück, ihr Gonadotropingehalt normalisiert sich wieder (HOHLWEG 1931, SCHOELLER).

3. Einfluß der Sexualhormone (Oestrogene, Androgene)

Über die Wirkung der *Oestrogene* auf die Hypophyse sind wir besser unterrichtet als über die der Androgene. Oestrogene hemmen in kleinen und mittleren Dosen bei der *Ratte* die Bildung und Abgabe von FSH und erhöhen die Abgabe von LH. Diese 1934 von Hohlweg beschriebene Eigenschaft (Hohlweg-Effekt) wurde später von vielen bestätigt. Unter Gewichtsanstieg erfolgt die Umwandlung des Ovars in Gelbkörper, eine Reaktion, die beim hypophysektomierten Tier ausbleibt (Guinet, Bradbury). Fortgesetzte Verabreichung senkt den Gonadotropingehalt bei männlichen und weiblichen Ratten beträchtlich (Meyer).

Die wirksamen Dosen sind sehr klein. Bei parabiotisch vereinigten Ratten (ein Partner kastriert, einer hypophysektomiert) hemmen schon 0,009 μg α-Oestradiol, gemessen am Ovarialgewicht des nicht kastrierten Partners, während erst 0,5—0,7 μg das Uterusgewicht anregen (Byrnes). Die Ausbildung der Kastrationshypophyse kann bei weiblichen Tieren mit 0,025 μg Oestradiolbenzoat pro Tag bzw. 2 μg pro Woche (Hohlweg 1934) verhindert werden. Verabreicht man hohe Dosen von Oestrogenen, dann wird der Gehalt an Gonadotropin der Hypophyse völlig vernichtet (beim Affen mit 100 μg Oestradiol). Aus diesen und ähnlichen Beobachtungen schließt man, daß bei Mäusen, Ratten und Affen schon die physiologischerweise vom Ovar gebildeten Oestrogene Bildung und Abgabe der hypophysären Gonadotropine drosseln.

Auch beim *Menschen* hemmen die Oestrogene stark. Rowlands u. Mitarb. (1940) konnte dies durch Implantation menschlicher Hypophysen von behandelten und nichtbehandelten klimakterischen Frauen direkt nachweisen. Die wirksamen Dosen sind nicht einheitlich. 0,1 mg Diäthylstilboestrol kann die Ausscheidung der Gonadotropine erhöhen, 0,5 mg bessern wohl klimakterische Ausfallserscheinungen, senken aber die Gonadotropinausscheidung nicht signifikant, erst unter 1 mg sinkt sie ab, ab 3 mg rasch, bei 10 mg täglich verschwinden sie völlig aus dem Urin. Zwei bis drei Wochen nach Absetzen sind die alten Werte wieder erreicht (Tokuyama, Heller 1944). 5 mg Oestradiolbenzoat senkt die Gonadotropinausscheidung beim Turner-Syndrom signifikant. Der Anstieg nach kleinen Dosen ist wahrscheinlich durch die vermehrte Abgabe von LH bedingt (Hohlweg-Effekt). Einzelne Frauen verhalten sich selbst viermal 10 mg Oestradiolbenzoat gegenüber refraktär (Finkelstein, Heller 1939, Segaloff 1954). Diäthylstilboestrol hemmt am stärksten, konjugierte Oestrogene, die Equine nur $^1/_2$, Oestradiol nur $^1/_5$ so stark (Tokuyama).

Bei *männlichen Kastraten* hemmen etwa dieselben Oestrogendosen wie bei weiblichen. Die *Wirkung der Androgene* ist gewichtsmäßig wesentlich geringer. 100 μg Testosteronpropionat erhält bei kastrierten Ratten das Gewicht von Prostata und Samenblasen, während sich die Hypophyse zur Kastrationshypophyse umwandelt. Nach Gans (1953, 1959) erniedrigten 100 μg Testosteronpropionat die erhöhten Serumgonadotropine der kastrierten männlichen Ratte eindeutig, und zwar sowohl bestimmt als FSH als auch als ICSH. 2 μg Oestradiolbenzoat hat dieselbe Wirkungsstärke. Bei Leghorn-Kapaunen erhalten 0,5 bis 10 μg Testosteron pro Tag das Wachstum des Kammes. Die Hypophyse solcher Tiere enthält pro Gramm Gewicht aber schon dieselbe hohe Menge an gonadotropem Hormon wie die unbehandelter Kastraten. Testosteron scheint mehr die Abgabe, Oestradiol mehr die Bildung zu hemmen (van Rees).

Bei klimakterischen Frauen sind größere Dosen nötig als bei männlichen Kastraten. 25 mg jeden zweiten Tag vermindert nur um 50% (Buchholz). Andere sahen die Gonadotropine bei klimakterischen Frauen, die wegen Mammacarcinom dreimal 100 mg Testosteronpropionat pro Woche erhalten, erst nach zehn Wochen verschwinden. Vorwiegend anabol wirkende Derivate des Testosterons, wie 2-Methyl-androstan-17β-ol-3-on hemmen die Ausscheidung weniger 9α-fluor-11β-hydroxy-17α-methyltestosteron (Fluoxymesteron) nur in geringem Maße, obwohl die Wirkung auf die Carcinommetastasen erhalten ist. Hemmung der hypophysären Gonadotropine scheint keine Voraussetzung für die anticancerogene Wirksamkeit eines Androgens zu sein.

Auch beim männlichen Kastraten sind Testosterondosen — 10—15 mg Testosteronpropionat täglich —, die die Kastrationszeichen zur Rückbildung bringen (normale Prostata, Samenblase, normaler Haarwuchs, normales Ejaculat usw.) nicht imstande, die erhöhte Ausscheidung von Gonadotropinen zu senken (McCULLAGH 1948, LARICHE), erst 20 mg und mehr sind allmählich wirksam (CATCHPOLE 1939, 1940, 1942, NATHANSON 1939, SALMON, SHORR). Beim Klinefelter-Syndrom normalisieren erst unverhältnismäßig hohe Testosteronmengen die Harngonadotropine. 150 mg Testosteronpropionat pro Woche hemmt im allgemeinen nicht, selbst 300 mg Testosteronpropionat pro Woche sind noch unsicher (McCULLAGH).

Damit stimmt die Beobachtung überein, daß die Gonadotropinausscheidung bei normaler Funktion der Leydigzellen stark erhöht sein kann. Die Diskrepanz der Hormondosis, die die hypophysären Gonadotropine hemmt, zu der androgenwirksamen, hat schon lange die Vermutung nach einem zweiten Keimdrüsenhormon aufkommen lassen.

Neben dem Testosteron sind eine ganze Reihe von Vorstufen und Derivaten auf ihre hemmende Wirkung untersucht. Pregnenolonacetat, 17α-Hydroxyprogesteron, Androst-5-en-3β-ol-17-on-acetat (Dehydroisoandrosteronacetat). Androsta-4,6-dien-3-17-dion und wasserlösliche Extrakte aus 25 g Hodengewebe sind unwirksam (MORTIMORE), die vorwiegend anabol wirkenden Derivate des Testosterons verhalten sich verschieden.

4. Bedeutung des „zweiten" Keimdrüsenhormons (X-Hormon, Inhibin)

Schon 1923 haben MOTTRAM und CRAMER festgestellt, daß die Hypophyse von Ratten, deren Samenepithel durch Röntgenbestrahlung zerstört wurde, das Aussehen einer Kastrationshypophyse annimmt. Werden solche Tiere parabiotisch mit weiblichen Ratten verbunden, dann tritt als Folge der vermehrten Gonadotropinbildung ein Daueroestrus ein (WITSCHI). Verpflanzt man die Hoden von männlichen Ratten in die Bauchhöhle, dann nimmt die Hypophyse nach 75 Tagen das Aussehen einer Kastrationshypophyse an, nach 240 Tagen entwickelt sich eine Atrophie der Samenblasen und erst nach 400 auch eine solche der Prostata (NELSON 1934). Da die Kanälchen eines kryptorchen Hodens lange vor den interstiellen Zellen zugrunde gehen, darf man aus dieser zeitlichen Differenz schließen, daß die Entwicklung der Kastrationshypophyse auf eine Degeneration der Tubuluszellen zurückgeht. GATZ hat daher vorgeschlagen, die Bezeichnung Kastrationszellen durch Sterilitätszellen zu ersetzen. Auch beim Menschen ist die Gonadotropinausscheidung bei Atrophie der Kanälchen und erhaltener Leydigzellfunktion erhöht, so beim doppelseitigen Kryptorchismus, der Kanälchenatrophie nach Mumps und anderen Infektionskrankheiten, beim Klinefelter-Syndrom und Vitamin E-Mangel. Bei leichteren und auch schwereren Formen der Oligospermie ist sie dagegen normal.

Man hat daher ein zweites Keimdrüsenhormon, das „Inhibin", auch als X-Hormon bezeichnet, postuliert (McCULLAGH 1953, HOWARD 1950), das in den Kanälchen entsteht und das Bildung und Abgabe des FSH in der Hypophyse hemmt. Man glaubte, das Inhibin sei in wäßrigen Hodenextrakten enthalten. doch konnte diese Angabe nicht bestätigt werden.

Es ist immer noch strittig, wem der hemmende Effekt zukommt, dem Keimepithel oder den Sertolizellen. Die Befunde einer erhöhten Gonadotropinausscheidung sind bei den verschiedenen Krankheitsbildern des Menschen nicht einheitlich. Das nimmt bei einer mit so vielen Fehlern behafteten Methode nicht wunder. Auch erlaubt die einfache Hodenbiopsie, auf die man sich im allgemeinen stützen muß, keine sichere Aussage über die Verfassung des gesamten Kanälchensystems. DEL CASTILLO (1947) hat in dem von ihm beschriebenen Syndrom (Sertoli cells only) normale Gonadotropinwerte im Urin gefunden. Nachuntersuchungen solcher Fälle ergaben aber auch eine erhöhte Ausscheidung (NELSON 1934). Bei der Kanälchenschädigung nach Orchitis, Röntgenbestrahlung, Vitamin E-Mangel, bleiben die Sertolizellen häufig erhalten, obwohl die Gonadotropine erhöht sein können. Eine konstante und starke Erhöhung findet sich dagegen bei der Sklerosierung der Kanälchen, wobei sowohl das Keimepithel als auch die Sertolizellen zugrunde gegangen sind, so daß die klinischen Betrachtungen mehr für die Sertolizellen als Bildungsstätte sprechen (HOWARD 1950).

In der letzten Zeit hat man den Oestrogenen des Hodens die Rolle des Inhibins zugeschrieben (FORBES). Wie DICZFALUSY (1954) festgestellt hat, enthält die Samenflüssigkeit sowohl Oestron als auch Oestriol in freier Form. Obwohl die Frage des Bildungsortes der Oestrogene zugunsten der Leydigzellen entschieden ist, so erscheint es doch möglich, daß das Keimepithel durch Speicherung der Oestrogene, durch Umwandlung in stärker hypophysär hemmende Formen an der Regulation teilnimmt. Die Oestrogene können aber das „Inhibin" nicht ganz ersetzen, da die Gonadotropinausscheidung auch in den Fällen von Kanälchenschwund erhöht ist, die mit einer normalen Ausscheidung von 17-Ketosteroiden und Oestrogenen einhergehen.

HELLER und NELSON (1945) nehmen an, daß die Höhe der Gonadotropinausscheidung im wesentlichen davon abhängt, wieviel von den Hypophysenhormonen vom Hodengewebe adsorbiert, verbraucht oder inaktiviert wird. Nach dieser Verbrauchstheorie sezerniert der Hypophysenvorderlappen für gewöhnlich etwa konstante Mengen Gonadotropin. Ein überwiegender Teil wird vom Hodengewebe bei der Bildung der Keimzellen und der Hormone verbraucht. Die Hormone des Hodens, vorwiegend die Oestrogene, weniger die Androgene, können in der Regulation mithelfen, sie hemmen stärker, aber nur, wenn sie in größeren Mengen vorhanden sind. Bei Verlust des Hodens oder Schädigung der Kanälchen oder der Leydigzellen werden die Gonadotropine nicht mehr utilisiert, die Ausscheidung erhöht sich.

Wie man sieht, ist die feinere Regulation der Gonadotropinbildung beim männlichen Organismus nicht geklärt. Fest steht, daß die normale Androgen-, Oestrogen- und Inhibinbildung die Gonadotropinsekretion in Grenzen hält. Ob dabei niedrige Dosen der Androgene nur die ICSH-Bildung hemmen (GREEP 1950) und erst unphysiologisch hohe auch das FSH, niedrige Dosen der Oestrogene nur FSH hemmen, die ICSH-Bildung dagegen anregen und erst hohe Dosen beide vermindern, ist nicht geklärt. Die meisten Untersuchungen sind mit einem einzelnen Hormon, mit Oestrogen oder Testosteron oder Progesteron angestellt, einer Versuchsanordnung, wie sie dem Physiologischen nicht entspricht. Vorläufig muß man sich mit der Annahme begnügen, daß das Keimepithel, und zwar wahrscheinlich sowohl die unreifen Keimzellen als auch die Sertolizellen, durch Bildung eines eigenen Wirkstoffes an der Regulation der Bildung und Abgabe der Gonadotropine im Hypophysenvorderlappen beteiligt sind. Das „Inhibin" steht vermutlich mit dem FSH im Gleichgewicht. HOWARD (1950) nimmt an, daß es gleichzeitig die ICSH-Bildung anregt, ähnlich wie kleine Oestrogendosen die LH-Aktivität beim weiblichen Tier stimulieren. Fehlt das Inhibin, dann erhöht sich Bildung und Ausscheidung des FSH, während ICSH normal bleiben oder sich erhöhen kann. Mit der Zeit können die FSH-bildenden Zellen offenbar die ICSH-Bildner überwuchern und dadurch einen sekundären Eunuchoidismus auslösen (HOWARD 1950).

5. Bedeutung des Zentralnervensystems

Der Einfluß des *Zentralnervensystems* auf die Funktion der Gonade der Säuger tritt am deutlichsten bei der Auslösung der Ovulation durch die Kohabitation bei Kaninchen, Frettchen und Katzen in Erscheinung. 10—12 Std nach dem Coitus oder nach elektrischer Reizung des Uterus erfolgt durch die Abgabe von luteotropem Hormon der Follikelsprung. Die Ovulation kann auch durch elektrische Reizung der Kerne des Tuber cinereum (NOWAKOWSKI 1950) und des Infundibulums (mediane Eminenz) bzw. des Nucleus amygdaloideus ausgelöst werden (EVERETT 1956) ebenso durch Instillation von adrenergischen oder cholinergischen Substanzen in die Hypophyse selbst oder in die Portalgefäße (SAWYER).

Die Abhängigkeit der gonadotropen Funktion des Hypophysenvorderlappens von Teilen des Zwischenhirns ist in den letzten Jahren durch zahlreiche Untersuchungen bei verschiedenen Tierarten (Ratten, Hunde, Enten u.a.) sichergestellt worden. Erst nachdem man dazu überging, die Trennung des Hypophysenstiels durch Einlage von in Wachs getränkten Papierstückchen, Stanniol u.ä. zu sichern, entwickelte sich nach der Stieldurchtrennung regelmäßig eine Atrophie aller vom Vorderlappen abhängigen peripheren innersekretorischen Drüsen, also der Keimdrüsen, der Nebennieren und der Schilddrüse (GREEP 1951, HARRIS 1948, WESTMAN). Der Vorderlappen der Hypophyse fällt einer teilweisen bindegewebigen Umwandlung anheim. Als beweisend werden die Ergebnisse der Transplantation von Hypophysen angesehen, wie sie zuerst von HARRIS und JACOBSOHN (1952) vorgenommen wurden. Transplantation von Hypophysen in andere Organe führt zu einem weitgehenden Schwund der Hypophyse und zu einer Atrophie der peripheren Hormondrüsen. Bei der Transplantation in die vordere Augenkammer (BENOIT) bleiben die Zellen des Vorderlappens erhalten. Trotzdem sind die Keimdrüsen solcher Tiere stark geschwunden, die Nebennieren sind aber noch imstande, auf gewisse Reize zu reagieren. Bei Transplantation der Hypophyse unter die Nierenkapsel bleibt die Sekretion von luteotropem Hormon erhalten, während die von FSH und LH völlig aufhört. Die LTH-Sekretion ist also unabhängig vom ZNS. Bei Transplantation von Hypophysen neugeborener Ratten unter den Temporallappen ihrer hypophysektomierten Mütter blieben die Gonaden funktionslos. Nur wenn die Hypophysen direkt unter die mediane Eminenz, also unter das Infundibulum gelegt werden, nehmen sie die Funktion auf und das innersekretorische System bleibt funktionstüchtig (BENOIT, EVERETT 1954, HARRIS 1952).

Diese Befunde werden allgemein als Beweis für eine Reizübertragung aus dem Zwischenhirn auf den Hypophysenvorderlappen angesehen, da nur bei erhaltener anatomischer Verbindung die Funktion des Vorderlappens erhalten bleibt oder sich wieder einstellt.

Einzelne Beobachtungen aus der menschlichen Pathologie (BAILEY 1922, CAMUS, SMITH 1944) machten wahrscheinlich, daß im Gebiet des Zwischenhirns eine Schaltstelle vorhanden ist, von der aus die gonadotrope Partialfunktion der Hypophyse gesteuert ist. Systematische Untersuchungen der Spatzschen

Schule (BUSTAMENTE, DIEPEN, GAUPP) lokalisierten diese Schaltstelle in das
mediale Tuberfeld, den Nucleus infundibularis und Nucleus principalis tuberis.
Bei Zerstörung dieses Gebietes bleibt bei infantilen Kaninchen die Sexualreifung
aus, bei ausgewachsenen atrophieren die Hoden. Bei Ratten führen verschiedene
lokalisierte Schädigungen des Zwischenhirns zur Atrophie der Keimdrüsen, so
im vorderen (BENOIT, GREER, HILLARP 1955), im mittleren (McCANN) und im
hinteren (BOGDANOVE, SOULAIRAC) Hypothalamus. Die Schäden in der medianen
Eminenz liegen so nahe am blutführenden Hypophysenstiel, daß eine Mangel-
durchblutung der Adenohypophyse als Ursache der Genitalatrophie nicht sicher
ausgeschlossen werden kann. Man konnte bis jetzt die Gebiete des Zwischenhirns, das nervöse und humorale Reize aus der Peripherie und aus dem Zentralnervensystem entgegennimmt, verarbeitet und auf humoralem Wege zum Vorderlappen weitergibt, nicht genau lokalisieren. Offenbar bestehen bei den einzelnen
Tierarten ziemliche Unterschiede.

Nach Zerstörung von Teilen des vorderen Hypothalamus, besonders in der
Gegend des Nucleus paraventricularis und der Area praeoptica tritt bei Meer-
schweinchen und Ratten ein Daueroestrus ein (BROOKHART, DEY 1942, 1943,
HILLARP). Diese Gegend interferiert mit der Bildung des Luteinisierungshormons.
Doppelseitige ausgedehnte Schäden im Nucleus infraopticus und Nucleus para-
ventricularis selbst bedingen bei Enten eine schwere Gonadenatrophie (BENOIT).
Neuerdings wird für FSH ein Hemmungs- und Anregungszentrum postuliert.

Die Übermittlung der hypothalamischen Impulse auf den Vorderlappen erfolgt nicht auf nervösem, sondern auf *humoralem Weg.*

Die arterielle Versorgung des Hypophysenvorderlappens geschieht vorwiegend
über mehrere Arteriae hypophyseae superiores aus der intrakraniellen Carotis
bzw. der Arteria communicans posterior. Diese Arterien ziehen zum Teil im
Hypophysenstiel (Trichterlappen bzw. Pars infundibularis), teils im Subarach-
noidalraum abwärts zum Vorderlappen und verzweigen sich hier in einem weit-
maschigen Capillarnetz, das die Zellen umspinnt.

Die Länge des Trichterlappens, dem nach hinten das Infundibulum folgt,
wird durchzogen von dünnwandigen Gefäßen, die aus Zweigen der Arteriae
superiores entspringen. Von ihnen aus strahlen Capillarschlingen in das Infundibulum ein, die SPATZ als „Spezialgefäße" benennt. Das Blut sammelt sich
wieder in den Portalgefäßen, die sich in einem zweiten Capillarnetz im Vorderlappen aufteilen und diesen mit Blut versorgen. Die Verbindung zwischen Hypophyse und dem Hypothalamus wird durch diese Spezialgefäße hergestellt, die
in das Infundibulum oder in die mediane Eminenz des Tuber cinereum als ge-
schlossene Schlingen einstrahlen. Hier werden sie umsponnen von zahlreichen
markreichen gomorinegativen Nervenfasern, die aus den hypophysennahen
Teilen des Zwischenhirns stammen. In dieser *adeno-neurohypophysären Kontakt-
fläche* (SPATZ) erfolgt nach der gegenwärtigen Auffassung der wichtige humorale
Stoffaustausch. Man nimmt an, daß sekretorische Produkte der vorderen Zwi-
schenhirnkerne über diese neurovasculäre Verbindung zum Vorderlappen trans-
portiert werden. Die Natur der hypothalamischen Trägersubstanz ist nicht
bekannt.

D. Sexualhormone
I. Allgemeine Wirkung der Steroidhormone

Das griechische Wort „Hormao", ich errege, wurde 1905 von STARLING für
solche direkt in das Blut abgegebene Sekrete geprägt, die als „chemical mes-
sengers" wirken und die ihre Eigenschaften an einer vom Entstehungsort ent-

fernten Stelle entfalten. Sein Gedanke war dabei, die regulatorische Funktion bestimmter Verbindungen von anderen Arten der Reizübertragung zu unterscheiden.

Die Klasse der Substanzen, die als *Steroide* (I) bezeichnet werden, ist in Tier- und Pflanzenwelt weit verbreitet und schließt die Sterole, die Gallensäuren, die herzaktiven Aglykone, die Sapogenine, die Steroidalkaloide und Provitamin D_3 ein.

Da über die Funktion dieser natürlich vorkommenden Steroide verhältnismäßig wenig bekannt ist, wird der Begriff der Steroide in Biologie und Medizin auf die Steroidhormone beschränkt. Diese umfassen die Androgene, die Oestrogene, die progestionalen Hormone, die Mineralocorticoide und die Glucocorticoide.

Androgene und Oestrogene sind Wuchsstoffe, die ihre Wirkung besonders an den primären und sekundären Geschlechtsorganen entfalten. Durch Eingreifen in den Zellstoffwechsel und durch Bereitstellung besonderer Bausteine schaffen sie die Voraussetzung für das Wachstum der Endorgane.

Die Androgene haben einen starken Einfluß auf den Stoffwechsel und die Funktion von Epithelzellen, die Oestrogene fördern mehr die Zellteilung, beide steigern das Wachstum von Drüsen und des Bindegewebes. Weder die Androgene noch die Oestrogene sind geschlechtsspezifisch, da beide im männlichen und weiblichen Organismus physiologisch sind und dort spezifische Wirkungen entfalten.

Die biologische Wirkung ist abhängig von Zahl und Stellung der OH- und O-Gruppen im Molekül. Die Gewebe besitzen spezifische Enzyme, die die Funktionsgruppen oxydieren und reduzieren und das Hormon damit inaktivieren. Die Aktivität und Verteilung dieser Enzyme wechselt nicht nur in den verschiedenen Geweben derselben Species, sondern auch im selben Gewebe der verschiedenen Species. KOCHAKIAN (1956) hat die Hypothese aufgestellt, daß die Aktivität der verschiedenen Androgene von den Metaboliten abhängig ist, die in den einzelnen Geweben gebildet werden. Sie ist in den Zellen am stärksten, in denen die Abbaufermente, also besonders die Dehydrogenasen, fehlen.

Über den Angriffsort und die Wirkungsweise der Steroidhormone im Stoffwechsel der Zellen ist wenig bekannt. Kastration und Verabreichung von Androgenen ändern die Aktivität verschiedener Fermente in verschiedenen Organen, man hat aber noch keine Vorstellung, an welcher Stelle des Intermediärstoffwechsels sie ihre primäre Wirkung entfalten.

Da Cholesterin in großer Menge in die Zelloberfläche eingelagert ist und die Steroide ähnliche chemische Substanzen sind, hat man angenommen, daß die Steroidhormone durch Einlagerung in die Zelloberfläche die Durchlässigkeit der Zellmembran für bestimmte Stoffe ändern und dadurch die Steuerung der Zellfunktion in die Hand nehmen. Änderung der Durchlässigkeit der Zellmembran scheint aber mehr eine Eigenschaft der Eiweißhormone (Insulin, Gonadotropine, ACTH u.a.) zu sein (SAMUELS 1949). Neuere Untersuchungen machen wahrscheinlich, daß die Steroidhormone direkt an bestimmten Enzymsystemen angreifen. VILLEE u. Mitarb. hatten gefunden, daß Oestrogene, inkubiert mit Zellen von menschlicher Placenta, bei der Anwesenheit von Isocitrat die Reduktion von DPN und die Oxydation des zugeführten Isocitrates zu α-Oxyglutarat stimulieren. Sie nehmen an, daß die Oestrogene eine spezifische DPN-Isocitratdehydrogenase der Placenta aktivieren. Oestradiol-17 β ist in diesem Versuch in einer Konzentration von 10^{-8} wirksam, Testosteron erst bei 15 μg. TALALAY u. Mitarb. erweiterten diese Versuche und gaben eine andere Erklärung. Die Anregung der Reduktion von DPN durch Oestradiol-17 β wird bei Gegenwart von Isocitrat aufgehoben, wenn man den Placentaextrakt fraktioniert, durch

Zugabe von katalytischem TPN aber wieder herstellt. Was als einfache Stimulierung einer DPN-abhängigen Isocitratdehydrogenase erschien, ist in Wirklichkeit das Zusammenwirken eines DPN-abhängigen Isocitratdehydrogenase-
systems auf ein Pyridinnucleotid-Transhydrogenasesystem, das durch Oestrogen
aktiviert wird. Die Autoren machen darauf aufmerksam, daß viele Stoffwechselreaktionen, die von den Steroidhormonen beeinflußt werden, wie die Beschleunigung des Einbaues von Aminosäuren in Eiweiß, von Acetat in Fettsäuren, die
Bildung von Fructose u.ä., von Fermentsystemen durchgeführt werden, die
TPNH-gebunden sind. Sie nehmen an, daß sich das Hormon an das Enzym
anlagert und interpretieren die Aktivität der DPN-TPNH-Transhydrogenase als
wechselnde Dehydrierung und Hydrierung des Steroidmoleküls, wobei das Steroid
durch Umwandlung von einem Steroidalkohol in ein Steroidketon als Wasserstoff-
überträger wirkt.

$$H^+ + TPNH + Oestron \rightleftarrows TPN^+ + Oestradiol\text{-}17\beta$$

$$Oestradiol\text{-}17\beta + DPN \rightleftarrows Oestron + DPNH + H^+$$

Der Oxydo-Reduktionsmechanismus der Oestrogene als Co-Faktoren von Trans-
hydrogenasen ist theoretisch auch auf andere Steroidhormone übertragbar, z. B.

$$Androstendion \rightleftharpoons Testosteron$$
$$Androstandion \rightleftharpoons Androsteron$$
$$Cortison \rightleftharpoons Cortisol$$
$$Progesteron \rightleftharpoons 20\alpha\text{-Hydroxy-4-pregnen 20-on}$$

Ob diese in vitro-Untersuchungen an mehr oder weniger gereinigten Enzymsystemen auf die sich in der Zelle abspielenden Vorgänge übertragen werden dürfen erscheint fraglich, nachdem die Oxydo-Reduktion bei den biologisch hoch
aktiven synthetischen Oestrogenen chemisch nicht vorstellbar ist (Marrian;
Hübener u. a.).

Die Theorie von Hübener, die annimmt, daß die Steroidhormone als sog.
Enzym-Induktoren bzw. Enzym-Repressoren wirken, bedarf noch der weiteren
Bearbeitung.

Zahlreiche Untersuchungen des letzten Jahrzehnts haben ergeben, daß das
Enzymmuster einer Zelle nicht gleichmäßig zusammengesetzt ist, sondern sich
je nach den Stoffwechselbedürfnissen ändert. Die Neubildung von Enzymen
wird induziert. Die Übertragung der Information zur Enzymneubildung ist ein
komplizierter Vorgang, der nach den gegenwärtigen Kenntnissen durch drei Gene
koordiniert wird, ein Regulator-Gen (DNS) steuert mit Hilfe eines Repressors
(Apo-Repressor) die Aktivität eines Operator-Gens. Das Operator-Gen wiederum
steigert die Bildung einer spezifischen Ribonucleinsäure, die sog. Messenger-
Ribonucleinsäure, die ihre Information von den Genen des Zellkerns, den Des-
oxyribonucleinsäuren erhält. Induktoren können den Apo-Repressor hemmen,
Co-Repressoren seine Wirkung verstärken. Im ersteren Fall spricht man von
Enzyminduktion, im letzteren von Enzym-Repression. Als Induktoren bzw.
Co-Repressoren sind unter anderem Kohlenhydrate, Steroide und Aminosäuren
bekannt. Die in der Zelle vorhandenen Aminosäuren werden zunächst zu Amino-
acyl-AMP (Adenosin-5-Monophosphat) aktiviert, danach wird die aktivierte
Aminosäure auf lösliche Ribonucleinsäure übertragen. Aus den aktivierten
Aminosäuren bilden dann die Ribosomen, die vorwiegend aus Ribonucleotiden
entstehen, Enzymproteine.

Hübener stellt die Enzyminduktion als wesentliche Wirkungsweise der
Nebennierenrindensteroide auf Grund folgender Beobachtungen zur Diskussion.
Im Experiment kann durch Antimetaboliten und Hemmstoffe der Proteinsynthese

und durch Antimetaboliten der Robinucleinsäure-Synthese die Glykogenbildung in der Leber nach Cortisolgabe verhindert werden. Weiter fand er eine qualitative und quantitative Korrelation zwischen der durch Cortisol ausgelösten Glykogenbildung einerseits und dem Anstieg, d. h. der Induktion zweier Leberenzyme andererseits. Die Gluconeogenese und die Aktivität der induzierten Enzyme setzen erst voll ein, wenn die Nebennierenrindenhormone in der Leber bereits nicht mehr nachweisbar sind. Bei den Androgenen wird eine ähnliche Diskrepanz zwischen Lebenszeit und der Wirkungsdauer beobachtet. Testosteron 4-^{14}C reichert sich zunächst in den Erfolgsorganen, z. B. der Samenblase, an, es ist jedoch bereits wieder verschwunden, wenn die biologische Wirkung, d. h. der Anstieg des Aminosäureeinbaues in Proteine einsetzt. Auch die Wirkungsdauer der Oestrogene überdauert ihre Anwesenheit und Lebenszeit im Organsubstrat beträchtlich. Diese Diskrepanz läßt sich zwanglos durch Enzyminduktion erklären. Das einmal induzierte Enzym bleibt über viele Stunden, ja Tage in der Zelle erhalten, unabhängig von der Anwesenheit oder Lebenszeit des Induktors. Ihrer biologischen Wirkungsweise nach müssen Androgene und Oestrogene vorwiegend Enzymmuster bzw. Enzymketten induzieren, die die Aminosäuren- und Eiweißsynthese regulieren.

II. Struktur und Nomenklatur der Steroide

Steroidhormone besitzen alle den 1,2-Cyclopentanphenanthren-Ring, sie unterscheiden sich von den Sterinen dadurch, daß sie an C 17 keine aliphatische Seitenkette, sondern höchstens eine meist hochoxydierte 2-Kohlenstoffkette besitzen.

Im Steroidmolekül sind die Ringe B/C und die Ringe C/D immer in Transstellung vereinigt. Die Methylgruppen an den Ringverbindungen A/B und C/D stehen aus der allgemeinen Ebene hervor und werden als anguläre Methylgruppen bezeichnet. Alle Konfigurationen im Molekül werden auf diese angulären Methylgruppen bezogen. Diejenigen, die auf derselben Seite liegen, werden mit dem griechischen Buchstaben Beta (β)-Cis bezeichnet und sind mit einer ausgezogenen Valenzlinie mit dem Ring verbunden. Diejenigen, die auf der Gegenseite liegen, werden mit Alpha (α)-Trans bezeichnet und gestrichelt mit den Ringen verbunden. Die C-Atome der einzelnen Ringe werden durchnumeriert, ebenso die der Seitenketten (I).

I. Grundstruktur der Sterine

Die Nomenklatur bezieht sich nie auf den Cyclopentanphenanthren-Ring, sondern auf Verbindungen mit der gleichen Gesamtkonfiguration, den gleichen angulären Methylgruppen und Seitenketten, also auf die Grundformen Androstan (II), Ätiocholan (III), Oestran (IV) und Pregnan (V). Androstan und Ätiocholan unterscheiden sich nur in der Lage des H-Atoms am C 5.

Die Hormone unterscheiden sich von den Grundformen durch zusätzliche O-Gruppen an einzelnen C-Atomen und durch Doppelbindungen in den Ringen. Eine Hydroxylgruppe am 11 C-Atom steht immer in β-Stellung, während die Hydroxylgruppe am 17 C bei den Verbindungen, die eine Kohlenstoffseitenkette haben, immer in α-Stellung angeordnet ist. Die Hydroxylgruppen (C—OH) werden mit dem Suffix-ol, die Ketogruppen (C=O) mit dem Suffix-on, die Aldehydgruppe mit al bezeichnet und mit der Nummer des C-Atoms, mit dem sie im Ringsystem in Verbindung steht, versehen und nach der Grundform angeordnet, wobei ol immer vor on steht, also z.B. Δ^5-Androsten-3β-ol-17-on Die moderne Tendenz geht dahin, daß wissenschaftliche Benennungen nicht mehr als *ein* Suffix haben sollen, alle anderen Substituenten werden als Präfixe der Benennung vorangestellt, also nicht Δ^5-Androsten-3β-ol-17-on, sondern 3β-Hydroxy-5-androsten-17-one = Dehydroepiandrosteron (VI).

Doppelbindungen zwischen aufeinanderfolgenden C-Atomen werden mit der Nummer des ersten C-Atoms gekennzeichnet, 5-Androsten, früher mit Δ versehen. Doppelbindungen zwischen nicht aufeinanderfolgenden C-Atomen werden mit beiden Nummern — die zweite Nummer in Klammern — bezeichnet, z.B. $\Delta^{5\,(10)}$.

II. Androstan   III. Ätiocholan   IV. Oestran   V. Pregnan
(19 C-Steroid)   (19 C-Steroid)   (18 C-Steroid)   (21 C-Steroid)

Fällt eine anguläre Methylgruppe weg, dann erhält die Verbindung das Präfix Nor (no radical), wobei die Lage mit der entsprechenden Nummer gekennzeichnet wird, z.B. 19-Nor-Testosteron. Neben den wissenschaftlichen Bezeichnungen sind für die meisten Steroide Trivialnamen im Gebrauch, die wegen der raschen Zunahme neuer synthetischer Verbindungen langsam ausgemerzt werden sollen.

VI. 3β-Hydroxy-   VII. 3α-Hydroxy-
5-Androsten-17-on   Androstan-17-on
Dehydroepiandrosteron   Androsteron

Oft gebrauchte Bezeichnungen sind noch: Desoxy = Fehlen einer sonst üblichen Hydroxylgruppe, Desoxo = Fehlen einer sonst üblichen Ketogruppe, Anhydro = Wegnahme von H_2O, Dihydro, Tetrahydro usw. = Absättigung einer oder mehrerer Doppelbindungen, Dehydro = Einführung einer Doppelbindung durch Wegnahme von zwei H-Atomen.

Isomere sind Verbindungen, bei denen die an der Verknüpfungsstelle der einzelnen Ringe stehenden H-Atome ober- oder unterhalb der Molekülebene liegen, z.B. Androsteron und Ätiocholanolon (5α bzw. 5β).

Als Epimere werden Verbindungen bezeichnet, die sich nur in der sterischen Struktur unterscheiden. Von Oestriol kennt man z.B. die Epimere 16-Epioestrol, 17-Epioestrol, 16,17-Epioestrol, wobei das Präfix Epi bedeutet, daß die Orientierung der OH-Gruppen am 16 C bzw. 17 C von der des Oestriols abweichen.

III. Darstellung und Biosynthese der Androgene

Der Göttinger Physiologe Berthold beobachtete, daß die Folgen der Kastration von Hähnen ausbleiben, wenn man einen Hoden an einer anderen Körperstelle wieder einpflanzt und vermutete schon 1849, daß dem Hoden neben seiner exkretorischen auch eine innersekretorische Leistung zukommt. Erst viel später wurde die innersekretorische Funktion dieses Organs durch zahlreiche experimentelle Untersuchungen bestätigt. Nach Entfernung des Organs atrophieren die primären und sekundären Genitalorgane bei geschlechtsreifen Tieren und Menschen, während die Ausbildung beim Infantilen unterbleibt. Reimplantation oder Verabfolgung von Gesamtextrakten heben die Ausfallserscheinungen wieder auf. Der erste eindeutige Beweis für die stoffliche Natur dieser Wirkungen wurde 1927 von dem Arbeitskreis um MOORE und KOCH erbracht.

Nachdem DOISY in den USA und BUTENANDT in Deutschland 1929 reines Follikelhormon aus Schwangerenharn gewonnen hatten, isolierten BUTENANDT und TSCHERNING 1931 aus 25000 Liter Männerharn 15 mg Androsteron. Ihre hypothetische Formel besagte, daß es sich um ein Steroidgerüst mit einer Keto- und einer Hydroxylgruppe handeln müsse (3α-Hydroxy-androstan-17-on) (VII). Androsteron (VII) war damit das erste isolierte männliche Androgen. RUZICKA u. Mitarb. haben es 1934 aus Cholesterin synthetisiert. 1935 gelang LAQUEUR die Isolierung des eigentlichen männlichen Sexualhormons Testosteron aus Hoden von Stieren.

In der Folge wurden noch weitere Androgene aus Männerurin gewonnen, so von BUTENANDT 1934 Dehydroepiandrosteron, später Androstandion, Androstendion, Androstanolon, 5-Androstendiol, 11β-Hydroxyandrostendion und die Isomeren des Androsterons, die entsprechenden Ätiocholanolone.

Biologisch gesehen sind *Androgene* Verbindungen, die im Versuch am Säuger die spezifischen Gewebsstrukturen der primären und sekundären Geschlechtsorgane aufrechterhalten und nach der Kastration wiederherstellen. Chemisch gesprochen sind Androgene Steroide, die sich von der Grundform Androstan (5α) (II) ableiten. Sie bilden die einfachste Gruppe der Steroidhormone. Im Gegensatz zu den Nebennierenrindensteroiden, den C_{21}-Steroiden, sind es Steroide mit 19 C-Atomen — C_{19}-Steroide — sie haben keine Seitenkette am C_{17}, sondern nur Sauerstofffunktionen am C_3 und C_{17} und eine Doppelbindung im Ring A zwischen C_4 und C_5. Viele dieser Verbindungen sind im biologischen Versuch nur schwach wirksam. Jedes Androgen ist also doppelt zu definieren: als chemische Verbindung und als spezifisch biologischer Stoff. Die Androgene sind so einfach gebaut, daß sie sowohl als Abbauprodukte komplizierter gebauter Steroide, besonders der Nebennierenrindenhormone und deren Vorstufen dienen, aber auch Durchgangsstadien in der Biosynthese anderer Hormone sein können. Dies erschwert, wie man später sieht, die Deutung der Ergebnisse von Hormonanalysen der Androgene und ihrer Abbauprodukte beträchtlich.

1. Vorkommen der Androgene

Androgene wurden gewonnen aus Hoden, Nebennieren und Ovar. Neben biologisch androgenaktiven Steroiden wurden aus allen Drüsen auch inaktive Substanzen isoliert. Das natürliche Androgen *Testosteron*, 17β-Hydroxy-4-androsten-3-on (VIII) ist nachgewiesen im Hoden, Ovar und Nebennieren. Die Tagesproduktion ist nicht sicher bekannt, FUKUSHIMA u. Mitarb. (1959) schätzen sie auf 17 mg/24 Std.

Die wichtigsten anderen aus Drüsen isolierten Steroide mit Androgenstruktur sind:

4-Androsten-3,17-dion (IX), isoliert aus menschlichen und tierischen Hoden, menschlichen und tierischen Nebennieren und aus Ovar, biologisch ein schwaches Androgen. Tagesproduktion nicht bekannt.

Dehydroepiandrosteron, 5-Androsten-3β, 17β-diol (DEA) (VI), nachgewiesen in großen Mengen in Nebennieren, in kleinsten auch im Hoden und Ovar, biologisch sehr schwaches Androgen. Tagesproduktion nicht sicher bekannt, LIE-BERMANN (1952) schätzt sie auf 25 mg.

11β-Hydroxy-4-androsten-3-17-dion (X), isoliert aus menschlichem und tierischem Nebennierengewebe, Endprodukt der Androgensynthese in der Nebenniere, biologisch nur ein schwaches Androgen. Tagesproduktion nicht bekannt.

VIII. 17β-Hydroxy-4-Androsten-3-on Testosteron

IX. 4-Androsten-3, 17-dion

X. 11β-Hydroxy-4-Androsten-3,17-dion

XI. 4-Pregnen-3, 11, 17 trion-Adrenosteron

4-Androsten-3,11,17-trion (Adrenosteron) (XI), in geringer Menge isoliert aus Nebennieren, starke androgene Wirkung.

16-Androsten-3α-ol und sein 3-Epimer, nur im Hodengewebe gefunden, biologisch nicht untersucht.

In den letzten Jahren konnten aus Hoden und Ovar zusätzlich eine Reihe von C_{21}-Steroiden — 2-Kohlenstoffkette an C_{17} — isoliert werden, die in der

XII. 3β-Hydroxy-5-Pregnen-20-on Pregnenolon

XIII. 4-Pregnen-3,20-dion Progesteron

XIV. 17α-Hydroxy-Progesteron

Nebenniere schon lange bekannt sind und dort als Zwischenprodukte in der Synthese der Cortisole fungieren. Es sind:

3β-Hydroxy-5-pregnen-20-on (Pregnenolon) (XII), biologisch ohne androgene Eigenschaften.

4-Pregnen-3-20-dion (Progesteron) (XIII), das natürliche Hormon des Corpus luteum.

17-Hydroxy-4-androsten-3-20-dion (17α-Hydroxyprogesteron) (XIV), beide haben nur am menschlichen Fet androgene Wirkung.

a) Hoden

Testosteron (17β-Hydroxy-androst-4-en-3-on) das stärkste bis jetzt bekannte natürliche Androgen, ist auch das wichtigste des Hodens. Der menschliche Hoden enthält pro Gramm Gewebe nur $5 \mu g$ (BRADY 1951), der von Kälbern $0,4$—$9 \mu g$, von Stieren 1—$6 \mu g/g$ (LINDNER), das Venenblut der Spermatica des Menschen hat eine Konzentration von $0,4$—$1,6 \mu g/cm^3$ (LUCAS), im Alter Abfall auf $0,025 \mu g/cm^3$ (HOLLANDER 1941). 5000 E menschliches Choriongonadotropin erhöhen beim Hund die Menge von $0,2 \mu g/cm^3$ auf $2,2 \mu g/cm^3$ (BRINK-JOHNSEN 1957). DORFMAN konnte mit der besonders empfindlichen Methode der fermentativen Umwandlung von Testosteron in Oestradiol und Oestron, im mensch-

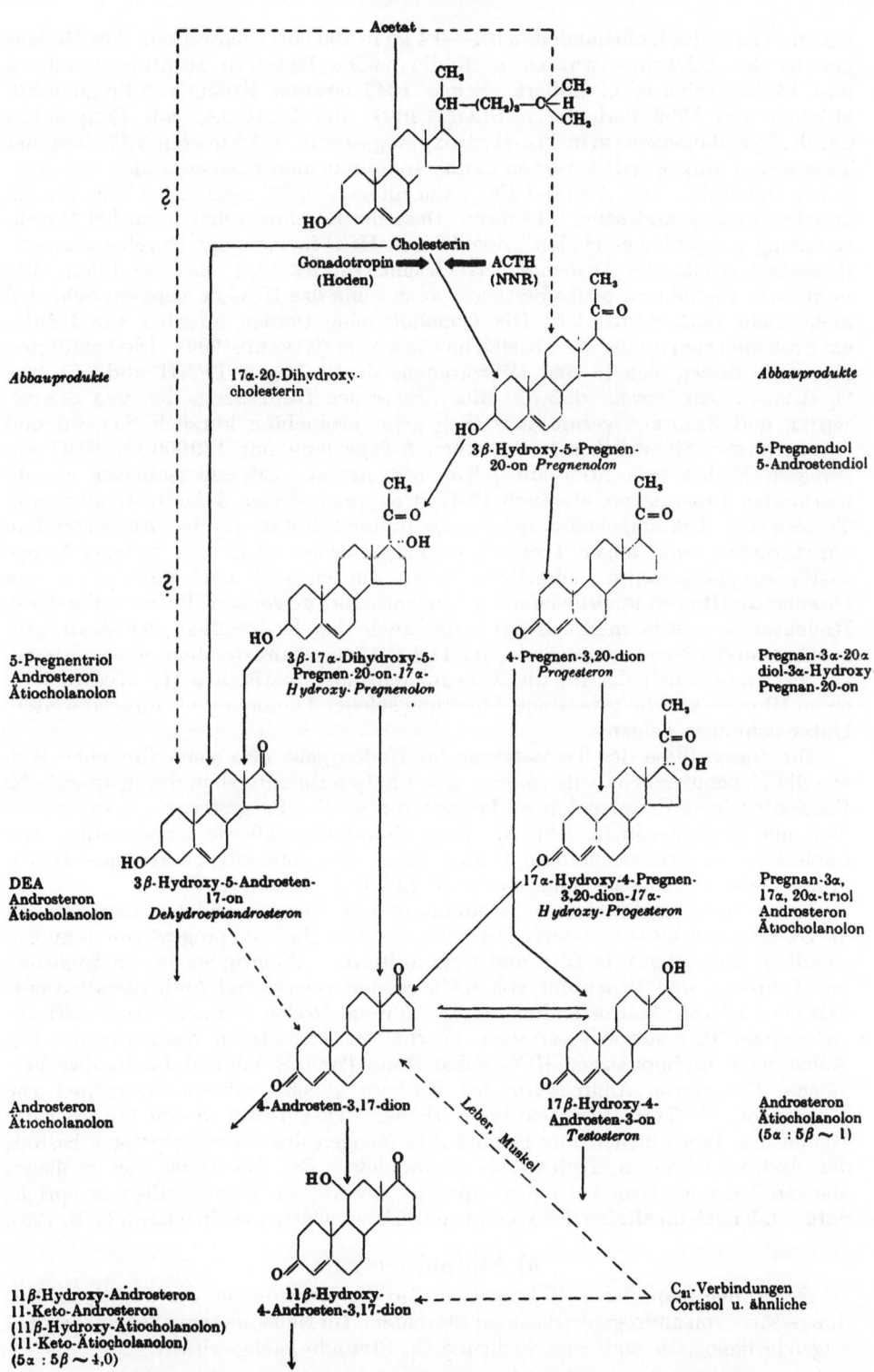

Abb. 2. Schema der Biosynthese der Androgene. —— Hauptwege; ----- Nebenwege

lichen Plasma des Unbehandelten 0,1—0,4 μg in 100 cm³ nachweisen. Aus Hodengewebe des Schweines wurden noch die beiden Isomeren 16-Androsten-3α-ol
und 16-Androsten-3β-ol isoliert. Schon 1943 gewann Ruzicka 5-Pregnen-3β-
ol-20-on und 1956 berichteten Slaunwhite und Samuels, daß Progesteron
durch Hodenhomogenate in 17α-Hydroxyprogesteron, 4-Androsten-3,17-dion und
Testosteron umgewandelt werden kann. Inkubiert man Hodenschnitte von Menschen und Ratten mit Acetat-1-C¹⁴, dann bildet sich C¹⁴-markiertes Testosteron.
daneben auch 4-Androsten-3,17-dion. Dasselbe Ergebnis erhält man bei Durchströmung menschlicher Hoden. Zugabe von HCG in vitro zur Durchströmungs-
flüssigkeit erhöht die Ausbeute beträchtlich (Brady 1951, Savard 1952). Die
vermehrte Produktion bleibt bestehen, auch wenn das HCG im venösen Schenkel
nicht mehr nachweisbar ist. Die Gonadotropine werden offenbar wie Insulin
als Proteohormon an der Zelloberfläche adsorbiert (Savard 1960). Die beteiligten
Fermente finden sich in den Mikrosomen, sie benötigen TPNH und teilweise
O₂ (Lynn). Den Beweis, daß die Biosynthese des Testosterons den von Slaunwhite und Samuels vermuteten Weg geht, erbrachten kürzlich Savard und
Goldzieher. Sie durchströmten einen 6 Tage lang mit 130000 IE HCG an-
geregten Hoden vom Stier am 7. Tag mit Acetat-1-C¹⁴ und isolierten sowohl
markiertes Progesteron als auch 17-Hydroxyprogesteron, 4-Androstendion und
Testosteron. Die eingebaute spezifische Radioaktivität war bei Androstendion
am stärksten, dann folgen Testosteron, Progesteron und in sehr geringer Menge
17-Hydroxyprogesteron. Dieselben Stufen wurden auch nach Inkubation von
Gewebsschnitten eines virilisierenden Hodentumors gewonnen. Bei einem anderen
Hodentumor wurde merkwürdigerweise auch das Endprodukt der Androgensynthese in der Nebennierenrinde, das 11β-Hydroxyandrostendion, nachgewiesen.
Ob die Anwesenheit der für die Nebennierenrinde spezifischen 11β-Hydroxylase
einen Hinweis auf die genetische Ableitung solcher Tumoren gibt, müssen weitere
Untersuchungen zeigen.

Die Biosynthese des Testosterons im Hoden geht also einen ähnlichen Weg
wie die Nebennierenrindenhormone. Aus Cholesterin entstehen durch spezifische
Fermentsysteme Pregnenolon = Progesteron = 17α-Progesteron = Androstendion und Testosteron (s. Abb. 2). Man nimmt an, daß die Umwandlung von
Cholesterin in Pregnenolon im Hoden durch das gonadotrope Hormon ICSH,
in der Nebennierenrinde dagegen durch ACTH gesteuert wird.

Unter einer hochdosierten Behandlung mit Choriogonadotropinen können
die Zwischenprodukte und deren Derivate, also 17α-Hydroxyprogesteron, 4-Andro-
stendion, Androsteron in Blut und Urin auftreten. Wichtig ist die Beobachtung
von Lindner, daß Venenblut von Kälberhoden vorwiegend Androstendion enthält (Testosteron:Androstendion = 0,7), während Hoden von erwachsenen Stieren
vorwiegend Testosteron sezernieren (Verhältnis Testosteron:Androsteron = 15).
Selbst nach dreimonatiger HCG-Behandlung (2000 E täglich) bleibt das Verhältnis Testosteron:Androsteron bei Kälbern gleich, während ausgewachsene
Tiere sofort die Testosteronsekretion erhöhen. Dies deutet darauf hin, daß der
Hoden des Jugendlichen nur beschränkte Mengen des Fermentsystems besitzt,
die Androstendion in Testosteron umwandeln. Der Nachweis von größeren
Mengen DEA im Urin bei einem operativ bestätigten Leydigzelltumor spricht
dafür, daß auch im Hoden der Weg über DEA beschritten werden kann (s. S. 773).

b) Nebennierenrinde

Neben den männlichen Keimdrüsen sind die Nebennieren die wichtigste Bildungsstätte von androgenwirksamen Steroiden. Im Nebennierenvenen*blut* wurden
folgende biologisch androgen wirkende C₁₉-Steroide nachgewiesen:

Dehydroepiandrosteron (DEA), (3β-Hydroxy-androst-5-en-17-on), *β-Androst-4-en-3,17-dion* und das Endprodukt der Synthese *11β-Hydroxy-androst-4-en-3,17-dion*. Aus *Gewebe* konnten noch Androsteron (4-Androsten-3,11,17-trion), Androstan-3β-11β-diol-17-on und kleine Mengen von Testosteron (ANLIKER) gewonnen werden. Durchströmt man Nebennieren von Rindern mit radioaktivem Acetat, dann erscheinen im Nebennierenvenenblut markiertes 4-Androsten-3,17-dion und 11β-Hydroxy-4-androsten-dion (DORFMAN). Werden embryonale Nebennieren des Menschen mit *Progesteron-4-C14* inkubiert, dann entstehen ebenfalls 17-Hydroxy-progesteron und 4-Androstendion (SOLOMON 1961). Wird normales Nebennierengewebe des Menschen mit markiertem *Acetat* inkubiert, dann kann in der umgebenden Flüssigkeit Dehydroepiandrosteron, 4-Androstendion und 11β-Hydroxy-androstendion festgestellt werden (DORFMAN 1957). Testosteron selbst ist bis jetzt bei Inkubation und Durchströmungsversuchen normaler Nebennieren nicht nachgewiesen, wohl aber ist es aus virilisierenden Geschwülsten der Frau isoliert. Das physiologische Endprodukt der Androgene der Nebennierenrinde ist das 11β-Hydroxy-4-androsten-3,17-dion, von dem nur kleine Mengen ins Blut abgegeben werden. Von den Vorstufen erscheint DHA in größerer, 4-Androstendion in kleinerer Menge im Blut, alle sind nur schwache Androgene. So besitzt Androstendion beim Menschen nur etwa 3—6% der Stärke des Testosterons. Die Kastrationsfolgen werden durch die Nebennierenrinde nicht ausgeglichen, alle Androgene der Nebennierenrinde werden als 17-Ketosteroide ausgeschieden und stellen die Hauptmasse derselben dar.

Die Biosynthese der Androgene der Nebenniere ist nicht voll geklärt. Der früheren Folge (1) über Progesteron mit den Stufen Acetat—Mevalonsäure—Cholesterin—Pregnenolon—Progesteron—17α-Hydroxyprogesteron, 11-Dehydro-isoandrosteron bzw. direkt Androstendion und 11β-Hydroxyandrostendion wurde ein zweiter Weg über 17α-Pregnenolon, Dehydroepiandrosteron, 4-Androstendion und 11β-Hydroxyandrostendion zur Seite gestellt (2) (HECHTER, PINCUS, GALLAGHER, DORFMAN, SAMUELS u. a.) und neuerdings von DORFMAN durch den direkten Weg von Cholesterin über 20α-Hydroxycholesterin, 20α, 17α-dihydroxycholesterin, Dehydroisoandrosteron zu Androstendion ergänzt (3). Dieser dritte Weg soll der in der Nebennierenrinde meist beschrittene sein, während (1) und (2) wenig begangen werden (s. Abb. 2). Von hier ist es nur ein kleiner Schritt zum Testosteron, das für die Nebennierenrinde unphysiologisch ist. Auch der direkte Weg vom Acetat zum Dehydroepiandrosteron wird diskutiert. Auch Oestrogene können bei Inkubation in vitro mit Nebennierenrindengewebe gewonnen werden. Aus 4-Androstendion entsteht über 19-Hydroxy-4-androsten-dion, 18-Hydroxy-4-androstendion und Oestron.

Es ist wahrscheinlich, daß das Cholesterin für alle Steroidhormone die wesentlichste und wichtigste Grundsubstanz darstellt. WERBIN und LE ROY (1954, 1955) verabreichten gesunden Menschen markiertes Cholesterin (C^{14} und H^{3}) und isolierten aus dem Urin Tetrahydrocortison, Tetrahydrocortisol, 11-Ketoätiocholanolon, Androsteron und Ätiocholanolon. Die Metaboliten im Urin hatten das errechnete Verhältnis von radioaktivem C und radioaktivem H, so daß die direkte Ableitung der Hormone aus Cholesterin ohne vorherigen Abbau zu kleineren Bruchstücken wahrscheinlich ist. Bei der Durchströmung von Kalbsnebennieren mit markiertem Acetat enthält das isolierte Cortisol und 11-Desoxycortisol das radioaktive Kohlenstoffatom am C_{20}, nicht am C_{21}. Auch daraus ist der Schluß berechtigt, daß diese Steroide über Cholesterin entstehen. Die Synthese aus Acetat unter Umgehung von Cholesterin wird von allen Biochemikern für möglich gehalten.

c) Ovarium

Neben ihrer oestrogenen Wirkung haben Gesamtextrakte aus Ovarien auch geringe androgene Eigenschaften. Gibt man Vögeln, besonders Hühnern, Choriongonadotropin, dann fängt der Kamm an zu wachsen. Erinnert sei an die Tierversuche von HILL, der Ovarien auf die Ohren von kastrierten männlichen Mäusen transplantierte und danach ein Wachstum von Samenblasen und Prostata feststellte, ein Experiment, das vielfach wiederholt wurde und das auch bei Ratten gelingt. Es scheint, daß hier allein die Erniedrigung der Gewebstemperatur die Hormonsynthese zugunsten der Androgene verschiebt.

Bei der Frau ist der Hirsutismus und der Virilismus als Ausdruck einer vermehrten Androgenproduktion eine verhältnismäßig häufige Erscheinung. Selten ist die Ursache in einer Hyperplasie oder in einem Tumor der Nebennierenrinde zu suchen, viel häufiger geht die Androgenproduktion vom Ovar aus, wobei sich neben gut- und bösartigen Tumoren besonders die polycystische Hyperplasie (Stein-Leventhal-Syndrom) als Ursache findet.

Der Nachweis von Testosteron in Ovarialextrakten von gesunden Tieren und Menschen ist bis jetzt noch nicht gelungen. Dagegen konnten ZANDER u. Mitarb. aus Follikeln und Corpora lutea des Menschen nicht nur Progesteron und 17α-Hydroxyprogesteron, sondern auch das Androgen 4-Androsten-3,17-dion, das im Hoden als Vorstufe des Testosterons dient, in einer Konzentration von $0,6\,\mu g/g$ isolieren (SAVARD 1961). Vorher schon hatten SOLOMON u. Mitarb. nach Inkubation von Rinderovarien mit Progesteron-4-C^{14}, 17α-Hydroxyprogesteron und 4-Androstendion nachgewiesen. Bei Inkubation von Gewebsschnitten menschlicher Ovarien mit Progesteron konnten dieselben Produkte festgestellt werden. Bei den zahlreichen in vitro-Untersuchungen mit normalen Ovarien wurde Testosteron nie gefunden. Nur KASE, FORCHIELLI und DORFMAN gelang vor kurzem bei Inkubation normaler menschlicher Ovarien mit 17α-Hydroxyprogesteron-4-C^{14} und Progesteron-7-H^3 die Isolierung von Androstendion und kleinen Mengen Testosteron. Die Konversion zu Androstendion betrug 23%, zu Testosteron 1,7—2,3%. Diese in vitro-Versuche können mit der Funktion des Ovars in situ nicht ohne weiteres verglichen werden, sie zeigen aber, daß nicht nur Ovarialtumoren, sondern auch normales Eierstockgewebe alle zur Testosteronbildung nötigen Fermente besitzen. Das natürliche Androgen des Ovars ist das biologisch schwach wirksame Androstendion. Wie oben erwähnt, wird es als 17-Ketosteroid ausgeschieden. Die Höhe der 17-Ketosteroidausscheidung ändert sich bei der Frau durch die Kastration nicht. Nach Verabreichung von hohen Dosen Choriongonadotropin an Frauen steigen die 17-Ketosteroide im Plasma nicht an, während der Mann mit einer Erhöhung von Androsteron reagiert. Zwischen dem Plasma des Großkreislaufs und dem direkt aus der V. ovarica entnommenen Blut besteht aber ein Unterschied von $130 \pm 57,8\,\mu g/$ 17-Ketosteroid zugunsten des Ovarblutes. In vitro kann der Beweis für die Testosteronproduktion auch bei virilisierenden Ovarialtumoren erbracht werden. ZANDER u. Mitarb. (1958), SAVARD u. Mitarb. (1961) inkubierten Gewebsschnitte eines Arrhenoblastoms mit Progesteron-4-C^{14} und isolierten in der Inkubationsflüssigkeit neben 17α-Hydroxyprogesteron und Androstendion auch Testosteron. Sowohl beim Stein-Leventhal-Syndrom als auch bei den meisten Fällen von virilisierenden Ovarialtumoren ist die 17-Ketosteroidausscheidung nicht oder nur wenig erhöht. Dies läßt darauf schließen, daß in diesen Fällen Testosteron und nicht das natürliche Androgen des Ovars das Androstendion produziert wird. Die Bildung von 3—5 mg Testosteron ist an der 17-Ketosteroidausscheidung nicht faßbar, da nur etwa 40% in Form der 17-Ketosteroide den Körper ver-

lassen, eine Menge, die in der physiologischen Schwankungsbreite des Einzel-
menschen untergeht. Wäre das schwache Androgen Androstendion die Ursache
des Virilismus, dann müßte es in großen Mengen produziert werden und würde
dann an der starken Erhöhung der 17-Ketosteroide faßbar (DORFMAN).

Weitere in vitro-Untersuchungen haben dann ergeben, daß das physiologische
Androgen des Ovars, das 4-Androsten-3,17-dion ein Zwischenprodukt der Oestro-
gensynthese darstellt.

d) Abbauprodukte der Corticoide

Eine weitere Möglichkeit der Bildung von biologisch androgen wirksamen Steroiden ist durch den Abbau im peripheren Gewebe eines Teiles der von den Nebennieren unter normalen Verhältnissen ins Blut abgegebener 11-Desoxyverbin-
dungen zu Androsteron und Androstan-3,17-dion gegeben. Als Ausgangsprodukte
sind besonders 17α-Hydroxyprogesteron, das im Plasma der Nebennierenrinden-
zellen in großer Menge vorhanden ist, und 17α-, 21α-Dihydroxyprogesteron
(11-Desoxycortisol) zu erwähnen. Wird 11-Desoxycortisol in vitro mit Leber-
gewebe inkubiert, dann lassen sich in der Inkubationsflüssigkeit 4-Androstendion,
Androsteron und Androstan-3,17-dion nachweisen. Unter physiologischen Bedingungen werden nur geringe Mengen dieser C_{21}-Verbindungen ins Blut abgegeben, bei Störungen der Steroidsynthese, wie z. B. bei Blockierung der 11β-
Hydroxylase, erscheinen sie aber in beträchtlicher Menge im Nebennierenvenenblut.

e) Der sog. X-Stoff

LAQUEUR hat 1935 aus Hodengewebe Fraktionen erhalten, die für sich allein
unwirksam sind, die aber die Wirkung des Testosterons, Dehydroisoandrosterons
und einiger anderer verwandter Steroide auf die Vesiculardrüsen steigern. Am
Kapaunenkamm wirken diese Stoffe nicht synergistisch. LAQUEUR vermutete,
daß es sich hierbei um höhere organische Säuren handelt, wie sie MIESCHER
aus Hoden isoliert hat. Verabreicht man Propionsäure, Palmitinsäure allein,
so sind sie völlig unwirksam, wird Testosteron zugefügt, so steigert sich dessen
Wirkung um das 2—3fache. Der X-Stoff soll 100mal stärker wirken als alle
bekannten Säuren, Näheres ist nicht bekannt.

IV. Biosynthese der Oestrogene

Die Vermutung, daß die Oestrogene aus Androgenen entstehen, wurde zum
erstenmal von ZONDEK (1929) geäußert. BUTENANDT und KUDZUS wiesen 1935
nach, daß 4-Androsten-3,17-dion und Testosteron eine schwache oestrogene
Wirkung zukommt, eine Beobachtung, die inzwischen wiederholt bestätigt wurde,
sie nahmen 4-Androstendion als die natürliche Vorstufe der Oestrogene an.
1955 gelang MEYER in vitro die Umwandlung von 4-Androsten-19-ol-3,17-dion
in Oestron nach Zusatz von Enzymen aus der Placenta und der Follikelflüssigkeit
des Ovars.

BAGGETT u. Mitarb. (1956) inkubierten menschliches Ovarialgewebe mit Testo-
steron-3-C^{14}. Dabei blieben 70% der Radioaktivität in Form des Testosterons
erhalten, der größte Teil der verbleibenden fand sich als 4-Androsten-3,17-dion,
1,2% als Oestradiol. WOTIZ (1956) konnte nach Inkubation von Ovarialgewebe einer Frau in der Menopause mit Testosteron Oestradiol, Oestron
und Oestriol feststellen, während das Ovar direkt nach der Menstruation Testosteron nicht umwandeln kann.

BAGGETT inkubierte C^{14}- Testosteron mit menschlicher Placenta, Hengsthoden und mit Gewebe eines Nebennierencarcinoms mit femininen Zügen des Trägers und

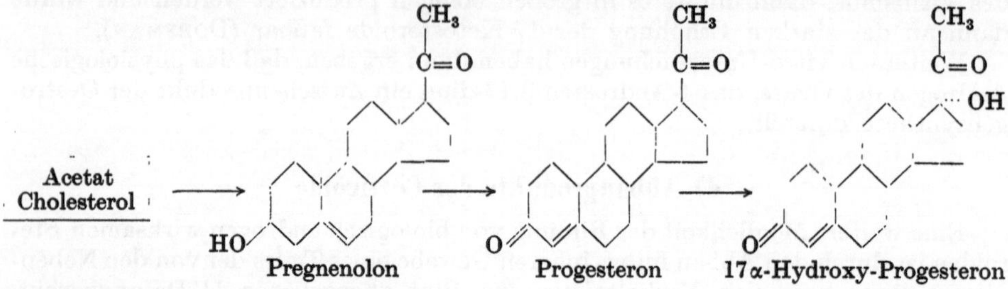

isolierte daraus C^{14}-oestrogene Stero-ide. Die Ausbeute aus Nebennieren- und Hodengewebe war gering, aus Placentagewebe dagegen groß. Die Placenta des Hundes kann 4-Andro-stendion-3,17 und 19-Hydroxy-4-androstendion in Oestron umwan-deln. A. S. MEYER hat schon 1955 vermutet, daß 19-hydroxylierte Ver-bindungen ein Zwischenprodukt zwi-schen den neutralen C^{19}-Steroiden und den aromatisierten C^{18}-Steroiden darstellen. Die Aromatisierung von Testosteron erfolgt z.B. mit Mito-chondrien aus Placentagewebe in vitro bei Anwesenheit von TPNH (RYAN 1959). Aus 4-Androstendion-(3,17) entsteht zuerst 19-Hydroxy-4-androstendion, dann 18-Hydroxy-androstendion und Oestron (Abb. 3). Das Ausmaß dieser Umwandlung ist in den einzelnen Geweben sehr ver-schieden. In der Placenta erfolgt sie rasch und vollständig, so daß Inter-mediärprodukte nicht faßbar sind. Im Ovar ebenfalls, aber nicht ganz so rasch und vollständig, während von Hodengewebe und Nebennieren-tumor nur kleine Mengen zu Oestro-genen konvertiert werden. Die Hauptaufgabe dieser Organe liegt in der Bildung der C^{19}- und C^{21}-Steroide (BAGGETT 1959). Kürzlich fand RYAN einen zweiten Mechanismus, 16α-Hy-droxy-5-androsten-3β,17β-diol wur-de durch Placentamikrosomen über

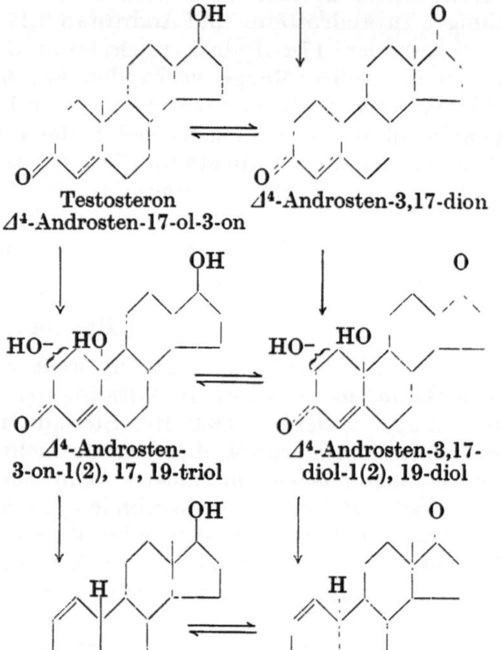

Abb. 3. Biosynthese der Oestrogene über Androgene (DORFMAN)

16α-Hydroxy-testosteron und 16α-Hydroxy-oestron zu Oestriol umgewandelt. Die Aromatisierung von Androstendion bzw. Testosteron kann dennoch sowohl über eine Hydroxylierung am C_{19}, als auch am C_{16} erfolgen.

V. Gemeinsame Biosynthese der Steroidhormone

SOLOMON (1956) und SAVARD vermuteten als erste, daß die Steroidsynthese in allen steroidproduzierenden Organen — Nebennieren, Hoden, Ovar — denselben Weg geht, aber je nach der Menge und Art der vorhandenen Enzyme zu verschiedenen Endprodukten führt. Während die ersten Stufen in den einzelnen

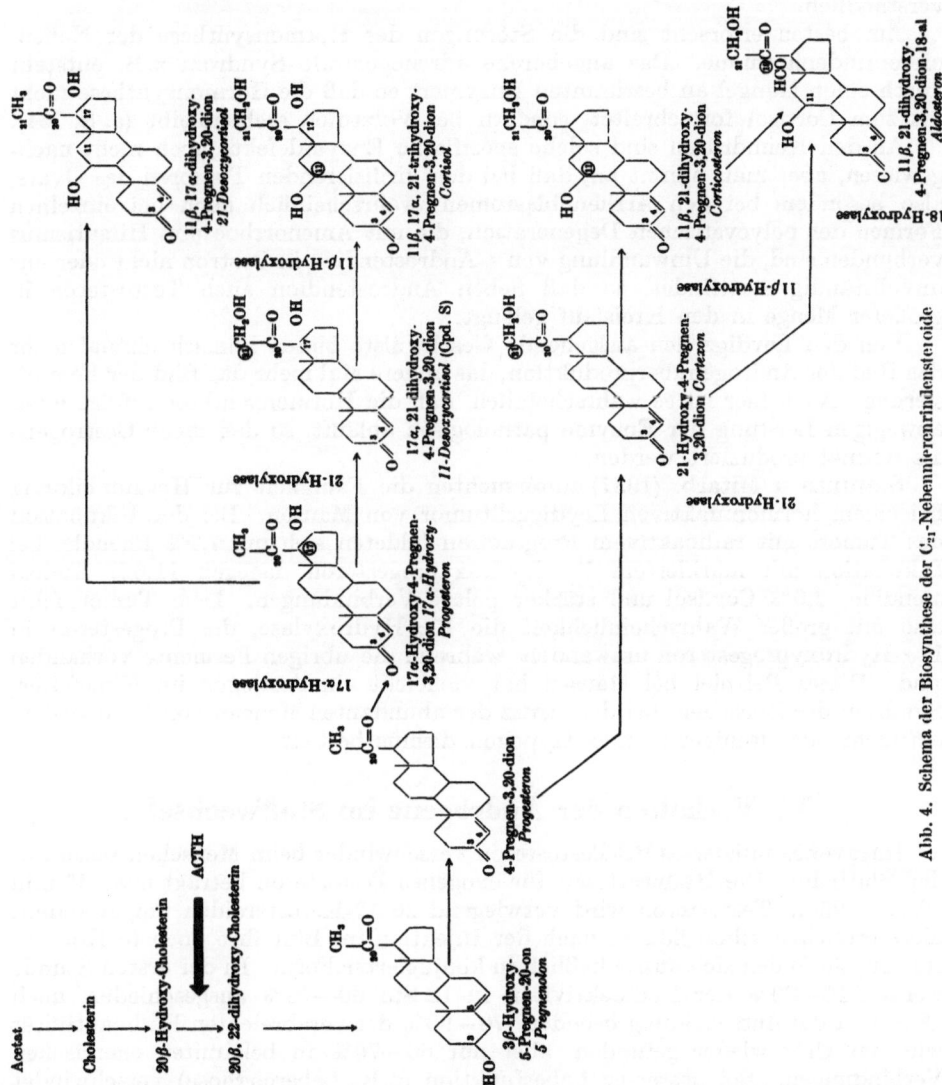

Abb. 4. Schema der Biosynthese der C_{21}-Nebennierenrindensteroide

Organen noch strittig sind (Acetat—Cholesterin—Pregnenolon—Progesteron) oder vom Acetat direkt unter Umgehung von Cholesterin und Pregnenolon, ist für die Androgene der Nebennierenrinde und des Hodens und für die Oestrogene des Ovars das 4-Androstendion als Zwischenglied sichergestellt. Die verschiedenen Wege der Biosynthese sind aus Abb. 2—4 zu ersehen. Die gleichen potentiellen Möglichkeiten der drei innersekretorischen Organe sind ein biologischer Beweis für die enge genetische Verwandtschaft der drei Gewebsarten und erklären die unter pathologischen Bedingungen mögliche gleichartige Dysharmonie der Hormonproduktion. Hyperplasie oder echte Tumoren der drei Organe können einmal mehr Androgene, das andere Mal mehr Oestrogene produzieren, je nach der Aktivierung oder Blockierung der Fermentsysteme. Nur auf diesem Wege ist das bunte und immer wechselnde klinische Bild der Erkrankung dieser Drüsen verständlich.

Am besten erforscht sind die Störungen der Hormonsynthese der Nebennierenrindenhormone. Das angeborene adrenogenitale Syndrom z.B. entsteht durch einen Mangel an bestimmten Enzymen, so daß die Hormonsynthese nicht bis zum Cortisol fortschreitet, sondern bei Vorstufen stehenbleibt (s. S. 764).

An den Keimdrüsen sind solche spezifische Enzymdefekte noch nicht nachgewiesen, aber man nimmt an, daß bei den virilisierenden Tumoren des Ovars, also besonders bei den Arrhenoblastomen, wahrscheinlich auch bei einzelnen Formen der polycystischen Degeneration, die mit Amenorrhoe und Hirsutismus verbunden sind, die Umwandlung von 4-Androstendion in Oestron nicht oder nur unvollständig stattfindet, so daß neben Androstendion auch Testosteron in größerer Menge in den Kreislauf gelangt.

Von den Leydigzellen ausgehende Geschwülste bieten klinisch einmal mehr das Bild der Androgenüberproduktion, das andere Mal mehr das Bild der Feminisierung. Auch hier ist es wahrscheinlich, daß die Hormonsynthese infolge einer abwegigen Leistung der Enzyme pathologisch abläuft, so daß mehr Oestrogene als normal produziert werden.

SAMUELS u. Mitarb. (1957) untersuchten die Fähigkeit zur Hormonbildung bei einem hormoninaktiven Leydigzelltumor von Mäusen. Bei der Inkubation des Tumors mit radioaktivem Progesteron bildeten sich nur 7,7% Phenole, bei Inkubation mit markiertem 17α-Hydroxyprogesteron dagegen 11,6% Androstendion, 2,6% Cortisol und stärker polare Verbindungen. Dem Tumor fehlt also mit großer Wahrscheinlichkeit die 17α-Hydroxylase, die Progesteron in 17α-Hydroxyprogesteron umwandelt, während die übrigen Fermente vorhanden sind. Dieses Beispiel bei Mäusen hat vielleicht ein Analogon im Klinefelter-Syndrom des Menschen, bei dem trotz der abundanten Mengen von Leydigzellen ein mehr oder weniger starker Hypogonadismus besteht.

VI. Verhalten der Androgene im Stoffwechsel

Intravenös injiziertes ^{14}C-Testosteron verschwindet beim Menschen rasch aus der Blutbahn. Die Halbwertszeit für exogenes Testosteron beträgt etwa 17 min (WEST 1956). Testosteron wird vorwiegend zu 17-Ketosteroiden umgewandelt. diese erreichen schon 20 min nach der Injektion im Blut ihre höchste Konzentration, sie finden sich ausschließlich in konjugierter Form. In der ersten Stunde werden 15—20% der Radioaktivität, in 12 Std 60—70% ausgeschieden, nach 48 Std ist die Ausscheidung beendet. 70—90% der verabreichten Radioaktivität wird im Urin wieder gefunden, aber nur 60—70% in bekannten chemischen Verbindungen. Bei gestörter Leberfunktion (z.B. Lebercirrhose) verschwindet Testosteron ebenso rasch aus dem Blut, die Umwandlung in 17-Ketosteroide erfolgt aber etwas langsamer, ebenso die Ausscheidung.

Tierversuche an Hunden, Kaninchen und Ratten haben dieselben Ergebnisse gebracht. Mit Ausnahme von Leber und Prostata kann Testosteron-^{14}C in allen Geweben nachgewiesen werden, besonders im Körperfett, aus dem es nach einigen Stunden wieder verschwunden ist. Auch nach Entfernung von Leber und Niere verschwindet die Hauptmenge des injizierten Testosterons rasch aus dem Blut.

Tabelle 2. *Tagesproduktion, Konzentration des Nebennierenvenenblutes und des peripheren Blutes an C 19- und C 21-Steroiden, die ganz oder teilweise als 17-Keto(Oxo-)Steroide ausgeschieden werden* (P = Plasma), 1) = Bestimmung chemisch, 2) = Bestimmung mit Isotopen

Hormone	Geschätzte Tagesproduktion 1) chemisch 2) Isotopenverdünnungsmethode	Gehalt der NN-Vene in (100 ml)	Gehalt des peripheren Venenblutes (100 ml)	Ausgeschieden als 17-Keto-(Oxo-)Steroide	Spezifische Abbauprodukte
Testosteron	17 mg chemisch (FUKUSHIMA) 1) ♂ 4—11,8 mg ♀ 0,9—2,8 mg } 2)		0,1—0,4 μg 1) ♂ 0,1—0,98 μg ♀ 0,02—0,26 μg 2) (DORFMAN u. Mitarb. 1964) ♂ 0,70 μg ♀ 0,18 μg 2) (BÜRGER u. Mitarb. 1964)	Androsteron 80% Ätiocholanolon 90% ♂ 1,158% ♀ 0,773% als testosteron (2) (MIGEON)	5α-Androst-16-en 3α-ol? (DORFMAN) ♂ 1,3 mg ♀ 0,45 mg
4-Androstendion	18 mg 1) (DORFMAN)	32 μg 1)	Androsteron 1) ♂ 25,0 ± 10,7 μg (P) (MIGEON) 17,3 + 0,9 μg (P) (EIK-NES)	Androsteron Ätiocholanolon	keine bekannt
Dehydroepiandrosteron	♂ 15—50 mg ♀ 12—25 mg } 2) (REYMANN u. Mitarb.)	+	Dehydroepiandrosteron 48,2 ± 15,1 μg (P) (MIGEON) 34,9 + 0,7 μg (P) (EIK-NES)	Androsteron Ätiocholanolon	Dehydroepiandrosteron 0,5—1,68 mg (HENI u. GÖBEL) kleine Mengen 6-Androsten-3β, 16α, 17β-triol ?
11β-Hydroxy-androstendion	2 mg 1) (FUKUSHIMA u. Mitarb.) 7,4 mg 1) (DORFMAN)	84 μg 1)	nicht nachgewiesen	11β-Hydroxyandrosteron 11-Keto-Androsteron (11β-Hydroxyätiocholanolon 11-Keto-Ätiocholanolon) 5β:5α 0,2	3α,11β-dihydroxy-androsteron-17-on
17-Hydroxy-progesteron		+		kleine Mengen als Andro-steron und Ätiocholanolon	Pregnan-3α, 17α, 20α-triol 0,2—2,0 mg (BONGIOVANNI)
11-Desoxycortisol	2,6 mg 1) (DORFMAN)		Spuren	kleine Mengen als Andro-steron und Ätiocholanolon	Pregnan-3α, 17α-21-triol-20-on Pregnan-3α, 17α, 20β, 21-tetriol

Tabelle 3. *Produktion, Gehalt des NN-Venenblutes, des peripheren Plasmas und Abbauprodukte der C 21-Steroide der Nebennierenrinde (Mensch)*

Ausgangssubstanzen	Tagesproduktion (Isotopenverdünnungsmethode in mg)	Gehalt der NN-Vene (100 mg)	Gehalt des peripheren Venenblutes (Plasma) (100 mg)	Ausgeschieden als 17-Ketosteroid	Spezifische Abbauprodukte
Cortisol	$15{,}7 \pm 5{,}6$ (PRUNTY u. Mitarb. 1963) $21{,}3 \pm 1{,}5$ (VERMEULEN u. Mitarb. 1964) ♀ $16{,}1 \pm 0{,}8$ (PINCUS u. Mitarb. 1964)	320—880 μg (PINCUS, u. Mitarb.)	8—14 μg (SAMUELS, SWEAT u. a.) 0,3—1,2 μg nicht proteingebunden (MILLS)	11β-Hydroxyätiocholanolon und 11-Keto-Ätiocholanolon (8—9%) 11β-Hydroxyandrosteron 2% 11-Ketoandrosteron, Spuren	Tetrahydrocortisol 1,5—3 mg Tetrahydrocortison 2,6—5 mg Cortisol ⎫ 3 mg Cortolon ⎭ Allotetrahydrocortisol 0,1 bis 1,8 mg (FUKUSHIMA, GUIGNARD DE MEYR u. Mitarb.)
Corticosteron	3 mg (PETERSON) 3,6 mg (VERMEULEN)	170—240 μg (PINCUS u. Mitarb.)	4,3 μg (SWEAT) (1963)	ganz geringe Beträge	Pregnan-3α, 21-ol-11,20-dion Pregnan-3α, 11β,21-triol-20-on
11-Desoxycortisol (Cpd S)		77—128 μg (LUETSCHER u. Mitarb.)	3,6 μg (LUETSCHER)	Androsteron, kleiner Teil als Ätiocholanolon (fällt nicht ins Gewicht)	Pregnan-3α-17α-(20β)-20α, 21-tetrol Pregnan-3α, 17α, 21-trihydroxy-20-on
21-Desoxycortisol		kleine Mengen nachgewiesen		kleine Anteile als 11-Keto-ätiocholanolon 11-Ketoandrosteron	Pregnan-3α, 11β, 17α, 20α-(20β)-tetrol Pregnan-3α, 17β, 20α-(20β)-triol-11-on
Aldosteron	77 μg (FLOOD u. Mitarb.) 200 μg (WETTSTEIN) 120—140 μg (TAIT u. Mitarb.)	2,5—5 μg (FARRELL) (chemisch)	0,03—0,16 μg (WETTSTEIN) 0,04—0,08 μg (PETERSON, TAIT 1962)	nicht	freies Aldosteron 0,2% Δ4-3-oxokonjugate 14% Tetrahydroaldosteron 35—45% Allotetradihydroaldosteron 20—25%
Progesteron	0,6 mg (NNR) (FARRELL u. Mitarb.)	3,6 μg (SCHORR)	~5 μg normal (Frau), 4—45 μg in Schwangerschaft (ZANDER u. Mitarb.)	nicht	Pregnan-3α, 20α-diol Pregnan-3α-ol-20-on

Während bei Ratten nach oraler oder intramuskulärer Verabreichung 30 bis 35% der Radioaktivität im Harn und 65% im Kot erscheint, spielt beim Menschen der enterohepatische Kreislauf keine Rolle. Bei Menschen mit kompletter Gallenfistel wird nur 0,1—0,7% der Radioaktivität in der Galle gemessen.

Nach oraler Verabreichung erfolgt beim Menschen die Ausscheidung radioaktiver Produkte im Harn ebenso rasch wie nach intravenöser Injektion. Die orale Unwirksamkeit des Testosterons ist also nicht durch schlechte Resorption, sondern durch die rasche Inaktivierung in der Leber bedingt.

Ein großer Teil der Steroide, sowohl der konjugierten, als auch der nichtkonjugierten, wird im Blut an Plasmaeiweißkörper gebunden Die Hormone der Nebennierenrinde, Cortisol, sind wie Eisen oder Kupfer zu 87,5—97,5% an einen spezifischen Eiweißkörper, das Transcortin, fest gebunden (DAUGHADAY 1958a, MILLS 1961, SANDBERG 1959). Man glaubt, daß nur der nicht eiweißgebundene Anteil in das Gewebe eindringt, gebundenes und ungebundenes stehen in einem labilen Gleichgewicht. Der unverhältnismäßig hohe Cortisonspiegel während der Schwangerschaft und bei oestrogenbehandelten Trägern eines Prostatacarcinoms findet seine Erklärung in der beträchtlichen Erhöhung des Transcortins, die im Gefolge der endogenen Überproduktion oder nach Verabreichung von natürlichen und synthetischen Oestrogenen eintritt. Transcortin vermehrt sich unter der Oestrogengabe um das 2—3fache, entsprechend auch die Gesamtmenge des zirkulierenden Cortisols. Da die Bindung fest ist, treten keine Erscheinungen eines Hypercorticoidismus auf. Transcortin bindet die übrigen Corticoide in abnehmender Affinität, 11-Desoxycortisol, Corticosteron, Prednisolon, Desoxycorticosteron, Cortison, Progesteron, Aldosteron.

Injiziert man Mäusen 1 mg Testosteron-4-^{14}C, dann findet sich die stärkste Radioaktivität 15 min bis 4 Std nach der Injektion am Albumin und den α-Globulinen. Zugabe von 4-C^{14}-Testosteron zu Blutplasma in vitro bestätigt die Bindung an Albumin. Auch mit Hilfe der Ultrafiltration und der fraktionierten Eiweißfällung kann man die Eiweißbindung der Androgene und Oestrogene nachweisen. Androgene sind vorwiegend an die Albumine und die α_1-Globuline, die Oestrogene und Progesteron an die β-Globuline gebunden, die Bindung ist nur locker, sie ist umgekehrt proportional zur Zahl der polaren Gruppen.

VII. Abbau der Androgene

Die einzelnen Stufen des Androgenabbaus sind durch zahlreiche Inkubationsexperimente mit den verschiedensten Geweben weitgehend aufgeklärt, der größte Teil der beteiligten Fermente und deren Wirkungsbedingungen ist bekannt (KOCHAKIAN 1958). Inkubation von Testosteron mit Rattenleberstückchen führt zur Umwandlung in Δ^4-Androstendion und Epitestosteron. Umgekehrt kann auch Androstendion zu Testosteron und Epitestosteron umgewandelt werden. Auch Nierengewebe, Prostata, Ovarialcarcinom, menschliches Serum, können Testosteron zu 4-Androstendion umwandeln. Das beteiligte Enzym ist die 17β-Hydroxysteroid-Dehydrogenase, die sowohl mit DPN als auch mit TPN reagiert (s. Tabelle 2 und 3).

Infolge ihres hohen Gehaltes an aktiven Dehydrogenasen dehydrieren Leber und Niere alle Steroide mit einer 17-Hydroxylgruppe zu 17-Ketoverbindungen (KOCHAKIAN 1958), mit Ausnahme der künstlich geschaffenen, die am C_{17} zusätzlich einen Alkylrest tragen. Auch die entgegengesetzte Reaktion, die Umwandlung von Androsteron, Ätiocholanolon und Dehydroepiandrosteron zu 17β-Hydroxysteroiden ist in vitro möglich. Leber und Milz oxydieren auch die 3-Hydroxygruppe und die 3,17-Dihydroxysteroide zu den entsprechenden Diketonen.

Die Doppelbindung zwischen C_4 und C_5 wird von Leber von Ratten und Meerschweinchen und von Nierengewebe reduziert. Citrat oder Isocitrat dienen als oxydierbare Substanz und TPN als Wasserstoff- und Elektronenträger.

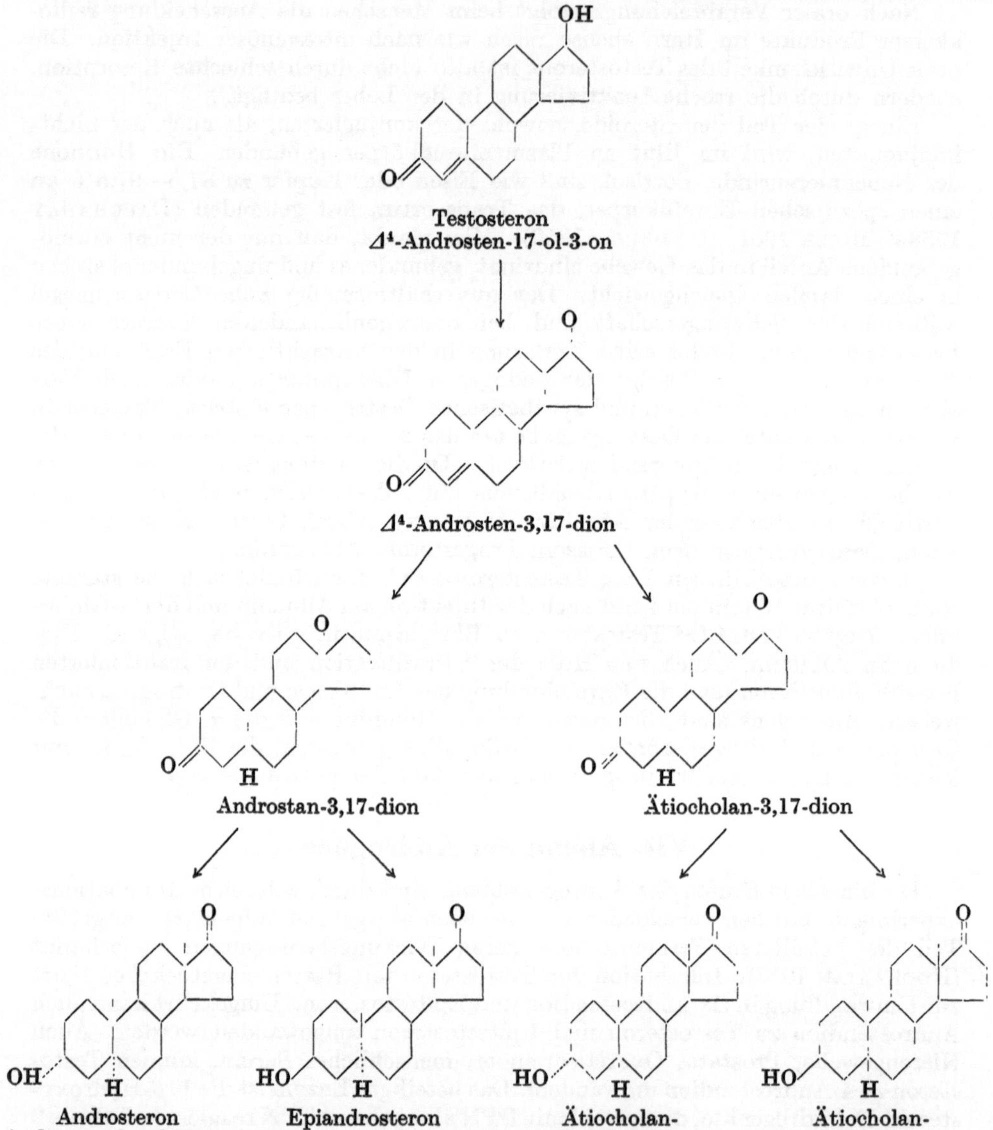

Testosteron
Δ^4-Androsten-17-ol-3-on

Δ^4-Androsten-3,17-dion

Androstan-3,17-dion

Ätiocholan-3,17-dion

Androsteron
Androstan-3α-ol-17-on

Epiandrosteron

Ätiocholan-3α-ol-17-on

Ätiocholan-3β-ol-17-on

Abb. 5. Abbau des Testosterons nach Dorfman

Bei allen in vitro-Untersuchungen ist es Kochakian nach Zusatz von Androgenen zu den einzelnen Ansätzen nicht gelungen, Oestrogene in nachweisbarer Menge im peripheren Gewebe festzustellen. Entweder besitzt dieses nicht die Fähigkeit, Androgene in Oestrogene umzuwandeln, oder die entstandenen Mengen sind so klein, daß man sie mit den gegenwärtigen Methoden nicht erfassen kann.

Die Leber bindet Testosteron und die meisten bekannten Steroide an Glucuron-säure und Schwefelsäure und macht sie dadurch wasserlöslich und harnfähig.

Die aktiven biologischen Hormone Testosteron und 4-Androstendion werden unter normalen Bedingungen nicht im Urin ausgeschieden, nur nach parenteraler Verabreichung von großen Dosen erscheinen kleine Mengen unverändert.

Ort der Zerstörung ist, wie oben ausgeführt, vorwiegend die Leber. Implantiert man Hoden an Körperstellen, von denen aus das Venenblut die Leber passiert, dann verhütet die Reimplantation die Kastrationsfolgen bei der Ratte nicht. Pflanzt man dasselbe Hodenstück danach subcutan ein, dann regenerieren sich Prostata und Samenblasen wieder.

Die Fähigkeit der Leber zur Inaktivierung von Testosteron wird durch Schädigung mit Tetrachlorkohlenstoff, Formiat, Eiweißmangel, Hunger u.ä. nicht beeinflußt. Neben der Leber ist die Niere am aktivsten, aber auch alle anderen Gewebe sind zum Abbau befähigt.

Nach den Richtlinien von DORFMAN (1958) werden C_{19}-Steroide, die eine $\varDelta_4$-Ketogruppe im Ring A besitzen und ein zusätzliches Sauerstoffatom am C_{17} tragen, bei C_4 und C_5 unter der Bildung einer etwas höheren 5β- (Ätiocholanolon)

XV. 3α-Hydroxy-Ätiocho-lan-17-on Ätiocholanolon

XVI. 11-Desoxycortisol (Cpd. S)

XVII. 3α-11β-dihydroxy-Ätiocholan-17-on-11β-Hydroxyätiocholanolon

als 5α-Fraktion (Androsteron) reduziert (Verhältnis von 5β zu 5α zwischen 1,5 und 2,0). C_{19}-Steroide, die eine $\varDelta$4-3-Ketogruppe im Ring A besitzen und zusätzlich ein Sauerstoffatom am C_{11} *und* am C_{17} tragen, werden am C_4 und C_5 unter der Bildung einer größeren Menge 5α- als 5β-Verbindungen reduziert. Die O-Gruppen an C_{11} und an C_{17} können im Stoffwechsel nicht abgebaut werden, sie bleiben als Keto- oder Hydroxylgruppen erhalten (GALLAGHER 1958). Die Primärhormone und ihre Derivate werden in der Leber sehr rasch an Säuren, besonders an Glucuronsäure, Schwefelsäure und an noch nicht bekannte gebunden, dadurch inaktiviert und harnfähig gemacht.

Die wichtigsten Umwandlungsprodukte des *Testosteron* (VIII) sind (s. Abb. 5): Androsteron (VII) (3α-Hydroxy-5α-androstan-17-on) und Ätiocholanolon (XV) (3α-Hydroxy-5β-androstan-17-on). 80—90% von markiertem Testosteron werden als Androsteron und Ätiocholanolon ausgeschieden (GALLAGHER 1958). Daneben findet man kleine Mengen von Androstan-3α-17β-dion, Ätiocholan-3α-ol-17-on, Ätiocholan-3α-17β-dion, Ätiocholan-3β-ol-17-on. Das Verhältnis von 5β:α ist = 1.

Wie Markierungsversuche ergeben haben, wird ein kleiner Anteil des Testosteron nicht als 17-Ketosteroide ausgeschieden, sondern als 16α-Hydroxytestosteron, 6β-Hydroxytestosteron, 2β-Hydroxytestosteron, 6β-Hydroxyandrostendion. Aus Androstendion entstehen kleine Mengen von 19-Hydroxyandrostendion, 6α,11β-Dihydroxyandrostendion, 6β-Hydroxyandrostendion, 6α-Hydroxyandrostendion, 11β-Hydroxyandrostendion.

Die Metaboliten des *4-Androsten-3,17-dion* entsprechen denen des Testosteron, da beide Verbindungen leicht ineinander übergehen.

Unter dem Einfluß von Desmolasen entstehen im peripheren Gewebe, hauptsächlich in der Leber, aus einem Teil der C_{21}-Steroide der Nebenniere C_{19}-Steroide. Der Mechanismus ist grundsätzlich derselbe wie bei der Biosynthese der Androgene im Hodengewebe, nur daß der Vorgang in umgekehrter Richtung abläuft. Aus 17α-Hydroxyprogesteron und 11-Desoxycortisol (XVI) (Compound S) wird 4-Androsten-3,17-dion, das seinerseits wieder zu Androsteron und Ätiocholanolon abgebaut wird (s. Tabelle 2).

Unter der Wirkung derselben Desmolasen entsteht in der Leber aus einem kleinen Anteil des *Cortisols* und *Cortisons* 11β-Hydroxyätiocholanolon (XVII), 11-Ketoätiocholanolon (XVIII) und 11β-Hydroxyandrosteron (XIX) bzw. 11-Ketoandrosteron (XX). Der größere Anteil besteht aus dem 5β-Typ, also

XVIII. 3α-Hydroxy-Ätiocholan-11, 17-dion-11-Ketoätiocholanolon

XIX. 3α, 11β-Dihydroxy-Androstan-17-on-11β-Hydroxyandrosteron

XX. 3α-Hydroxy-Ätiocholan-11, 17-dion-11-Ketoandrosteron

den Ätiocholanolonen (5β:5α=8,5—9,0) (DORFMAN 1958). Nach Verabreichung von markiertem Cortisol werden 18% der Gesamtmenge als oxygenierte 17-Ketosteroide ausgeschieden.

Demgegenüber wird die Endstufe der Androgene der Nebennierenrinde, das 11β-Hydroxyandrostendion, vorwiegend zu 5α-Verbindungen, also zu 11β-Hydroxyandrosteron und 11-Ketoandrosteron und nur zu kleinem Teil zu den entsprechenden Isomeren abgebaut. Verhältnis von 5β:5α = 0,19 (DORFMAN 1958). Nach Verabreichung von markiertem 11β-Hydroxy-4-androstendion isolierten BRADLOW und GALLAGHER 80% der injizierten Menge wieder aus dem Urin. 69% davon bestanden aus der 5α-Verbindung 11β-Hydroxyandrosteron, 14,5% aus den 11-oxydierten Ätiocholanolonen (5β:5α = 0,21) (s. Tabelle 3 und Abb. 2).

VIII. 17-Ketosteroide (17-Oxo-Steroide)

Die Hauptmasse der 17-Ketosteroide im Urin besteht aus Androsteron, Ätiocholanolon und Dehydroepiandrosteron. Obwohl diese Metaboliten schon vor über 20 Jahren isoliert wurden, sind unsere Kenntnisse über ihren Ursprung im einzelnen noch keineswegs endgültig.

Wie aus Abb. 2 hervorgeht, in der nur die wichtigsten Primärsteroide eingetragen sind, können sich Androsteron, Androgene und Ätiocholanolon aus einer ganzen Reihe von Muttersubstanzen ableiten.

Unklarheiten bestehen insbesondere noch über die Menge des produzierten Testosterons und des 4-Androstendions und über den Anteil, den diese beiden biologisch aktivsten Steroide am Gesamtpool des Androsterons und Ätiocholanolons ausmachen. Testosteron und 4-Androstendion werden wohl vorwiegend im Hoden gebildet, in kleinen Mengen aber auch in den Nebennieren.

Beim Gesunden ist der Anteil des *Testosterons* am ausgeschiedenen Androsteron und Ätiocholanolon und damit an den Gesamt-17-Ketosteroiden nicht feststellbar. Das Verhältnis der 5β:5α-Metaboliten, das für Testosteron = 1 ist, gibt keinen Hinweis, da Androsteron und Ätiocholanolon sich auch aus Vorstufen der Nebennierenhormone mit anderem Verhältnis der 5β:5α-Verbindungen ableiten. Die täglich produzierte Testosteronmenge ist daher bis heute noch nicht sicher bekannt, FUKUSHIMA und SLAUNWHITE schätzen sie auf etwa 17 mg, andere errechnen ∼ 10 mg (s. Tab. 2). Der Anteil des Testosterons an den Gesamt-17-Ketosteroiden wird mit 2—4 mg angegeben, eine Menge also, die in der täglichen physiologischen Schwankung der 17-Ketosteroidausscheidung desselben Menschen untergeht (s. Tabelle 2).

Normalerweise werden nur kleine Mengen von Androsteron und Ätiocholanolon als Metaboliten der Vorstufen der Nebennierenhormone, also von 17-Hydroxycortexon (Compound S), von 11-Desoxycorticosteron (Cortexon) und von 17α-Hydroxyprogesteron ausgeschieden. In Fällen pathologischer Hormonproduktion kann ihr Anteil dagegen hoch sein. Erfaßt wird er nur durch gleichzeitige Bestimmung der Hauptmetaboliten dieser Steroide, also von Tetrahydro S, Pregnantetrol, Pregnantriolon und Pregnantriol (s. Tabelle 2 und 3).

Die größte Unsicherheit besteht bezüglich des *Deshydroepiandrosterons* (DEA) (3β-Hydroxy-Δ₅-steroid), dessen täglich produzierte Menge ebenfalls nicht sicher bekannt ist. LIEBERMAN u. Mitarb. (1959) schätzen sie auf den hohen Wert von 25 mg. Im Plasma findet es sich in so hoher Konzentration wie kein anderes Steroid (25—60 μg auf 100 ml) MIGEON u. PLAGER), 80 μg (OERTEL und EIK-NES). Untersuchungen mit tritium-markiertem DEA ergaben, daß alle wichtigen 17-Ketosteroide: DEA selbst, Androsteron und Ätiocholanolon in radioaktiver Form im Urin erscheinen (s. Tabelle 2). DEA ist wahrscheinlich ein wichtiges Muttersteroid von Androsteron und Ätiocholanolon. DEA stammt vorwiegend aus 3β,17α-Dihydroxy-pregn-5-en-20-on, also 17α-Hydroxypregnenolon. Bei direkter Bestimmung schwanken die Werte für Dehydroepiandrosteron im Urin beim Mann zwischen 0,1 und 8,8 mg, bei der Frau zwischen 0,0 und 6,4 mg. Nur ein Teil wird als 3β-Hydroxysteroide ausgeschieden. Dazu gehören als größte Masse DEA selbst und kleine Mengen von 5-Androsten-3β, 16α, 17β-triol, 5-Androsten-3β, 17β-diol. Ein Teil des DEA macht eine ähnliche Umwandlung wie Oestron via 16α-Hydroxyoestron in Oestriol durch (FOTHERBY).

Die Ausscheidung der einzelnen Anteile der 17-Ketosteroide durch die Niere geschieht verschieden rasch, so beträgt die renale Clearance für Androsteron 20—24 ml Plasma/min, für Dehydroepiandrosteron 2,0—2,8 ml Plasma/min. Probenacid senkt die Clearance von Androsteron auf 2,5 ml Plasma/min. Androsteron wird also vorwiegend in den Tubuli sezerniert. Die verschieden große renale Clearance von Androsteron und Dehydroepiandrosteron ist mit ein Grund für die hohe Konzentration des Dehydroepiandrosterons im Plasma (BONGIOVANNI 1957).

Wenn schon unter normalen Bedingungen der Anteil der einzelnen Steroide an den Einzelfraktionen der 17-Ketosteroide nicht sicher feststeht, dann um wieviel mehr in pathologischen Fällen, wenn es gilt, einen Hirsutismus und Virilismus der Frau, eine Pubertas praecox eines Jungen, die Feminisierung eines erwachsenen Mannes, einem bestimmten innersekretorischen Organ — Nebennierenrinde, Ovar, Hoden — zuzuordnen.

Ein weiterer Unsicherheitsfaktor ist in der Funktion der Leber als zentrales Organ des Steroidabbaues gegeben. Grobe Defekte führen zum weitgehenden Unvermögen, 17-Ketosteroide zu bilden, sichtbar daran, daß bei allen schweren Allgemeinerkrankungen die Höhe der 17-Ketosteroidausscheidung stark sinkt, obwohl die Nebennierenrinde normale Hormonmengen produziert. Bei feineren Defekten oder bei Partiärstörungen der Funktion, z.B. unter Thyroxingabe, kann sich das Verhältnis von Androsteron:Ätiocholanolon verschieben oder die Bindung an Glucuronsäure leiden.

1. Chemische Bestimmung

17-Ketosteroide entstehen beim Abbau der Androgene, der Oestrogene und der Corticosteroide. Aus den Oestrogenen bilden sich saure, phenolische Steroide, die sich durch Alkali abtrennen lassen. Zurück bleiben die sog. „neutralen 17-Ketosteroide", im klinischen Sprachgebrauch einfach als 17-KS bezeichnet.

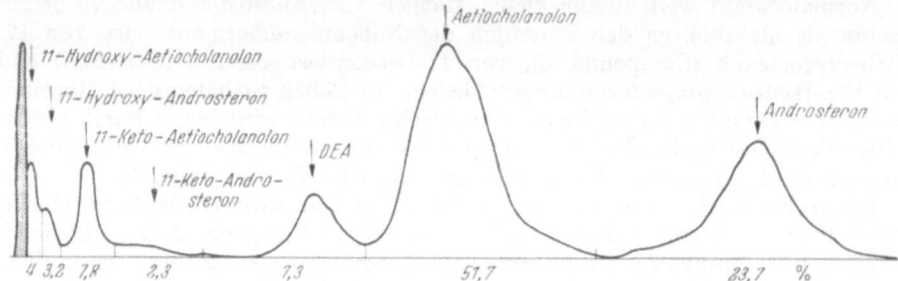

Abb. 6. 28jähriger Mann, Normalfall, 17-Kerosteroide: 7,51 mg/24 Std, Papierchromatographische Trennung der 17-Ketosteroide nach Giradbehandlung

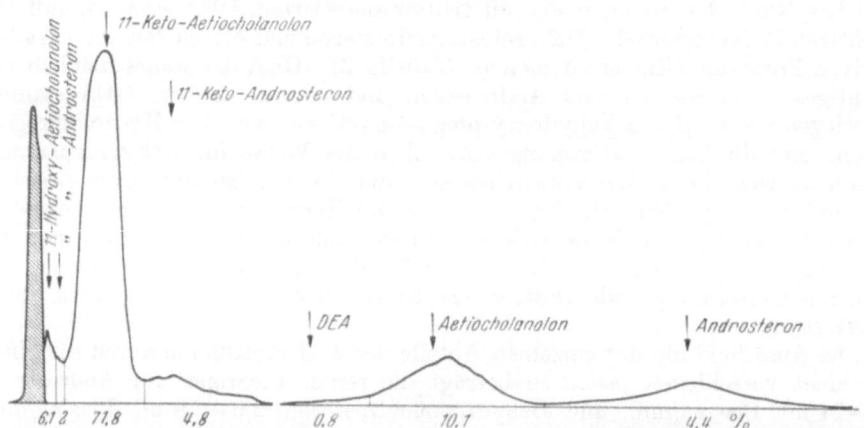

Abb. 7. Fünfjähriger gesunder Junge, 17-Ketosteroide: 0,588 mg/24 Std. Papierchromatographische Trennung; Stark erniedrigte Androgenfraktion (Androsteron, Ätiocholanolon und DEA) bei starker Vermehrung der Cortisol-metaboliten (11-Keto- und 11-Hydroxy-Ätiocholanolon). Vgl. Nr. 11 Cushing Syndrom des Erwachsenen

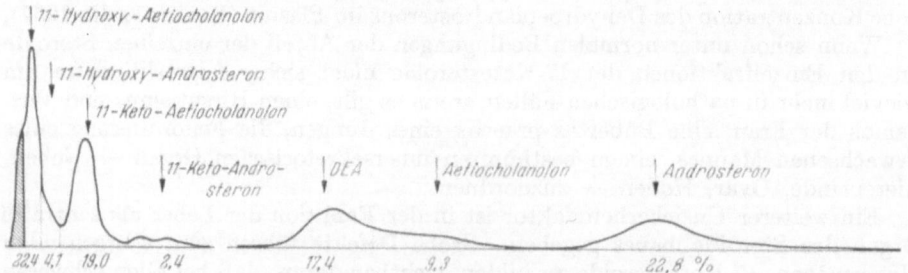

Abb. 8. Benignes NNR-Adenom (reines Cushing-Syndrom) 17-Ketosteroide 5,58 mg/24 Std. Chromatogramm; starke Vermehrung von 11-Keto- und 11-Hydroxy-Aetiocholanolon

Diese Fraktion enthält etwa 50 Verbindungen, der größte Teil liegt in wasser-
löslichen Konjugaten mit Glucuronsäure und Schwefelsäure vor. Durch die
Hydrolyse und Reinigung entstehen eine Reihe von Artefakten. Die 17-Keto-
steroide sind zu $^2/_3$ Abbauprodukte der Hormone der Nebennierenrinde und nur
zu $^1/_3$—$^1/_4$ der Hormone des Hodens. Sie werden bestimmt mit Hilfe der Zimmermannschen Reaktion, bei der eine neben einer Methylgruppe liegende Ketogruppe
(CH_2CO, Methylenketon) in alkalischer Lösung mit Dinitrobenzol unter Bildung
eines voilettroten Farbstoffes mit maximaler Absorption bei 530 mμ reagiert.
Die stärkste Reaktion geben die 17-Ketoverbindungen, 3- und 20-Ketoverbin-
dungen tragen zu einem kleinen Teil an der Farbgebung bei, ihre Farbintensität
beträgt nur $^1/_8$ derjenigen der 17-Ketosteroide. Die Gesamtneutralfraktion erfaßt
auch einen Teil der Urinchromogene. Zuverlässig sind auch die Werte der ketonischen
Neutralfraktion, die man mit Hilfe des Girard-Reagens T von den Nichtketonen
abtrennen kann. Mit Digitonin lassen sich die 3α- und β-17-Ketosteroide voneinander trennen. Steroide mit der 3β-Hydroxykonfiguration gehen mit Digitonin eine unlösliche Verbindung ein. Der größte Teil der 3β-Fraktion wird vom
Dehydroepiandrosteron und Iso-androsteron ausgemacht (10—25%). DEA kann
auch mit der Methode von DIRSCHERL-ALLEN direkt erfaßt werden (Blaufärbung
mit konzentrierter Schwefelsäure). PINCUS (1947) hat eine Reaktion angegeben
(Erhitzen mit essigsaurer $SbCl_3$-Lösung), die Androsteron und seine Isomeren
nachweist. Viele Laboratorien arbeiten mit etwas voneinander abweichenden
Vorschriften, so daß die Ergebnisse stark schwanken (Normalwerte des Mannes
aus Literatur 9,0—22,6 mg). Die allgemeine Übernahme der vom Medical Research
Council (London) (Committee on Clin. Endocrin.) 1951 empfohlenen Standard-
ausführung würde die Möglichkeit des Vergleichs der Werte der einzelnen Laboratorien zulassen.

Es ist das große Verdient von DINGEMANSE (1946), mit Hilfe der Säulen-
chromatographie die Auftrennung der 17-Ketosteroide in die einzelnen Fraktionen vorgenommen zu haben. Die Verfahren sind in der Zwischenzeit durch
Verwendung der Elutionschromatographie (LAKSHMAN und LIEBERMAN) und die
Papierchromatographie (BEAULIEU, GÖBEL u. Mitarb.) wesentlich verbessert worden. Letztere erlauben die gesonderte Bestimmung der wichtigsten Komponenten, und zwar von Androsteron, Ätiocholanolon, Dehydroepiandrosteron,
11-Ketoandrosteron, 11-Ketoätiocholanolon, 11-Hydroxyandrosteron, 11-Hydr-
oxyätiocholanol (GÖBEL u. HENI) (s. Tabelle 4 und Abb. 6—8).

a) Gehalt des Urins

Die Ausscheidung der 17-Ketosteroide ist abhängig vom Alter, vom Geschlecht,
von der Körperverfassung und von der momentanen körperlichen und psychischen
Belastung. Die beste Zusammenfassung der unübersehbaren Literatur haben
DORFMAN und SHIPLEY (1956) gegeben.

In den ersten Lebenstagen liegt die Ausscheidung mit 1,1—1,5 mg recht hoch,
sie fällt in den folgenden Tagen rasch ab. Kinder scheiden in den beiden ersten
Lebensjahren nur geringe Mengen aus (0,3—1 mg). Um das 7.—9. Lebensjahr
steigt die Ausscheidung rasch und gleichmäßig an und erreicht bei Männern
gegen das 30., bei Frauen gegen das 25. Lebensjahr den höchsten Gipfel (HAM-
BURGER 1948) (Abb. 9).

Die Normalwerte des Erwachsenen schwanken beim Mann zwischen 6 und
25 mg, bei der Frau zwischen 3 und 22 als untere und obere Grenzwerte. Infolge
der verschiedenen Hydrolyse- und Extraktionsverfahren sind die Schwankungen

Tabelle 4. *Auftrennung der Gesamt-17-Ketosteroide*

	Säulenchromato-graphie und spektrographische Identifizierung (Dobriner)	Säulenchromato-graphie und infra-rotspektrographische Identifizierung (Planten u. Birkl)	Säulenchromato-graphie mit Äthanol-Benzolgemisch (Kellie u. Wade)
Androsteron	3,5 mg	62,8—66,6%	2,93—4,08
Ätiocholanol	4,9 mg	62,8—66,6%	4,10—6,20
Dehydroepiandrosteron . .		5,8—8,5%	0,81—2,14
11β-Hydroxy-Androsteron .	1,0 mg	nicht nachgewiesen	0,16—0,58
11-Keto-Androsteron . . .		nicht nachgewiesen	0,02—0,16
11-Hydroxy-Ätiocholanolon		nicht nachgewiesen	0,09—0,56
11-Keto-Ätiocholanolon . .	0,8 mg	7,1—11,2%	0,55—1,35
Androstandion			
Acetate			
Gesamt	10,0 mg	100%	11,87—13,52

bei den einzelnen Autoren recht beträchtlich (Mason 1950). Die Girard-Trennung gibt wegen der Eliminierung unspezifischer Chromogene etwas niedrigere Werte. Der höchste Gipfel liegt während der Nacht und in den frühen Morgenstunden (Pincus 1947). Der Tagesrhythmus ist nicht endogen, sondern ist Folge der verschieden starken Belastung.

Die Schwankungen bei ein und demselben Individuum können bei ambulantem Urinsammeln recht beträchtlich sein. Chou und Wu errechnen $\pm 20\%$, Drekter etwas weniger als 30%, Miller u. Mitarb. 5,5%. Hamburger (1948) hat bei einem 44jährigen gesunden Mann die Ausscheidung 6 Jahre lang täglich geprüft, er fand Schwankungen zwischen 9 und 16,4 mg in 24 Std bei einem Mittelwert von 11,83; mit zunehmendem Alter sank die Ausscheidung nur geringfügig ab, von 12,2 auf 11,1. Die individuelle Schwankung wird geringer, je ruhiger sich die Untersuchten verhalten, bei Bettruhe sind es aber immer noch 1—4 mg.

Vor der Pubertät leiten sich die 17-Ketosteroide wahrscheinlich gänzlich aus der Nebennierenrinde ab. Auch der Anstieg während des Wachstumsalters ist vorwiegend durch das Wachstum und die Entwicklung der Nebenniere, die sich proportional zur Körpermasse vergrößert, bedingt. Der stärkere Anstieg des Mannes gegenüber der Frau um die Pubertät wird auf die zusätzliche Androgenbildung in den Leydigzellen zurückgeführt. Man muß aber bedenken, daß die Nebenniere des erwachsenen Mannes größer ist als die der Frau und mehr 17-Ketosteroide liefert (Dorfman 1956).

Der Gipfel wird um das 30. Lebensjahr erreicht. Von da ab erniedrigt sich die Ausscheidung, zwischen 50 und 60 liegt sie um 9 mg, über 80 um 2—3 mg (Hamburger 1948, McCullagh 1953, Dorfman 1956, Zondek 1934). Die Neigung der Kurve verläuft bei Mann und Frau etwa gleich, Hamburger findet bei der Frau zwischen 35 und 50 eine gewisse Abflachung (Abb. 9). Es sollte zur Ausschaltung von Chromogenen grundsätzlich die Girardtrennung angewandt werden.

b) Gehalt des Plasmas

Neuerdings wurden die 17-Ketosteroide auch im Plasma bestimmt. Die Hauptkomponenten sind Dehydroepiandrosteron und Androsteron. Beim Mann stammen sie aus der Nebennierenrinde und den Keimdrüsen, bei der Frau aus der Nebennierenrinde. Sie folgen einem täglichen Rhythmus und sind wie die 17-Ketosteroide im Urin altersabhängig. Nach dem 40. Lebensjahr fallen sie rasch ab und sind im 70. Lebensjahr nicht mehr nachzuweisen.

= 17-Oxosteroide des Urins in die Einzelkomponenten (24 Std)

Papierchromatographische Trennung (JAYLE u. Mitarb.)		Papierchromatographische Aufteilung nach Girard-Trennung (GÖBEL u. HENI)	
♂	♀	♂ (20—40 Jahre)	♀ (20—40 Jahre)
< 50 Jahre			
2—4 mg	1—3 mg	1,5 mg ± 0,66	1,42 mg ± 0,46
3—6 mg	2—4 mg	2,91 mg ± 1,13	2,63 mg ± 0,75
3—6 mg	2—5 mg	0,53 mg ± 0,47	0,36 mg ± 0,22
1—2 mg	1 mg	0,27 mg ± 0,18	0,23 mg ± 0,13
Spuren	Spuren	0,13 mg ± 0,06	0,14 mg ± 0,1
Spuren	Spuren	0,22 mg ± 0,14	0,21 mg ± 0,11
1—2 mg	1 mg	0,52 mg ± 0,40	0,53 mg ± 0,28
		0,13 mg ± 0,13	0,17 mg ± 0,15
		0,49 mg ± 0,4	0,49 mg ± 0,4
10—20 mg	7—14 mg	6,70 mg/24 Std ± 2,36	6,18 mg/24 Std ± 1,6

Normalwerte: *Androsteron* 25,0 µg ± 10,7 (MIGEON u. Mitarb.), 17,3 ± 0,9 (EIK-NES u. Mitarb.), 20,7 µg (GÖBEL u. Mitarb.), Dehydroepiandrosteron 48,2 ± 15,1 (MIGEON 1957), 57,5 ± 10,5 µg (EIK-NES u. Mitarb.), 43,0 µg (GÖBEL u. Mitarb., 1958).

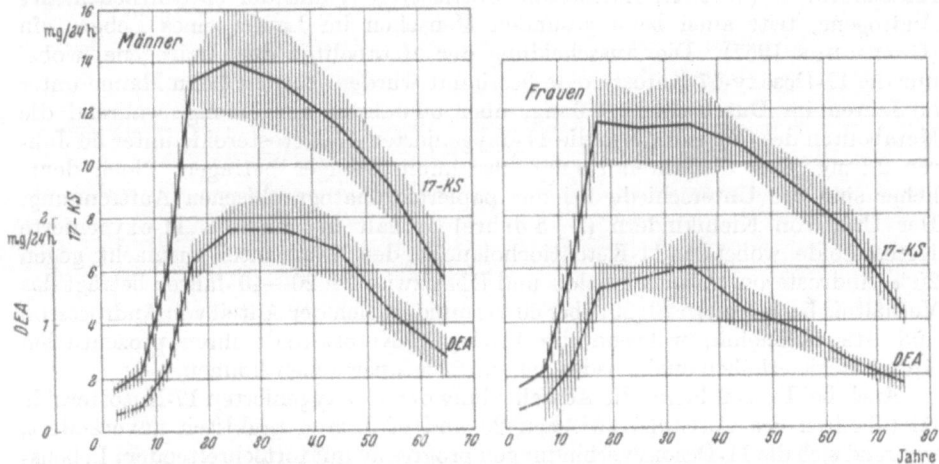

Abb. 9. Altersmäßige Verteilung der 17-Ketosteroide und des DEA bei Mann und Frau

Unter 1000 E HCG steigt Androsteron beim Mann nach 2—4 Std deutlich an, während DEA nur seinen physiologischen Rhythmus verliert (EIK-NES u. Mitarb.). Frauen zeigen keine Änderung. Das Mehr stammt wahrscheinlich aus den Leydigzellen.

Die Gesamt-17-Ketosteroide betragen im Plasma nach GARDNER bei Männern 40—130 µg in 100 ml, nach TAMM u. Mitarb. 101,1 µg, nach RAVERA bis zum 40. Lebensjahr 71,0 µg, über 40 Jahren 28 µg/100 ml.

2. Bedeutung der 17-Ketosteroidausscheidung

Nach den gegenwärtigen Vorstellungen der ACTH-Wirkung — Stimulierung der Umwandlung von Cholesterin in Pregnenolon — und der Biosynthese der Nebennierenrindenhormone (s. Abb. 4) müßte sich die Produktion der Cortisole und der Androgene der Nebennierenrinde immer gleichsinnig ändern.

Verschiedene Beobachtungen machen aber wahrscheinlich, daß die Bildung der Androgene und der Corticoide der Nebennierenrinde nicht nur unter pathologischen, sondern auch physiologischen Bedingungen auseinandergeht. Der Mechanismus der verschieden starken Produktion der beiden großen Gruppen ist nicht bekannt. Wenn man das ACTH als einziges tropes Hormon der Nebennierenrinde anerkennt, dann muß die Ursache in der wechselnden Aktivität der Enzyme der Nebennierenrinde liegen, die zur Bildung der beiden Gruppen führt. Untersuchungen mit synthetisch hergestellten Bruchstücken des ACTH stärken die Ansicht derjenigen, die mehrere ACTH-Arten mit verschiedener biologischer Wirkung annehmen.

a) Abhängigkeit von Geschlecht und Lebensalter

Besonders charakteristisch ist die Verschiebung des Verhältnisses der 11-Oxy-(Cortisolabkömmlinge) zu den 11-Desoxy-Metaboliten (Androgene und Cortisolvorstufen) der Nebennierenrinde bei den echten Hyperplasien. Die klinische Äußerung reicht von der reinen Form des Morbus Cushing mit der isolierten Überproduktion von Cortisol mit allen Übergängen bis zur reinen Form des Virilismus mit der isolierten Überproduktion der Androgene der Nebennierenrinde. Eine ähnliche quantitative Verschiebung der unentbehrlichen Nebennierenrindenhormone (Cortisol, Aldosteron, Corticosteron) und der entbehrlichen, der Androgene, tritt auch beim gesunden Menschen im Laufe seines Lebens ein (Gallagher 1957). Die Ausscheidung der Metaboliten der Androgene, wobei nur die 11-Desoxy-17-Ketosteroide bestimmt wurden, beträgt beim Manne unter 50 Jahren im Durchschnitt 8,6 mg, über 50 Jahren nur 4,4 mg, während die Metaboliten des Cortisols, also die 11-oxygenierten 17-Ketosteroide unter 50 Jahren 2,1 mg, über 50 Jahren 1,8 mg, also kaum weniger betragen. Noch deutlicher sind die Unterschiede bei der papierchromatographischen Auftrennung. Der Urin von Kleinkindern (2—5 Jahre) enthält bis zu 80% 11-oxygenierte Ketosteroide, wobei das 11-Ketoätiocholanolon den Hauptanteil ausmacht, gegen 20% Androsteron, Ätiocholanolon und DEA zwischen 20—40 Jahren beträgt das Verhältnis bei Männern 20:80, über 60 vermindert sich der Anteil von Androsteron und Ätiocholanolon, während die 11-Oxy-17-Ketosteroide ihren prozentualen Anteil stark erhöhen und wieder bis zu 80% ausmachen können. Auch bei Frauen bleibt die Ausscheidung der 11-oxygenierten 17-Ketosteroide (Metaboliten des Cortisols) zwischen 20 und 60 Jahren praktisch unverändert, während sich die 11-Desoxyverbindungen progressiv mit fortschreitendem Lebensalter vermindern. Den wesentlichsten Anteil an dieser Verminderung haben die Androgene der Nebennierenrindenhormone. Mit zunehmendem Alter verschiebt sich also sowohl beim Mann als auch bei der Frau die Sekretionsleistung der Nebennierenrinde, indem die Produktion von Cortisol und Aldosteron gleich bleibt, die der Androgene aber progressiv vermindert wird (Gallagher 1957).

b) Abhängigkeit von Allgemeinerkrankungen

Während man in den Anfangsjahren nach der Entdeckung und Einführung der Zimmermannschen Reaktion in die Klinik aus der Erniedrigung und der Erhöhung der Ausscheidung weitgehende Schlüsse gezogen hat, werden die Ergebnisse heute viel kritischer bewertet. Besonders die Erniedrigung ist vieldeutig und erlaubt ohne zusätzliche Hormonuntersuchungen anderer Art weder die Annahme einer Nebennieren- noch Hodeninsuffizienz.

Eine der ersten Erkrankungen, bei der eine starke Erniedrigung der 17-Ketosteroidausscheidung im Urin auffiel, war die primär chronische Polyarthritis in fortgeschrittenem Stadium (DAVIDSON 1947, HENCH, MARTI 1951, VENNING 1951). Die Annahme einer Nebennniereninsuffizienz mußte wieder aufgegeben werden, nachdem man feststellte, daß die 17-Ketosteroide bei allen chronischen Erkrankungen, die mit einer starken Gewichtsabnahme verbunden sind, also chronische Entzündungen des Mesenchyms, chronische Leukosen, metastasierende Carcinome, chronische kardiale Dekompensation, progrediente Tuberkulose u. a. bis auf $^1/_3$—$^1/_2$ des Normalen erniedrigt sein können, ohne daß die Nebennieren autoptisch atrophisch waren oder degenerative Zeichen boten. Die Bestimmung des Plasmacortisols und die Ausscheidung der Cortisolmetaboliten ergab dann später normale Werte. Testung mit ACTH erhöht das Plasmacortisol und die Urinmetaboliten wie beim Gesunden, während die 17-Ketosteroide bei diesen Kranken einen nicht signifikanten Anstieg erfahren. Diese Diskrepanz kann Folge der verschiedenen Reaktionsweise der beiden Haupthormongruppen der lebenswichtigen Cortisole und nicht lebenswichtigen Androgene sein, sie kann auch mit einem andersartigen Abbau der Androgene bei diesen chronisch Kranken zusammenhängen. In zahlreichen Untersuchungen wurden die 17-Ketosteroide bei Leberkranken sowohl bei der Lebercirrhose als auch bei der frischen Hepatitis epidemica beträchtlich vermindert gefunden, obwohl in diesen Fällen das Plasmacortisol und dessen Anstieg auf ACTH normal waren (NELSON 1952). Die in ihrer Funktion geschädigte Leber ist offenbar nicht mehr imstande, die Steroidhormone in normaler Art und Weise abzubauen. Dies gilt für die Oestrogene, deren Ausscheidung erhöht ist und in gewissem Umfange auch für Corticoide. Zuerst leidet die Bindung der Metaboliten an Glucuronsäure, die durch ein besonderes Fermentsystem der Leber vollzogen wird. Der Gesunde scheidet mindestens 50% der 17-Ketosteroide in gebundener Form aus, bei der Lebercirrhose sind es nur 10—30%. Von parenteral verabreichtem Testosteronpropionat (25 mg) können beim Gesunden 40—60% wieder als 17-Ketosteroide im Urin erfaßt werden, beim Lebergeschädigten erhöhen sich die 17-Ketosteroide entweder gar nicht oder es erscheinen nur 4—15% des verabreichten Hormons im Urin (BIRKE 1953, WEST 1956).

Wie schwierig die Verhältnisse in Wirklichkeit sind, zeigt eine Beobachtung von BRADLOW, der bei Menschen mit Hypothyreose nach Verabreichung von Testosteron eine beträchtliche Vermehrung der Ausscheidung von Ätiocholanolon gegenüber Androsteron feststellte. Das normale Verhältnis der $5\beta:5\alpha$-Verbindungen von 1 steigt bei der Hypothyreose bis auf 8:1 an.

Nach Thyroxin normalisiert sich das Verhältnis wieder. Erzeugt man bei einem gesunden Menschen durch die Verabreichung von Trijodthyronin eine Hyperthyreose, dann verschiebt sich das Verhältnis von Ätiocholanolon und Androsteron zugunsten von Androsteron auch ohne zusätzliche Testosterongabe. Die üblichen Leberfunktionsprüfungen, wie die Takatasche Reaktion, Thymolreaktion, Bromsulfaleinprobe, Fermentbestimmungen wie SGOT, LAP, fallen dabei normal aus und trotzdem ist der Abbau von Testosteron deutlich verändert. Diese Beobachtung unterstreicht die Wichtigkeit der Funktion der peripheren Organe, insbesondere der Leber für den Abbau zu 17-Ketosteroiden und zeigt, wie vorsichtig man auch in der Deutung der vom Normalen abweichenden Befunde der chromatographischen Auftrennung der 17-Ketosteroide sein muß.

Eine ähnlich unvollständige Auskunft geben die 17-Ketosteroide während einer akuten *schweren Belastung* des Gesamtorganismus. Unter einem operativen Eingriff steigen sie in den ersten 24—48 Std über die obere Grenze des Normalen, fallen am 3.—5. Tag auf unternormale Werte ab, um dann im Laufe von weiteren 10 Tagen langsam den Ausgangswert zu erreichen. Chronisch Kranke oder Schwerkranke, die eine niedrige Ketosteroidausscheidung haben, reagieren auf den Stress einer Operation häufig nicht mit einem Anstieg der 17-Ketosteroide, obwohl die Cortisonmetaboliten ein normales Ansprechen der Nebenniere auf die Belastung anzeigen (Mason 1950). Ähnlich nichtssagend ist die 17-Ketosteroidausscheidung unter einer schweren körperlichen Anstrengung. Hierbei ist die Ausscheidung nur in den ersten Stunden erhöht und fällt trotz Fortsetzung der körperlichen Tätigkeit auf normale, ja sogar unternormale Werte ab. Bei Untrainierten soll sie gleich bleiben oder von Anfang an absinken.

Das ungenügende Ansprechen der Androgenproduktion der Nebenniere wird ganz offensichtlich bei der Testung mit ACTH in Form der intravenösen achtstündigen Dauerinfusion von 20 E oder unter 40 E eines guten Deportpäparates intramuskulär. Einmalige ACTH-Gabe erhöht die 17-Ketosteroidausscheidung bei einem größeren Vergleichsgut gesunder Menschen nicht signifikant, erst am 2. Tag ist die erhöhte Ausscheidung verwertbar, ganz im Gegensatz zum raschen Anstieg der 17-Hydroxycorticoide. Die 17-Ketosteroidausscheidung eignet sich nicht zur Funktionsprüfung der Nebennierenrinde mit ACTH.

c) Abhängigkeit von der Funktion des innersekretorischen Systems

α) Hypophysenvorderlappen

Die voll ausgeprägte Hypophysenvorderlappeninsuffizienz ergibt die niedrigsten Werte, da hier sowohl der Anteil aus den Nebennieren als auch der aus dem Hoden bzw. Ovarium wegfällt. Ausscheidung von 1 mg und darunter ist immer verdächtig auf eine echte hypophysäre Insuffizienz. Der Anstieg unter ACTH erfolgt, abhängig von Schwere und Dauer der Erkrankung, nicht selten erst nach mehrmaliger ACTH-Gabe. Im Chromatogramm sind alle Einzelfraktionen gleichmäßig vermindert. Eine normale 17-Ketosteroidausscheidung schließt eine Hypophysenvorderlappeninsuffizienz aus. Funktionierende Adenome der Hypophyse gehen mit einer Erhöhung der 17-Ketosteroidausscheidung einher, wenn die Nebennieren in die Stimulierung miteinbezogen sind, besonders also beim Morbus Cushing und bei einem Teil der Kranken mit Akromegalie.

β) Nebennierenrinde

Bei völliger Zerstörung beider Nebennieren, Morbus Addison, sind die 17-Ketosteroide immer stark erniedrigt, bei Frauen stärker als bei Männern, da die Ovarien nichts beisteuern. Eine normale oder an der unteren Grenze des Normalen liegende 17-Ketosteroidausscheidung schließt das Vorliegen einer echten Nebennierenrindeninsuffizienz aber nicht aus, da eine gewisse Basisfunktion erhalten bleiben kann, erst das Unvermögen des Anstiegs auf wiederholte ACTH-Gabe beweist den anatomischen Defekt. Zur feineren Diagnostik benützt man besser die Metaboliten des Cortisols als die der Androgene.

Bei der Hyperplasie und den hormonaktiven Tumoren geht die 17-Ketosteroidausscheidung dem klinischen Bild weitgehend parallel. Reine Formen des Cushing-Syndroms, die durch die alleinige Vermehrung der Glucocorticoidproduktion bedingt sind, zeigen normale Werte. Je mehr dagegen die Virilisierung im klinischen Bild hervortritt, um so stärker ist die Ausscheidung erhöht. Die einfache Hyperplasie erreicht dabei Werte bis zu 60 mg, Tumoren bis über 1000 mg pro Tag. Bei einem großen Teil der Tumoren ist die Ausscheidung der β-Fraktion, besonders das Dehydroepiandrosteron, stark erhöht. Bei Hyperplasie und bei Tumoren können auch große Mengen der Vorstufen des Cortisols im Urin nachgewiesen werden. Die charakteristischen Veränderungen des angeborenen adrenogenitalen Syndroms sind auf S. 767 beschrieben.

Bei einem Teil der Fälle mit adrenalem Virilismus und bei Tumoren ist die Ausscheidung des *Dehydroepiandrosterons* besonders stark erhöht. Dieses Steroid, das direkt aus einer Vorstufe des Pregnenolons oder aus Pregnenolon entstehen kann, fällt vorwiegend dann vermehrt an, wenn eine absolute oder relative Insuffizienz der Kondensationsenzyme die Produktion von Pregnenolon stört oder wenn die 3β-ol-Dehydrogenase oder die 4-5-Isomerase, die Pregnenolon in Progesteron umwandeln, insuffizient ist. Bis jetzt hat man das vermehrte Auftreten von DEA als beweisend für eine Dysfunktion der Nebennierenrinde angesehen, nach neueren Beobachtungen kann es sich offenbar auch aus dem Ovar oder dem Hoden herleiten (s. Abb. 10).

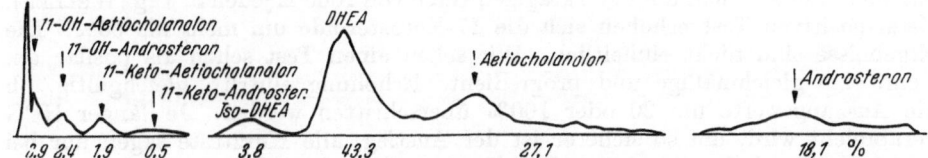

Abb. 10. Chromatogramm der 17-Ketosteroide von einem Leydigzelltumor. Isolierte Vermehrung des DEA (Fall 1)

γ) Keimdrüsen (Choriogonadotropintest)

Beim Vollkastraten wird die Ausscheidung verschieden angegeben, McCullagh u. Mitarb. (1948) finden bei fünf Eunuchen nur 50% des Normalen, Callow u. Mitarb. bei elf Eunuchen im Rahmen des Normalen liegende Werte. Im Vergleich zu einer Gruppe Gesunder desselben Alters sind die 17-Ketosteroide im Durchschnitt etwas vermindert (Callow 1938). Hamilton (1954) veröffentlichte kürzlich Untersuchungen an 52 Kastraten im Alter zwischen 23 und 81 Jahren. Die Mittelwerte liegen mit 12,55 mg in 24 Std gegen 15,1 mg der Kontrollen recht hoch. In der Altersklasse zwischen 20 und 30 Jahren ist der Unterschied nicht signifikant, 16,11 mg bei Kastraten und 16,74 mg bei den Kontrollen! Dies rührt von einer ungeklärt hohen Ausscheidung — über 20 mg —, die sechs der neun Kastraten dieses Lebensalters aufwiesen. Auch beim Kastraten fällt die Ausscheidung mit zunehmendem Alter ab, nach dem 50. Lebensjahr unterscheiden sie sich nicht mehr von den Kontrollen. Im Chromatogramm sind Androsteron und Ätiocholanolon stärker vermindert als DEA und die oxygenierten Derivate. Scott und Vermeulen untersuchten zehn Männer mit Prostatacarcinom vor und nach der Kastration. Bei allen fielen die Ketosteroide nach der Kastration deutlich ab und stiegen dann langsam wieder an, teilweise sogar auf höhere Werte als vor der Kastration. Dieses Verhalten kann nicht mit einer kompensatorischen Hypertrophie der Nebenniere erklärt werden, wie sie bei verschiedenen Laboratoriumstieren nach Kastration angegeben wird. Bei den Carcinomträgern verbesserte sich der Allgemeinzustand nach der Entfernung der Testes, dies allein erklärt die Normalisierung.

Dieselben Ergebnisse erhält man bei den verschiedenen Formen des Hypogonadismus. Bei völligem Ausfall der Hodenfunktion können die 17-Ketosteroide durchaus im Normalbereich liegen, besonders wenn man einen Einzelfall betrachtet. Vergleicht man dagegen eine größere Gruppe von schwerem Hypogonadismus mit denselben Altersstufen, dann ergibt sich, wie beim echten Kastraten, eine geringe, aber signifikante Verminderung. Leichtere Formen der Hodeninsuffizienz unterscheiden sich von den Kontrollen nicht. Mit Hilfe der 17-Ketosteroidausscheidung kann man also weder den Ausfall der inkretorischen

Hodenfunktion beweisen noch ausschließen, geschweige eine feinere Differenzierung des Ausmaßes der Insuffizienz treffen. Man ist daher schon frühzeitig, ähnlich wie bei der Nebennierenrinde, zur Prüfung der Funktion durch Gonadotropine übergegangen.

Der *Choriongonadotropintest* kann eine Aussage über die Ätiologie einer Insuffizienz geben. Beim sekundären Hypogonadismus wird HCG die atrophischen Leydigzellen entfalten und zur Funktion bringen. Bei einer primären Hodeninsuffizienz gelingt es nicht, die geschädigten, funktionsuntüchtigen oder fehlenden Leydigzellen anzuregen, die 17-Ketosteroide steigen nicht an. Der Test ist besonders wertvoll beim Kryptorchismus und beim Hypogonadismus Jugendlicher, wenn die Probeexcision kein klares Ergebnis bringt.

Die Durchführung des Testes wird verschieden gehandhabt. Zuverlässige Ergebnisse erhält man mit der 14tägigen Gabe von 1000 E jeden 2. Tag (Weller). Beim positiven Test erhöhen sich die 17-Ketosteroide um mehr als 60%. Die Ergebnisse sind nicht einheitlich. Wir sehen einen Test schon als positiv an, wenn eine gleichmäßige und progrediente Erhöhung eintritt, gleichgültig, ob die Ausgangswerte um 30 oder 100% überschritten werden. Je länger HCG verabreicht wird, um so sicherer ist der Anstieg, alle Kurzteste sagen nur bei positivem Ergebnis etwas aus. Der Test eignet sich nicht zur feineren Funktionsdiagnostik, da die Reaktion der Leydigzellen ausgesprochen träge ist.

Landau u. Mitarb. (1959) geben z.B. 5000 E über 4 Tage verteilt und finden beim Gesunden eine Erhöhung zwischen 3 und 14 mg, sie geben auch eine Erhöhung von Pregnantriol, ein Metabolit des 17α-Hydroxyprogesterons um 1,3 mg im Durchschnitt an. Hibbit verabreichte HCG in Form einer Dauerinfusion von 8 Std, zwei Tage lang, täglich 10000 E. Bei 14 Testen beträgt die Erhöhung am 1. Tag nur 3 mg, am 2. Tag 6 mg, sie fehlte beim Kastraten. Wie Maddock (1952) u.a. gezeigt haben, ist der Anstieg der Oestrogene unter HCG prozentual viel stärker als der der 17-Ketosteroide. Die allgemeine Verwendung der Oestrogene im HCG-Test scheitert aber vorläufig noch an der technisch schwierigen chemischen Bestimmung, die nur in Speziallaboratorien vorgenommen werden kann.

Eine echte, durch erhöhte Produktion von hypophysären Gonadotropinen ausgelöste, über das physiologische Maß hinausgehende Testosteronproduktion im Hoden ist nicht sicher bewiesen. Wohl hat man klinisch bei einzelnen Formen der Akromegalie den Eindruck einer übermäßigen Androgenität, aber mit Hilfe der 17-Ketosteroidausscheidung sind keine signifikanten Abweichungen von der Norm zu fassen. ICSH-produzierende Adenome mit dem histologischen Bild der Leydigzellhyperplasie sind nicht bekannt, obwohl sie ebenso vorkommen müssen wie die Adenome der anderen spezifischen Zellarten der Hypophyse. Die Schwierigkeit der Feststellung beruht einmal in der nicht signifikanten Erhöhung der 17-Ketosteroidausscheidung, selbst bei Verdoppelung der Testosteronproduktion, zum anderen in der Unwirksamkeit des vermehrt zirkulierenden Testosterons am voll ausgebildeten männlichen Organismus. Eine vermehrte hypophysäre Androgenproduktion ist daher nur faßbar, wenn sie vorzeitig, also vor der Pubertät erfolgt (Pubertas praecox). Die 17-Ketosteroidausscheidung bleibt dabei unter der des Erwachsenen.

Anders bei den echten Tumoren der Leydigzellen. Hier können die 17-Ketosteroide stark erhöhte Werte erreichen (s. S. 772).

Wenig Sicheres weiß man darüber, ob auch in den Leydigzellen, ähnlich wie in der Nebennierenrinde, ein Fermentmangel der ersten Stufen der Testosteronsynthese, also der 17β-Hydroxylase oder der 3β-Dehydrogenase vorkommt. Das einzige bis jetzt bekannte Beispiel ist die *kongenitale Lipoidhyperplasie* der

Nebennieren von PRADER und SIEBENMANN, bei der offenbar nicht nur eine Synthesestörung in der Nebennierenrinde, sondern auch im Hoden, vielleicht zwischen Cholesterin und Pregnenolon oder Pregnenolon und Progesteron vorliegt. Da die neugeborenen Knaben dieser Art ein weibliches äußeres Genitale trotz männlichem Gonadengeschlecht haben, müssen die Androgene schon während der embryonalen Differenzierung der Geschlechtsorgane fehlen. Daß solche Enzymdefekte vielleicht nicht so ganz selten sind, zeigt ein von GUINET (1954) beschriebener Leydigzelltumor mit Gynäkomastie, wobei die 17-Ketosteroide, die Oestrogene und Gonadotropine im Urin normal waren und sich nur eine starke Vermehrung der Pregnandiolausscheidung feststellen ließ. Die starke Hyperplasie der Leydigzellen beim Klinefelter-Syndrom bei gleichzeitigen Zeichen eines Hypoandrogenismus läßt ebenfalls an einen solchen partiellen Enzymdefekt denken.

δ) Schilddrüse

Beim schweren und länger dauernden Myxödem ist die Ausscheidung deutlich erniedrigt, zwischen 3 und 6 mg bei Männern und 2 und 4 mg bei Frauen; Werte unter 2 mg sahen wir nur bei der Hypophysenvorderlappeninsuffizienz. Die Angaben in der Literatur, daß die Kompensation des Myxödems durch Schilddrüsenhormon die 17-Ketosteroidausscheidung nicht normalisiert, kann ich nicht bestätigen. Solche Fälle erwecken den Verdacht einer hypophysären Insuffizienz.

Leichte bis mittelschwere Formen des Hyperthyreoidismus zeigen eine normale Ausscheidung, bei schweren ist sie deutlich vermindert. Die Androsteronausscheidung ist deutlich höher als die des Ätiocholanolons.

IX. Darstellung und Biosynthese der Oestrogene

Oestrogene wurden zum erstenmal 1927 von ASCHHEIM und ZONDEK aus dem Urin von schwangeren Frauen nachgewiesen und fast gleichzeitig und unabhängig voneinander von DOISY (1929), BUTENANDT (1929) und LAQUEUR kristallisiert dargestellt.

Die Oestrogene sind C_{18}-Steroide mit drei Doppelbindungen im Ring A. Eigenschaften und Verhalten im Spektrum entsprechen einem Phenol mit einem aromatischen Kern. Synthese s. S. 667.

XXI. Oestron   XXII. Oestradiol   XXIII. Oestriol

Die wichtigsten im Urin ausgeschiedenen Oestrogene sind:

a) *Oestron*, 1,3,5(10)-Oestratrien-3-ol-17-on (XXI), nachgewiesen in Harn, Blut, Placentagewebe und Ovarium.

b) *Oestradiol*, entsteht durch Hydrierung der Ketogruppe am C_{17}=1,5,3(10)-Oestratrien-3,17β-diol (XXII), nachgewiesen in Harn, Blut, Placenta, Ovarium, Hoden.

c) *Oestriol*, das Hydrat = 1,3,5(10)-Oestratrien-3,16α-17β-triol (XXIII), nachgewiesen in Harn, Blut und Placenta, nicht im Ovar.

Die Hälfte der ausgeschiedenen Oestrogene besteht aus Oestriol, die andere Hälfte verteilt sich gleichmäßig auf Oestron und Oestradiol-17β, normales Verhältnis Oestriol:Oestron+17β-Oestradiol = 1.

Daneben sind kleine Mengen von 16-Epioestriol, 16α-Hydroxyoestron, 16-Oxooestradiol-17β, 16β-Hydroxyoestron, 16-Oxooestron, 2-Methoxyoestron, 18-Hydroxyoestron isoliert worden. Man weiß noch nicht sicher, wie diese verschiedenen Steroide im Abbau aufeinanderfolgen. Die Vorstellungen von DICZFALUSY sind in Abb. 11 dargestellt.

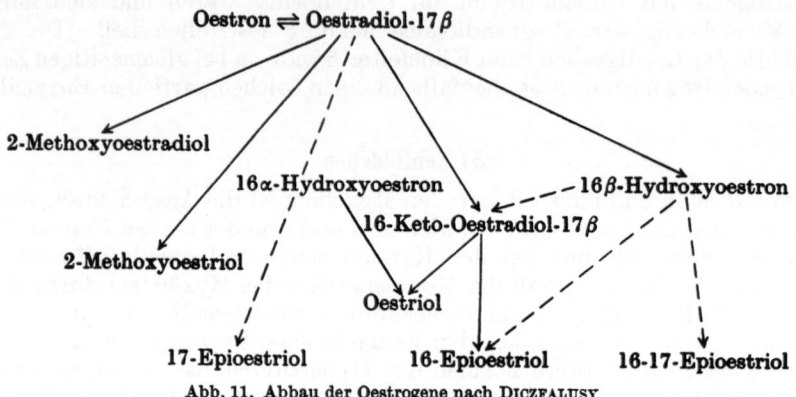

Abb. 11. Abbau der Oestrogene nach DICZFALUSY

1. Vorkommen

a) Ovarium

Die wichtigste Quelle ist das Ovarium. Als Bildungsstätte werden sowohl die Granulosazellen, die Thecazellen (ZODNEK 1927) und auch die interstitiellen Zellen (McARTHUR, CHARNY 1940) diskutiert. *Oestradiol-17β* ist wahrscheinlich das eigentliche Ovarialhormon.

Follikelflüssigkeit und Gelbkörper enthalten große Mengen von Oestradiol-17β und Oestron, nicht aber Oestriol. Der Gelbkörper soll in 24 Std 200—300 μg produzieren.

b) Placenta

Im *Placentagewebe* des Menschen fand DICZFALUSY 1961 pro Kilogramm Feuchtgewicht 31,3 μg Oestron, 170,2 Oestradiol-17β und 314,6 μg Oestriol.

Die biologisch im Allen-Doisy-Test bestimmten Aktivitäten weichen erheblich von den chemisch bestimmten ab. Ein reifer Follikel enthält 8—12 ME, die Placenta auf 0,1 g 1 ME, die gesamte also für 500 g 5000 ME, der Urin von Frauen je nach Aufarbeitung 70—300 ME, in den letzten Schwangerschaftsmonaten 12000 ME (ZONDEK 1934). Die chemische Bestimmung ergibt bei der Frau 20—85 μg Gesamtoestrogenausscheidung pro Tag. Die gesamte im Blut befindliche Menge wird in etwa 6 min umgesetzt (endogener Turnover) (PEARLMAN 1957).

c) Hoden

Oestrogene wurden im Urin und im *Hoden* verschiedener Species festgestellt. So ist seit langem bekannt, daß sich aus dem Hoden von Hengsten Oestrogene in höherer Konzentration als aus Ovarien von Stuten extrahieren lassen (BEALL, DEULOFEU, HÄUSSLER). Der Harn dieser Tiere enthält mit 100000—250000 ME je Liter sogar mehr Oestrogene als der von trächtigen Stuten. Beim Hund, seltener beim Menschen, entwickeln sich feminisierende Hodentumoren mit hoher Oestrogenproduktion. Die Ableitung dieser Geschwülste aus den Sertolizellen (TEILUM) wird in den letzten Jahren mit Recht bezweifelt, sie entwickeln sich aus den Leydigzellen. BEALL gelang 1940 die chemische Identifizierung von Oestron und Oestradiol-17β in Hengsthoden, er errechnete auf 20 kg Gewebe 0,36 mg Oestron und 0,21 mg Oestradiol. Auch aus menschlichem Hoden wurde Oestradiol-17β isoliert. Hodentumoren können besonders hohe Oestrogenaktivität besitzen, so gewannen MARTI und HEUSSER aus 180 g Tumorgewebe die große Menge von 14 mg Oestradiol-17β. Der gesunde Mann scheidet zwischen 2 bis 29 μg Gesamtoestrogene im Urin aus, die in 24 Std produzierte Menge wird mit 20—50 μg errechnet. Für das normale Hodengewebe ist der Bildungsort der Oestrogene in den Leydigzellen sichergestellt. MADDOCK und NELSON (1952) stellten beim Mann unter großen Dosen von Choriongonadotropin (5000 E dreimal wöchentlich 47—65 Tage lang) ein Ansteigen der Oestrogene im Urin um das 5—16fache fest, während sich die 17-Ketosteroide als Maß der Androgenproduktion nur etwa verdoppelten. Histologisch entwickelt sich dabei eine starke Hyperplasie der Leydigzellen, während die Kanälchen Degenerationszeichen aufweisen und die Sertolizellen unverändert bleiben.

RABINOWITZ (1955) konnte nach Inkubation von Hodenhomogenaten mit markiertem Acetat markiertes 17β-Oestradiol isolieren. Als weiterer Beweis für die Oestrogenbildung kann der Oestrogengehalt des tierischen und menschlichen Spermasan gesehen werden. So fand DICZFALUSY (1953) in 1 Liter Sammelsperma von Männern 60 μg Oestron, 60 μg Oestradiol-17β und 30 μg Oestriol.

d) Nebennierenrinde

Man hat die *Nebennierenrinde* auch als akzessorische Geschlechtsdrüse angesprochen. Diese Ansicht gründet sich auf die Beobachtung, daß bei kastrierten Ratten durch die Injektion konzentrierter Nebennierenextrakte ein Oestrus erzeugt werden kann. Bei bestimmten Mäuse- und Rattenstämmen entstehen in der Nebennierenrinde nach der Kastration gonadotropinabhängige Androgene und Oestrogene produzierende Geschwülste (COREY 1934, 1941). Beim erwachsenen Nager oder Mensch kann die Nebennierenrinde keine einzige Erscheinung der Kastration ausgleichen. Der direkte Nachweis von Oestrogenen ist bis jetzt in Homogenaten von normalem Nebennierengewebe des Menschen nicht gelungen. Das menschliche Nebennierenvenenblut weist aber eine höhere Oestrogenkonzentration auf als das periphere Venenblut (8 μg gegen 2 μg/ml Plasma). Im Harn von kastrierten Frauen konnten zahlreiche Untersucher oestrogene Aktivität feststellen, während nach zusätzlicher Adrenalektomie keine oder nur noch kleinere Mengen ausgeschieden werden. WEST u. Mitarb. (1958) finden unter der Verabreichung von ACTH bei Kastratinnen einen deutlichen Anstieg der Oestrogenausscheidung.

Endlich konnte man in vitro-Versuchen nachweisen, daß Nebennierenrindengewebe aus 19-Hydroxyandrostendion Oestrogene bilden kann (MEYER 1955).

Die meisten Autoren nehmen an, daß die *normale Nebenniere* von Mann und Frau kleine Mengen von Oestrogenen produziert und in den Kreislauf abgibt, und zwar vorwiegend 18-Hydroxyoestron und 18-Hydroxyoestradiol-17β (MARRIAN 1957). Über die Bedeutung dieser Oestrogenproduktion im Stoffwechsel ist nichts bekannt.

Dagegen ist in *pathologischen* Fällen sowohl bei der Nebennierenhyperplasie als auch bei Nebennierengeschwülsten, der Nachweis von Oestrogenen in zahlreichen Fällen gelungen. Die bei Tumoren im Urin ausgeschiedene Menge war zum Teil sehr hoch, über 3000 ME pro Liter (Savard 1958), 2600 μg im 24 Std-Urin, 70 g Tumorgewebe enthielten 280 mg Oestronäquivalente (Higgins).

Seltener als die Carcinome produzieren auch gutartige Adenome der Nebennierenrinde Oestrogene. Klinisch handelt es sich bei Frauen nicht immer um feminisierende Geschwülste, sondern wie in einem Fall von Jailer (1948) um einen vorwiegend virilisierenden Nebennierentumor einer Frau, die 176 mg 17-Ketosteroide und 296 μg Oestrogene in 24 Std ausschied.

Die einfache Hyperplasie der Nebenniere verhält sich verschieden. Während die angeborenen Formen meist eine erhöhte Ausscheidung aufweisen (Jayle), zeigen die erworbenen meist keine Vermehrung.

e) Umwandlung von Androgenen zu Oestrogenen

Steinach hat 1936 nach Verabreichung von Androgenen bei Ratten und Menschen einen Anstieg der biologisch getestete Oestrogenaktivität des Urins festgestellt. Nathanson (1941) konnte aus dem Urin von kastrierten Frauen, die wegen metastasierendem Brustkrebs mit Testosteron behandelt wurden, Oestron, Oestradiol-17β und Oestriol im Urin nachweisen. Da bei diesen Untersuchungen die Nebennierenrinde als Quelle nicht ausgeschlossen war, gaben West u. Mitarb. (1956) wegen metastasierendem Mammacarcinom ovarektomierten und adrenal-ektomierten Frauen täglich 200 mg Testosteron. Unter der Erhaltungsdosis von 75 mg Cortisol konnten keine Oestrogene im Urin nachgewiesen werden, nach zusätzlicher Testosterongabe in 24 Std 17,2—24,1 μg Oestron, 16,3—25,5 μg Oestradiol-17β, während Oestriol fehlte. Die Höhe der Umwandlung ist nicht nennenswert, doch sei daran erinnert, daß die Gesamtoestrogenausscheidung der gesunden Frau zum Teil niedriger liegt! Wird durch hohe Testosterondosen das Wachstum von oestrogenabhängigen Tumoren begünstigt, dann kann die Ursache in der Umwandlung in Oestrogene beruhen, über deren Ausmaß im abnormalen peripheren Stoffwechsel nichts bekannt ist. Wichtig ist, daß auch aus den Vorstufen der Androgene der Nebennierenrinde, also aus DEA, Pregnenolon, ja sogar aus Cortisol, wahrscheinlich auch zeitweise aus den anabol wirkenden Derivaten des Testosterons in der Leber Oestrogene entstehen können. Die Leber besitzt dieselben Fermentsysteme wie die Keimdrüsen, das Zwischenglied von den Androgenen zu den Oestrogenen ist wahrscheinlich 4-Androstendion.

f) Exogene Quellen

In der Natur finden sich eine Reihe oestrogenartig wirkender Substanzen in der Kohle, Erdöl, Schiefer, Moor und Asphalt sowie in vielen tierischen und pflanzlichen Nahrungsmitteln. In vielen Ländern werden Oestrogene zur Aufzucht von Schlachttieren, Rindern, Schweinen und Hühnern verwendet. Der Gehalt des Fleisches soll so gering sein, daß keine Schädigung eintreten kann (Birke 1953, Bulbrook). Das Palmkernöl enthält als natürliches Nahrungsmittel Oestron. Hopfen gehört zu den oestrogenreichsten Pflanzen, während Sojabohnen, Rhabarber, Kartoffeln, Petersilie nur geringe Mengen enthalten. Bei normaler Kost soll der Mensch im Durchschnitt 2—20% der im Körper täglich gebildeten Oestrogenmenge exogen aufnehmen (Hohlweg 1952). Die Angaben stammen aus früherer Zeit. Man muß auch immer daran denken, daß eine Reihe von Medikamenten eine geringe oestrogenartige Wirkung besitzt, die besonders bei verzögerter Inaktivierung und Ausscheidung bei defekter Leberfunktion Symptome machen können. Dazu gehören Digitalis, Vitamin D, Lecithin, Lakritze, Ichthyol.

2. Verhalten im Stoffwechsel

Nach Injektion von markierten Oestrogenen findet sich anfangs der größte Teil der Radioaktivität an den Erythrocyten (14—32%) (MIGEON 1959). Bei der Leberpassage wird etwa die Hälfte rasch an Glucuronsäure und Sulfate und unbekannte Ester gebunden. Die konjugierten Metaboliten erreichen schon 15—30 min nach der Injektion im Plasma ihren Höchstwert (SANDBERG). Die Halbwertszeit nach intravenöser Injektion von freiem Oestradiol und Oestron beträgt 70 min. Während früher die Anreicherung im Uterus nicht feststellbar war, ergaben neue Untersuchungen von JENSEN und JACOBSON (1961) mit Tritium markiertem Oestradiol und Oestron an unreifen Ratten verschiedenes Verhalten der einzelnen Organe. 2—6 Std nach der Injektion von 0,1 μg Oestradiol sind im Uterus 50—150 $\mu\mu$g nachweisbar. Uterus und Vagina unterscheiden sich von Leber, Niere, Muskel, Nebenniere in denen sich das Oestradiol ebenfalls anreichert dadurch, daß das radioaktive Steroid im Uterus eine höhere Konzentration erreicht, und sich hier noch zu einer Zeit anreichert, in der die anderen Gewebe schon eine abfallende Tendenz zeigen. Der größte Teil des radioaktiven Materials besteht im Uterus aus freiem Oestradiol, während in der Leber eine Mischung von Steroiden vorhanden ist und ein beträchtlicher Teil eiweißgebunden und wasserlöslich ist. Die Oestrogene verhalten sich also im „End-Organ" anders als in den Geweben, in denen sie abgebaut werden. Ein Teil der konjugierten unf dreien Oestrogene sind im Plasma an Albumin gebunden, und zwar Oestradiol am stärksten, Oestron und Progesteron wesentlich weniger. Die Bindungskräfte sind beträchtlich geringer als die zwischen Cortisol und Transcortin (SLAUN-WHITE und SANDBERG; DAUGHADAY u. a.). Die Bedeutung dieser Eiweißbindung ist nicht geklärt. Man vermutet, daß die Steroide dadurch weniger leicht diffundieren und langsamer durch die Glomerula filtriert werden.

In den ersten 4 Std erscheinen 12%, in 12 Std 33%, in 96 und 120 Std etwa 80% markierter Oestrogenderivate im Urin. Auch nach 120 Std ist die Ausscheidung noch nicht ganz beendet (SANDBERG).

Die Ursache dieser verzögerten Ausscheidung ist wahrscheinlich in einem enterohepatischen Cyclus zu sehen. Nicht nur bei Hunden, sondern auch beim Menschen mit Gallengangfisteln erscheinen etwa 40% der Radioaktivität in der Galle. Die Oestrogene der Galle sind zu einem kleinen Teil an Glucuronid, zum größeren an nicht bekannte Säuren gebunden. Hydrolyse bei p_H 1 ergibt die größte Ausbeute. Da sich im Stuhl nur 7% der Radioaktivität nachweisen lassen, muß ein enterohepatischer Kreislauf bestehen (SANDBERG). Die gebundenen Oestrogene werden im Darm wieder gespalten und erneut der Leber angeboten. Diese bindet jetzt einen Teil an Glucuronsäure, der dann im Urin erscheint, der größere Teil wird an andere Säuren gebunden und wieder mit der Leber in den Darm ausgeschieden. Dieser wiederholte Kreislauf ist die Ursache für die langsame und verzögerte Ausscheidung der Radioaktivität. Steroide, wie die Corticoide und Androgene, die rasch im Urin erscheinen, werden nur in ganz geringer Menge in der Galle nachweisbar.

Oestradiol-17β und Oestrol gehen leicht ineinander über, beide können in geringer Konzentration in fast allen tierischen Geweben nachgewiesen werden, ein Teil wird zu Oestriol umgewandelt, das nicht mehr zurückverwandelt werden kann (BROWN 1956, DICZFALUSY 1956, SCHILLER).

ZONDEK hat zum erstenmal festgestellt, daß Leberbrei Oestron zu inaktivieren vermag, eine Beobachtung, die in der Zwischenzeit von vielen Untersuchern bestätigt wurde. Nach LIEBERMAN u. Mitarb. können 1500 g menschlicher Leber 11,4 g Oestradiol-17β pro Tag zu unwirksamen Metaboliten, die nur zu einem kleinen Teil bekannt sind, umwandeln.

Diese Fähigkeit der Leber geht auch aus den bekannten Implantationsversuchen von Ovarien in das portale Gefäßgebiet hervor. Implantiert man kastrierten Nagern Ovarien in die Milz oder in das Mesenterium, so bleiben die Tiere im Anoestrus, der Uterus atrophiert, obwohl die Oestrogensekretion anhält und riesige Ovarien, ja sogar Geschwülste, entstehen. Werden diese Ovarien in die Subcutis transplantiert, so beginnt bald wieder der normale Oestrus (BISKIND). Das der Leber unter Umgehung des Allgemeinkreislaufes direkt zufließende Oestrogen wird vollständig inaktiviert. Zusätzliche parenterale Verabreichung von Oestrogenen oder Hypophysektomie verhindert die Größenzunahme des in die Milz transplantierten Ovars.

In Tierversuchen verliert die Leber nach Schädigung mit Tetrachlorkohlenstoff und anderen leichten Giften, ja sogar schon im Hunger und bei eiweißfreier Kost, die Fähigkeit zur Inaktivierung. Die Beobachtungen beim Menschen sind widersprechend. Während bei leberkranken Frauen die biologisch bestimmte

Tabelle 5. *Konzentration der Oestrogene im Plasma* (100 ml) *und Tagesausscheidung im Urin* (D = Durchschnitt)

			Oestron μg	Oestradiol μg	Oestriol μg
		Plasma			
OERTEL	Papierchromatographie Colorimetrie	Frau	0,4—1,5	0,3—0,9	0,1—0,7
PREEDY u. AITKEN	Fluorimetrie	Frau	0,11	0,07	0,19
OERTEL	Papierchromatographie Colorimetrie	gravide Frau	3,5—7,5	1,9—4,1	2,1—3,9
PREEDY u. AITKEN	Fluorimetrie	Mann	0,07	0,07	0,15
		Urin			
BROWN	Colorimetrie	Mann	3—8,2	0—6,3	0,8—11 D 10 μg
BROWN	Colorimetrie	Frau	4—23	0—14	0—72 D 50 μg

Oestrogenausscheidung meist erhöht gefunden wird, gelingt dieser Nachweis mit den chemischen Methoden nur in schweren Formen oder nach Verabreichung hoher Oestrogenmengen (LYNGBYE).

Von 1 mg parenteral injiziertem Oestron oder Oestradiol konnte BROWN (1956) bei der gesunden Frau 27—59% als Oestriol und Oestradiol wieder im Urin nachweisen. Nach Injektion von Oestriol erscheinen 80% wieder als Oestriol im Urin. Die Ausscheidung wird erst im Laufe von 2—4 Tagen wieder normal. Nach Gabe von markiertem Oestradiol findet man 65—80% der Radioaktivität im Urin wieder (BEER, SANDBERG).

3. Ausscheidung

Die Oestrogenausscheidung bei Kindern ist bis zum 9.—10. Lebensjahr bei beiden Geschlechtern gleich (um 30 IE in 24 Std). Knaben steigen nur langsam etwas an, während sich die Ausscheidung bei Mädchen ab dem 11.—12. Lebensjahr stark bis auf Werte über 350 IE in 24 Std erhöht (NATHANSON 1941). Die chemisch bestimmten Werte betragen bei *Mädchen* im Alter zwischen 9 und 11 Jahren 0,9 μg Oestron, 0,5 μg Oestradiol und 1,0 μg Oestriol, für *Knaben* 0,6 μg Oestron, 1,1 μg Oestradiol und 0,2 μg Oestriol (PERSSON).

Bei der geschlechtsreifen *Frau* wechselt die Ausscheidung mit dem Cyclus, sie ist am niedrigsten nach der Periode, am höchsten um die Zeit der Ovulation und sinkt bis zum Eintritt der Menstruation langsam ab. Postmenstruell enthält der Urin: Oestron 2,8 μg, Oestradiol 0,7 μg, Oestriol 4,7 μg, zur Zeit der Ovulation: Oestron 20,1 μg, Oestradiol 7,9 μg, Oestriol 30,9 μg (BROWN) (s. Tabelle 5).

Wie die 17-Ketosteroide, steigen auch die Oestrogene im *Urin* bis etwa zum 30. Lebensjahr noch etwas an, um von da bis zum 50. langsam, von da an rascher abzufallen.

Bei *Männern* sind die Angaben je nach der angewandten Methodik verschieden. BROWN findet eine Gesamtmenge von 10 μg, die sich verteilt: Oestron 3—8 μg, Oestradiol 0—2 μg, Oestriol 1 μg. AITKEN und PREEDY erhalten mit der fluorimetrischen Methode: Oestron 2—4 μg, Oestradiol 2 μg, Oestriol 2 μg pro Tag. Im Alter fallen die Oestrogene weniger stark ab als bei den Frauen (Abb. 9).

Tabelle 6. *Herkunft und ungefähre Produktion von Oestrogenen im Organismus von Männern und nichtschwangeren Frauen. (Schätzung aus Ausscheidungsuntersuchungen und Bestimmungen des Oestrogengehaltes verschiedener Nahrungsmittel.) (Aus* DICZFALUSY *und* LAURITZEN 1961)

Herkunft	Oestrogen	Ungefähre Menge (μg/d)
Ovarien	17 β-Oestradiol, Oestron	50—300 je nach Cyclusphase
Hoden	17 β-Oestradiol	10—40
Nebennieren	Oestron (?)	10—40
Periphere Umwandlung aus Progesteron . .	Oestron	wahrscheinlich sehr kleine Mengen
Periphere Umwandlung aus Corticosteroiden	11 β-Hydroxy-17 β-oestradiol, Oestriol (?), 16-Epioestriol (?)[1]	keine quantitativen Angaben vorhanden, aber wahrscheinlich sehr kleine Mengen
Periphere Umwandlung aus Androgenen . .	17 β-Oestradiol, Oestron	niedrige Umwandlungsrate (0,05—0,5 %)
Nahrung	Steroide und nichtsteroide Verbindungen mit Oestronaktivität	10—300 ME/d (ungefähr 1—30 μg Oestronäquivalente) je nach Kostform[2]

[1] Von CHANG und DAO postuliert. Bisher nicht nachuntersucht.
[2] Sehr approximative Werte, teilweise auf veralteten Untersuchungen beruhend.

Biologisch bestimmt, findet PINCUS (1955) eine gleichmäßige Höhe zwischen 9—13 RE = 4,5—6,5 μg Oestronäquivalente in allen Altersgruppen.

Im *Blut* sind die mit den biologischen Methoden bestimmten Werte bei den einzelnen Autoren sehr unterschiedlich. 100—200 ME = 10—20 μg Oestronäquivalente (SIEBKE, FRANK). OERTEL findet mit der Brownschen Methode bei nicht Schwangeren 0,4—1,5 μg Oestron, 0,3—0,9 μg Oestradiol, 0,1—0,7 μg Oestriol (100 ml) (s. Tabelle 5).

DICZFALUSY u. Mitarb. u.a. (1957) messen dem Quotienten Oestriol: Oestron + Oestradiol (normal = 1:1) eine große Bedeutung bei. Normalerweise wird das C_{16}-substituierte Oestriol nicht im Ovar gebildet, sondern es entsteht erst als Umwandlungsprodukt im Stoffwechsel. Störungen desselben können unter Umständen durch eine Änderung des Quotienten angezeigt werden. Nach mehrtägiger Gabe von Oestrogenen steigt der Quotient bis auf 7:1 an.

Zur Errechnung der Gesamttagesproduktion ist man auf die Messung der Ausscheidung nach Injektionen und Implantationen von Oestrogenen und auf den biologischen Versuch des Schleimhautaufbaues von Kastraten, und ähnliche, in ihrer Gesamtheit schwer übersehbare Prüfungen angewiesen. Die in der Tabelle 6 angegebenen Werte dürfen daher nur als ungefähre Maße angesehen werden.

4. Synthetische Oestrogene

Die natürlichen Oestrogene haben ihre stärkste Wirksamkeit bei parenteraler Verabreichung, oral werden sie wohl resorbiert, erleiden aber wegen der raschen Inaktivierung in der Leber einen erheblichen Wirkungsverlust. Die in der Therapie gebräuchlichen synthetischen Oestrogene sind dagegen oral meist ebenso stark wirksam wie parenteral, da die Leber diesen Fremdkörper nur allmählich inaktivieren kann (s. Tabelle 7). Die chemische Struktur hat bei einem Teil der synthetischen Produkte mit den natürlichen nichts mehr gemein. Die meisten sind bifunktionell und haben die allgemeine Konfiguration $HO \cdot Aryl \cdot OH$ bzw. $HO \cdot Aryl \cdot Alkyl \cdot OH$. Trotzdem ist ihre biologische Wirkung praktisch gleich der der natürlichen Oestrogene. Experimentell sind besonders die Stilbene geprüft. Im Vaginalverhornungstest, im Uteruswachstumstest, Brustdrüsenwachstumstest, im Hypophysenhemmtest unterscheiden sie sich nicht. Auch der Einfluß auf den Stoffwechsel der Steroidhormone,

Tabelle 7. *Abhängigkeit der oestrogenen Dosis (kastrierte Ratte) von der Art der Zufuhr* [Hohlweg: Zbl. Gynäk. 71, 330 (1949)]

	Wirksame Dosis (μg)		
	parenteral	oral	Verhältnis parenteral/oral
Oestron	0,83	50	1:60
Oestriol	10	10	1:1
17β-Oestradiol . . .	0,1	40	1:400
17-Äthinyl-oestradiol	0,12	30	1:250
Diäthylstilboestrol .	0,5	2,5	1:5
Dienoestrol-acetat .	0,8	1,2	1:1,5

Tabelle 8.
Vergleichbare Dosen der verschiedenen Oestrogene beim Mensch. (L. S. Goodman und A. Gilman: The Pharmacological Basis of Therapeutics, Macmillan Company 1958, New York) [1]

Art der Verabreichung	Präparate	Niedrige Dosierung mg	Mittlere Dosierung mg	Hohe Dosierung mg
Oral	Diethylstilbestrol (1)	0,1—0,5	1,0—3,0	3,0
	Diethylstilbestrol Dipropionat (1)	0,1—0,5	1,0—3,0	5,0
	Hexestrol (1)	0,3—1,5	3,0—10,0	15,0
	Mestilbol (1)	0,3—1,5	3,0—10,0	15,0
	Promethestrol Dipropionat (1)	0,5—2,5	5,0—15,0	
	Estrol (1)	0,2—1,0	1,0—2,0	
	Estrogene Substanzen (H_2O-löslich) (1)	0,625	1,25—2,5	
	Benzestrol (1)	0,5—1,0	2,0—5,0	
	Dienestrol (1)	0,2—1,0	3,0—5,0	5,0
	Ethinyl Estradiol (1)	0,02—0,05	0,2—0,2	0,2
	Chlorotrianisen (1)	6,0—12,0	24,0—48,0	
Intramuskulär	Estradiol (1)	0,02—0,05	0,1—0,2	
	Estradiol Benzoat und Dipropionat (2)	0,05—0,1	0,1—0,2	
	Estron (1)	0,1—0,5	1,0—3,0	
	Estrogene Substanzen (1)	0,1—0,5	1,0—3,0	
	Diethylstilbestrol Dipropionat (2)	0,1—0,5	1,0—3,0	
Vaginal	Estron (1)	0,2	0,5	
	Estrogene Substanzen (H_2O-löslich) (1)	0,2	0,5	
	Benzestrol (1)		0,5	
	Diethylstilbestrol (1)	0,1	0,5	

(1) täglich; (2) dreimal pro Woche.

[1] Mit Genehmigung des Verlages.

des Schilddrüsenhormons, auf Grundumsatz, Sauerstoffverbrauch und Blutlipoide ist derselbe. In letzter Zeit ist man auf Verbindungen gestoßen, die nur noch Partiarfunktionen der ursprünglichen Oestrogene besitzen.

Therapeutisch werden wegen ihrer starken Oestrogenwirkung angewandt (s. Tabelle 8):

17α-Äthinyl-17β-Oestradiol = 17α-Äthinyl-Oestra-1,3,5(10)-trien-3,17β-diol. Parenteral besitzt es dieselbe Wirkung wie Oestradiol, oral ist es zehnmal stärker aktiv. Als stärkstes orales Oestrogen wird es praktisch nur in Form von Tabletten angewandt.

Dioxydiäthylstilben (Stilboestrol) ähnelt nur formal dem Oestradiol, oral gut wirksam.

Dioxydiäthylstilbendiphosphat, intravenös injizierbar.

Hexoestrol, oral und parenteral etwa gleich wirksam.

Dienoestron, angewandt in Form von Tabletten oder als wäßrige Suspension.

Eine weitere Gruppe gehört zur Reihe der α,β,β-Triaryl-äthylenderivate. Erwähnenswert ist hier das *Chlorotrianisen* = 1,1,2-Tri-para-anisyl-2-chlor-äthylen, das sich in seiner Struktur gänzlich von den Oestrogenen unterscheidet, biologisch aber noch eine typische, wenn auch schwache oestrogene Wirkung besitzt.

3-Methoxy-16α-methyl-1,3,5(10)-estatrien-16β, 17β-diol = Mytatriendiol, hat nur noch schwache oestrogene Eigenschaften, besitzt aber eine kräftige Stoffwechselwirkung, es senkt die Blutlipoide, besonders das Cholesterin, die Calciumbilanz wird positiv, Stickstoffretention ist nicht sicher festgestellt. Die Anwendung bei Frauen verspricht einen günstigen Einfluß auf die Osteoporose.

5. Antioestrogene

Die Androgene werden vielfach zu Unrecht als Antioestrogene bezeichnet. Die Wirkung von Testosteron ist dosisabhängig. Am Rattenuterus wirken niedere Dosen synergistisch mit Oestradiol und steigern das Uteruswachstum, hohe Dosen verhindern die Verhornung des Vaginalepithels und den Austritt von Leukocyten, der durch Oestron oder Oestriol erreicht wird.

Auch Progesteron hemmt die Wirkung der Oestrogene auf die Uterusschleimhaut, besonders die von Oestron (s. unter Progesteron). Bezüglich des Drüsenkörpers der Mamma ist eine ausgesprochen kongruente Wirkung beider Steroide zu verzeichnen.

Die progestional wirkenden 19-Nor-testosterone sind starke Antioestrogene, besonders das 17α-Äthyl-19-nor-testosteron. Die progestionalen Eigenschaften gehen den antioestrogenen nicht parallel, wie das 2-Methallyl-19-nor-testosteron zeigt, das wohl eine sehr starke progestionale, aber nur eine geringe antioestrogene Wirkung besitzt.

Schwache Oestrogene können die Wirkung biologisch aktiver hemmen. Geringe Änderungen am Molekül der synthetischen Oestrogene führt zu Verbindungen mit ausgesprochen antioestrogenen Eigenschaften. Dazu gehört Dimethylstilboestrol (ALBERT 1958), Äthylstilboestrol, Propylstilboestrol, Butoestrol (EMENS 1960). Auch dem Nichtsteroidoestrogen Chlorotrianisen ähnliche Verbindungen wie das MRL/41 (1-[p-(β-diäthylaminoäthoxy)-phenyl]-1,2-diphenyl-2-chloro-äthylen) und MER 25 wirken als leichte Antoioestrogene. Die Hemmung kann im Allen-Doisy-Test festgestellt werden, sie fehlt im Mitose- und im metabolischen Oestrogentest (EMMENS). Die Ergebnisse der Tierversuche dürfen nicht ohne weiteres auf den Menschen übertragen werden. Während MRL/41 bei der Ratte die Fruchtbarkeit und Gonadotropinproduktion hemmt, konnte bei anovulatorischen amenorrhoischen Frauen die Ovulation ausgelöst werden.

Diese kompetitiven Oestrogenantagonisten hätten beim Menschen ein weites Anwendungsfeld, wenn man die Wirkung der endogen gebildeten Oestrogene ausschalten will, so bei oestrogenabhängigen Geschwülsten, bei der isosexuellen Pubertas praecox des Mädchens, bei feminisierenden Geschwülsten des Mannes, bei der Hyperfollikulinämie der Frau. Die bis jetzt synthetisierten Derivate erwiesen sich beim Menschen als unsicher und bedingen nicht tragbare Nebenerscheinungen (Anorie, Erbrechen, Tremor, Ataxie). Beim Menschen wurden Derivate mit günstiger Stoffwechselwirkung versucht, wie Acytatriendol (positive Ca-Bilanz, Cholesterinsenkung) und Triparanol (MER 29) (Hemmung der Cholesterinsynthese). Die Biosynthese des Cholesterins wird durch Triparanol nur unvollständig blockiert, im Blut erscheint ein zweites Sterin (bis zu 30%), das 24-Dehydrocholesterin (Desmosterol), das mit den in der Klinik üblichen Bestimmungsmethoden (Digitoninfällung, Oxydation, Eisenchlorid) mitbestimmt wird und das im Stoffwechsel ähnlich gehandhabt wird wie Cholesterin selbst. Bei längerer Gabe wird die Synthese der Steroidhormone gestört.

X. Progesteron und Gestagene

Die ersten Beobachtungen einer humoralen Wirkung des Gelbkörpers stammen von L. Fraenkel, der 1902 bei Kaninchen kurz vor der Befruchtung das aus dem geplatzten Follikel entstandene frische Corpus luteum entfernte und feststellte, daß darauf die Einbettung des Eies in die Uterusschleimhaut unterblieb. Wird der Gelbkörper im Anfang der Schwangerschaft entfernt, so kommt es zum Abort oder zur Resorption der Frucht.

Das Hormon wurde fast gleichzeitig 1934 von Butenandt und Westphal. von Allen und Wintersteiner, von Hartmann und Wettstein und von Slotta u. Mitarb. dargestellt.

Es handelt sich um ein $C_{21} \alpha\beta$ ungesättigtes Diketon, ein 4-Pregnen-3,20-on (XIII), das aus Stigmasterin, aus Pregnandiol, aus Cholesterin, aus Dihydroandrosteron und besonders aus Sapogenien hergestellt werden kann. 1 IE entspricht 1 mg kristallinem Progesteron.

Die biologische Auswertung erfolgt nach dem Corner-Allen- bzw. Clauberg-Test.

Corner-Allen-Test. Weibliche Kaninchen werden 4—8 Std nach der Paarung kastriert. Die zu untersuchende Substanz wird den Tieren 5 Tage lang parenteral verabreicht. Am 6. Tag wird die Uterusschleimhaut histologisch untersucht. Eine Kanincheneinheit (KE) ist diejenige Menge, welche dieselbe Umwandlung der proliferierten Schleimhaut in die pseudogravide bewirkt wie 1 mg Progesteron.

Clauberg verwendet mit Follikelhormon vorbehandelte junge Kaninchen und nimmt die sekretorische Umwandlung der Uterusschleimhaut unter dem zu prüfenden Hormon als Test. Bei subcutaner Verabreichung lassen sich 0,6 mg, bei intrauteriner 0,7 μg Progesteron nachweisen. Eine Kanincheneinheit etwa 0,6 mg Progesteron.

Hooker-Forbes-Test. Hier wird nach bestimmten Kernveränderungen in den Stromazellen des Endometriums der kastrierten Maus gesucht. Minimaldosis bei subcutaner Injektion 125 μg, bei intrauteriner 0,002 μg. Da 17α-Hydroxyprogesteron, das an der Uterusschleimhaut keine progestionalen Eigenschaften hat, 60mal stärker wirkt als Progesteron, kann es sich nur um eine unspezifische Reaktion handeln.

Neben dem eigentlichen Corpus luteum-Hormon besitzt eine ganze Reihe anderer Steroide progesteronartige Wirkung. Dazu gehören besonders Testosteron, 17α-Methyltestosteron, das Androstendion und Desoxycorticosteron. Gegenüber dem Progesteron benötigt man von diesen Steroiden die 3—50fache Dosis.

In neuerer Zeit wurde eine Reihe von oral wirksamen Derivaten des Testosterons mit Progesteronwirkung hergestellt, so das 17α-Äthinyltestosteron (Pregneninolon), das parenteral $1/_3$ so stark wie Progesteron, oral dagegen viel stärker wirkt. Das 17α-Äthinyl-19-nor-testosteron, ein oral stark wirksames Gestagen, zeigt in allen biologischen Testen die typische Progesteronwirkung. Andere sind das 17α-Äthyl, bzw. das 17α-Methyl-19-nor-testosteron. Einführung einer Methylgruppe in 6α-Stellung wie beim 6α-Methyl-17α-hydroxyprogesteron erhöht den Wirkungsgrad bei parenteraler Gabe beträchtlich (10,5mal wirksamer als Progesteron). Eine ähnlich hohe gestagene Wirkung besitzt 1-Methyl-17α-äthinyl-19-nortestosteron.

1. Vorkommen und Verhalten im Stoffwechsel

Progesteron wird unter der Einwirkung von Prolactin vom Corpus luteum in der zweiten Hälfte des Cyclus sezerniert. Im Grafschen Follikel kurz vor der Ovulation wurden 49.4 μg, im Corpus luteum während des 2. und 3. Schwangerschaftsmonates 26—56 μg. am Ende der Schwangerschaft 6—10.4 μg/g Gewebe festgestellt (ZANDER 1954). Im Laufe der Schwangerschaft geht die Progesteronbildung auf die Placenta über, Ausscheidung am Ende zwischen 190—280 μg (ZANDER). Im Plasma der Frau beträgt der Gehalt nicht mehr als 5 μg/100 ml (s. Tabelle 3).

Im Ovarium ist das Progesteron ein normales Endprodukt der Hormonsynthese. Nach den histochemischen Untersuchungen von TAYLOR an Ratten wird es nicht nur vom lutealen Gewebe, sondern auch von den Theca- und interstitiellen Zellen gebildet. In der Nebennierenrinde und im Hoden ist Progesteron nur eine Zwischenstufe, im peripheren Blut des Mannes ist es nicht nachgewiesen. ICSH (LH) stimuliert den Follikelsprung und die Bildung des Corpus luteum, aber erst durch Prolactin (luteotropes Hormon, LTH) wird die Progesteronproduktion angeregt. Inwieweit dieser bei den Nagern nachgewiesene Regulationsmechanismus auch für den Menschen Gültigkeit hat, ist nicht sicher bekannt.

Injiziertes markiertes 4-C_{14}-Progesteron wird ziemlich fest an Serumalbumin gebunden. Die Halbwertszeit von exogenem liegt zwischen 4,9—11,5 min, die Umsatzgeschwindigkeit des endogen gebildeten wird auf 3,3 min geschätzt (PEARLMAN). Nur $1/_3$ der Radioaktivität erscheint im Urin. Die Inaktivierung erfolgt vorwiegend in der Leber. Das Hormon ist wirkungslos, wenn Kristalle in das Mesenterium oder in die Milz implantiert werden. Inkubiert man Progesteron mit Ratten- oder Kaninchenleber, dann verschwindet die für die α,β-ungesättigten Ketone charakteristische Absorption bei 240 mmμ (SAMUELS 1949). Die hauptsächlichsten Metaboliten des Progesterons sind das Pregnan-3α, 20α-diol=Pregnandiol und Pregnan-3α-ol-20-on. Nach intramuskulärer Injektion oder oraler Gabe werden nur 10—15% als Pregnandiol im Urin ausgeschieden. Dieser Betrag erhöht sich bei fortgesetzter Verabreichung auf 25—30%. Im Urin der Frau ist Pregnandiol nur in der zweiten Cyclushälfte nachweisbar (2—5 mg) (MARRIAN 1949), es fehlt beim Mann. Progesteron wird nicht zu 17-Ketosteroiden abgebaut.

2. Biologische Wirkung

Die wichtigste Wirkung entfaltet das Hormon an der Uterusschleimhaut. Nach vorangegangener Proliferation durch Follikelhormon wird die Schleimhaut durch Progesteron drüsig umgewandelt. Läßt man zur Zeit der Eieinbettung einen Fremdkörperreiz auf die Uterusschleimhaut einwirken, dann bilden sich die sog. Deciduome, das einnistende Ei wirkt offenbar als Fremdkörper (placenta-

698   F. HENI:

ähnliche Neubildungen). Bei kastrierten Frauen kann man durch nacheinander-
folgende Verabreichung von Follikelhormon und Progesteron eine Menstruationsblutung auslösen. Nach KAUFMANN benötigt man zum Aufbau der Schleimhaut
65 mg Oestradioldipropionat und 200 mg Progesteron. Auch die Schleimhaut
der Eileiter wird zur Proliferation angeregt.

Unphysiologisch hohe Dosen von Progesteron während der ersten Cyclusphase
unterdrücken die Eireifung und die Ovulation. Hohe Dosen hemmen in der
Hypophyse die Abgabe des Luteinisierungshormons (LH, ICSH) und wahrscheinlich auch des Follikelreifungshormons (FSH), da das Ovar bei monatelanger
Behandlung von Affen völlig atrophisch wird. Keinen Einfluß hat Progesteron
dagegen auf die Abgabe des Prolactins (LTH, lactogenes Hormon), das die Progesteronproduktion im Gelbkörper stimuliert. Progesteron ist das einzige bis jetzt
bekannte Steroidhormon, bei dem der sog. „feed-back Mechanismus" keine Gültigkeit hat.

Eine wichtige, therapeutisch noch zu wenig angewandte Eigenschaft des
Progesteron ist die Aufhebung der spezifischen Oestrogenwirkung auf Uterusschleimhaut und Vaginalepithel.

Gibt man zu 1 KE Progesteron — d.h. eine Menge, die die mit Oestrogenen
vorbehandelte Uterusschleimhaut des kastrierten Kaninchens in die sekretorische
Phase umwandelt — gleichzeitig 10 RE Follikelhormon, dann unterbleibt die
Umwandlung völlig. 0,02 mg Oestradiol heben die Fähigkeit zur Bildung von
Deciduomata von 1,5 mg Progesteron auf. Drei KE Progesteron verhindern die
Verhornung des Vaginaepithels der Maus durch 1 ME Follikelhormon, ebenso
die Öffnung der Vaginalmembran infantiler Mäuse durch Oestrogene. Hohe Doesen
hemmen das Wachstum des Uterus und verhindern die durch Oestrogengabe
im Kaninchenuterus entstehenden Fibromyome und Fibroide in der Bauchhöhle.
Dieser gegenseitige Antagonismus ist ein direkter, er wird nicht über die Hypophyse gesteuert und kommt den neuen synthetischen Progestinen in verstärktem
Maße zu.

Die Wirkung im Stoffwechsel ist gering. Progesteron erhöht bei hypophysektomierten Ratten die Wasserausscheidung, fördert den Aufbau von Knorpeln
und Knochen bei jungen Meerschweinchen, außerdem soll es bei kastrierten
Ratten eine Hypertrophie der Langerhansschen Inseln induzieren. Im Serum
steigert es die Aktivität der Cholinesterase beträchtlich.

E. Biologische Wirkung der Sexualhormone
I. Androgene Eigenschaften der Androgene

Zur Prüfung der biologischen Eigenschaften der Androgene stehen verschiedene Testverfahren zur Verfügung, die Aufschluß geben über die spezifischen
androgenen Eigenschaften und über die unspezifischen Wirkungen im Stoffwechsel. Am häufigsten angewandt werden:

1. Spezifische Teste

Der *Kapaunenkammtest*. Das Wachstum des Kammes von Leghornhähnchen
beginnt zwischen dem 10. und 15. Lebenstag, es fällt mit der Entwicklung der
Hoden und mit dem Auftreten von Gonadotropin in der Hypophyse zusammen.
Parenterale oder lokale Verabreichung von Testosteron bedingt eine vorzeitige
Entwicklung des Kammes. Der ausgebildete Kamm des erwachsenen Hahns
bildet sich nach Kastration oder nach Entfernung der Hypophyse bis zur Größe
desjenigen von weiblichen Hühnern zurück. Die Atrophie wird durch Verab-

reichung von Testosteron verhindert. Wahrscheinlich ist das ICSH das verantwortliche hypophysäre Hormon (NALBANDOR, BREUEMAN).

Tabelle 9. *Wirksamkeit männlicher Sexualhormone in verschiedenen Testen* (Nach W. DIR-SCHERL: „Die männlichen Sexualhormone". In Fermente, Hormone, Vitamine, Bd. II, 1960, Georg Thieme-Verl. Stgt., S. 325)[1]

	Inernat. Kapauneneinheit (intramuskuläre Injektion)	Percutane Kapauneneinheit	Mäuseeinheit im Vesiculardrüsentest	Ml.-E. (Colchinin-Mitosen-Test)
	μg	μg	μg	μg
Testosteron (4-Androsten-17β-ol, 3-on)	15	1—2	100	10
Androstendion (4-Androsten-3,17-dion).	100	0,2	350	500
Dehydro-epi-androsteron (5-Androsten-3β-ol 17-on)	300	—	> 1000	500
Androsteron (Androstan-3α-ol, 17-on)	100	2	> 2000	2000
Epi-Androsteron (Androstan-3β-ol-17-on)	700	15—20	1000	
Androstandion (Androstan-3,17-dion)	125	—	—	—
Ätiocholan-3β-ol-17-on und 17-Dihydroverbindungen		100 wirkungslos	> 2000	2000

[1] Mit Genehmigung des Verlages.

Vor der Pubertät der Tiere besteht das Corium des Kammes vorwiegend aus einem dichten fibrösen Bindegewebe. Mit der Pubertät entsteht ein lockeres Bindegewebe mit reichlich intercellulärer Grundsubstanz. Diese verhält sich färberisch metachromatisch, sie besteht vorwiegend aus Mucopolysacchariden und enthält Hyaluronsäure, Glucosamin und wahrscheinlich Chondroitinschwefelsäure. Der Einbau von markiertem $S_{35}O_4$ wird unter der lokalen Einreibung von Testosteron meßbar gesteigert. Wahrscheinlich werden die Fibroblasten des Bindegewebes durch Testosteron zur Bildung der Polysaccharide angeregt (MANCINI).

Vesiculardrüsentest von LÖWE *und* VOSS. Die Vesiculardrüsen sondern ein Sekret ab, das bei Tieren nach erfolgter Paarung zu einem Tropfen gerinnt. Nach Kastration wird die Drüse kleiner, das Drüsenepithel bildet sich zurück, die Sekretion versiegt. Zufuhr androgen wirksamer Stoffe bringt die Drüse wieder zum Wachstum. Wichtiger als die

Tabelle 10. *Vergleich der relativen Wirkung der Androgene im Samenblasentest jugendlicher Ratten und im Kapaunen-Kammtest* (Testosteron = 100 %). (R. J. DORFMAN und R. A. SHIPLEY: Androgens New York. John Wiley & Sons, 1956)[1]

	Relative Wirkung	
	Samenblasentest	Kapaunenkamm
4-Androsten-17-ol-3-on-Testosteron .	100	100
Androstan-17-ol-3-on	200	75
17-Methylandrostan-3,17-diol	50	50
Androstan-3,17-diol	33	75
4-Androsten-3,17-dion	20	12
Androstan-3,17-dion	14	12
5-Androsten-3,17-diol	14	3
Androstan-3,17-diol	10	2
Androstan-3-ol-17-on (Androsteron) .	10	10
Androstan-3-ol-17-on-Epiandrosteron .	7	12
5-Androsten-3,17-dion	5	3
17-Methyl-5-Androsten-3,17-diol (Methylandrostendiol)	3	16
5-Androsten-3-ol-17-on (Dehydroepiandrosteron)	3	2

[1] Mit Genehmigung des Verlages.

Gewichtszunahme ist die mikroskopische Messung der Zellhöhe und die Anzahl der Mitosen, die man durch Colchicin quantitativ sichtbar machen kann.

Musculus levator ani-Test. Nach Kastration bildet sich bei der Ratte die Muskulatur des Beckenbodens zurück. Verabreichung von Testosteron entwickelt sie wieder normal. Diese myotrope Eigenschaft des Testosterons wird über den Angriff im Eiweißstoffwechsel erklärt und als Maß der *anabolen* Wirksamkeit eines Steroids gewertet, obwohl die Ratte das einzige Tier ist, bei dem die Atrophie dieser Muskelgruppe eintritt.

Prostatatest. Am häufigsten verwandt wird die Größenzunahme der Prostata der kastrierten Ratte. Besonders empfindlich reagiert der ventrale Anteil der Prostata, dessen gewichtsmäßige Zunahme einen besseren Anhalt gibt als das Gesamtgewicht der Prostata.

Tabelle 11. *Androgene Wirkungsstärke verschiedener Steroide im Kapaunenkammtest* (Nach W. R. Nes: Steroid Hormones. In Medicinal Chemistry, S. 757, London: Interscience Publishers) [1]

Verbindung	Aktivität in I.U. [2]
Testosterone	15
17-Methylandrostan-17β-ol-3-one	15
Androstan-17β-ol-3-one	20
Androstane-3α, 17β-diol	20—25
17α-Methyltestosterone	25—30
5-Androstene-3α, 17β-diol	35
17-Methylandrostane-3α, 17β-diol	35
17α-Äthyltestosterone	70—100
Androsterone	100
5,6-Dehydroandrosterone	100
4-Androstene-3,17-dione	120
Androstane-3,17-dione	125
4,6-Androstadien-17β-ol-3-one	200
4-Androsten-3β-ol-17-one	150—200
Dehydroepiandrosterone	200
Androstan-17α-ol-3-one	300
Androstane-3α, 17α-diol	350
17-Epitestosterone	400
Androstane-3β, 17β-diol	500
5-Androstene-3β, 17β-diol	500
3-Epiandrosterone	700
13-Epiandrosterone	> 1000 oder inaktiv
Testan-3α-ol-17-one (etiocholanolone)	> 1000 oder inaktiv
3β-Chloro-5-androsten-17-one	> 1000 oder inaktiv
Testane-3α, 11β-diol-17-one	> 1000 oder inaktiv
4-Androsten-6β-ol-3,17-dione	> 1000 oder inaktiv
4-Androsten-6α-ol-3,17-dione	> 1000 oder inaktiv

[1] Mit Genehmigung des Verlages.
[2] Eine I.U. entspricht der Menge eines Steroids, die dieselbe Reaktion am Kamm hervorruft wie 100 μg Androsteron.

Die Schwierigkeit der Beurteilung der androgenen und anabolen Eigenschaften der natürlichen und der abgewandelten Androgene liegt darin, daß die Steroide in verschiedenen Testverfahren verschieden starke Wachstumsimpulse entfalten. Ein typisches Beispiel geben Testosteron und Dehydroepiandrosteron, wenn sowohl das Wachstum der ventralen Prostata als auch der Samenblasen der kastrierten Ratte als Test verwendet werden. 4 mg Testosteron erhöhen das Gewicht beider Organe um etwa das 7fache, während 4 mg Dehydroepiandrosteron das Gewicht der Prostata um das 3fache erhöht, auf die Samenblasen aber beinahe ohne Wirkung ist. Auch bei anderen Verbindungen ist das Wirkungsverhältnis Prostata: Samenblasen häufig nicht = 1.

Noch größere Unterschiede ergeben sich beim Vergleich des Hahnenkammtestes mit dem Prostata- bzw. Samenblasentest (vgl. Tab. 9—11).

Bei den synthetischen Androgenen gibt es Verbindungen, die an Rattenorganen deutlich androgen wirken, am Hahnenkamm ganz versagen. Bis jetzt hat man keine sichere Korrelation eines Testes am Tier zu den androgenen Eigenschaften beim Menschen feststellen können, so daß die experimentelle Prüfung eines Präparates auf möglichst breiter Basis erfolgen muß.

Beim Menschen scheint die Prüfung der *Talgdrüsenfunktion* eine einfache Möglichkeit zu eröffnen. Eine wichtige Eigenschaft der Androgene ist die Stimulierung des Wachstums der Talgdrüsen der Haut im Gesicht. Bis zur Pubertät sind sie nur rudimentär ausgebildet, erst mit der Pubertät wachsen sie stark. 5 mg Methyltestosteron oral führen beim präpuberalen Jungen im Laufe von 2 Wochen zu einem starken Wachstum der Talgdrüsen. STRAUSS u. Mitarb. schlagen vor, einfach mit Hilfe eines Filtrierpapiers, das über die Stirne geklebt wird und in dem nach 3 Std der Fettgehalt bestimmt wird, die Talgabsonderung zu messen.

Die biologische Androgenaktivität des Urins des Menschen wird vorwiegend durch Androsteron, das etwa $1/6$—$1/10$ so stark wirkt wie Testosteron, bestimmt. DEA und 11-Hydroxyandrosteron tragen nur wenig dazu bei. Die Ätiochloanolone sind unwirksam. Da sich der Gehalt des Urins an Androsteron während des Lebens beträchtlich ändert, ist die biologische Aktivität von 1 mg 17-Ketosteroid in verschiedenen Lebensaltern verschieden groß. Der Index — IE Androgene pro Milligramm 17-Ketosteroid — beträgt beim männlichen Geschlecht: bis 8 Jahre 0,2; bis 18 Jahre 2,9; bis 39 Jahre 3,7; bis 59 Jahre 3,4; bis 75 Jahre 2,9, beim Eunuchen 1,4. Bei Frauen zwischen 20—39 Jahre 3,6, zwischen 55—75 Jahre 1,8 (HAMILTON 1954).

Bei der biologischen Prüfung von Urinextrakten am Kapaunen findet CALLOW im Männer- und Frauenurin 26—29 IE je Liter, GALLAGHER (1937) im Tagesurin von Männern 63—69 IE, von Frauen 13—46 IE, bei kastrierten Männern 1—3,5 IE. Die biologischen Teste sind, abgesehen von speziellen Fragestellungen, ganz aufgegeben worden.

2. Wirkung auf die männlichen Genitalorgane

a) Hoden

Die Wirkung der Androgene auf den Hoden ist abhängig vom Lebensalter, in dem die Hormonbehandlung begonnen wird, von der angewandten Dosis, von der Art des Androgens, von der Dauer der Behandlung und von der Tierart, an der das Androgen getestet wird.

MOORE und PRICE (1937) fanden, daß sich die Hoden von jungen Ratten nach Injektion von Hodenextrakten verkleinern, es treten degenerative Veränderungen am Keimepithel auf. Sie sprachen die Vermutung aus, daß die Hemmung des Wachstums und der Entwicklung des Hodens unter den Androgenen auf eine Hemmung der Bildung und Abgabe von gonadotropem Hormon im Hypophysenvorderlappen zurückgeht, eine Annahme, die später von SELYE und FRIEDMANN; ZAHLER experimentell bestätigt wurde.

Die zahlreichen Untersuchungen der folgenden Jahre brachten etwas widersprechende Ergebnisse. Gibt man *Ratten* vor dem 40. Lebenstag Testosteron oder Androsteron oder Testosteronpropionat in der Dosis von 0,05—2,5 mg. dann nimmt das Hodengewicht deutlich ab, bei den niedrigen Dosen stärker als bei den hohen (—27 bis —72%). Die Spermiogenese ist arretiert und es treten degenerative Veränderungen am Keimepithel auf. Bei hohen Dosen (3 mg) reifen dagegen Spermatogonien zu Spermatozoen aus. Wenn die Behandlung statt um den 20. erst nach dem 60.—80. Lebenstag begonnen wird, sind die Veränderungen geringer, die Gewichtsabnahme des Hodens beträgt bei kleinen Dosen nur noch 15—24%, die Struktur ist wenig verändert (MOORE 1937, 1958, KORENCHERSKY, RUBINSTEIN). Hohe Dosen (3—10 mg) erhöhen sogar das Gewicht und regen die Tubuli an, die Spermiogenese bleibt erhalten.

Die Dosisabhängigkeit der Wirkung der Androgene auf das Kanälchenepithel ist ganz ausgesprochen. Man kann allgemein sagen, daß niedrige Dosen eine Kanälchenatrophie und starke Gewichtsabnahme hervorrufen. Unter hohen Dosen bleibt das Gewicht erhalten, es kann sich sogar etwas erhöhen, die Spermiogenese verläuft normal, immer sind aber die Leydigzellen atrophisch.

SELYE und FRIEDMANN (1941) unterschieden als erste die beiden wesentlichen Eigenschaften des Testosterons: Hemmung der Gonadotropinbildung im Hypophysenvorderlappen und Anregung der Spermiogenese. Die Hemmung des Hypophysenvorderlappens ist bei mittleren und hohen Dosen ausgeprägt, sie fehlt bei niedrigen, die spermiogenetische ist dagegen gebunden an hohe. Je nach der Empfindlichkeit der verwandten Tierart sind kleine Dosen wirkungslos (bei Ratten unter 0,01 mg Testosteron), sie hemmen weder den Vorderlappen, noch regen sie die Spermiogenese an. Mittlere Dosen (0,01—1,0 mg) hemmen nur die Gonadotropinbildung, hohe (über 1,0 mg Testosteron) hemmen die Gonadotropinbildung ebenso, regen aber darüber hinaus die Spermiogenese direkt an. Eine Bestätigung dieser Ansicht brachte die Implantation von Testosteron in das Hodengewebe (HOHLWEG 1946).

Wenn man eine Hormonmenge in den Hoden implantiert, die bei der hypophysektomierten Ratte nicht ausreicht, um die Spermiogenese zu erhalten, dann bleiben die Kanälchen in der Umgebung des Implantates voll funktionstüchtig. Eine größere Dosis gesunden Ratten implantiert, erhält die Spermiogenese im implantierten Hoden, während der nichtimplantierte atrophiert. Die Gewichtsunterschiede sind beträchtlich, 80 mg gegen 350 mg (HOHLWEG 1946). Auch nach der Hypophysektomie enthalten die Kanälchen um das Implantat reife Spermatozoen.

HOHLWEG u. Mitarb. erweiterten die früheren Implantationsversuche. Die Hoden von Ratten wurden durch zweimal 50 mg Dienoestroldiacetat pro Woche 11 Wochen lang, zur völligen Atrophie gebracht (Hodengewicht 56 mg gegen 327 mg). Wird den Tieren in einen Hoden 3 mg Testosteron implantiert, dann erholt sich im Laufe einiger Wochen die Spermiogenese praktisch vollkommen, Libido, Potenz und Fertilität dieser Rattenmännchen werden normal. HOHLWEG bezeichnet daher das ICSH und das Testosteron als die eigentlichen gametokinetischen Hormone, nicht das FSH.

Die stimulierende Wirkung der Androgene auf die Kanälchen wird besonders deutlich bei *hypophysektomierten* Tieren. NELSON (1937), WALSH, CUYLER und McCULLAGH konnten mit Androsteron die Atrophie der Kanälchen verhindern, während die Leydigzellen sich stark verkleinerten. In Versuchen von NELSON (1937) blieb die Spermiogenese noch 178 Tage nach der Hypophysektomie erhalten. Er konnte mit 3 mg Testosteron die Spermiogenese sogar wieder bis zu den Endstadien in Gang bringen, wenn die Androgenverabreichung erst 28 Tage nach der Hypophysektomie erfolgte. Die Tiere verhielten sich wie normale Ratten und zeugten gesunde Nachkommen. Neben Testosteron und Androsteron sind besonders Androstandion, Androstendion und Dehydroepiandrosteron spermiogenetisch wirksam (NELSON und MERCKEL). In den Ludwigschen Untersuchungen zu dieser Frage war der Kanälchendurchmesser etwas kleiner als normal, das Gewicht des Hodens gegenüber den Kontrollen erniedrigt und die Spermiogenese in den einzelnen Kanälchen unterschiedlich fortgeschritten. Die nicht ganz vollwertige spermiogenetische Wirkung der Androgene beim hypophysektomierten Tier zeigen auch Versuche von MASSON (1945) an jugendlichen Tieren. 40—60 g schwere Ratten wurden 10 Tage lang mit 2 mg Androgenen behandelt. Dabei erhöhte sich das Hodengewicht wohl von 300 mg zur Zeit der Hypophysektomie auf 381 mg unter Δ_5-Androstendiol-13β,17β-dipropionat, auf 364 mg unter 17-Methyltestosteron, auf 310 mg unter Testosteron, gegenüber unbehandelten, nicht hypophysektomierten Tieren mit einem Hodengewicht von 878 mg blieb das Hodenwachstum aber erheblich zurück. Pregnenolon war nicht, DHEA praktisch nicht wirksam. Für den völlig normalen Ablauf der Spermiogenese scheint eine ausreichende FSH-Stimulierung unerläßlich. In den bisherigen Untersuchungen ist besonders der Zeitfaktor in der Reifung der einzelnen Entwicklungsphasen nicht berücksichtigt worden.

Verabreichung von *Oestrogenen* in höheren Dosen wirkt auf den Hoden wie die Entfernung der Hypophyse. Die Atrophie der Leydigzellen und der Kanälchen schreitet rasch fort. SELYE und FRIEDMANN konnten die Kanälchenatrophie durch gleichzeitige Gabe von 1 mg Testosteron verhindern. Die Oestrogene wirken demnach nicht direkt auf den Hoden, sondern nur indirekt über die Hemmung der Gonadotropine.

Gibt man Androgene oder Oestrogene zusammen mit hypophysären Gonadotropinen, dann bleiben atrophische Veränderungen an den Hodenstrukturen aus (BOTTOMLEY und FOLLEY 1938 a, b).

Die spermiogenetischen Eigenschaften der Steroide gehen den eigentlichen androgenen — geprüft an Gewicht der Prostata und Samenblasen — nicht parallel (NELSON 1937). So verhalten sich z.B. Androstendiol (cis) und Methylandrostendiol in bezug auf den Hoden gleich, während das Gewicht der Samenblasen bei ersterem nur 25,1 mg, beim letzteren 152 mg beträgt. Der Dosiswirkungsunterschied der parenteral verabreichten Androgene und der physiologisch in den Leydigzellen gebildeten ist darin begründet, daß die in den Leydigzellen gebildeten die Kanälchen direkt in hoher Konzentration umspülen, im allgemeinen Kreislauf aber so stark verdünnt sind, daß die Hypophyse nicht oder nur wenig gehemmt wird. Parenteral gegebenes wird im Blut rasch verdünnt, so daß nur bei sehr hohen Dosen in den Hodenkanälchen die spermiogenetisch wirksame hohe Konzentration erreicht wird.

Der Mechanismus der spermiogenetischen Wirkung der Androgene ist nicht geklärt. TONUTTI (1955 b) unterscheidet die *Kontaktwirkung* von der Fernwirkung. Er nimmt an, daß die Androgene die Feinstruktur und Permeabilität der Kanälchenwand, die von maßgeblicher Bedeutung für die Ernährung des Samenepithels ist, erhalten bzw. wiederherstellen. Es würde sich demnach um eine unspezifische Wirkung handeln.

b) Rebound-Phänomen

Beim *Menschen* liegen erst seit wenigen Jahren größere Erfahrungen über die Wirkung des Testosterons vor.

1939 beobachtete HECKEL, daß sich nach Behandlung eines Mannes mit Testosteronpropionat eine Azoospermie entwickelte. Erst 1950 haben dann HELLER u. Mitarb. ausgedehnte Untersuchungen an Freiwilligen durchgeführt, wobei Hodenbiopsien vor der Testosteronbehandlung, am Ende derselben und 6—17 Monate danach gemacht werden konnten. Nach täglicher Injektion von 25 mg Testosteronpropionat über 24—91 Tage fanden sie bei acht Männern ein völliges Verschwinden der Leydigzellen, eine beträchtliche Verkleinerung des Durchmessers der Kanälchen, eine schwere Reifungshemmung der Spermiogenese mit Abstoßung des Keimepithels und eine beträchtliche Sklerohyalinose der Basalmembran und der Tunica propria. Acht Männer, denen 3—7 Tabletten zu je 75 mg Testosteron implantiert worden waren, zeigten geringere Veränderungen. Sechs Monate nach Absetzen des Testosterons war eine gewisse Erholung eingetreten. Bei fünf konnten noch nach 17 Monaten Probeexcisionen gemacht werden. Jetzt waren die Schäden völlig abgeklungen, ja bei jedem einzelnen war die Hodenstruktur besser als zu Beginn der Therapie. Nicht nur Leydigzellen und die Spermatogenese war wieder normal, sondern auch die Hyalinisierung, die die Kanälchen vorher zeigten, war verschwunden (*Rebound-Phänomen*).

Zahlreiche Autoren haben seither über die hochdosierte Testosterongabe beim Menschen berichtet. Heckel und McDonald behandelten 64 wegen Oligospermie, von denen 36 verfolgt werden konnten. 23 zeigten das Rebound-Phänomen, einer erst nach 72 Wochen, fünfmal wurde die Ehefrau gravid, bei zweien erreichte die Zahl der Spermatozoen nicht mehr den Ausgangswert. Charny berichtet 1959 über 168 ein- und mehrmals behandelte sterile Männer mit Spermienzahlen von 0—20 Mill./cm$_3$. Im Gesamten besserten sich 20,2% (mindestens 20 Mill. Spermatozoen je Kubikzentimeter), 73,3% blieben gleich oder stiegen nur wenig an, bei 6,5% wurden die Ausgangswerte nicht mehr erreicht, zwei bekamen eine Azoospermie. Testosteron wurde zweimal wöchentlich in der Dosis von 50—75 mg oder als Depot — 300 mg alle 14 Tage — bis zu einer Gesamtdosis um 2700 mg gegeben. Nach 1500 mg verschwinden die Spermatozoen aus dem Ejaculat, bei Ausgangswerten unter 5 Mill. schon nach 1000 mg. Zwei Monate nach Beendigung treten die Spermien wieder auf, in Einzelfällen erst nach 3 Monaten, um rasch anzusteigen, häufig über den Ausgangswert, aber nur bei 20,2% über 20 Mill./cm^3 bei 40% normal beweglichen, d.h. über die Mindestmenge eines eben Fertilen. Der Anstieg hielt im Durchschnitt 2 Monate an. Die wiederholte Kur erreicht manchmal mehr als die einmalige. Von neun sprachen vier auf eine zweite Kur, von den fünf restlichen zwei auf eine dritte gut an. Die Indikation zur Testosteronkur darf nicht allein aus der Analyse des Ejaculates erfolgen, sondern es muß bioptisch vorher sichergestellt sein, daß es sich um eine reversible Veränderung handelt. Fälle mit verringertem Kanälchendurchmesser, intratubulärer Sklerose, Hyalinisierung, Fibrose der Basalmembran und des peritubulären Gewebes haben eine ungünstige Prognose und sollten nicht behandelt werden, da die Gefahr der Azoospermie gegeben ist (Charny 1959).

Heller sah eine Steigerung der Spermiogenese bei 19%, McDonald bei 21%, das sind hohe Zahlen, wenn man die schlechte Ausgangslage in Betracht zieht. Heinke und Tonutti behandelten 19 Patienten mit durchschnittlicher Dosis von 1200 mg Testosteronönanthat in etwa 9 Wochen. In etwas weniger als der Hälfte der Fälle trat Azoospermie mit nachfolgender Steigerung der Spermatogenese ein. Bei den übrigen fiel wohl die Spermienzahl ab, der Wiederanstieg blieb aber aus oder ging nur zögernd und in geringem Ausmaß vonstatten. Zweimal fehlte der Abfall der Spermien, einmal erfolgte trotzdem ein deutlicher Anstieg. Die Testosterondosen, die zu einer Azoo- oder Oligospermie führten, waren bei den einzelnen Menschen verschieden. Nach den bioptischen Untersuchungen erholt sich die Funktion der Leydigzellen vor derjenigen des Samenepithels. Neben der Änderung der Zahl der Spermien führt die Testosteronzufuhr auch zu einer Änderung im Cytogramm.

Wie im Tierexperiment hemmt Testosteron auch beim Menschen die Bildung und Abgabe von FSH und ICSH in der Adenohypophyse. Es entsteht ein sekundärer Hypogonadismus temporärer Art mit Inaktivierung der Leydigzellen und Erlöschen der spermiogenetischen Aktivität der Kanälchen. Ihr Durchmesser verkleinert sich, die Wand verdickt, nur Spermatogonien und einzelne Spermatocyten bleiben erhalten. Die Sertolizellen treten stark hervor, sowohl ihre Kerne als auch ihre faserigen Plasmaleiber werden in das Lumen hineingezogen (Heinke und Tonutti). Diese regressive Phase, die durch eine Azoospermie gekennzeichnet ist, wird nach einigen Wochen von einer progressiven abgelöst, in der die Spermiogenese wieder voll, ja sogar in vermehrtem Maße wieder aufgenommen wird (Rebound-Phänomen). Der plötzliche Wegfall der künstlichen Testosterongabe senkt den endogenen Androgenspiegel praktisch auf Null, da die Leydigzellen in der Zwischenzeit atrophisch geworden sind. Das Hypophysenzwischenhirnsystem reagiert darauf mit einem langanhaltenden Anstieg der Gonadotropinproduktion, der die progressive Phase auslöst.

Die beim Menschen verwandten Dosen liegen zwischen 25 mg täglich, 75 mg zweimal wöchentlich, 300 mg Depot alle 14 Tage über Monate. Azoospermie tritt nach einer Gesamtmenge von 1000—1800 mg Testosteronpropionat ein.

Vergleicht man diese Dosen mit den im Tierexperiment gegebenen, dann bewegt man sich nur in den niedrigen, die über die Hypophyse sowohl die ICSH- als auch die FSH-Abgabe hemmen, während die Kontaktwirkung noch fehlt. Um die Spermiogenese direkt zu beeinflussen, wären — verglichen mit der Ratte (200 g Gewicht 3—10 mg Testosteronpropionat) — bei einem 70 kg schweren Menschen 1050—3500 mg täglich notwendig. Das Rebound-Phänomen kann auch mit Choriongonadotropin und mit den Oestrogenen ausgelöst werden.

c) Prostata

Nach Kastration bildet sich die *Prostata* bei der Ratte, dem Meerschweinchen und dem Menschen zurück, bei den Nagern nur, wenn sie nach der sexuellen Reifung und nach der Involution der X-Zone der Nebennierenrinde vorgenommen wird.

MOORE, GALLAGHER und KOCH haben als erste gezeigt, daß diese Involution bei Meerschweinchen, Ratten und Affen durch die Verabreichung von Androgenen verhindert werden kann.

Beim Menschen beginnt die Prostata mit dem Penis zu wachsen. Die Drüse vergrößert sich anfangs nur langsam und erreicht erst gegen Ende der Pubertät ihre volle Größe. Unter dem Einfluß der Androgene entfalten sich die Drüsen- alveolen, das Epithel erhöht sich, Sekretgranula treten auf, der Golgiapparat wird sichtbar, das Epithel beginnt zu sezernieren.

Bei der Ratte besteht die Prostata aus gefalteten Alveolen, die in ein lockeres bindegewebiges Stroma eingebettet sind. Die Acini wechseln stark an Größe, das Epithel ist säulenartig angeordnet und sitzt einer Basalmembran auf. Die runden oder ovalen Kerne haben einen gut färbbaren Nucleolus, der an der Basis sitzt. Zwischen dem Kern und dem Lumen liegt eine leuchtend helle Zone, die mit der Lage des Golgi-Apparates zusammenfällt. Hier vollziehen sich die ersten Zeichen der Kastration.

Vier Tage nach Entfernung beider Hoden treten die ersten Erscheinungen auf. Der Durchmesser der Acini verringert sich, das sekretorische Epithel flacht etwas ab, Veränderungen, die man noch nicht auf den Ausfall der Androgene beziehen kann. Aber am vierten Tag ist die helle Aera über dem Zellkern nur noch schwach zu sehen oder in der Mehrzahl der Zellen schon ganz verschwunden. Nach 10 Ta- gen sind die Erscheinungen stärker ausgeprägt, der Durchmesser der Acini hat weiter abgenommen, das Epithel ist beträchtlich niedriger geworden und das intertubuläre Bindegewebe erscheint vermehrt.

Schon nach 20 Tagen ist das Endstadium erreicht, das Epithel hat nur noch die Hälfte oder ein Drittel der Höhe der Kontrollen, das Cytoplasma ist blaß, zeigt Vacuolen, die Kerne sind klein, liegen eng aneinander, die Nucleolen fehlen. Im Gegensatz dazu ist das interacinöse Bindegewebe vermehrt, wahrscheinlich nur als Folge der Schrumpfung des Epithels.

In seinen ersten Untersuchungen hat MOORE selbst hergestellte Extrakte aus Hodengewebe zum Wiederaufbau des Gewebes benützt. Mit diesen und mit Testosteron konnte er die Folgen der Kastration durch laufende Injektion ver- hindern und eine völlig atrophische Prostata — 30—100 Tage nach der Kastra- tion — in etwa 20 Tagen wieder auf den normalen Stand bringen. Der ventrale

Prostatalappen ist besonders empfindlich auf die Androgene. Seine Gewichtszunahme beim infantilen und hypophysektomierten Tier wird daher zur Bestimmung des ICSH verwendet, beim kastrierten zur Festlegung der Wirkungsstärke
von Testosteron und seiner Derivate. Beim Menschen ist die palpatorisch leicht
feststellbare Größe und Konsistenz der Prostata bis zum 45. Lebensjahr ein
guter Maßstab der Androgenproduktion. Bis zur vollen Entwicklung des Organs
beim Kastraten vergehen Monate.

HUGGINS hat beim Hund durch eine einfache operative Maßnahme die Möglichkeit zur genauen quantitativen und qualitativen Erfassung des Prostatasekretes geschaffen. Die normale Sekretionsrate bleibt in der Gefangenschaft
wochenlang ungefähr gleich, die in Gefangenschaft beobachtete Hodenatrophie
ist beschränkt auf das Keimepithel und beeinflußt die innere Sekretion und das
Prostatasekret nicht. Die Menge des Prostatasekretes beim ausgewachsenen
Hund ist unabhängig von der Größe der Drüse. Nach Kastration sinkt die
Sekretion rasch ab, die sistiert nach 7—23 Tagen vollständig. Durch Testosteron-
Propionat kann sie wieder hergestellt werden. Wenn die Prostata wieder aufge-
baut ist, genügen beträchtlich kleinere Mengen von Androgenen, um sie zu erhalten.

d) Samenblasen

Auch die *Samenblasen* erleiden regressive Veränderungen. Größe, Gewicht,
grober anatomischer Bau sind keine befriedigenden Indicatoren, wohl aber die
Größe und Struktur der Epithelzellen selbst. Normalerweise sind die Zellen
hoch und schmal (25—$35\,\mu$) mit einem großen, ovalen, basal liegenden Kern.
Lumenwärts liegen im Protoplasma stark lichtbrechende und gleichmäßig verteilte sekretorische Granula.

Schon 2 Tage nach der Kastration ist die Zellhöhe auf $11\,\mu$ reduziert, mit
Hämatoxilinfärbung sieht man keine Spur von Sekretionsgranula mehr. Diese
verschwinden schon im Laufe von 24 Std. Die Reduktion der Zellhöhe, Schwund
des Zellkerns, Verlust des Golgi-Apparates setzen sich fort, bis nach 10 Tagen
das Endstadium des Gewebsschwundes erreicht ist. Verabreichung von Hodenextrakten oder von Testosteron stellt die Drüse, das Epithel und die Zellstruktur
wieder völlig her. Schon 10 Std nach Testosterongabe ist die O_2-Aufnahme des
Epithels gesteigert.

Bei kastrierten Tieren steht die Höhe des Epithels, die Zahl der Mitosen,
Größe und Gewicht des Organs in strenger Abhängigkeit von der Menge des
zugeführten androgenen Hormons und der Dauer seiner Einwirkung. Die Reak-
tion der Samenblasen ist daher einer der besten biologischen Teste zum Nachweis der Androgenwirksamkeit eines Steroids (BURROWS 1945; LÖWE). Bei der
Maus hat das Organ zur Zeit der Pubertät seine größte Empfindlichkeit. Das
Sekret der Samenblasen bildet die Hauptmenge des Ejaculates, sein wichtigster
Bestandteil ist Fructose, die von den Spermien als Energiespender benötigt wird.
Volumen und Fructosegehalt können unter bestimmten Voraussetzungen als Maß
der Androgenproduktion verwendet werden (MANN 1946 und 1954). Gibt man
kastrierten Ratten oder Mäusen Androgene in einer Dosis, die das atrophische
Epithel nicht anregen, dann werden diese wirksam, wenn gleichzeitig Oestrogene
zugefügt werden (BIDDULPH, SELYE 1941). Beim Menschen entfalten sich die
Samenblasen mit dem ersten Beginn der Pubertät. Das Organ scheint, wie bei
Mäusen, um diese Zeit besonders androgenempfindlich zu sein.

e) Vas deferens, Epididymis

Vas deferens, Epididymis, Cowper-Drüse und die präputialen Drüsen atrophieren nach der Kastration. Im Nebenhoden und im Ductus deferens erniedrigt

sich die Höhe des Epithels, die Cilien degenerieren, der Kanälchenquerschnitt verengt sich. Im Nebenhoden vermehrt sich das Bindegewebe, im Vas deferens atrophieren die Muskelschichten. Auch die Cowperschen Drüsen und die Präputialdrüsen atrophieren nach der Kastration und können durch Androgene wieder angeregt werden (SHAY, ZUCKERMAN 1938). Die Oestrogene wirken auch an diesen Geweben vorwiegend auf das Stroma, während das Epithel der Ausführungsgänge verhornt und metaplasiert.

f) Fermente und Sekrete

Das Epithel der Prostata des Erwachsenen enthält große Mengen einer *Phosphatase* mit stärkster Aktivität bei pH 5,0, daneben geringe Mengen einer alkalischen. Während der Kindheit und im Jugendalter ist die Konzentration sehr gering, erst mit der Pubertät steigt der Gehalt an, nach Kastration verschwindet das Ferment. Verabreichung von Testosteron normalisiert wieder. Die sekretorische Leistung der Drüsenzellen steht in direkter Abhängigkeit vom Gehalt an saurer Phosphatase und diese wiederum von der Höhe der zirkulierenden Androgene. Unter Oestrogengabe vermindert sich der Gehalt ebenso stark wie nach der Kastration (MANN 1947 u. 1954; MACLEOD, HUMPHREY 1948 u. 1949).

Dauernde Vermehrung der sauren Phosphatase im Blut findet sich nur bei Metastasierung eines Prostatacarcinoms in die Knochen und die Lymphknoten (HUGGINS u. Mitarb. 1940). Vorübergehende Erhöhungen des Serumtiters kann auch nach Operationen, Palpation und Verletzungen der Prostata vorkommen.

Die alkalische Phosphatase wird im Knochen gebildet, sie ist ein Maßstab für die Umbauvorgänge im Knochen. Ihre Vermehrung ist nicht spezifisch für das Prostatacarcinom, sie kann aber bei ausgedehnten osteoblastischen Metastasen beträchtlich erhöht sein. Nach Kastration und nach Verabreichung von Oestrogenen sinkt die saure Phosphatase rasch auf normale Werte ab, während die alkalische sich vorübergehend erhöht, um erst später wieder abzusinken. Dieses Verhalten wird seit den Arbeiten von HUGGINS (1940) als Maßstab für die Wirksamkeit der Behandlung des Prostatacarcinoms genommen. Erhöht sich eine schon vorher hohe alkalische Phosphatase unter der therapeutischen Gabe von Diäthylstilboestrol, dann kann dies als Bestätigung für das Vorliegen eines Prostatacarcinoms gewertet werden. Normale Phosphatasewerte schließen ein metastasierendes Prostatacarcinom nicht aus, die Erhöhung findet sich in etwa 60%. Neuerdings wird gesagt, daß die Verfolgung der Serum-Aldolase zuverlässiger sei.

Im Sekret der Prostata findet sich noch die *Citronensäure* in hoher Konzentration. Diese ist ebenfalls abhängig von der Androgenproduktion. Die Prostata enthält außerdem eine Reihe von proteolytischen Fermenten, von denen das *Fibrinolysin* klinisch das wichtigste ist. Bei metastasierenden Prostatacarcinomen kann es in großer Menge in die Blutbahn gelangen und eine schwere hämorrhagische „Diathese" mit dem Bild einer Afibrinogenämie vortäuschen.

Das Epithel der *Samenblasen* bildet *Fructose*, den Energiespender der Spermatozoen, *Ergothionin*, eine seltene Aminosäure und mehr alkalische als saure Phosphatase. Die Produktion dieser Stoffe ist ebenfalls von der Höhe des Testosteronspiegels abhängig, NOWAKOWSKI u. a. benützen den Gehalt des Ejaculates an Fructose als biologisches Maß der Androgenproduktion. In Prostata und Samenblasen steht noch der Gehalt an Succindehydrogenase und Succinoxydase in Abhängigkeit von der Androgenkonzentration des Blutes (DAVIS u. Mitarb.).

Wenig erforscht ist die Bedeutung des autonomen Nervensystems für die Funktion des Epithels von Prostata und Samenblasen. Abgesehen davon, daß mit Adrenolytika und Ganglienblockern behandelte Hochdruckkranke über Abnahme oder Verlust von Libido und Potenz klagen, kann auch die Sekretion von Prostata und Samenblasen völlig versiegen.

3. Wirkung auf die weiblichen Genitalorgane
a) Uterus und Adnexe

Die Atrophie des *Uterus* nach der Kastration kann bei Ratten und anderen Nagern durch Gabe von 1 mg Testosteronpropionat in Grenzen gehalten werden. Im Myometrium entwickeln sich umschriebene Bezirke mit Fibrosierung, nach längerer Gabe entstehen Fibromyome. Unter hohen Dosen (über 2 mg) entwickeln sich bei kastrierten, mit Oestrogenen vorbehandelten Ratten typische progestionale Schleimhautveränderungen (MAZER). Bei einigen synthetischen Testosteronderivaten ist diese progestionale Eigenschaft sehr verstärkt. In der Menopause löst Testosteron eine Verhornung des Vaginalepithels aus, wie sie normalerweise nur durch Oestradiol zu erreichen ist.

An den *Fallopschen Tuben* wird der Tonus und die Kontraktilität erhöht. Die nach Kastration eintretende Atrophie der präputialen Drüsen wird verhindert. Die Paraurethraldrüsen, das Analogon der Prostata des Mannes bei der Frau, sind gegenüber Androgenen empfindlicher als gegenüber Oestrogenen.

Die Klitoris vergrößert sich unter der Anwendung synthetischer Androgene und der pathologischen Mehrbildung von endogenen. Neben Testosteron sind auch Androsteron, 4-Androstendion, 5-Androstendiol und Dehydroepiandrosteron wirksam.

Der Einfluß auf das *Brustdrüsengewebe* wechselt je nach den eingehaltenen Versuchsbedingungen. Mit großen Dosen kann die Sekretion der lactierenden Mamma in wenigen Stunden unterbrochen werden. So genügen bei der Frau 50—100 mg Testosteronpropionat, um im Laufe von 24—48 Std die Lactation beträchtlich zu hemmen. Dauerbehandlung mit mittleren Dosen führt das Drüsengewebe zur Atrophie.

Die *synergistische Wirkung* des männlichen und des weiblichen Keimdrüsenhormons auf die Genitalorgane ist bei den kleinen Nagern und sonstigen Laboratoriumstieren besser untersucht als beim Menschen. KORENCHEVSKY u. Mitarb. (1940) konnten in zahlreichen Experimenten zeigen, daß bei der männlichen und weiblichen Ratte ein völlig normaler Genitaltrakt nur bei gleichzeitiger Verabreichung von männlichem und weiblichem Hormon aufgebaut wird.

Verschiedene experimentelle Beobachtungen weisen darauf hin, daß kurzdauernde Behandlung mit Testosteron in kleinen bis mittleren Dosen die Sekretion des Hypophysenvorderlappens in dem Sinne ändert, daß mehr FSH als LH abgegeben wird. Die einmalige Gabe von 1—10 mg Testosteron regt bei jugendlichen Ratten und Mäusen die Follikelreifung an. Beim Menschen ist diese Wirkung nicht gesichert.

b) Ovarium

Behandelt man Nager über mehrere Wochen und Monate, dann entwickelt sich eine Atrophie des *Ovars*. Follikelreifung und Ovulation sistieren, die Cyclen hören auf, die Zahl der interstitiellen Zellen geht zurück und das Gewicht des Ovars vermindert sich. Die Atrophie erreicht man bei der Ratte mit 1 mg Testosteronpropionat täglich über eine Woche, beim Meerschweinchen mit 4 mg täglich, bei der Maus mit 0,02 mg täglich, bei Affen mit 25 mg zweimal in der Woche und bei der Frau mit 150 mg oder mehr pro Woche. Unter 50 mg Testosteronpropionat pro Woche bleibt der Cyclus im allgemeinen unbeeinflußt.

Gibt man in der präovulatorischen Phase im Laufe von 8—14 Tagen sehr hohe Dosen — 600—1000 mg —, dann wird die Ovulation und die Ausbildung eines Corpus luteum verhindert. In der postovulatorischen wird dagegen die Funktion des Corpus luteum nicht beeinflußt.

Die Ursache des Funktionsausfalls des Ovars beruht in der Blockierung der Gonadotropinsekretion des Vorderlappens. Wie der Hoden, so behält auch das Ovar seine Reaktionsfähigkeit auf parenteral zugeführtes Gonadotropin unter der gleichzeitigen Gabe von Androgenen (CARTER u. Mitarb., LAQUEUR u. Mitarb. 1942: PARKES u. ZUCKERMAN 1938; PAPANICOLAOU u. Mitarb. 1939; ROBSON, ZUBLIN).

II. Oestrogene Eigenschaften der Oestrogene

1. Spezifische Teste

Der gebräuchlichste Test baut sich auf der spezifischen Wirkung des Follikelhormons, die Vaginalschleimhaut von Nagern zur Proliferation zu bringen, auf. Die celluläre Proliferation wird automatisch in die Verhornung übergeführt. Diese Eigenschaft benützt der bis jetzt fast ausschließlich zur Prüfung angewendete Allen-Doisy-Test. Eine Mäuseeinheit (ME) entspricht der Menge Oestrogen, die bei 50% kastrierter Mäuse ein reines Schollenstadium in der Vagina (Oestrus) herbeiführt, eine Ratteneinheit (RE) der Menge, die bei kastrierten Ratten den Oestrus auslöst. 24 Std nach Einbringen von Oestrogenen in die Vagina oder nach parenteraler Verabreichung sind die Mitosen des Epithels erheblich vermehrt, ihre Zunahme läßt sich nach Colchicingabe genau bestimmen. Dieser Mitosetest von MARTIN und CLARINGBOLD (1958a) ist ebenso spezifisch wie der Allen-Doisy-Test, aber viermal genauer und zehnmal empfindlicher als dieser. Das proliferierte Epithel reduziert 2-3-5-Triphenyltetrazoliumchlorid zu Formazan, das sich leicht aus der Schleimhaut auswaschen und colorimetrisch bestimmen läßt (EMMENS u. Mitarb. 1958 u. 1960). Dieser Tetrazoliumtest ist gleich empfindlich wie der Mitosetest. Bei der Frau kann die Einwirkung der Oestrogene am Verhalten der Epithelien der Vagina festgestellt werden (PAPANICOLAOU 1936).

2. Wirkung auf die weiblichen Genitalorgane

a) Uterus

Am Uterus bewirken die Follikelhormone eine starke Vergrößerung des Organs und die Proliferation der Uterusschleimhaut. Bei infantilen Ratten nimmt das Uterusgewicht nach Injektion von 0,5 g Oestradiol im Laufe von 24 Std um 120% zu. Auch bei der kastrierten Frau wird das Uteruswachstum und die Proliferation der Schleimhaut angeregt. Nachfolgende Behandlung mit Corpus luteum-Hormon (Progesteron) wandelt die Proliferationsphase in die Transformationsphase um. Eine ME und eine RE sind sehr kleine Einheiten. Um das Wachstum des Uterus und der Uterusschleimhaut bei Ratten und Mäusen zu erreichen, ist die 10—100fache, ja sogar 200fache Menge notwendig. Daraus geht hervor, daß der Schwellenwert der einzelnen Erfolgsorgane verschieden groß ist. Wie bei den anderen Hormonen, bestehen auch beträchtliche Unterschiede in der Stärke der Wirkung bei den einzelnen Tierarten.

Obwohl die Oestrogene im Gewebe verhältnismäßig gleichmäßig verteilt sind, wirken sie sich doch nur auf ganz spezifische Organe und Gewebssubstrate aus. Das Ansprechen des Uterus auf eine Oestradiolkonzentration von 2×10^{-9} M in vitro ist ohne die Annahme spezifischer Receptoren nicht verständlich. Ausführliche Übersichten haben SZEGO (1953) und ROBERTS (1953a) und PINCUS (1955b) gegeben.

ROBERTS und SZEGO (1953b) finden im Uterus zuerst eine Hyperämie, dann eine Steigerung der Permeabilität der Uteruscapillaren und Aufnahme von extracellulären Elektrolyten und Wasser (Induktionsphase). Die erste Phase, die „Akkumulationsphase", reicht von der 6. bis zur 24. Std und ist charakterisiert durch den Anstieg der Ribonucleinsäure (RNA), der mit einer Vermehrung des Eiweißgehaltes verbunden ist. Die Zunahme der Desoxyribonucleinsäure spiegelt die Zunahme der Zellen und die Steigerung der mitotischen Aktivität wider. Erst in den letzten Jahren konnte die Steigerung des Einbaues von Aminosäuren in Eiweiß bewiesen werden. Die einmalige Gabe von 10 μg Oestradiol erhöht den Einbau von Glycin-2-C 14 in den ersten 12 Std stark, nach 20 Std sinkt er wieder ab, eine zweite und dritte Injektion erhöhen den Einbau weiter. Neben Glycin sind auch Alanin, Serin, Lysin, Tryptophan geprüft.

In den ersten 4 Std ist sowohl die aerobe als auch die anaerobe Glykolyse gesteigert, ohne daß mehr Sauerstoff verbraucht wird. Erst in der RNA-Akkumulationsphase erhöht sich die Atmungsgröße mit der Glykolyse. In den ersten Stunden wird also der Tricarbonsäurecyclus nicht in Anspruch genommen. Bemerkenswert ist auch die Steigerung der Umwandlung von Acetat in Cholesterin, die nach 20 Std das 30fache beträgt, auch die Synthese der Fettsäuren wird erhöht.

Nach Kastration ist der Gehalt an Ribonucleinsäure (RNA) sehr niedrig. Schon 6 Std nach Verabreichung von Oestradiol steigt er rasch an, auch der Einbau von radioaktivem Sauerstoff in Thimin und Uridin, von radioaktivem CO_2 in Adenin erhöht sich auf über 150% des Ausgangswertes.

Bei der Präzisierung dieser verschiedenartigen Wirkungen im Stoffwechsel des wachsenden Uterusgewebes hat man den Einfluß von Oestradiol auf einzelne Fermentsysteme genauer untersucht. Die Serin-Aldolase, die Serin in Glycin umwandelt, erhöht ihre Aktivität beträchtlich. In Uterus und Placenta wird nach Zugabe von Oestriol die lösliche phosphornucleotidgebundene Isocytricdehydrogenase angeregt (MUELLER). In vitro sind hierbei schon 0,001 γ Oestradiol pro Kubikzentimeter Inkubationsmedium wirksam. Das Enzym ist nicht an Mikrosomen angeheftet, sondern liegt frei im Protoplasma. Oestradiol-17α, Stilboestrol wirken als Inhibitoren. Neben Oestradiol-17β hat Oestriol die stärkste stimulierende Eigenschaft auf das Ferment. Während VILLEE annimmt, daß die Oestrogene die Isocytricdehydrogenase nur aktivieren und dadurch den Ablauf der Reaktion Isocytrat + oxydiertes DPN $\rightleftarrows$ reduziertes DPN + Alpha-Ketoglutarat + CO_2 in Richtung des Alpha-Ketoglutarat verschieben, haben neuere Untersuchungen von TALALAY eine direkte Teilnahme des Steroides im Sinne eines Coenzyms an der Reaktion wahrscheinlich gemacht (s. S. 658).

Die proliferative Wirkung der Oestrogene am Vaginalepithel und am Endometrium kann durch Androgene gehemmt werden, das Verhältnis Oestrogen zu Androgen muß jedoch mindestens 1:30 bis 1:50 betragen. Diese Eigenschaft macht man sich bei der Behandlung der Endometriose und der Mastopathia chronica cystica zunutze. Testosteron hemmt auch die Wachstumswirkung des Oestradiols auf den Uterus.

b) Tuben

Die Oestrogene begünstigen den Transport des Eies in den Tuben, höhere Dosen führen zur Hyperämie, zur Schleimhautproliferation und zum Wachstum der Tuben.

c) Ovarium

Die Wirkung auf das Ovar ist abhängig von der Dosis. Die normale Reifung der Follikel erfolgte nur bei Anwesenheit kleinster Mengen. Unter der Einwirkung etwas höherer Dosen vollzieht sich präovulatorisch eine Änderung der Gonadotropinsekretion, indem die Hypophyse etwas mehr LH abgibt. Dadurch wird das Follikelwachstum deutlich gefördert. Hohe Dosen hemmen dagegen Abgabe und Bildung der gonadotropen Hormone (s. hypophysäre Gonadotropine, S. 652). Den Oestrogenen kommt aber noch eine direkte Wirkung auf das Ovar zu, indem auch beim hypophysektomierten Tier die Granulosazellen der Follikel zur Zellteilung angeregt werden und eine geringe Gewichtszunahme eintritt. Eine solche direkte Einwirkung der Hormone auf ihre Produktionsstätten unter Umgehung der Hypophyse scheint für andere Hormone wie die Corticoide zuzutreffen.

d) Brustdrüsen

Zusammen mit Progesteron und dem hypophysären Prolactin bewirken die Oestrogene die Proliferation der Brustdrüsen. Beim hypophysektomierten Tier ist zur Auslösung der Lactation noch die zusätzliche Gabe von Nebennierenrindenhormonen erforderlich. Die Oestrogene stimulieren besonders das Wachstum der Gänge, beim Menschen in geringem Umfang auch der Läppchen. Die volle Entwicklung der Drüsenläppchen erfolgt aber nur unter der gleichzeitigen Verabreichung von Progesteron. Auch bei dem mit Oestrogen behandelten Prostatiker proliferieren vorwiegend die Ausführungsgänge, die Drüsenläppchen selbst nur wenig. Das Gewebswachstum erfolgt auch beim kastrierten und adrenalektomierten oestrogenbehandelten Mann.

3. Wirkung auf die männlichen Genitalorgane

Unter der *hetero*sexuellen Wirkung der Sexualhormone versteht man den Einfluß auf das andere Geschlecht, also die Wirkung der Androgene im weiblichen, der Oestrogene im männlichen Organismus. Man hat diese Eigenschaften auch als „paradoxe" bezeichnet. Nachdem aber beide Sexualhormone sowohl im männlichen als auch im weiblichen Organismus physiologisch sind, sollten diese Begriffe nicht mehr gebraucht werden.

Die Reaktionsfähigkeit der einzelnen Tierarten ist verschieden, sie ist außerdem abhängig vom Lebensalter, vom Kastrationsalter und von der Art des verwandten Oestrogens.

a) Hoden

Verabreichung mittlerer und kleinerer Dosen von Oestrogenen führt bei männlichen Tieren zu einer weitgehenden Atrophie der Gonaden, es schwinden sowohl das Kanälchenepithel als auch die Leydigzellen. Mit 10 μg Oestradiolbenzoat wöchentlich erreicht die Hodenatrophie bei ausgewachsenen Ratten in 2 Monaten ihren Höhepunkt (HOHLWEG 1934). Prostata und Samenblasen atrophieren ebenfalls, das Stroma vermehrt sich. Ursache ist die Hemmung der Gonadotropinbildung, von FSH und ICSH. Diese hormonale Kastration wird vielfach beim Schlachtvieh zur Verbesserung des Fleisches und Erhöhung des Körpergewichtes angewandt. Bestimmte Mäusestämme entwickeln nach mehrmonatiger Oestrogenbehandlung Tumoren der interstitiellen Zellen, nach viermonatiger Gabe von 0,05—0,25 mg Diäthylstilboestrol in 76%, nach 9 Monaten in 100%. Diese Tumoren sind auf oestrogenbehandelte Tiere transplantabel, sie metastasieren und bilden Androgene, sie entstehen also aus den Leydigzellen.

GARDNER (1937) nahm als Ursache eine gesteigerte ICSH-Produktion an, deren Entstehungsmechanismus durch die Langzeitversuche von HOHLWEG (s. Regulation, S. 649) eine Erklärung findet.

Bei Menschen liegen zahlreiche Befunde über die Auswirkung der Oestrogene vor (HOWARD u. Mitarb. 1950; LYNCH, HELLER u. NELSON 1948a). Eine ausführliche Darstellung hat DE LA BALZE (1954b) gegeben. Der Ablauf ist ziemlich einheitlich. Fast gleichzeitig atrophiert das Kanälchenepithel, bildet sich eine peritubuläre Sklerose mit Hyalinisierung aus und verschwinden die normalen Leydigzellen des Erwachsenen. DE LA BALZE teilt die Schäden in drei Grade ein. Der *erste* Schweregrad besteht in einer Dissoziierung und Abstoßung des Kanälchenepithels. Die Sertolizellen scheinen aktiviert und enthalten mehr

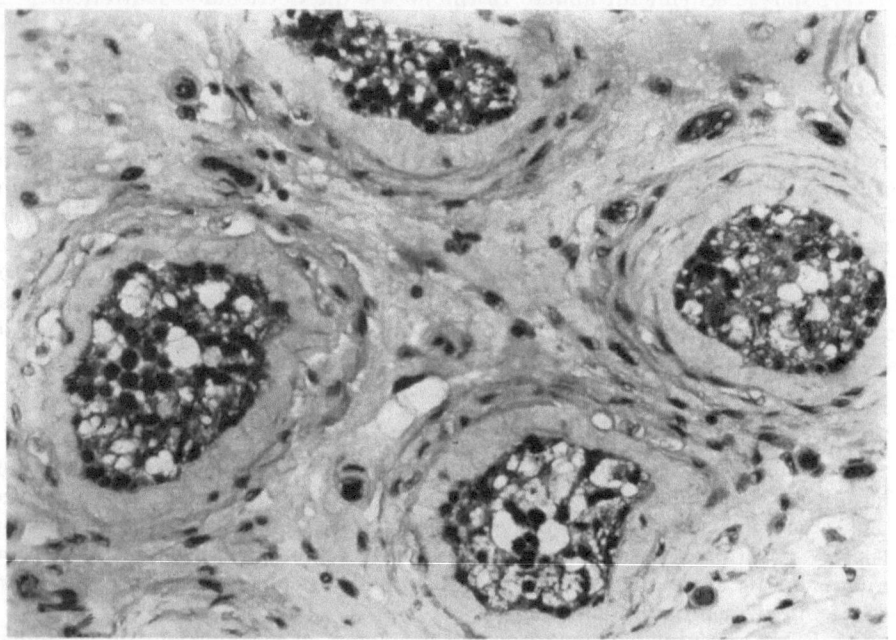

Abb. 12. 69jähriger Mann. Vor 3 Jahren Prostatacarcinom operativ entfernt, laufend Cyren. 4 Wochen vor dem Tod noch 100 mg Diaethyloxystilben implantiert. Kanälchen stark verkleinert mit sehr dicker Wand, nur Sertolizellen und einzelne Spermatogonien, keine sichere Leydigzellen. (Hämatoxylin-Eosin, 300fach)

Lipoide und Glykogen. Die Basalmembran verdünnt sich, während sich die Fasern etwas verdicken und die Fibroblasten vermehren. Die Leydigzellen schwinden, zeigen Kernpyknose, nehmen eine fusiforme Gestalt an und werden Fibroblasten immer ähnlicher. Daneben vermehren sich die typischen Fibrocyten und Fibroblasten des Interstitiums. Schon 8—11 Tage nach Behandlungsbeginn kann man die ersten Veränderungen feststellen, das Vollbild des ersten Stadiums ist nach etwa 30 Tagen erreicht.

Im *zweiten Stadium* nimmt die Spermiogenese weiter ab, der Kanälchendurchmesser wird kleiner, die Sertolizellen atrophieren. Die Tubuluswand verdickt sich weiter. Die Tunica propria zeigt alle Grade der fibrillären Verdickung (Fibrose) bis zur zellarmen Verdichtung (Sklerose) und Homogenisierung (Hyalinose). Die unreifen Bindegewebszellen nehmen zu und werden in die hyaline Masse einbezogen. Die Leydigzellen werden immer fibroblastenähnlicher, Lipoide und Cholesterinester bleiben erhalten, der Ascorbinsäuregehalt ist vermindert.

Die Mastzellen sind vermehrt. Die kleinen Arterien zeigen erhebliche Intima-verdickungen. Dieses Stadium wird zwischen dem 30. und 70. Behandlungstag erreicht (s. Abb. 12).

Das *dritte Stadium* bietet Besonderheiten. Nach zweijähriger Behandlung mit täglich 50 mg zeigen die Kanälchen eine intensive Hyalinose, selbst die Sertoli-zellen sind weitgehend verschwunden. In einzelnen Kanälchen ist noch eine mangelhafte Spermiogenese sichtbar. Das Interstitium ist vollgefüllt mit zahl-reichen Zellen eines völlig neuen Types. Sie sind mittelgroß, polygonal oder rund mit großem Kern und dichtem Chromatin. Das Cytoplasma zeigt teilweise Vacuolisierung. Alle Zellen enthalten kleine eosinophile Granula und mäßige Mengen von Lipoiden und Cholesterinestern. Einzelne Zellgruppen sehen aus wie unreife Leydigzellen mit metachromatischem Cytoplasma, hypertrophem Kern und Nucleolen.

Die Ursache der Leydigzellhyperplasie ist nicht geklärt, sie hat ihre Parallelen in den oben erwähnten Tierversuchen und bei der Lebercirrhose des Menschen. Wahrscheinlich wird die anfänglich gehemmte Gonadotropinproduktion über-kompensiert, so daß zum mindesten ICSH in vermehrtem Maße entsteht, wie es schon GARDNER angenommen hat. Das Geschehen kann mit dem Rebound-phänomen verglichen werden.

Diese Beobachtungen geben keinerlei Hinweis auf die physiologische Bedeu-tung der unter normalen Verhältnissen in den Leydigzellen gebildeten Oestrogene, die die Kanälchen ebenso umspülen wie die Androgene. Nach Untersuchungen von ELERT haben die Oestrogene eine gewisse spermiogenetische Wirkung. Er injizierte 4 Tage lang täglich 2,5 mg Oestradiolmonobenzoat in den rechten Hoden geschlechtsreifer Ratten. Der linke zeigte nach 21 Tagen eine erheblich geschädigte Spermiogenese. Im rechten waren die Mitosen der Spermatogonien und Spermatocyten I und die Spermatocyten I selbst deutlich vermehrt. Die spermiogene Wirkung ist nicht spezifisch, da Spermatogonien und Spermato-cyten I auch bei hypophysektomierten Tieren erhalten bleiben. Wahrscheinlich wird, ähnlich wie bei den Androgenen, nur die Durchblutung und Permeabilität der Wand verbessert.

b) Prostata

LACASSAGNE (1933) verabreichte Mäusen 5 Monate lang Oestrogene und fand eine beträchtliche Vergrößerung der dorsalen Prostatalappen mit Urinretention und der Ausbildung einer Hydronephrose. Diese ersten Beobachtungen wurden von zahlreichen anderen Autoren bestätigt. BURROWS (1935) zeigte dann, daß sich das Wachstum nicht nur auf den dorsalen Lappen beschränkte, sondern auf alle Prostatalappen übergriff und daß vorwiegend Veränderungen am fibro-muskulären Anteil der Prostata und weniger an den epithelialen Zellen eintreten.

Bei der *Ratte* findet man eine starke Atrophie des Epithels der gesamten Prostata und eine mäßige Zunahme des bindegewebigen Anteils, während das Epithel im Hinterlappen metaplasiert und das Bindegewebe sich stark vermehrt. Beim *Affen* entwickelt sich eine squamöse Metaplasie des Epithels im Bereich des Utriculus masculinus und der Urethra, ein Schwund der Drüsenzellen und eine deutliche Zunahme des fibromuskulären Anteiles aller Prostatalappen (KOREN-CHERSKY 1934). Dasselbe Verhalten zeigt der *Hund* mit Umwandlung des Epithels in ein squamöses Plattenepithel, besonders an den Ausführungsgängen der Pro-stata, am Uterus masculinus, am Urethraanteil, während sich das fibromuskuläre Stroma der Drüse vermehrt (VAN WAGENEN, PAKES 1935, COURRIER). Die Gesamtgröße der Prostata kann sich wegen der ausgedehnten Epithelmetaplasie, der Retention von käsigem Detritus trotz des Schwundes des epithelialen Anteiles stark erhöhen (Huggins 1940, de Jongh).

Huggins u. Mitarb. (1940) untersuchten die sekretorische Leistung nach dem von ihnen entwickelten Verfahren beim Hund. Verabreichung von Oestrogenen bringt die Sekretion praktisch zum Erliegen. Erhalten kastrierte Hunde, deren Sekretion durch tägliche Injektion von 10 mg Testosteronpropionat wieder normalisiert war, zusätzlich Stilboestrol, so sinkt die Sekretion in Abhängigkeit von der verabreichten Oestrogendosis ab. 0,1 — 0,2 mg haben keinen Einfluß, 0,4 mg hemmen etwas, 1 mg dagegen stark. Es besteht also ein Antagonismus der beiden Hormone in ihrer direkten Wirkung auf die Epithelzelle der Prostata. Wie die histologische Untersuchung des Organs zeigt, heben sich die Hormone gegenseitig nicht auf, sondern die Zellen zeigen die Einwirkung beider. Die Gesamtgröße der Prostata ist mäßig vermindert, in den hinteren Lappen findet sich die für die Oestrogene charakteristische Plattenepithelmetaplasie, während das Epithel der Acini an Höhe wohl abnimmt, aber kubisch bleibt.

Die Veränderungen nach synthetischem Oestrogen beim *Menschen* — z. B. Stilboestrol — sind grundsätzlich dieselben wie beim Tier. Die Schleimhautzellen zeigen eine beträchtliche Metaplasie in Richtung auf ein desquamierendes und verhornendes Epithel. Gleichzeitig vergrößern sie sich, werden vacuolig, so daß man an das Epithel der Talgdrüsen erinnert wird, ganze Lumina der Acini können mit diesen hyperplastischen Zellen ausgefüllt sein. Die Epithelmetaplasie ist ungleichmäßig verteilt, in großen Teilen der Drüse vorhanden, sie ist nicht nur auf die Ausführungsgänge, den Colliculus seminalis und die Pars prostatica der Urethra beschränkt. Das übrige Epithel atrophiert stark. Der fibromuskuläre Anteil der Drüse ist vermehrt. Das Ausmaß des Umbaues ist abhängig von Dosis und Dauer der Oestrogenbehandlung. Ein ähnliches histologisches Bild zeigt der Fet ab dem sechsten Monat und der Neugeborene. Das Epithel ist teilweise stark hyperplastisch und metaplasiert, es besteht aus großen, hellen Zellen, die die Lumina völlig ausfüllen können. Diese Veränderungen beruhen wahrscheinlich auf der Überschwemmung des Fet mit placentären Oestrogenen.

Hamburger und Halvorsen, Pincus u. Mitarb. (1955a) u. a. fanden die Ausscheidung der Oestrogene beim Menschen während des gesamten Lebens etwa gleich hoch, während die Androgene nach dem 40. Lebensjahr beträchtlich abnehmen. Laqueur, de Jongh u. Zuckermann (1951) u. a. nahmen daher an, daß das Überwiegen der Oestrogeneinwirkung auf die Prostata im höheren Lebensalter mit eine Ursache für die benigne Prostatahypertrophie darstelle, besonders auch, da sich die ersten Veränderungen der benignen Hypertrophie, multizentrische aglanduläre Knötchen, im stark oestrogenempfindlichen periurethralen fibromuskulären Gewebe zwischen Blasenhals und Colliculus seminalis entwickeln. Jakobsen (1951) untersuchte die Prostata von 75 Männern zwischen 60 und 88 Jahren. 50 zeigten das gewöhnliche Bild der senilen Prostata. Bei 10 ergab die systematische Suche umschriebene Metaplasien und Hypertrophien des Epithels im Sinne des desquamierenden Epithels, ein Teil der Lumina war völlig obliteriert. Die Veränderungen sind lange nicht so stark ausgeprägt wie unter künstlicher Verabreichung von Oestrogenen, sie zeigen aber an, daß sich die Oestrogene wahrscheinlich infolge der Verschiebung des Verhältnisses zu den Androgenen am Organ auswirken können.

Die Frage, ob die benigne Prostatahypertrophie eine endokrine Erkrankung ist oder nicht, wird heute allgemein abgelehnt, obwohl bei Kastraten weder eine Prostatahypertrophie oder ein Prostatacarcinom, noch ein Uterusmyom oder Carcinom, noch eine glandulär cystische Hypertrophie der Mamma, noch ein Mammacarcinom vorkommt. Die normale Entwicklung des Gewebes und die volle Funktion der Drüsen sind wohl Voraussetzung, aber nicht Ursache der benignen und malignen Geschwülste sagt BUTENANDT.

Die Verabreichung von Sexualhormonen hat keinen Einfluß auf die gewebliche Struktur der Prostatahypertrophie. Durch Androgene ändert sich das histologische Bild nicht, unter Oestrogenen entwickeln sich nur die typischen Epithelmetaplasien, auch die Kastration ist wirkungslos.

c) Samenblasen und Ductus deferens

Gibt man kastrierten Ratten Oestron, dann erhöht sich das Gewicht der Samenblasen gegenüber den Kontrollen. Histologisch findet man eine Hypertrophie der glatten Muskulatur mit Zunahme des Bindegewebes, während das Epithel wenig unbeeinflußt bleibt. Wie bei der Prostata, metaplasiert es an den Ausführungsgängen; auch Epididymis und Ductus deferens reagieren mit einer Bindegewebsvermehrung.

Injiziert man kastrierten Ratten Testosteron-Propionat in einer Dosis, daß sich Prostata und Samenblasen nicht voll entwickeln, dann führt die Zugabe von Oestrogenen zum Wachsen des fibromuskulären Anteils mit weiterer Gewichtszunahme und Normalisierung der Struktur der Drüse. Wahrscheinlich nehmen auch beim Mann die im Hoden gebildeten Oestrogene am Aufbau der sekundären Geschlechtsdrüsen teil. *Physiologische Dosen der beiden Hormone wirken synergistisch, hohe Dosen dagegen gegensinnig.*

Die Wirkung der Oestrogene ist also mehrschichtig. Einmal hemmen sie die Wirkung der Gonadotropine in der Adenohypophyse und heben damit die Produktion der Androgene und Oestrogene in den Leydigzellen auf, sie haben denselben Effekt auf das Epithel wie die Kastration. Der Begriff der „hormonalen Kastration" ist nicht ganz richtig, da die Oestrogene selbst auf die sekundären Geschlechtsorgane einwirken und eine Metaplasie des Epithels und eine Zunahme des fibromuskulären Stromas der Drüsen auslösen. Steht das Epithel gleichzeitig unter der Wirkung von Androgenen, dann sind sehr hohe Oestrogendosen notwendig, um die Funktion der Drüsenzellen auszulöschen, aber selbst mit höchsten Dosen atrophiert das Epithel nicht so vollständig wie nach der Kastration.

III. Stoffwechselwirkung der Androgene und Oestrogene
1. Eiweißstoffwechsel (anabole Wirkung)

Neben der spezifischen Wirkung der Sexualhormone auf die primären und sekundären Geschlechtsorgane steht die auf den Eiweißstoffwechsel des Organismus, die auch unter dem Begriff der *anabolen*, der eiweißaufbauenden Wirkung zusammengefaßt wird. Diese wurde zum erstenmal von KOCHAKIAN und MURLINS (1935) festgestellt. Sie fanden, daß Extrakte aus männlichem Urin und Testosteron bei kastrierten Hunden stickstoffretinierend wirken. Stickstoff wird auch nach Entfernung der Hypophyse, der Nebennieren und des Pankreas einbehalten, d. h., der Effekt wird nicht durch andere innersekretorische Drüsen vermittelt, er ist eine echte, integrierende Eigenschaft der androgenen Hormone. Die Einsparung erfolgt fast ausschließlich durch Abnahme der Harnstoffausscheidung, während sich die Ammoniakausscheidung wenig ändert und die Stickstoffausscheidung im Stuhl nicht beeinflußt wird. Die Stickstoffretention wird nicht von einer Erhöhung des Harnstoffes im Blut begleitet, hohe Testosterondosen führen sogar zu einer vorübergehenden Abnahme desselben. Erhöhung der

Testosterondosis und verlängerte Behandlung steigert bei Hunden die Stickstoff-retention nicht über ein erreichbares Maß (maximale Stickstoffretention 0,05 g pro Kilogramm Körpergewicht und Tag). Nach Absetzen des Hormons wird die Bilanz negativ, doch geht nur ein Teil des einbehaltenen Stickstoffes wieder verloren.

Bei kastrierten Tieren erleiden die Skeletmuskulatur, Leber, Milz, Nieren und der Knochen einen deutlichen Gewichtsverlust, der durch Testosteron wieder ausgeglichen wird. Die Stickstoffretention ist beim kastrierten Tier viel stärker als beim normalen. Beim Kastraten und eunuchoiden Menschen stehen die Körperzellen offenbar in einem dauernden Eiweißdefizit, das nur durch Testo-steron ausgeglichen werden kann (HANSEN 1946 u. 1949).

Die *trophische Gewebswirkung* wurde besonders von KOCHAKIAN und seinen Mitarbeitern untersucht. Die verschiedenen Gewebe reagieren verschieden stark, es bestehen auch erhebliche Unterschiede zwischen den einzelnen Species. So schwindet beim *Meerschweinchen* die Muskelmasse und der Gehalt des Muskels an Myosin und Actomyosin nach Kastration beträchtlich. Besonders empfindlich ist der Musculus temporalis. Testosteron stellt das ursprüngliche Muskelgewicht wieder her. Der M. temporalis reagiert schon auf kleinere Testosterondosen als die übrige Skeletmuskulatur. Bei der *Ratte* nimmt das Gesamtgewicht der Skeletmuskulatur nach der Kastration nicht oder nur wenig ab, Myosin und Actomyosingehalt bleiben gleich, nur die Muskulatur des Beckenbodens verliert beträchtlich an Masse. Zu diesem Muskelkomplex gehört auch der M. levator ani, der sich leicht präparieren läßt und dessen Restitution nach Kastration vielfach als Maß der myotrophen Wirkung der Androgene verwendet wird. Bei der *Maus* sind die Nieren besonders androgenempfindlich. Der erhöhte Stickstoffgehalt nach Testosteronbehandlung kastrierter Mäuse gegenüber den Kontrollen findet sich vorwiegend in den Nieren, in Prostata und Samenblasen. Die Gewichts- und Massenzunahme dieser Organe ist mit einer Vermehrung des Eiweißgehaltes ver-bunden, sie wird als Ausdruck der anabolen Eigenschaften der Androgene ange-sehen.

KOCHAKIAN u. Mitarb. haben schon frühzeitig erkannt, daß die Stärke der androgenen und anabolen Eigenschaften der androgenen Steroide nicht parallel geht. Sie fanden die Trennung der beiden biologischen Eigenschaften besonders ausgesprochen im Androstan-3α, 17β-diol, im 17-Methylandrostan-17β-ol und im 17-Methylandrosten-3β-17β-diol. Dadurch, daß man die anabole Wirkungs-stärke eines Androgens mit der androgenen in eine rechnerische Beziehung setzt, lassen sich die einzelnen Androgene in ihrer anabolen Wirkungsstärke miteinander vergleichen. Es zeigt sich dabei, daß die anabolen Eigenschaften der einzelnen Androgene bei den einzelnen Tierarten verschieden stark sind, je nachdem, ob die myotrophe Wirkung auf den M. temporalis des Meerschweinchens oder auf den M. levator ani bei der Ratte, oder die renotrophe Wirkung bei der Maus mit derjenigen auf die akzessorischen Geschlechtsorgane, also besonders die Samen-blasen und die Prostata in Beziehung gesetzt wird. Die Suche nach dem Steroid mit dem günstigsten Verhältnis von myotropher zu androgener Wirkung ist noch nicht abgeschlossen. Ein günstiges Wirkungsverhältnis kommt in jedem Falle durch eine Abnahme der Androgenwirkung und nicht durch eine Zunahme der anabolen Eigenschaften zustande. Die wichtige Schlußfolgerung aus den Kocha-kianschen Versuchen, daß der Trennung der beiden biologischen Eigenschaften am besten bei niedrigen oder physiologischen Dosen feststellbar ist, während exzessive Dosen und die kontinuierliche Anwendung dieser Steroide die andro-gene Wirksamkeit immer stärker hervortreten läßt, scheint wenig bekannt (s. S. 728—731).

Von den natürlichen androgenen Steroiden der Nebennierenrinde hat Androsten-3,17-dion eine deutliche anabole Stoffwechselwirkung, während 11 β-Hydroxyandrostendion die Stickstoff- und Phosphorbilanz wenig ändern, die Calciumbilanz wird von beiden nicht beeinflußt (PECKET u. Mitarb.).

Beim Menschen ist die eiweißanbauende Wirkung besonders beim M. Cushing, der Akromegalie, der senilen Osteoporose, der hormonalen Osteoporose, beim Hypogonadismus geprüft. 5 mg Testosteron-Propionat täglich sind schon wirksam, eine maximale Retention erreicht man mit 25—50 mg täglich. REIFENSTEIN (1958) berichtet z. B. über einen 72jährigen Mann mit seniler Osteoporose, der unter 125—150 mg Testosteron-Propionat oder 40—100 mg Methyltestosteron per os täglich 30—40 mg pro Kilogramm Körpergewicht Stickstoff, 3,2—4,8 mg pro Kilogramm Phosphor und 0,25—4,6 mg pro Kilogramm Calcium retinierte. Besonders wirksam sind die Depot-Präparate des Testosterons, so wurden nach Injektion von 350 mg Testosteron-Önanthat im Laufe von 30 Tagen 50 g Stickstoff, 1,5 g Phosphor, 1,5 g Calcium einbehalten. Erkrankungen mit allgemeinem oder lokalisiertem Gewebseiweißverlust aus nicht hormonaler Ursache reagieren geringer, ja die Stickstoffretention kann, wie bei Kranken mit schwerer juveniler Osteoporose unbekannter Ursache oder bei Eiweißresorptionsstörungen, ganz ausbleiben.

REIFENSTEIN fand auch unter der Verabreichung der *Oestrogene* eine Stickstoffretention z. B. während einer Periode von 5—15 Tagen bei täglicher Gabe von 1,66 mg Oestradiolbenzoat 16 mg N pro Kilogramm Körpergewicht und Tag. KNOWLTON u. Mitarb. konnten bei sexuell unterentwickelten Männern und Frauen und bei gesunden Frauen mit Oestrogenen eine Stickstoffretention erreichen, nicht bei gesunden Männern. Die Wirkung der Oestrogene ist viel geringer und unsicherer als die der Androgene und beschränkt sich auf bestimmte Gewebe, wie Uterus, Brustdrüsen, sie ist keine allgemeine Stoffwechseleigenschaft. Im Vergleich zum Natrium wird die Calcium- und Phosphorbilanz stärker positiv. Die direkte Anregung der Osteoblasten ist nicht bewiesen. Hohe Dosen wirken ausgesprochen katabol (STERNBERG u. Mitarb., ALBBRIGHT 1940 u. 1941).

Nach Kastration nehmen bei Ratten und Menschen die Serumalbumine und die α_1-Globuline etwas ab. Beim Gesunden hat Testosteron keinen Einfluß auf die Bluteiweißbildung, dagegen wurde wiederholt beobachtet, daß Anabolica bei Eiweißmangelsyndromen eine Vermehrung der Albumine gebracht hat, β- und γ-Globuline können auf übernormale Weise ansteigen.

Hier ist noch bemerkenswert, daß Testosteron auch scheinbar hormonal unabhängig erscheinende Reparationsvorgänge des Gewebes beeinflußt. KOWALEWSKI u. Mitarb. verfolgten bei normalen und kastrierten Ratten den Einbau von S 35 in künstlich gesetzte Knochenfrakturen. Unter der Verabreichung von Testosteron und Nor-Testosteron ist die Aufnahme von S 35 gesteigert, beim Kastrierten stärker als bei den Kontrollen. Die Autoren vermuten eine Anregung der Synthese von Chondroitin-Schwefelsäure im kollagenen Gewebe in Heilung. begriffener Knochenbrüche, ähnlich wie in den Fibrocyten des Hahnenkamms.

Die Art der Wirkungsweise der Steroide auf den Eiweißstoffwechsel ist nicht sichergestellt, Steigerung der Eiweißsynthese (anabol) und die Verminderung des Eiweißabbaues (antikatabol) werden diskutiert. Untersuchungen mit markierten Aminosäuren sprechen mehr für die Erhöhung der Eiweißsynthese. Da auch beim hungernden Menschen unter Testosteron-Propionat die Ausscheidung von Stickstoff, Kalium und Phosphor etwas abnimmt, während der Gewichtsverlust nicht aufgehalten wird, der hohe Umsatz sich nicht ändert, nehmen BUTLER u. Mitarb. (1945) an, daß Testosteron doch auch antikatabole Eigenschaften hat. Durch Hormonbehandlung wird außerdem der biologische Wert des Nahrungseiweißes verändert. Das minderwertige Eiweiß aus Mais erhält bei Ratten unter Testosteron den Wert von Lactalbumin, dagegen sinkt unter Cortison der Wert des Lactalbumins auf den der Gelatine ab. Als dritter Faktor kommt also noch die verbesserte Ausnützung des Nahrungseiweißes hinzu, während die Resorption nicht beeinflußt wird.

2. Kreatinstoffwechsel

Die *Kreatinausscheidung* steht in enger Beziehung zur Muskelmasse des Körpers, zum Alter und zum Geschlecht. Jugendliche und Kastraten weisen eine beträchtliche Spontankreatinurie auf, sie scheiden parenteral verabreichtes Kreatin zum größten Teil unverändert wieder aus, während der erwachsene Mann dagegen fast vollständig Kreatinin daraus bildet. Ein Kreatin-Kreatinin-Quotient von 70 im Kindesalter sinkt beim Erwachsenen auf 2,6—10,2 ab (WILDER). Nach Testosteron sinkt die Kreatinausscheidung bei jugendlichen Tieren (Ratten, Affen), beim Kind und männlichen Kastraten stark ab, zugeführtes Kreatin erscheint nicht mehr im Urin. Bei Kindern mit Muskeldystrophie ist Testosteron wirkungslos, während die hohe Ausscheidung der Hyperthyreose und des M. Addison zurückgeht (MEYER 1955). WILKINS u. Mitarb. (1941) und DORFMAN u. SHIPLEY (1956) beobachteten, daß alkylierte Androgene wie 17-Methyltestosteron und andere C 17-Substituierte, die Kreatinausscheidung im Urin beträchtlich erhöhen. Der Effekt tritt nach einer Latenzzeit von 4—6 Tagen ein, steigert sich bis zum 3.—6. Monat und kann während der ganzen Behandlungsdauer auf dieser Höhe erhalten bleiben. Man nimmt an, daß Methyltestosteron und ähnliche Derivate sowohl die Synthese als auch die Speicherung von Kreatin erhöhen, Testosteron dagegen besonders die Speicherungsfähigkeit (STOKES u. Mitarb.). KOCHAKIAN erklärt die Unterschiede dagegen durch die verschieden starke Wirkung auf die Kreatinsynthese.

3. Fettstoffwechsel

Oestrogene verhüten die Verfettung der Leber von Ratten, die ohne lipotrope Substanzen ernährt werden. Der Angriffsort liegt wahrscheinlich extrahepatisch.

Die geringere Häufigkeit des Coronarinfarktes der menstruierenden Frau gegenüber dem Mann desselben Alters und die Häufung der Infarkte bei Frauen nach dem Klimakterium haben schon lange die Vermutung erweckt, daß die Oestrogene einen Einfluß auf den Fett- und Cholesterinstoffwechsel ausüben. Viele Untersuchungen brachten negative Ergebnisse, aber im allgemeinen nimmt das Blutcholesterin bei ausreichender Dosierung ab, während die β-Lipoproteide und Phosphorlipoide etwas ansteigen. Auch bei Diäthylstilboestrol behandelten Prostatikern wurde eine geringe Erhöhung der Phosphorlipoide und Verminderung des Gesamtcholesterins festgestellt, das Verhältnis Cholesterin: Phosphorlipoide sinkt deutlich ab. Wegen der starken Nebenwirkungen auf Hypophyse, Keimdrüsen und Uterus konnte diese günstige Eigenschaft therapeutisch wenig ausgenützt werden. Bei weiterer Suche ist man auf Derivate von Chlortrianisene gestoßen, die als Oestrogenantagonisten keine spezifischen Wirkungen mehr besitzen, den Cholesterinspiegel durch Verminderung der Cholesterinsynthese jedoch beträchtlich senken können (MRL 41, MER 25). Statt Cholesterin werden aber je nach der Lokalisation der Blockierung der Biosynthese Vorstufen mit mehr oder weniger starken „Fett"eigenschaften im Körper angehäuft. Die vollständige Blockierung der Cholesterinsynthese gefährdet die Biosynthese der Steroidhormone.

4. Elektrolyt- und Wasserhaushalt

THORN und HARROP (1937) berichteten als erste nach Verabreichung von *Testosteron* über eine Vermehrung des Blutvolumens, eine geringe Erhöhung des Natriums, des Chlors und des Kaliums im Serum. Der gesunde Mensch schwemmt nach 4—6 Tagen den größten Teil der einbehaltenen Flüssigkeit wieder aus. Die individuelle Reaktion ist sehr verschieden. Bei Behandlung von Eunuchoiden können vorübergehend harmlose Ödeme auftreten. Vorsichtig sei man bei älteren Menschen mit schlechter Herzleistung, Ödemneigung und manifester oder latenter Niereninsuffizienz. Dosen über 25 mg Testosteron können vorhandene Ödeme verstärken, das Blutvolumen vermehren, Blutdrucksteigerung und ein Lungenödem auslösen. Natrium und Wasser werden im distalen Tubulus vermehrt rückresorbiert, Kalium mit Wasser zum Aufbau des neuen Eiweißes verwendet und intracellular eingelagert. Die anabolen Derivate des Testosterons wirken in höheren Dosen gleich.

Die *Oestrogene* wirken beträchtlich stärker als Testosteron. Beim weiblichen Organismus wird das Wasser besonders im Uterus und in der Gegend der Vulva angelagert. Die prämenstruelle Wasserretention soll auf die erhöhte Oestrogen-Produktion zu dieser Zeit zurückgehen.

Beim gesunden Menschen kann man durch die Verabreichung von 15—50 mg eines kurzwirkenden Oestradiolesters eine Gewichtszunahme bis zu 2 kg erzeugen, der Höhepunkt wird nach 7—10 Tagen erreicht. Das Plasmavolumen ändert sich wenig, das Wasser wird vorwiegend im interstitiellen Gewebe abgelagert. Bei manifester und latenter Herzinsuffizienz, bei eingeschränkter Nierenleistung kann die Retention beträchtliche Ausmaße annehmen und mit allgemeinen Anasarka, Blutdrucksteigerung und Hungerödem verbunden sein, „Cyrenödeme" des Prostatacarcinomträgers.

Der Angriffspunkt ist unklar. Neben einer Erhöhung des antidiuretischen Effektes des Hypophysenhinterlappenhormons wird eine vermehrte Capillar-durchlässigkeit, eine Änderung der Zellmembran mit Erhöhung der K-Konzentration im Zellinnern, der Na-Konzentration im Extracellularraum diskutiert.

Die Steigerung des Knochenwachstums, die Besserung der hormonalen und der senilen Osteoporose ist, wie erwähnt, nicht nur durch eine Vermehrung der eiweißhaltigen Grundsubstanz, sondern auch durch die verbesserte Einlagerung von *Calcium* und *Phosphor* in den Knochen bedingt. Die Stickstoffretention geht mit einer Retention von Calcium und Phosphor parallel, wobei sich die Plasmawerte dieser Elektrolyte nicht verändern. Die Oestrogene wirken stärker als die Androgene. Etwa 6 Tage nach Oestradiol nimmt die Calcium- und Phosphorausscheidung ab, erreicht aber erst nach 30 Tagen ihr Maximum. Erhöhte Serumphosphorwerte sinken ab, die alkalische Phosphatase wird nicht beeinflußt. Testosteron-Propionat in der Dosis von 25—50 mg, Methyltestosteron 40—100 mg täglich, Oestradiol-Benzoat 3,32—1,66 mg jeden dritten Tag intramuskulär und Diäthyl-Stilboestrol 1—1,5 mg täglich per os sind etwa gleich stark wirksam.

Der Einfluß auf die *Citronensäureausscheidung* ist gegensätzlich, sie wird durch Testosteron vermindert, durch Oestrogene vermehrt, durch die Kombination neutralisiert (WHEDON). Bei allen Menschen mit Steindiathese, besonders bei Bildung von Calciumsteinen, muß dies beachtet werden, da die Citronensäure im Urin die schwer löslichen Calciumsalze besser in Lösung hält. WHEDON u. Mitarb. schlagen in solchen Fällen vor, eine notwendige Testosteronbehandlung immer mit Oestrogenen im Verhältnis 20—30:1 zu kombinieren.

5. Innersekretorische Organe

a) Hypophyse

Kleine Mengen von Oestrogenen fördern die Abgabe des LH bzw. des ICSH, größere hemmen die Produktion aller Gonadotropine (s. S. 640). Man vermutet, daß nach kurzdauernder Gabe zunächst eine Sperre der Hormonausschwemmung und erst nach längerer Einwirkung eine Hemmung der Produktion stattfindet (BROWN u. Mitarb. 1953). Hypophysen von mit Oestradiol behandelten Frauen enthalten weniger Gonadotropine als die unbehandelter Personen (ROWLANDS u. Mitarb. 1940).

Werden Oestrogene nach längerdauernder Verabreichung abgesetzt, dann setzt eine überschießende Bildung der Gonadotropine ein (Desensibilisierungseffekt, Rebound-Phänomen, Depletion-Effekt, s. S. 650).

Bei langdauernder Verabreichung tritt bei Ratten und Mäusen ein Gewichtsverlust aller innerer Organe, in der Reihenfolge Herz, Leber, Gehirn, Lungen, Milz, Schilddrüse, Thymus, Pankreas, Nebenniere ein. Man vermutet, daß bei diesen Tieren nicht nur die Gonadotropinproduktion, sondern auch die des Wachstumshormons und des thyreotropen Hormons gehemmt wird. Die bei kastrierten Nagern in der Hypophyse auftretenden Kastrations- oder Siegelringzellen bilden sich unter Oestrogenen rasch zurück. Beim Menschen sind die Veränderungen uncharakteristisch, manchmal findet sich eine Zunahme der Eosinophilen und eine Abnahme der Neutrophilen und Basophilen, es kann aber auch jede Veränderung fehlen (TONUTTI 1960).

b) Nebennierenrinde, Cortisolplasmaspiegel, Transcortin

Die sich vielfach widersprechenden Untersuchungen an Tieren geben kein einheitliches Bild. Nach Kastration männlicher Ratten erhöht sich das Nebennierengewicht, histologisch hypertrophieren alle Zonen mit Ausnahme der Glomerulosa, bei weiblichen Tieren reagiert die Nebenniere nicht. Verabreichung von Testosteron verhindert die Hypertrophie. Bei infantilen und kastrierten männlichen Mäusen bringen die Androgene die sog. X-Zone zum Verschwinden und vermindern die Breite der Zona glomerulosa (DEANSLY u. PARKES 1036; MARTIN 1930). Die nach Kastration eintretende Hypertrophie der Nebenniere ändert das Erscheinungsbild der Kastration bei Ratten und Mäusen in keiner Weise. Die viel diskutierte Hypothese der kompensatorischen Hypertrophie der Nebennierenrinde als Ausgleich der verlorenen androgenen und oestrogenen Bildungsstätte entbehrt der sicheren Unterlage. Beim Menschen erhöht sich die Ausscheidung der 17-Ketosteroide nach der Kastration nicht, hohe und höchste Mengen von HCG haben beim Kastraten keinen Einfluß auf die 17-Ketosteroidausscheidung. Trotzdem müssen zwischen beiden Organen gewisse Wechselbeziehungen bestehen. Bei Inzucht-Mäusen der Stämme DBA/2 WyDi und CE/WyDi entwickelt sich eine Hyperplasie der Nebennierenrinde, aus der in hohem Prozentsatz Neoplasmen entstehen, wenn die Tiere 1—3 Tage nach der Geburt kastriert werden. Kurze Zeit danach wachsen die sekundären Geschlechtsmerkmale. In der Hypophyse entwickeln sich basophile Knoten. Hypophysektomie, aber auch Verabreichung von Oestrogenen verhindert die Ausbildung der Geschwülste (BROWN u. Mitarb. 1953).

Bei Nagern hypertrophieren die Nebennieren unter Zufuhr von Oestron, Oestradiol oder von Oestriol beträchtlich. Cholesterin- und Ascorbinsäurekonzentration nehmen ab, die Zona glomerulosa und fasciculata verbreitern sich und zeigen histologisch und histochemisch Zeichen einer vermehrten Aktivität. Nach

Entfernung der Hypophyse sind die Oestrogene wirkungslos, sie stimulieren also die Abgabe von ACTH. Bei einzelnen Mäusestämmen entwickeln sich unter dieser Stimulierung metastasierende Nebennierentumoren. Auch beim Menschen ist die Vergrößerung der Nebenniere nach langdauernder Oestrogengabe sichergestellt (TONUTTI).

Erst in den letzten Jahren konnte der merkwürdige Befund der starken Erhöhung der 17-Hydroxycorticoide im Plasma während der Gravidität geklärt werden. MARTIN und MILLS (1958b) hatten schon einen Zusammenhang mit der übermäßigen Bildung von Oestrogenen in der Gravidität vermutet. Auch künstliche Verabreichung von Oestrogenen erhöht den 17-Hydroxycorticoidspiegel des Plasmas von Mann und Frau beträchtlich, die Ausscheidung der Metaboliten des Cortisols bleibt normal. Gibt man einem Kranken mit M. Addison, der auf eine bestimmte Menge von Cortisol eingestellt ist, Oestrogene, dann steigt auch hier das Plasmacortisol an. Dieser erhöhte Cortisolspiegel hat keine biologische Wirkung, denn weder unter der intensiven Oestrogenbehandlung des Prostatacarcinoms, noch während der Gravidität entsteht das Bild des M. Cushing, noch fallen die Bluteosinophilen ab, noch entstehen in der Hypophyse die für die Überdosierung von Cortison charakteristischen Crookeschen Zellen (ROBERTSON u. Mitarb.).

Der Anstieg des Cortisols im Plasma unter 0,5 mg Äthinyloestradiol pro Tag ist beträchtlich, z. B. von 14 auf 59 μg-% nach 39 Tagen Therapie, von 17 auf 47 μg-% nach 21 Tagen, von 12 auf 56 μg-% nach 40 Tagen, von 11 auf 50 μg nach 18 Tagen. Die Nebennierenrindenhormone Cortisol, Corticosteron finden sich im Blut in zwei verschiedenen physikochemischen Zuständen, ungebunden und fest gebunden an einen spezifischen Eiweißkörper das *Transcortin*. Man nimmt an, daß nur der ungebundene Anteil in die Zellen eindringen kann. Die Oestrogene erhöhen entweder die Menge des corticoidbindenden Plasmaproteins, das Transcortin oder sie machen an diesem Eiweißkörper zusätzliche Bindungsplätze frei. Folge dieser vermehrten Bindung ist eine verlängerte Halbwertszeit des Cortisols, ein verlangsamter Abbau in der Leber und eine verminderte Ausscheidung der Metaboliten im Urin. Die 17-Ketosteroide sind davon nicht betroffen. Aldosteron ist nur locker gebunden.

c) Schilddrüse und ihre Hormone, PBJ, TBP

Schon 1948 war aufgefallen, daß während der Schwangerschaft eine Erhöhung des eiweißgebundenen Jods (PBJ) eintritt. Es blieb lange unklar, warum diese Vermehrung nicht von einem Hyperthyreoidismus begleitet ist. Später fand man, daß unter der Verabreichung von Oestrogenen nicht nur das PBJ, sondern auch das thyroxinbindende Protein (TBP) ansteigt.

Die erste Wirkung des Oestrogens besteht nach ENGBRING und ENGSTROM in einer Erhöhung der *thyroxinbindenden Kapazität des Serums*. Diese erfolgt unabhängig von der Funktion der Schilddrüse und unabhängig von der Menge des zur Verfügung stehenden Thyroxins. Als Folge davon steigt die Konzentration des zirkulierenden Thyroxins und des PBJ des Plasmas, selbst bei Menschen ohne Schilddrüse, die auf eine bestimmte Menge Schilddrüsenhormon eingestellt sind. Wie beim Cortisol erhöht sich die Halbwertszeit für Thyroxin, wahrscheinlich weil der Gradient zwischen Plasma und Gewebe als Folge der Vermehrung des TBP verändert wird. Der Thyroxinverbrauch sinkt ab. Trotz erhöhtem Hormonjod im Plasma zirkuliert wegen der erhöhten Bindungskapazität der Plasmaeiweißkörper weniger freies Hormon. Die Abgabe von thyreotropem Hormon wird gesteigert, die Schilddrüse wird aktiviert, doch wird der größte Teil des abgegebenen Hormons wieder an Proteine gebunden und dadurch wirkungslos, langsamer verbraucht und inaktiviert. Der Grundumsatz erniedrigt sich etwas. Ob diese Ereignisfolge nur durch die Erhöhung der Bindungskapazität des Plasmas in Gang gebracht wird, ist noch nicht geklärt.

Die Veränderungen unter *Testosteron* sind nicht so eindrucksvoll. Bei Männern und Frauen findet man eine konstante Abnahme des eiweißgebundenen Jods (PBJ) im Serum, während die Abnahme der thyroxinbindenden Kapazität (TBP) nur in einem Teil der Fälle feststellbar ist. Bei der Hypothyreose ist diese Abnahme deutlicher als beim Euthyreoten. Mit der Abnahme des PBJ und des TBP ist eine vorübergehende Erhöhung des freien Thyroxins und ein gesteigerter Hormonverbrauch in der Gewebsperipherie mit Erhöhung des Grundumsatzes verbunden. Die Ausschläge sind geringgradig, aber nachweisbar. Als Folge des erhöhten Thyroxinspiegels im Blut wird die Abgabe von thyreotropem Hormon gebremst und die Leistung der Schilddrüse gedrosselt, die Aufnahme von J^{131} sinkt.

Der Einfluß des Testosterons auf die Schilddrüsenökonomie ist demjenigen der Oestrogene also gerade entgegengesetzt, der Einfluß der Androgene ist aber beträchtlich geringer als der der Oestrogene.

6. Einzelne Organe

a) Nieren

Es wurde schon erwähnt, daß unter *Testosteron* der Eiweißgehalt des Nierengewebes ansteigt. Bei *Mäusen* und *Ratten* vermindert sich das Nierengewicht nach Kastration beträchtlich, es wird durch Verabreichung von Testosteron wieder normalisiert, während das Nierengewicht von *Kaninchen, Hamstern* und *Meerschweinchen* durch die Kastration nicht beeinflußt wird. Hohe Testosterondosen erhöhen das Nierengewicht normaler Mäuse und Ratten über das Normale hinaus. Die Vergrößerung ist durch eine Hypertrophie der Tubuluszellen im distalen und im proximalen Teil der Tubuli contorti bedingt. Im Experiment wird die Sekretionsleistung der Tubuli durch Testosteron gesteigert, die Resistenz gegenüber Sublimat erhöht (Heinke u. Tonutti, Selye, Feyel). Bei Mäusen nehmen Teile der epithelialen Bowmanschen Kapsel kubische Gestalt an. *Oestrogene* bedingen nur eine leichte Hypertrophie der proximalen und distalen Tubuluszellen und der Bowmanschen Kapsel. Bei unphysiologisch hohen Dosen entsteht das Bild der schweren toxischen Nephrose.

Die Anwendung von Testosteron und seinen Derivaten bei chronischen Erkrankungen der Nieren des Menschen, besonders solchen des tubulären Systems, hat keine eindeutigen Ergebnisse gebracht. Die vorübergehende Harnstoffsenkung im Plasma bei der akuten tubulären Insuffizienz ist nicht entscheidend, das geschädigte Tubulusepithel ist offenbar weniger androgenempfindlich als das gesunde.

b) Speicheldrüsen

Die experimentellen Ergebnisse sind nicht einheitlich. Die von Lacassagne (1940a) bei kastrierten Mäusen und Ratten festgestellte Gewichtsabnahme der Submaxillaris und Parotis wird von Kochakian (1955) nicht bestätigt. *Testosteron* erhöht das Gewicht dieser Drüsen beim kastrierten und nichtkastrierten Tier. Das Epithel der Ausbildungsgänge wird kubischer.

c) Leber

Kleine und mittlere *Oestrogen-Dosen* erhöhen das Gesamtgewicht der *Leber* durch Hypertrophie und Wassereinlagerung. Fettgehalt und Synthese von

Cholesterin sind vermindert (ROSENMAN u. Mitarb.). Der Gehalt der Cholinesterase ist bei weiblichen Nagern 5—8mal größer als bei männlichen Tieren, er sinkt nach Entfernung der Ovarien ab. Verabreichung von Oestrogenen an männliche Tiere erhöht die Cholinesterase, auch die β-Glucuronidase nimmt zu. Hohe Dosen begünstigen die Leberverfettung.

d) Herz und Gefäßsystem

Am *Herzen* ist die Wirkung beider ähnlich, die der Oestrogene aber in jeder Hinsicht schwächer als die der Androgene. Am Tier beobachtet man eine beschleunigte Resynthese von Milchsäure zu Glykogen, eine Verkürzung der Anspannungszeit, eine Verlängerung der Austreibungs- und der Überleitungszeit. Ein geschädigter Herzmuskel reagiert nicht mehr auf Sexualhormone.

Die gefäßerweiternde Wirkung der Oestrogene betrifft in besonderem Maße das Versorgungsgebiet der A. ovarica. Die Hyperämie am Uterus geht der Stoffwechselwirkung voraus und wird durch Atropin blockiert. Wahrscheinlich wird sie durch Freisetzung des Vagusreizstoffes Acetylcholin hervorgerufen (REYNOLD). Die Erweiterung der Capillaren und Venolen tritt in abgeschwächter Form auch in anderen Gefäßgebieten, besonders in der Haut, im Gehirn und am Herzen ein, sie wird in der Behandlung von Durchblutungsstörungen dieser Organe benützt. Testosteron wirkt viel schwächer als Oestrogen.

e) Haut, Bindegewebe, Knochen

Ein Teil der Wirkung der *Oestrogene* auf die *Haut* geht wahrscheinlich auf die hyperämisierende Wirkung zurück. Die Zahl der Mitosen wird erhöht und die Zellproliferation und Regeneration beschleunigt, dadurch verdickt sich die Epidermis. Diese proliferative Wirkung zeigt sich auch in den Schleimhäuten der Nase und des Mundes. Selbst beim alten Menschen verdickt sich die atrophische Haut wieder.

Hohe Dosen von Oestrogenen führen zu einer ähnlichen Pigmentierung wie in der Schwangerschaft, so daß man das Chloasma uterinum als oestrogenbedingt ansieht. Die Pigmentzunahme an bestimmten Hautteilen, besonders an den äußeren Genitalien, den Brustwarzen, der Linea alba erfolgt auch beim Mann.

Im *Bindegewebe* verstärken sich unter Oestrogenen die kollagenen Fasern, die Grundstruktur wird durch Erhöhung des Gehaltes an Hyaluronsäure, Chondroitinschwefelsäure und von Mucoitinschwefelsäure verstärkt (BURROWS 1949, KOCH u. Mitarb., PECK u. Mitarb.). Das Bindegewebe lagert mehr Wasser ein, die Zahl der Fibrocyten, Fibroblasten und Histiocyten nimmt zu. Testosteron wirkt gleichsinnig, aber schwächer.

Der Einfluß der Ovarialhormone auf den *Knochen* unterscheidet sich grundsätzlich von dem der Androgene. Bei jugendlichen Tieren beobachtet man unter Oestrogen-Gabe eine Hemmung des Längenwachstums, eine Beschleunigung der Knochenreifung und eine Verdichtung der Knochen, das Wachstum der langen und der platten Knochen hört auf, die Ossifikationszentren entwickeln sich vorzeitig, auch der Epiphysenschluß erfolgt vorzeitig. Bei Mädchen fehlt der Wachstumsstoß der Pubertät, mit der Menarche hört das Längenwachstum auf. Man nimmt an, daß die Oestrogene die Osteoblasten stimulieren, die Einlagerung von Calcium, Phosphor und Stickstoff in die Knochenmatrix begünstigen und dadurch die Knochenreifung bewirken.

Nach Kastration bzw. in der Menopause vermindert sich die Osteoblastentätigkeit. Bleibt dabei die der Osteoklasten gleich, dann resultiert eine Knochenresorption mit Entkalkung. Daß die Osteoporose bei Frauen früher und häufiger auftritt als bei Männern, erklärt man durch den vorzeitigen und weitgehenderen Ausfall der Gonadenfunktion.

Die alleinige hormonale Ätiologie der *Osteoporose* des höheren Lebensalters — Abnahme der Androgen- und Oestrogenproduktion bei Gleichbleiben der Cortisolproduktion und damit Verschiebung des Gleichgewichtes der „anabolen" und „katabolen" Hormone — ist umstritten. Zusätzliche Faktoren, wie unzureichende Mengen von Kalk in der Nahrung, Störung der Calciumresorption, des Citronensäurestoffwechsels, vermehrte Calciumausscheidung, sind vielfach wesentliche Komponenten. Die Albrightsche These der verminderten Bildung der Knochenmatrix konnte mit Isotopenuntersuchungen bis jetzt nicht bestätigt werden, so daß heute wieder mehr die vermehrte Knochenresorption als Folge einer negativen Ca-Bilanz als Ursache der Osteoporose diskutiert wird. Behandlung mit Testosteron und anabolen Steroiden ist häufig erfolglos, Besserung der Knochenstruktur röntgenologisch nicht erwiesen. Das kann nicht allein daran liegen, daß der Knochen 30% seines Kalkgehaltes verloren oder zugelegt haben muß, bevor im Röntgenbild die veränderte Struktur sichtbar wird.

Die Erfolge sind bei kombinierter Therapie mit Androgenen bzw. anabolen Steroiden und Oestrogenen, die Reifenstein zum erstenmal empfohlen hat, besser als bei alleiniger Androgengabe, wahrscheinlich wegen des stärkeren Einflusses der Oestrogene auf die Ca-Bilanz. Hutchins u. Mitarb. (1959) behandelte 66 Frauen 2—8 Jahre mit Oestrogenen und Androgenen (OestradiolBenzoat 0,25 mg täglich oder Ethinyloestradiol 0,005 mg täglich, oder Hexoestrol 0,001 mg täglich, dazu Methyltestosteron 3,5 mg täglich bzw. NorandrostenolonPhenylpropionat 50 mg alle 8 Wochen, wobei die Oestrogene alle 6 Wochen für 14 Tage unterbrochen wurden). Als Maß der Wirkung benützte er wie Albright das Aufhalten der Abnahme der Körpergröße in der Menopause. Diese beginnt etwa 6—8 Jahre nach der Menopause und ist nach 9—12 Jahren am stärksten, mit höherem Lebensalter wird sie wieder geringer. Die prophylaktische Steroidbehandlung in der Menopause verhinderte in all seinen Fällen die Abnahme der Körpergröße. Bei Frauen, die erst nach Eintritt eines Größenverlustes behandelt wurden, wurde das weitere Fortschreiten erst nach etwa zweijähriger Hormonbehandlung aufgehalten. Befundänderungen in der röntgenologisch feststellbaren Dichte der Wirbelsäule traten nicht ein!

Eine weitere Besserung der Ergebnisse wird nach unseren Erfahrungen mit der zusätzlichen oralen Gabe von Ca-Salzen (Ca-Lactat, Ca-Gluconat) erreicht.

IV. Testosteron und Derivate, anabole, progestionale Steroide

Im Gegensatz zu den Nebennierenrindensteroiden Cortisol und seinen Derivaten wird die biologische Aktivität des Testosterons durch Änderungen des Moleküls nur wenig verändert. So besitzt Dihydrotestosteron noch $^3/_4$ der Wirkung, Verlagerung der Doppelbindung von C 4 nach C 1 vermindert die Stärke nur um die Hälfte, Einführung einer Methylgruppe an C 17 macht das Steroid oral wirksam, die androgene Eigenschaft bleibt stark, auch Verschiebung der Doppelbindung von C 4 nach C 5 mit Reduktion der 3-Ketogruppe ist ohne großen Einfluß, Umwandlung der 3β- in eine 3α-Hydroxylbindung erhöht sogar die Wirksamkeit. Dagegen vermindert sich die Androgenität beträchtlich, wenn die 17β-Hydroxylgruppe zu einer Carbonylgruppe oxydiert oder in eine 17α-Hydroxylgruppe umgewandelt wird. Die 17β-Hydroxylgruppe bestimmt die biologische Aktivität der natürlichen Androgene.

Eine Reihe von neuen Verbindungen wurde durch Entfernung der Methylgruppe am C 19 oder durch Umlagerung an C 1 geschaffen (Tabelle 12). *19-Nor-*

Testosteron (XXIV) ändert seine Eigenschaften gegenüber Testosteron völlig. Aus dem stärksten Androgen wird ein starkes Gestagen, während die androgenen Eigenschaften auf 30%, beim *19-Nor-Androstendion* sogar auf 20% des ursprünglichen sinken. Wird die 19-Methylgruppe des Testosterons nach C 1 verschoben, wie beim 1-Methyl-19-Nortestosteron, dann sinkt die Aktivität noch weiter. Zusätzliche Einführung einer Alkylgruppe am C 17 (Methyl, Äthyl, Äthenyl) steigert die anabolen Eigenschaften, vermindert die androgenen und erhöht die progestionalen stark.

Alle Überlegungen über die Bindung der androgenen und anabolen Eigenschaften an bestimmte Struktureinheiten des Moleküls macht die Entdeckung von DORFMAN zunichte, daß auch das 2-acetyl-7-oxo-1,2,3,4, 4a,4b,5,6,7,9,10,10 a-dodecahydrophenantren (Verbindung Ro 2-2739) androgene und anabole Eigenschaften haben kann (TYLER 1960). Bei der kastrierten Ratte erhöhen 100 mg des Phenantrenderivates, subcutan gegeben, das Gewicht der Prostata, Samenblasen und des M. levator ani um 80—90%. Auch das Wachstum des Kammes von Hühnern wird bei direktem Auftragen angeregt. In Parabioseversuchen ist die Hemmung der Gonadotropinproduktion etwa zehnmal so stark wie die androgene auf Samenblasen und Prostata. Verglichen mit Testosteron beträgt die relative androgene Wirksamkeit im Kammtest etwa $^1/_{100}$ und im Samenblasentest $^1/_{400}$. Die anabolen Eigenschaften sind etwas stärker als die androgenen.

Ein anderes Derivat mit fünfgliedrigen Kernen, der Diäthylester, der $\alpha\beta$-dicyclopentanon-2,2′-äthan-1,1′-dicarbonsäure, soll in der Dosis von 15 μg bei Ratten androgen wirken.

Tabelle 12. *Einfluß der Demethylierung am C 19 auf die androgene Wirksamkeit*
(Nach W. R. NES: In Medicinal Chemistry, S.758. London: Interscience Publishers [1]

Verbindung	I.U.[2]	D-Homosteroide 19-Nor-derivate
Androsteron	100	100
Androstan-3β-ol-17-on .	770	150
Androstane-3,17-dion .	130	100
Androstane-3β, 17β-diol	500	160
Androstane-3α, 17β-diol	900	500
4,5α-Dihydrotestosteron	20	25
4-Androstene-3,17-dion	130	45
Testosteron	15	25
17-Epitestosteron . . .	400	250
17α-Methyltestosteron .	27	15
17β-Methyltestosteron .	Inaktiv	

[1] Mit Genehmigung des Verlages.

[2] Relative Androgenaktivität. Eine I.U. entspricht der Menge des geprüften Steroids, das dieselbe androgene Wirkung besitzt wie 100 μg Androsteron. Eine Verminderung der I.U. entspricht einer Erhöhung der Wirksamkeit.

XXIV. 19-Nortestosteron

1. Testosteron und Ester

JUNKMANN macht darauf aufmerksam, daß viele Effekte der Sexualhormone in der Anregung von Wachstumsvorgängen bestehen, die sich durch Steigerung der Dosierung nicht beliebig beschleunigen lassen. Zur Erzielung einer günstigen Wirkung gibt es eine optimale Anflutgeschwindigkeit, die möglichst gleichmäßig erhalten bleiben soll. Das Optimum würde durch eine kontinuierliche Infusion erreicht werden, eine Maßnahme, die sich zeitlich nur beschränkt durchführen läßt.

Das *reine Testosteron* wird intravenös gegeben zu 63% in den ersten 24 Std als 17-Ketosteroide im Urin ausgeschieden. Bei oraler Verabreichung ist die Resorption vollständig, die Inaktivierung erfolgt aber sehr rasch, so daß die Wirkungsstärke nur $^1/_6$ bis $^1/_{20}$ des intramuskulär gegebenen beträgt. Die sublinguale Verabreichung ist der oralen nur wenig überlegen.

Gebräuchlich ist heute noch die *percutane* Verabreichungsart. Die Resorption durch die Haut erfolgt verhältnismäßig langsam, so daß die Wirkung etwas protrahiert ist. Freies Testosteron wird langsamer resorbiert als das Propionat.

Auch die subcutane *Implantation* von gepreßten Tabletten wird noch verwendet. ESKAMILLA und LISSER errechneten aus 200 mg Tabletten von Methyltestosteron eine tägliche Resorption von 3,5 mg oder 0,87%. HOWARD und JEWETT verwandten 200 mg Tabletten von Testosteronpropionat. Sie fanden anfangs eine starke Resorption, die etwa 3 mg pro Tablette erreicht, nach Bildung einer Kapsel um den Fremdkörper aber auf 0,5—1 mg pro Tag absinkt. Der Nachteil der Implantation ist die häufige Ausstoßung ohne daß eine bakterielle Infektion hinzugetreten ist. Die Entwicklung der langwirkenden Ester des Testosterons hat die Implantation von Tabletten überflüssig gemacht. Tabletten von 100 mg Gewicht sind etwa 6 Monate wirksam. Von der Implantation in den Hoden ist man ganz abgekommen.

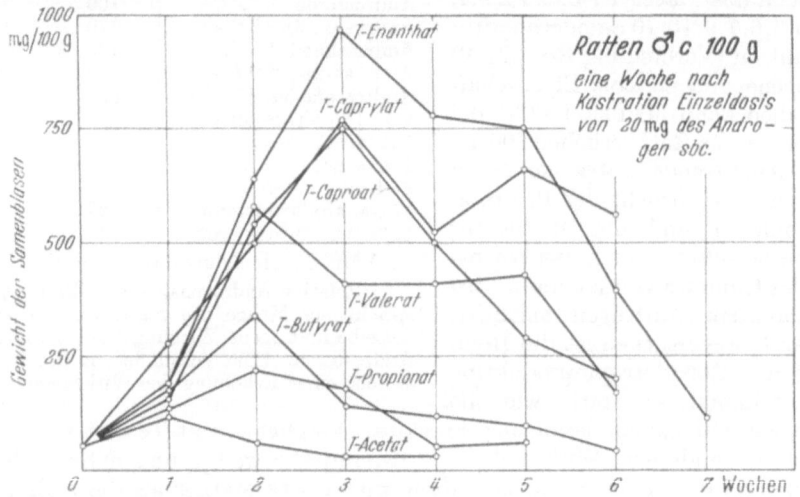

Abb. 13. Wirkungsdauer und Intensität verschiedener Testosteronester. (Nach JUNKMAN)

Wirkungsstärke und Wirkungsdauer des Testosterons kann durch Veresterung mit verschiedenen Fettsäuren erheblich gesteigert werden.

Veresterung von Androgenen und anderen Steroidhormonen natürlicher und künstlicher Provenienz bedingt eine Verlängerung der Wirkungsdauer und eine Erhöhung der Wirkungsstärke (s. Abb. 13). Bis heute ist die Ursache hierfür noch nicht geklärt. Anfangs hatte man angenommen, daß die Resorption verzögert erfolgt. Prüfung mit markierten Produkten zeigte aber, daß die Radioaktivität am Ort der Injektion rasch verschwindet. Die Wirkungsdauer geht nicht mit der in vitro feststellbaren Hydrolysedauer parallel. Dagegen nimmt die Spaltbarkeit durch Leberhomogenate in vitro mit zunehmender Länge der Fettsäurekomponente ab (DIRSCHERL), ebenso die Verseifbarkeit durch alkoholische KOH. Die frühere Ansicht von JUNKMANN, daß diese Verbindungen als Ester wirken, ist auch heute noch nicht widerlegt.

Man hat versucht, die *Wirkungsdauer* der einzelnen Verbindungen durch die Bestimmung der *17-Ketosteroidausscheidung* zu erfassen. Nach einmaliger Injektion von 100—200 mg Testosteronpropionat können 22—72%, im Durchschnitt 44% des Hormons in Form der erhöhten 17-Ketosteroidausscheidung im Urin wiedergefunden werden. In den ersten 24 Std sind die 17-Ketosteroide am stärksten erhöht, die Hauptmenge wird in den ersten 2—3 Tagen ausgeschieden. Bei Verabreichung von Testosteronpropionat in Form einer Kristallsuspension (200 bis 500 mg) wird die höchste Ketosteroidausscheidung nach 3—5 Tagen erreicht, sie bleibt mindestens 9—11 Tage hoch. Die als 17-Ketosteroide wiedergewonnene Menge des Testosterons schwankt zwischen 27 und 50%. Eine gleichmäßig erhöhte 17-Ketosteroidausscheidung, die eine gleichmäßige Resorption und Wirkung anzeigt, erreicht man nur bei täglicher Gabe von Testosteronpropionat intramuskulär (HAMBURGER 1948). Für die Ester mit Depotwirkung gibt die Verfolgung der 17-Ketosteroidausscheidung keinen Aufschluß über Stärke und Dauer der Wirkung. DICZFALUSY und CASSMER konnten nach Injektion von Testosteronoenanthat nur 6,9%, nach Testosteron-Hexoxyphenyl-Propionat nur 4,8% der verabreichten 200 mg wiederfinden. Die Ergebnisse an Laboratoriumstieren dürfen nicht einfach auf den Menschen übertragen werden, da nicht nur das Ansprechen der einzelnen Tierarten untereinander, sondern auch des Menschen im Vergleich zu den Laboratoriumstieren verschieden ist. Bei der Behandlung des Menschen selbst ist wiederum der Entwicklungsgrad, das Lebensalter, die Reaktionsfähigkeit der Geschlechtsorgane von wesentlicher Bedeutung.

Mit der Veresterung der Steroidhormone kann nicht nur eine Verlängerung der Wirkungsdauer, sondern auch eine *Änderung der biologischen Eigenschaften* verbunden sein. Das erste Beispiel dieser Art war die Veresterung von 17α-Hydroxyprogesteron. Das unveresterte Steroid, das bei Nagern als schwaches Androgen wirkt, ist beim Menschen, selbst in höchsten Dosen, völlig wirkungslos. Veresterung mit Caproinsäure gibt dem 17α-Hydroxyprogesteron die Eigenschaften

XXV. Testosteronpropionat

eines stark wirkenden Progesteron. Diese Beobachtung zog eine rasche Entwicklung nach sich und war der Ausgangspunkt für die zahllosen Versuche, durch Änderung und Neuanlagerung von Seitenketten, schließlich auch durch Wandlungen im Molekül von Testosteron, Progesteron und den Oestrogenen, eine Änderung der biologischen Eigenschaft der Ausgangssubstanz zu erzielen. Die wichtigsten Derivate dieser Art werden im nächsten Abschnitt besprochen. Das Bemühen der Biochemiker ist dabei, die mehrschichtigen Eigenschaften der Hormone auf ganz bestimmte Stoffwechselvorgänge zu beschränken.

Testosteronpropionat (XXV), der am häufigsten verwendete Ester, wird rasch resorbiert und inaktiviert, so daß seine Wirkung nur 1—2 Tage anhält. Bei Injektion über 15 mg steigt die 17-Ketosteroidausscheidung deutlich an. Die Wirkungssteigerung gegenüber dem reinen Testosteron beträgt das Zehnfache. Testosteronpropionat wird immer dann gegeben, wenn es darauf ankommt, in kurzer Zeit eine möglichst starke Wirkung zu erreichen. Die mittlere Dosis zur Behandlung des schweren Hypogonadismus liegt in den ersten 3 Monaten bei dreimal 50 mg pro Woche, später bei dreimal 25 mg.

Testosteronphenylpropionat. Wirkungsdauer von 6—10 Tagen. Die mittlere Dosierung zur Behandlung des schweren Hypogonadismus beträgt 50 mg alle 4—5 Tage.

Testosteronisobutyrat in Form von Mikrokristallen. Wirkungsdauer von 14 bis 18 Tagen. Mittlere Dosierung zur Behandlung des schweren Hypogonadismus 50 mg alle 14 Tage.

Testosteronoenanthat. Wirkungsdauer 3—4 Wochen, mittlere Dosierung zur Behandlung des schweren Hypogonadismus 250 mg alle 3—4 Wochen.

Testosteroncaprionat. Wirkungsdauer 3—4 Wochen.

Testosteron-p-hexoxyphenylpropionat hat die längste Wirkungsdauer aller bekannten Ester (4—6 Wochen).

Ganz allgemein haben die langwirkenden Ester den Nachteil, daß während des ersten und letzten Viertels zu wenig Hormon zirkuliert. Man mischt sie daher gerne mit rascher wirkenden Verbindungen, so mit Testosteronpropionat und Phenylpropionat oder gibt im letzten Drittel Methyltestosteron per os hinzu.

2. Oral wirksame Androgene

Methyltestosteron. 17α-Methyltestosteron (XXVI) besitzt bei oraler Gabe etwa die doppelte Wirkung des freien Testosterons. Sein Vorzug liegt in seiner *peroralen Wirksamkeit.* In Form von Linguetten ist es etwa halb so stark wie Testosteronpropionat intramuskulär. Die Methylierung am C_{17} erschwert die Inaktivierung durch die Leber. In der Dauerbehandlung benötigt man etwa die 2—3fache Dosis des intramuskulär gegebenen Testosteronpropionats. Nach eigenen Erfahrungen eignet sich das Derivat nicht zum Aufbau der primären und sekundären Sexualorgane beim präpuberalen und postpuberalen Kastraten,

XXVI.
17α-Methyltestosteron

XXVII. 9α-Fluor-11β-Hydroxy-17α-Methyltestosteron-
Fluoxymesteron

10—15 mg täglich können aber die Organfunktion erhalten, mit 30 mg täglich tritt bei Frauen ein Virilismus auf.

9α-Fluor-11β-Hydroxy-17α-Methyltestosteron, Fluoxymesteron (XXVII) (Ultandren bzw. Halotestin), seit 1957 in die Therapie eingeführt, ist ebenfalls oral

wirksam. Im Tierversuch ist es gegenüber oralem Methyltestosteron im Samenblasentest 9,5mal, im Musculus laevator ani-Test etwa 20mal so stark wirksam. Wie Methyltestosteron verwendet man es zweckmäßigerweise nur bei leichteren Formen des Hypogonadismus, während man die schweren erst mit Depottestosteron ausgleicht und dann mit 7,5—10 mg Fluoxymesteron fortfährt (HERR, HERSHBERGER). Eine wichtige Indikation geben Kinder bzw. Halbwüchsige mit retardiertem Wachstum und mäßigem Hypogonadismus. Die starken anabolen Eigenschaften steigern das Linearwachstum und die Gewichtszunahme, ohne daß bei 0,15 mg/kg androgene Nebenerscheinungen auftreten. Erst Dosen über 0,25 mg/kg machen auch die androgenen Eigenschaften des Präparates bei Kindern sichtbar. Zur Virilisierung kommt es bei Frauen, die mehr als 10 mg über längere Zeit erhalten. Die Behaarung im Gesicht, den Extremitäten und am Stamm nimmt zu, die Stimme vertieft sich, die Haut wird fett und ölig, bei jüngeren Frauen kann sich eine Acne und eine Alopecie des Kopfhaares entwickeln (LARON). 10 mg täglich sind zur Behandlung des echten Klimakterium virile zu empfehlen.

3. Derivate mit stärkeren anabolen Eigenschaften

Bei einer Reihe von Indikationen sind die *anabolen* Eigenschaften des Testosterons für die Behandlung wichtiger als die androgenen. In den letzten Jahren wurden Derivate des Testosteron, Androstan und Androstadien entwickelt, die stärkere *anabole* als androgene Eigenschaften besitzen (HERSHBERGER, SAUNDERS).

Bei höherer Dosierung und längerer Verabreichung zeigen aber alle auch noch die androgenen Eigenschaften der Muttersubstanzen, so daß bei Frauen und Kindern eine Virilisierung eintritt. Im unteren Dosisbereich überwiegt bei den meisten der anabole Effekt den androgenen stark, bei hohen und höchsten entspricht wie beim Testosteron der androgene dem anabolen. Bei einem Teil sind die *progesteronartigen* Eigenschaften des Testosterons so verstärkt, daß sie vorwiegend als Progestine bzw. Gestagene Anwendung finden. Auch diese Derivate besitzen in hohen Dosen noch androgene und anabole Eigenschaften, so daß immer mit Nebenerscheinungen gerechnet werden muß (s. S. 715).

Die klassische Testung eines anabolen Steroids besteht seit den Untersuchungen von KOCHAKIAN und MURLIN in der Bestimmung der Bilanz für Stickstoff und andere Eiweißkonstituenten. Wegen des großen Aufwandes wird im allgemeinen die Fähigkeit, das Wachstum des Musculus laevator ani der kastrierten männlichen Ratte anzuregen. verwandt. Diese myotrophe Wirkung soll der im Stickstoffhaushalt parallel gehen.

Die im Musculus laevator ani-Test (SELYE 1958, HERSHBERGER) an der kastrierten Ratte wirksame Dosis wird zu der im Samenblasentest errechneten androgenen Wirkungsdosis in Beziehung gesetzt und als *„anaboler Wirkungs-quotient"* bezeichnet. Zur Prüfung der anabolen Qualitäten sollte aber immer auch die Stickstoffbilanz und die Kompensation des durch Prednisone oder durch Dihydrotachysterin künstlich katabol gemach-

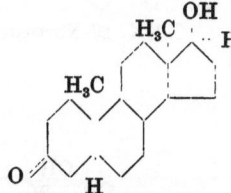

XXVIII. 17α-Methyl-
5-Androsten-3β, 17β-diol

XXIX. 17β-Hydroxy-
Androstan-3-on

ten Stoffwechsels herangezogen werden. Eine vollständige Prüfung der androgenen Qualitäten muß die Virilisierung von Feten mit einschließen.

Wie Testosteron, stimulieren die anabolen Steroide auch die Knochenreifung und das Längenwachstum von Kindern beiderlei Geschlechts.

Die Hemmung der *Gonadotropinbildung* der einzelnen Derivate ist unterschiedlich stark. In Parabioseversuchen an Mäusen (männliches Tier kastriert, weibliches normal) finden KINCL u. Mitarb. keine Parallelität von androgener und antigonadotroper Wirkungsstärke, letztere entspricht eher der myotrophen.

4-Chlor-17α-Methyl-19-Nortestosteron und 2-Methyl-17β-hydroxy-19-nor-androstan-3-on hemmen stark und haben stark myotrophe Eigenschaften, während Samenblasen und Prostata kaum angeregt werden. 17α-Methyl-17β-hydroxy androstan-3-on hat im Vergleich zu seinen geringen androgenen und anabolen Eigenschaften eine unverhältnismäßig starke hypophysenhemmende Wirkung und wäre das geeignete Steroid für die Behandlung der echten Pubertas praecox. Beim Menschen beginnt die Gonadotropinausscheidung bei oraler Gabe von 30 mg 17-Methyl-19-Nortestosteron täglich nach 8 Tagen abzusinken und fällt langsam auf nicht mehr meßbare Werte. 30 mg täglich hemmen beträchtlich stärker als 300 mg Testosteronpropionat pro Woche (ZANOW). Auch die anderen alkylierten 19-Nortestosteronderivate hemmen kräftig.

Androstan-3,17-diol, Androstan-17β-ol, 3-on (XXIX), 17α-Methyl-5-Andro-sten-3,17-diol (XXVIII) waren die ersten Derivate, bei denen die anabole Stoffwechselwirkung gegenüber der androgenen stärker hervortrat (RUZICKA, HENDERSON).

Androstan-17β-ol, 3-on (XXIX) = Anaboleen bzw. Stanolon wird beim Menschen verwandt.

17α-Äthyl-19-Nor-Testosteron = Noräthandrolon = Nilevar. Nilevar besitzt
gegenüber Methyltestosteron gesteigerte anabole Eigenschaften, es ist aber auch
noch ein kräftiges Androgen, so daß das Verhältnis anabol: androgen, Methyltestosteron = 1 gesetzt, nur 1,75 beträgt (Suchowsky). 20 mg per os senken die
Stickstoffausscheidung deutlich, 50 mg maximal. 25—50 mg kehren die negative
N-Bilanz nach Frakturen oder chirurgischen Eingriffen um. 0,5 mg täglich
erhöht bei Kindern die Wachstumsrate, ohne das Genitale zu beeinflussen,
1 mg täglich wirkt dagegen androgen (Gordan). Bei Frauen wächst bei 50 mg
täglich nach 5—7 Wochen ein Bart.

HELLER fand, daß sich die anabole Wirkung bei Eunuchen deutlich von der
androgenen abtrennen läßt. Nach mehrmonatiger Gabe von 15 mg und mehr

XXX. 19-Nortestosteronphenylpropionat

XXXI. 17α-Methyl-17β-Hydroxy-
Androsta-1,4-dien-3-on-
Methandrostenolon

XXXII. 4-Hydroxy-17α-
Methyltestosteron

XXXIII. 4-Chlor-
Testosteron-acetat

XXXIV. 1-Methyl-1-Andro-
sten-17β-ol, 3-on-acetat

können bei Frauen Zeichen einer Virilisierung auftreten (WILKINS 1941). Dosen
über 30 mg sind auch progestional wirksam, sie erhöhen die Körpertemperatur,
verhindern die Menstruation oder bedingen Abbruchsblutungen. Das Derivat verursacht häufig Übelkeit und Erbrechen, selten auch einen cholostatischen Ikterus.

17β-Phenyl-19-Nor-Testosteron-Propionat (XXX) = Durabolin ist oral nur
wenig wirksam und muß intramuskulär gegeben werden. Das Verhältnis der
anabolen zu androgenen Wirkung beträgt bei Ratten 2,4 Testosteronpropionat = 1
gesetzt (Suchowsky). 50 mg alle 18—20 Tage wirken beim Menschen deutlich
anabol und heben die katabole Eigenschaft von 35 mg Prednison auf. Die
Stickstoff- und Phosphorbilanz wird positiv, die Wirkung auf den Calcium-
haushalt ist gering. Bis zu 50 mg alle 14 Tage hat keine progestionale Wirkung.
Dagegen treten die androgenen Eigenschaften bei höherer Dosierung deutlich
hervor. 20 mg und mehr pro Woche kann bei Frauen nach längerer Behandlungsdauer (12—15 Wochen) deutliche Virilisierungserscheinungen auslösen (Acne,
Hirsutismus, tiefe Stimme). Ältere Frauen nehmen häufig deutlich an Gewicht
zu, bekommen ein rotes Rundgesicht wie beim Morbus Cushing und klagen
über Hitzewallungen. Beim Menschen stehen also die androgenen Eigenschaften
des Präparates dem des Testosteronpropionates wenig nach.

17α-Methyl-17β-Hydroxy-androsta-1,4-dien-3-on, Methandrostenolon = Δ_1-17α-Methyl-Testosteron (**XXXI**) (Dianabol), hat im Hahnenkammtest nur 0,7% der Aktivität von Testosteronpropionat. Der anabole Wirkungsquotient beträgt 20, Testosteronpropionat = 1 (LISTER). Beim Menschen wirken 5 mg per os stickstoffretinierend, das Optimum liegt bei 10—15 mg täglich. Längere Verabreichung von 15—20 mg kann bei Frauen mittleren und höheren Alters zu Acne, Hirsutismus, zu starker Gewichtszunahme mit cushingähnlicher Verteilung, zu Vollmondgesicht, Gesichtserythem und Verstärkung der Behaarung Veranlassung geben. Bei Neigung zu Wasserretention (kardialer, renaler Insuffizienz, Lebercirrhose) können Ödeme und Blutungssteigerung auftreten.

4-Hydroxy-17α-Methyl-Testosteron (**XXXII**) = Oranabol wirkt im Tierexperiment am Musculus laevator ani-Test etwa dreimal so stark anabol wie Methyltestosteron, am Samenblasentest etwa halb so stark androgen. Bis zur Dosis von 20 mg treten beim Menschen keine androgenen Nebenwirkungen ein.

4-Chlor-Testosteronacetat (**XXXIII**) = Steranabol wirkt nur intramuskulär. Der anabole Wirkungsquotient, gemessen an der Ratte, beträgt gegenüber Testosteronpropionat 11,0 (SUCHOWSKY). Das Derivat ist also vorwiegend ein Anabolicum.

1-Methyl-1-Androsten-17β-ol-3-on-Acetat (**XXXIV**) = Primobolan oder das Oenanthat = Primobolan-Depot intramuskular. An der Ratte beträgt die androgene Wirkung im Samenblasentest $^1/_{10}$ der des Testosteronpropionats, die Stimulierung des Gewichtes des Musculus laevator ani ist 4,5mal stärker. Der anabole Wirkungsquotient ist gegenüber Testosteronpropionat 24,4 (SUCHOWSKY). Beim Menschen erreicht man mit 20 mg Acetat intramuskulär alle 2 Tage oder mit 100 mg Depot alle 14 Tage eine tägliche Stickstoffretention von 2—4 g, auch die Calcium- und Phosphorbilanz wird bei diesen Dosen positiv. Während 10 mg Testosteronpropionat täglich intramuskulär bei Spätkastraten Ejaculatvolumen und Fructosegehalt normalisieren, erreicht man dies erst mit 40 mg Primobolan intramuskulär täglich (SUCHOWSKY).

Laufend kommen neue mehr anabol wirkende Präparate auf den Markt, doch alle besitzen noch eine androgene Komponente und müssen vorsichtig dosiert werden.

4. Derivate mit progestionalen Eigenschaften, Gestagene

In den letzten Jahren wurde auch eine Reihe von neuen Gestagenen in die Therapie eingeführt. Neben den bei der Besprechung des Progesterons schon erwähnten 17α-Hydroxyprogesteron-Acetat und Capronat, dem 17α-Äthinyl-Testosteron, das auch als Pregneninolon bezeichnet wird, sind es besonders die Derivate des 19-Nor-Progesteron und 19-Nortestosteron, die starke progestionale Eigenschaften besitzen, so 17α-Methyl-19-nortestosteron und 17α-Äthenyl-19-nortestosteron = Noräthisteron.

Die synthetischen Progestine wirken biologisch nicht ganz gleich wie Progesteron. Nach Aufbau der Uterusschleimhaut durch Oestrogene entwickeln sich die Drüsen geringer als das Stroma, so daß bei hohen Dosen ein deciduaähnliches Gewebe entsteht, „starre Sekretion". Werden die Derivate während der Proliferationsphase verabreicht, dann wird die Ovulation über die Hemmung der Gonadotropinbildung unterdrückt und der normalerweise in der zweiten Cyclusphase eintretende Anstieg des Pregnandiols bleibt aus, eine Gravidität tritt nicht ein. Daß es sich tatsächlich um echte Progestine handelt, zeigt die antagonistische Wirkung gegenüber den spezifischen Eigenschaften der Oestrogene. So verhindern sie in größerer Dosis die proliferative Wirkung der Oestrogene auf das Endometrium, das durch Oestrogene ausgelöste Wachstum des

Eileiters von Kücken und die durch Oestrogene auslösbaren Fibromyome des Uterus von Meerschweinchen. Die synthetischen Präparate wirken pro Gewichtseinheit im allgemeinen oral viel stärker als das ursprüngliche Progesteron intramuskulär. Sie eignen sich daher nicht nur zur Behandlung von Menstruationsstörungen, sondern besonders zur Verhinderung der Ovulation. In einigen Ländern werden zur Zeit Großversuche zum Zwecke der Geburtenregulierung durchgeführt. Man kombiniert dabei die Progestine mit kleinen Oestrogendosen. Bewährt hat sich die Gabe von 2,5—5 mg Norethynodrel und 0,10 mg des 3-Methyl-äther des Äthinyloestradiol vom 5.—25. Tage (PINCUS, TYLER 1959) oder von 4 mg Äthenyl-Nortestosteron-Acetat und 0,06 mg Äthinyloestradiol vom 5.—24. Cyclustag (PEETERS). Die nach Unterbrechung eintretende Blutung entspricht etwa einer normalen Menstruationsblutung.

Alle sich vom Testosteron oder Androsteron ableitenden Derivate besitzen neben ihren progestionalen auch noch androgene Eigenschaften, die bei den 19-Nortestosteronen noch etwa 30—50%, bei den 19-Norandrostendionen noch 15—30% der Ausgangsubstanz betragen. Im Tierexperiment und am Menschen ist 17α-Methyl-19-Nortestosteron ein etwa halb so starkes Androgen wie Testosteronpropionat, während 17α-Äthinyl-Nortestosteron, 17α-Äthinyltestosteron im Samenblasentest nur schwach wirken. Am empfindlichsten reagieren Feten, wenn die Mütter diese synthetischen Progestine erhalten (s. S. 737). Die anabole Wirkung bleibt weitgehend erhalten, so entspricht z.B. 17α-Methyl-19-Nortestosteron dem Testosteronpropionat.

5. Ausscheidung der 17-Alkylderivate

Schon vom oral wirksamen 17-Methyltestosteron war bekannt, daß sich die 17-Ketosteroidausscheidung im Urin bei der Verabreichung dieses Steroids bei Menschen und beim Tier nicht erhöht. Ratten scheiden methyl-markiertes Methyltestosteron und Methylandrostendiol (HYDE) ebenso rasch aus wie Testosteron. In der Ausatmungsluft fehlt nach Unterbindung der Gallengänge jedoch jegliche Radioaktivität, die Methylgruppe wird also nicht zu CO_2 abgebaut.

Bei Verabreichung von 4-C^{14}-markiertem 17α-Hydroxyprogesteron-17α-Capronat (HPC) sind die Hauptausscheidungsprodukte in der sauren und phenolischen Fraktion enthalten, während die neutrale nur geringe Mengen von Radioaktivität aufweist. Bei der Bebrütung von HPC mit Rattenleberhomogenaten wird der Ring A reduziert, es entsteht Allopregnan-3β, 17α-diol-20-on-17α-Capronat und eine kleine Menge von Pregnan-3α, 17α-diol-20-on, 17α-Capronat (WIENER). Die Veresterung mit Capronsäure am C_{17} wird nicht entfernt, so wie das JUNKMANN bei den veresterten Testosteronen schon immer vermutet hat.

LANGECKER findet nach Verabreichung von 17α-Äthinyl-19-Nor-Testosteron (Noräthisteron) einen beträchtlichen Teil von Metaboliten, die noch die Äthinylgruppe tragen. Die fehlende Desalkylierung beeinträchtigt auch den fermentativen Angriff an der 4-3-Ketogruppe. Die gesamte als Ketone und Alkohole im Urin wiedergewonnene Menge beträgt nur 2,6—4,55% des oral verabreichten Noräthisteron. 0,02—0,1% werden als Äthinyloestradiol ausgeschieden. In 1-Stellung methylierte Verbindungen können offenbar durch die 1a-Hydroxylase nicht angegriffen werden, so daß die Aromatisierung und Umwandlung in Oestrogene ausbleibt.

Der Organismus ist also nicht imstande, die am C_{17} veresterten Steroide zu spalten und als 17-Ketosteroide auszuscheiden, selbst bei höchsten Dosen bleibt ein Anstieg aus. Der Abbau dieser synthetischen Derivate ist im einzelnen noch nicht bekannt, ein kleiner Teil verläßt den Körper in Form von phenolischen C_{18}-Steroiden (LANGECKER).

V. Nebenwirkungen der Steroidtherapie

1. Allgemeine

a) Ödeme und Blutdrucksteigerung

Vermehrte Retention von Wasser und Natrium ist eine häufige Begleiterscheinung der Androgen- und Oestrogentherapie. Bei Herz- und Nierengesunden wird nach einigen Tagen die vermehrt einbehaltene Flüssigkeit in Form einer Harnflut wieder ausgeschieden. Bei älteren Menschen mit geschädigtem Herzen, latenter oder manifester Niereninsuffizienz wird das Wasser dagegen in das subcutane Gewebe, besonders im Bereich des Gesichtes, an den Händen, an den Beinen eingelagert, ohne daß im Anfang eindrückbare Dellen zurückbleiben. Die meisten oestrogenbehandelten Prostatacarcinomträger sind an ihrem vollen, aufgedunsenen Gesicht zu erkennen. Anfangs müssen die Kranken genau beobachtet werden — tägliche Gewichtskontrolle und Blutdruckmessung —, da die Erhöhung des Blutvolumens Blutdrucksteigerung mit Insuffizienz des Herzens und Lungenödem herbeiführen kann. Strenge salzlose Kost, Verabreichung von Diuretica, die Kochsalz ausschwemmen, wie die Thiazide, Diamox und vorsichtige Digitalisierung verhindern in den meisten Fällen ernstere Komplikationen und erlauben auch die Dauertherapie bei Herzgeschädigten.

b) Magen-Darmkanal

Die orale Verabreichung natürlicher und synthetischer Oestrogene, Androgene, anaboler und gestagener Steroide löst bei einem Teil der Kranken Übelkeit, Appetitlosigkeit, Erbrechen, Leibschmerzen und Durchfälle aus. Die Ursache ist nicht recht klar, psychogene Momente müssen ausgeschlossen werden. Manchmal muß die Behandlung wegen der Heftigkeit der Beschwerden vorübergehend unterbrochen werden, bei parenteraler Therapie sind gastritische Symptome seltener. Schwerwiegende Komplikationen wie Ulcera, Blutungen kommen nur bei entsprechender Disposition vor.

c) Hypercalcämiesyndrom

Eine unangenehme Komplikation bei Behandlung des metastasierenden Mamma- und Prostatacarcinoms mit Androgenen oder Oestrogenen ist die Hypercalcämie. Meistens sind mehrere Faktoren am Entstehen beteiligt. Zerstörung des Knochens durch osteolytische Metastasen setzt verhältnismäßig viel Calcium frei. Die Calciumausscheidung ist vermehrt, der Calciumspiegel bleibt bei den Kranken lange Zeit normal oder ist nur mäßig erhöht, eine Organschädigung bleibt aus. Zusätzliche Bettruhe verstärkt die Ca-Mobilisierung aus dem gesunden Knochen, Verabreichung von Androgenen und Oestrogenen vermindert die Calciumausscheidung im Urin. Die resultierende Hypercalcämie bleibt aber geringgradig und meist harmlos. Das schwere Bild des Hypercalcämiesyndroms entwickelt sich offenbar nur, wenn unter der Oestrogen- und Androgenbehandlung eine rasche Ausbreitung des Tumors im Knochen einsetzt und dadurch plötzlich große Ca-Mengen anfallen. Dieses Ereignis ist häufig am Ansteigen der alkalischen Phosphatase im Serum vorauszusehen.

Die klinischen Erscheinungen sind denjenigen des akuten Hyperparathyreoidismus sehr ähnlich. Übelkeit, Anorexie, Erbrechen, Bluteindickung, Durchfall, Hyponatriämie, Hypochlorämie treten ein, die Kranken werden dösig, komatös, der Blutdruck fällt ab, der Harnstoff steigt an. In den verschiedensten Organen, vorwiegend an Stellen mit niedrigem p_H, wird Kalk abgelagert, besonders in den Nieren, Magen, Lunge, aber auch im Myokard, Leber, Skeletmuskulatur und Arterien. In vielen Organen entwickeln sich Nekrosen. Die akute tubuläre Insuffizienz ist die eigentliche Todesursache. Die Feststellung dieser Komplikationen im ersten Anfangsstadium ist schwierig, da leichte Symptome auch durch die Grundkrankheit oder durch die Hormonbehandlung selbst hervorgerufen sein können.

Die Behandlung verlangt ein sofortiges Absetzen der Hormongabe und Bekämpfung der Exsiccose mit hyposmotischen Kochsalzlösungen. Die Hypercalcämie selbst wird durch intravenöse Infusion von 2,5%igem Natriumcitrat — 250 cm³ alle 4 Std intravenös so lange gegeben, bis sich das Bewußtsein aufhellt — bekämpft. Dadurch werden die schwer löslichen Ca^{++}-Ionen in lösliche schwach ionisierte Calciumcitrationen abgebunden und die Konzentration des ionisierten Calciums im Blut vermindert. Die Bestimmung des Blutcalciums erfaßt diese Änderung nicht. Unter Umständen wird die Anwendung der künstlichen Niere erforderlich (KENNEDY 1953a, b, LÜHRS, PFEFFER, SWYER 1950).

d) Antikörperbildung gegen Steroide

Vorwiegend französische Autoren (GILBERT-DREYFUS) vertreten die Ansicht, daß die Sexualhormone, besonders die Oestrogene, aber auch Progesteron, allergische Reaktionen hervorrufen können. Man nimmt an, daß die Hormone mit Eiweißkörpern eine Bindung eingehen und dadurch zu Halbantigenen werden. Die Antikörper sollen nicht nur gegen den Eiweißanteil, sondern auch gegen das Steroid gerichtet sein. Als Symptome werden angeführt: Kopfschmerzen, Übelkeit, Erbrechen, lokalisierte Exantheme, Rötungen der Haut und Schleimhäute, Juckreiz, Asthmaanfälle, Migräne und vasomotorische Reaktionen der verschiedensten Art. Der Beweis für die Deutung dieser Symptome als Überempfindlichkeitsreaktion ist nicht sicher erbracht, ebenso sind die Erfolge der Desensibilisierung umstritten.

e) Leberschädigung, cholostatischer Ikterus

In einzelnen Fällen ist bei Menschen nach langdauernder Verabreichung von synthetischen *Oestrogenen* beim Prostatacarcinom über Leberparenchymschäden berichtet worden. GUMBRECHT und LOESER erzeugten im Tierexperiment mit hohen Oestrogendosen an Ratten Lebernekrosen und Verfettungen. TAUPITZ hat diese älteren Befunde noch einmal überprüft und einen Unterschied zwischen den synthetischen und den natürlichen Oestrogenen in ihrer Wirkung auf die Leber festgestellt. Diäthyldioxystilben in der Menge von 1—3,5 mg/kg führt bei Ratten nach 14 Tagen in 60% zu einer deutlichen Verfettung und Vacuolisierung der Leberzellen. Die alkalische Phosphatase in den Leberzellen ist vermehrt und ungleichmäßig verteilt, im Serum steigt sie an, Gesamtcholesterin und die Cholesterinester fallen ab. Die Vermehrung dieses Fermentes entspricht den Befunden nach toxischer Schädigung der Leber mit Äthylalkohol und ähnlichen Giften und ist ein Ausdruck der Zellschädigung (TAUPITZ 1959). Die Abnahme des Cholesterins und der Cholesterinester nach synthetischen Oestrogenen ist wiederholt auch beim Menschen beobachtet worden. Im Gegensatz dazu macht das natürliche Oestradiol keine Verfettung, die alkalische Phosphatase des Serums nimmt ab, während der Cholesterinspiegel keine signifikante Änderung zeigt (TAUPITZ 1960). Beim Menschen liegen systematische Untersuchungen über die Funktion der Leber unter langdauernder Oestrogengabe nicht vor.

Testosteron und seine Ester beeinträchtigen die Funktion der Leber nicht. Dagegen ist nach Verabreichung der am C_{17} substituierten 17α-Derivate — zum erstenmal nach 17α-Methyltestosteron — das Auftreten eines *cholostatischen Ikterus* beschrieben worden. Es ist nicht das hohe Angebot des Hormons durch die Pfortader, das die Leber schädigt, da die Toxikose auch bei parenteraler Verabreichung auftritt (Foss). Man schreibt heute die Leberschädigung einer spezifischen Eigenschaft der am C_{17} ein Alkyl tragenden Steroide zu, die die Leber nicht wie die anderen Steroide handhaben kann. Die 19-Norverbindungen scheinen toxischer als die 19-methylierten Steroide.

Trotz der großen Verwendung dieser Testosteronderivate sind die Schäden doch verhältnismäßig selten. Foss und SIMSON konnten bis 1959 nach Methyltestosteron nur 42 Fälle mit einem Todesfall in der Literatur finden, eine kleine Zahl, wenn man sie mit der häufigen Verwendung dieses Derivates in Beziehung bringt. Neuerdings wurde auch bei Anwendung der 17-alkylierten Nortestosterone über dieselben Schäden berichtet.

Der Ikterus tritt meist erst nach mehrmonatiger Behandlung auf, in seltenen Fällen schon nach 10—20 Tagen. Die Kranken klagen zuerst über Appetitlosigkeit, Erbrechen, Unruhe, über eine Lethargie, nach einigen Tagen folgt die Gelbfärbung der Haut mit hellen Stühlen und auffallend starker Braunfärbung des Urins. Neben dem Bilirubin, das im Blut rasch hohe Werte annehmen kann, findet man eine Erhöhung der alkalischen Serumphosphatase und der Serumglutaminsäure-Oxalessigsäure-Transaminase (SGOT) bis auf 500 und mehr. Wir sahen auch regelmäßig eine Vermehrung der LAP, während die SGPT normal blieb.

Der Verlauf ist im allgemeinen günstig, der Ikterus kann nach Absetzen des Steroids in 8—14 Tagen zurückgehen, bei schweren Formen hält er aber 4—8 Wochen an. Die Prognose ist gut, vorausgesetzt, daß zusätzliche Schäden ferngehalten werden. Histologisch findet sich das Bild des sog. „cholostatischen Ikterus". Man versteht darunter ein Phänomen, das durch eine Störung des Gallenflusses hervorgerufen wird (POPPER und SCHAFFNER 1957). Histologisch sind die intralobulären Gallengänge erweitert und vielfach mit Gallenthromben ausgefüllt. Die Leberzellen nehmen im späteren Verlauf Gallenpigment auf, ebenso die Kupfferschen Sternzellen. Das Bild ist dasselbe wie beim Verschlußikterus, nur daß die großen Gallengänge nicht erweitert sind. Die Leberzelle selbst ist nicht geschädigt, entzündliche Infiltrate in den portalen Feldern fehlen oder sind nur gering ausgeprägt. Die Ursache des gestörten Galletransportes ist nicht bekannt. Man vermutet eine Erhöhung der Viscosität der Galle, reichliche Thrombenbildung behindert den Abfluß. Auch eine Störung der Permeabilität der Gallengänge wird diskutiert.

Guten Aufschluß geben einige neuere Untersuchungen mit regelmäßiger Kontrolle der Leberfunktion. KORY (1959) verabreichte 47 Patienten 25—50 mg Dianabol über 6 Monate. 35 dieser Kranken, d.h. 74%, zeigten eine Erhöhung der Bromsulfaleinretention, die bei 50 mg täglich beträchtlich höher war als bei 25 mg. Bei 7 dieser Kranken, die leberpunktiert werden konnten, ergab die histologische Untersuchung keine Cholostase. SCHAFFNER beobachtet bei der täglichen Gabe von 60 mg Norethandrolon (Nilevar) über 3—5 Wochen in 60% eine Erhöhung der SGOT, aber nur bei 4 von 24 Patienten bioptisch eine Cholostase, obwohl alle 24 erhöhte Transaminasen im Serum hatten. WYNN u. Mitarb. sahen klinisch keine toxischen Erscheinungen nach Dianabol, das sie zum Teil in sehr hohen Dosen (25—50 mg, ein Patient 26 Tage lang 100 mg, anschließend noch 198 Tage 75 mg) gaben, auch nicht bei Kranken mit vorher schon vorhandener Leberfunktionsstörung. Sie finden die klassischen Funktionsteste wie

Bilirubin, alkalische Phosphatase, Thymoltrübung, Thymolflockung, Serum-
elektrophorese, Urobilinogen ungestört. Nur SGOT und der Bromsulfaleintest
(BSP) zeigten Abweichungen. 70% aller Behandelten hatten zu irgendeinem
Zeitpunkt eine vermehrte Retention von BSP (Höchstwert 34%). Trotz Fortführung der Behandlung sank diese in allen Fällen bis auf einen wieder auf normale Werte ab. Bei einem Drittel der Patienten war die SGOT erhöht, bei
hohen Dosen häufiger als bei niedrigen. Nach Aussetzen fällt SGOT rasch ab,
trotz Weitergabe des Hormons erreicht sie nach einiger Zeit wieder normale
Werte. Auch nach unseren Erfahrungen geht der Ausfall des Bromsulfaleintestes
(BST) mit den übrigen Leberfunktionsproben nicht parallel. Der Ausscheidungs-
mechanismus des Bromsulfaleins ist ein ganz spezifischer Vorgang, an dem
mehrere Fermentsysteme beteiligt sind, so daß der alleinige pathologische Ausfall
dieser Probe nicht als Leberschädigung aufgefaßt werden darf. Unter der Behandlung mit hohen Dosen (30 mg) 17-Methyl-Nortestosteron (Gestagen) sind
die Zeichen der Gallenabflußstörung noch eindeutiger (FELDMAN). Bei zehn von
elf Behandelten erhöhte sich das Bilirubin bis auf 3,2 mg, wenn mehr als 4200 mg
verabreicht war, ebenso das Cholesterin, während die Bewegung der Phosphatasen
und von Bromsulfalein in diesen Fällen wegen der ausgedehnten Metastasierung
in Knochen und Leber nicht zu verwerten ist. Beim Gesunden vermindert sich
unter 17-Methyl-Nortestosteron die Ausscheidungsfähigkeit für den Farbstoff
schon nach 2 Wochen.

Im ganzen gesehen ist der cholostatische Ikterus eine seltene Komplikation
der Hormonbehandlung. Ob er bei jedem am C_{17} substituierten Testosteron,
Androsteron, Progesteron oder Oestrogen auftreten kann, ist noch nicht geklärt.
Bei Verwendung kleiner und mittlerer Dosen ist das Risiko gering, sind hohe
notwendig, dann gibt man besser am C_{17} nicht alkylierte Derivate. Bei höheren
Dosen und längerer Behandlung wird man in jedem Falle die Transaminasen,
Hydrogenasen und Phosphatasen neben dem Bromsulfalein verfolgen, aber nur
bei übermäßigem Anstieg die Behandlung unterbrechen. Wichtiger ist es, den
subjektiven Beschwerden, wie Übelkeit, Appetitlosigkeit, Erbrechen, allgemeines
Abgeschlagensein, Hautjucken, sein Augenmerk zu schenken, dies sind die
sichersten Vorboten der Cholostase.

Therapeutisch hat sich die Verabreichung von Prednisonen, im Anfang 20 bis
30 mg, bewährt, da dadurch der Gallenfluß rascher in Gang kommt. Daneben
ist es wichtig, jeden zusätzlichen Schaden fernzuhalten und schon prophylaktisch
für eine calorisch ausreichende eiweiß- und kohlenhydratreiche Kost zu sorgen.
Die sog. „Leberschutzbehandlung" ist nicht nötig.

2. Spezifische

a) Virilisierung durch Androgene, anabole und gestagene Steroide

Frauen sind gegenüber der Einwirkung von androgenwirksamen Steroiden
verschieden empfindlich. Zeichen des Hirsutismus und des *Virilismus* treten
im Klimakterium und nach Kastration früher und mit kleineren Dosen auf
als im gebärfähigen Alter. Besonders das vermehrte Wachstum der Lanugobehaarung im Gesicht, weniger am Stamm und an den Extremitäten ist dabei
störend. Eine ausgesprochene Virilisierung des Körperbaues ist selbst bei Verwendung hoher und höchster Dosen von Androgenen sehr selten. Bei Mädchen
und jüngeren Frauen wird dagegen frühzeitig die Tätigkeit der Talgdrüsen erhöht,
Gesicht, besonders die Stirne und die Kopfhaut erhalten ein fettiges und öliges
Aussehen. Es entwickelt sich eine sehr störende Acne, besonders im Gesicht,

auf Rücken und Brust, aus der sekundäre Pyodermien und Furunkulosen entstehen können. In einem Bericht von KENNEDY (1953a) über 82 Frauen, die wegen Mammacarcinom wöchentlich dreimal 50 mg Testosteronpropionat erhielten, zeigte sich als erste Erscheinung eine Heiserkeit der Stimme, die mit der Dauer der Behandlung zunimmt, die Stimmbänder verdicken sich, die Stimme wird tiefer, zwei Drittel der Behandelten waren davon betroffen. 22% klagten über einen ausgeprägten Haarverlust und bekamen Alopecien, 45% gaben eine Zunahme der Libido an, die Klitoris kann sich vergrößern. Im allgemeinen bessert sich das Wohlbefinden, doch sind bei älteren Frauen depressive Verstimmungen nicht selten. Klimakterische Ausfallserscheinungen wie Hitzewallungen und Schweißausbrüche können sich erheblich verstärken.

Die individuelle Empfindlichkeit gegenüber Androgenen ist sehr verschieden. 200—400 mg Testosteronpropionat oder eine entsprechende Dosis eines anabolen Derivates während eines Cyclus führen im allgemeinen zu keinen Nebenerscheinungen (ZENZEN). Die Angaben der einzelnen Autoren sind jedoch sehr verschieden, so wurde schon bei 200 mg über Virilisierungserscheinungen berichtet. Die kräftigen androgenen Eigenschaften der anabolen Nortestosterone zeigt z.B. das 17-Methyl-19-Nortestosteron. 30 mg täglich per os entsprechen bei klimakterischen Frauen 300 mg Testosteronpropionat pro Woche. Beim 17-Nortestosteron bekamen sieben, beim Testosteron acht Frauen von 20 behandelten einen Hirsutismus, eine tiefe Stimme, Acne und Klitorishypertrophie (FELDMAN), fünf von dreizehn nach Beendigung der 17-Nortestosterongabe eine oestrogene Abbruchsblutung.

Bei der Behandlung metastasierender Carcinome wird das Testosteron und seine Derivate oft so hoch dosiert, daß die Bildung der Gonadotropine in der Hypophyse blockiert wird, obwohl deren Verminderung keine Vorbedingung für die anticancerogene Wirksamkeit eines Steroids ist. Die Hypophysenblockade wird erst mit Dosen ab 500 mg Testosteronpropionat oder einem entsprechenden Esterderivat erreicht. Vor dem Klimakterium führen diese Dosen zu einer Hemmung der Follikelreifung und mit der Zeit zu einer schweren Atrophie des Ovars.

Man hat versucht, die Virilisierung der Frau durch die Kombination von männlichen und weiblichen Hormonen hintanzuhalten, dies gelingt jedoch nicht vollständig. Nach MASTERS soll jedoch eine Mischung von Androgenen und Oestrogenen im Verhältnis von 30:1 (mg) die androgenen Eigenschaften mildern, bei einer Mischung im Verhältnis von 20:1 sollen sie bei älteren Frauen „neutralisiert" werden können.

Erst spät wurde erkannt, daß Mißbildungen im Sinne der Vermännlichung (Pseudohermaphroditismus feminus) am äußeren Genitale weiblicher Neugeborener durch Verabreichung von Androgenen, Gestagenen und sogar von Oestrogenen während der Gravidität entstehen können. Die erste Beschreibung von ZANDER stammt schon von 1952, aber erst durch die weite Verbreitung der synthetischen Gestagene häuften sich die Fälle in den letzten Jahren. Die Frauen wurden wegen drohendem Abort, Pruritus, Erbrechen, allgemeiner Körperschwäche, Osteoporose, Alopecie, Mastodynie oder wegen Geschwülsten behandelt. Erhielten die Mütter die Hormone nach der 6., aber vor der 13. Schwangerschaftswoche, dann waren bei den weiblichen Neugeborenen die Labioscrotalfalten verschmolzen, Urethra und Vagina mündeten in einem Urogenitalsinus, in extremen Fällen an der Spitze einer stark vergrößerten Klitoris, die Wolffschen Gänge waren — soweit dies untersucht werden konnte — im Gegensatz zu behandelten Tieren nicht stimuliert. Wurde die Behandlung erst nach der 13. Schwangerschaftswoche begonnen, dann fand sich nur eine deutlich vergrößerte Klitoris und große Labia majora. Die Häufigkeit dieser Mißbildungen wird sehr verschieden angegeben. Bongiovanni u. Mitarb. ermittelten bei 650 mit Äthinyl-Testosteron oder Äthinyl-Nortestosteron behandelten Graviden eine Rate von 0,3%, Jakobsen bei 53 mit Äthinyl-Nortestosteron behandelten 34%! Am häufigsten findet sich 17α-Äthinyltestosteron, 17α-Äthinyl-Nortestosteron, Progesteron, 17α-Oxyprogesteron erwähnt. Verhältnismäßig häufig wurden Mißbildungen auch bei kombinierter Behandlung mit Androgenen und Oestrogenen (Äthinyl-Nortestosteron und Oestrogene) beobachtet, ja selbst nach alleiniger Gabe von Stilboestrol (5—50 mg täglich).

Erst auf Grund dieser Beobachtungen am Menschen hat man die maskulinisierende Wirkung der Derivate an Tieren geprüft (Phoenix). Die einzelnen Arten reagieren verschieden. Die Steroide sind unwirksam, solange die Entwicklung des Genitale noch nicht eingesetzt hat. Der unterste Genitaltrakt ist am empfindlichsten, so daß in allen Fällen die Maskulinisierung des äußeren Genitales und des Urogenitalsinus recht ausgeprägt war. Bei den meisten Tierarten entwickelten sich auch die Wolffschen Gänge, ohne daß sich die Müllerschen zurückbildeten, es entsteht also das typische Bild des künstlichen Pseudohermaphroditismus feminus, wie es seit den Versuchen von Dantschakoff bekannt ist. Im intrauterinen Virilisierungstest sind 6-Methyl-17α-Hydroxyprogesteronacetat, 17α-Äthinyl-Testosteron, 17α-Äthinyl-Nor-Testosteron, 17α-Äthinyl-19-Nor-Δ 5(10)-Androsten-17β-ol-3-on in Dosen wirksam, wie sie zur Auslösung der gestagenen Eigenschaften bei der Frau erforderlich sind. Die androgenen Eigenschaften im Samenblasen- und Hahnenkammtest gehen mit der Stärke der Virilisierung des Feten nicht parallel.

Eine wesentliche Ursache dieser abnormen Reaktion beruht in der besonderen Empfindlichkeit des Fet gegenüber den Androgenen (Jost 1947), so daß im intrauterinen Virilisierungstest Steroide noch androgene bzw. virilisierende Eigenschaften zeigen, die mit anderen biologischen Prüfungen nicht erfaßt werden können, wie z.B. die Oestrogene.

Neuerdings werden Kinder und Jugendliche mit verzögerter Rekonvaleszenz nach Infektionskrankheiten, mit Resorptionsstörungen des Magen-Darmkanals, mit Magerkeit und chronischem Appetitmängel u. ä. ziemlich kritiklos mit anabolen Steroiden behandelt. Der Einfluß auf das *Längenwachstum* ist bei längerer Behandlung sehr zu beachten. 0,1—0,3 mg/kg Körpergewicht 17-Nortestosteron regen bei Kindern und Jugendlichen von 4—15 Jahren das Längenwachstum deutlich an. Man darf annehmen, daß bei längerdauernder Behandlung und insbesondere bei Behandlung Jugendlicher um die Zeit der Pubertät wie durch Testosteron der Epiphysenschluß vorzeitig erfolgen kann. Dabei ist auch die Gefahr der Auslösung einer *vorzeitigen Pubertät* mit Wachstum der Körper- und Schambehaarung, Vergrößerung des Genitales, Tieferwerden der Stimme u. ä. gegeben.

b) Feminisierung durch Ovarialhormone

Der Urologe steht manchmal vor der Entscheidung, Frauen im geschlechtsreifen Alter oder im Klimakterium mit *Ovarialhormonen* zu behandeln. Die wichtigsten und schwersten Nebenerscheinungen sind dabei *Uterusblutungen* als Folge der Proliferation der Schleimhaut. Eine Blutung aus dem Endometrium tritt auf, wenn der Hormonspiegel im Blut bei proliferierter Schleimhaut rasch absinkt. Eine solche sog. Entzugsblutung oder Abbruchsblutung kann nach einer kurzdauernden, aber überschwelligen Behandlung mit Oestrogenen eintreten. Solche Blutungen sind im allgemeinen nur geringfügig, kurzdauernd und werden praktisch nie bedrohlich.

Wird länger als über 6—8 Wochen behandelt, dann besteht bei dem stark proliferierten und hyperplastischen Endometrium die Gefahr einer Dauerblutung auch ohne daß an der Oestrogendosis etwas geändert wird. Der gleichbleibende Oestrogenspiegel reicht eines Tages nicht mehr aus, um die Gefäßversorgung der gewucherten Schleimhaut zu gewährleisten. Als Folge eines relativen Oestrogenmangels beginnen Blutungen aus oberflächlichen Nekrosen, die auch nach Absetzen der Oestrogenzufuhr nicht zum Stehen kommen. Die starken und langandauernden Metrorrhagien können zu erheblichen Blutverlusten und bei älteren Menschen zu Schäden führen. Die intramuskulär injizierbaren Oestrogenpräparate sind im allgemeinen in der Dosis so abgestimmt, daß Dauerblutungen ausbleiben. Am besten dosierbar ist die orale Verabreichung, die — wenn es die Grundkrankheit erlaubt — alle 3—4 Wochen für 4—6 Tage unterbrochen wird, um die harmlose Entzugsblutung einzuleiten und dadurch die schwere Dauerblutung zu verhüten.

Eine genügend hohe Dosis innerhalb der ersten 8—10 Tage des Cyclus verhindert die Ausschüttung von FSH und damit die Reifung eines Follikels und die Ovulation. Diese *Hemmung der Ovulation* wird ohne die starke Proliferation des Endometriums auch durch hohe Progesterondosen und besonders durch die progestional wirkenden 19-Norsteroide erreicht. Gleichmäßige Verabreichung über Monate führt zu einer Atrophie des Ovars, während die cyclusgerecht unterbrochene Behandlung die Keimdrüse nicht zum Schwinden bringt. Um trotz gehemmter Ovulation cyclusähnliche Blutungen beizubehalten, müssen die Norsteroide mit kleinen Oestrogendosen kombiniert werden. PINCUS u. Mitarb. fanden auf Puerto Rico die Kombination von 2,5 mg Norethynodrel und 0,075 bis 0,1 mg des 3-Methyläthers von 17α-Äthinyl-oestradiol als Antikonzipiens im 5—25 Tage-Regime am besten wirksam. Die „Menstruationsblutung" dauert kürzer und fließt weniger als eine normale. Nebenerscheinungen wie Übelsein, Erbrechen, Magenschmerzen, Kopfdruck und -schmerz, Schmerzen im Becken und eine empfindliche Brust seien vorwiegend psychogen.

Die hochdosierte Oestrogenbehandlung des Prostatacarcinoms führt in 20 bis 40% der Fälle zu einer Schwellung der Brustdrüse. Zuerst macht sich eine Überempfindlichkeit der etwas prominierenden Brustwarzen geltend, später wächst das Fettgewebe zusammen mit dem Drüsenkörper, bis sich eine deutliche *Gynäkomastie* entwickelt hat. Der Drüsenkörper erreicht eine Größe von 5—7 cm im Durchmesser und 2—3 cm in der Dicke. Lactation ist selten, kommt aber vor. Zusätzliche Gabe von Testosteron, selbst im Verhältnis von 20:1, verhindert das Drüsenwachstum nicht. Die Gesamtdosen bis zum Auftreten der ersten Erscheinungen schwanken zwischen 15 und 60 mg Oestradiolbenzoat. Allmählich verliert sich die starke Empfindlichkeit, das Spannungsgefühl nimmt ab und die meisten Männer fühlen sich nicht weiter gestört. Die Wirkung der Oestrogene ist bei der geschlechtsreifen Frau gering. Selbst unter der hochdosierten Oestrogenbehandlung von Mammacarcinomträgerinnen vergrößert sich die Brustdrüse nur in einem ganz kleinen Teil der Fälle.

Die Oestrogene ändern bei Frauen den Behaarungstyp nicht, Männer verlieren einen Teil der *Körperbehaarung*, die Schamhaargrenze wird horizontal, Genital-, Achsel- und Bartbehaarung vermindern sich, bleiben aber erhalten. Dies ist keine direkte Wirkung der Oestrogene, sondern Folge der Hemmung der Gonadotropinproduktion und der eigenen Androgenbildung.

Unangenehm kann die manchmal eintretende *Hautpigmentierung* werden. Menschen, die leicht Pigmente bilden, sind stärker betroffen als helle Typen. Bestimmte Körperpartien wie Brustwarzen, Warzenhof, Linea alba, äußeres Genitale, mechanisch beanspruchte Hautpartien und Gesicht werden bevorzugt.

Im Gesicht ist die Pigmentierung meist grobfleckig und hat Ähnlichkeit mit dem Chloasma uterinum.

Beim Mann wird die *Psychosexualität* durch Oestrogene empfindlich gestört. Höhere Dosen führen zum völligen Verlust von Libido und Potenz, einmal sah ich eine paradoxe Reaktion. Die Oestrogenbehandlung von Sittlichkeitsverbrechern ist keine absolut sichere Methode. Testosteronpropionat in hohen Dosen erhöht bei 40—60% der Frauen die Libido, während die androgenwirksamen Nortestosterone wohl die Klitoris zum Wachstum anregen, aber die Psyche nicht stimulieren sollen.

VI. Bedeutung des männlichen Keimdrüsenhormons für Entwicklung und Wachstum

Die Wirkung der Androgene ist in gewissem Umfange abhängig vom *Lebensalter*. Alle Gewebe, die eine besondere Empfindlichkeit gegenüber den Sexualhormonen haben, besitzen diese schon intrauterin. Mit zunehmendem Alter scheint sich das Reaktionsvermögen einzelner Organe zu verstärken. Die Prostata einer jungen Ratte spricht vom 1.—14. Lebenstag zunehmend stärker auf dieselbe Dosis von Testosteron an, dann ist ein Maximum erreicht. Samenblasen und Koagulationsdrüsen reagieren am 26. Lebenstag am stärksten. Man nimmt an, daß sich auch beim Menschen die Pubertät aus zwei Faktorengruppen zusammensetzt, einmal aus der Zunahme der Testosteronproduktion, die nach Dorfman u. Mitarb. (1956) schon beim Kleinkind in geringer Menge vorhanden ist, die sich aber um die Zeit der Pubertät, also zwischen dem 11.—15. Lebensjahr auf das 5—7fache erhöht. Der andere Faktor ist die wachsende Empfindlichkeit der sekundären Geschlechtsorgane. Diese Empfindlichkeit ist nicht nur abhängig von der Erreichung eines bestimmten Reifegrades des Gewebes, sondern auch vom Zentralnervensystem und von den anderen innersekretorischen Drüsen, besonders der Schilddrüse. Mit zunehmendem Alter soll die Empfindlichkeit des Gewebes wieder abnehmen.

1. Skelet

Das komplizierte Geschehen des Längenwachstums steht unter dem Einfluß des somatotropen Hormons, des Schilddrüsenhormons und der anabolen Wirkungskomponente der Androgene.

Das *Schilddrüsenhormon* hat schon in den ersten Lebensjahren einen wesentlichen Einfluß auf Wachstum und Entwicklung aller Körpergewebe. Es verstärkt die Wirkung des STH entweder durch Anregung der STH-Bildung oder durch Katalysierung der Stoffwechselreaktionen im Gewebe. Darüber hinaus hat es aber auch eine direkte Wirkung auf die Knochenreifung. Die Bildung der Knochenkerne erfolgt bei schilddrüsenlosen Tieren verzögert und abwegig, indem multiple kleine Kerne in den Epiphysen auftreten, die verspätet zusammenfließen (Kretinenhüfte). Der hypothyreote Zwerg hat andere Körperproportionen wie der hypophysäre.

Das Wachstumshormon STH (HGH) übernimmt erst im 3.—4. Lebensjahr die Führung. Vor dem 4. Lebensjahr ist das Hormon für das Körperwachstum nicht erforderlich. Gemzel (1959) hat STH in Hypophysen menschlicher Feten im 5. Graviditätsmonat nachgewiesen. Almquist u. Mitarb. finden den Sulfation-Faktor (SF) — gemessen wird die S35-Aufnahme von Knorpelgewebe — als Maß der Aktivität des STH schon in den ersten Lebensmonaten im Blut (0,6 SF). Im 4. Lebensjahr erfolgt ein kräftiger Anstieg auf 1 E, die mit Schwankungen bis ins Alter von 70 Jahren erhalten bleibt. Die Maxima liegen im 8. und 15. Lebensjahr, die Minima im 6.—12. und 4. Lebensjahr.

STH stimuliert besonders den proliferierenden Epiphysenknorpel und fördert damit die Chondrogenese, also vorwiegend das Längenwachstum. Unter seinem Einfluß ist das Wachstum ein gleichmäßiges. Bleiben die Androgene um die Zeit der Pubertät aus (Eunuchismus), dann wächst der Betroffene langsam weiter. Da die Knochenreifung stark verzögert ist (3.—4. Jahrzehnt), verlängert sich die Wachstumsperiode erheblich. Es resultiert letztlich ein Hochwuchs mit bestimmten Skeletproportionen, auch normalwüchsige Eunuchoide haben eunuchoide Proportionen. Epiphysen, die sich normalerweise erst nach der Pubertät schließen, wie die Beckenrandapophyse, können zeitlebens offenbleiben.

Die *androgenen* und anabolen Steroide stimulieren sowohl die endochondrale als auch die endostale *Knochenbildung* und fördern damit sowohl das Längen- als auch das Dickenwachstum des Skelets. ALBRIGHT nimmt an, daß die Osteoblasten zur Ablagerung der Knochenmatrix angeregt werden. Die Androgene erhöhen plötzlich die Wachstumsrate und induzieren den für die Pubertät charakteristischen Wachstumsstoß. Gleichzeitig fördern sie aber auch die Knochenreifung, sie beschleunigen die Ossifikation des Epiphysenknorpels und damit den Schluß der Epiphysenfugen und bringen das Wachstum damit zum Abschluß. Die Wachstumssteigerung erfolgt auch beim hypophysektomierten Tier, sie ist also unabhängig vom STH. Ist ein Organismus vor Erreichung seiner puberalen Körpergröße einer hohen Androgenwirkung ausgesetzt (Pubertas praecox), dann wird vorübergehend die Wachstumsrate wie zur Zeit der Pubertät erhöht, gleichzeitig reift der Knochen und der Epiphysenschluß erfolgt vorzeitig. Das Ergebnis ist ein Minderwuchs. Mit der Steigerung des Längenwachstums geht eine rasche Gewichtszunahme parallel, die vorwiegend auf die Entwicklung der Muskulatur zurückgeht.

2. Genitalorgane

Wie früher erwähnt, differenziert sich die indifferente Genitalanlage nur unter dem Einfluß der in der Embryonalzeit in den Leydigzellen gebildeten Androgene in männlicher Richtung. Während der Pubertät regen diese wiederum spezifisch das Wachstum des Genitalapparates an und sind auch später verantwortlich für die Erhaltung seiner Funktion.

Penis und Scrotum vergrößern sich vor der Pubertät nur wenig. Mit Beginn der Androgenbildung wächst der Penis sowohl in der Länge, später auch in der Dicke. Bei vielen Säuglingen und Kindern sind Präputium und Glans noch miteinander verbacken und lösen sich erst mit der Androgenproduktion. Glatte und quergestreifte Muskeln vergrößern sich, die Beckenbodenmuskulatur hypertrophiert, besonders der Musculus levator ani, der Tonus des Musculus detrusor vesicae wird gesteigert. Während der Pubertät ist die Größe des Penis ein guter und einfacher Maßstab der Androgenbildung. Auch das *Scrotum* macht eine ganz charakteristische Wandlung durch, so daß man die Phase der Pubertätsentwicklung daran ablesen kann. Beim Kind hat es die Form einer Kuppel. Mit der Pubertät verlängert es sich, während die Basis noch eng bleibt. Gegen Ende der Pubertät bildet sich die Tunica dartos aus, die dem Scrotum seine Contractilität verleiht. Zugleich pigmentiert sich Scrotum und Penis. Jetzt erst verbreitert sich auch die Basis und die beim Kind deutlich hervortretende Raphe mediana verwischt sich. Die Contractilität der Tunica dartos ist gebunden an die Anwesenheit von Androgenen.

Bei Ratten, Mäusen und Meerschweinchen bilden sich Penis und Scrotum ausgewachsener Tiere nach der Kastration teilweise zurück. Das Erektionsvermögen schwindet weitgehend, jedoch nicht gänzlich. Bei Ratten liegen Beobachtungen vor, daß nicht nur hormonale, sondern auch mechanische Faktoren

für die Entwicklung des Scrotums wichtig sind. Entfernt man mit der Kastration Hoden und Nebenhoden, dann atrophiert das Scrotum und entwickelt sich
nach Androgenbehandlung nicht mehr. Beläßt man dagegen die Epididymis
oder legt statt dessen kleine Glasstäbchen ein, dann entwickelt sich das Scrotum
unter Testosteron wieder normal. Dieser mechanische Faktor mag der Grund
sein, weshalb beim einseitigen Kryptorchismus der leere Scrotumteil immer
weniger entwickelt ist als der gesunde und weshalb beim Menschen nach Kastration durch Entfernung beider Hoden das Scrotum kleiner ist als beim hypophysären Eunuchismus, bei dem die Leydigzellfunktion ganz erloschen ist, die
Hoden aber im Scrotum liegen. Bei fehlender Androgenbildung atrophieren die
Tunica dartos und der Musculus cremaster, der Cremasterreflex erlischt. Einfluß
auf Hoden, Prostata, Samenblasen, weibliche Genitalorgane s. S. 711.

3. Haut

Wie alle Körpergewebe, so besitzt auch die *Haut* und ihre Anhangsgebilde
bei jedem einzelnen Individuum bestimmte Wachstumspotenzen. Diese werden
von den Androgenen voll zur Entfaltung gebracht, darüber hinaus sind die
Sexualhormone wirkungslos. Wenn die Fähigkeit zur Pigmentbildung schlecht
ist, Haarfollikel in bestimmten Körpergegenden nicht angelegt sind, dann können
die Androgene auch nicht wirksam werden.

Mit der Pubertät nimmt die Pigmentbildung der Haut zu, besonders im
Bereich des Scrotums, des Perineums, der Linea alba und an der Brustwarze.

Die Schweiß-, Duft- und *Talgdrüsen* entfalten sich erst zur Zeit der Pubertät
vollständig. Besonders die Talgdrüsen werden stimuliert. 99% aller Jungen
bekommen zwischen 13 und 20 eine Acne, der Gipfel liegt um 18 Jahre.

Die Entwicklung des *Haarkleides* erfolgt in konstanter Reihenfolge. Zuerst
erscheinen an der Peniswurzel einige wenige glatte Härchen. Etwa zur gleichen
Zeit werden die Lanugohaare an den Streckseiten von Arm und Bein dicker,
die Schamhaare werden langsam dichter, breiten sich auf den Unterbauch aus
und beginnen sich zu kräuseln. Der Bart fängt an der Oberlippe und an den
Wangen unter den Ohren an zu wachsen. Erst spät breiten sich die Schamhaare auf das Scrotum, das Perineum und auf den Unterbauch aus. Die Begrenzung bleibt lange horizontal. Die Achselbehaarung folgt etwa ein Jahr
nach Beginn der Pubesbehaarung. Die endgültige Körperbehaarung ist erst
Mitte bis Ende der zwanziger Jahre voll ausgebildet, ihr Ausmaß wird durch
die Konstitution bestimmt, ihre volle Entwicklung ist nicht möglich ohne die
Sexualhormone. Kastraten zeigen nur an der Peniswurzel einige glatte Haare,
ebenso einige wenige an den Streckseiten der Arme und Beine, während die
Behaarung im Gesicht, der Achsel und am Rumpf fehlt.

Zum Bild des Hypogonadismus gehört ein dichtes Kopfhaar, das in die Stirne
hereinzuwachsen scheint (Pelzmütze). Gegen Ende der Pubertät tritt das Kopfhaar an beiden Schläfen unter einer Winkelbildung zurück. Diese Calvitis frontalis bildet sich nur bei Anwesenheit der Androgene aus. Ein Kastrat bekommt
keine Glatze.

4. Kehlkopf

Mit Beginn der Pubertät wächst der *Kehlkopf* in allen Proportionen, das
Organ tritt am Hals als Adamsapfel hervor, Stimmbänder und Stimmritze werden
größer und der Stimmwechsel vollzieht sich allmählich, wobei die Stimmlage
in der Regel eine Oktave tiefer als vorher liegt. Auch der Kehlkopf des Kindes
und der der Frau wächst unter Testosteron, die Stimme wird rauher und tiefer.

Nach Ausschalten der pathologischen Androgenquelle bildet sich der Kehlkopf nur unvollständig zurück, bei Frauen bleibt die Stimme tiefer.

5. Brustdrüse

Während der Pubertät kommt es zu einer Vergrößerung und Schwellung des Warzenhofes und der *Brustdrüse*. Man tastet eine feste, flache, zwei- bis drei-markstückgroße, empfindliche, gut verschiebbare, mit der Mamille ver-bundene Masse.

Die *Makromastie* ist physiolo-gisch, sie ist zwischen 14 und 15 Jahren am stärksten ausgebildet und verschwindet 1—2 Jahre später spon-tan wieder. Bei etwa 1% bleibt sie bis ins Erwachsenenalter bestehen. Die Ursache ist nicht bekannt, wahr-scheinlich sind es die Androgene, die das Wachstum stimulieren, da man eine Vergrößerung der Drüse auch bei Behandlung eines Eunuchoiden mit Testosteron beobachtet.

Bei einem kleinen Teil entwickelt sich die Brustdrüse zu einem kasta-nien- bis faustgroßen Organ, nicht selten einseitig. Auch in diesen Fällen bildet sich die Drüse spon-tan wieder zurück. Hier muß eine besondere Empfindlichkeit des Drü-senkörpers vorliegen (Abb. 14).

Zwischen der Nasenschleimhaut und der Genitalsphäre bestehen ge-wisse Verbindungen, die man nur unvollständig kennt. Injektion von Testosteron führt zu einem perivas-culären Ödem und einer vermehrten Flüssigkeitssekretion in bestimmten Teilen der Nasenschleimhaut (HA-MILTON 1937).

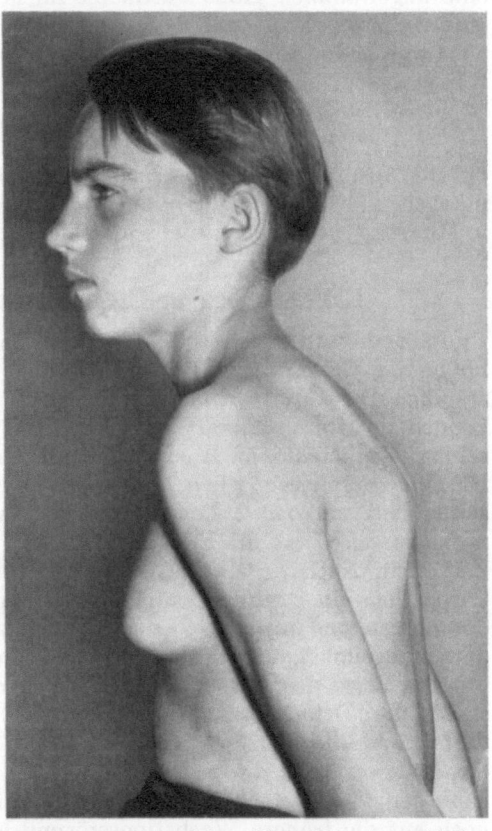

Abb. 14. H. M., 15 Jahre. Körperlich gut entwickelter Junge. Beginn der Pubertät mit 12$^{1}/_{2}$ Jahren. Seit 1 Jahr Wachstum beider Brustdrüsen, Genitale normal. Harn-gonadotropine 26 MEU, chromatinnegativ

6. Maskuline Körperprägung

Die *maskuline Prägung* des menschlichen Körpers wird durch die besondere Gestaltung des Skelets, der Muskulatur, des subcutanen Fettgewebes, der Haut und ihrer Anhangsgebilde bestimmt. Diese Gewebe werden in ihrer besonderen Bildung wesentlich durch die androgenen Hormone bestimmt. Man nimmt an, daß die anabolen Eigenschaften des Testosterons und nicht die Androgene dafür verantwortlich sind, ohne dafür aber sichere Beweise zu haben.

Besonders ausgesprochen ist der Einfluß auf die Entwicklung der *Körper-muskulatur*. Beim Mann erfahren die Rumpf- und Gliedmaßenmuskeln erst mit der Pubertätsentwicklung ihre charakteristische Form. Es handelt sich um eine echte Muskelhypertrophie, wie sie auch unter körperlichem Training eintritt.

Besonders sinnfällig ist der Einfluß der Androgene auf die Muskelentwicklung bei der Pubertas praecox, der Pseudopubertas praecox, der Nebennierenrinden-hyperplasie und dem weiblichen Pseudohermaphroditismus bzw. dem adreno-genitalen Syndrom der Frau.

Hamilton (1948b) beschrieb die charakteristische *Fettverteilung* beim Eu-nuchen. Das Fettgewebe häuft sich besonders am Bauch, über der Symphyse, um die Brustdrüsen, an den Hüften und im Rücken an. Autoptisch findet man eine ungewöhnlich große Fettmasse im Mesenterium. Die Gestaltung des sub-cutanen Fettpolsters und besonders der Unterschied zwischen Mann und Frau wird durch die Sexualhormone bedingt (Nathanson u. Wilson 1943a).

VII. Symptome des Androgenmangels

Die Ausprägung des klinischen Bildes ist nicht nur vom Grad des Androgen-mangels abhängig, sondern auch vom Zeitpunkt des Auftretens. Hamilton u. Mitarb. (1942) haben die umfassendste Beschreibung gegeben.

1. Präpuberaler Eunuchismus und Eunuchoidismus

Fällt die Androgenproduktion vor Beginn der Pubertät aus, dann unter-bleibt der Gestaltwandel vom Kind über den Jüngling zum Mann. Der voll-ständige Defekt ist an der kindlichen Ausbildung des Genitales leicht zu er-kennen, er wird als *Eunuchismus* bezeichnet. Infolge des verspäteten Epiphysen-schlusses entsteht ein Hochwuchs mit charakteristischen Körperproportionen. Einzelne Epiphysen, wie z.B. die des Radius und der Ulna, schließen sich nicht selten erst um das 3. Lebensjahrzehnt, andere wie die des Ileumrandes, die normalerweise erst im Erwachsenenalter verschwinden, bleiben unbeschränkte Zeit offen. Auch die Wirbelsäulenepiphysen schließen sich verspätet. Der Wirbel-körper hat ein zweites Ossifikationszentrum in Form einer dünnen Platte an der oberen und unteren Fläche. Bei verspätetem Schluß entstehen als Folge der unregelmäßigen Ossifikation fleckförmige Verkalkungen am oberen und unteren Rand des Wirbelkörpers. Bei Überbelastung kommt es leicht zu Arro-sionen und Deformierungen der Wirbelkörper, besonders im Bereich der Brust-wirbelsäule, die identisch sind mit denen der *Scheuermannschen Krankheit.* Mit der Zeit verlieren die röntgenologischen Veränderungen ihr charakteristisches Aussehen. Nur eine Kalkarmut und die niedrigen, flachen Wirbelkörper weisen noch auf die frühere Wachstumsstörung hin.

Die *Körpergröße* des Kastraten ist nicht immer anormal hoch, wohl aber sind die Körperproportionen mit dem Überwiegen der Unterlänge gegenüber der Oberlänge, der Spannweite gegen die Körpergröße, der Beckenbreite gegen die Schulterbreite charakteristisch. Für den Eunuchen sind lange Extremitäten, lange und grazile Hände und Finger, Füße und Zehen typisch. Erst seit man in den letzten Jahren das Skelet regelmäßig röntgenologisch untersucht, wird der Befund einer *Osteoporose* häufiger erhoben. Die Röhrenknochen sind dünn, die Corticalis verschmälert, die Spongiosa vergröbert, besonders die Wirbelsäule kann erhebliche Veränderungen aufweisen (vgl. Abb. 15). Nowakowski (1954) fand bei 62 Kranken mit Hypogonadismus in über 50% eine Osteoporose, die vom 36. Lebensjahr ab gehäuft auftrat. In höherem Alter ist die Arthrose und Spondylose häufiger und schwerer als beim Bevölkerungsdurchschnitt. Die Ur-sache sehen Albright (1958) in der ungenügenden Ablagerung der eiweißhaltigen Knochenmatrix infolge des Ausfalls der wichtigsten anabolen Stoffwechselhormone des Erwachsenen. Die gebildete Knochengrundsubstanz verkalkt in normaler

Weise, aber die Gesamtmenge an Osteoid, die zur Verkalkung zur Verfügung steht, ist geringer.

Die *Muskulatur* ist schlecht entwickelt, das Muskelrelief tritt nicht hervor, die körperliche Leistung ist eingeschränkt, die Kreatinausscheidung abnorm hoch.

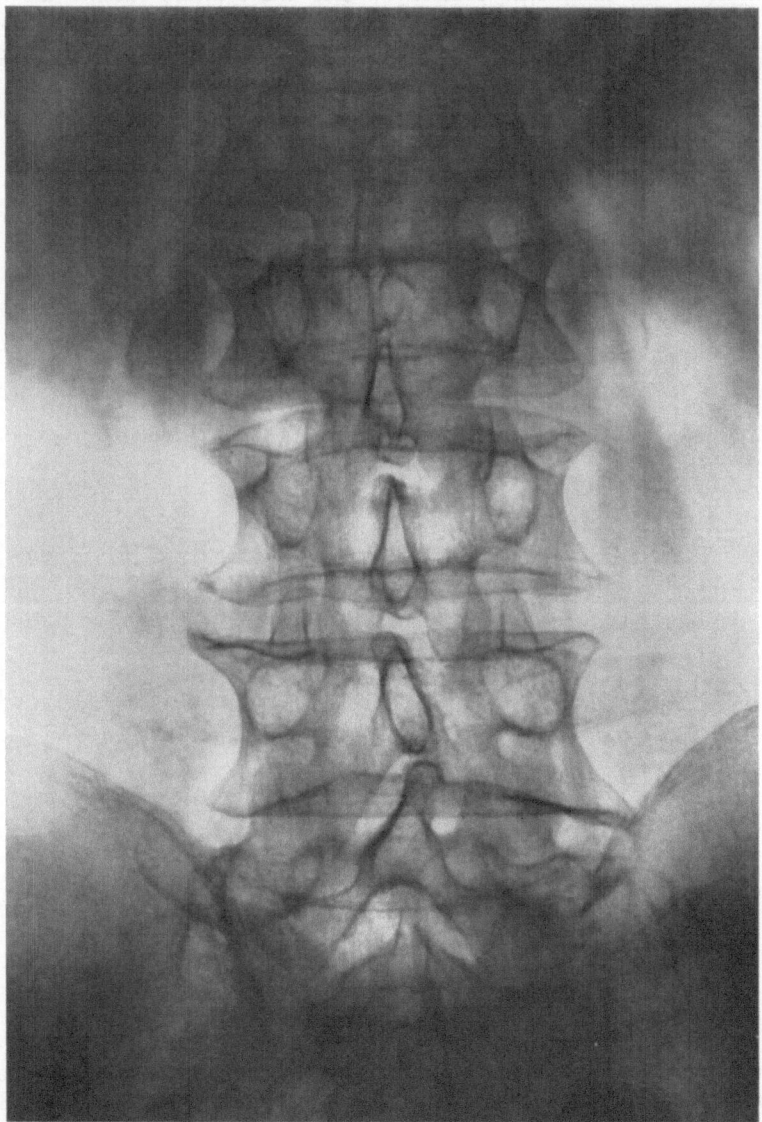

Abb. 15. Röntgenbild der Wirbelsäule eines 48jährigen Kastraten durch Kriegsverletzung, schwere Osteoporose mit degenerativen Randwülsten

Charakteristisch ist die *abnorme Fettverteilung*. Das Fettgewebe ist besonders im Bereich der Hüften, am Unterbauch, an den Oberschenkeln und an der Brust angehäuft. Infolge der schlechten Muskel- und Knochenentwicklung wiegen Eunuchoide und Eunuche meist weniger als gleichaltrige Kontrollen (HAMILTON u. Mitarb. 1942). Junge, körperlich tätige Eunuche sind nicht fettsüchtig. Wie andere Formen der Fettsucht, ist auch die „Kastrationsfettsucht" ein calorisches Problem.

Die *Haut* ist trocken, pastös, dünn, schlecht durchblutet, pigmentarm und erinnert an ein Myxödem. Das schwammige, ungeprägte, bartlose Gesicht gibt den Eunuchen ein kindliches Aussehen. Die Haut altert rascher als normal, so daß sich um das 40. Jahr das Gesicht mit vielen feinen Runzeln überzieht (vgl. Abb. 16). Talg- und Schweißdrüsen bleiben unterentwickelt. Der Bart-

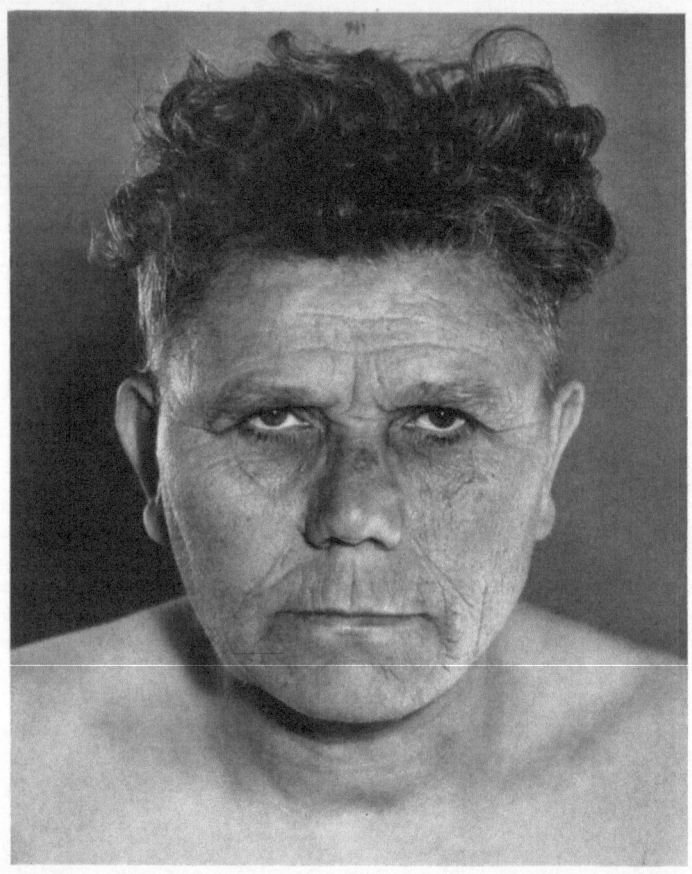

Abb. 16. G. E., 45 Jahre. Unbehandelter Kastrat durch Verletzung im 30. Lebensjahr

wuchs fehlt vollständig, während sich eine ganz geringe glatte Schambehaarung entwickeln kann, die sonstige Körperbehaarung fehlt. Jegliche stärkere Scham- und Achselbehaarung spricht gegen den völligen Ausfall der inkretorischen Hodenfunktion. Das Kopfhaar ist dagegen überreichlich und reicht weit in die Stirn (Pelzmütze). Die Calvitis frontalis bleibt aus, eine Glatze ist ganz ungewöhnlich.

Bei vielen Eunuchen ist der *Grundumsatz* deutlich erniedrigt (—5% bis —20%), während die Speicherungsfähigkeit der Schilddrüse für J^{131} normal oder etwas erhöht ist. PBJ ist normal. Ein herabgesetzter Grundumsatz darf nicht im Sinne einer begleitenden Hypothyreose aufgefaßt werden.

Erniedrigung des Hämoglobins und der Zahl der Erythrocyten um 10—15% sind beim unbehandelten Kastraten immer vorhanden. Schon bei einer geringen Eigenproduktion an Testosteron fehlt die *normochrome Anämie*.

Die Ursache des erhöhten Serumcholesterins ist nicht bekannt, man bringt damit das vorzeitige Auftreten der degenerativen Gefäßveränderungen in Verbindung.

Die Funktion der Nebennierenrinde ist normal.

Das äußere *Genitale* bleibt so klein wie bei einem 6—8jährigen. Das Scrotum ist kaum entwickelt, Prostata und Samenblasen können nicht getastet werden, ihre Sekretion fehlt. Libido und Potenz fehlen. Die charakteristischen Eigenschaften des Eunuchen — er ist argwöhnisch, mißtrauisch, verschlossen, unbeständig. ängstlich und neigt zur Hypochondrie — entstehen aus dem Gefühl der Unterwertigkeit und sind nicht Folge des Hormonmangels.

Bei unvollständigem Ausfall der inkretorischen Hodenfunktion vor Beginn oder während der Pubertät — *präpuberaler* oder *puberaler Eunuchoidismus* — sind die Symptome nur in abgeschwächter Form vorhanden. Die meisten Erfolgsorgane sprechen schon auf kleine Testosterondosen an, doch bleibt die Entwicklung unvollständig. Hoden, Penis, Scrotum, Prostata und Samenblasen bleiben kleiner als normal, ihre Funktion ist unterwertig. Achsel- und Schambehaarung. auch die Extremitätenbehaarung bildet sich verhältnismäßig gut aus, während der Bartwuchs immer dürftig bleibt, auch wenn eine deutliche Calvitis frontalis vorhanden ist. Die normale Entwicklung des Skelets und der Muskulatur verlangt die volle Menge von Testosteron. Den präpuberalen Eunuchoidismus kann man daher noch im späteren Leben nach erfolgreicher Behandlung an den eunuchoiden Körperproportionen. dem Überwiegen der Unterlänge gegenüber der Oberlänge erkennen.

2. Postpuberaler Eunuchismus und Eunuchoidismus

Erfolgt der Ausfall der Keimdrüsenfunktion erst nach Abschluß der Pubertät — *postpuberaler Eunuchismus* —, dann sind die klinischen Zeichen viel geringer ausgeprägt. Da bis zur Zeit der Kastration das Skeletsystem und die übrigen Organe voll entwickelt und normal ausgebildet waren, bleiben sie mit Ausnahme der spezifischen Organe erhalten. Der eunuchoide Habitus fehlt, Penis und Scrotum bleiben etwa gleich groß, die Runzelung fehlt. Auch die Größe des Kehlkopfs bleibt erhalten, so daß die Stimme nur wenig höher wird. Prostata und Samenblasen atrophieren, Libido und Potenz erlöschen.

Die schlecht durchblutete *Haut* ist weich und hat reichlich subcutanes Fett, die individuelle Prägung des Gesichts verwischt sich. Der Rückgang der Behaarung ist beträchtlich. Achsel-, Scham- und Körperbehaarung fallen aber nicht vollständig aus, auch der Bartwuchs bleibt in gewissem Umfang, aber die Wachstumsgröße der Haare nimmt erheblich ab.

Am Skelet ist der Aufbau des Osteoids gestört, so daß vorzeitig eine Osteoporose auftritt (ALBRIGHT 1958) (vgl. Abb. 15).

Die Ausbildung der Muskulatur ist abhängig von der körperlichen Tätigkeit, die Menge des Fettgewebes von der calorischen Bilanz. Direkt nach der Kastration sind vasomotorische Erscheinungen. wie Hitze, Schwitzen, Wallungen, Schweißausbrüche, Herzklopfen, Unruhe, häufig. Sie verschwinden nach einigen Monaten auch ohne Behandlung. Man bringt sie mit dem plötzlichen Entzug der Hormone in Zusammenhang.

Die Zeichen des teilweisen Verlustes der androgenen Funktion — *postpuberaler Eunuchoidismus* — sind sowohl im somatischen, psychischen und sexuellen Verhalten nur geringgradig. Manchmal ist es nicht sicher möglich, Involutionserscheinungen von physiologischen Varianten und Altersveränderungen abzugrenzen. Bei jüngeren Menschen gibt die Größe der Prostata und der Bartwuchs einen gewissen Anhalt. 17-Ketosteroid- und Oestrogenausscheidung ist unverändert. In diesen Fällen ist die Funktionsdiagnostik der männlichen Adnexe — Bestimmung der Fructosekonzentration im Sperma — wertvoll.

F. Pubertät und ihre Störungen

Die normale Pubertätsentwicklung vollzieht sich bei der Betrachtung einer größeren Zahl von Menschen innerhalb einer weiten Variationsbreite, die durch individuelle, familiäre und rassische Faktoren reguliert, aber auch durch die Ernährung und durch Krankheiten beeinflußt wird. Bei der Mehrzahl der Knaben liegt der Reifungsbeginn zwischen dem 12. und 13. Lebensjahr (OSTER). Als unterste Grenze einer noch normal anzusehenden Pubertät bei Knaben nennt SECKEL (1950) 9 Jahre. Nach den Untersuchungen von LENZ und ORT (1959) an Hamburger Gymnasiasten ist der Pubertätsbeginn 1957 gegen 1877 nur um ein Jahr vorverlegt, während die körperliche Entwicklung vor Einsetzen der Pubertät heute gegenüber früher deutlich fortgeschritten ist. Das Längenwachstum der heutigen 11—13jährigen übertrifft das der Gleichaltrigen vor 1900 um 2—3 Jahreswachstumsraten. Diese Acceleration der Wachstumsvorgänge vor der Pubertät ist in allen untersuchten Ländern (Schweden, Schweiz, Dänemark, England, Italien, USA) etwa gleich. Die Kinder sind mit Beginn der Pubertät 5—10 cm größer als früher. Der absolute Größengewinn am Ende der Wachstumsperiode beträgt in Deutschland 5 cm. Die 1957 für die Bundeswehr im Alter von 19,6 Jahren Gemusterten sind im Durchschnitt nur 5 cm größer als die des kaiserlichen Heeres 1894 (HORSTER). Die Wachstumskurve flacht sich nach der Pubertät rascher ab.

Mit der Pubertät steigert sich das Längenwachstum beträchtlich und erreicht eine jährliche Zuwachsrate von 10—12 cm, gleichzeitig wächst die Muskulatur und die inneren Organe vergrößern sich proportional, nur Thymus und lymphatisches System bilden sich zurück.

Die zeitliche Folge der wichtigsten Ereignisse des Pubertätsgeschehens sind in der Tabelle 13 zusammengestellt, die einer Arbeit von PRADER (1957) entnommen ist. Das Erwachsenenalter wird durch die Sekretion der gonadotropen Hormone ausgelöst. Es ist bis heute unbekannt, warum die Regulationszentren im Zwischenhirn plötzlich anfangen, humorale Reize an den Vorderlappen abzugeben. Man vermutet, daß mit dem Ingangkommen der Gonadotropinsekretion die Bildung des STH in der Hypophyse vermindert wird, so daß mit der Pubertät die Sexualhormone die einzigen wichtigen anabolen Stoffwechselhormone darstellen.

Die normalen *Körperproportionen*, besonders das Verhältnis von Stamm zu Extremitätenlänge, sind weitgehend von der Einwirkung der Androgene abhängig. Im allgemeinen wird die Unterlänge mit der Oberlänge und der Spannweite verglichen. Bei der Geburt beträgt das Verhältnis von Ober- zu Unterlänge 1,7:1. Die Beine wachsen beträchtlich rascher als der Rumpf, so daß im Alter von 10—11 Jahren die beiden Verhältnisse etwa gleich sind. Diese Proportion bleibt bei regelrechter zeitlicher Folge der Entwicklungsvorgänge mit kleinen Schwankungen bis zum Erwachsenenalter bestehen. Je größer die Kinder vor Eintritt der Pubertät geworden sind, um so mehr überwiegt die Unterlänge die Oberlänge. Ein 185 cm großer, zu normaler Zeit gereifter Erwachsener kann also „eunuchoide"

Körperproportionen aufweisen. Beim Erwachsenen verhält sich Obermaß zu Untermaß zur Hälfte der Spannweite wie 1:1:1. Beim hypothyreotischen Minderwuchs betrifft die Wachstumsverzögerung Ober- und Unterlänge in etwa demselben Maße, so daß der Index immer bei 1 bleibt. Bei den schwereren Formen des Eunuchoidismus wachsen dagegen wie im Kindesalter unter der reinen STH-Wirkung die Extremitäten rascher als der Rumpf, so daß ein Übergewicht der Unterlänge und der Spannweite im Vergleich zur Oberlänge und der Körpergröße resultiert (WILKINS 1950).

Bei der normal ablaufenden Entwicklung schreiten chronologisches Alter und Knochenalter gleichmäßig voran. Bei den vielen Störungsmöglichkeiten der Pubertät kann eine Dissoziation dieser beiden Größen eintreten. Der Zeitpunkt

Tabelle 13. *Zeittafel der Pubertätsentwicklung beim Knaben.* [Nach PRADER (1958a)]

Alter Jahre	Somatische Merkmale	Hormonbefunde im Urin
vor 10	Infantile Verhältnisse: Testesvolumen etwa 1 cm³	17-Ketosteroide unter 1 mg/Tag: Gonadotropine (FSH) nicht nachweisbar
11	Testes, Penis und Prostata beginnen zu wachsen	17-Ketosteroide 1—4 mg/Tag
12—13	Wachstum des Kehlkopfes; erste Pubes; Zunahme des Längenwachstums, erstes Daumensesambein, beginnende Sekretion der Talgdrüsen	FSH wird nachweisbar
13—14	Testes (etwa 5 cm³). Penis und Prostata wachsen stark, leichte Brustdrüsenschwellung	17-Ketosteroide 3—8 mg/Tag, FSH 4—26 ME pro Tag
14—15	Stimmbruch; Axillarbehaarung; Pubesbegrenzung noch weiblich; beginnende Schnauzbehaarung; stärkere Brustdrüsenschwellung	
15	Reife Spermatozoen	17-Ketosteroide höher als beim Mädchen
16—17	Acne; zunehmende Körper- und Gesichtsbehaarung, Stirn-Haargrenze männlich; Pubesbegrenzung männlich; Rückgang der Brustdrüsenschwellung	
18—19	Epiphysenschluß und Wachstumsstillstand; Testes 12—25 cm³	17-Ketosteroide 10—20 mg/Tag, FSH 4—26 ME pro Tag

des Pubertätseintrittes ist viel enger an die Skeletreife als an das chronologische Alter gebunden (GREULICH u. Mitarb. 1942). Die Knochenentwicklung wird an Hand der Röntgenbilder des Skeletsystems beurteilt. Die Knochenherde im Knorpel treten an den einzelnen Knochen in bestimmter Reihenfolge auf. Auch hier gibt es beträchtliche individuelle Schwankungen, so daß mehrere Knochen zur Beurteilung herangezogen werden müssen. Die genaueste Darstellung der normalen Verhältnisse haben GREULICH und PYLE (1950) gegeben. Die Festlegung des Knochenalters läßt einen gewissen Schluß für die zeitliche Voraussage des Pubertätseintrittes zu. Entspricht das Knochenalter bei einem 15jährigen dem eines 13jährigen, dann kann man mit dem Eintritt der Pubertät im nächsten Jahr rechnen. Ist die Knochenreife stärker verzögert, dann läßt die Pubertät noch länger auf sich warten. Das Wachstum der Hoden ist zeitlich der erste Vorgang. Ihre Größenzunahme beruht fast ausschließlich auf der Längen- und Dickenzunahme der Samenkanälchen. Die Leydigzellen erscheinen normalerweise um das 10. Lebensjahr (CHARNY 1957c).

I. Pubertas tarda

Man versteht darunter das nicht zeitgerechte Einspielen der Gonadotropin-bildung in einem an sich normalen endokrinen System (Tonutti 1960). Da alle Kinder vor der Pubertät klinisch das Bild des präpuberalen Eunuchoidismus bieten, kann man im Einzelfall nicht entscheiden, ob es sich um eine einfache verzögerte Pubertätsentwicklung handelt oder um einen echten Defekt in der Anlage des Hodens oder des Hypophysenzwischenhirns. Kinder, die bis ins 14. Lebensjahr noch keine Anzeichen einer Entwicklung zeigen, muß man einer eingehenden Untersuchung unterziehen.

1. Mit Störung der Knochenreifung

Man trennt zwischen zwei Gruppen. Bei der einen bleibt die Knochenreifung hinter dem chronologischen Alter zurück. Diese Kinder sind auch im Längen-wachstum zurückgeblieben und haben eine schlechte allgemeine Körper- und Kräfteverfassung. Neben der mangelnden Gonadotropinproduktion liegt auch eine ungenügende Produktion von Wachstumshormon vor. Bei der anderen entspricht das Knochenalter dem Lebensalter. Hier handelt es sich um einen alleinigen Mangel an Gonadotropinen.

Bei der ersten Gruppe sind es *chronische Erkrankungen* der verschiedensten Art, deren Folgen sich im wachsenden Organismus viel schwerwiegender aus-wirken als beim Erwachsenen. Mangel an hochwertigen Aminosäuren bedingt ungenügende Bildung der Hypophysenvorderlappenhormone, besonders der Gonadotropine, aber auch des Wachstumshormons und selten des thyreotropen Hormons. Chronische Erkrankungen der Leber, der Nieren, Herzfehler mit erheb-licher Sauerstoffuntersättigung, Anämien, Resorptionsstörungen des Magen-Darmkanals, Hunger, Diabetes mellitus und chronische Infektionskrankheiten finden sich als Ursache. Inwieweit der Mangel an Baustoffen die einzelnen Gewebe selbst in ihrem Ansprechen auf die Hypophysenvorderlappenhormone weniger empfindlich macht, ist noch ungenügend untersucht. Bei einem be-gleitenden Mangel an Schilddrüsenhormon kommt das noch produzierte Wachs-tumshormon (STH) an den Epiphysen nicht zur vollen Wirkung. In solchen Fällen ist die Knochenentwicklung besonders stark verzögert.

Die Prognose ist abhängig von der Grundkrankheit. Kann diese, wie z. B. bei der konstitutionellen hämolytischen Anämie mit Sphärocytose, durch die Entfernung der Milz günstig gestaltet werden, dann blühen die Betreffenden auf und holen in wenigen Monaten nach, was sie in Jahren versäumt haben. Kann die Grundkrankheit nicht nachhaltig gebessert werden, dann entwickeln sich die Betroffenen doch allmählich, die Kranken behalten aber dauernd die Züge eines leichteren präpuberalen Eunuchoidismus. Man kann die Reifung durch die Verabreichung von Choriongonadotropinen beschleunigen und vervoll-ständigen und damit häufig auch die Grundkrankheit günstig beeinflussen. Bei unheilbaren Krankheiten wird man von Anfang an Testosteron vorziehen.

Bei einem kleinen Teil der ersten Gruppe kann man keine allgemeine Ursache für die verspätete Pubertät finden. Differentialdiagnostisch müssen dabei echte Formen des sekundären Hypogonadismus in Betracht gezogen werden. Es sei daran erinnert, daß intra- und suprasellärе Tumoren auch bei eingehender Unter-suchung der Diagnostik entgehen können und daß chronische Entzündungen der Hypophyse, die im Kindesalter meist von den Meningen auf Hypophyse, Hypophysenstiel und Schädelbasis übergreifen und nur selten primär in Hypo-physe oder Zwischenhirn lokalisiert sind, unter dem Bild der Pubertas tarda verlaufen können. Demgegenüber stehen Jugendliche, die ohne sichtbaren Grund nur langsam wachsen und sich nicht entwickeln, bei denen man eine ungenügende Produktion von STH annimmt. Während des Pubertätsalters zwischen 13 und 16 Jahren kann die Abtrennung unüberwindliche Schwierigkeiten machen, je älter die Betreffenden sind, um so wahrscheinlicher wird der organische Defekt. Bei Fehlbildungen der Keimdrüsen selbst ist die Knochenreifung bis ins Pubertätsalter (11—13 Jahre) normal und differiert erst später mit den normalen Kontrollen. In der Differentialdiagnose hilft außerdem der Choriongonadotropintest, doch muß die Verabreichung von Gonadotropinen nicht selten länger als 14 Tage durchgeführt werden, da die üblicherweise verwandten 7000 E nicht ausreichen, um die Entfaltung und Funktionsaufnahme völlig hypoplastischer Leydigzellen zu gewährleisten. Die Bestimmung der Gonadotropine im Urin gibt manchmal ebenfalls keine sicheren Ergebnisse, da die hohe Ausscheidung, die für den primären Hypogonadismus des Erwachsenen so charakteristisch ist, im Pubertätsalter nur zögernd aufgenommen wird.

Bei den reinen Formen der Pubertas tarda handelt es sich meist um magere, im Wachstum zurückgebliebene, körperlich und geistig aber recht lebendige Jungen, die während der ganzen Kindheit schon immer etwas dürftig und zart gewesen sind. Bei den schweren Fällen entspricht das Genitale des 14—16jährigen einem 8—10jährigen Kind, die Hoden sind noch ganz weich und man erkennt keine Spur einer beginnenden Reifung.

Bei den leichteren Formen ist das Genitale mitgewachsen und hat Größe und Form eines 10—12jährigen vor Beginn der Pubertät, der Hoden hat an Konsistenz zugenommen und ist nicht mehr so weich wie im Kindesalter. Bei genauer Untersuchung findet man auch schon die ersten Reifungszeichen, die Schweiß- und Duftdrüsen der Achselhöhlen, Talgdrüsen der Stirn nehmen ihre Funktion auf, man sieht einige Härchen an der Peniswurzel und erfährt von den Angehörigen, daß der Junge im letzten Jahr mehr gewachsen ist als in den vorausgehenden.

Häufige Ursache ist offenbar die ungenügende Produktion von Wachstumshormon, das sowohl für das Knochenalter als auch für die Reifung der Sexualregion des Zwischenhirns verantwortlich ist. In den schweren Fällen tritt eine selbständige Verzögerung der Gonadotropine aus unbekannter Ursache hinzu. Der Schweregrad dieser Fälle kann häufig — keineswegs immer — mit Hilfe der röntgenologischen Bestimmung des Knochenalters festgestellt werden. Ist die Knochenreifung stärker zurückgeblieben (>2 Jahre), dann muß die Prognose mit Vorsicht gestellt werden. Ist die Reifung dagegen nur um 1—2 Jahre verzögert, dann darf im allgemeinen mit einer spontanen Pubertät gerechnet werden. Eine weitere Möglichkeit bietet der Gonadotropintest. Je rascher der Anstieg der Oestrogen- und 17-Ketosteroidausscheidung im Urin eintritt, um so früher wird auch die spontane Aufnahme der Gonadotropinbildung erfolgen.

Vielfach hört man in der Familienvorgeschichte, daß auch der Vater oder sonst ein naher Verwandter ein Spätentwickler gewesen ist, so daß man in Ruhe abwarten könnte.

2. Mit normaler Knochenreifung

Die zweite Gruppe ist dadurch charakterisiert, daß Körpergröße und Knochenalter den Verhältnissen zu Beginn der normalen Pubertät entsprechen. Ein Teil dieser Kinder ist normalgewichtig, hat normal entwickelte Muskulatur und bietet keine Zeichen sonstiger innersekretorischer Störungen. Andere sind körperlich dürftig und schwächlich, Röntgenaufnahmen des Skelets zeigen dann aber eine in die physiologische Schwankungsbreite fallende Knochenreife. Man erkennt diese günstig gelagerten Fälle auch daran, daß die Größe des Genitales und der Hoden dem präpuberalen Entwicklungszustand und nicht dem eines Kindes unter 10 Jahren entspricht. Bei einigen hat die Hodengröße schon etwas zugenommen, ohne daß sichere Zeichen der Geschlechtsreifung erkennbar sind. Die Biopsie deckt in solchen Fällen verhältnismäßig gut entwickelte Kanälchen mit reifendem Samenepithel auf, während die Leydigzellen noch praktisch fehlen und keine Aktivitätszeichen vorhanden sind (ALBERT u. Mitarb. 1953). Die Aufnahme der FSH-Produktion geht in diesen Fällen der des ICSH unter Umständen beträchtlich voraus. Die normale Knochenreifung zeigt an, daß die Produktion des Wachstumshormons (STH) eine normale ist, daß ein wesentlicher Faktor der verspäteten Gonadotropinbildung wegfällt.

Die Ursache der verzögerten Gonadotropinproduktion bei der unkomplizierten Pubertas tarda ist nicht bekannt, bei der günstigen Prognose muß man sie noch als physiologische Variante der normalen Pubertätsentwicklung ansehen. Die Fälle mit isoliertem, irreparablem Defekt der gonadotropinbildenden Zellen der Adenohypophyse sind in der Allgemeinpraxis so selten, daß man sie nicht in den Kreis seiner Überlegungen aufzunehmen braucht.

3. Pseudodystrophie

Die größte Masse dieser Gruppe machen die fettsüchtigen Jungen aus, die wegen „Drüsenstörungen" den Arzt aufsuchen, der dann entscheiden soll, ob es sich um einen schwerwiegenden Defekt im Sinne der Dystrophia adiposo genitalis, um ein cushingartiges Krankheitsbild oder nur um eine verzögerte Pubertät bei einem Fettsüchtigen, also um eine *Pseudodystrophie* handelt (siehe Abb. 17—19). Die Häufigkeit dieser Jugendlichen beiderlei Geschlechtes hat in den letzten Jahren beträchtlich zugenommen. Ein Teil dieser Kinder ist von Jugend auf übergewichtig und fett, andere nehmen erst vor der Pubertät, also vor der letzten Streckperiode, an Gewicht zu. Die Fettverteilung ist eine gleichmäßige, sie betrifft Hüften, Brust, Nacken, Rücken, Gesicht, Oberarme, Oberschenkel und Unterschenkel in gleicher Weise, es fehlt also das Freibleiben oder das mindere Befallensein der Extremitäten. Obwohl die Muskulatur normal entwickelt ist, sind die Kinder körperlich wenig leistungsfähig und ermüden rasch. Läßt man sie hungern, dann werden sie unruhig, klagen über Kopfschmerzen, fangen an zu schwitzen, sie können schwere hypoglykämische Anfälle bekommen. Etwa die Hälfte hat nicht nur eine Störung des Appetits, sondern auch des Durstempfindens. Dursten wird noch schlechter toleriert als hungern. An Bauch, Brust, Oberschenkel und Oberarmen können reichlich schmale und breitere, meist frischrote Striae distensae vorhanden sein. Diese weisen wohl auf eine aktive Nebennierenrinde hin, sind aber bei den jugendlichen Menschen kein Zeichen einer schwerwiegenden Überfunktion der Nebennierenrinde im Sinne des Morbus Cushing. Man beobachtet sie nur bei rascher Gewichtszunahme, sie blassen sofort ab, wenn das Gewicht stehenbleibt, um bei einem neuerlichen Schub an anderer Stelle erneut aufzutreten. Alte blasse neben frischen roten Striae sind immer ein Zeichen für den schubweisen Verlauf der Gewichtszunahme.

Man vertritt heute vielfach die Ansicht, daß jede Fettsucht ein rein calorisch energetisches Problem und keine Stoffwechselstörung und keine hormonale Dysfunktion als Ursache hat. Das träge und phlegmatische Wesen dieser Fettsüchtigen begünstigt die positive Bilanz. Schon von Jugend an wird der Appetit anerzogen und das ganze Leben über beibehalten. Die übermäßige Calorienzufuhr verlangt aber eine Umstellung des innersekretorischen Systems, damit das nicht Verbrauchte auf Depot gelegt werden kann, wobei besonders die Bauchspeicheldrüse (Insulin), die Nebennierenrinde, vielleicht auch der Hypophysenhinterlappen beteiligt sind. Beim Versuch, sich untercalorisch zu ernähren, verhindert die Hypoglykämie das Durchhalten, der in Richtung Fettbildung eingestellte Stoffwechsel, die sog. lipomatöse Tendenz, fordert ihre Rechte.

Auf der anderen Seite weist die Störung des Appetits und des Sättigungsgefühles, die gleichzeitig vorhandene Störung des Durstempfindens auf eine funk-

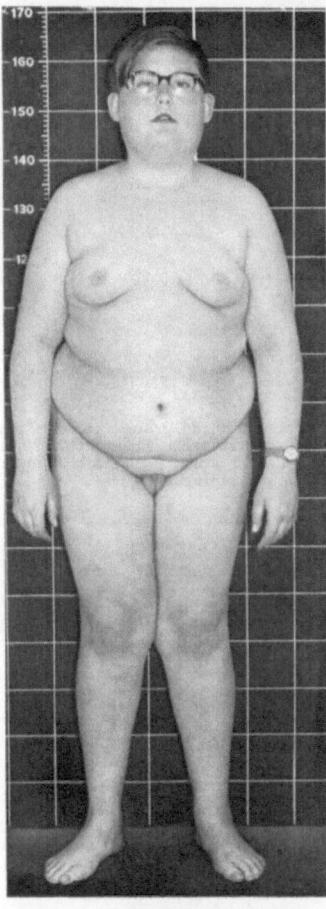 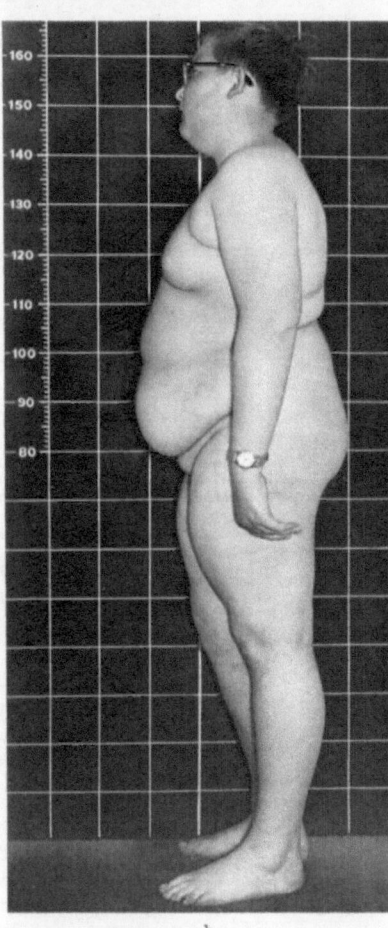

Abb. 17. 17jähriger Junge mit schwerer Adipositas und Pubertas tarda. Keine echte Gynäkomastie. X-Beine. Epiphysenlösung am Humeruskopf beidseits, Gonadotropine negativ

tionelle Schädigung des Zwischenhirns hin, wobei dann die Verzögerung der Pubertät nur eine Teilerscheinung dieser Zwischenhirnschwäche wäre. Das viel diskutierte, aber nie sicher nachgewiesene Fettstoffwechselhormon des Hypophysenvorderlappens ist noch nicht gänzlich ad acta gelegt.

Ein wichtiges Unterscheidungsmerkmal gegenüber der echten Dystrophia adiposogenitalis ist die normale, ja häufig übernormale Körpergröße dieser Fettsüchtigen. Die gleichzeitige Beeinträchtigung anderer Vorderlappenfunktionen bei organischen Prozessen des Hypophysenzwischenhirnsystems wirkt sich immer auch auf das Längenwachstum aus. Die pseudodystrophen Kinder übertreffen

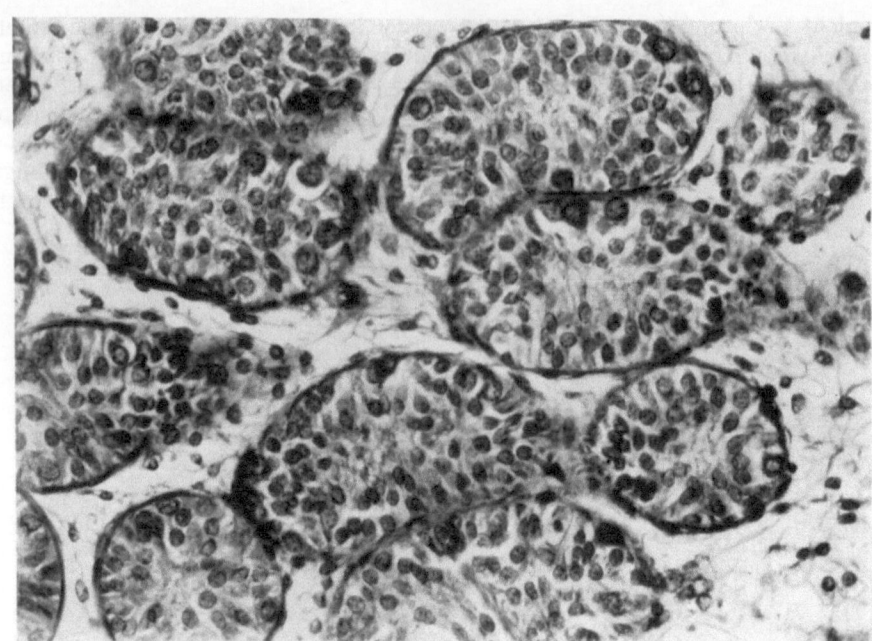

Abb. 18. Hodenbild desselben Jungen (Abb. 17) mit idiopathischer Pubertas tarda, Kanälchen sehr klein und durchweg ohne Lumen. Die Differenzierung zu Sertolizellen ist überall eingetreten, Spermatogonien sind in zahlreichen Kanälchen, Spermatocyten nur in einzelnen zu erkennen. Das Zwischengewebe ist sehr locker und enthält nur unreife Zwischenzellen (Vergrößerung 140 fach)

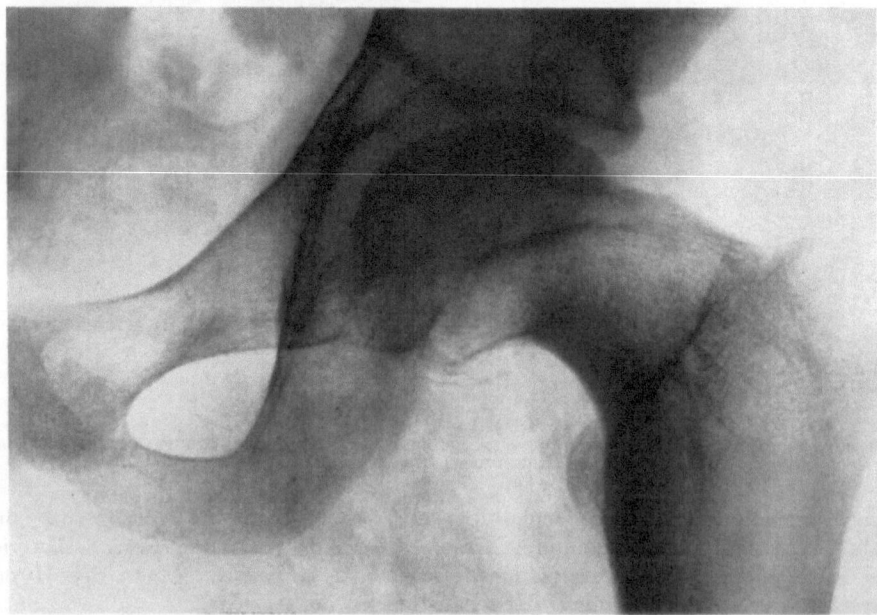

Abb. 19. Linkes Hüftgelenk desselben Jungen (Abb. 17). Epiphysenlösung vom Typ Perthes

ihre Altersgenossen an Körperlänge, der „Gigantismus" schließt eine echte Dystrophia adiposogenitalis aus. Röntgenologisch ist die Knochenreifung normal, bei einem Teil der Fälle sogar überstürzt.

Es ist nicht ganz einfach, den objektiven Entwicklungsgrad bei diesen Dicken festzulegen, da man wegen des vielen Fettes die wirkliche Größe des Penis und der Hoden schlecht beurteilen kann und auch durch die Körpermasse in den Proportionen irregeführt wird. Bei einem Teil der Kinder fehlt kein echtes Zurückbleiben der Entwicklung.

Die Untersuchung ergibt normale oder an der unteren Grenze des Normalen liegende Werte für den Grundumsatz, eine normale Fähigkeit der Schilddrüse für Speicherung von radioaktivem Jod, die 17-Ketosteroidausscheidung entspricht der Körpergröße und nicht der Sexualentwicklung, die Gonadotropine fehlen jedoch im Urin.

Die *Prognose* der Pubertas tarda ist im überwiegenden Teil der Fälle gut. Plötzlich mit 15, 16 oder 17 Jahren fangen die Jungen auch ohne Behandlung an, sich spontan zu entwickeln und sind nach 2—3 Jahren nicht mehr wiederzuerkennen.

Eine Einschränkung ist notwendig. Die Häufigkeit von Defekten des Kanälchenapparates scheint beträchtlich größer als bei Kindern, die sich zur normalen Zeit entwickeln. Dies geht einmal aus dem höheren Prozentsatz des ein- und doppelseitigen Kryptorchismus bei Menschen mit Pubertas tarda hervor, zum anderen ist, worauf besonders CHARNY (1957c) aufmerksam macht, die tubuläre Insuffizienz in Form der schweren Reifungshemmung des Samenepithels bei verzögerter Pubertät häufiger als sonst. In 30% von 500 bioptisch untersuchten sterilen Männern läßt die Vorgeschichte eine verzögerte Pubertät vermuten (CHARNY 1957c). Ob bei den Fettsüchtigen die erhöhte Innentemperatur des Scrotums gegenüber einem normalgewichtigen Jungen von Bedeutung ist, weiß man nicht. Solche Dysgenesien des Samenepithels weisen auf eine dritte Möglichkeit der verzögerten Pubertät hin, auf eine Reifungsstörung des Hodens selbst, der wohl zur Entwicklung fähig ist, diese aber erst nach längerdauernder Einwirkung der Gonadotropine in Angriff nimmt. Man wird diese dritte Gruppe erst sicher abtrennen können, wenn die Methoden der Gonadotropinbestimmung im Urin so verbessert sind, daß auch kleine Mengen sicher bestimmbar sind. Die histologische Untersuchung eines bioptisch entnommenen Hodenstückchens zeigt in solchen Fällen einen ungleichmäßigen Reifungsgrad der einzelnen Kanälchen. CHARNY (1957c) gibt ein charakteristisches Beispiel.

21jähriger junger Mann, wurde zum erstenmal mit 15 Jahren wegen Fettsucht und Hypogonadismus untersucht, war damals 158 cm groß und wog 75 kg. Keine Körperbehaarung, kleiner Penis, normal gebildetes Scrotum, Hodengröße 1,5 cm. Die Biopsie ergab einen Entwicklungsgrad wie bei einem 11—12jährigen, wobei aber zwei verschiedene Typen von Tubuli auffielen. Ein Teil ist angefüllt mit undifferenzierten Zellen, der andere ist in der Reifung etwas weiter fortgeschritten. In diesen sieht man einige Spermatogonien und einige primäre Spermatocyten, es besteht eine deutliche Sklerosierung des intertubulären Gewebes. Keine Behandlung, spontane Entwicklung vom 16. Lebensjahr an. Jetzt mit 21 Jahren verheiratet, wiegt bei 175 cm Größe 76 kg, rasiert sich täglich, äußeres Genitale normal, die Größe des Hodens im Längsdurchmesser 4 cm. Im Spermiogramm fehlen die Spermien gänzlich. Die histologische Untersuchung zeigt Kanälchen mit kleinerem Durchmesser und stark vermindertem Zellgehalt. Man sieht nur Spermatogonien und einige primäre Spermatocyten, weiter schreitet die Differenzierung nicht. Das Zwischengewebe ist gut entwickelt, zahlreiche Leydigzellen.

Obwohl also die volle Entwicklung spontan eingetreten ist und damit die Fähigkeit zur Gonadotropinbildung erwiesen ist, reift das Keimepithel nicht. Die Ursache liegt mit großer Wahrscheinlichkeit in einem angeborenen Defekt des Epithels und nicht in einer mangelnden FSH-Bildung.

Die Beurteilung des Einzelfalles ist schwierig. Die Methoden der Gonadotropinbestimmung sind bei den kleinen Mengen, die nachgewiesen werden sollen, mit ziemlichen Fehlerquellen belastet. Die 17-Ketosteroidausscheidung erfährt schon vor der Pubertät, etwa um das 8.—11. Lebensjahr, einen kräftigen Anstieg, der etwa dem Längenwachstum parallel geht (Adrenarche), so daß die Schwankungsbreite um die Zeit der Pubertät viel größer ist als beim Erwachsenen. Die Grenze zum Pathologischen ist schwer zu bestimmen. Von diesen beiden Methoden darf man also keine wesentliche Unterstützung erwarten. Der einfache negative Choriongonadotropintest (siebenmal 1000 E) schließt die Entwicklungsfähigkeit des Hodens nicht aus. Man richtet sich am besten nach der Knochenreife, der Körpergröße, der Hodengröße und nach der Familienanamnese.

Erfahrungsgemäß erreicht die größte Zahl der Jugendlichen mit verzögerter Reifung auch ohne Behandlung volle Maturität. Je größer die Differenz in der Entwicklung zu ihren gleichaltrigen Kameraden aber wird, um so leichter entwickeln sich Minderwertigkeitskomplexe, die den Betreffenden das ganze Leben belasten können. Diejenigen mit normaler Knochenreifung und normalem Längenwachstum, also besonders die Fettsüchtigen, wachsen weiter und bekommen eunuchoide Körperproportionen. Das leicht deformierte Skelet begünstigt das Auftreten von Überlastungsschäden im Sinne des Morbus Perthes, des Scheuermann (juvenile Kyphose), von X-Beinen, Reifungsstörungen des Skelets, die bei einer rechtzeitig einsetzenden Androgenproduktion vermeidbar sind oder nur geringe Grade erreichen.

4. Behandlung

Aus den eben genannten Gründen beginnen wir die Behandlung mit Beginn des 15. Lebensjahres, bei übernormal großen Jungen schon im 14. Lebensjahr. Implantation tierischer Hypophysen oder Verabreichung von Extrakten aus solchen ist wirkungslos, da die einzelne Hypophyse zu wenig Wirkstoff enthält und verhältnismäßig rasch Antikörper gegen das injizierte Fremdeiweiß gebildet werden. Die mit oralen Hypophysenpräparaten, besonders mit Hyphobion beschriebenen Erfolge sind Selbsttäuschungen. Am zweckmäßigsten ist die Verabreichung von Choriongonadotropin (HCG). Die in den Leydigzellen gebildeten Androgene (Testosteron) bedingen eine Desensibilisierung der Sexualregion des Zwischenhirns und leiten die Aufnahme der eigenen Gonadotropinproduktion ein. Man testet zuerst die Wirksamkeit von kleinen Dosen, dreimal 500 E pro Woche, steigert in Abständen von 4 Wochen um 500 E bis auf dreimal 1500 E und gibt diese Menge so lange, bis Zeichen der Androgenbildung faßbar oder sichtbar werden. Man verfolgt die 17-Ketosteroidausscheidung, die einen Anstieg erfährt, da die Empfindlichkeit der Leydigzellen um die Zeit der Pubertät am größten ist, registriert die Funktion der Schweiß- und Talgdrüsen und prüft Größe und Konsistenz der Hoden in regelmäßigen Abständen. Die Dosis von dreimal 1500 E (pro Woche) wird erst auf zweimal 1500, zweimal 1000, zweimal 500 reduziert, wenn Penis und Scrotum gewachsen sind und Pubes und Achselbehaarung erscheinen. Bei zu früher Unterbrechung reift die Sexualregion im Zwischenhirn nicht und der spontane Fortgang der Entwicklung bleibt aus.

Die Behandlungsdauer ist individuell verschieden. Bei einem Teil genügt ein Anstoß von 6—8 Wochen, um die physiologischen Vorgänge einzuleiten, bei anderen muß man monatelang therapieren. Es ist zweckmäßig, die Behandlung, alle Vierteljahr für 2—3 Wochen zu unterbrechen. Bleibt die 17-Ketosteroidausscheidung in der zweiten Woche gleich hoch wie unter der Behandlung dann darf man annehmen, daß die Hypophyse die Gonadotropinbildung aufgenommen hat, fällt sie ab, dann muß weiterbehandelt werden. Denselben Einblick erhält man mit der Bestimmung der Uringonadotropine, sind sie 14 Tage nach der Unterbrechung nachweisbar oder auf normale Höhe angestiegen, dann kann man die Behandlung abbrechen.

Vielfach erinnert die blasse, trockene, abschilfernde Haut dieser retardierten Jugendlichen an das gleichzeitige Vorliegen einer Hypothyreose. Geringe Verminderungen des Ruheumsatzes bis zu 7% sind häufig, ohne daß eine echte Hypothyreose vorhanden wäre. Nur bei Fettsüchtigen, die mit untercalorischer Ernährung allein nicht abnehmen, ist die Verabreichung von Thyreoidin indiziert. Man gibt Thyreoidea sicca 0,1—0,3 g oder wegen der leichteren Dosierbarkeit Trijodthyronin in der Dosis von 40—80 γ. Thyreoidin hat keinen Einfluß auf die Pubertätsentwicklung, aber jedes Kilogramm verlorenes Körpergewicht steigert die Leistung des zentralen Motors, es ist wie wenn das Fett die Gonadotropinproduktion hemmt. Verabreichung von Androgenen — Testosteron und seine Ester — ist unzweckmäßig, weniger wegen der damit verbundenen Hemmung der hypophysären Gonadotropinproduktion — diese erfolgt in gewissem Umfang auch durch die selbstgebildeten Androgene —, sondern wegen der fehlenden Anregung des Samenepithels, die durch HCG bei der lokalen Bildung des Testosterons in den Leydigzellen erreicht wird (s. S. 646). Man sollte alles vermeiden, was die Reifung des Samenepithels behindert. Aus diesem Grunde darf man auch der gegenwärtig bei Zurückbleiben im Wachstum, bei Unterernährung, bei Appetitmangel u. a. propagierten Anwendung der anabolen Steroide (s. S. 729) nicht kritiklos folgen. Alle diese Steroide hemmen auch die Gonadotropinproduktion in der Hypophyse und bei der nicht bekannten Empfindlichkeit des Hypophysenzwischenhirnsystems zu Beginn der Pubertät sollte man jeden groben Eingriff unterlassen.

Wir verwenden die *Anabolica* in den Fällen, die schon eine gewisse Entwicklung zeigen, bei denen die Pubertät aber unverhältnismäßig langsam und verzögert abläuft, die in der Knochenreifung deutlich zurückgeblieben sind, und bei allen Jugendlichen mit isolierten Wachstumsstörungen einzelner Knochen (Perthes, Scheuermann). Ihr Vorteil liegt in der spezifischen Anregung des Epiphysenwachstums, der Knochenreifung und der Reifung der Sexualregion, wobei die niedrigste noch wirksame Dosis die richtige ist (s. S. 738). Bei zu früher Anwendung, also vor dem Pubertätsalter, besteht wie bei der vorzeitigen Verabreichung oder Eigenproduktion von Testosteron, die Gefahr der vorzeitigen Pubertätsauslösung, denn die trophische Gewebswirkung des Testosterons, auch die auf die Reifung der Sexualregion (s. Pubertas praecox) kommt nicht seiner androgenen, sondern der anabolen Wirkungskomponente zu. Man muß die mit Anabolica behandelten Kinder sorgfältig beobachten und beim geringsten Zweifel die Gonadotropinausscheidung zur Entscheidung heranziehen.

II. Pubertas praecox

Bei Knaben spricht man von Pubertas praecox, wenn puberale Reifungsmerkmale vor dem 10. Lebensjahr auftreten. Die *echte* ist durch eine vorzeitige Aufnahme der Gonadotropinproduktion durch die Hypophyse bedingt, die *Pseudo-Pubertas* praecox durch eine vorzeitige, autochthone Bildung von androgenen Hormonen. Die Störung ist bei Mädchen etwa dreimal häufiger als bei Knaben. Übersichten stammen von SECKEL (1950), JOLLY (1955a), ROYER, RIVRON, WILKINS (1950), NOVAK, HAIN (1947a) u.a. ROYER und RIVRON haben bis 1957 250 männliche Fälle zusammengestellt. 41% gehören der sog. idiopathischen Form an, bei 33% liegt eine cerebrale Ursache vor, bei 20% handelt es sich um Erkrankungen der Nebennierenrinde, nur 6% sind durch Tumoren des Hodens selbst bedingt. Novak nimmt an, daß sogar 90% und mehr aller Fälle von Pubertas praecox der idiopathischen Form angehören, da diese Fälle in den letzten Jahren nicht mehr mitgeteilt werden. Die Kranken bleiben gesund und wachsen zu normalen, aber kleinwüchsigen Erwachsenen heran und bieten keine besonderen Probleme. Den Eltern der betroffenen Kinder fällt meist das anormal große Genitale auf. Die Vergrößerung des Penis, das Wachstum des Scrotums, die wachsende Pubesbehaarung sind die ersten Zeichen einer vermehrten Androgenproduktion. Die Keimdrüsen verhalten sich verschieden. Bleiben sie kindlich klein und symmetrisch, während nur der Penis wächst, dann handelt es sich um eine extragenitale Androgenvermehrung. Wachsen sie gleichmäßig symmetrisch und nehmen eine normale Konsistenz an, dann liegt die Ursache in einer Vermehrung der Gonadotropinbildung. Eine Asymmetrie in der Hodengröße endlich weist auf eine lokale Geschwulst in einem Hoden hin. Ein gutes Maß für die Menge der Androgenbildung ist die Größe der Prostata und der Samenblasen.

Im weiteren Verlauf treten bestimmte Reifemerkmale besonders hervor. Das sind besonders die Entwicklung der Terminalbehaarung, das Wachstum der Prostata, das Tieferwerden der Stimme. Bei stärkerer Androgenproduktion entwickelt sich die Skeletmuskulatur vorzeitig, so daß die Kinder schon mit 3 bis 4 Jahren einen athletischen Körperbau aufweisen. Eine besondere Bedeutung kommt der vorzeitigen Entwicklung des Skeletsystems zu. Tonutti u. Mitarb. machen darauf aufmerksam, daß bei der vorzeitigen Androgeneinwirkung ein Skelet mit völlig anderer Ausgangslage vorliegt. Je nach Lebensalter sind einzelne Knochenkerne überhaupt noch nicht angelegt und die Epiphysenfugen stehen weit offen. In diesen Fällen bewirkt der vorzeitige Androgeneinfluß eine unzeitgemäße und überstürzte Knochenreifung mit erheblich verfrühtem Auftreten der noch fehlenden Knochenkerne. Zugleich wird das Längenwachstum durch einen überhöhten jährlichen Zuwachs stark beschleunigt. Dadurch eilt das Knochenalter dem chronologischen Alter weit voraus, die Patienten sind wesentlich größer als ihre Alterskameraden. Die überstürzte Knochenreifung verursacht jedoch auch einen vorzeitigen Schluß der Epiphysenfugen und verkürzt damit die für das Wachstum zur Verfügung stehende Zeit, es resultiert daher ein Minderwuchs. Die Entwicklung des Gebisses steht nicht unter der Kontrolle der Keimdrüsen und entspricht dem Lebensalter.

Auch die geistige und seelische Entwicklung richtet sich nach dem Lebensalter. Schwierigkeiten in der Erziehung treten auf, wenn die Diskrepanz zwischen körperlicher und geistiger Entwicklung zu groß ist. Das vorzeitige Auftreten von sexuellen Regungen kommt vor (Stutte); Jolly (1955a) vermerkt dies dreimal bei 19 Fällen, Royer u. Mitarb. einmal bei 15. Manche Kinder sind reizbar und aggressiv, andere wiederum ängstlich und mehr depressiv.

1. Echte Pubertas praecox

Die echte Pubertas praecox beruht in der vorzeitigen Aktivierung der Gonadotropinbildung des Hypophysenvorderlappens. Die Anregung geht nie vom Vorderlappen selbst aus, sondern von einer vorzeitigen Aktivierung des Sexualzentrums im vorderen Zwischenhirn. Die Ursache ist meist unbekannt — idiopathisch, seltener wird sie durch Erkrankungen des Zwischenhirns hervorgerufen.

a) Idiopathische oder konstitutionelle Form

Bei der *idiopathischen* oder *konstitutionellen* Form (Novak) unterscheidet man eine inkomplette und eine vollständige Art. Bei der ersteren sind die Zeichen der Reifung wenig ausgeprägt. Die Biopsie zeigt nur eine geringe Entwicklung der Kanälchen ohne Spermatocyten oder Spermatozoen, während das Zwischengewebe besser entfaltet ist und die 17-Ketosteroide sich mehr dem Normalen nähern. Offenbar wird in diesen Fällen zuerst ICSH gebildet. Dem entspricht die geringe Gonadotropinausscheidung. Meistens handelt es sich nur um ein Durchgangsstadium zur vollständigen Form. Der Verlauf ist protrahiert.

Bei der *kompletten Form* entwickelt sich der Hoden normal, die Kanälchen enthalten reife Spermatozoen, das Interstitium ist voll entwickelt, die Pubertät wird zum Abschluß gebracht, 17-Ketosteroid- und Oestrogenausscheidung entsprechen dem 12—14jähriger, ebenso die Gonadotropinausscheidung, nie erreichen sie übernormale Werte.

Diese idiopathische Form ist bei Mädchen viel häufiger als bei Knaben. Familiäres Vorkommen ist verhältnismäßig häufig beobachtet und wird zur Differentialdiagnose verwendet (NOVAK, RUSH u. Mitarb., SIGRIST, GARDINER-HILL, HAIN 1947a). Der bekannteste Stammbaum umfaßt 27 Fälle, alle bei Männern, die sich über vier Generationen einer Familie verteilen (RUSH u. Mitarb.).

Die Pubertätsentwicklung beginnt im allgemeinen nach dem 3.—4. Lebensjahr, bei Mädchen sind aber zahlreiche Fälle schon in früherem Alter beschrieben. Von 310 Mädchen waren 70 vor dem 14. Lebensjahr und 18 zwischen dem 5. und 10. Jahr gravide. Aus Peru wurde ein Mädchen berichtet, das mit 8 Monaten menstruierte und mit $5^1/_2$ Jahren durch Sectio caesaria entbunden wurde (NOVAK, SIGRIST). Die Diagnose der idiopathischen Form darf nur nach Ausschluß von organischen cerebralen Störungen gestellt werden. Die Hormonproduktion in Hypophyse und Gonaden überschreitet die Höhe derjenigen von Erwachsenen nicht.

Die Ursache ist unbekannt. Wegen des familiären Vorkommens vermutet man, daß genetische Faktoren die vorzeitige Reifung des Sexualzentrums auslösen (NOVAK). Ob hyperplastische Veränderungen im Tubergebiet, wie sie im nächsten Abschnitt erwähnt sind, auch das anatomische Substrat dieser idiopathischen Formen sind, ist nicht geklärt.

Irgendwelche neurologischen Phänomene oder Zeichen einer gestörten geistigen Entwicklung fehlen. Naturgemäß kann die Diagnose erst nach mehrjähriger Beobachtung gestellt werden, da benigne Tumoren unter Umständen jahrelang benötigen, um Symptome zu machen. Die Prognose ist gut. NOVAK hat auf die Bedeutung der richtigen psychologischen Führung hingewiesen.

b) Organische Gehirnerkrankungen

Seit der Zusammenstellung von LANGE-COSACK unterscheidet man in der deutschen Literatur zwei Hauptgruppen.

α) Hyperplastische Mißbildungen des Tuber cinereum

Hierbei handelt es sich um kirschkern- bis hühnereigroße tumorartige Gebilde des ventralen Hypothalamus. Im Tumorgewebe kommen zahlreiche ausgereifte Nervenzellen und Nervenfasern vor. Ein Teil dieser Geschwülste wurde als Astrocytome oder Gliome gedeutet, doch können auch in diesen Fällen nervöse Strukturen festgestellt werden, die an den Bau des Tuber cinereum erinnern. Der erste Fall dieser Art wurde von DRIGGS und SPATZ beschrieben. Es handelte sich um einen $3^1/_2$jährigen Jungen, der bei seinem Tod einen körperlichen Entwicklungszustand eines 15—16jährigen hatte. Hypophyse, Zirbeldrüse, Nebennieren, Keimdrüsen waren intakt. Als Ursache fand sich ein vom Tuber cinereum in die Basalzisterne herabhängendes Gebilde von Kirschgröße, das bei seiner

geringen Ausdehnung keine Druckwirkung auf den sonst völlig intakten Hypothalamus ausgeübt hat. Histologisch fand sich eine hyperplastische Mißbildung
mit massenhaft Nervenzellen und Nervenfasern.

McCullagh u. Mitarb. (1951) berichten über einen $6^{1}/_{2}$jährigen Jungen, der
schon Ende des 1. Lebensjahres wegen einer Vergrößerung des Genitales auffiel
und mehrmals untersucht wurde. Der Junge wuchs und entwickelte sich ohne
abnorme Symptome bis zum Alter von $5^{1}/_{2}$ Jahren rasch. Zu dieser Zeit traten
epileptische Anfälle mit nachfolgenden Dämmerzuständen auf. Mit $6^{1}/_{2}$ Jahren
entsprach die körperliche Entwicklung einem 12—13jährigen. Acne, kräftige
Muskelentwicklung, normal großer Penis, normal große Hoden, palpable Prostata,
starke Pubesbehaarung waren vorhanden. 17-Ketosteroidausscheidung um 2 mg
in 24 Std bei mehrmaliger Bestimmung zweimal unter 1 mg, Uringonadotropine
— Methode von Gorbman (ME) — beträchtlich erhöht, zwischen 52 und 202 MU,
im Gegensatz zu 13—105 MU des normalen Erwachsenen. ICSH — bestimmt
an der hypophysektomierten Ratte durch Gehalt an alkalischer Phosphatase
der Prostata — betrug 4 E gegenüber 4—8 E des gesunden Erwachsenen. Mikroskopisch bestand das Bild einer normal aktiven Spermiogenese. Der Junge starb
mit 9 Jahren durch Ertrinken. Im Tuber cinereum wurde ein Hamartom von
1,5 cm Durchmesser gefunden.

In anderen Fällen ist der Befund ähnlich, sie werden in der Literatur zum
Teil auch unter dem Begriff der *tuberösen Sklerose* zusammengefaßt (Hooft
u. Mitarb., Krabbe 1922, Seckel u. Mitarb. 1949, Meyer u. Mitarb. 1930,
Schmalz).

In der Zusammenstellung von Lange-Cosack (1950) (6 Mädchen, 12 Knaben)
hatten 4 Kinder schon bei der Geburt ein abnorm großes Genitale und unmittelbar
nach der Geburt setzte die überstürzte allgemeine und genitale Entwicklung ein.
Bei 10 Fällen begannen die ersten Krankheitserscheinungen bereits im 1. Lebensjahr, bei 5 bis zum Abschluß des 4. Lebensjahres, das späteste Manifestationsalter lag bei 7 Jahren. Neurologische Erscheinungen wie Gangunsicherheit,
Kopfschmerzen, Hirndruckerscheinungen, Stauungspapille sind häufig. Die Kinder starben, bevor sie das 10. Lebensjahr erreicht hatten, an interkurrenten
Infektionen, ein Teil im Anschluß an operative Eingriffe. Lange-Cosack (1950)
rechnet zu dieser Gruppe auch Fälle von Astrocytomen und Gliomen, die von
verschiedenen Autoren veröffentlicht sind und in denen histologisch keine Nervenzellen oder nervenfaserartige Strukturen erwähnt sind.

Als Ursache dieser Form der Pubertas praecox wird die vorzeitige Aufnahme
der Tätigkeit des Sexualzentrums, das in den hyperplastischen, tumorartig
gewucherten Nervenstrukturen des vorderen Hypothalamus angenommen wird,
vermutet (Lange-Cosack 1950).

β) Tumoren des Hypothalamus

Die zweite Gruppe umfaßt *Tumoren des Hypothalamus* und andere organische
Gehirnerkrankungen. Beobachtet wurden Kraniopharyngiome, Gliome, Astrocytome, Ependymome, Ganglioneurome, Neurofibrome, Infundibulome, Pinealome. Die Lokalisation der Geschwülste ist sehr verschieden, ein Teil liegt im
vorderen Hypothalamus, andere im caudalen Gebiet der Mamillarregion, wieder
andere in der Gegend der Zirbeldrüse. Diese Geschwülste können in jedem
Lebensalter zu wachsen beginnen, im allgemeinen beginnt die Pubertätsentwicklung jedoch erst zwischen dem 6. und 10. Lebensjahr (Lange-Cosack 1950).
Besonderes Interesse haben schon immer die Zirbeltumoren gefunden (Reilly,
Marburg). Für die Ansicht, daß vom Corpus pineale hemmende Impulse ausgehen, die bei seiner Zerstörung wegfallen. hat man keine sicheren experimentellen

Beweise. Von 56 Kindern mit Zirbeltumoren wiesen nur 21 eine vorzeitige Pubertät auf. Einfache Zerstörung der Epiphyse macht keine Pubertas praecox (KRABBE 1922, WEINBERGER u. Mitarb.).

Verhältnismäßig häufig findet sich die Pubertas praecox auch bei nicht geschwulstartigen Krankheitsprozessen des Gehirns, besonders beim *Hydrocephalus internus*, aber auch nach Ablauf von Encephalitiden im Gefolge von Mumps, Masern, Keuchhusten, bei der tuberkulösen Meningitis, der Arachnitis der hinteren Schädelgrube. Diese Formen sind die weitaus häufigsten.

LANGE-COSACK (1950) sieht die Ursache dieser zweiten Gruppe in einer Druckwirkung auf das Tuber cinereum, wodurch eine vorzeitige Impulsauslösung im Sexualzentrum eintreten soll. Als wichtigstes gemeinsames Charakteristicum besteht in diesen Fällen ein Hydrocephalus internus des 3. Ventrikels. WEINBERGER und GRANT nehmen dagegen an, daß im caudalen Gebiet der Mamillarregion ein Hemmzentrum liegt, bei dessen Ausschaltung das Tubergebiet die Überhand gewinnt und vorzeitig Reize zur Gonadotropinbildung an die Hypophyse abgibt. Auch diese Theorie ist eine Hypothese, die der Bestätigung bedarf, da nicht alle Tumoren im hinteren Hypothalamus eine Pubertas praecox verursachen.

Im ganzen gesehen ist die Ursache dieser cerebralen Formen letzten Endes ungeklärt. Die erste Gruppe ist möglicherweise durch eine vermehrte Produktion der physiologischen humoralen, die Gonadotropinproduktion der Adenohypophyse anregenden Substanzen des Zwischenhirns bedingt. Bei der zweiten Gruppe ist der Wegfall hemmender Einflüsse auf das Sexualzentrum am wahrscheinlichsten, wobei unklar ist, welche Teile des Hypothalamus bzw. des Gehirns hierfür von größter Bedeutung sind.

Die Prognose dieser Fälle ist ungünstig, da die Kranken meist an den Folgen des chronischen Hirndrucks sterben.

Therapie. Kommt eine operative Behandlung (Tumorentfernung, Kompensation eines Hydrocephalus) nicht in Betracht, bleibt der Versuch der Hemmung der Gonadotropinsekretion durch androgen, oestrogen und anabol unwirksame Derivate der androgenen oder oestrogenen Steroide, bei denen die Hemmung der Gonadotropinbildung noch erhalten ist. Mit MRL/41 (Chloramiphen) und 17α-Methyl-17β-hydroxy-androstan-3-on (GREENBLATT u. Mitarb.) hat man bis jetzt keine guten Ergebnisse gehabt, es ist aber nur eine Frage der Zeit, bis bessere Hypophysenblocker gefunden werden.

c) Albright-Syndrom

Das Albright-Syndrom kommt bei Mädchen viel häufiger vor als bei Knaben. Seine Charakteristica sind:

1. die polyostitische-fibröse Dysplasie des Knochens, die sich durch Schmerzen in den Extremitäten anzeigt und eventuell zu Spontanfrakturen führen kann. Röntgenologisch sieht man große cystische Aufhellungen im Becken und den Extremitätenknochen. wobei meist ein Entwicklungsstrahl stärker betroffen ist als der andere. An der Schädelbasis sind umschriebene Knochenverdichtungen häufig;

2. eine intensive fleckige Pigmentierung der Haut, die im Bereich der Knochencysten meist am stärksten ausgeprägt ist und

3. eine meist im frühen Kindesalter beginnende, aber langsam fortschreitende vorzeitige sexuelle Entwicklung, deren Ursache nicht bekannt ist (echte Pubertas praecox). Die erwachsenen Träger dieser Anomalie sind minderwüchsig, Kleinwuchs ist dagegen selten.

2. Pseudopubertas praecox

a) Leydigzelltumoren

Bis 1955 hat Jolly 16 Fälle, Bishop u. Mitarb. bis 1959 25 Fälle, vorwiegend aus der englisch-amerikanischen Literatur, zusammengestellt. Die Zeichen der Pubertät entwickelten sich im Alter von $1^3/_4$—9 Jahren, beim größten Teil zwischen dem 3. und 6. Lebensjahr.

Die Größe der Geschwülste wechselt zwischen 1,2 und 12 cm, meist sind sie etwa kirschgroß, gelbbraun, gut abgegrenzt, selten wachsen sie infiltrierend in die Umgebung. In einem Fall war der Tumor maligne, das Kind starb mit 9 Jahren. Der Tumor kann anfangs so klein sein, daß keine Hodenvergrößerung auffällt. Der gesunde Hoden bleibt klein und infantil. Verlauf beim Erwachsenen s. unter Hodentumoren.

Histologisch finden sich solide Geschwülste mit gleichmäßig ausgereiften großen, vieleckigen, leberzellähnlichen Leydigzellen mit reichlich acidophilem und granulärem Cytoplasma. In einigen Fällen waren auch Reincke-Kristalle vorhanden. Die Unterscheidung von der tumorartigen Leydigzellhyperplasie ist nicht immer einfach (Warren und Olshausen 1943).

Bemerkenswert ist das Auftreten von ausreifenden Kanälchen in der direkten Umgebung des Tumors. Ihr Durchmesser kann beträchtlich vergrößert sein, im Innern sieht man die basalen Stadien der Spermiogenese bis zu den Spermatocyten. Entfernt vom Tumor liegende Kanälchen sowie diejenigen der anderen Seite, bleiben dagegen im infantilen Zustand. Schmidt und Tonutti deuten diesen Befund als direkte Nachbarschaftswirkung der Androgene.

Die vorzeitige Androgeneinwirkung führt wie bei anderen Formen der Pubertas praecox zu einem beschleunigten somatischen Wachstum. Der Unterschied zwischen dem wirklichen Knochenalter und dem Lebensalter kann sehr beträchtlich sein, so in den Fällen von Jolly (1955a) $2^4/_{12}$ gegen 6—7 Jahre, von Schmidt und Tonutti $5^2/_{12}$ gegen 12—13, von Jungck $8^6/_{12}$ gegen 17.

Klinisch sind die Kinder gewöhnlich kräftig gebaut, haben eine gut entwickelte Muskulatur, eine gut entwickelte Schambehaarung, während Achsel-Gesichts- und Körperbehaarung zurückbleiben. Der Stimmbruch tritt früh ein. Drei Fälle hatten eine Gynäkomastie. Die Stärke der Androgenbildung zeigt die Größe des Penis und der Prostata.

Die Hälfte der von Bishop (1960) zusammengestellten Kinder zeigten auch Symptome einer vorzeitigen psychosexuellen Entwicklung. Zum Teil sind sie ausgesprochen aggressiv und schwer erziehbar.

Die *Hormonausscheidung* ist wenig untersucht. Die höchsten Werte für die 17-Ketosteroide bei Kindern berichten Bishop u. Mitarb. mit 550 mg, Florentin und Rauber mit 182 mg, Sandblom (1948) mit 64 mg, immer ist sie aber höher als dem Lebensalter entspricht (5—10 mg bei einem $5^2/_{12}$ Jahre alten Jungen (Schmidt u. Tonutti), 2,9 mg bei einem $5^6/_{12}$ Jahre alten Jungen (Jolly 1955a) und 25,7 bei einem $8^6/_{12}$jährigen Jungen (Jungck u. Mitarb. 1954). Die 17-Ketosteroide bestehen vorwiegend aus Androsteron, Ätiocholanolon, während DEA im Verhältnis zur Höhe der Gesamt-17-Ketosteroidausscheidung niedrig ist (Cook u. Mitarb.). Diese geringe Beteiligung des DEA spricht für den testiculären Ursprung der 17-Ketosteroidvorstufen.

Die Prognose ist günstig, da die Diagnose infolge der Pubertas praecox frühzeitig gestellt wird und Metastasierung nur bei langem Bestehen eintritt. Wilkins (1950) berichtet über diffuse Hodenvergrößerungen als Folge von hyperplastischem versprengtem Nebennierengewebe bei der angeborenen Nebennierenhyperplasie (AGS). Die Differentialdiagnose kann durch den Cortisontest getroffen werden.

Nach Entfernung des Tumors bilden sich die Zeichen der vorzeitigen Entwicklung nicht immer zurück. Dies berichten ROWLANDS u. Mitarb. (1929) bei einem 11jährigen, SOMERFORD bei einem $12^1/_2$jährigen, HUFFMANN bei einem 8jährigen, WERNER u. Mitarb. (1942) bei einem 7jährigen, JUNGCK u. Mitarb. (1954) bei einem $8^1/_2$jährigen. SANDBLOM vermerkt bei einem $4^1/_2$jährigen Jungen ein Wachstum des gesunden Hoden nach Entfernung des tumortragenden, ebenso JUNGCK. Dem entspricht auch ein unvollständiger Rückgang der 17-Ketosteroidausscheidung. So berichten THAMDRUP von einem 7jährigen Kind, das vor der Operation 40 mg 17-Ketosteroid, nach der Operation immer noch 5,3 mg 17-Ketosteroid, SANDBLOM von einem 3jährigen Kind, das vor der Operation 50—60 mg, nach $1^1/_2$ Jahren noch 17 mg 17-Ketosteroid ausschied. SCHMIDT und TONUTTI fanden in ihrem Falle vor der Operation 5—10 mg, direkt nach der Operation 2,8—4 mg und 3 Jahre danach im 8. Lebensjahr 9,6—12,3 mg. In diesem Fall war auch die Gonadotropinausscheidung im Urin mit 20 MUE gleich derjenigen eines Erwachsenen.

TONUTTI u. Mitarb. erwähnen zwei besonders instruktive Fälle von WILKINS und CARA (1954). Bei zwei Knaben im Alter von 6—9 Jahren mit isosexuellem adrenogenitalem Syndrom, die ein Knochenalter von 11—14 Jahren erreicht hatten, wuchsen nach Einleitung der Cortisontherapie rasch beide Hoden. 6—15 Monate nach Beginn der Cortisonbehandlung waren zahlreiche große und gut differenzierte Leydigzellen sowie weitgehend entfaltete Kanälchen vorhanden. Ein $4^3/_4$ Jahre alter Junge mit einem androgenbildenden Nebennierenrindentumor hatte ein Knochenalter von 12 Jahren erreicht, tägliche 17-Ketosteroidausscheidung 360 mg. Nach Exstirpation des Tumors wuchsen die Hoden rasch. Im histologischen Bild waren die Leydigzellen entfaltet und die Spermiogenese vollständig. SCHMIDT und TONUTTI berichten über einen $5^1/_2$jährigen Jungen mit Leydigzelltumor mit einem Knochenalter von 12—13 Jahren, der schon vor der Operation eine geringe, aber feststellbare Gonadotropinausscheidung aufwies und in beiden Hoden entfaltete Leydigzellen zeigte. Die 17-Ketosteroidausscheidung betrug 5—10 mg. Trotz der Androgenproduktion des Tumors war die gonadotrope Hypophysenfunktion in Gang gekommen, aus einer Pseudopubertas war eine echte Pubertas geworden. Hierbei ist nach TONUTTI das Vorauseilen der somatischen Entwicklung gegenüber dem chronologischen Alter entscheidend. Es eilt offenbar nicht nur das Knochen- und Skeletalter voraus, sondern auch die Reifung des Hypophysenzwischenhirnsystems, in dem der Mechanismus der Gonadotropinsekretion verankert ist. Dieses erlangt im Zuge der durch die Androgene beschleunigten somatischen Entwicklung Funktionsbereitschaft, wenn der Organismus ein Knochenalter von etwa 13 Jahren erreicht hat. Die Hypophyse vermag dann in gleicher Weise wie bei der physiologischen Pubertät die Gonadotropinsekretion aufzunehmen. Im allgemeinen kommt diese nicht in Gang, solange übermäßig große Androgenmengen produziert werden. Sobald aber der Androgenspiegel nach Exstirpation eines Tumors oder nach Cortisonbehandlung einer Nebennierenrindenhyperplasie absinkt, erfolgt der Start der Gonadotropinsekretion. Voraussetzung ist lediglich, daß die durch das Knochenalter von etwa 13 Jahren charakterisierte somatische Reifung des Organismus zu diesem Zeitpunkt erreicht ist. Das Hodengewebe entwickelt sich von da an normal weiter.

Dies erklärt, warum in vielen Fällen nach Entfernung des Leydigzelltumors die Entwicklung trotzdem weiter fortschreitet, und zwar um so rascher, je näher das Knochenalter des Betreffenden dem eines 13jährigen liegt und um so langsamer, je unreifer die Knochenentwicklung ist.

b) Kongenitale Nebennierenhyperplaise (KNH),
angeborenes adrenogenitales Syndrom (AGS)

Eine weitere Form der Pseudopubertas ist durch die übermäßige Produktion von androgenen Steroiden in der Nebennierenrinde bedingt. Diese kann auf einer kongenitalen Anomalie der Steroidsynthese beruhen oder aber im späteren Leben durch androgenproduzierende Tumoren erworben werden.

Die Häufigkeit der angeborenen Form wird in der amerikanischen Bevölkerung auf 1:78000 Neugeborene geschätzt. Das weibliche Geschlecht ist bei weitem bevorzugt.

Die kongenitale Nebennierenhyperplasie (KNH) tritt nicht selten bei Geschwistern auf, während in der Aszendenz der Betroffenen keine Erkrankungen vorkommen (WILKINS 1952b). Man vermutet einen recessiven Erbgang. Die Erkrankten sind also wahrscheinlich homozygot und ihre gesunden Eltern und ein Teil ihrer gesunden Geschwister heterozygot.

Die Ursache besteht in einer Störung der Hormonsynthese in der Nebennierenrinde. Das natürliche Nebennierensteroid Cortisol wird als Folge eines Enzymmangels nur noch in ungenügender Menge produziert. Dadurch fällt die Hemmung der ACTH-Produktion im Hypophysenvorderlappen weg. Die nachweisbare Mehrproduktion führt zu einer beträchtlichen Hyperplasie beider Nebennieren. Dadurch wird in den meisten Fällen doch eine beinahe normale Cortisolbildung erreicht, so daß Zeichen einer manifesten Nebenniereninsuffizienz fehlen. Daneben fällt aus den Vorstufen des Cortisol eine große Menge androgen wirkender Metaboliten an. Bei männlichen Individuen entsteht das Bild der Pseudopubertas praecox, das WILKINS als Macrogenitosomia praecox bezeichnet, da die Hodenreifung ausbleibt. Kinder weiblichen Geschlechts kommen mit dem Bild des *Pseudohermaphroditismus femininus* zur Welt. Neben der Bildung von Androgenen ist auch die der Oestrogene beträchtlich erhöht. Dieser übermäßige Anfall von Sexualhormonen hemmt Bildung und Abgabe der Gonadotropine in der Adenohypophyse, so daß die reguläre Pubertät ausbleibt und die Entwicklung der Keimdrüsen auch beim Erwachsenen auf infantiler Stufe stehenbleibt.

Anatomisch sind beide Nebennieren gleichmäßig stark vergrößert, wobei die Hyperplasie vorwiegend die Zona reticularis betrifft (JONES 1954), auch die Glomerulosa kann daran teilnehmen. Bei einigen Fällen, die an einem Salzmangelsyndrom gestorben sind, war die Glomerulosa nicht sicher nachweisbar (WILKINS 1950).

Die vermehrte Androgenproduktion beginnt schon im Fetalleben. Trotzdem ist bei der Geburt der Penis nur in wenigen Fällen vergrößert. Den Müttern fällt das Wachsen des Genitales erst mit 3—4 Jahren auf. Von da an schreitet die Entwicklung rasch fort. Penis und Prostata können mit 4—6 Jahren die normale Größe erreicht haben, Scham- und Achselbehaarung sind voll ausgebildet, die Stimme wird tief, Erektionen sind häufig. Im Gegensatz dazu bleiben die Hoden klein und unreif. Die Samenkanälchen sind völlig unentwickelt, Leydigzellen fehlen. In seltenen Fällen ist die Hodengröße normal oder sogar übernormal. Hier deckt die Biopsie ein versprengtes hyperplastisches Nebennierenrindengewebe im Hoden auf (WILKINS 1950).

Daneben ist die Beschleunigung des Körperwachstums und der Knochenentwicklung die auffälligste Erscheinung. Schon gegen Ende des 1. Lebensjahres hat man in einigen Fällen röntgenologisch eine beschleunigte Reifung des Knochens feststellen können. Der Unterschied zwischen Knochenalter und Lebensalter wird immer stärker, so daß mit 6—9 Jahren ein Knochenalter von 11—14 Jahren erreicht sein kann. Bis zum 10. Lebensjahr sind die Jungen ihren Altersgenossen an Körpergröße und Muskelentwicklung beträchtlich voraus. Von da an wachsen sie wegen des vorzeitigen Epiphysenschlusses nicht mehr weiter. Als Erwachsene erreichen sie eine Körpergröße zwischen 145 und 160 cm, sie sind auffallend gedrungen gebaut (vgl. Abb. 20 a—c).

WILKINS (1950), dem man die wichtigsten Beobachtungen verdankt, hat mehrere Verlaufsformen beschrieben.

1. Die *kompensierte Form*, die sich ungefähr im Hormongleichgewicht befindet, da die kompensatorische Hypertrophie der Nebennierenrinde eine etwa normale Cortisolbildung erlaubt.

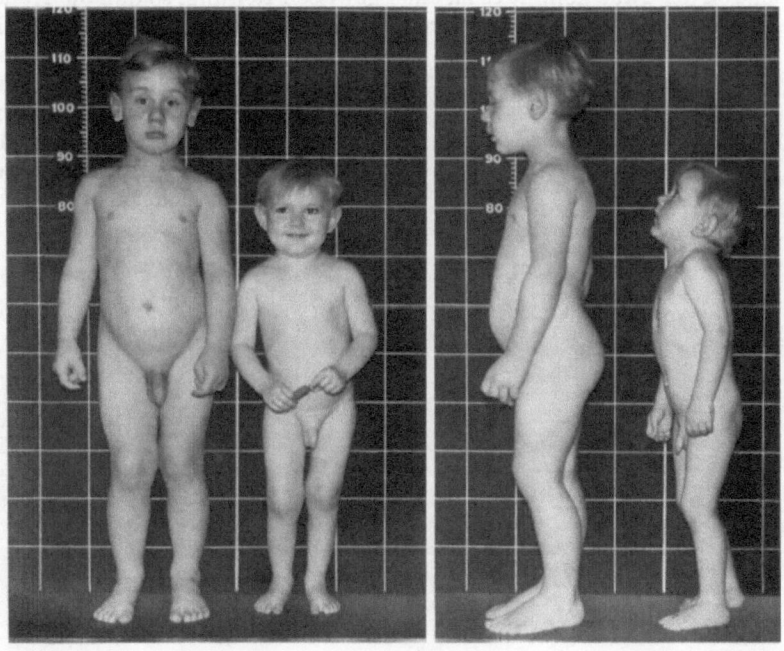

a

Abb. 20 a—c. F. W., 3jährig, Größe 115 cm (Soll 92 cm), Gewicht 24,1 kg (Soll 19,1 kg). Daneben gleichaltriger gesunder Junge. Seit 1 Jahr rasches Körper- und Genitalwachstum, kräftige Muskulatur, fleischiges Gesicht. Größenalter 5jährig, Knochenalter 7jährig, Zähne machen Entwicklung nicht mit. 17-Ketosteroide: 5,3 bis 6,1; DEA 1,8 mg, Pregnandiol 0,6 mg. Nach Cortisongabe: 17-Ketosteroide 2,3 bis 4 mg, Pregnandiol negativ. Diagnose: Makrogenitosomia praecox bei angeborener Nebennierenhyperplasie. (Kinderklinik Tübingen)

2. In einem Drittel aller Fälle geht das AGS mit einem Salzverlust einher — Debré-Fibiger-Syndrom — *(salzverlierende Form)*. Früher starben solche Kinder in den ersten Lebensmonaten an einer Exsiccose. Das Blut ist eingedickt, Natrium und Chlor sind vermindert, Kalium stark erhöht, die Bicarbonatkonzentration niedrig. Zum Unterschied von der einfachen Pylorusstenose ist die Chlorausscheidung im Urin normal. WILKINS (1950) hat in diesen Fällen die Bildung eines besonderen salzdiuretisch wirkenden Hormons angenommen.

3. Seltener ist die KNH bei Kindern und Erwachsenen mit einer beträchtlichen Blutdrucksteigerung verbunden *(hypertensive Form)*. Auch bei diesen beiden Unterformen ist die Androgen- und Oestrogenproduktion stark erhöht, so daß das klinische Bild von einer Pseudopubertas praecox begleitet ist.

Beim *erwachsenen Manne* ist die Diagnose der angeborenen Nebennierenrindenhyperplasie schwierig. Solche Menschen kommen wegen Sterilität zur Untersuchung oder werden zufällig entdeckt. Die Ausbildung der sekundären

Geschlechtsmerkmale ist normal, meist besteht eine intensive Behaarung und schon in jungem Alter eine erhebliche Glatzenbildung. Die Muskulatur ist kräftig entwickelt, es fällt aber die geringe Körpergröße von 145—160 cm auf. Der Ausfall der inkretorischen Hodenfunktion wird durch die Nebennierenrinden-androgene verdeckt. In der Anamnese erfährt man von der vorzeitigen Pubertät. Beide Hoden sind klein, atrophisch, weich. Bei Einlagerung von versprengtem Nebennierengewebe können sie beinahe normal groß erscheinen (WILKINS 1950). Die Hodenreifung bleibt in schweren Fällen auf frühkindlicher Stufe stehen, meist ist die Differenzierung der Spermatogonien und Sertolizellen eingetreten. In einem Teil der Fälle kommt es zu einer gewissen Reifung, so daß die Kanälchen Spermatocyten und einige reife Spermien enthalten können. Bei Frauen ist die FSH-Ausscheidung teilweise normal gefunden worden. In höherem Alter kann sich eine beträchtliche Hyalinisierung der Kanälchen entwickeln, die sich trotz Normalisierung der Hormonproduktion durch Cortison nicht mehr zurückbildet (NIKOLOWSKI).

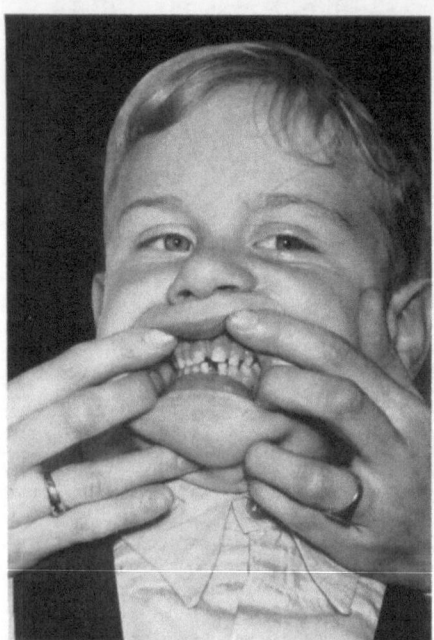

Abb. 20b

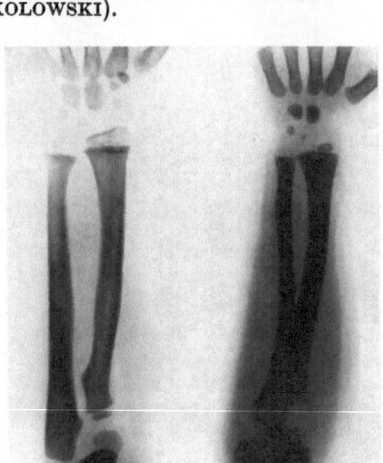

Abb. 20c

Wohl den ersten Fall eines Erwachsenen haben NOWAKOWSKI und PÜSCHEL beschrieben. Ein seit 2 Jahren kinderlos verheirateter 25jähriger Mann kommt wegen Sterilität zur Untersuchung. Dabei ergibt sich eine völlige Azoospermie. In der Anamnese erfährt man, daß der Kranke im 1. Lebensjahr wegen eines kaum stillbaren Erbrechens in einem Krankenhaus gewesen war. Ab dem 2. Lebensjahr hat er sich körperlich rasch entwickelt und überragte im 3. Lebensjahr seine Altersgenossen bereits um Kopflänge. Im 4. Lebensjahr bemerkten die Eltern das Wachstum der Schambehaarung und eine abnorme Größe des Penis. Mit 5 Jahren war er 141 cm groß, hatte deutlich entwickelte Pubes, während die Achselbehaarung noch fehlte. Die Stimme hatte schon begonnen zu mutieren. Beide Hoden sind nur pflaumen-kerngroß, während die 8 cm lange Penis stark entwickelt ist. Mit 25 Jahren betrug die Körpergröße 160 cm, das Gewicht 72 kg, der Körperbau ist gedrungen und muskulös, die Behaarung unauffällig, Penis und Scrotum normal entwickelt, beide Hoden sind jedoch nur bohnengroß, derbelastisch. Prostata über kastaniengroß und prall. Die bioptische Untersuchung des linken Hodens zeigt kleine Kanälchen ohne Lumen. Das Samenepithel besteht fast nur aus Spermatogonien und Sertolizellen, nur hie und da sind einige Mitrosen"zu erkennen. Leydigsche Zwischenzellen fehlen. Das histologisches Bild entspricht dem eines präpuberalen Hodens. Hormonausscheidung: 17-Ketosteroide zwischen 11,39—37,7 mg, β-Fraktion zwischen 21,8 und 60,2%, Gonadotropine nicht nachweisbar. Nach Verabreichung von Cortison sinkt die 17-Ketosteroidausscheidung auf normale Werte.

Die Vermutung einer Störung des Hormonaufbaues wurde durch den Nachweis von großen Mengen Pregnan-3α, 17α, 20α-triol, Pregnandiol und 17α-Hydroxy-Pregnanolon im Urin nahegelegt (BUTLER 1937, LIEBERMAN 1945, MASON 1945, VENNING 1959, BONGIOVANNI 1959). Die meisten Fälle scheiden große Mengen dieser C_{21}-methylierten Intermediär- und Abbauprodukte, also 21-Desoxyverbindungen, die einen Mangel der Hydroxylierung am C_{21}-Atom nahelegen, im Urin aus. 16 solcher 21-Desoxyverbindungen sind bis heute bei der KNH isoliert worden (BONGIOVANNI 1959).

Die Aufdeckung der Biosynthese der Nebennierenrindenhormone durch HECHTER, DORFMAN, SAMUELS u.a. machte klar, daß der Mechanismus der Störung in einer Blockierung der Umwandlung von 17α-Hydroxyprogesteron (17α-Hydroxy-4-pregnen-3,20-dion), in 17α-21-dihydroxy-4-pregnen-3,20-dion = 11-Desoxycortisol oder Substanz S beruht, daß also die 21-Hydroxylase mehr oder weniger insuffizient ist.

α) Kompensierte Form

Der Enzymdefekt ist bei der kompensierten Form kein vollständiger, denn hier ist die Ausscheidung der Cortisolmetaboliten normal oder nur wenig vermindert, ebenso die von Aldosteron. Das neue Gleichgewicht wird durch den Anfall großer Mengen nicht hydroxylierter C_{21}-Verbindungen und deren Abbauprodukte erkauft. Aldosteron wird in normaler Menge produziert.

Da normalerweise die C_{21}-Hydroxylierung der C_{11}-Hydroxylierung vorausgeht, hatte man lange angenommen, daß bei *schwerem Defekt* auch die Hydroxylierung am C_{11} nicht mehr möglich ist. FINKELSTEIN u. Mitarb. (1957), COX u. FINKELSTEIN konnten dann aber in einem typischen Fall, ebenso wie später GALLAGHER (1957a) und BONGIOVANNI (1959), FUKUSHIMA u. Mitarb. (1959) Derivate des 21-Desoxy-Hydrocortison (17α, 11β-dihydroxy-4-pregnen-3,20-dion) isolieren. 12 mg 11-Ketopregnantriol und 4 mg 11-Hydroxy-pregnantriol wurden bei einer Gesamtmenge von 65 mg Pregnantriol in einem Fall nachgewiesen (GALLAGHER 1957a).

Bei Verabreichung von 21-Desoxyhydrocortison-4-C^{14} entstehen sowohl beim KNH (CAH) als auch beim Gesunden dieselben Metaboliten, nämlich 44—51% 11-Ketopregnan 3α, 17α, 20α-triol, 10% Pregnan-3α, 11β, 17α, 20α-tetrol, 7—12% 3α, 17α-Dihydroxypregnan-11,20-dion, 8% Pregnan-3α, 11β, 17α, 20β-tetrol, 11-Ketopregnan-3α, 17α, 20β-triol und 20-Ketopregnan-3α, 11β, 17α-triol. Die Umwandlung in die 17-Ketosteroide 11-Ketoätiocholan-3α-ol, 17-on, 11-Ketoandrosteron und 11β-Hydroxyandrosteron betrug nur je 0,2—0,4% (FUKUSHIMA 1959).

Nicht Pregnantriol, das auch bei Tumoren der Nebennieren gefunden wird und nach ACTH-Gabe im Urin Gesunder erscheint, ist der charakteristische Metabolit der kompensierten Form, sondern Pregnantriolon (FINKELSTEIN u. SCHOENBERGER, COX u. FINKELSTEIN).

In vitro-Untersuchungen (BONGIOVANNI 1958) mit isolierten Nebennieren solcher Kranken bestätigten den Defekt des C_{21}-Hydroxylierungssystems. Während die Substanz S zu Hydrocortison umgewandelt werden konnte, wurde 17α-Hydroxy-progesteron weder am C_{11} noch am C_{21} hydroxyliert.

β) Hochdruckform

Die seltenere, durch den begleitenden Hochdruck charakterisierte Form scheidet große Mengen von Metaboliten des 17, 21-Dihydroxy-4-pregnen-3,20-dion = 11-Desoxycortisol = Substanz S aus, und zwar Pregnan-3α, 17α, 20α(20β),

21-tetrol und Tetrahydro S, während die C_{11}-oxygenierten Metaboliten stark
vermindert sind oder ganz fehlen. Auch die Corticosteronsynthese ist unvollständig. Dafür wird das Intermediärprodukt Desoxycorticosteron (DOC) vermehrt in den Kreislauf abgegeben. Man nimmt an, daß vorwiegend DOC, weniger
das Cpd. S die Hypertension bedingt. Hier liegt also ein Defekt der 11-Hydroxy-
lierung nicht der 21-Hydroxylierung vor (EBERLEIN 1956, JAILER u. Mitarb. 1955),
Cortisol, Corticosteron und Aldosteron werden nur noch unvollständig gebildet.

γ) Salz-Wasserverlust

Der progressive Salz-Wasserverlust mit Hyperkaliämie der dritten Form
kann nur durch massive Dosen von Desoxycorticosteron korrigiert werden,
während ACTH-Gabe die Na-Diurese verstärkt. WILKINS (1957) vermutet schon
lange, daß diese Kinder einen natriumdiuretisch wirkenden Faktor, einen Anta-
gonisten zum Aldosteron, vermehrt produzieren. Die Kinder scheiden in den
ersten Lebensjahren viel Pregnantriol, 17α-Hydroxy-pregnanolon und 11-Keto-
pregnantriol aus. Über das Verhalten der Aldosteronausscheidung ist man sich
noch nicht klar. Während Kinder ohne Salzverlust Cortisolmetaboliten in etwa
normaler Höhe ausscheiden, fehlen diese beim Salzverlust-Syndrom weitgehend.
Man nimmt hier daher einen *kompletten* Defekt der 21-Hydroxylase an (EBER-
LEIN u. BONGIOVANNI 1958, ROSEMBERG u. Mitarb.). Bei einem Teil gleicht sich
dieser Defekt mit zunehmendem Alter spontan aus, die Kinder gehen in die
kompensierte Form über. Verschiedentlich wurde im Urin solcher Kinder eine
Substanz isoliert, die im Experiment eine Na-Diurese auslöst und bei der neben-
nierenlosen Ratte sogar die Na-retinierende Wirkung von DOC aufhebt (ROSEM-
BERG u. Mitarb. 1960a). Ob diese mit dem Na-diuretischen Faktor von NEHER
u. Mitarb. (3β, 16α-Dihydroxy-allopregnan-20-on) identisch ist, ist nicht geklärt.

Vieles spricht dafür, daß die Enzymstörung nicht nur verschiedene Grade
aufweist, sondern daß auch verschiedene Fermente gleichzeitig betroffen sein
können. Man steht wahrscheinlich erst am Anfang einer Entwicklung.

MIGEON und GARDNER (1952) fanden in 13 Fällen von KNH — 10 weiblichen und 3 männlichen — die Ausscheidung der *Oestrogene* im Urin deutlich
erhöht. Im Alter zwischen $3^1/_2$ und $18^1/_2$ Jahren betrug sie 62,6—212 μg in
24 Std, bei einem Kind von wenigen Monaten 26,5 μg (Normalwerte fluorimetrisch:
Kinder 5—15 μg, Erwachsene 20—45 μg). Bei den Tumoren der Nebennierenrinde ist die Ausscheidung nicht höher, sie sinkt aber nach Verabreichung von
Cortison im Gegensatz zur Hyperplasie nicht ab.

Bei allen Formen ist auch die Ausscheidung der *17-Ketosteroide* stark erhöht.
Sie stammen nur zu einem kleinen Teil aus den Metaboliten der C_{21}-Steroide
17α-Hydroxyprogesteron, 11-Desoxycortisol (als Ätiocholanolon und Androsteron) und dem 21-Desoxycortisol (als 11-Ketoätiocholanolon, 11-Ketoandro-
steron), sondern vorwiegend aus den natürlichen Androgenen der Nebennierenrinde, dem Androstendion und 11β-Hydroxyandrostendion, während sich das
Dehydroepiandrosteron (DEA) verschieden verhält (s. Abb. 21 und 22). Die
vermehrte reaktive ACTH-Produktion erhöht in der hyperplastischen Nebenniere
die Produktion der normalen Androgene in demselben Verhältnis wie die der
Vorstufen der C_{21}-Steroide.

Bis heute ist noch nicht ganz geklärt, welche Steroide bei diesem Krankheitsbild eigentlich als Androgene wirken und das Bild der Pseudopubertas
praecox bzw. des Pseudohermaphroditismus femininus hervorrufen. Wahrscheinlich sind es weniger die Metaboliten des 17α-Hydroxy-progesteron und des
Cpd. S, die man früher verantwortlich machte, sondern DEA, 4-Androstendion

und 11β-Hydroxy-4-androstendion, also die natürlichen Androgene der Nebennierenrinde, die im wesentlichen als Androsteron, 11β-Hydroxy- und 11-Ketoandrosteron im Urin erscheinen. Inkubation von Nebennierengewebe eines KNH mit markiertem Acetat ergab einen geringen Anfall von 17α-Hydroxyprogesteron, während beträchtliche Mengen von DEA, 4-Androstendion und 11β-Hydroxy-androstendion im Verhältnis 17:1:3 gebildet wurde, wobei der Weg über DEA wahrscheinlicher ist als der über 17-Hydroxyprogesteron (BLOCH u. Mitarb.). Ohne die Annahme einer gleichzeitigen Insuffizienz der 3β-Dehydrogenase und der 4-5-Isomerase sind die hohen 17-Ketosteroidwerte nicht erklärbar.

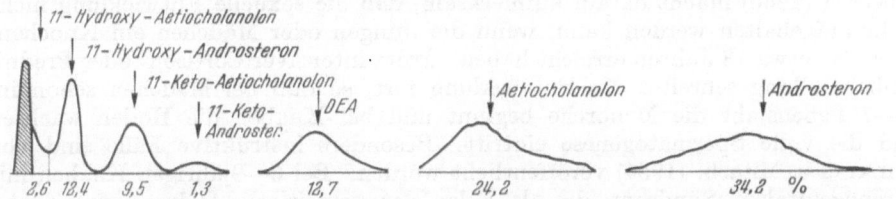

Abb. 21. 16jähriges Mädchen, angeborenes adrenogenitales Syndrom (17-Ketosteroide: 58,3 mg/24 Std). Chromatogramm kräftige Vermehrung von 11-Keto-Aetiocholanolon und 11-Hydroxy-Androsteron als Stoffwechselprodukte von 11β-Hydroxy-Androstendion und 21-Desoxycortisol

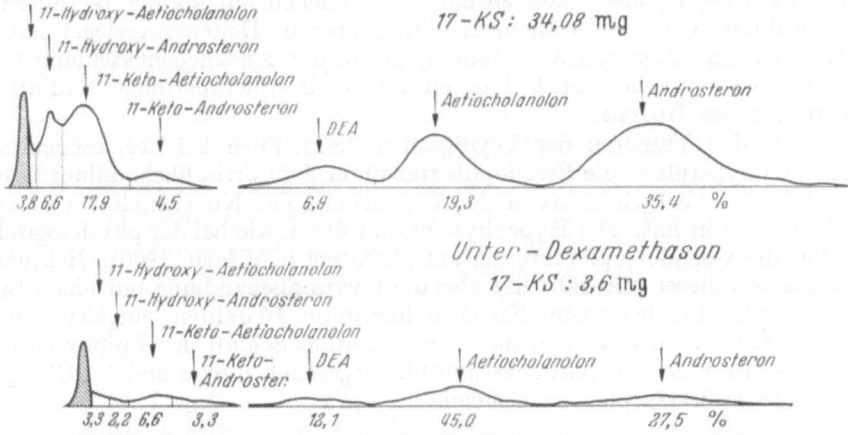

Abb. 22. Angeborenes adrenogenitales Syndrom (HCL-Hydrolyse) Chromatogramm der 17-Ketosteroide, vor und unter Dexamethason, starke Vermehrung von 11-Keto-Aetiocholanolon und 11-Hydroxy-Androsteron als Stoffwechselprodukte von 21 Desoxycortisol und 11β-Hydroxy-Androstendion. Normalisierung unter Dexamethason

δ) Behandlung

Unter der von BARTTER u. Mitarb. (1952), WILKINS u. Mitarb. (1952b) u.a. eingeführten Behandlung mit Cortisol und seinen Derivaten, durch die der angeborene Enzymdefekt der Nebennierenrinde künstlich ausgeglichen wird, normalisiert sich die Funktion der Nebennierenrinde. Die übermäßige ACTH-Bildung fällt auf normale Werte und die Hormonsynthese läuft wieder in normalen Bahnen. Pregnantriol, Pregnantriolon, Pregnantetrol verschwinden aus dem Urin. Die Ausscheidung der 17-Ketosteroide läßt sich durch die laufende Verabreichung der Prednisone auf normale Werte einstellen. Mit dem Wegfall der vermehrten Androgen- und Oestrogenproduktion in der Nebenniere regularisiert sich die Bildung der Gonadotropine, so daß die Keimdrüsen anfangen zu wachsen und sich zu entwickeln (WILKINS 1952b). Bei Frauen ist wiederholt der Eintritt der Gravidität beobachtet, bei Männern wird der histologische Aufbau

des exkretorischen und inkretorischen Anteils des Hodens normal, auch die
Zahl der Spermatozoen im Ejaculat normalisiert sich. Die notwendige Cortisondosis schwankt zwischen 25 und 100 mg per os, für Prednison zwischen 15 und
25 mg. Die Behandlung muß dauernd erfolgen, da der Enzymdefekt in der
Nebenniere durch die Cortisonbehandlung nicht geändert wird.

Nur wenn die Diagnose im Kleinkindesalter gestellt wird, kann die Beschleunigung des Wachstums und der Knochenentwicklung und damit der gesamten
körperlichen Entwicklung aufgehalten und in normale Bahnen gelenkt werden.
Schon vorhandene männliche Geschlechtsmerkmale bilden sich selten zurück.
Tonutti (1960) macht darauf aufmerksam, daß die sexuelle Entwicklung nicht
mehr aufgehalten werden kann, wenn die Jungen oder Mädchen ein Knochenalter von etwa 13 Jahren erreicht haben. Trotz intensiver Cortison- oder Predni-
sonbehandlung schreitet die Entwicklung fort, so daß bei Mädchen schon im
6.—7. Lebensjahr die Menarche beginnt und bei Knaben die Hoden wachsen
und die volle Spermatogenese eintritt. Besonders instruktive Fälle sind von
Wilkins u. Mitarb. (1954) veröffentlicht worden. Bei 6—9jährigen Knaben mit
adrenogenitalem Syndrom, die als Folge der vorzeitigen Androgeneinwirkung
ein Knochenalter von 11—14 Jahren erreicht hatten, ergab die bioptische Untersuchung 6—12 Monate nach Beginn der Cortisonbehandlung große, normal
differenzierte Leydigzellen, weit entfaltete Kanälchen mit kompletter Spermiogenese, während vor der Cortisonbehandlung infantile Hoden vorgelegen hatten.
Bei Kranken im Alter von 3—4 Jahren, die in der Knochenentwicklung 9 bis
$10^1/_2$jährigen entsprachen, blieb dagegen die Cortisontherapie ohne Einfluß auf
die Struktur des Hodens.

Wie bei den Tumoren der Leydigzellen, kann auch bei der kongenitalen
Nebennierenhyperplasie die Pseudopubertas unter der Cortisonbehandlung in eine
echte Pubertas übergehen, wenn der Organismus ein Knochenalter von etwa
13 Jahren erreicht hat. Die Hypophyse nimmt dann, wie bei der physiologischen
Pubertät, die Gonadotropinsekretion auf (Tonutti u. Mitarb. 1960). Bei männlichen Trägern dieser Anomalie hat also die Cortisonbehandlung nur einen Sinn,
wenn sie frühzeitig, bei einem Knochenalter unter 10 Jahren, eingeleitet wird.
Nur dann kann man erwarten, daß der vorzeitige Schluß der Epiphysenfugen
mit dem Sistieren des Längenwachstums hinausgeschoben wird und der Übergang
in die echte Pubertas praecox ausbleibt.

G. Hormonproduzierende Geschwülste des Erwachsenen

I. Hodentumoren

Nach Gilbert und Hamilton (1940) machen die Hodentumoren 1,5—2%
aller malignen Geschwülste des Mannes aus. Dixon und Moore (1952) errechnen
in der amerikanischen Armee für die Jahre 1940—1947 2,88 Hodengeschwülste
auf 100000 Soldaten, davon sind 96,5% embryonaler Art. Unter 1000 Hodentumoren befanden sich 1,2% Leydigzelltumoren.

Einige Beobachtungen sprechen für die Beteiligung hormonaler Faktoren an
der Tumorentstehung (Twombly 1947, 1950). Durch Injektion von Zink oder
Kupfersalzen in den Hoden von Hähnen können Teratome ausgelöst werden,
aber nur im Frühjahr, wenn das innersekretorische System aktiv ist oder unter
der gleichzeitigen Injektion von Hypophysenvorderlappenhormonen (Bagg 1957).
Verabreichung von Oestrogenen über mehrere Monate löst bei einem bestimmten

Mäusestamm hormonaktive, metastasierende maligne Leydigzelltumoren aus (HOOKER 1940, BONSER 1940). Implantation von infantilen Hoden in die Milz von kastrierten Ratten führt in einem beträchtlichen Teil der Tiere zu tumorartigen Wucherungen der Leydigzellen (TWOMBLY 1949). Beim Menschen sind maligne Hodentumoren vor der Pubertät und nach dem 50. Lebensjahr selten, der Hauptgipfel liegt zwischen dem 30. und 40. Lebensjahr. Diese Häufung könnte für eine Mitbeteiligung hormonaler Faktoren sprechen, auch das stärkere Befallensein des kryptorchen Hodens (11% von 7000 malignen Hodentumoren betrafen kryptorche Hoden) (GILBERT u. Mitarb. 1940) bzw. 13,3% (TWOMBLY 1947) bzw. 11% von 345 intraabdominell gelegene Hoden von männlichen Pseudohermaphroditen (GILBERT u. Mitarb. 1940), obwohl in diesen Fällen neben der Mehrproduktion der Gonadotropin auch dysgenetische Faktoren eine Rolle spielen.

Praktisch alle Hodentumoren sind maligne und leiten sich von embryonalen Zellen des Hodens ab. Keine Einheitlichkeit besteht jedoch bezüglich der Zuordnung der einzelnen Geschwülste zu bestimmten embryonalen Gewebsteilen.

Der gleichförmige Ablauf der Biosynthese der Steroidhormone im Hoden und im Ovar macht verständlich, daß Geschwülste, die sich histologisch sehr gleichen, das eine Mal mehr Androgene, das andere Mal mehr Oestrogene, das dritte Mal nur hormonal inaktive Vorstufen produzieren, gleichgültig, ob sie aus dem Hoden oder dem Ovar stammen.

1. Seminome

Die häufigste Geschwulst ist das Seminom, das von den primordialen Keimzellen (FRIEDEMAN 1946) bzw. von den Spermatocyten (R. MASSON 1946) abgeleitet wird. Die Hormonausscheidung ist meist normal, ein Teil der Kranken scheidet vermehrt Gonadotropine vom Typ des FSH, wenige auch Choriongonadotropine aus (HAMBURGER u. Mitarb. 1941, TWOMBLY 1947). Die erhöhte FSH-Ausscheidung bleibt nach der Tumorentfernung bestehen und ist hypophysären Ursprungs.

Bei diesen sich rasch ausbreitenden malignen Geschwülsten kommt es frühzeitig zu regressiven Veränderungen des Samenepithels, besonders deutlich unter der Röntgenbestrahlung oder einer cytostatischen Behandlung, so daß die vermehrten hypophysären Gonadotropine mit dem Wegfall der physiologischen Hemmung erklärt werden, der Nachweis von Choriongonadotropinen spricht für einen embryonalen Tumor vom Typ eines Teratoms, auch wenn dieser histologisch als Seminom imponiert, da die Choriongonadotropine nur vom Tumor selbst stammen können (TWOMBLY 1947).

2. Embryonale Teratome

Die choriongonadotropinproduzierenden Geschwülste gehören zur Gruppe der *embryonalen Teratome*. Je nach dem entartenden Gewebsanteil spricht man vom embryonalen Carcinom, vom chorialen Carcinom, embryonalen Adenocarcinom, von gemischten Epitheliomen, Terato-Carcinomen, vom Goniom und vom Chorionepitheliom. Solche embryonale Mischgeschwülste entstehen selten auch in anderen Organen.

Besonders HAMBURGER und GODTFREDSEN (1941), TWOMBLY (1947) sowie FRANCIS haben eingehende Untersuchungen über die Gonadotropinausscheidung vorgenommen. Meist handelt es sich um Gonadotropine vom Typ des ICSH, also um HCG, seltener um FSH. Die Geschwülste produzieren um so mehr Hormon, je mehr chorionepitheliomatöse Anteile im Primärtumor oder in den

Metastasen vorhanden sind, am geringsten ist die Ausscheidung bei den Carcinomen. Die Choriongonadotropine sind aus dem Tumor extrahierbar, ihr Fehlen spricht nicht gegen das Vorliegen eines malignen Teratoms. Bleibt nach Entfernung eines Tumors die Ausscheidung hoch oder steigt sie erneut nach vorübergehendem Abfall an, dann sind mit Sicherheit Metastasen vorhanden. Für die vermehrte Ausscheidung der hypophysären Gonadotropine hat man keine rechte Erklärung.

Die Androgen- und Oestrogenausscheidung ist wenig untersucht (WARREN 1945, HAMBURGER u. GODTFREDSEN 1941, TWOMBLY 1947). Die Oestrogene sind häufiger vermehrt, besonders wenn große Mengen von Choriongonadotropin produziert werden, auch Pregnandiol wurde vermehrt gefunden (TWOMBLY 1947). Die 17-Ketosteroidausscheidung verhält sich verschieden. Ein Teil der Fälle hat eine doppelseitige Gynäkomastie. Die Sexualhormone stammen wahrscheinlich aus den Leydigzellen der gesunden Seite. Hier kann eine echte Hyperplasie des Zwischengewebes vorhanden sein, die zum erstenmal von DIXON und MOORE (1952) beobachtet wurde. UMIKER (1954) berichtet über 36 Patienten, von denen 10 eine ausgesprochene, 11 eine wahrscheinliche Hyperplasie der Leydigzellen hatten. Die Tumoren waren histologisch unreif und hatten trophoblastische Elemente. Ob in den Teratomen selbst Sexualhormone gebildet werden können, ist ungewiß.

Kranke mit solch hormonaktiven Hodentumoren können sich bis gegen das tödliche Ende trotz ausgedehnter Metastasierung in verschiedenen Geweben in verhältnismäßig gutem Allgemeinzustand befinden. Ursache ist wahrscheinlich die vermehrte Produktion der Sexualhormone.

3. Geschwülste der Leydigzellen

Zusammenstellungen stammen von NATION (1944), MELICOW (1949), DALGAARD und HESSELBERG (1957) und BISHOP u. Mitarb. (1960).

Bei den 94 Fällen von DALGAARD u. Mitarb. (1957) zeigt die Altersverteilung zwei Maxima, eines zwischen 5—10 Jahren, das zweite zwischen 30—35 Jahren. Der jüngste Patient war 2 Jahre und 6 Monate alt, der älteste maligne Tumor 82 Jahre.

Durch die Entwicklung einer Pseudopubertas praecox wird die Diagnosestellung im Kindesalter leicht gemacht (s. dort). Beim Erwachsenen fehlen endokrine Erscheinungen in zwei Drittel aller Fälle (TWOMBLY u. Mitarb. 1949). Das Hauptsymptom ist die *Gynäkomastie*, selten nehmen Libido und Potenz ab, Zunahme der Behaarung wird nicht berichtet. Die Dauer der Erkrankung schwankt zwischen 2 Monaten und mehreren Jahren.

Im Urin ist die 17-Ketosteroidausscheidung nicht immer erhöht, in einzelnen Fällen wird sie sogar als vermindert angegeben. Die höchsten Werte berichtet VENNING (1952) mit 980—1040 mg/24 Std. In einem eigenen Fall betrug die Ausscheidung 13—20 mg/24 Std, bemerkenswert war hier der hohe Anteil von DEA (s. Abb. 10). Auch die Oestrogenausscheidung kann beträchtlich erhöht sein, so berichten GILBERT-DREYFUSS u. Mitarb. (1957) über einen gutartigen Leydigzelltumor mit einer Oestrogenausscheidung von mehr als 1000 E im Liter, POWELL (1938), HERMANN (1958) berichten ebenfalls über erhöhte Werte im Urin, auch ein eigener Fall schied etwas mehr aus. HUNT und BUDD (1939) isolierten 20 ME Oestrin aus 1,73 g Tumorgewebe, LAUFER und SULMANN 1000 IE pro Gramm. Die Gynäkomastie wird mit der erhöhten Oestrogenproduktion in Zusammenhang gebracht, so daß man auch bei normalen Oestrogenausscheidungen eine erhöhte Oestrogenproduktion annehmen darf. Wichtig ist ein Fall von GUINET (1957), bei dem weder die 17-Ketosteroide noch die Oestrogene vermehrt waren, sich aber eine stark erhöhte Pregnandiolausscheidung fand als Zeichen, daß die Biosynthese der Hormone auf früher Stufe (Progesteron ?) stehengeblieben ist. Diese Beobachtung erklärt das häufige Fehlen aller innersekretorischen Zeichen. Die Gonadotropinausscheidung ist wenig untersucht und teilweise normal, teilweise erniedrigt gefunden.

Die Größe des Tumors wechselt von etwa erbsengroßen Gewebsteilen bis zu mehreren Zentimetern Durchmesser. Die Geschwülste sind meist rundlich oder oval, häufig haben sie eine ausgesprochene Kapsel. Der übrige Hodenanteil ist bei großen Tumoren komprimiert. Die Farbe wird als braun-gelb, gelb-braun, rot-braun, grün-braun, schwarz und dunkel beschrieben.

Histologisch sind die Befunde einheitlich. Charakteristisch sind gleichmäßig gereifte große, polyedrische, leberzellähnliche Leydigzellen mit reichlich acidophilem und granulärem Cytoplasma. In einigen Fällen waren Reincke-Kristalle vorhanden. In den echten Geschwülsten fehlen die Überbleibsel von Kanälchen ganz. Beim Erwachsenen ist die Atrophie des gesunden Hodens nicht deutlich, obwohl eine Sterilität mit Azoospermie bestehen kann. In einem eigenen Fall bestand eine Hemmung der Spermiogenese.

Die Tumoren sind meist sowohl klinisch als auch histologisch benigne. In der Serie von DALGAARD (1957) werden aber doch neun als maligne beschrieben. Das Durchschnittsalter der

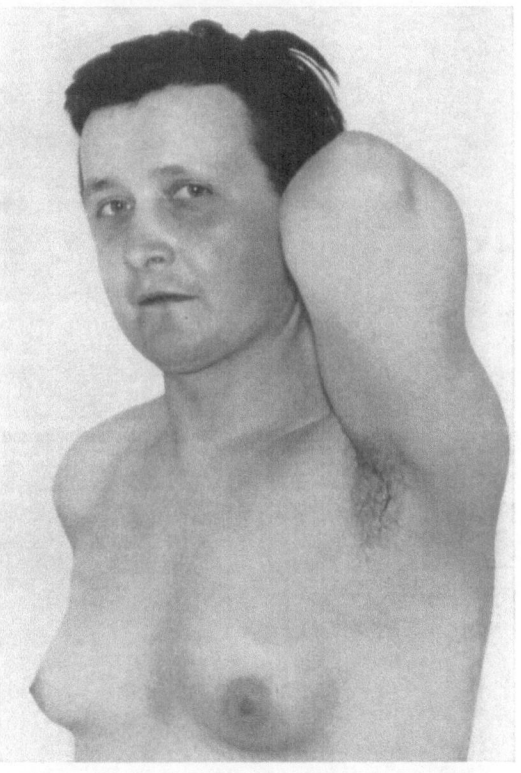

Abb. 23. 34jähriger Mann mit Leydigzelltumor, Gynäkomastie

malignen Formen liegt mit 55,3 Jahren erheblich höher als das der gutartigen. Zur Tumorentfernung wird im allgemeinen die Semikastration empfohlen.

Ein Beispiel ist folgendes:

Fall 1. J. K., 34jähriger Mann (vgl. Abb. 23—25).
In der Familie keine Besonderheiten.
Acht Geschwister, von denen sechs leben, einer ist gefallen, eine Schwester an Diphtherie gestorben. Frau gesund, ebenso zwei eigene Kinder.
Früher nicht besonders krank bis auf mehrere Unfälle.
Anfang 1959 bemerkt er eine rasch zunehmende Anschwellung beider Brüste. Zunächst hat er nur einen harten, kleinen Knoten getastet, der dann auf Druck oder Berührung schmerzhaft wurde. Mit der Zeit wurde der Knoten größer und etwas weicher und mehr empfindlich. Libido und Potenz haben sich nicht verändert. Bartwuchs und Achselbehaarung, weniger die Schambehaarung, sind etwas zurückgegangen.
84 kg, 176 cm. Körperbehaarung schlecht ausgebildet, nur wenig Haare auf der Brust, mäßige Achselbehaarung, Barthaare nur an Kinn und auf der Oberlippe, weibliche Begrenzung der Schambehaare, ziemlicher Fettansatz im Bereich des Rumpfes.

Beide Drüsenkörper der Brust sind etwa kleinkinderfaustgroß, auf Druck deutlich empfindlich, sie bestehen aus festem Drüsengewebe (s. Abb. 23).

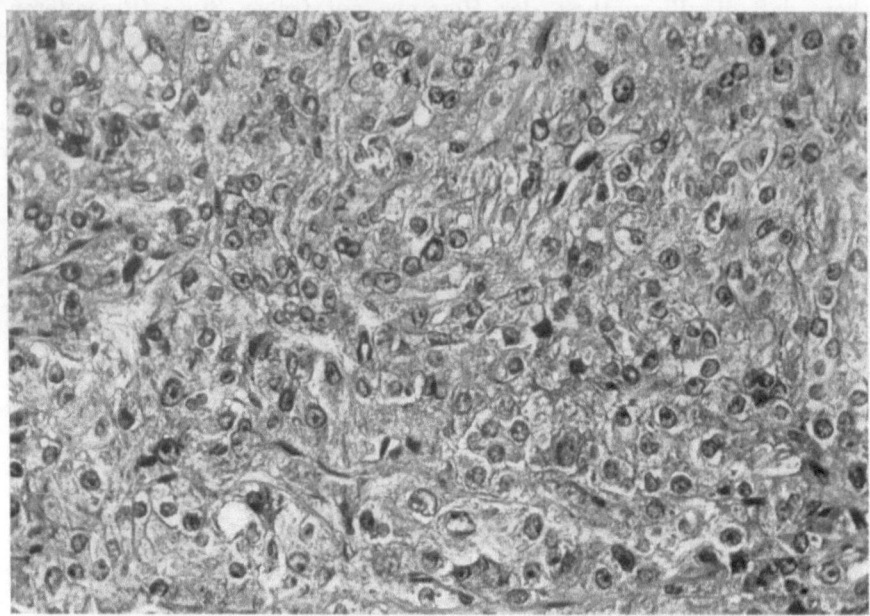

Abb. 24. Teilansicht des Tumors (Beschreibung s. Text). (Hämatoxylin-Eosin, 300fach)

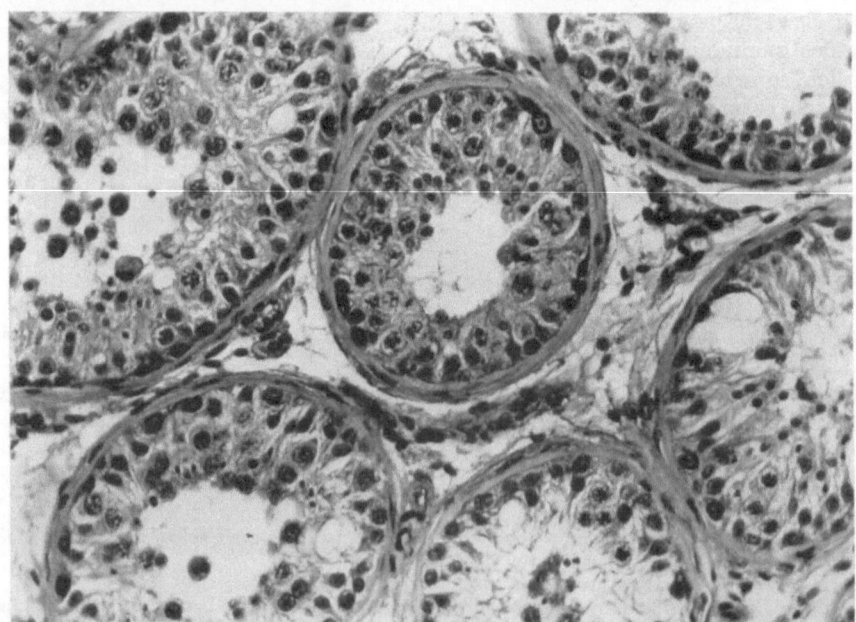

Abb. 25. Bild aus dem den Leydigzelltumor umgebenen Hodengewebe. Kanälchendurchmesser verkleinert, Wand
verdickt, dürftige nur bis Spermatocyten I gehende Spermiogenese, spärliche und wenig entwickelte Leydigzellen,
(Hämatoxylin-Eosin, 300fach).

Genitale: Penis normal, beide Hoden sind normal groß, Konsistenz etwas weich und
nachgiebig, wenig empfindlich. Am oberen Pol des linken sitzt ein etwa pfennigstückgroßer,
runder, derber Knoten.

17-Keto 13—20 mg. Chromatographie: starke Erhöhung von DEA (s. Abb. 10). Oestrogen-ausscheidung: 85—112 μg. 17-Hydroxycorticoide 7,2 und 8,0 mg.

Revision des linken Hodens und Entfernung, nachdem an seinem oberen Pol ein kirsch-großer Tumor von gelblich-brauner Farbe festgestellt wurde. Histologischer Befund von Prof. TONUTTI: Das Gewebe besteht aus unregelmäßigen Zellplatten. In gut fixierten Ab-schnitten ist zu erkennen, daß es sich um große epitheloide Zellen handelt, die scharf ab-gegrenzt sind. Die Zellen enthalten einen großen, verhältnismäßig chromatinarmen Kern mit einem in der Regel sehr großen Nucleolus. Das Cytoplasma ist fein granuliert, häufig bleibt in Kernnähe ein heller Bereich von den Granula frei. An anderen Stellen sind die Zellen unregelmäßig gestaltet, manchmal auch fibrocytenähnlich ausgebreitet, auch mehr-kernige kommen häufig vor. Das Tumorgewebe ist durch eine verhältnismäßig dicke Kapsel von angrenzendem Hodengewebe getrennt. Diagnose: Leydigzelltumor (vgl. Abb. 24).

Hoden: Kanälchen mit kleinem Durchmesser, ausgesprochene Wandverdickung, ver-hältnismäßig weites Lumen, sehr dürftige Spermiogenese, die in den meisten Kanälchen nur bis zu den Spermatocyten I. Ordnung geht. Leydigzellen spärlich und wenig diffe-renziert. Mäßiger sekundärer Hypogonadismus als Folge des hormonaktiven Leydigzell-tumors (vgl. Abb. 25).

Drei Monate nach der Tumorentfernung hatte sich die Gynäkomastie deutlich, aber noch nicht vollständig zurückgebildet.

Die Leydigzelltumoren stehen in enger Beziehung zu den *Hiluszelltumoren des Ovars*, die BERGER (1923) zum erstenmal beschrieb. GERMAN und HUT konnten 1961 zwölf Fälle aus der Literatur zusammenstellen. Die Hiluszellen sind Reste des Markanteils der Gonadenanlage, sie sind noch zur Bildung von Androgenen fähig. Die Tumoren bestehen aus großen blassen Zellen, die den sympathischen Nervenzellen ähnlich sehen ("sympathico cells").

Bei den Frauen entwickelt sich ein Hirsutismus mit Alopecie und vorzeitiger Amenorrhoe, selten eine maskuline Stimme oder Clitorishypertrophie. Die in den meisten Fällen normale 17-Ketosteroidausscheidung weist darauf hin, daß die Tumoren hochwirksame Androgene, also wahrscheinlich Testosteron selbst produzieren.

4. Geschwülste der Sertolizellen

PICK beschrieb 1905 beim männlichen Pseudohermaphrodismus einzelne und auch multiple Adenome in ektopischen Hoden. Er nannte sie Adenoma tubulare testicularii ovarii, da sie Ähnlichkeit haben mit bestimmten Ovarialtumoren.

Das Adenom besteht histologisch aus einem Gewebe mit kanälchenartigem Bau und entspricht dem tubulären Adenom des Ovars. Die kleinen Kanälchen sind mit prismatischen Zellen ausgekleidet, die Ähnlichkeit mit Sertolizellen haben. Die Kanälchen sind meist sehr klein und kommen besonders in krypt-orchen Hoden und beim Pseudohermaphroditen vor. Die Verteilung von tubulären und mesenchymalen Anteilen wechselt von Fall zu Fall. Die Tumoren bilden keine Hormone (HUGGINS 1945).

Die Existenz *von hormonproduzierenden Tumoren*, die sich aus den *Sertoli-zellen* ableiten, ist heute sehr fraglich geworden. Mitbeeinflußt durch die ent-wicklungsgeschichtliche Ableitung der einzelnen Zellarten in Hoden und Ovar von WITSCHI (1951) — die Granulosazellen sollen den Sertolizellen, die Theca-zellen den Leydigzellen entsprechen — hat man vielfach angenommen, daß Tumoren mit überwiegender Oestrogenproduktion aus den Sertolizellen bestehen (TEILUM 1946, HUGGINS 1945). Die Oestrogenbildung dieser Geschwülste wurde häufig aus der Entwicklung einer Gynäkomastie abgeleitet, seltener aus der direkten biologischen oder chemischen Bestimmung der ausgeschiedenen Hor-mone. Den ersten Tumor dieser Art beschrieb TEILUM (1946) bei einem 53jährigen Manne mit einer erheblichen Gynäkomastie und Impotenz. Der Tumor war abgekapselt, intensiv gelb gefärbt und maß 6:4:3 cm. Sein histologischer Aufbau war nicht einheitlich. Einige Bezirke hatten die Charakteristica eines Androblastoms mit Differenzierung in Richtung der virilisierenden Arrhenoblastome des Ovars, andere bestanden aus tubulären oder alveolären Gewebsteilen, die TEILUM von den Sertolizellen ableitet. Diese sehr seltenen Androblastome sind Analoge der Arrhenoblastome, es sind Tumoren, die wie fetale Hoden aussehen und in drei verschiedenen Entwicklungsstadien vorkommen (DIXON u. MOORE 1952).

Solche feminisierende Tumoren sind bei Hunden verhältnismäßig häufig. HUGGINS und MOULDER (1945) fanden bei fünf solcher Geschwülste den Oestrogengehalt im Tumor stark erhöht. Die Tumoren sind in Läppchen aufgeteilt, die teilweise solide Hodenkanälchen enthalten, in anderen sind sertoliartige Zellen palisadenförmig angeordnet. Leydigzellen fehlen. Der Aufbau erinnert an das Adenoma tubulare des Hodens (BERTRONG u. Mitarb. 1949, GREULICH u. BURFORD 1936, ZUCKERMAN 1937).

Beim Menschen sind feminisierende Geschwülste außerordentlich selten. 1949 sammelte LEWIS u. Mitarb. vier Fälle aus der Literatur und fügte einen eigenen hinzu. GOODWIN (1954) berichtet über einen weiteren. Die feminisierenden Eigenschaften bestehen meist im Auftreten einer mehr oder weniger starken Gynäkomastie, nur in einem Teil ist die vermehrte Oestrogenausscheidung im Urin nachgewiesen. Sowohl der Tumor von GOODWIN als auch der von LEWIS wurde von verschiedenen Untersuchern, denen die histologischen Präparate vorgelegt wurden, verschieden eingeordnet, teils als Sertolizelltumor, teils als Leydigzelltumor. Man ersieht daraus die Schwierigkeit der Differenzierung nach rein morphologischen Gesichtspunkten.

II. Tumoren der Nebennierenrinde

Die mehrfachen Aufgaben der Nebennierenrinde, die in den verschiedenen Endprodukten der Hormonsynthese ihren Ausdruck findet — Hydrocortison, Aldosteron, Androgene, Oestrogene — bedingt bei den hormonaktiven Geschwülsten verschiedene klinische Syndrome, die *Pseudopubertas praecox* bei Knaben, die *Virilisierung* bei Frauen bei Produktion von Androgenen, *Feminisierung* bei Knaben und die Pseudopubertas praecox bei Mädchen bei Produktion von Oestrogenen, das *Cushing-Syndrom* bei Produktion von Hydrocortison und den *Aldosteronismus* bei Produktion von Aldosteron.

Tumoren produzieren selten ganz isoliert nur Androgene oder Oestrogene oder Hydrocortison, sondern meist eine Mehrzahl von Hormonen und deren Vorstufen mit besonderer Bevorzugung einer Art. Der Nachweis einer erhöhten Oestrogenausscheidung bei virilisierenden Geschwülsten, einer erhöhten 17-Ketosteroidausscheidung bei feminisierenden ist daher etwas häufiges. Viele dieser Tumoren bilden auch gewisse Mengen von Hydrocortison, so daß das normale Nebennierengewebe, insbesondere die kontralaterale Seite, atrophiert. Die operative Entfernung des Tumors darf daher nur unter der ausreichenden Gabe von Hydrocortison erfolgen, auch wenn klinisch keine Zeichen eines Cushing-Syndroms also einer Stoffwechselstörung vorhanden sind. Meist handelt es sich um rasch wachsende, früh metastasierende Geschwülste, seltener um Adenome, deren Abgrenzung gegen die Umgebung häufig unscharf ist.

WILKINS hat bis zum Jahre 1948 etwa 68 Nebennierentumoren bei Kindern unter 10 Jahren gesammelt. 51 davon betrafen Mädchen, 17 Knaben. Von den Mädchen bilden 29 vorwiegend Androgene mit dem Symptomenbild des adrenogenitalen Syndroms, 22 vorwiegend Hydrocortison mit den Symptomen des Cushing ohne Virilisierung.

1. Androgenproduzierende Nebennierenrindentumoren

Nebennierentumoren gehen bei Kindern entweder mit einer exzessiven Fettsucht oder mit den Zeichen einer vermehrten Androgenproduktion, also der *Pseudopubertas* einher. Bei Knaben ist der Typ des infantilen Herkules häufiger als bei Mädchen. Mischformen mit dem Cushing-Syndrom oder das reine Cushing-Syndrom selbst sind bei Kindern immer durch Geschwülste bedingt. Bei 17 Knaben mit Nebennierentumoren verliefen 4 als Cushing-Syndrom, 12 als Pseudopubertas praecox, 1 unter den Zeichen der Feminisierung (WILKINS 1948).

Das Bild des Cushing-Syndroms kann bei Knaben von den Zeichen einer vorzeitigen sexuellen Entwicklung begleitet sein (WILKINS 1948, BERDINELLI 1952). Im Beginn der Erkrankung steht meist die zunehmende Fettsucht des Gesichtes, des Nackens, der Brust, des Bauches und der Flanken mit einem mäßigen Hirsutismus und verhältnismäßig geringer Genitalhypertrophie im Vordergrund. Später tritt dann die vorzeitige Sexualentwicklung hinzu. Die vorzeitige körperliche und sexuelle Entwicklung kann auch als erstes Symptom auftreten. Die Zeichen der vorzeitigen Sexualreifung sind unterschiedlich ausgeprägt, sie können beträchtliche Ausmaße annehmen.

Die Hoden bleiben für gewöhnlich klein und unreif, im Gegensatz zu der isosexuellen Pubertät. Die Sertolizellen können differenziert sein, Leydigzellen fehlen. Die Entwicklung des Samenepithels kann bis zu den Spermatocyten fortschreiten (WILKINS 1948, 1954, SOBEL u. Mitarb. 1951, FORDYCE, MAINZER, LISSER 1933), einmal war eine reife Spermatogenese nachweisbar (LISSER 1933). Wenn die Kinder ein Knochenalter von 12—13 Jahren erreicht haben, beginnt offenbar wie bei der angeborenen Nebennierenhyperplasie die endogene Gonadotropinproduktion.

Beim *erwachsenen Manne* sind Nebennierentumoren außerordentlich selten. Sie verlaufen unter dem Bild eines Morbus Cushing, wobei ein verstärktes Wachstum der Körperbehaarung eine vermehrte Androgenproduktion vermuten läßt. Gleichzeitig geben die Kranken ein Schwinden von Libido und Potenz an, die Hoden verlieren an Konsistenz und können ziemlich atrophisch werden. Die Tumoren lassen sich von der Hyperplasie beim Erwachsenen nach dem klinischen Bild nicht unterscheiden.

Nur die selteneren großen Tumoren machen Lokalsymptome und können durch die Palpation erfaßt werden. Die von Kindern und Jugendlichen wiegen im allgemeinen weniger als 100 g. Histologisch besteht der gesamte Tumor aus nebennierenähnlichen Zellen, wobei das Cytoplasma infolge des Lipoidgehaltes eine starke Vacuolisierung aufweisen kann. Das Bild ist im allgemeinen sehr einheitlich, obwohl die Zellgröße beträchtlich wechseln kann (JONES u. SCOTT).

Hormonausscheidung. Ein wichtiges Charakteristicum ist die stark erhöhte 17-Ketosteroidausscheidung, meist über 100 mg, in einigen Fällen über 1000 mg. CALLOW hat 1938 zum erstenmal Dehydroepiandrosteron, ein 3β-Hydroxy-17-ketosteroid isoliert. Die starke Vermehrung des DEA ist ein wichtiges Unterscheidungsmerkmal gegen die kongenitale Hyperplasie. Es sind auch eine Reihe von Hormonvorstufen aus dem Urin isoliert worden. Abgegrenzte Adenome und maligne Geschwülste, die klinisch das Bild des reinen Cushing-Syndroms zeigen, können ohne Erhöhung der Gesamt-17-Ketosteroide einhergehen. Man sieht dann bei der Chromatographie eine beträchtliche Vermehrung der 11-oxygenierten 17-Ketosteroide, ähnlich dem durch einfache Nebennierenhyperplasie hervorgerufenen Cushing-Syndrom (s. Abb. 26). Starke Vermehrung von DEA kommt auch bei der einfachen Hyperplasie vor, wenn das klinische Bild des Hirsutismus vorhanden ist (s. Abb. 27).

Die Oestrogene verhalten sich verschieden. Bei virilisierenden Nebennierengeschwülsten von Frauen können sie beträchtlich vermehrt sein (FRANK 1933,
MASON u. KEPLER 1945, WEST u. Mitarb. 1958), sowohl Oestron als auch Oestriol
wurden isoliert. Da auch Kranke mit angeborener Nebennierenhyperplasie hohe
Oestrogenwerte im Urin ausscheiden, kann die Differentialdiagnose nicht ausschließlich auf Grund der Oestrogenausscheidung getroffen werden.

Die *Differenzierung* gegenüber der angeborenen Nebennierenhyperplasie ist
bei Kindern und Jugendlichen mit Hilfe des *Cortisontestes* im allgemeinen nicht
schwierig. Bei Geschwülsten fällt die 17-Ketosteroidausscheidung unter Cortison-
besser Prednisongabe nicht ab, unter ACTH steigt sie im allgemeinen nicht an.

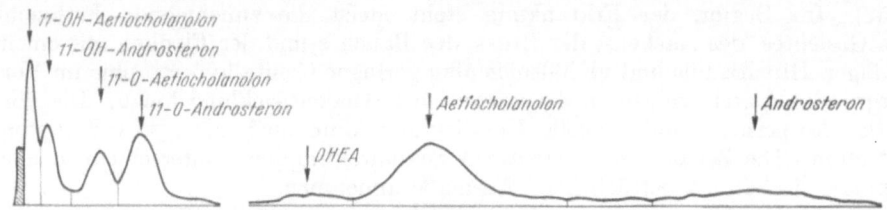

Abb. 26. Chromatogramm einer 24jährigen Frau mit M. Cushing und Hirsutismus. 17-Ketosteroide: 22,3 mg
24 Std, Porter-Silber-Chromogene 18,6 mg/24 Std. Deutliche Vermehrung von 11-Hydroxy-Aetiocholanolon,
etwas weniger von 11-Keto-Aetiocholanolon als Folge der vermehrten Cortisolproduktion, aber auch von 11-Keto-
und 11-Hydroxy-Androsteron als Metaboliten von 11-Hydroxy-Androstendion

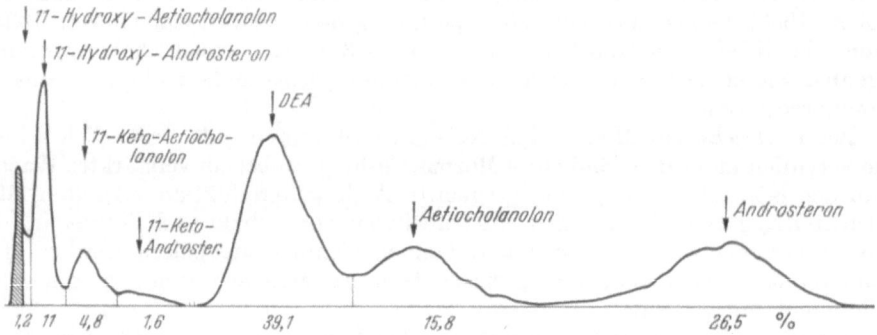

Abb. 27. 32jährige Frau, erworbene NNR-Hyperplasie (Hirsutismus). 17-Ketosteroide: 20,37 mg/24 Std. Chromatogramm: abnorme Vermehrung von Dehydroepiandrosteron und 11-Hydroxy-Androsteron

Neuerdings wurde aber über einige Nebennierentumoren berichtet, bei denen
sich unter ACTH sowohl die 17-Ketosteroide als auch die 17-Hydroxycorticoid-
ausscheidung erhöhte. Auch Tumorzellen können auf ACTH empfindlich sein.
Keinesfalls findet man aber die völlige Normalisierung der 17-Ketosteroidaus-
scheidung unter Dexamethason oder einem anderen Prednisolon, wie sie für die
kongenitale Nebennierenhyperplasie so charakteristisch ist. Bei Erwachsenen
mit dem klinischen Bild des Cushing-Syndroms — hervorgerufen durch eine
doppelseitige Hyperplasie — fallen sowohl der Cortison- als auch der ACTH-Test
nicht selten zweifelhaft aus. Da kleine Tumoren durch die präsacrale Darstellung
mit Stickoxydul nicht erfaßt werden, diese Methode wegen der starken Fettmasse überhaupt große Fehlerquellen hat, wird die endgültige Diagnose manchmal
erst intra operationem gestellt. Die operative Entfernung der Geschwülste ist
nicht ungefährlich, da die kontralaterale Nebenniere häufig atrophisch ist. Die
Prognose ist schlecht. RAPAPORT stellte 1952 52 operierte Fälle (Frauen und
Männer) zusammen. Von 37, die den operativen Eingriff überlebten, starben 7
nach kurzer Zeit an Metastasen oder lokalen Rezidiven, von den verbleibenden

30 überlebte 1 Kind 5 Jahre; 5 1—5 Jahre; 9 weniger als 1 Jahr, von den restlichen 15 konnte nichts in Erfahrung gebracht werden. Die direkte Operationsmortalität ist heute durch Hydrocortisonprophylaxe erheblich gesunken, die
Gesamtprognose hat sich dadurch nicht verbessert. Die Tumoren sind gegen
Androgene und Oestrogene insensibel.

2. Oestrogenproduzierende Nebennierenrindentumoren

28 bis 1956 veröffentlichte Fälle bei Männern sammelten HIGGINS, BROWNLEE
und MANZ. Sie verteilen sich zwischen 5 und 59 Jahren, 3 waren unter 25 Jahre
alt, 21 im 3. Jahrzehnt, 4 im 5. Jahrzehnt. WALLACH u. Mitarb. stellten 1957
34 Fälle zusammen.

Wichtigstes Symptom ist die *Gynäkomastie*, die in allen Fällen vorhanden
war, sie ist in über der Hälfte auch das erste Symptom der Erkrankung. Die
Vergrößerung der Brust erfolgt meist symmetrisch, Unterschiede zwischen rechts
und links kommen vor. In 8 von 28 Fällen wurden die Barthaare dünn und es
entstand eine horizontale Begrenzung der Schambehaarung, bei den übrigen
war keine Änderung der Körperbehaarung eingetreten. Verminderung von Libido
und Potenz wird in einem Drittel der Fälle geklagt. In 21 von 29 Fällen wird
eine leichte oder stärkere Atrophie der Hoden, die histologisch das Bild des
sekundären Hypogonadismus zeigt, erwähnt, auch der Penis kann an Größe
abnehmen (WALLACH u. Mitarb.). Die Prostata atrophiert nicht, einmal war sie
unauffällig, zweimal eher vergrößert und fest. Das Cushing-Aussehen ist wenig
ausgeprägt. Sieben Kranke waren fettsüchtig, 2 zeigten einen gestörten Kohlen-
hydrathaushalt, bei 6 war die Haut stärker pigmentiert, einer hatte Striae
purpureae, 2 eine Acne, 4 eine deutliche Erhöhung des Blutdruckes. 20 der
28 Geschwülste waren palpabel, 17 der 20 palpablen Geschwülste bösartig. In
16 von 17 Untersuchten war das intravenöse Pyelogramm diagnostisch eindeutig.

Feminisierende Nebennierentumoren muß man differentialdiagnostisch immer
erwägen, wenn sich bei Erwachsenen eine *Gynäkomastie* entwickelt. Abtrennung
von der Pubertätsmakromastie, der Gynäkomastie des Klinefelter-Syndroms und
anderen hypergonadotropen Formen des Hypogonadismus ist leicht, von palpablen
Hodentumoren ebenfalls, von versteckt liegenden Leydigzelltumoren dagegen
sehr schwierig. In 5 Fällen waren die 17-Ketosteroide stark, in 3 mäßig erhöht,
in 8 normal. Im Falle von HIGGINS u. Mitarb. schwankte die Ausscheidung
zwischen 150 und 600 mg. DEA war in 2 Fällen stark erhöht, Pregnandiol in
den Fällen von HIGGINS u. Mitarb., JONES u. SCOTT, MASON u. ENGSTROM (1950).

Bei 12 von 14 Untersuchten erwies sich die Oestrogenausscheidung deutlich
erhöht, bis 6200 μg bei HIGGINS. In 70 g Tumorgewebe konnte er 280 mg Oestrogene (Kober-Reaktion), 4 mg Pregnandiol und 3,1 mg 17-Ketosteroid nachweisen.

Pathologisch-anatomisch waren 19 Fälle maligne, 6 benigne (HIGGINS u. Mitarb.). Histologisch findet man zwei Zelltypen, die einen sehen aus wie die Zellen
der Zona reticularis, die anderen erinnern an Zellen der Fasciculata. Die Prognose
ist abhängig von der Struktur des Tumors. Nach Entfernung eines benignen
bilden sich alle Symptome rasch zurück. Bösartige haben meist im Zeitpunkt
der Operation schon Metastasen gesetzt.

Den einzigen Fall bei einem männlichen Kind haben WILKINS u. CARA (1954)
berichtet.

Dabei handelt es sich um einen $4^1/_2$jährigen Knaben, der im 6. Lebensmonat eine Gynäkomastie bekam. Bei der Aufnahme in das John Hopkins-Hospital war er $4^8/_{12}$ Jahre alt,
er kam wegen eines gebrochenen Armes. Die beidseitige Gynäkomastie war das einzige
Symptom des Nebennierentumors. Daneben fand sich eine Vergrößerung der Prostata,
eine leichte Eosinophilie, Gesamt-17-Ketosteroidausscheidung mit 4,1 mg erhöht, Knochen-

alter 10 Jahre. Oestrogene im Urin leicht vermehrt. Bei der Exploration wurde ein links-
seitiger Nebennierentumor von Erdnußgröße entdeckt und entfernt. Histologisch erschien
der Tumor als benignes Adenom. Heilung.

Ein anderer von SIMPSON und JOLL beschriebener Fall betrifft einen 34jährigen Arzt,
bei dem sich die Brust ab 1932 vergrößerte, im August 1933 nahmen Libido und Potenz
ab, das Genitale wurde kleiner, Gewichtsschwankungen. Im Juli tastete man über der
linken, tiefstehenden Niere eine Resistenz. Es wurde ein großer, maligner Tumor operativ
entfernt. Die vorher stark erhöhte Oestrogenausscheidung verschwand nach der operativen
Entfernung des Tumors. Zwei Monate nach der Operation hatten Körpergewicht und Kräfte-
zustand wieder zugenommen, die Brust hatte sich verkleinert, das Genitale vergrößert.
Libido und Potenz besserten sich wieder, ohne ganz normal zu werden. Im März 1935 zeigte
sich die Brust wieder voll entwickelt, Penis und Testis atrophierten wieder, auf dem Abdomen
hatten sich deutliche Striae distensae entwickelt. Körper- und Bartbehaarung blieben
unverändert. In den folgenden Monaten nahm das Körpergewicht zu, die Impotenz wurde
vollständig und im April 1936 entdeckte man Metastasen in der Leber. Der Kranke starb
im Juni 1936.

Neben dem Hoden wurde versprengtes Nebennierengewebe auch selten in der
Leber festgestellt. Davon ausgehende Geschwülste können ebenfalls eine Pseudopubertas praecox auslösen. PENDEL u. SCHERLACHER berichten über zwei der-
artige Fälle. Bei einem 5jährigen Jungen entwickelte sich eine Pubertas als
Folge einer Metastasierung eines orangegroßen Tumors der Leber, der im Alter
von 17 Monaten entfernt worden war. Ein anderer zeigte mit $2^9/_{12}$ Jahren einen
Virilismus mit Symptomen eines Morbus Cushing, 17-Ketosteroidausscheidung
12,2 bzw. 9,8 mg. Nach Entfernung des Tumors aus der Leber verschwanden
die klinischen Zeichen des Virilismus, die 17-Ketosteroidausscheidung fiel auf
0,5 mg ab.

Histologisch bestehen die Geschwülste aus ziemlich großen Zellen, die ähnlich
wie die der Zona fasciculata angeordnet sind. Das Cytoplasma enthält feine
Granula und ist manchmal schaumig.

H. Sekundärer Hypogonadismus (hypogonadotroper Eunuchismus und Eunuchoidismus)

Der sekundäre oder hypophysäre Hypogonadismus ist durch die fehlende
oder mangelhafte Bildung der Gonadotropine in der Adenohypophyse bedingt.
Die Störung betrifft meist beide gonadotrope Hormone, also FSH und ICSH
gemeinsam, in seltenen Fällen nur das ICSH. Das klinische Bild ist sehr variabel
und von verschiedenen Faktoren abhängig. Angeborene Defekte und Erkrankungen, die bis zur Pubertät erworben werden, bedingen das Bild des präpuberalen
Hypogonadismus. Der vollständige Ausfall der Gonadotropine beim Erwachsenen bringt sowohl die inkretorische als auch die spermiogenetische Hodenfunktion zum Erlöschen, einfache Verminderung kann mehr das FSH oder das
ICSH betreffen. Dadurch entstehen wechselnde Bilder, die histologisch nur
schwer von primären Formen des Hypogonadismus und von exogenen Schäden
abzutrennen sind. In- und suprasselläre Tumoren, Entzündungen der Adenohypophyse bedingen anfangs häufig einen isolierten Ausfall der gonadotropen
Partialfunktion, der meist mit einer verminderten Produktion von FSH beginnt
und erst später in den totalen Verlust übergeht. Sind alle Funktionen der Hypophyse betroffen, oder sind zusätzlich Funktionsbereiche des Zwischenhirns mit
einbezogen, dann entstehen sehr komplexe Krankheitsbilder, bei denen der Hypogonadismus in den Hintergrund tritt.

Charakteristisch ist die fehlende oder stark erniedrigte *Gonadotropinausscheidung*. Die verschiedenen Methoden haben verschiedene Normalwerte, so daß
man eine einheitliche untere Grenze nicht angeben kann. Leichte Formen der

primären Dysgenesie der Hodenkanälchen gehen nicht ganz selten mit einer Pubertas tarda einher, so daß noch im Alter von 16—18 Jahren die Gonadotropine erniedrigt sein können. Kombinationen von defekter Gonadotropinproduktion und Dysgenesie des Hodens erscheinen möglich, sind aber bis jetzt anatomisch noch nicht bestätigt.

I. Histologie
1. Präpuberale Form

Es liegen zahlreiche und eingehende *histologische Untersuchungen* vor (CAHILL u. Mitarb. 1938, FORD u. Mitarb. 1959c, 1961, HOWARD u. Mitarb., NELSON 1953b, SNIFFEN u. Mitarb. 1950b, TONUTTI 1955b, TILLINGER). Die *präpuberalen Formen* zeigen das charakteristische Bild des frühkindlichen Hodens. Die kleinen Kanälchen bestehen aus lumenlosen dünnen Schläuchen, die undifferenzierte Sertolizellen und unreife Spermatogonien enthalten. Die Zellen sind manchmal in 2—3 Schichten angeordnet. Die Kerne der Sertolizellen sind dicht und ohne Nucleolen, die Spermiogonien erscheinen als runde, helle Zellen ohne Reifungszeichen. Die Kanälchenwand selbst ist dünn und zart und bietet keine Zeichen einer Sklerose. Das interstitielle Gewebe ist zellreich und enthält viele Fibrocyten, Leydigzellen fehlen. Ein wesentliches Charakteristicum der präpuberalen Formen ist das Fehlen der Kanälchensklerose bzw. Hyalinose. Wenn keine Aktivierung eintritt, soll der undifferenzierte Zustand immer bestehenbleiben (SNIFFEN u. Mitarb. 1950b). Schwierigkeiten in der Zuordnung bereiten die Fälle, die CHARNY unter dem Begriff der „schweren Hypoplasie" führt. Hier ist der Kanälchendurchmesser noch kleiner, die ein- bis dreischichtigen Zellreihen bestehen aus ganz undifferenzierten Zellen mit chromatinreichen Zellen ohne Nucleolen, Spermatogonien fehlen gänzlich. Das Zwischengewebe ist sehr locker und sehr zellarm, die fibrocytenähnlichen Zellen sind unreif (Abb. 55, 57). Der Gonadenaufbau ist unreifer als zu irgendeinem Zeitpunkt der postembryonalen Entwicklung, so daß diese Fälle im allgemeinen als Defektbildungen angesehen und in die Gruppe der Dysgenesie des Hodens eingereiht werden. Die eigenen Fälle dieser Art — 25-, 32-, 43jährig — schieden keine Gonadotropine aus, so daß ein zusätzlicher hypophysärer Defekt angenommen werden müßte. Wir halten es aber für möglich, daß Kanälchen und Interstitium bei völligem Fehlen der Gonadotropine von Geburt an im Laufe der Jahre degenerieren und sich dann von den angeborenen Dysgenesien weder anatomisch noch funktionell unterscheiden.

Der Gonadotropindefekt ist häufig nicht vollständig. Außerdem sind gegenwärtig die meisten Kranken, bevor sie zur Biopsie kommen, mit Testosteron oder HCG anbehandelt. In diesen Fällen ist der histologische Befund recht variabel. SNIFFEN u. Mitarb. (1950b) machen folgende Unterteilungen:

Neben der schweren Hypoplasie zeigt ein Teil der Kranken eine gewisse Vergrößerung des Kanälchendruckmessers, eine gewisse Reifung der Sertolizellen und eine geringe spermatogene Aktivität, während die Entwicklung der Leydigzellen fehlt. In diesen Kanälchen sieht man neben primitiven Spermatogonien eine bestimmte Zahl primärer Spermatocyten (vgl. Abb. 28). Bei einer dritten Gruppe fallen reife Sertolizellen und eine ziemlich aktive Spermiogenese auf, die bis zu den Spermatozoen reicht, die Gesamtzellzahl ist aber beträchtlich vermindert. Leydigzellen fehlen auch hier. Von 92 Kranken mit hypogonadotropem Eunuchoidismus findet NELSON (1953b) die erste Gruppe in 75 Fällen, die zweite in 8 und die dritte in 9. Bei der zweiten und dritten Gruppe muß

man annehmen, daß eine gewisse FSH-Sekretion vorhanden ist. Manchmal ist
die Tunica verdickt und in den äußeren Schichten haben sich elastische Fasern
abgelagert. Das Interstitium kann auch abnorme Leydigzellen enthalten. Diese
liegen meist einzeln, haben eine mehr längliche Gestalt mit Plasmaausläufern,
einen kleinen Zellkern mit dichter Chromatineinlagerung (TONUTTI 1943). Geringe
Reifung ist durch eine teilweise Stimulierung durch die Gonadotropine bedingt.
Wenn diese wieder zurückgeht, treten in der Kanälchenwand regressive Erscheinungen auf. Eine verdickte Tunica propria kann sich unter Behandlung
mit Choriongonadotropin oder Testosteron wieder zurückbilden (SNIFFEN u. Mit-

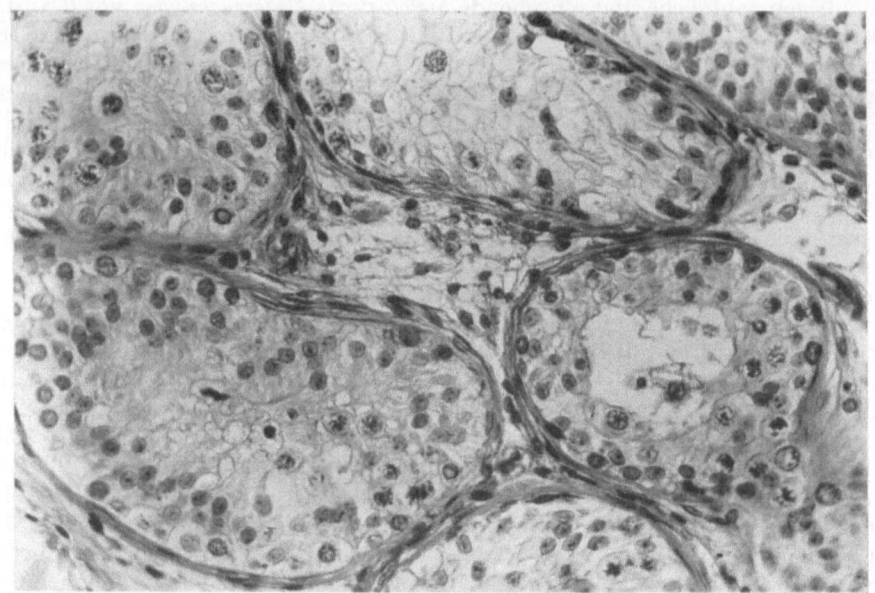

Abb. 28. 26jähriger Mann, idiopathischer hypogonadotroper Eunuchoidismus präpuberaler Art. Vor 2 Jahren
1 Jahr lang mit Testosteron Depot-Präparaten behandelt. Tubuli durchweg von kleinem Durchmesser, Tunica
propria überall beträchtlich verdickt, viele Tubuli enthalten vorwiegend Sertolizellen, nur in einzelnen finden sich
Spermatogonien und Spermatocyten I. Ordnung. Zwischengewebe ziemlich zellreich, keine reifen Leydigzellen
zu erkennen, auch unreife Leydigformen sind nur spärlich vorhanden. Gonadotropine im Urin nicht sicher nachweisbar. Einjährige Behandlung mit HCG bringt keine Vergrößerung der Hoden (bohnengroß). (Hämatoxylin-
Eosin, 300fach)

arb. 1950b), eine Beobachtung, die in der Pathologie keine Parallele hat. Wird
die Behandlung abgebrochen, dann verdickt sich die Tunica propria wieder
(SNIFFEN u. Mitarb. 1950b).

2. Postpuberale Form

Versiegt die Gonadotropinbildung erst, nachdem die normale Ausbildung des
Hodengewebes erfolgt war *(postpuberale Form)*, dann ist der Ablauf ziemlich
uniform.

Die erste sichtbare Erscheinung besteht in der Verminderung der spermato-
genen Aktivität. Die Keimzellen werden abgestoßen, meist bis zu den primären
Spermatocyten (Bild des „spermiogenic arrest"). In diesem Stadium fehlen noch
alle anderen Erscheinungen, auch die Verdickung der Tunica propria. Die Leydigzellen sehen noch normal aus. Später entwickelt sich eine schwere Hypospermatogenese, schließlich bleiben nur noch einige wenige sich teilende Keimzellen übrig.
Gleichzeitig häufen sich in den Sertolizellen feine Lipoidtropfen an. Der Durch-

messer der Kanälchen schwindet langsam, während sich die kollagenen Fasern
in der Tunica propria vermehren, erscheinen auch viele elastische Fasern in der
peritubulären Zone. Im Interstitium vermehrt sich das Kollagen. Die Zahl der
sklerosierten Kanälchen und der Kollagengehalt des Interstitiums wechseln von
Fall zu Fall, manchmal tritt hier ein eosinophiles granuläres Präcipitat auf.
In der Folge schwindet der Kanälchendurchmesser weiter, das Lumen wird
vom schaumigen Cytoplasma der Sertolizellen ausgefüllt. Die Kerne der Sertolizellen bleiben lange unverändert, sie bilden eine gleichmäßige Linie an der Basis
der Zellen. Oft sind noch einige primäre, oft mehrkernige Keimzellen vorhanden,
die entlang der Basalmembran liegen. Die Spermatogenese geht aber nicht mehr

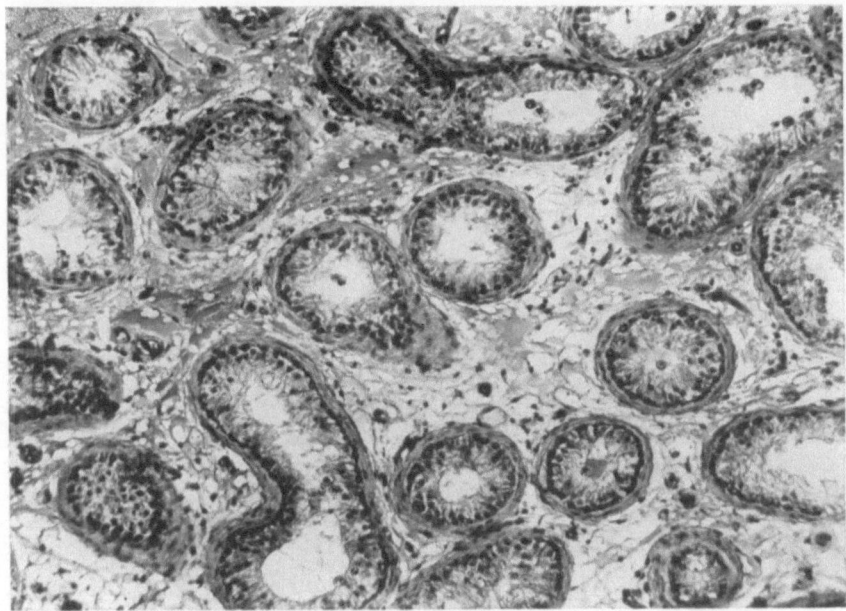

Abb. 29. 45jähriger Mann mit suprasellärem Tumor, verkleinerte Kanälchen mit verdickter Wand, Sertolizellen
treten stark hervor, reichlich Spermatogonien, einzelne Spermatocyten. Zwischengewebe feinfaserig, verdickte
Gefäßwände, ganz vereinzelt unreife Leydigzellen. (Hämatoxylin-Eosin, 120fach)

über diese Formen hinaus. Die Fibrillen der Tunica propria verdicken sich immer
mehr, auch die peritubulären Bindegewebslamellen vermehren sich, vorwiegend
durch die Ablagerung elastischer Fasern, beträchtlich (vgl. Abb. 29).

Mit der Entwicklung einer schweren Hypospermiogenese oder einer schweren
Atrophie der Kanälchen sind auch die Leydigzellen atrophisch geworden. Ihre
Zahl ist vermindert, die groben cytoplasmatischen Granula verschwinden, Verteilung und Zahl der Vacuolen im Cytoplasma sind anormal, der Zelldurchmesser
verkleinert sich, auch die Zellkerne schwinden und werden pyknotisch, die
Pigmentgranula sind vermehrt. Das Interstitium verdichtet sich durch Kollagen-
einlagerung, die Wand der Arteriolen ist verdickt (vgl. Abb. 30).

Die reichliche Vermehrung der Bindegewebsfasern der Kanälchenwand stört
ihrerseits wiederum die Ernährung des Samenepithels, so daß im Endstadium
nur noch Kanälchenschatten übrigbleiben (TONUTTI). Das Lumen der Kanälchen
ist durch die fibrilläre Tunica obliteriert, die Basalmembran ist verschwunden,
die Kanälchen werden begrenzt durch eine Schicht mehrerer Lagen von peritubulären elastischen Lamellen. Das stark kollagen umgewandelte interstitielle

Gewebe enthält nur noch Fibrocyten (SNIFFEN 1950b, CAHILL 1942, TONUTTI, HELLER u. NELSON 1948a) (vgl. Abb. 31). Das wichtigste Charakteristicum der erworbenen hypophysären Atrophie ist die Bindegewebsverdickung der Kanälchenwand. War das Kanälchen einmal entfaltet, dann kann es seinen unreifen Zustand nicht mehr annehmen, sagt SNIFFEN.

Die Endstadien sind leicht zu diagnostizieren. Die Befunde sind schwerer einzuordnen, wenn nur ein partieller Verlust der Gonadotropinbildung vorhanden

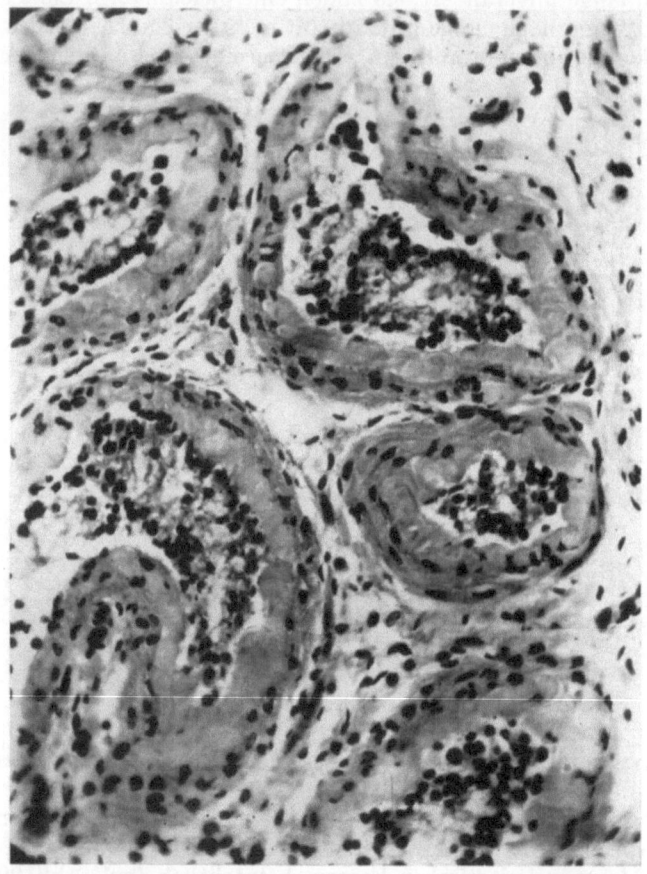

Abb. 30. 48jähriger Mann, verheiratet, zwei Kinder, 1939—1944 Infanterist. Erste Zeichen der Hypophysenvorderlappeninsuffizienz vor 3 Jahren, gestorben an (Gehirnödem bei hühnereigroßem Kraniopharyngeom). Gleichmäßig verkleinerte Kanälchen mit verdickter Wand, vorwiegend Sertolizellen, nur vereinzelt Spermatogonien enthaltend, Interstitium faserreiches Bindegewebe, keine Leydigzellen. (Hämatoxylin-Eosin, 300fach)

ist oder wenn eine Behandlung mit Gonadotropinen vorausging. Die Abtrennung gegen gewisse Formen des primären Hypogonadismus ist dann nicht sicher möglich. Veränderungen der Leydigzellen sind in diesen Fällen meist eindeutiger als die der Kanälchen (TILLINGER, TONUTTI).

Der Nachweis zusätzlicher endokriner Störungen der von der Hypophyse abhängigen Drüsen erleichtert die Diagnose sehr. Während man in der Bewertung von Ausfallserscheinungen des Zentralnervensystems, besonders des Zwischenhirns, sehr zurückhaltend sein soll.

Der Erfolg der Verabreichung von *Choriongonadotropin* mit der Erhöhung der 17-Ketosteroid- und Oestrogenausscheidung gibt eine weitere Bestätigung.

Die Dosis von siebenmal 1000 E im Laufe von 14 Tagen, wie sie WELLER vor-
schlägt, ist nach unseren Erfahrungen nicht immer ausreichend. Manche Kranke
müssen länger und mit höheren Dosen behandelt werden. Unter der Gabe von
5000 E täglich — wie sie GILBERT-DREYFUSS (1957) empfiehlt — können wiederum
auch Formen des primären Hypogonadismus, z.B. des Klinefelter-Syndroms,
positiv reagieren. Überzeugende Besserungen therapeutischer Art erreicht
man nur beim sekundären Hypogonadismus. Bleibt die 17-Ketosteroid- und
Oestrogenausscheidung, die Hodengröße, die Sexualentwicklung auch nach
Unterbrechung der HCG-Behandlung erhalten, dann hat es sich nur um eine
Pubertas tarda gehandelt.

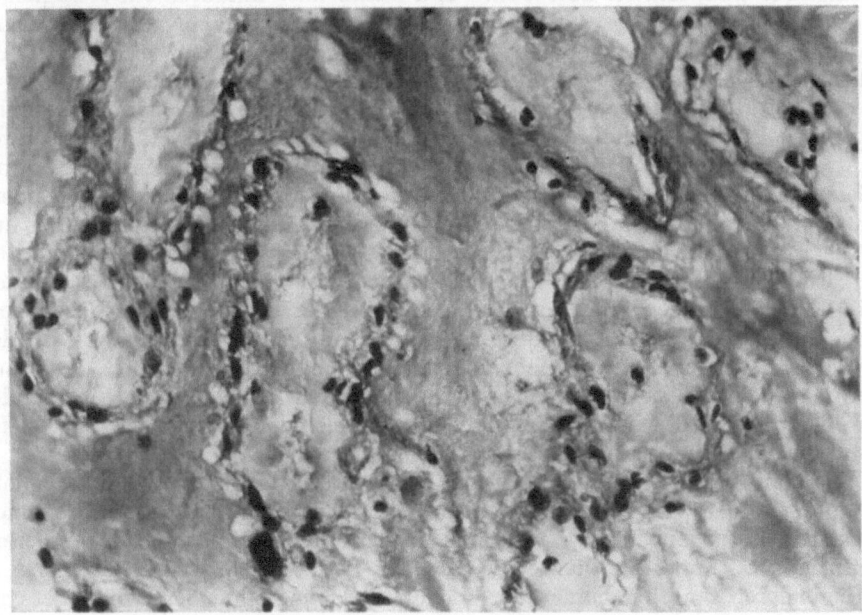

Abb. 31. 52jähriger Mann mit Hypophysenvorderlappeninsuffizienz bei Adenom, erste Symptome vor 15 Jahren,
Kanälchen völlig atrophisch, nur außen einfache Lage von Fibrocyten. Intertubulär einige fibrocytenähnliche
Zellen, keine Leydigzellen. (Hämatoxylin-Eosin, 300fach)

Die Häufigkeit ist je nach dem Krankengut der einzelnen Untersucher sehr
verschieden. NELSON (1953a) findet den sekundären Hypogonadismus in 62%,
ALBERT u. Mitarb. in 25%, TILLINGER in 31% ihres gesamten Krankengutes.

II. Klinik

1. Panhypopituitarismus

Das Vollbild der Hypophysenvorderlappeninsuffizienz ist durch den Ausfall
sämtlicher tropen Hormone und des somatotropen Hormons charakterisiert.
Beim Erwachsenen entwickelt sich ein komplexes klinisches Bild, das gekennzeichnet ist durch einen Hypogonadismus, eine Hypothyreose und einen Hypo-
corticoidismus. Das Vollbild wird im allgemeinen erst nach Jahren erreicht.
Die Diagnose ist nicht schwierig, wenn man daran denkt, daß stärkere Gewichtsabnahme, Anorexie, Asthenie, nicht zum unkomplizierten Verlauf gehören. Das
Körpergewicht ist meist normal, ein Teil ist sogar übergewichtig. Die Funktionsstörung der Nebennierenrinde tritt klinisch wenig hervor, sondern wird erst

durch spezielle Untersuchungen, besonders durch die Prüfung der Insulinempfindlichkeit und der Steroidausscheidung erfaßt. Die Kranken fallen auf durch
myxödematöse Züge, die Haut ist trocken, blaß, gedunsen, die Körperbehaarung
hat abgenommen, und zwar sowohl die Achsel- und Schambehaarung als auch
die Körper- und Gesichtsbehaarung. Meist sind auch die Augenbrauen reduziert.
Der Funktionsausfall der Nebenniere ist kein vollständiger, eine gewisse Basisleistung bleibt erhalten, so daß die gefährlichen Störungen des Wasserhaushaltes
der primären Nebenniereninsuffizienz ausbleiben. Die begleitende Hypothyreose
auf der anderen Seite erniedrigt den Bedarf an Nebennierenhormon beträchtlich.
Dies ist der Grund, weshalb die Kranken müde, antriebsarm und im ganzen
verlangsamt sind, daß sie aber Jahre und Jahrzehnte hindurch ein erträgliches
Leben führen können. Die Lebenserwartung ist verhältnismäßig gut. Die Kranken sind aber immer gefährdet, da sie keinerlei Funktionsreserven besitzen, um
Mehrbelastungen durch eine Mehrbildung von Corticoiden abzufangen.

Dieser totale Funktionsausfall, auch *globale Insuffizienz* genannt, ist ohne
eingehende Funktionsprüfung des innersekretorischen Systems klinisch schwer
abzutrennen von der sog. *Partiarinsuffizienz*. Man versteht darunter einen unvollständigen Ausfall der Funktion, woran einzelne trope Hormone mehr, andere
weniger teilnehmen. Diese partielle Insuffizienz ist in den meisten Fällen nur
das Anfangsstadium einer weitergehenden Entwicklung, die mit dem Fortschreiten
des pathologisch-anatomischen Prozesses in der Globalinsuffizienz endet. Selten
bleibt sie über längere Zeit bestehen, noch seltener bildet sie sich durch eine
Regeneration des Hypophysengewebes wieder zurück. Der Übergang von der
partiellen in die globale Insuffizienz vollzieht sich unmerklich. Vielfach diagnostiziert man rein klinisch wegen des verhältnismäßig guten Allgemeinzustandes
nur eine partielle Insuffizienz, obwohl die eingehende Funktionsprüfung dann
doch eine totale oder eine Globalinsuffizienz ergibt.

Unabhängig von der Ursache ist der *Hypogonadismus* häufig das erste objektive inkretorische Symptom. OBERDISSE fand bei 104 chromophoben Adenomen
64mal den Hypogonadismus, 11mal die Hypothyreose, 9mal die Nebenniereninsuffizienz als erstes Zeichen. Die Ursache beruht wahrscheinlich einmal in
der besonderen Empfindlichkeit der die Gonadotropine bildenden Zellen, der sog.
„Gonadotrophs", zum anderen aber wahrscheinlich in einer zusätzlichen Druckschädigung des vorderen Hypothalamus bei sich suprasellär ausbreitenden Geschwülsten und Entzündungen.

Die Ausfallserscheinungen der Keimdrüsen sind je nach Alter die eines leichteren oder schwereren präpuberalen oder postpuberalen Hypogonadismus. Im
Erwachsenenalter also Rückgang der Sekundärbehaarung, Abnahme der Hodengröße, Schwund der Prostata, Schwund der Muskulatur, vorzeitige Osteoporose,
während Stimme und Größe des äußeren Genitales unverändert bleiben. Bei
Kindern ist der präpuberale Eunuchoidismus Teilerscheinung eines Infantilismus.

Das *bioptische Bild* entspricht im allgemeinen der Schwere der Vorderlappeninsuffizienz. Zuerst wird die Spermiogenese geschädigt, dann verdichten sich
Basalmembran und peritubuläres Gewebe, die Leydigzellen verkleinern sich und
verschwinden schließlich ganz (s. Histologie). Bei 7 von 20 Fällen, meist mit
chromophoben Adenomen, war das Biopsiebild normal (McCULLAGH 1950).

Die *Ursache* der Vorderlappeninsuffizienz des Mannes sind vorwiegend intrasellär gelegene Geschwülste. Am häufigsten handelt es sich dabei um das *chromophobe Adenom*, das etwa ³/₄ aller Neubildungen der Hypophyse ausmacht. Die
chromophoben Zellen sezernieren selbst keine Wirkstoffe, so daß sich die Symptomatologie vorwiegend aus der Größe der Geschwülste, die das umliegende Gewebe
durch Druck schädigen, erklärt. Sie sind meist gutartig und vergrößern sich

langsam, so daß Jahre vergehen, bis sich das typische Krankheitsbild entwickelt. Nur 13,5% wachsen rein intrasellär, die übrigen dehnen sich supra- und parasellär aus (Tönnis u. Mitarb.). Meist werden Menschen zwischen dem 40. und dem 60. Lebensjahr betroffen, es ist jedoch kein Lebensalter ausgenommen. Vom chromophoben Adenom trennt man neuerdings das *Mischtypadenom* ab. Auch große eosinophile und basophile Adenome können durch Druck die übrige Hypophyse schädigen und von einem Hypogonadismus begleitet sein.

Verhältnismäßig häufig sind auch intraselläre *Kraniopharyngiome*, die ebenfalls die Tendenz zur Ausbreitung nach oben hinten besitzen. Als weitere Ursachen kommen in Betracht: Cystenbildungen, wahrscheinlich als Folge von Nekrosen, chronische Entzündungen wie Tuberkulose, Boecksches Sarkoid, Aktinomykose, Pilzerkrankungen, Lues, Speicherkrankheiten, rezidivierende Embolien, Nekrosen unbekannter Ätiologie mit dem Endbild der Fibrose, lokalisierte Arachnoiditis, entzündliche Gefäßprozesse, Aneurysmen, metastatische Absiedlungen von Carcinomen, besonders der Bronchien, Schilddrüse und Prostata, Lymphogranulomatose und granulomatöse Entzündungen unbekannter Ätiologie.

Für die *Diagnose* ist eine genaue Aufnahme des endokrinen Status und eine genaue Funktionsprüfung der einzelnen innersekretorischen Organe notwendig. Die 17-Ketosteroidausscheidung ist viel stärker vermindert als beim primären Hypogonadismus, ebenso die der 17-Hydroxycorticoide. Uringonadotropine fehlen in schweren Fällen, in leichteren liegen sie unter den Normalwerten. Elektrolytwerte des Serums und des Urins sind im allgemeinen normal, Störungen treten nur nach Belastung auf. Der Nüchternblutzucker ist vermindert, besonders charakteristisch ist die übermäßige Empfindlichkeit gegenüber Insulin. Die orale Zuckerbelastungskurve verläuft abgeflacht, doch ist dies kein spezifisches Symptom. Der Grundumsatz ist erniedrigt, die Jodspeicherungsfähigkeit der Schilddrüse stark herabgesetzt, Cholesterin im Blut oft erhöht. Hämoglobin und Zahl der Erythrocyten sind mäßig vermindert, es besteht eine normochrome, selten eine leicht makrocytäre Anämie.

Diese Untersuchungsergebnisse müssen durch Funktionsprüfungen der einzelnen peripheren Hormondrüsen ergänzt werden, nur so läßt sich der Grad der Insuffizienz genauer bestimmen.

Die *Prognose* ist abhängig von der Ätiologie. In Ruhe und ohne körperliche Tätigkeit sind die Kranken nicht gefährdet, bei irgendwelchen Belastungen, fieberhaften Krankheiten, Unfällen, operativen Eingriffen usw. können sie nicht mit der notwendigen Mehrbildung von Nebennierenrindenhormon reagieren und geraten in einen Schockzustand oder in eine Hypoglykämie, Gefahren, die sich heute durch rechtzeitige Erhöhung der Cortisondosis leicht vermeiden lassen.

Handelt es sich um Geschwülste ohne Wachstumstendenz, dann kann man abwarten und einfach die Insuffizienz behandeln. Greift der Tumor auf die Umgebung über, dann ist ein aktives Vorgehen angezeigt. Die Operationsmortalität liegt etwa bei 10% (Tönnis u. Mitarb., Krayenbühl). Die Röntgenbestrahlung brachte früher keine guten Ergebnisse und war mit Schäden wie Kolliquationsnekrosen und Opticusatrophie belastet. Bei der heutigen Bestrahlungstechnik mit der Möglichkeit der genauen Einstellung des Mittelpunktes eines Pendelfeldes kommt man mit kleinen Feldgrößen aus, so daß Schädigungen des umgebenden Gewebes vermieden werden können (Breit, Decker u. Lauter). Wir ziehen eine solche Pendelbestrahlung als erste Maßnahme der Operation vor, insbesondere, da sich gezeigt hat, daß auch bestrahlte Geschwülste nicht schwieriger zu operieren sind als unbestrahlte (Decker u. Lauter).

Die Behandlung der inkretorischen Insuffizienz mit glandotropen Hormonen hat nur theoretische Bedeutung. In der Praxis gibt man die peripheren

Hormone. Dabei ist es wichtig, nicht mit dem Schilddrüsenhormon anzufangen, da die Steigerung des Stoffwechselumsatzes die Nebennierenrindeninsuffizienz erst manifest macht. Man beginnt immer mit 2—3mal 25 mg Cortison-Acetat in Form von Tabletten per os, gibt nach 8—14 Tagen zusätzlich 0,1—0,3 Thyreoidea sicca oder 40—60 γ Trijodthyronin hinzu und vervollständigt die Behandlung durch die Injektion von 200—400 mg eines langwirkenden Testosteronesters alle 3—4 Wochen. Die zusätzliche Gabe von Testosteron bessert die Arbeitsfähigkeit und die Anämie dieser Menschen beträchtlich, verhindert eine schwerere Osteoporose und den vorzeitigen Muskelschwund. Im Alter über 60 Jahre kann Testosteron durch eines der mehr anabol wirkenden Derivate ersetzt werden.

2. Hypopituitarismus mit Zwischenhirnbeteiligung

Eine Mitbeteiligung des Zwischenhirns am klinischen Bild der Vorderlappeninsuffizienz ist auf zweierlei Weise möglich. Entweder kann ein Prozeß von der Hypophyse selbst über den Hypophysenstiel auf das vordere Zwischenhirn übergreifen oder aber ein suprasellär im vorderen Zwischenhirn sich entwickelnder Tumor oder eine Entzündung führt zu einer Beeinträchtigung der Funktion des Hypophysenvorderlappens. Dies ist durch direkte Schädigung, durch Druck und durch Beeinflussung der Blutversorgung möglich, oder durch eine Unterbrechung der Verbindung zwischen vorderem Zwischenhirn und dem Hypophysenvorderlappen und endlich durch Schädigung der Areale des Zwischenhirns, die zur Anregung der Hypophysentätigkeit notwendig sind. In den meisten Fällen ist der Funktionsausfall des Hypophysenvorderlappens kein vollständiger, so daß das Bild der Globalinsuffizienz nicht eintritt. Im Vordergrund steht auch hier der Ausfall der gonadotropen Hypophysenfunktion. Entwickelt sich der Tumor vor der Pubertät, dann ist häufig auch das Wachstum beeinträchtigt und es entsteht das Bild des hypophysären Zwergwuchses. Meist erfährt auch die Funktion der Schilddrüse eine gewisse Beeinträchtigung, während die der Nebennierenrinde weitgehend erhalten bleibt.

Zu den rein inkretorischen Symptomen treten solche neurologischer Art, die durch die Lokalisation des Tumors in der vorderen Schädelgrube bedingt sind, außerdem vegetative Ausfalls- und Reizerscheinungen des Hypothalamus, wie ein Diabetes insipidus, eine Polydipsie, übermäßig gesteigerter Appetit, Polyphagie, Freßsucht führen zu beträchtlichen Gewichtszunahmen. In anderen Fällen besteht eine Anorexie, so daß die Kranken hochgradig abmagern. Ungeklärte Fieberperioden, Zustände von Somnolenz, Schweißausbrüche, Störungen des Elektrolythaushaltes, besonders eine Hypernatriumämie vervollständigen das Bild.

a) Kraniopharyngiom

Der häufigste Vertreter dieses Syndroms ist das *Kraniopharyngiom,* nach dem chromophoben Adenom die häufigste intrakranielle Geschwulst. Sie betrifft etwa 4,3% aller intrakraniellen Neubildungen (BAILEY u. Mitarb. 1951). Es handelt sich um kongenitale Tumoren, die aus dem Hypophysengang entstehen. Zellreste finden sich in $^3/_4$ aller Hypophysen von Erwachsenen, sie liegen zum Teil im vorderen, zum Teil im oberen Anteil, auch in der Pars infundibularis. Durch die Rotation der Rathkeschen Tasche gelangen sie an die Oberfläche des Infundibulums. Entwickelt sich das Kraniopharyngiom aus Zellresten im Vorderlappen selbst, dann entsteht ein intrasellärer Tumor, entwickelt er sich aus Zellresten der Pars infundibularis, dann entsteht ein suprasellär gelegener Tumor, der sich meist von unten nach oben hinten ausbreitet. Von 158 von

BAILEY u. Mitarb. (1951) gesammelten Fällen waren 20 unter 10 Jahre alt,
66 unter 20 Jahre, während sich die übrigen 72 gleichmäßig zwischen dem 20.
und dem 60. Lebensjahr verteilten. Häufig läßt sich die Anamnese über Jahre
zurück verfolgen. Es ist nichts Seltenes, daß solche Menschen über ein Jahrzehnt
und länger intermittierend leichte Symptome zeigen und dann ziemlich plötzlich,
meist bei Hinzutreten einer anderen körperbelastenden Erkrankung, dekompen-
sieren.

b) Tumoren des Zwischenhirns

Besonders interessant sind Defekte des *Zwischenhirns*, die mit einem Hypogonadismus einhergehen. Ein solcher fand sich bei 19 der 60 Tumoren der
Statistik von BAUER (12 Männer, 7 Frauen). Bei dreien war der Hypothalamus
praktisch völlig zerstört, bei 13 nur zu $1/3$—$2/3$, bei einem Fall nur ein kleiner Teil
der medianen Eminenz. 16mal waren Tumoren die Ursache — 8 Kraniopharyngiome, 2 Infundibulome, 2 Pinealome, 1 Angiom, 1 Cyste im 3. Ventrikel, 2 nicht
identifizierte Geschwülste — dreimal nur entzündliche Veränderungen. Die
Tumoren waren vorwiegend im vorderen Hypothalamus, besonders in der Tuber-
und Infundibulargegend lokalisiert. 16 hatten Schädigungen am Boden des
3. Ventrikels verursacht. Sehr wichtig ist die Feststellung, daß bei 16 Kranken
die Hypophyse 14mal makroskopisch normal war, 7mal fehlte auch histologisch
jegliche Veränderung, so daß in diesen Fällen der Hypogonadismus mit großer
Wahrscheinlichkeit nicht durch eine direkte Schädigung des Hypophysenvorderlappens, sondern durch eine solche des vorderen Zwischenhirns bedingt ist.
Selten findet sich ein Hydrocephalus internus als Folge entzündlicher Verkle-
bungen.

3. Dystrophia adiposogenitalis (Fröhlich-Syndrom)

1901 berichtete FRÖHLICH über einen 14 Jahre alten Jungen, der an heftigen
Kopfschmerzen und Erbrechen litt, rasch an Gewicht zugenommen hatte und
bei dem sich eine fortschreitende Abnahme der Sehkraft des linken Auges ein-
stellte. Es bestand eine Adipositas bei geringem Minderwuchs, der Penis war
normal, die Hoden klein, Achsel- und Schambehaarung fehlten. Bei der Operation
fand sich ein intrakranieller Tumor, wahrscheinlich ein Kraniopharyngiom, dessen
cystitischer Inhalt abgesaugt wurde. 1900 hatte BABINSKI über eine junge Frau
berichtet, die an einem Hypophysentumor litt und einen Hypogonadismus aufwies. ERDHEIM hat 1904 vermutet, daß die Fettsucht des sog. Fröhlich-Syndroms
auf einer Verletzung oder einer Reizung einer Region an der Basis des Gehirns
beruht. Erst die experimentellen Untersuchungen von CAMUS und ROUSSY,
HEINBECKER u.a., BAILEY und BREMER, HETHERINGTON, RANSON u.a. brachten
die Klärung. Beidseitige Zerstörung der ventromedialen Kerne des Zwischenhirns
führt bei Tieren als Folge einer Polyphagie zu einer schweren Adipositas. Die
Einbeziehung des vorderen Zwischenhirns in die Zerstörung bedingt zusätzlich
einen Hypogonadismus.

In der oben erwähnten Zusammenstellung von BAUER über 60 Fälle von
organischen Erkrankungen des Hypothalamus, von denen 51 durch Neoplasmen,
7 durch Entzündungen und 2 durch degenerative Veränderungen hervorgerufen
waren (Arteriosklerose, tuberöse Sklerose), bestand 19mal ein Hypogonadismus.
15 dieser organischen Zwischenhirnkranken hatten eine Adipositas, 11 waren
abgemagert. Es ist bekannt, daß im Experiment auch eine Minderung des
Appetits durch Zerstörung von Zwischenhirngewebe ausgelöst werden kann.

Beim Menschen darf die Dystrophia adiposogenitalis nur angenommen werden, wenn eine erhebliche *Adipositas* neben einem präpuberalen *Hypogonadismus* vorhanden und eine *organische Erkrankung* des Zwischenhirns nachweisbar ist. Meistens handelt es sich um Tumoren, wobei das Kraniopharyngiom an erster Stelle steht, aber auch Meningeome, Gliome, Cholesteatome, granulomatöse Entzündungen und postencephalitische Veränderungen, Hydrocephalus internus und andere hypophysäre Störungen kommen in Betracht.

Der Begriff der Dystrophia adiposogenitalis, des Fröhlich-Syndroms, ist in den letzten Jahrzehnten viel mißbraucht worden, indem man adipöse Jungen und Mädchen mit Pubertas tarda mit diesem Namen belegte. Diese Durchgangsstadien der Entwicklung bezeichnet man am besten als *Adiposogigantismus* und vermeidet die Ausdrücke *Pseudo-Fröhlich-Syndrom* und *Pseudodystrophie.* Es kann nicht scharf genug betont werden, daß die Diagnose Fröhlich-Syndrom auf organische Erkrankungen des Hypophysenzwischenhirnsystems beschränkt bleiben muß. Im Gegensatz zum Adiposogigantismus ist beim Morbus Fröhlich das Längenwachstum und die Knochenreifung gehemmt.

Das *Biopsiebild* ist das des Gonadotropinmangels mit infantilen Hoden. Wenn vorübergehend eine gewisse Entwicklung stattgefunden hatte, kann die Kanälchenwand etwas verdickt sein. Wenn die Ursache chirurgisch angehbar ist, kann der Zustand der Kranken verbessert werden. Sonst bleibt nur die Ersatzbehandlung wie bei der Vorderlappeninsuffizienz.

4. Dystopie des Hypophysenhinterlappens

Eine seltene Ursache eines Hypopituitarismus ist die angeborene Dystopie des Hypophysenhinterlappens (Prisel 1920). Hedinger und Hürzeler haben kürzlich 16 Fälle aus der Literatur zusammengestellt, von denen 7 endokrine Störungen hatten, besonders Kleinwuchs und Hypopituitarismus. Der Infantilismus wird dreimal erwähnt und war auch in dem Fall von Hedinger vorhanden. 21jähriger Mann, 145 cm groß, mit Vollmondgesicht, eunuchoiden Proportionen und schwerem Hypogonadismus. Histologisch sind beide Hodenanteile unterentwickelt, die Kanälchenwand etwas verdickt. Gewicht: Hoden 3 g, Nebennieren zusammen 7 g, Schilddrüse 10 g, Hypophyse 0,2 g. Die Hypophyse bestand nur aus Vorderlappengewebe mit relativer Vermehrung der eosinophilen Anteile. Der Hinterlappen war an die Hirnbasis, in die Gegend des Infundibulums in Form eines kleinen Knötchens, das mit einem fadenartigen Fortsatz mit dem Hypophysenvorderlappen in Verbindung stand, verlagert. Histologisch ist die Struktur des Hinterlappengewebes normal. Der Hedingersche Fall hatte noch zahlreiche Mißbildungen anderer Organe, besonders der Nieren und des Herzens (Septumdefekt). Ursache der endokrinen Ausfälle ist nicht die fehlende Verbindung des Hinterlappens mit dem Vorderlappen, sondern eine gestörte Verbindung des Hypophysenvorderlappens mit dem vorderen Zwischenhirn. Klinisch imponieren die Kranken wie ein Fröhlich-Syndrom.

5. Hypophysärer Zwergwuchs

Der Begriff des Infantilismus hat in früheren Jahrzehnten eine große Rolle gespielt. 1871 beschrieb Lorain und sein Schüler Faneau de la Cour den Infantilismus mit folgenden Worten: « caracterisée par la débilité, la gracilité et la petitesse du corps, par une sorte d'arret de développement qui porerait plûtot sur la masse de l'individu que sur un appareil spécial: en un mot des sujets atteints d'une juvénilité persistante qui retarde indefiniment chez eux l'établissement intégral de la puberté». PALTAUF hat 1891 einen infantilen Zwerg ohne ätiologische Klärung beschrieben.

Später wurde der Begriff des Infantilismus verschieden gebraucht. CONRAD bezog ihn nur auf die physische und psychische Sexualkonstitution, andere bezeichnen damit sowohl das Stehenbleiben des Gesamtorganismus, als auch das seiner Teile auf einer Durchgangsstufe der Entwicklung (NOBEL u. Mitarb.). Wenn man unter Infantilismus eine mehr oder weniger schwerwiegende Hemmung der somatischen *und* sexuellen Entwicklung bei Erhaltenbleiben einer kindlichen Erscheinung über das Pubertätsalter hinaus versteht (KRABBE 1919, GOLDZIEHER 1939, ZONDEK 1926), dann handelt es sich um einen Symptomenkomplex, der mit dem *hypophysären Zwerg- bzw. Minderwuchs* gleichgesetzt werden kann. Ursächlich liegt ihm ein Mangel an somatotropem und gonadotropem Hormon oder eine noch komplexere hypophysäre Insuffizienz zugrunde.

a) Funktionelle Insuffizienz

Die hypophysäre Insuffizienz kann eine *funktionelle* sein, ausgelöst durch chronische erschöpfende Krankheiten wie Resorptionsstörungen, Vitaminmangel, Unterernährung, Nephrose, exsudative Enteropathie, hämolytischer Ikterus, chronische Niereninsuffizienz, chronische infektiöse Prozesse u.a., wobei der Eiweiß- bzw. der Aminosäuremangel für die Bildung der hypophysären Hormone, die vorwiegend die Gonadotropine und das STH betreffen, verantwortlich gemacht wird. Diese Formen, auf die BRISSAUD zum erstenmal hingewiesen hat, sind im allgemeinen leichterer Natur, sie gleichen sich nach Behebung der Ursache von allein aus (s. bei Pubertas tarda).

b) Organische Erkrankungen

Die zweite Gruppe umfaßt die *organischen Erkrankungen* der Adenohypophyse oder des Zwischenhirns. Als Ursache findet man Tumoren, besonders das Kraniopharyngiom, so daß diese Gruppe auch einfach als Tumorform bezeichnet wird; es kommen aber auch Mißbildungen der Hypophyse und alle oben erwähnten Ursachen der Hypophysenvorderlappeninsuffizienz des Erwachsenen in Betracht. Häufig ist die Hypophysenfunktion nicht vollständig erloschen, zum mindesten in den ersten Krankheitsjahren. Die Wachstumsstörung beginnt meist erst nach dem 6. Lebensjahr, der Hypogonadismus ist präpuberaler Art. Beim kompletten Gonadotropinausfall bleiben die Zellen der Kanälchen undifferenziert, die Wand zart, das Interstitium zellarm. Die Bilder sind von angeborenen Defekten der Hodenanlage nur schwer zu unterscheiden. Im klinischen Aspekt lassen sich zwei Typen abtrennen. Der eine entspricht dem Bild der *Dystrophia adiposogenitalis* (s. dort), der andere ist der magere, untergewichtige, im Wachstum stark zurückgebliebene Junge, bei dem die Pubertätsentwicklung ausbleibt und der meist in der Kachexie stirbt. Die Diagnose ist leicht zu stellen, wenn cerebrale Symptome vorhanden sind, die auf eine organische Erkrankung hinweisen. Fehlen diese, dann ist die Abtrennung von der idiopathischen Form sehr schwierig, da in Schilddrüse und Nebennierenrinde eine Basisfunktion erhalten bleiben kann, deren Starre den üblichen Testen entgeht. Der Verlauf ist abhängig von der Ursache. Manchmal gelingt die Entfernung eines Tumors und damit die Heilung. Nicht selten bleibt der Tumor im Wachstum stehen, die Hypophysenfunktion erholt sich teilweise und es entwickelt sich ein stationärer Zustand. Die Kranken wachsen langsam weiter und erreichen schließlich mit 30 Jahren doch noch eine Körpergröße um 150 cm. Sie haben aber eunuchoide Körperproportionen und einen mehr oder weniger starken Hypogonadismus, wobei das histologische Bild an den Kanälchen infolge der wechselnden Einwirkung der Gonadotropine das eines erworbenen hypogonadotropen Hypogonadismus mit Sklerohyalinose sein kann. Kleinwuchs, noch offene Epiphysenfugen, nicht ossifizierte Randleisten an den Wirbelkörpern mit 30 Jahren, flache, niedrige Wirbelkörper, Rundrücken, Coxa vara weisen dann auf den präpuberalen Beginn hin. Das Leben dieser Menschen ist nur bedroht, wenn eine Belastung von ihnen gefordert wird (Unfall, Operation, Fieber, Hunger, schwere körperliche Anstrengung u.a.), der die Nebennierenrinde nicht nachkommen kann. Bei *unvollständigem Ausfall* der Hypophysenfunktion finden sich alle Übergänge bis zur einfachen verzögerten Pubertät.

c) Idiopathische Form

Interessanter ist eine dritte Form des hypophysären Zwergwuchses, bei der eine Schädigung der Hypophyse und des Zwischenhirnsystems nicht nachgewiesen werden kann, der sog. *idiopathische hypophysäre Zwergwuchs*. Ablauf und Bild sind typisch. Die Kinder werden meist erst im Alter von 6—8 Jahren zur Beobachtung gebracht. Bei der Geburt ist die Körpergröße normal, die Wachstumsperiode der ersten Lebensjahre verläuft unauffällig. Erst ab dem 3.—4. Lebensjahr bleiben sie im Wachstum zurück, während die geistige Entwicklung normal weiter läuft. In der Schule sind sie immer bei weitem die kleinsten, mit 12 bis 14 Jahren erreichen sie eine Größe von 115—125 cm, sie neigen zur Körperfülle und haben ein schwammiges Puppengesicht. Charakteristisch sind ein großer Kopf, ein verhältnismäßig langer Rumpf, kurze Extremitäten mit kurzen, plumpen Händen und Füßen, ein fetter Rumpf, das Fehlen jeglicher Behaarung, eine schlecht entwickelte Muskulatur, während die körperliche Leistungsfähigkeit auffallend gut ist. Es besteht ein kompletter präpuberaler Eunuchismus, der unbehandelt bis ans Lebensende fortbesteht. Klinische Zeichen einer Hypothyreose oder einer Nebenniereninsuffizienz bestehen nicht. Kinder und Erwachsene sind geistig meist rege, manche arbeiten sich beruflich hoch, obwohl sie körperlich unproportioniert bleiben.

Von früher Jugend an bleibt die Reifung des *Skeletes* gegenüber dem Lebensalter zurück, später kann der Unterschied 10—20 Jahre betragen. Unbehandelt wachsen sie bis ins 30. und 40. Lebensjahr langsam weiter und erreichen dadurch noch eine Körpergröße um 150 cm. Um das 30. Lebensjahr verlieren sie ihr jugendliches, frisches Aussehen und altern rasch. Das Gehirn entwickelt sich normal, der Kopf erscheint daher lange unverhältnismäßig groß, die Schädelnähte schließen sich regelrecht, das Gebiß entwickelt sich normal. Die Größe der inneren Organe entspricht der Körpergröße. Das wichtigste diagnostische Merkmal des hypophysären Zwergwuchses gegenüber allen anderen Formen ist das starke Zurückbleiben der Skeletreifung als Folge des Fehlens des Wachstumshormons.

Die Ursache des idiopathischen hypophysären Zwergwuchses ist unbekannt, angenommen wird neben dem alleinigen Fehlen der Produktionsstätten des STH auch ein funktioneller Ausfall anderer Hypophysenfunktionen.

Bei der *Funktionsprüfung* der einzelnen endokrinen Drüsen sind die Ergebnisse nicht einheitlich. Bei der größeren Zahl ist der Grundumsatz mäßig erniedrigt (—2 bis —15%), die Speicherung von J^{131} ist in vier eigenen Fällen normal. Bierich findet sie bei sechs erniedrigt. Die Erniedrigung des Grundumsatzes ist nicht stärker als bei den schweren Formen des primären Hypogonadismus, so daß ein Mangel an thyreotropem Hormon damit nicht bewiesen ist.

Die Nebennierenrinde verhält sich in vier eigenen Fällen normal. Die Ausscheidung der 17-Ketosteroide und der Cortisolmetaboliten ist absolut erniedrigt, sie entspricht aber der geringen Körpergröße. Unter ACTH erfolgt ein prompter und ausreichender Anstieg. Die oft vorhandene mäßig erhöhte Insulinempfindlichkeit kann auf das Fehlen des Wachstumshormons zurückgehen.

Gonadotropine sind im Urin nicht feststellbar. BIERICH, M. M. MARTIN u. WILKINS nehmen in ihren Fällen neben der Wachstumsstörung und dem Hypogonadismus auch eine Störung der Schilddrüsen- und Nebennierenrindenfunktion an, obwohl die Abweichungen von dem Verhalten gleich großer Individuen nicht eindeutig sind.

Das *histologische* Bild entspricht dem sekundären Hypogonadismus. Beide Hodenanteile bleiben infantil. Im Interstitium fehlen die beim einfachen sekundären Hypogonadismus zahlreichen Bindegewebszellen. In den unentwickelten Kanälchen degenerieren in höherem Alter die Spermiogonien, die Kanälchenwand kann dann eine gewisse Hyalinisierung zeigen.

Man weiß schon lange, daß die Verabreichung von Choriongonadotropin oder von Testosteron bei einem Teil der Fälle nicht nur auf die Entwicklung der sekundären Geschlechtsmerkmale, auf die Entwicklung der Muskulatur, auf das Längenwachstum, sondern auch auf die Entwicklung der Hoden eine günstige, manchmal ganz überraschende Wirkung hatte (ALBRIGHT 1947, DORFF, GORDON, HORSTMANN, LURIE, NOWAKOWSKY u. ASSMANN 1957b, TALBOT u. SOBEL, THOMPSON 1944, WELLER, PRADER 1954), eine Beobachtung, die mit der Annahme einer alle Funktionen der Adenohypophyse betreffenden Störung nicht vereinbar ist. WELLER und TONUTTI konnten bei einem ihrer Kranken durch Verabreichung von Choriongonadotropin, bei einem anderen durch Testosteron, den normalen Längenspurt, wie er durch die Pubertät ausgelöst wird, künstlich erzeugen und die Reifung des Skeletsystems auslösen. Nachdem die Kranken unter der systematischen Hormonbehandlung ein Knochenalter von 12—14 Jahren erreicht hatten, wurden Gonadotropine im Urin nachweisbar und die eigene Hypophyse nahm ihre reguläre gonadotrope Leistung auf. Nach Absetzen der Gonadotropine bzw. der Testosteronbehandlung schritt die Pubertätsentwicklung weiter und vollendete sich. Das bioptische Bild des Hodens entsprach dann dem eines gesunden Erwachsenen.

Die Körpergröße der Behandelten bleibt kleiner als normal, da der Wachstumsstoß der künstlichen Pubertät bei einem entsprechend kleineren Organismus einsetzt. TONUTTI und FETZER (1956b) geben nachstehende Deutung des Geschehens.

Es ist bekannt, daß das Zwischenhirn oder übergeordnete Gehirnteile den Anstoß zur Gonadotropinproduktion erst geben, wenn sie einen gewissen Reifungszustand erreicht haben, der dem der Skeletreifung parallel geht. Diese Gewebsreifung erfolgt normalerweise unter der anabolen Wirkung des somatotropen Hormons. Fehlt dieses, dann bleibt mit der Gewebsreifung auch die der Sexualregion im Zwischenhirn aus und es entsteht das Bild des idiopathischen Zwergwuchses, der durch einen Minderwuchs und einen schweren sekundären Hypogonadismus charakterisiert ist. Der idiopathische hypophysäre Zwergwuchs ist also ein einfacher Defekt der STH-Produktion.

Die anabole Wirkung des Testosterons kann offenbar die des STH ersetzen und die Reifung der Sexualregion erreichen. Einige Beobachtungen in der Literatur (PRADER 1954, 1957) sprechen dafür, daß diese Reifung im späteren Leben auch spontan erfolgen kann. Die Gruppe der idiopathischen Formen darf wahrscheinlich nicht ganz mit dem einfachen Mangel an STH gleichgesetzt werden. MARTIN und WILKINS (1958) berichten bei einem Teil ihrer Fälle über schlechte

Ergebnisse der Testosteronbehandlung. Sie gaben 200—400 mg Oenanthat mehrere Jahre alle 3—4 Wochen und erreichten ein rasches Längenwachstum, eine Gewichtszunahme, eine beträchtliche Verbreiterung der Knochenbälkchen, eine gute Muskelentwicklung, die Stimme wurde tiefer, Genitale und Prostata wuchsen. Das Ausmaß der Virilisierung blieb aber nicht nur hinter der Norm, sondern auch hinter dem, was bei Patienten mit primärem testiculärem Hypogonadismus erreicht werden kann, zurück. Das Wachstum der Haare im Gesicht, der Achsel- und Schamhaare ist sehr dürftig, die Prostata bleibt klein, der Ge-

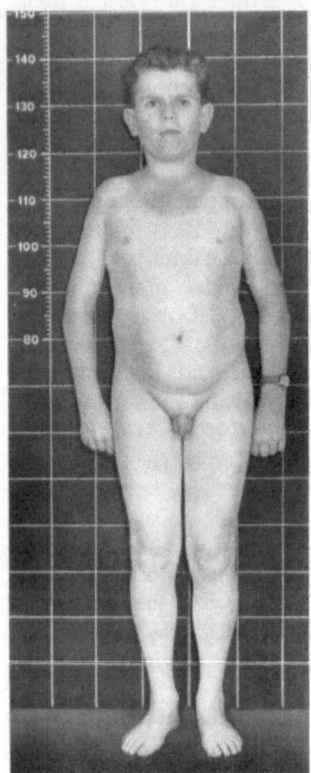

sichtsausdruck wird reifer, doch behalten die Kranken ihr rundes Gesicht und ihr jugendliches Aussehen. Eine spontane Entwicklung der Keimdrüsen unterblieb. Das Wachstum erfolgte in den ersten 6—12 Monaten rasch und verflachte sich dann. Keiner der Patienten erreichte über 158,8 cm, eine Reihe nur 152,4 cm. Beim Vergleich mit einem 45jährigen nie behandelten mit 154,9 cm scheint es fraglich, ob die Testosteronbehandlung an der endgültigen Körpergröße etwas ändert.

d) Behandlung

Auch die bisherigen Ergebnisse der *Behandlung mit Wachstumshormon* scheinen eine Unterteilung notwendig zu machen. Die Verwendung von tierischen Produkten hat sich nicht bewährt. Erst seit man seit einigen Jahren Wachstumshormon aus menschlichen Hypophysen gewinnt, sind die Ergebnisse etwas besser. Hutchings berichtet über ein $11^1/_2$jähriges Mädchen, das in Körpergröße und Entwicklung einem $8^3/_4$jährigen entsprach, das er mit einem nach Li gewonnenen STH-Präparat behandelte. Bei täglicher Gabe von 5 mg wurde Stickstoff, Natrium, Kalium, Phosphor einbehalten. Eine anfänglich negative Calciumbilanz wurde später positiv. Während einer neunmonatigen Behandlung nahm die Körpergröße um 9 cm zu,

Abb. 32. Hypophysärer Zwergwuchs, 27jährig, nach unterschwelliger Testosteronbehandlung. Keinerlei Behaarung. Infantiles Genitale, aber kräftige Muskulatur (Fall 2)

während das Kind in den Jahren vorher jährlich nur um 3 cm gewachsen war. Lipsett behandelte vier Kranke zwischen 6 und 17 Jahren mit täglich 5—10 mg STH, *ohne* daß eine Steigerung des Wachstums eingetreten ist. Die Stickstoffbilanz wurde im Gegensatz zum normalen Kind oder zum Erwachsenen nicht positiv. Lipsett nimmt an, daß die Bilanz nur in den Fällen positiv wird, die mit einer Steigerung des Epiphysenwachstums reagieren. Man könnte demnach in kurzfristigen Behandlungsperioden die Reaktion eines Kranken prüfen und wäre nicht gezwungen, die umständliche STH-Behandlung unnötigerweise über Monate fortzuführen. Die mangelnde Wirkung des Wachstumhormons hängt wahrscheinlich mit zusätzlichen Störungen anderer Hypophysenvorderlappenfunktionen zusammen, so daß sich in diesen Fällen die Kombination mit Thyreoidin, Testosteron bzw. anabolen Steroiden empfiehlt.

Fall 2. J. M., 27jährig. Hypophysärer Zwergwuchs (vgl. Abb. 32). Beide Eltern normal groß, desgleichen fünf Geschwister, Mutter war bei der Geburt 39 Jahre alt, er ist das fünfte Kind. Das nächste Kind entwickelte sich normal.

Bei der Geburt 50 cm groß. Lernte Ende des ersten Lebensjahres gehen und im gleichen Alter wie seine Geschwister sprechen. Erst mit 5 Jahren ist der Mutter aufgefallen, daß ihr Junge im Wachstum zurückblieb, sie hat ihn von dieser Zeit an regelmäßig gemessen und die Notizen darüber aufgehoben. Ab dem achten Lebensjahr bis vor 2 Jahren regelmäßig Thyreoidin eingenommen, ohne daß dadurch das Wachstum beschleunigt worden wäre. Zwischen 10 und 16 Jahren wiederholt Gesamtextrakte des Hypophysenvorderlappens, Implantationen von Kalbshypophysen, Injektion von Hypophysenbreien von Tieren ohne irgendeinen Erfolg. Mit 21 Jahren Beginn mit einer unterschwelligen Behandlung mit Choriongonadotropin und Depot-Testosteron. Erst in den zwei letzten Jahren (25jährig) höhere Dosierung (250 mg Testosetronoenanthat alle 4 Wochen).

21jährig, 122 cm, 31,5 kg, gedrungen, adipöser Rumpf, pastöses Gesicht (Abb. 35).

Genitale: Entspricht einem 8—10jährigen, Penis 3 cm, beide Testes im Scrotum, kleinbohnengroß und weich. Prostata nicht zu tasten.

GU —7%, Insulinempfindlichkeit 2 E intravenös negativ.

ACTH intravenös 8 Std 10 E Abfall der Eo —96%.

17-Ketosteroide 3,4 3,2, 3,6 mg, Porter-Silberchromogene 4,1, 4,8; unter ACTH Anstieg auf 12,4 mg.

Uringonadotropine bei 24 MEU negativ.

Knochenalter entspricht etwa einem 9jährigen (vgl. Abb. 34).

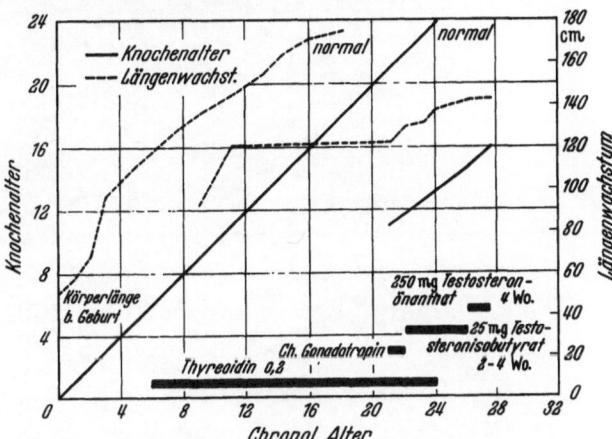

Abb. 33. Wachstumskurve eines 27¹/₂jährigen hypophysären Zwergwuchses (Fall 2)

In den folgenden Jahren regelmäßige Kontrollen (vgl. Wachstumskurve 33).

27jährig, Körpergröße 143 cm, Gewicht 39 kg.

Kräftigere Muskulatur, Gesichtszüge jetzt besser ausgeprägt.

GU +11%, reichlich Fett am Rumpf. Keine Sekundärbehaarung, keine Pubes, keine Achselbehaarung (vgl. Abb. 36).

Genitale: Penis 4 cm, an der Wurzel ziemlich breit, beide Hoden nur wenig über bohnengroß und in der Konsistenz ziemlich fest. Knochenalter 16—17jährig. Fortführung der Testosteronbehandlung.

29jährig, Größe 1,45 m, Gewicht 39,5 kg, Genitale wie früher, Prostata jetzt eben tastbar, Knochenalter 16—17jährig. Urin: Gonadotropine nach 4wöchiger Behandlungspause negativ.

Beurteilung: Hypophysärer Zwergwuchs mit normaler Funktion der Nebenniere, vermindertem Grundumsatz trotz Behandlung mit kleinen Thyreoidindosen seit der Jugend. Ab 21 Jahren unterschwellige Behandlung mit Testosteron (25 mg Perandren M alle 2—4 Wochen) und Choriongonadotropin zweimal 500 E pro Woche über ein halbes Jahr ohne nennenswerte Reifung des Genitales, aber trotzdem stetige Zunahme der Körpergröße und langsam fortschreitende Reifung des Skeletes. Mit 29 Jahren sind die Epiphysenfugen noch alle weit offen. Nach Erreichen der Körpergröße von 142 cm hochdosierte Testosteronbehandlung, die keine raschere Skeletreifung und kein rascheres Wachstum auslöst.

Der Kranke lehrt, daß schon kleine Hormondosen die Wachstumsrate deutlich steigern. Trotz einer Größenzunahme von 22 cm sind die Epiphysen noch weit offen. Gonadotropinsekretion kommt nicht in Gang.

Die Verabreichung von *Schilddrüsenhormon* über Jahre bringt weder eine Änderung des puppenhaften Aussehens, noch eine Steigerung der Wachstumsrate, noch eine Reifung des Skelets. Die hohen Dosen, die diese Menschen ohne Nebenerscheinungen ertragen, schließt eine begleitende Nebennierenrindeninsuffizienz aus. Auch Cortison bzw. Prednison sind völlig wirkungslos. Die einzige erfolgversprechende Behandlung besteht gegenwärtig in der Verabreichung von *Choriongonadotropin* oder von *Testosteron* bzw. von *anabolen Steroiden*. Es ist schwer, den Zeitpunkt des Behandlungsbeginnes festzulegen, da diese Menschen spontan langsam weiterwachsen und jeder vor der Auslösung der künstlichen Pubertät erreichte Zentimeter ein Gewinn an endgültiger Körpergröße darstellt.

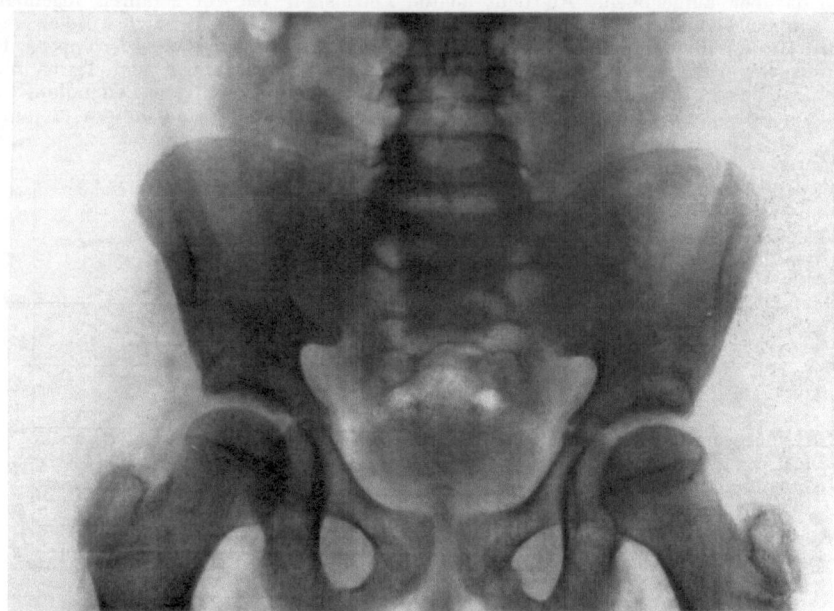

Abb. 34. Beckenübersicht des Kranken im Alter von 21 Jahren (Fall 2)

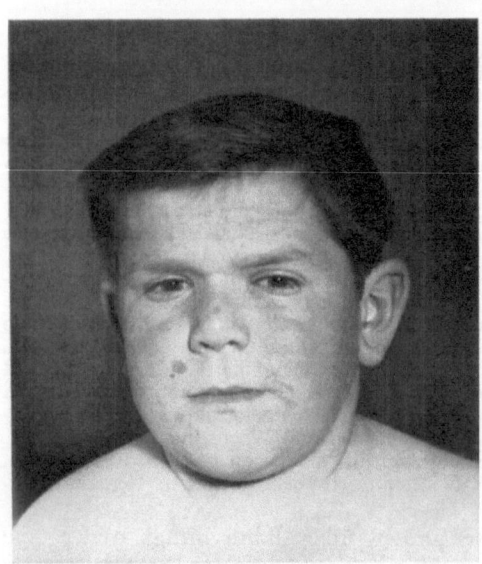 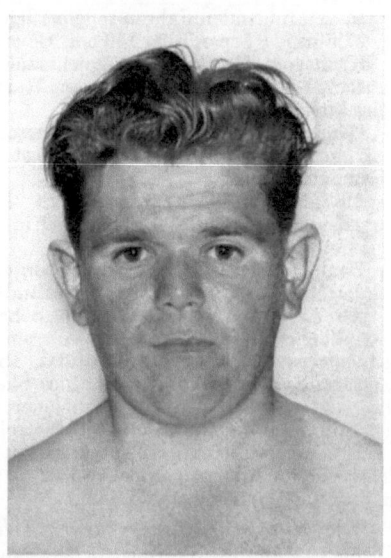

Abb. 35. Hypophysärer Zwergwuchs. Pastöses Rundgesicht mit 21 Jahren

Abb. 36. Differenziertes Jungmännergesicht nach niedrig dosierter Testosteronbehandlung mit 27 Jahren (Fall 2)

Im allgemeinen beginnt man im Alter von 10—12 Jahren und behandelt so intensiv, daß im Laufe von 3—4 Jahren die Knochenreifung Gleichaltriger erreicht wird. Vom kostspieligen Choriongonadotropin benötigt man wöchentlich mindestens dreimal 1500 E, anfangs sogar dreimal 3000 E. Da nach den Beobachtungen von Tonutti (1956b) Testosteron nicht schadet, kann man von den wesentlich billigeren Depotpräparaten monatlich 150—300 mg geben. Bei dieser intensiven Behandlung wird die rasche und intensive Entwicklung des Genitales als störend empfunden. Eigene Erfahrungen mit den *anabolen Steroiden* machen es wahrscheinlich, daß ihre Anwendung dieselben Ergebnisse hat, wie die des Testosterons, so daß man heute die Behandlung früher, schon mit 5—6 Jahren, beginnen kann und bei niedriger Dosierung die vorzeitige Genitalentwicklung nicht fürchten muß. Wenn ein Knochenalter von etwa 13—14 Jahren erreicht ist, wird die Behandlung unterbrochen. Sind Gonadotropine im Urin nachweisbar, dann wartet man ab, fehlen sie noch, dann wird die Behandlung mit Testosteron fortgesetzt.

Wir haben den Eindruck, daß im Gegensatz zum Testosteron bei den Anabolica das Längenwachstum nicht hinter der Skeletreifung zurückbleibt. Da die Reifung des Hypophysenzwischenhirnsystems der anabolen Partiarfunktion des Testosterons zukommt, darf man erwarten, daß unter den anabolen Steroiden dieselbe Spontanentwicklung der Gonaden eintreten kann wie unter Testosteron.

Die Gruppe des idiopathischen hypophysären Zwergwuchses zerfällt demnach in *zwei Formen*. Eine, bei der die Produktion der Gonadotropine nur funktionell gestört ist. In diesen Fällen bringt die Behandlung mit Testosteron, anabolen Steroiden oder mit Choriongonadotropinen das Gewebe zur Reifung, auch die Sexualregion im Zwischenhirn, so daß die Adenohypophyse die Gonadotropinproduktion aufnimmt und die Gonaden sich entwickeln. Bei der zweiten Form fehlen nicht nur die Produktionsstätten des Wachstumshormons, sondern auch der Gonadotropine. Trotz künstlich erzeugter Reifung des Zwischenhirns durch anabole Steroide kann die Gonadotropinproduktion nicht aufgenommen werden, die Entwicklung der Gonaden bleibt aus. Je mehr Produktionsstätten troper Hormone der Adenohypophyse defekt sind, um so unwahrscheinlicher wird die idiopathische Form und um so wahrscheinlicher ist die organische Ursache der Hypophysenvorderlappeninsuffizienz.

6. Idiopathischer Hypogonadismus

a) Hypogonadotroper Eunuchoidismus

Es gibt einen selektiven Defekt der Gonadotropinproduktion in der Adenohypophyse, dessen Ursache unbekannt ist. Der Defekt kann vollständig und unvollständig sein. Diese Form wird von Howard (1950) als „idiopathischer Eunuchoidismus" mit niedrigem FSH, von Heller und Nelson (1945) als „hypogonadotroper Eunuchoidismus" bezeichnet.

Familiäres Vorkommen ist vereinzelt beobachtet. Roth (1947) beschreibt vier Brüder einer Familie mit schwerem hypogonadotropem Hypogonadismus, histologisch mit dem Bild des unterentwickelten Hodens mit teilweiser Sklerosierung der Kanälchen, erniedrigter Gonadotropinausscheidung und einfacher Degeneration der Retina ohne Pigmentierung, mit zusätzlicher Opticusatrophie in einem Fall. Er rechnet diese Kranken zum Laurence-Moon-Biedl-Syndrom, obwohl die typische Retinitis pigmentosa fehlt. Nur ein Kranker war adipös und hatte eine ganz erhebliche Gynäkomastie.

Overzier (1956) beschreibt zwei Brüder mit dem Bild des schweren präpuberalen Eunuchoidismus, 17-Ketosteroide um 5 mg, GU —24%, histologisch das Bild des unentwickelten Hoden, fehlende Gonadotropinausscheidung, aber Gynäkomastie. Sechsmonatige Behandlung mit 5000 E CHG wöchentlich führt zu einem mäßigen Wachstum des äußeren Genitale, beide Hoden werden deutlich größer. 17-Ketosteroide jetzt 9,5 mg, GU +1%.

Le Marquand (1954) berichtet über eine Familie, in der von sechs Kindern drei männliche und zwei weibliche einen Hypogonadismus hatten. Die Männer sprachen auf Behandlung mit Gonadotropin gut an.

Biben und Gordan (1955) berichten über zwei Familien. In der ersten waren von sechs Geschwistern drei Brüder, in der zweiten von drei Geschwistern ein Bruder und eine Schwester betroffen.

Kombination mit anderen Anomalien, wie sie bei Turner-Syndrom, Kallman-Syndrom, Laurence-Moon-Biedl-Syndrom vorkommen, erwecken den Verdacht auf einen primären Hypogonadismus (s. dort).

Jugendliche Kranke dieser Art kann man von der Pubertas tarda nicht abtrennen. Erst die wenig erfolgreiche Behandlung erweckt mit 18—20 Jahren den Verdacht auf eine schwerwiegendere Störung. Durch die vorausgegangene Verabreichung von Choriongonadotropin oder Testosteron ist das Hodenbild manchmal verändert, so daß kein ursprünglicher präpuberaler Hoden mehr vorliegt. Im allgemeinen zeigen die Kranken das Bild eines schweren präpuberalen, seltener eines puberalen Eunuchoidismus. Hoden und äußere Genitale entsprechen dem eines Kindes vor oder zu Beginn der Pubertät, Gonadotropine fehlen im Urin, die Prostata ist nicht feststellbar, die Schambehaarung ist dürftig. Körper- und Bartbehaarung fehlen. Häufig besteht ein eunuchoider Hochwuchs, eine mäßige Adipositas mit femininer Fettverteilung, die Muskulatur ist schlecht entwickelt, die Haut blaß, trocken und etwas gedunsen, die Reifung des Skeletsystems verzögert, die geistige Entwicklung normal. Ein- und beidseitiger Kryptorchismus sind nicht selten. Auch eine Gynäkomastie kommt vor. Ausfälle anderer Hypophysenfunktionen oder gar pathologische Veränderungen im suprasellären Gebiet schließen die idiopathische Form aus. Es sei hervorgehoben, daß isolierte schwere Formen des Androgenmangels mit einer deutlichen Erniedrigung des GU einhergehen können, die sich nach alleiniger Behandlung mit Testosteron ausgleicht. Auch eine gewisse Insulinüberempfindlichkeit kann bestehen, während die Funktion der Nebennierenrinde immer normal ist. Wenn man weiß, wie lange der Ausfall der Gonadotropine bei organischen Erkrankungen des Hypophysenzwischenhirnsystems dem anderer troper Hormone vorausgehen kann und wenn man bedenkt, wie häufig die Objektivierung pathologischer Prozesse im Bereich des Hypophysenzwischenhirnsystems intra vitam nicht gelingt, wird man mit der Diagnose des idiopathischen Eunuchoidismus zurückhaltend sein.

Das Syndrom hat verschiedene Spielarten, die durch den unvollständigen Ausfall der Gonadotropine bedingt sind. In einem Fall wird etwas FSH, im anderen etwas ICSH oder auch beides produziert. Der Hypogonadismus ist dann weniger stark ausgeprägt, aber von der präpuberalen Form. Gonadotropine werden im Urin nachweisbar. Das histologische Bild wechselt und bringt dann nicht immer eine sichere Entscheidung. Hier ist der Gonadotropintest und die intensive Gonadotropinbehandlung von großer Bedeutung. Deutliches Ansteigen der 17-Ketosteroide oder Oestrogene, Behebung des Hypoandrogenismus, Abfall der 17-Ketosteroide und der Oestrogene nach Unterbrechung der Therapie bestätigen dann die Diagnose.

Verwendet man die Choriongonadotropinbehandlung zur Diagnosestellung, dann muß sie mit hohen Dosen mindestens einen Monat lang durchgeführt werden. Gilbert-Dreyfuss (1957) empfiehlt täglich 5000 E; wir geben 1500 bis 3000 E jeden zweiten Tag. Je höher das Lebensalter, in dem die Behandlung begonnen wird, um so höhere Dosen sind erforderlich.

In einem Teil der Kranken mit präpuberalem Eunuchoidismus, die man im Alter von 16—18 Jahren als bleibende Defekte diagnostiziert hat, kommt nach einer oder mehreren intensiven Gonadotropinkuren doch noch die Eigenproduktion der Gonadotropine in Gang. Andere unvollständige Defekte gewinnen mit jeder Kur ein etwas höheres, bleibendes Plateau, ohne aber die volle Reifung zu erlangen. Diese Formen der Pubertas tarda kann man vor der Behandlung nicht sicher abtrennen. BARTTER (1952) klassifiziert diese doch noch auf die Behandlung ansprechenden Fälle als Pubertas tarda bzw. Eunu-

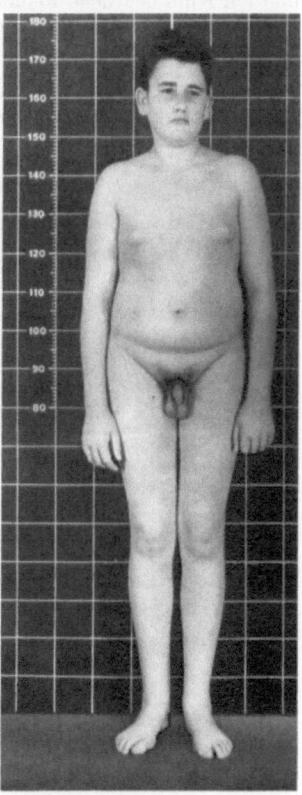

choidismus mit niedrigem FSH und gewisser Hodenentwicklung. Bei über 18jährigen haben wir den Eindruck, daß es ohne Behandlung spontan nicht mehr zu einer bleibenden Entwicklung kommt. Ein solcher Verlauf ist im Falle Nr. 3 dargestellt.

Bei seltenem vollständigem Defekt regt die Gonadotropingabe wohl die Androgenbildung an, die Pubertät kommt in Gang, der Penis wächst, die Pubes fangen an zu sprossen, aber das Fortschreiten der allgemeinen Reifung erfolgt nur langsam und zögernd. Die Hoden bleiben klein, da die Kanälchen nicht oder nur wenig reifen. Selbst bei intensiver Behandlung über 2—4 Jahre wird die Entwicklung nicht ganz zu Ende geführt, es bleiben deutliche Symptome des Hypoandrogenismus — mangelhafte Bart- und Körperbehaarung, unvollständiger Stimmbruch, infantiles Gesicht, mangelhafte psychische Reifung — dauernd bestehen. Da auch die mehrjährige Testosteronbehandlung wenig bessere Ergebnisse bringt, kann die Ursache nicht in einem unzureichenden Ansprechen der Leydigzellen beruhen. Wahrscheinlich ist das höhere Lebensalter, in dem erst mit einer intensiven Therapie begonnen wird — über 20 Jahre —, dafür verantwortlich zu machen. Die peripheren Gewebe sind nicht mehr so empfindlich gegen die Androgene wie im Pubertasalter, so daß jede Verzögerung des Therapiebeginns über das 16. Lebensjahr hinaus das Endergebnis beeinträchtigt.

Abb. 37. Ganzaufnahme D. R., 18-jährig (Fall 3). Idiopathische Pubertas tarda mit präpuberalem Hypogonadismus. Diskrepanz zwischen Hodengröße und Penis. Gynäkomastie. Histologisches Bild; vgl. Abb. 38.

ǀFall 3. D. R., 22jährig. Mit 10 Jahren schwerer Scharlach, später Typhus abdominalis, seither beträchtliche Gewichtszunahme, Entwicklung kam nur unvollständig in Gang.

Mit 16 Jahren zum erstenmal in ärztlicher Behandlung wegen Hypogonadismus. Jede Woche 3000 E Choriongonadotropin, im ganzen 30 Injektionen. Keine nennenswerte Änderung, ein halbes Jahr lang Methyltestosteron in Form von Linguetten.

Oktober 1958: Größe 174 cm, Oberlänge 84 cm, Unterlänge 90 cm. Gewicht 68,8 kg. Dicklich, schlecht entwickelte Muskulatur, leichte Kyphose der BWS, geringe Entwicklung der Scham- und Achselbehaarung, kein Bart. Mäßige Überlänge der Extremitäten. Beidseits beträchtliche Gynäkomastie mit Drüsenkörper von Fünfmarkstückgröße. Histologisch einfache Fibrosis mammae virilis (Abb. 37).

Genitale: Scrotum verhältnismäßig gut entwickelt. Die Hoden sind kleinwalnußgroß, fest, 3,3 cm lang, 2,1 cm breit. Im Verhältnis dazu ist der Penis mit 4,7 cm auffallend kurz, Prostata kleintaubeneigroß.

17-Ketosteroide: 12,3, 14,1 mg. Uringonadotropine negativ. Grundumsatz $\pm$ 0. J^{131}-Speicherung: Erste Stunde 8%, nach 6 Std 88%, nach 24 Std 100%.

Skeletsystem: mäßig retardierte Entwicklung.

Februar 1959 Hodenbiopsie (Prof. Tonutti): Tubuli sehr unterschiedliche Durchmesser, fast durchweg stark verkleinert. Tunica propria verdickt, dürftige Spermiogenese. Starkes Hervortreten der Sertolizellen. In einzelnen, allerdings spärlichen Kanälchen, sind alle Stufen der Spermiogenese vorhanden. Zwischengewebe: nur sehr kleine Gruppen reifer Leydigzellen auffindbar. Es besteht eine Spermiogenesehemmung und ungenügende Entfaltung der Zwischenzellen mit Verdacht auf ICSH-Mangel (Abb. 38).

Eine besondere Behandlung wird nicht durchgeführt. Trotzdem kommt es im Laufe eines Jahres zu einem Fortschreiten der Entwicklung.

Februar 1960: Stimme jetzt tief, im Gesicht wachsen an den Wangen, an den Oberlippen und am Kinn deutliche Flaumhaare. Muskulatur ist besser entwickelt, Hoden normal groß, Penis 6 cm, Prostata kleinkastaniengroß, Achsel- und Schambehaarung kräftig, aber noch keine vollständige Reifung.

17-Ketosteroide: 11,4, 13,2 mg. Uringonadotropine nicht sicher positiv.

Die mehrmals negative Gonadotropinausscheidung und das histologische Bild sprechen für einen sekundären Hypogonadismus, wobei der Mangel an FSH histologisch weniger aus-

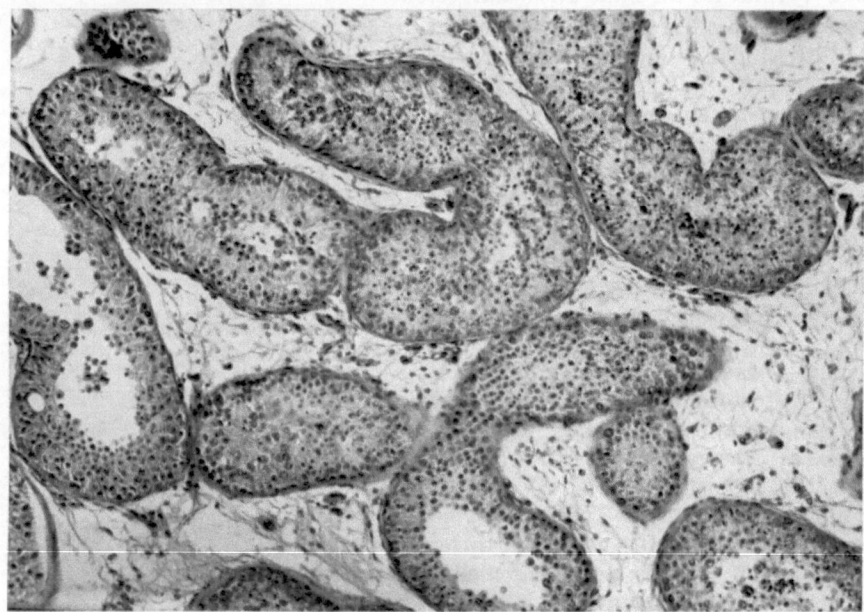

Abb. 38. D. R., 18jährig. Im Gegensatz zu der verhältnismäßig guten Entwicklung der Kanälchen sind die Leydigzellen kaum entfaltet. (Hämatoxylin-Eosin, 120fach) (Fall 3)

geprägt ist als der an ICSH. Die verdickte Tunica propria ist wahrscheinlich Folge der vorübergehenden Aktivierung der Leydigzellen durch HCG, die wieder aufgegeben worden war. Die Gynäkomastie paßt in keiner Weise zu dem negativen Gonadotropinbefund im Urin. Diagnose: Nur Pubertas tarda, wobei die FSH-Produktion jahrelang im Vordergrund stand.

b) Selektiver ICSH-Mangel. Hypogonadismus mit Spermiogenese

1953 beschrieben Pasqualini u. Mitarb., McCullach u. Mitarb. (1953) eine bis dahin nicht beachtete Form des Hypogonadismus, die durch eine inkretorische Hodeninsuffizienz bei weitgehender Erhaltung der Spermatogenese charakterisiert ist. In kurzer Folge wurden zahlreiche Fälle berichtet (Albert u. Mitarb. 1953, Conti, Landau 1953, Nelson 1953b, Nowakowsky u. Assmann 1957b, Tonutti 1956a und b). Bei diesen Menschen bestehen deutliche Zeichen eines präpuberalen Hypogonadismus trotz unerwartet großer Hoden, die histologisch ein entfaltendes Keimepithel mit reifen Spermien aufweisen; McCullagh u. Mitarb. (1953) sprechen daher auch vom „fertilen Eunuchen".

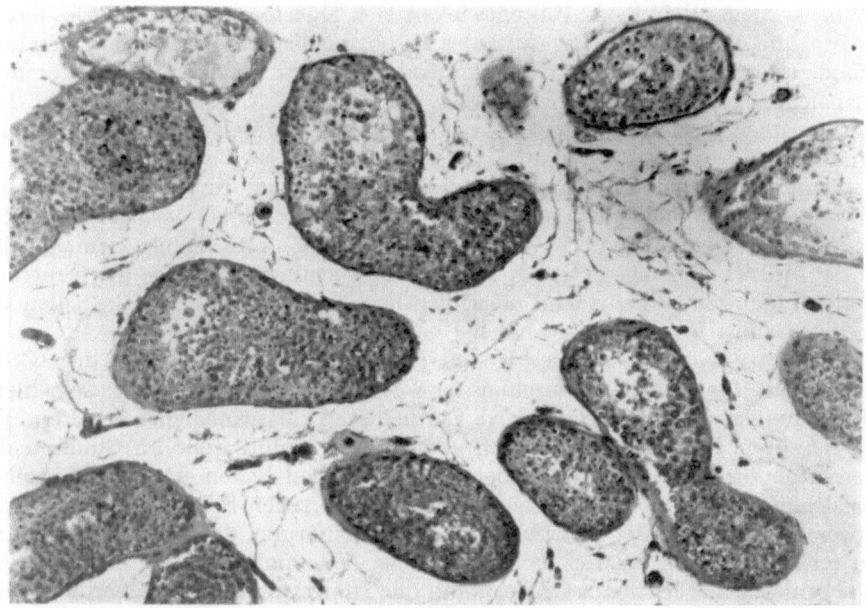

Abb. 39

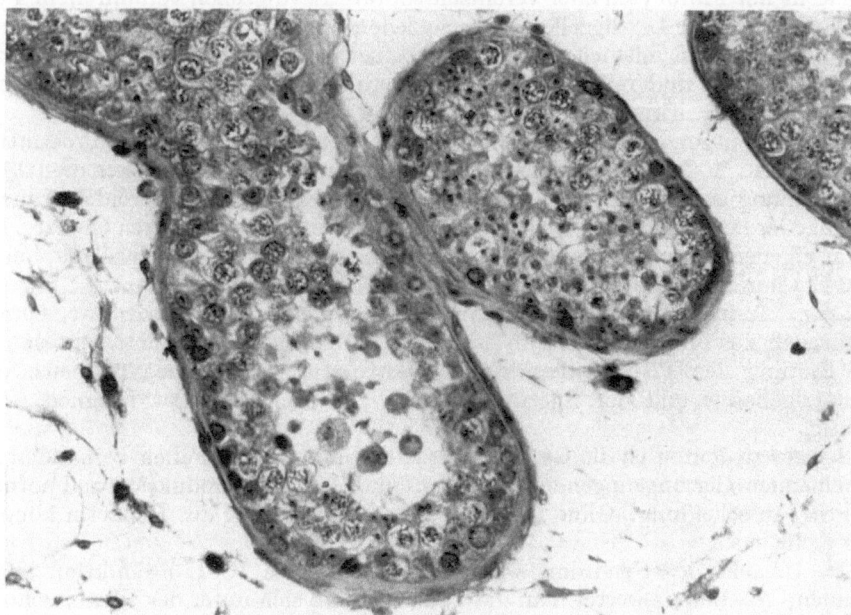

Abb. 40

Abb. 39 und 40. Kanälchen mit sehr kleinem Durchmesser, Tunica propria durchweg verdickt, Spermiogenese stoppt größtenteils bei den Spermatocyten I. Ordnung, in einigen Kanälchen sind alle Stadien vorhanden. Zwischengewebe außerordentlich faser- und zellarm („fertiler Eunuch"). (Hämatoxylin-Eosin 120- und 300fach) (Fall 4)

Die Kranken haben ausgesprochene eunuchoide Körperproportionen, schlecht entwickelte Muskulatur, häufig reichliches Fettpolster von femininer Verteilung, deutlich herabgesetzte Sekundär- und Geschlechtsbehaarung und oft ganz fehlende

Bartbehaarung. Bei einem Teil entwickelt sich eine Gynäkomastie. Die Größe der Prostata entspricht der Schwere des Hypogonadismus. Das äußere Genitale, besonders der Penis, ist klein und kontrastiert stark zu der wenig unter dem Normalen liegenden Größe der Hoden, die von fester Konsistenz sind. Der Hypogonadismus kann auch gering ausgeprägt sein, so daß nur der kleine Penis auffällt.

Wenn die Gewinnung eines Ejaculates möglich ist, findet man selbst bei schwerem Hypogonadismus einzelne reife Spermatozoen, bei geringeren Graden des Androgenmangels sind normale Spermienzahlen pro Kubikzentimeter berichtet. Die Gesamtmenge des Ejaculates ist vermindert, ebenso der Fructosegehalt. Libido und Potenz sind meist herabgesetzt. Einzelne Kranke sollen vor der Behandlung Kinder gehabt haben.

Der *histologische Befund* des Hodens ist abhängig vom Ausmaß der ICSH-Produktion. Der Kanälchendurchmesser wechselt, bei einzelnen ist er sehr klein, bei anderen normal. Das germinative Epithel ist in allen Kanälchen erhalten. Bei den schweren Formen sistiert die Spermiogenese größtenteils im Stadium der Spermatocyten erster Ordnung, aber auch in solchen Fällen erfolgt in einzelnen Kanälchen eine weitere Differenzierung bis zu den reifen Spermien. Bei weniger schweren Formen ist der Kanälchendurchmesser normal, das Keimepithel bis zu den reifen Spermien entwickelt, die gesamte Zellpopulation vermindert. Beim Hypogenitalismus schweren Grades kann die Tunica propria etwas verdickt sein.

Das Zwischengewebe ist faser- und zellarm und beim Schneiden sehr brüchig. Man sieht nur Fibrocyten oder vereinzelt solitäre Leydigzellen von unreifem Typ. Die Hypoplasie der Leydigzellen ist verschieden stark ausgeprägt, aber mit keiner histologischen oder histochemischen Färbemethode gelingt der Nachweis von wirklich aktiven und reifen Formen (Pasqualini 1953, McCullagh u. Mitarb. 1953, Tonutti u. Fetzer 1956 b) (vgl. Abb. 39 und 40).

Die Gesamtgonadotropinausscheidung ist normal, da die FSH-Produktion ungestört ist. McCullagh u. Mitarb. (1953) fanden bei einigen Kranken die ICSH-Ausscheidung erniedrigt. Auch die Ausscheidung der 17-Ketosteroide ist meist normal oder liegt selbst bei den schweren Formen nur an der unteren Grenze. Bei einem eigenen Kranken dieser Art erfolgte unter der sechstägigen Gabe von je 3000 E Choriongonadotropin ein Anstieg der 17-Ketosteroide von 6,1 mg auf 10,3 mg. Androsteron, das vorher im Plasma nicht nachweisbar war, betrug 6 Std nach der fünften Injektion 38,2 mg-%. Der Choriongonadotropintest mit der Prüfung der 17-Ketosteroide, der Oestrogene, des Spermavolumens, des Fructosegehaltes und der Spermienzahl ist zur Sicherung der Diagnose sehr wichtig.

Schwer zu deuten ist die Gynäkomastie, die in einzelnen Fällen vorhanden ist bei fehlender oder ungenügender Androgen- und Oestrogenproduktion und normaler FSH-Ausscheidung. Ohne Annahme einer Vermehrung des Prolactin kommt man nicht aus.

Als Ursache des Syndroms wird eine verminderte ICSH-Produktion angenommen. Als Beweis wertet man die Tatsache, daß sich unter der Verabreichung von Choriongonadotropin die Androgenbildung und die Reifung der Spermiogenese völlig normalisiert. Infolge des ICSH-Mangels, der in den klassischen Fällen angeboren ist, werden die Leydigzellen mit der Pubertät nicht oder ungenügend stimuliert. Zur Beurteilung der Schwere des ICSH-Mangels ist das klinische Bild wichtiger als das Aussehen des Zwischengewebes, da trotz eines nur leichten Hypogonadismus histologisch die Kriterien einer schweren Hypoplasie bestehen können. Dagegen gibt die Größe der Kanälchen einen besseren Anhalt für die Schwere des hormonalen Defektes. Die normale FSH-Ausscheidung zeigt an, daß die Kanälchen eine normale Menge von Hemmfaktoren produzieren auch in Fällen, bei denen die Leydigzellen völlig inaktiv sind. Dieses Syndrom spricht gegen die Ansicht, daß das sog. Inhibin mit den in den Leydigzellen produzierten Oestrogenen gleichzusetzen ist. In seiner vollen Ausprägung ist es außerdem ein Beweis für den Dualismus der hypophysären Gonadotropine und endlich dafür, daß das FSH allein für die Reifung des Samenepithels nicht ausreicht.

Zwei Beispiele:

Fall 4. W. H., 32jährig, 1959. Als Kind Masern, Diphtherie, sonst nicht krank.

Die Pubertät ist ausgeblieben. Mit 28 Jahren 150 cm groß, mit 32 Jahren 167 cm. Auch im letzten Jahr noch etwas gewachsen. Leicht ermüdbar, körperlich nicht leistungsfähig. Immer schlecht entwickelte Muskulatur, viel Fett an Bauch, Hüften, Brust, Oberschenkel, hat sich nie rasiert, nie eine Körperbehaarung gehabt, immer nur ganz wenig Schamhaare, keine Achselbehaarung. Als 20jähriger vorübergehende Testosteronbehandlung, fühlte sich körperlich wesentlich leistungsfähiger, auch Libido und Potenz nahmen zu, das Genitale wurde größer.

169 cm, Oberlänge 77 cm, Unterlänge 92 cm, Einhalbspannweite 87,5 cm, Gewicht 71,6 kg, reichliche Fettanhäufung im Bereich des Bauches und der Mammae, schlecht entwickelte Muskulatur, zarte, weiche, etwas pastöse Haut, erhebliche X-Beine, leichte Kyphose der Brustwirbelsäule, hohe Stimme, kaum ausgebildeter Kehlkopf.

Behaarung: wenige Schamhaare, fehlende Achsel-, Gesichts- und Körperbehaarung.

Genitale: Penis 5 cm, beide Hoden kleinkastaniengroß, feste Konsistenz, Prostata nur als bindegewebiger Strang zu tasten.

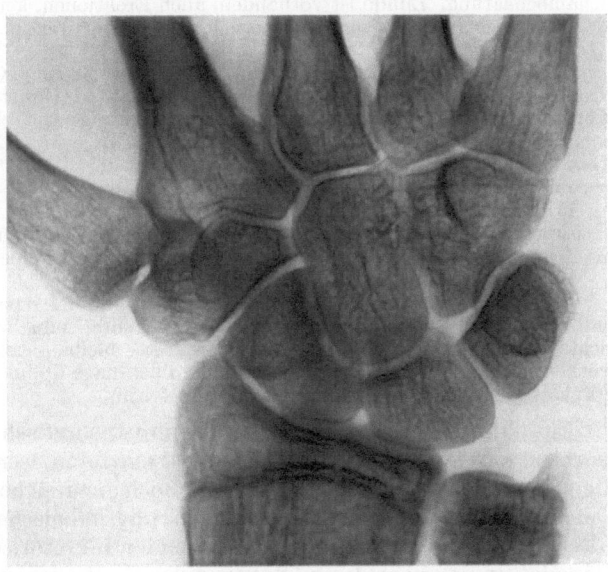

Abb. 41. „Fertiler Eunuch" (Fall 4). Als Zeichen des schweren präpuberalen ICSH-Mangels sind Radius- und Ulnaepiphyse bei dem 31jährigen Mann noch offen

Skelet: Radiusepiphyse noch offen (vgl. Abb. 41), Randleisten der Wirbelkörper noch sichtbar.

17-Ketosteroide: 4,9, 5,0, 5,6 mg. Porter-Silberchromogene 7,3, 7,9, 8,2 mg. Gonadotropine im Urin nicht sicher festzustellen.

Kernchromatine in Mundepithelien negativ.

Ejaculat nicht zu gewinnen.

Probeexcision aus dem rechten Hoden (Prof. Tonutti): Die Tubuli haben einen sehr kleinen Durchmesser, die Tunica propria ist durchweg verdickt. Das germinative Epithel ist in allen Kanälchen erhalten, die Spermiogenese sistiert jedoch großenteils im Stadium der Spermatocyten erster Ordnung, es finden sich jedoch in einigen Kanälchen auch die weiteren Stadien, insbesondere auch Spermien. Das Zwischengewebe ist außerordentlich faser- und zellarm. Die kleinen Arteriolen weisen teilweise eine verdickte hyalinisierte Wand auf. An Zellen finden sich im Zwischengewebe Fibrocyten und nur ganz vereinzelt solitäre Leydigzellen unreifen Types. *Diagnose:* hochgradige Reduktion der Spermatogenese, größtenteils Block bei Spermatocyten erster Ordnung. Reife Leydigzellen fehlen vollständig. ICSH-Mangel (Abb. 39 und 40).

Behandlung mit Choriongonadotropin dreimal 1000 E pro Woche über 6 Monate. Wesentliche subjektive Besserung, mäßige Zunahme der Achsel-, Scham- und Körperbehaarung. Kräftiges Wachstum des Penis, deutliches Wachstum beider Hoden, die nach 6 Monaten pflaumengroß sind und eine feste Konsistenz besitzen. Libido und Potenz normal, die Ehefrau erwartet ein Kind.

Ejaculat: 4 cm³, von normaler Konsistenz. Im Kubikzentimeter 61 Mill. Spermien, von denen $^2/_3$ eine normale Beweglichkeit besitzen.

Nach 6 Monaten Reduzierung der Dosis auf einmal 1000 E pro Woche. Darunter noch gutes Befinden, aber deutliche Abnahme von Libido und Potenz, Kleiner- und Weicherwerden der Hoden. Ejaculat nur 1 cm³, Spermienzahl 1,5 Mill.

Nach vorübergehendem Aussetzen der Behandlung Übergang auf Testosteron 200 mg Oenanthat alle 4 Wochen. Darunter kräftiger Anstieg von Libido und Potenz, die noch nie so stark gewesen ist wie jetzt. Wachstum der sekundären Geschlechtsmerkmale, der Körperbehaarung mit Ausnahme der Gesichtsbehaarung. Abnahme der Hodengröße, Ejaculat 6 cm³, 1,8 Mill. Spermien pro Kubikzentimeter.

Fall 5. C. F., 33jährig, 1958.

Früher nie krank. Beabsichtigt, sich zu verheiraten und möchte Klarheit über seinen sexuellen Zustand. Ihm selbst fällt auf, daß das Genitale zu klein ist. In der Jugend rasch gewachsen, auch noch im Alter von 25 Jahren etwas an Körpergröße zugenommen, Stimmbruch blieb aus, kein Bart gewachsen, Körperbehaarung sehr dürftig, ebenso Achsel- und Schambehaarung. Libido ist vorhanden, auch Erektionen, keine Pollutionen.

Fühlt sich frisch, gesund, körperlich und geistig wendig. Seit 2 Jahren Bürgermeister einer Gemeinde.

Größe 185 cm, Oberlänge 87 cm, Unterlänge 98 cm. Gewicht 92,3 kg. Eunuchoide Proportionen, kräftige Muskulatur, blasse Haut und Gesichtsfarbe, keine Behaarung am Körper, kein Bartwuchs, Achselbehaarung sehr gering, Schambehaarung dürftig. Fettanhäufungen im Bereich der Brust und am Bauch, geringe Gynäkomastie. Genitale: Penis 6 cm, Hoden kleinwalnußgroß, von ziemlich fester Konsistenz. Prostata flacher bindegewebiger Körper. Ejaculat nicht zu gewinnen.

17-Ketosteroide: 18,2, 14,6, unter ACTH 29,0 mg, Gonadotropine 24 MEU positiv. Probeexcision: Kanälchen stark verkleinert, Wand nicht verdickt, dürftige Spermiogenese, meist nur bis Spermatocyten erster Ordnung, einzelne Fibrocyten, keine Leydigzellen.

Diagnose: Wahrscheinlich fertiler Eunuch.

Behandlung mit Testosteronoenanthat 250 mg alle 4 Wochen. Wachstum der primären und sekundären Geschlechtsorgane, auch der Achsel- und Schambehaarung, nicht der Gesichts- und Körperbehaarung. Größe der Testes bleibt gleich. Nach Heirat HCG zweimal wöchentlich 1500 E. Beide Hoden werden größer, nach dreimonatiger Therapie wird Ehefrau gravide. Darauf wieder Übergang auf Testosteron.

Ein ähnliches histologisches Bild kann theoretisch bei angeborenem oder erworbenem Defekt der Leydigzellen selbst auftreten, wenn diese auf das in normaler Menge produzierte ICSH nicht oder nur noch unzureichend ansprechen. Ein solcher Defekt entwickelt sich wahrscheinlich physiologischerweise mit zunehmendem Alter und ist die Ursache der abnehmenden inkretorischen Leistung bei erhöhter Gonadotropinausscheidung (Nowakowski u. Assmann 1957 b).

Ob es bei jüngeren Menschen neben dem angeborenen auch eine erworbenen ICSH-Mangel gibt, ist nicht aufgeklärt. Kimmig (1955) deutet die Erniedrigung des Fructosegehaltes im Sperma bei normalen Spermienzahlen, normalem Aussehen und normaler Beweglichkeit der Spermien bei Menschen ohne irgendwelche Zeichen eines Hypogonadismus auf diese Weise.

Die Fructosekonzentration lag in seinen Fällen zwischen 280 und 500 γ/cm³ gegenüber einem Normalwert von 1500 γ/cm³. Diese Erniedrigung glich sich nach Verabreichung von Choriongonadotropin oder kleinen Dosen Methyltestosteron (10 mg) täglich aus (Nowakowski 1959). Die Bildung der Androgene in den Leydigzellen wäre in diesen Fällen ausreichend, um die Spermatogenese und die sekundären Geschlechtsmerkmale voll zu entfalten und zu erhalten, ungenügend aber, um die Fructoseproduktion in den Samenblasen auf normale Höhe zu bringen. Es sei daran erinnert, daß Prolactin das Ansprechen von Samenblasen und Prostata auf Androgene bessert (Pasqualini), möglicherweise liegt in diesen Fällen eine mangelhafte Prolactinproduktion vor.

Die *Behandlung* des Hypogonadismus mit Spermiogenese besteht in der Verabreichung von ICSH, also von HCG.

Darunter vermindern sich die Zeichen des Hypogonadismus, auch bei intensiver und langdauernder Behandlung bilden sie sich bei Beginn der Therapie im Erwachsenenalter nicht mehr völlig zurück. Wenn der Hoden vorher klein war, vergrößert er sich, die Spermiogenese, Menge des Ejaculats, Fructosegehalt normalisieren sich.

Die notwendige Dosis ist in den einzelnen Fällen verschieden, abhängig von der Schwere des Mangels. Bei zwei eigenen Kranken mit mittelschwerem Hypogonadismus waren dreimal 1000—1500 E HCG pro Woche ausreichend. Zahl der Spermien, Menge des Ejaculats, Libido und Potenz wurden im Laufe von 4—8 Wochen normal, die Partner konzipierten. Unter einmal 1000 E Choriongonadotropin pro Woche sank der Spermiengehalt rasch auf $1/_4$ ab. Theoretisch muß die HCG-Behandlung dauernd fortgesetzt werden, einmal weil die Leydigzellen nur durch HCG entfaltet bleiben, dann aber auch weil sich nach seinem Absetzen die voll entwickelten Kanälchen wieder zurückbilden und bei mehrfachem Hin und Her die Gefahr der Sklerosierung der Kanälchenwand gegeben ist. Testosterondepot gleicht den Hypogonadismus ebenso aus, vermindert in höheren Dosen jedoch durch Hemmung der Gonadotropinbildung die noch vorhandene Spermiogenese. Bei den hohen Kosten der HCG-Therapie ist die intermittierende Testosterontherapie aber unvermeidlich.

Die Angaben in der Literatur, daß kleine und mittlere Dosen Testosteron, so z. B. 25 mg Testosteronpropionat intramuskulär oder Methyltestosteron 10—24 mg per os (LANDAU 1953) den Gehalt der Spermatozoen im Ejaculat deutlich erhöhen, können wir nicht bestätigen. Bei zwei eigenen Fällen ging die durch HCG normalisierte Spermienzahl unter 150—200 mg Testosteron-Oenanthat, alle 4 Wochen rasch zurück.

c) Selektiver FSH-Mangel

Bei der Entwicklung von Geschwülsten der Adenohypophyse und des Zwischenhirns geht die Reifungshemmung des Samenepithels und die Atrophie der Kanälchen der Atrophie der Leydigzellen meist voraus (SNIFFEN u. Mitarb. 1950b, McCULLAGH u. Mitarb. 1953). Bei unvollständiger Entfernung der Hypophyse oder nach intensiver Röntgenbestrahlung kann ein selektiver FSH-Mangel entstehen. Diese Formen sind selten und meist nur Durchgangsstadien zu schwereren Defekten. Das histologische Bild ist das des Spermiogenese-Stopps auf der Stufe der Spermatocyten, selten auf der Stufe der Spermatogonien bei vorhandenen Leydigzellen. Man kann diese Veränderung künstlich durch die gleichzeitige Verabreichung von Choriongonadotropin und Testosteron, wie z.B. beim Rebound-Phänomen, auslösen. Unter der gehemmten Gonadotropinproduktion bleibt die Spermiogenese auf der Stufe der Spermatocyten stehen, während die Leydigzellen entfaltet bleiben. Man erhebt also denselben Befund des „spermiogenic arrest" wie bei infertilen Männern. Ob es eine idiopathische Form des isolierten FSH-Mangels mit Stehenbleiben der Spermiogenese auf der Stufe der Spermatocyten oder Spermatogonien bei normal entfalteten Leydigzellen gibt, erscheint möglich, ist aber nicht sichergestellt, da die Abtrennung von FSH und ICSH im Urin und damit die getrennte Bestimmung der beiden Hormone noch nicht durchführbar ist. Fälle mit undifferenziertem Samenepithel (HORNSTEIN) bei normalen Leydigzellen erwecken den Verdacht auf einen angeborenen Defekt des Kanälchenepithels.

7. Hemmung der Gonadotropinbildung durch Sexual- und andere Hormone

Wie früher besprochen, hemmt die Verabreichung höherer Dosen von Androgenen über längere Zeit beim Menschen Abgabe und Produktion der Gonadotropine im Hypophysenvorderlappen. Das einzige was bei der körperlichen Unter-

suchung auffällt, ist die verminderte Konsistenz des Hodens. Histologisch sind
die Folgen sehr deutlich, indem sowohl eine Atrophie der Leydigschen Zwischenzellen als auch der Samenkanälchen mit tubulärer Insuffizienz im Sinne der
Azoo- bzw. Oligospermie eintritt mit dem Bild des Spermiogenese-Stopps
(s. S. 774).

Vermehrt Androgene können beim Mann bei Tumoren der Leydigzellen und
der Nebennierenrinde anfallen. Entwickeln sich solche Geschwülste bei Jugendlichen, dann entsteht die Pseudopubertas praecox (s. dort).

Die Gonadotropinausscheidung ist im allgemeinen vermindert, bei langdauernder Androgeneinwirkung kann sie sich wieder normalisieren. Die 17-Keto-

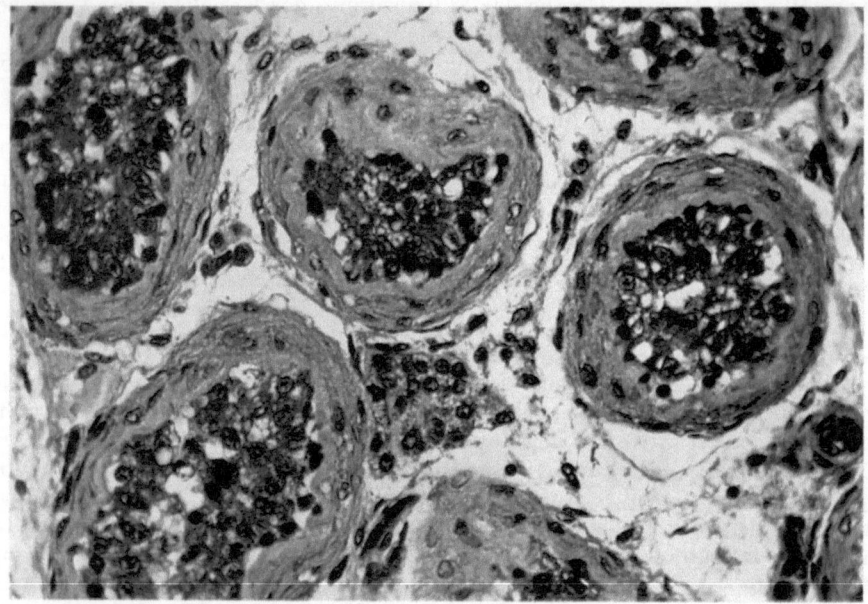

Abb. 42. 64jähriger Mann mit einer seit 2 Jahren rasch fortschreitenden Lebercirrhose. Tubuli stark verkleinert,
Wand beträchtlich verdickt, nur Sertolizellen und einzelne Spermatogonien, intertubuläres Gewebe faserarm, nur
sehr kleine Leydigzellen. (Hämatoxylin-Eosin, 300fach)

steroide sind normal oder erhöht. Ohne Hodenbiopsie ist eine sichere Diagnose
nicht möglich.

Auch der als Folge einer vermehrten *Oestrogeneinwirkung* eintretende Hypogonadismus ist durch die Hemmung der Gonadotropinbildung bedingt. Die
Atrophie betrifft sowohl die Samenkanälchen als auch die Leydigzellen, wobei
das histologische Bild verschiedene Phasen durchläuft (s. S. 711—713). Die Veränderungen sind reversibel, nach Aufhören der Oestrogeneinwirkung können sich
selbst schwere Veränderungen des Hodenparenchyms im Laufe von Monaten
wieder zurückbilden (SNIFFEN u. Mitarb. 1950b).

Eine pathologische Oestrogeneinwirkung beobachtet man häufig bei chronischen Erkrankungen der Leber, besonders der *Lebercirrhose* (s. Abb. 42.) Das
histologische Bild des Hodens gleicht ganz dem nach Verabreichung von Oestrogenen. Bei kurzer Krankheitsdauer finden sich nur die Zeichen einer Reifungshemmung der Spermiogenese auf verschiedenen Stadien, bei schweren und fortgeschrittenen Cirrhosen dagegen eine weitgehende bindegewebige Umwandlung
der Kanälchen und eine Atrophie der Leydigzellen (vgl. Abb. 42). In einigen

Fällen wurde eine ausgesprochene Hyperplasie der Leydigzellen beobachtet, die schon BARRELET (1912) aufgefallen ist und auch von anderen beschrieben wurde (LLOYD u. WILLIAMS 1948, RAVENNA 1940 und 1943).

Die Ursache der Hodenatrophie sieht man in einer Hemmung der Gonadotropinproduktion des Hypophysenvorderlappens. Alle fortgeschrittenen Lebercirrhotiker bieten Zeichen des sekundären Hypogonadismus mit Atrophie der Hoden, Abnahme der Scham- und Körperbehaarung, Schwund von Libido und Potenz, Verkleinerung der Prostata. Oft entwickeln sich auch klinische Zeichen eines Hyperoestrogenismus, denn die Gynäkomastie ist ein häufiges Symptom der Lebercirrhose (LEDERER, VOEGT u. WELLER). BARR und SOMMERS (1957) finden in 90% autoptisch Untersuchter Zeichen einer vermehrten Oestrogeneinwirkung auf die Brustdrüse und die Prostata. Die Prostatahypertrophie ist beim Cirrhotiker seltener als bei gesunden Gleichaltrigen, 30 gegen 53%. Palmar- und Plantarerythem werden auch mit dem erhöhten Oestrogenspiegel in Zusammenhang gebracht.

Die 17-Ketosteroidausscheidung ist stark vermindert. Da die Umwandlung der Androgene in harnfähige 17-Ketosteroide bei schwereren Leberschädigungen leidet, darf diese Erniedrigung nicht mit der Abnahme der Leydigzellfunktion gleichgesetzt werden. Die Uringonadotropine sind meist erniedrigt, in einigen Fällen wurden auch erhöhte Werte beobachtet.

Die letzte Ursache der erhöhten Zirkulation von Oestrogenen ist nicht geklärt. ZONDEK hat 1934 festgestellt, daß Oestron durch Leberbrei inaktiviert wird. Weiter fand man, daß die Implantation von Ovarien oder von Oestradioltabletten in das Mesenterium oder die Milz kastrierter weiblicher Mäuse die Kastrationsfolgen nicht ausgleicht, es entwickelt sich sogar eine Kastrationshypophyse. Man nimmt an, daß bei der Lebercirrhose die Inaktivierung der Oestrogene, besonders die Bindung an Schwefelsäure und Glucuronsäure gestört ist, doch konnten in vitro keine Unterschiede zwischen normalen Lebern und solchen von Cirrhotikern festgestellt werden. Auch die Ausscheidung der Oestrogene im Urin ist nicht einheitlich. BENNETT u. Mitarb. finden die Gesamtwerte normal, PINCUS u. Mitarb. (1951) dagegen immer erhöht.

Neben der verminderten Inaktivierung der Oestrogene wird auch eine gesteigerte Umwandlung von Androgenen zu Oestrogenen diskutiert. Letzten Endes ist es aber unklar, woher die Oestrogene stammen, denn wie sollen die ganz atrophisch gewordenen Leydigzellen noch Oestrogene produzieren?

Die Bilder der Leydigzellhyperplasie, wie sie selten zu sehen sind, können nur über eine vermehrte ICSH-Produktion erklärt werden, wie sie nach Desensibilisierung der Regulationszentren des Zwischenhirns auch im Experiment festzustellen ist (HOHLWEG 1953b). Ob darüber hinaus in der geschädigten Leber auch eine Bildung von Oestrogenen aus anderen Steroiden stattfindet, vielleicht aus DEA oder Androstendion der Nebennierenrinde, erscheint möglich.

Andere Hormone. Bei *Ausfall der Nebennierenrindenfunktion* durch Zerstörung des Nebennierengewebes bleibt die Funktion der Keimdrüsen lange unverändert. Bei schweren Formen klagen die Kranken über eine Abnahme von Libido und Potenz, doch ist dies mehr eine Folge des schlechten Gesamtzustandes, als die Folge einer echten inkretorischen oder spermiogenetischen Insuffizienz. Eine solche ist beim M. Addison nicht sicher nachgewiesen.

Die *Überfunktion der Nebennierenrinde*, der M. Cushing, dagegen bietet häufig eine funktionelle Keimdrüseninsuffizienz, besonders wenn gleichzeitig die Androgenproduktion in der Nebenniere vemehrt ist. Neben den Symptomen des M. Cushing besteht dabei eine beträchliche Zunahme der Körperbehaarung, eine Acne, der Muskelschwund ist mäßig, Libido und Potenz sind gestört. Bioptisch zeigt sich das Bild der vermehrten Androgenproduktion mit Hemmung der Gonadotropinbildung. Die reinen Cushingtypen mit alleiniger Cortisolüberproduktion sind dagegen bioptisch unauffällig.

Schilddrüse. Der sporadische Kretinismus, das angeborene und frühkindliche Myxödem sind gekennzeichnet durch geistige Defekte, durch Wachstumsstörungen und durch Anomalien der Genitalentwicklung. Besonders in die Augen springend ist die Wachstumsstörung. Aus dem Tierexperiment weiß man, daß das Wachstumshormon an den Epiphysen seine volle Wirkung nur bei Anwesenheit des Schilddrüsenhormons entfaltet. Die Knochenkerne treten verspätet auf, das Knorpelwachstum und die Kalkeinlagerung in den Epiphysen verläuft atypisch, der Epiphysenschluß erfolgt verzögert, so daß ein Minderwuchs mit kurzen, aber breiten Röhrenknochen resultiert. Im Bereich des Schenkelhalskopfes entstehen durch die Belastung häufig Nekrosen, die dann zum Bild der Kretinenhüfte führen. Menschen mit isolierter Athyreose bzw. schwerer Hypothyreose erreichen im allgemeinen eine Körpergröße um 150 cm. Bei den seltenen athyreotischen Zwergen mit wenig mehr als 1 m Körperlänge sind noch andere Defekte vorhanden.

Bei den unkomplizierten A- und Hypothyreosen verläuft die Entwicklung etwas verzögert, es wird aber ein normales Reifungsstadium erreicht. Sind beim Erwachsenen noch Zeichen eines Hypogonadismus vorhanden, dann ist dieser Folge einer zusätzlichen organischen Erkrankung des hypophysen Zwischenhirnsystems und nicht der einfachen Hypothyreose. In den meisten Fällen ist die Schilddrüsenfunktion nicht gänzlich erloschen. Hier findet sich die typische Wachstumsstörung in abgeschwächter Form. Die strenge Kongruenz der Pupertätsentwicklung mit der Knochenreifung, wie sie für den Gesunden so charakteristisch ist, gilt für die Hypothyreose nicht.

8. Exogene Ursachen

Unterernährung. Der Einfluß des *Eiweißmangels* ist im Experiment am besten untersucht. Bei jungen Mäusen und Ratten verhindert die Fütterung einer eiweißfreien Kost die Reifung der Hoden und der akzessorischen Sexualorgane (Horn 1955). *Junge* Ratten, die ohne Eiweiß aufgezogen wurden, hatten nach 30 Tagen ein Hodengewicht von 140 mg gegenüber 1695 mg ihrer Kontrollen, die 20% Casein erhalten hatten. Schon bei einem 6%igen Caseingehalt der Nahrung erhöht sich das Hodengewicht, die Spermatozoenbildung kommt in Gang, obwohl der Eiweißgehalt der Nahrung für das Körperwachstum unzureichend ist. *Ausgewachsene* Tiere sind viel widerstandsfähiger. Das Durchschnittsgewicht der Hoden von 25 Ratten, die 90 Tage eiweißfrei ernährt waren, betrug 1429 mg im Vergleich zu 3001 mg der Kontrollen, dabei war die Atrophie keineswegs gleichmäßig, sondern schwankte zwischen einer vollständigen und einem völlig normalen Verhalten (Leathem 1958). Auch einfache untercalorische Ernährung, also *Hunger*, verhindert beim wachsenden Organismus die Reifung der Reproduktionsorgane. Die Ursache sieht man vorwiegend in der verminderten Produktion der hypophysären Gonadotropine (Leathem 1958), da ihre Verabreichung die Hodenfunktion im Experiment normalisiert, selbst bei Fortführung der eiweißfreien Kost. Mangel an spezifischen Aminosäuren hat dieselbe Wirkung wie Eiweißmangel.

Dagegen ist der Gehalt der Hypophyse an Gonadotropin im Hunger und bei eiweißarmer bzw. -freier Kost recht unterschiedlich. Man fand Verminderung (Mason u. Wolfe 1930, Werner 1939), normale Werte (Marrian u. Parkes 1929) und Erhöhung (Maddock u. Heller 1947). Wahrscheinlich nimmt eine

Funktionsstörung der Leber, die die anfallenden Androgene und Oestrogene ungenügend inaktiviert, an dem Geschehen teil. Der erhöhte Gonadotropingehalt weist zum mindesten in einer Phase des Geschehens auf eine primäre Schädigung des Keimepithels hin.

STEFKO beschreibt bei Menschen, die im Hunger gestorben sind, eine Atrophie des Kanälchenepithels mit Phagocytose der Spermatoziden durch die Sertolizellen, OVERZIER sah das Kanälchenepithel vielfach abgestoßen, das Epithel ist von der Basalmembran durch ein Ödem abgehoben, das so stark sein kann, daß die Kanälchenlichtung ganz verschlossen ist. Das Samenepithel ist entweder einfach atrophisch oder man sieht das Bild der Hypospermiogenese. Das Zwischengewebe verhält sich verschieden, in leichteren Fällen ist es unverändert, in schweren können die Leydigzellen vermehrt sein.

ZUBIRÁN u. Mitarb. (1953) untersuchten 256 Männer, die an chronischer Unterernährung litten. 80% klagte über Verlust der Potenz. 85% über Verminderung der Libido, bei 73% waren die Hoden atrophisch. Teleangiektasien waren in 74% vorhanden. Gynäkomastie bei Krankenhausaufnahme in 20%. Die Gynäkomastie ist in der Phase der Erholung viel häufiger, und zwar dann, wenn gleichzeitig auch die Oestrogenausscheidung erhöht ist. Unterernährte gefangene Soldaten bekamen in hohem Prozentsatz 3—12 Wochen nach ausreichender Ernährung eine Gynäkomastie.

Die histologische Untersuchung von 89 Hoden zeigte eine Abnahme des Kanälchendurchmessers bei 54, eine verdickte Basalmembran in 56 Fällen, Abnahme der Höhe des Keimepithels in 75 Fällen, 34mal das Bild des „germinal cell arrest", 41mal fehlte die aktive Spermatogenese. Die Sertolizellen waren häufig vacuolisiert, die Leydigzellen klein, spärlich an Zahl, und in 63 Fällen mit braunem Pigment beladen. 25mal war eine diffuse oder fokale Fibrose vorhanden, 28 mal Rundzellinfiltrate. Die Produktion von FSH scheint früher gestört zu werden als die von ICSH.

Vitaminmangel. Nur bei geschlechtsreifen Ratten, Meerschweinchen und Schweinen führt künstlicher *Vitamin E-Mangel* zu irreparablen Schäden der Spermiogenese. Als erstes fällt die Einschränkung der Beweglichkeit der Spermien auf, später eine Azoospermie und eine Atrophie der Kanälchen. Die Ursache ist nicht sichergestellt. Vitamin E hemmt die *Hodenhyaluronidase* erheblich, so daß man eine plötzliche starke Vermehrung der Hyaluronsäure vermutet, die eine Schädigung des Keimepithels nach sich zieht. Als Folge der Kanälchendegeneration vermehrt sich sekundär der Gehalt der Adenohypophyse an gonadotropen Hormonen, doch sind diese Beobachtungen nicht einheitlich (P'AN u. Mitarb. 1949).

Auch beim schweren *Lactoflavin*- und *Pyridoxinmangel* ist eine gewisse Schädigung der Keimdrüsen bekannt. Vitamin B_6-Mangel führt im Experiment an der Ratte zu einer erheblichen Vermehrung der hypophysären Gonadotropine, besonders von FSH, wobei sowohl eine verminderte Abgabe als auch eine vermehrte Bildung diskutiert wird (WOOTEN u. Mitarb. 1955). Ob Vitaminmangel allein beim Menschen eine Hodenatrophie bewirken kann, ist nicht sichergestellt, da alle Vitaminmangelerkrankungen von einer Unterernährung oder von einer Eiweißmangelernährung begleitet sind. An sich sind Vitaminmangelschäden auch beim Mitteleuropäer nicht ganz selten, nicht als Folge einer Unterernährung, sondern als Folge von Resorptionsstörungen.

Nur beim jugendlichen Menschen stören *chronische Erkrankungen* der verschiedensten Art die rechtzeitige Aufnahme der Gonadotropinbildung. Die *Pubertas tarda* wird aber in jedem Falle nach Heilung der Grundkrankheit überwunden. Der erwachsene Mensch ist bedeutend weniger empfindlich.

Akute *schwere Belastungen* können zu einer vorübergehenden Abnahme der Gonadotropinsekretion führen (Selye 1945). Es soll in der Stress-Situation eine Umschaltung der Hypophysenfunktion eintreten, indem die vermehrte Abgabe von ACTH mit einer Drosselung der Abgabe von gonadotropem und thyreotropem Hormon beantwortet wird. Die Folge ist eine nur wenige Tage anhaltende Depression der Spermiogenese nach Operationen und anderen akuten Schäden. Bei schweren chronischen Krankheiten konnten wir keine Verminderung der Gonadotropinausscheidung feststellen.

III. Behandlung

1. Choriongonadotropin (HCG)

Man trifft vielfach die Auffassung, daß die alleinige Behandlung des hypogonadotropen Hypogonadismus, sei es der idiopathischen, sei es der organischen Formen, mit Choriongonadotropin (HCG) ohne nennenswerten Erfolg sei. Man erreicht eine Entfaltung der Leydigzellen, die die Androgenproduktion aufnehmen, primäre und sekundäre Geschlechtsmerkmale wachsen, aber trotz intensiver Behandlung wird bei den präpuberalen Formen keine Reifung der Kanälchen erreicht.

Jeder, der eine größere Zahl von Menschen mit präpuberalem Hypogonadismus konsequent mit HCG behandelt hat, sah schon unerwartete Besserungen in Fällen, die als echte idiopathische Formen aufgefaßt waren und histologisch das Bild des präpuberalen Hodens zeigten. Wenn bei solchen 17—22jährigen die Hoden doch noch anfangen zu wachsen, Gonadotropine im Urin nachweisbar werden und die Entwicklung auch nach Absetzen des HCG fortschreitet, dann kann es sich selbst bei älteren Messchen nur um funktionelle Störungen der Gonadotropinbildung gehandelt haben, um eine Pubertas tarda. Solche Fälle sind von Kinsell (1947), Hurxthal (1943), Bartter u. Mitarb. (1951), Heller und Nelson (1948b) u.a. mitgeteilt. Manchmal hat man den Eindruck, daß ohne die intensive HCG-Behandlung die Eigenproduktion der Gonadotropine nicht mehr in Gang gekommen wäre, daß also in diesen Fällen das Sexualzentrum unter der Einwirkung der Sexualhormone erst voll ausreifen muß, eine Ansicht, die man vorläufig nicht beweisen kann.

In eine zweite Gruppe sind Fälle einzuordnen, bei denen durch langdauernde und intensive HCG-Gabe eine Reifung der Leydigzellen und in gewissem Umfange auch des Samenepithels erreicht wurde, bei denen sich aber die Reifezeichen nach Unterbrechung der Behandlung wieder zurückbildeten. Hierher gehören die von Nielson u. Mitarb. (1956) veröffentlichten Fälle. Es handelte sich um 13 Kranke mit sekundärem Eunuchoidismus, von denen zehn der Gruppe der „idiopathischen" Formen zugehörten, zwei einen Panhypopituitarismus hatten und einer weder Gonadotropine noch 17-Ketosteroide im Urin ausschied. Vor der Behandlung ergab die Biopsie elfmal das Bild des präpuberalen Hoden, einmal eine gewisse Reifung des Samenepithels, zweimal eine verdickte Tunica propria. Behandelt wurde 15—72 Monate mit 5000—10000 iE HCG wöchentlich bzw. 14tägig. Die Änderung des Befundes wurde durch wiederholte Biopsien überprüft. Die vor der Behandlung immer erniedrigte 17-Ketosteroidausscheidung stieg während der Behandlung an und fiel nach Aufhören der Hormongabe als Zeichen des irreparablen Gonadotropindefektes wieder auf die alten Werte ab. Histologisch reiften die Leydigzellen aus, eine verdickte Tunica propria bildete sich zurück, auch die Kanälchen reiften in gewissem Umfange. Bei fünf von sieben Patienten konnten im Ejaculat während der Behandlung bewegliche Spermien nachgewiesen werden, jedoch nur einmal über 1 Mill. Alle Patienten bekamen vorübergehend eine Makromastie. Die zusätzliche Verabreichung von Methyltestosteron bei einem Teil der Fälle änderte am klinischen Bild nichts. BARTTER u. Mitarb. (1951) hatten schon früher über sechs Fälle mit erniedrigtem Uringonadotropin und völliger Unreife des Hodens berichtet, bei denen unter der HCG-Behandlung eine Reifung aller Hodenelemente einschließlich der Spermatocyten eintrat und in drei Fällen reife Spermatozoen nachgewiesen werden konnten. Nach Aufhören der Behandlung bildeten sich die Reifungserscheinungen wieder zurück.

Seit das Krankheitsbild des fertilen Eunuchen bekannt ist, hat man angenommen, daß es sich bei diesen erfolgreich allein mit HCG behandelten Fällen um den isolierten Defekt der ICSH-Produktion handelt. Nach den bioptischen Befunden trifft dies sicher nicht für alle Fälle, bei denen das Samenepithel angeregt wurde. zu. Ob aber diese erfolgreich behandelten Kranken nicht doch eine geringe Eigenproduktion von FSH hatten, die allein am Samenepithel nicht wirksam werden konnte — Bild des präpuberalen Hodens — ist nicht ausgeschlossen, wenn man die potenzierende Wirkung eines Gemisches von FSH und ICSH im Tierexperiment (s. bei hypophysäre Gonadotropine) in Betracht zieht. Eine solche unterschwellige Gonadotropinbildung ist mit den heutigen Nachweismethoden nicht zu erfassen. Der Erfolg wird um so besser sein, je weiter die Kanälchenreifung vor der Behandlung fortgeschritten ist, je mehr FSH spontan gebildet wird. In solchen Fällen kann man die volle Spermiogenese erreichen. Abbruch der HCG-Gabe führt aber zur Rückbildung der Hodenreifung.

Die Frage, ob beim Menschen mit HCG allein bei völligem Fehlen der eigenen Gonadotropinbildung eine Reifung des Samenepithels bis zu den Spermatozoen erfolgen kann, ist daher noch nicht entschieden, während das Ansprechen der Leydigzellen so oft beobachtet wurde, daß das Ausbleiben ihrer Reaktion als Ausdruck der minderwertigen Anlage der Zellen im Sinne der fehlenden Entwicklungspotenzen oder im Sinne der Unfähigkeit zur Hormonbildung (Fermentmangel) gedeutet werden kann.

Die postpuberalen Formen des hypogonadotropen Eunuchoidismus werden meist wegen des ausgedehnteren Defektes der Adenohypophyse von Anfang an kombiniert mit Testosteron, Cortison bzw. Prednison behandelt. Zunahme der 17-Ketosteroidausscheidung, Wachstum der Sekundärbehaarung und Vergrößerung der Prostata kann man aber leicht mit Dosen von dreimal 1500 E HCG pro Woche erreichen. Über die Rückbildung einer vorhandenen Kanälchenhyalinisierung weiß man wenig.

Die Dosierung wird verschieden gehandhabt: dreimal 1000 E pro Woche bis 5000 E pro Tag. Nach meinen Erfahrungen ist Steigerung der Dosis über 1000 E täglich ohne Wirkung, ja man hat sogar den Eindruck einer Wirkungsabschwächung, wenn 2000 E täglich überschritten werden. Da die Wirkungsdauer $2^1/_2$—3 Tage anhält (MADDOCK u. NELSON 1952) genügt die dreimalige Gabe pro Woche. Bei jüngeren Menschen benötigt man etwas weniger (dreimal 500—1000 E), bei älteren etwas mehr (dreimal 1500 E). Die Wirkung wird mit Hilfe der 17-Ketosteroid- bzw. Oestrogenausscheidung kontrolliert, die nach 8—14 Tagen ansteigt. Bei günstig reagierenden Fällen vergrößert sich nach 4—6 Wochen das Volumen des Hodens, Scrotum und Penis wachsen und langsam sprossen auch die Pubes. Die Volumenzunahme des Hodens ist immer ein Zeichen eines unvollständigen Gonadotropindefektes — geringe FSH-Produktion noch vorhanden —, die die eingeschlagene Behandlung erfolgversprechend macht. Bleibt eine Hodenvergrößerung auch nach 8—12 Wochen aus, dann sind die Aussichten für die Spermiogenese ungünstig. Man kann auch diese Fälle 8—12 Monate weiterbehandeln und für die endgültige Beurteilung den erneuten histologischen Befund zu Rate ziehen, doch steht der Aufwand in keinem Verhältnis zum Erfolg. Nach Erreichung einer genügenden Maskulinisierung wird die Dosis um ein Drittel oder die Hälfte verringert. Kranke, bei denen der Hoden unter der Behandlung wächst und das Samenepithel mitreift, wird man mit HCG allein zu Ende behandeln. Kranken, deren Hoden nicht größer geworden ist, gibt man nach 3—4 Monaten zusätzlich Serumgonadotropin. Erreicht man auch damit keine Volumenzunahme und bleibt das Epithel bei der bioptischen Kontrolle unbeeinflußt, dann geht man auf die reine Ersatzbehandlung mit Testosteron über.

2. Serumgonadotropin (PMSG)

Nachdem man lange Zeit vergebens die Entwicklung des Samenepithels mit HCG allein zu erreichen versucht hat, ist man in den letzten Jahren wieder auf die zusätzliche Verabreichung von Serumgonadotropin (PMSG) übergegangen. Endgültige Erfahrungen mit der kombinierten Behandlung liegen noch nicht vor. Die in früheren Jahren angewandten Präparate führten in kurzer Zeit zur Bildung von Antikörpern, so daß nicht nur das injizierte Serumgonadotropin, sondern auch die von der eigenen Hypophyse produzierten Gonadotropine inaktiviert wurden (s. S. 648). Diese Gefahr ist heute geringer, aber noch nicht ganz behoben. Man versucht die Antikörperbildung durch das Einlegen von zwei- bis dreiwöchigen Behandlungspausen und durch die Verabreichung von Prednisonen in der Dosis von 15—20 mg zu vermeiden.

GILBERT-DREYFUSS (1957) gibt beim hypogonadotropen Hypogonadismus beide Hormone in einer Spritze. Er mischt je 5000 iE HCG und 5000 iE SG, injiziert diese Menge täglich etwa 14 Tage lang, geht dann auf 3000 iE HCG und 1000—2000 iE SG zurück und gibt diese Dosis dreimal pro Woche über 3 Wochen des Monats. Nach zehntägiger Pause wird der Cyclus von neuem begonnen. Es ist fraglich, ob eine solch hohe Dosis mehr leistet als zwei- bis dreimal wöchentlich je 1000 E. Nach seinen Erfahrungen übertreffen die Ergebnisse dieser kombinierten Behandlung die alleinige HCG-Gabe beim sekundären Hypogonadismus beträchtlich. Das Volumen des Hodens nimmt deutlich zu, das Kanälchenepithel reift etwas, Spermatocyten erster Ordnung können auftreten. Es scheint, daß beim idiopathischen hypogonadotropen Eunuchoidismus mit unreifem Hodengewebe die Behandlungserfolge auch bezüglich der Anregung der Leydigzellen besser sind als mit der alleinigen HCG-Gabe. Daß bei Verwendung von menschlichem FSH in der Kombination mit HCG beim hypogonadotropen Eunuchoidismus eine normale Spermiogenese erreicht werden kann, haben HELLER und NELSON vor langen Jahren schon gezeigt.

Bei Oligo- und Hypospermien gibt man zweimal 500 bis zweimal 2000 E pro Woche und kombiniert die Behandlung mit HCG. Nach einem Vorschlag von HELLER und NELSON (1948b) sollte man durch eine hochdosierte und monatelang durchgeführte alleinige HCG-Behandlung das Zwischengewebe und das Kanälchenepithel zur höchsten erreichbaren Reifung gebracht haben, bevor man das artfremde Serumgonadotropin anwendet. Die Herstellung von FSH aus menschlichen Hypophysen ist heute in beschränktem Umfange möglich.

In den letzten 2 Jahren hat die Gewinnung von menschlichen Gonadotropin aus Hypophysen von Gestorbenen große Fortschritte gemacht, sie stehen in beschränktem Maße zur Anwendung zur Verfügung.

3. Testosterone

Neben den primären angeborenen oder erworbenen Schädigungen des Hodens ist auch der irreparable Defekt der Gonadotropinbildung in der Adenohypophyse eine wichtige Indikation für die Dauerbehandlung mit Testosteron. Es erfüllt hier die Aufgabe eines reinen Ersatzes. Man richtet sich in der Dosierung nach dem dort Gesagten.

Wie an anderer Stelle ausgeführt, ist die Abtrennung der organischen Schäden von funktionellen Störungen oft sehr schwierig und trotz eingehender Untersuchung im Einzelfall nicht immer sicher zu treffen. Dies mag die Ursache dafür sein, daß in der Literatur der früheren Jahre wiederholt über Fälle berichtet wurde, bei denen unter der Testosteronbehandlung eine Reifung der Keimdrüsen mit mehr oder weniger weitgehender Normalisierung der Spermiogenese eingetreten ist (HURXTHAL, KINSELL, PERLMAN 1949, PLUM, WERNER 1951). Der bemerkenswerte Fall von WERNER (1951) sei kurz angeführt: Ein 23jähriger Mann, 1938 mit den Zeichen eines präpuberalen Eunuchoidismus zum erstenmal untersucht, hatte eine Hodengröße von 0,5 × 0,5 cm bei weicher Konsistenz. Die Gonadotropinausscheidung war niedrig, die Knochenreife deutlich herabgesetzt. Der Kranke wurde mit Unterbrechungen anfangs mit dreimal 25 mg Testosteronpropionat intramuskulär wöchentlich, später mit Methyltestosteron per os 30—50 mg pro Tag bis 1949 behandelt und regelmäßig beobachtet. 1945 betrug die Hodengröße 1,5 × 1 × 0.5 cm. 1948 2.5 × 2 × 2 cm. 1949 fand sich bei der Biopsie der rechte Hoden praktisch normal, der linke zeigte eine verminderte Reifung der Spermatogenese. Uringonadotropin zwischen 10 und 80 E. Bei einer Zahl von 13 Mill. Spermatozoen im Kubikzentimeter und einem Ejaculatvolumen von 3 cm³ wurde die Ehefrau gravide. Nach den beigegebenen Bildern und der kleinen Hodengröße vor Beginn der Behandlung hat wahrscheinlich kein isolierter ICSH-Mangel vorgelegen. Eher muß man den Fall in die Gruppe des funktionellen hypogonadotropen Eunuchoidismus einordnen, bei dem sich nach einer lang und intensiv durchgeführten Testosteronbehandlung die Gonadotropinproduktion doch noch normalisierte, ein ungewöhnlicher, aber bei Betrachtung unter dem Gesichtspunkt der Hohlwegschen Desensibilisierung des zentralen Steuerungsmechanismus durch Testosteron kein ganz unmöglicher Erfolg.

Es ist undenkbar, daß in solch erfolgreich behandelten Fällen ein organischer Defekt der Gonadotropinproduktion bestanden hat, es erscheint aber möglich, daß es funktionelle Störungen der Gonadotropinproduktion gibt, die sich erst nach einer unverhältnismäßig langen und intensiven Testosteronbehandlung mit Choriongonadotropin oder Testosteron ausgleichen.

Von vielen wird die Verwendung des Testosterons bei leichteren und schweren Formen des sekundären Hypogonadismus, besonders auch bei der verzögerten Pubertät, abgelehnt, da das Testosteron die Gonadotropinproduktion in der Hypophyse hemmt. Man fürchtet, daß die Eigenproduktion der Gonadotropine dadurch überhaupt nicht mehr in Gang kommt. Nicht nur experimentelle Beobachtungen am Tier, sondern auch klinische am Menschen sprechen gegen diese Ansicht. Bei Verabreichung kleiner oder mittlerer Dosen von Testosteron erholt sich im Tierexperiment, wie HOHLWEG (1956) gezeigt hat, die Eigenproduktion des Hypophysenvorderlappens unter Testosteron wieder, präpuberal gegeben, wird sogar der Eintritt der Pubertät vorverlegt (BAHNER u. SCHWARZ). Gibt man Jugendlichen im Alter von 15—18 Jahren mit verzögerter Pubertät Testosteron, dann wird, wie mit HCG, die Pubertätsentwicklung in Gang gebracht. die Gonadotropinbildung also angeregt. Daß sich auch das Samenepithel dabei normal entwickelt, zeigen die Beobachtungen von TONUTTI u. Mitarb. (1960) bei der Behandlung des hypophysären Zwergwuchses. Testosteron führt beim ausgereiften Individuum über die Hemmung der Hypophyse zur Atrophie der Kanälchen und der Leydigzellen, die sich nach einigen Wochen wieder ausgleicht. Sind die Kanälchen und Leydigzellen gar nicht entwickelt, fehlt also die Gonadotropinproduktion noch, dann kann auch keine Hemmung und keine Hodenatrophie eintreten. Je schwerer also ein sekundärer Hypogonadismus ist, um so geringer sind die Schädigungsmöglichkeiten, je leichter, um so größer. Vor einem dauernden Schaden schützt in den meisten Fällen wahrscheinlich die Desensibilisierung der Zentren. Ob mit einem echten Rebound-Phänomen gerechnet werden kann, ist abhängig vom Ausmaß des Defektes der Sexualregion im Zwischenhirn bzw. in der Adenohypophyse. Je schwerer das klinische Bild des Androgendefektes ist, um so geringer sind auf lange Sicht gesehen die Erfolge der Gonadotropintherapie, sowohl mit HCG oder kombiniert mit PMSG. Eine Ausnahme macht nur der isolierte ICSH-Mangel, auf den das verhältnismäßig große Hodenvolumen hinweist. Es ist unzweckmäßig, solche Formen des funktionellen hypogonadotropen Eunuchoidismus ohne eindeutige Wirkung auf das Hodenvolumen länger als 4—6 Monate zu behandeln. Testosteron kann in solchen Fällen das Hodengewebe nicht schädigen, es verhindert auch nicht die spontane Aufnahme der Gonadotropinproduktion.

Je geringgradiger der Androgendefekt ist und je größer das erreichte Hodenvolumen ist, um so zurückhaltender sei man aber mit Testosteron. Diese Fälle behandelt man, wenn nötig, mehrere Jahre mit HCG, eventuell kombiniert mit PMSG, wobei die Dosis so niedrig gehalten werden soll, daß keine Hemmung der eigenen hypophysären Gonadotropinproduktion eintritt — nicht über 500 E täglich bzw. 3500 E wöchentlich. Nach den Beobachtungen von CHARNY scheint das in der Entwicklung begriffene Keimepithel besonders empfindlich gegenüber einer Unterbrechung der FSH-Einwirkung.

Die Hauptdomäne der Dauertherapie mit Testosteron sind die partielle und globale Hypophysenvorderlappeninsuffizienz aus organischer Ursache.

Eine wichtige Besonderheit ist bei der Behandlung des präpuberalen Eunuchoidismus noch zu beachten. Die Ansprechbarkeit der androgen abhängigen Gewebe wechselt mit dem Lebensalter, sie ist am größten um die Zeit der Pubertät, deutlich geringer beim Kind und beim Erwachsenen, noch stärker herabgesetzt im hohen Lebensalter. Die günstigste Behandlungszeit sind also die Jahre zwischen 14 und 20. Bei Menschen über 20 Jahre erreicht man selbst bei intensivster Therapie mit HCG oder Testosteron keine volle Ausprägung der sekundären Geschlechtsmerkmale mehr.

J. Primärer Hypogonadismus, hypergonadotroper Eunuchoidismus

Grundsätzlich unterscheidet man zwischen den angeborenen und erworbenen Formen, wobei mit zunehmender Erfahrung der Häufigkeit nach die angeborenen bei weitem überwiegen. Die Zuordnung erscheint einfach, da der Ausfall der Hodenhormone mit einer beträchtlichen Mehrbildung der hypophysären Gonadotropine beantwortet wird, die im Urin leicht nachgewiesen werden kann. Schwierigkeiten entstehen aber schon, wenn das Kanälchenepithel teilweise erhalten ist, da sich die Gonadotropinabgabe dabei normal verhalten kann und die Ausscheidung trotz der minderwertigen in- und exkretorischen Funktion vom Gesunden nicht abweicht (s. S. 644). Manche Fälle schwerer Hodenhypoplasie legen auch die Vermutung nahe, daß sowohl eine minderwertige Anlage des Hodengewebes als auch ein angeborenes Unvermögen oder eine Minderwertigkeit des zentralen Motors vorhanden ist, wobei anatomische Untersuchungen weder im Bereich des Zwischenhirns noch der Adenohypophyse nennenswerte Abweichungen vom Normalen ergeben haben.

Fehlt die Hodenanlage oder liegen frühembryonale, einem Verlust der Hoden gleichkommende Entwicklungsstörungen vor, dann ist die Diagnose einer angeborenen Mißbildung, einer schweren Gonadendysgenesie leicht. In den letzten

Jahren wurden aber eine Reihe geringgradiger Defekte des exkretorischen und inkretorischen Hodenanteils beschrieben, deren Abtrennung von erworbenen Schäden schwierig, ja nicht immer möglich ist. Die Auswirkung eines exogenen Schadens auf das Kanälchenepithel, die Kanälchenwand und das Zwischengewebe kann dasselbe morphologische Bild wie eine angeborene Dysgenesie haben, der Endzustand läßt die Ursache häufig nicht erkennen.

Die Annahme einer minderwertigen Anlage, die ganz verschiedene Grade aufweisen kann und die man unabhängig von ihrer Schwere zweckmäßig als Fehlbildung, *Dysgenesie*, bezeichnet, erscheint berechtigt bei familiärer Häufung, bei Kombination mit anderen Organdefekten, bei Kombination mit Erbkrankheiten, beim Ausbleiben der Reifung der Kanälchen oder des Zwischengewebes trotz normaler oder erhöhter Gonadotropinproduktion und bei starker Unterschiedlichkeit des Reifungsgrades der Kanälchen.

Man hat versucht, verschiedene Gruppen der angeborenen Hodendysgenesie aufzustellen. Man kann vom *klinischen Gesamtbild* ausgehen, den Hypogonadismus bzw. Eunuchoidismus nur im Rahmen anderer Organdefekte sehen und bestimmte Kombinationen von Mißbildungen zu einzelnen Syndromen zusammenfassen. So spricht man vom Hypogonadismus beim Ullrich-Turner-Syndrom des Mannes, beim Werner-Syndrom, beim Kallmann-Syndrom u. ä. Hier ist die Hodendysgenesie nur eines von mehreren möglichen Symptomen, keineswegs ein obligates und eines, das ganz verschiedene gestaltliche Ausprägung haben kann. Der Nachteil einer solchen Gruppierung besteht darin, daß atypische Fälle mit wenig Merkmalen und isolierte Formen der Hodendysgenesie nicht untergebracht werden können.

Eine andere Möglichkeit der Einteilung ist durch das *morphologische Bild* gegeben, wobei man die schwere Hypoplasie beider Gewebsanteile abtrennt von der Tubulusdegeneration mit Fibrosierung, der Keimzellaplasie und der einfachen Reifungshemmung des Samenepithels verschiedenen Schweregrades. Eine solche Ordnung wird der Vielfalt der Abnormitäten im Hodengewebe gerecht und erlaubt eine bessere Differenzierung und Unterteilung der Defekte. Sie würde bei Anwendung neuerer Methoden dazu beitragen, die gegenwärtige zu sehr vereinfachende und systematisierende Einteilung zu überwinden. Bei einer solchen, nur nach morphologischen Gesichtspunkten vorgenommenen Einteilung, geht aber wiederum das bunte klinische Bild mit seiner Vielzahl von Mißbildungen in anderen Organen gänzlich verloren. Es ist ein Charakteristicum der Hodendysgenesie, daß sie häufig mit anderen Organanomalien kombiniert ist, durch die wiederum ihre genetische Ursache unterstrichen wird. Bei familiärer Häufung dieser Fälle hat man schon immer an der genbedingten Ursache nicht gezweifelt. Sporadisch vorkommende Formen konnten erst in den letzten Jahren durch Chromosomenuntersuchungen mit Wahrscheinlichkeit ebenfalls als genbedingt erkannt werden, wobei die ungewöhnliche Entdeckung von *Anomalien der Geschlechtschromosomen* ein neues Ordnungsprinzip rechtfertigt, auch wenn sich später herausstellen sollte, daß diese Chromosomenanomalien nicht die letzte Ursache der minderwertigen Gonadenanlage und Entwicklung sind. Hier steht man erst am Anfang einer Entwicklung, die schon reiche Früchte getragen hat, aber auch viele neue Fragen aufwarf.

I. Anomalien der Geschlechtschromosome

Diese Entwicklung begann mit der Entdeckung eines sexuellen Dimorphismus der Struktur der intermitotischen männlichen und weiblichen Kerne durch BARR und BERTRAM (1949). Die Autoren wiesen zum erstenmal auf eine morphologische Differenz in den Kernen der Interphase bei Säugetieren verschiedenen Geschlechts hin und beschrieben in weiblichen Kernen eine spezifische Chromatinmasse, das Chromozenter, das als Geschlechtschromatinkörperchen bezeichnet wird und von dem man annahm, daß es nur in weiblichen Kernen vorkommt (Barr u. Bertram 1949).

Die Untersuchung des Geschlechtschromatins bei den einzelnen Formen der Fehlbildung der Keimdrüsen ergab dann den überraschenden Befund, daß beim Klinefelter- und beim Ullrich-Turner-Syndrom das chromosomale Geschlecht nicht mit dem gonadalen und nicht mit dem gonophoren übereinstimmen soll. Ein großer Teil der Kranken mit Klinefelter-Syndrom mit männlichem gonadalem und gonophorem Geschlecht zeigte ein weibliches Geschlechtschromatin, schien also genetisch weiblich und der größere Teil des Ullrich-Turner-Syndroms mit weiblichem gonophorem Geschlecht und Keimdrüsenresten war kernchromatinnegativ, schien also männlich.

Die Entwicklung neuer Techniken, die in Zellkulturen des Menschen die färberische Darstellung der Chromosomen erlaubt, brachte weitere Aufschlüsse. Es zeigte sich, daß Kranke mit Klinefelter-Syndrom mit positivem Geschlechtschromatin im Kern an Stelle von 46, 47 Chromosomen haben und daß das überzählige Chromosom mit großer Wahrscheinlichkeit ein zweites X-Chromosom darstellt (Ford u. Polani 1959a, Jacobs u. Strong 1959a, Court Brown 1960). Es handelt sich also um sog. XXY-Typen. Diese Kranken besitzen trotz ihrer XX-Chromosome männlich ausgebildete Gonaden, so daß man annimmt. daß das Y-Chromosom die Entwicklung der Gonaden in männlicher Richtung bestimmt (Einzelheiten s. Klinefelter-Syndrom, S. 828). Die mangelhafte Ausbildung der Gonaden mit dem Bild der medullären Dysgenesie ist — so vermutet man — dadurch bedingt, daß sich das Y-Chromosom gegen zwei, in einigen Fällen sogar gegen drei und vier weibliche X-Chromosome durchsetzen muß.

Umgekehrt fand man bei Trägern der Anomalie des Ullrich-Turner-Syndroms. bei denen die Keimdrüsen aus undifferenzierten Gewebsresten oder Rudimenten des Ovariums bestehen, nur 45 Chromosomen, es fehlt das Y-Chromosom, man spricht von den sog. XO-Typen. Auch hier ist man geneigt, die Ursache der Mißbildung der Gonaden in der Chromosomenanomalie zu sehen, obwohl bis jetzt ein verweiblichendes Gen auf den X-Chromosomen nicht sichergestellt ist.

Diese genetischen Anomalien der Geschlechtschromosomen geben aber gegenwärtig noch keine ausreichende Erklärung für die Entstehung der Gonadenmißbildung. Bei den wenigen bis jetzt chromosomal untersuchten Fällen dieser Art wurden schon jetzt Feststellungen getroffen, die die Bedeutung der Chromosomenanomalien für die Gonadenentwicklung einschränkt. Bei Mäusen ist seit längerer Zeit ein normal fruchtbarer Stamm bekannt, bei dem die weiblichen Tiere eine XO-Chromosomenkonstitution haben und innere und äußere Genitalien normal angelegt sind. Auch beim Menschen ist eine Frau mit XO-Konstitution beschrieben, die normal menstruierte und ein Kind geboren hat (Bahner u. Mitarb. 1960). Mit den gegenwärtigen Vorstellungen ist auch der von Bloise beschriebene Fall von männlichem Turner-Syndrom nicht in Einklang zu bringen, der im Zellkern chromatin negativ war, eine Chromosomenkonstitution von XO, ein männliches äußeres Genitale und einen hypoplastischen Hoden hatte. Ebenso schwierig zu deuten sind die Fälle von echtem Hermaphroditismus mit positivem Kernchromatin und normal weiblichen XX-Chromosomen in den Körperzellen, während die Gonaden sowohl weibliche als auch männliche Elemente besitzen. Man hilft sich mit der Annahme einer möglichen Mosaikstruktur, die Chromosomenformel der Gonaden sei in diesen Fällen XY, der Körperzellen XO, oder bei den echten Hermaphroditen hätten die weiblichen Teile der Gonade XX-, die männlichen XY-Konstitution, die Körperzellen könnten dann sowohl XX- oder XY-Chromosom haben.

Abgesehen davon, daß die Erklärung der Entstehung solcher Chromosomenmosaike erhebliche Schwierigkeiten bereitet, bleibt die Tatsache, daß dieselben schweren Mißbildungen der Keimdrüsen, also Rudimente und Kümmerformen oder schwere Formen der Tubulusdysgenesie bei Menschen beobachtet werden, bei denen chromosomales (genetisches) Geschlecht mit dem gonadalen und gonophoren übereinstimmt und Chromosomenanomalien fehlen. Die Entwicklungsstörung muß also auch noch andere Ursachen haben können als nur Anomalien der Geschlechtschromosome, es sei denn, man postuliere für diese Fälle heute schon, daß die Geschlechtschromosomen dieser Menschen trotz normaler Gestalt Defekte in den Genen haben, die für die Gonadenentwicklung verantwortlich sind (POLANI 1961 und HARNDEN u. JACOBS 1961).

Die Untersuchung der menschlichen Geschlechtschromosomen führte zur Aufstellung von drei Syndromen. Bei zweien war das klinische Bild schon lange bekannt. das dritte ist völlig neu. Jedes Syndrom hat verschiedene Varianten, die noch unvollständig untersucht sind.

Trisomie des X-Chromosoms (3 X-Syndrom). Bei minderbegabten und schwachsinnigen Frauen wurden 3 X-Chromosome festgestellt. Diese Frauen sind nicht steril, sie können normale Kinder haben. Man schätzt ihr Vorkommen auf 1% der weiblichen Minder

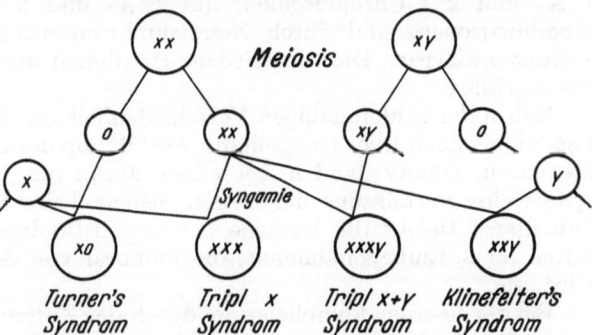

Abb. 43. Abnorme Geschlechtschromosomen bei bestimmten Syndromen. (Nach FERGUSON-SMITH). Ann. Intern. Med. **53**, 359 (1960)

begabten bzw. auf etwas unter 0,1% aller weiblichen Geburten. In den Zellen der Mundschleimhaut stellen sich 2 Geschlechtschromatinkörperchen dar. Einzelne Fälle hatten sogar 4 und 5 X-Chromosomen bzw. 3 und 4 Geschlechtschromatinkörper. Je größer ihre Zahl, um so größer scheint der geistige Defekt zu sein. Hypofertilität und vorzeitige Menopause zeigen die Minderwertigkeit der Keimdrüsen.

Trisomie von XXY. Beim Klinefelter-Syndrom war bekannt, daß etwa 80% trotz des männlichen gonadalen Geschlechts 1 Geschlechtschromosom im Kern besitzt. Die Aufklärung der Anomalie brachte erst die neue Technik der Chromosomenuntersuchung mit dem Nachweis der XXY-Chromosomenkonstitution. In letzter Zeit wurde über eine Reihe von Fällen mit Mosaikverhalten der Chromosomen mit 1 X-, mit 3 X-, ja mit 4 X-Chromosomen und einem zusätzlichen Y-Chromosom berichtet. Man schätzt, daß etwa 0,2% aller männlichen Geburten, etwa 1% aller minderbegabten Männer und etwa 3% aller sterilen Männer eine XXY-Chromosomenkonstitution oder ein Mosaik davon haben.

Monosomie von X. In seiner typischen Ausprägung hat das Ullrich-Turner-Syndrom nur 1 X-Chromosom (X0-Typus). Zusätzliche Anomalien sind häufig, besonders Mosaike von X0 und XX, auch X0 und XXX, ja sogar von X0 und XY, X0 und XYY.

Als Ursache der Mono- bzw. Trisomie wird eine Nondisjunktion angenommen (FORD) (Abb. 43). Dieser Begriff wurde aus den Beobachtungen an der Drosophila melanogaster übernommen, bei der nach Röntgenbestrahlung beide X-Chromosome in eine Zelle des endgültigen Eikernes überwandern können, während die andere Zelle kein X-Chromosom erhält. Eine solche Nondisjunktion wird als Ursache der Chromosomenanomalie des Klinefelter-, des Ullrich-Turner-Syndroms und des Mongolismus (Trisomie von 21) angesehen. Der Zeitpunkt der Teilungsstörung wird in die Reifungsperiode der Keimzellen während der ersten oder der zweiten *meiotischen* Teilung verlegt. Eine *somatische* Nondisjunktion ist beim Turner-Syndrom möglich. Aus der Häufigkeit der Farbenblindheit des chromatinpositiven Klinefelter-Syndroms (POLANI 1958, NOWAKOWSKI 1960) schließt man, daß die meisten Klinefelter-Fälle zwei genetisch verschiedene X-Chromosome haben und sich von einem Zygoten aus einem XX-Ei und einem Y-Spermium oder einem X-Ei und einem XY-Spermium herleiten können (POLANI 1958).

Die häufigste durch Nondisjunktion entstehende Chromosomenanomalie ist das XXY-Klinefelter-Syndrom, dann folgt das X0-Turner-Syndrom und nach den Feststellungen der letzten Jahre die Tripel-X-Frau. Auch die Entstehung der seltenen XXXY-Konstellation, Fälle mit 4 X- und 1 Y-Chromosom, mit 1 X- und 2 Y-Chromosomen, mit 2 X- und 2 Y-Chromosomen und andere Kombinationen, sind durch Nondisjunktion während der ersten und zweiten Teilung erklärbar. Die verschiedene Häufigkeit der einzelnen Anomalien ist noch nicht geklärt.

Neben der zahlenmäßigen Verschiedenheit der Geschlechtschromosomen wird neuerdings auch über mangelhafte Ausbildung der Chromosomen berichtet, selbst MUDAL u. OCKEY fanden bei einem Mann mit Muskeldystrophie und Hypospadie eine Verkürzung der langen Schenkel des Y-Chromosoms und vermuten daß dieser Defekt die Ursache der unvollständigen Vereinigung der Urethralfalten im 3. Embryonalmonat, die humoral von den Keimdrüsen aus induziert wird, sei.

Bei der überaus komplizierten, durch das Zusammenwirken mehrerer embryonaler Gewebe bestimmten Entwicklung der Keimdrüsen ist es auf der anderen Seite aber auch möglich, daß *Autosome* — also die Nichtgeschlechtschromosomen — und peristatische Faktoren Einfluß auf die Entwicklung nehmen können. Hier ist besonders die minderwertige Anlage des Cölomepithels und des Mesonephron anzuführen, aus denen sich der Rinden- bzw. der Markanteil der Gonade herleitet.

WITSCHI (1961) hat das Ergebnis seiner Versuche an Amphibien auf die Entwicklungsstörungen der menschlichen Keimdrüse übertragen. Er schreibt der Rinde und dem Mark eigene Organisatoren zu, die sich gegenseitig hemmend beeinflussen. Die Entstehung dieser Organisatoren ist abhängig von den primordialen Gonien, die in die undifferenzierte Drüse einwandern. Diese sind indifferent und entwickeln sich in der Rinde zum Follikel, im Mark zum Spermatozoon. Wird die Befruchtung von reifen Eiern bei Amphibien künstlich verzögert, dann zeigen die primordialen Keimzellen degenerative Veränderungen, sie vermehren sich nur langsam, es wandern nur wenig Gonien in die Keimfalte ein. Die geringe Zahl der entstehenden Follikel und Follikelzellen bildet dann nur einen schwachen Rindeninduktor, so daß der Markinduktor das Übergewicht gewinnt. Die Gonade entwickelt sich demzufolge als Hodengewebe. Die Zahl und die Entwicklungspotenz der einzelnen Gonien sind nach WITSCHI die wichtigsten Faktoren, die die Entwicklung einer Gonade bestimmen (GRUMBACH 1955, NELSON 1957, WITSCHI 1961).

Inwieweit auch peristatische Einflüsse auf den sich entwickelnden Embryo die Entwicklung der Keimdrüsen beeinflussen, ist nicht bekannt. Wenn man sich daran erinnert, wie viele genetisch bedingte Mißbildungen im Experiment durch Mangel an Sauerstoff, an Glucose oder Vitaminen in derselben Art und

Ausprägung phänokopiert werden, dann erscheint die Suche nach solchen schädigenden Einflüssen bei der Gonadendysgenesie des Menschen durchaus berechtigt, wobei im Einzelfall nicht entschieden werden kann, ob die abnormen Umweltfaktoren während der Entwicklung des Keimes die Mißbildung selbst hervorgerufen haben oder ob ein Gen mit geringerer Penetranz unter den besonderen Umweltsbedingungen manifest geworden ist.

II. Cytologie des chromosomalen Geschlechts

Trotz der noch ungeklärten Entstehung des Geschlechtschromatins ist die diagnostische Bedeutung so groß, daß entsprechende Untersuchungen nicht nur bei allen Anomalien des inneren und äußeren Genitales und bei allen Formen des präpuberalen Hypogonadismus, sondern auch bei Mißbildungen anderer Organe vorgenommen werden sollten.

GRAHAM und BARR (1952) glaubten anfangs, daß sich das Geschlechtschromatinkörperchen aus Teilen beider X-Chromosome mit positiver Heteropyknose ableitet, die im Interphasenkern dicht beieinanderliegen, daß es somit den morphologischen Ausdruck der normalen XX-Geschlechtschromosome des weiblichen Ruhezellkerns darstellt. Später machte man dann die Feststellung, daß Zellen mit der Formel XXX und XXXY nicht ein, sondern zwei normal große Körperchen, Zellen mit XXXX sogar drei besitzen. Ein Körperchen muß also sowohl von zwei als auch von einem X-Chromosom gebildet werden können. Gegenwärtig nimmt man an, daß das Geschlechtskörperchen den heteropyknotischen Anteil eines einzigen X-Chromosoms darstellt (STEWART 1959). Beim weiblichen menschlichen Feten wird in der Prophase einer Mitose nur eines der beiden X-Chromosome pyknotisch, das zweite X-Chromosom und das X-Chromosom der männlichen Zelle jedoch nicht. Dies ist der Grund, weshalb die männliche Körperzelle in der Ruhephase kein wirkliches Geschlechtschromatin aufweist.

Auch diese Auffassung trifft nicht mehr ganz zu. STEWART u. Mitarb. (1959) erhoben am Kanälchenepithel von sieben männlichen Individuen mit chromatinnegativen Körperzellen und der Chromosomenkonstitution XY bei 44 Autosomen den überraschenden Befund von chromatinpositiven Spermatogonien, primären und sekundären Spermatiden, wenn sich diese Zellen in der Prophase befanden. In einzelnen Zellen waren an der Membran neben dem Geschlechtschromatinkörperchen noch kleinere, feulgenpositive Strukturen sichtbar, aus denen man schließt, daß auch das Y-Chromosom während der frühen meiotischen Prophase darstellbar werden kann. In bestimmten Teilungsphasen der männlichen Zelle kann also das X-Chromosom pyknotisch werden und sich dann im Ruhekern heterochromatisch anfärben. Ähnliche Beobachtungen wurden bei Ratten gemacht (OHNO 1961).

Bei normalem Ablauf der Teilungsvorgänge der menschlichen Zellen ist die Deutung eines positiven Geschlechtskörperchens im Sinne eines weiblichen, heteropyknotischen X-Chromosoms berechtigt. Die Zahl der Chromatinkörperchen ist im allgemeinen um 1 kleiner als die Zahl der X-Chromosomen. 1 Chromatin entsprechen XX-, 2 Körperchen XXX-, 3 Körperchen XXXX-Chromosomen. Wechselnde Zahlen in derselben Zellart oder in verschiedenen Geweben sind verdächtig auf eine unterschiedliche Geschlechtschromosomenzahl, auf ein Mosaik. In Zweifelsfällen und bei pathologischem Ablauf der Kernteilung muß aber zur sicheren Entscheidung die Bestimmung des Chromosomensatzes herangezogen werden.

Die Häufigkeit eines positiven Geschlechtschromatins in Gewebsschnitten von Frauen wechselt je nach der angewandten Färbetechnik und der Art des Gewebes

zwischen 50 und 96%. Am besten läßt sich das Körperchen im Nervengewebe
(85%) (MOORE u. BARR 1953) und in den Membranen weiblicher Embryonen
(96%) (GRAHAM 1954) anfärben, die Durchschnittswerte verschiedener Gewebe
betragen nach BARR (1961) etwa 66% positive Kerne. In Präparaten von Männern
kann ein Chromozenter, das größer ist als andere Chromatinpartikel, aber im allgemeinen kleiner als das typische Geschlechtschromatin der Frau, in etwa 5%
der Kerne nachgewiesen werden. Die Spanne zwischen positiven männlichen und
positiven weiblichen Zellkernen ist also recht groß.

Die Form des Körperchens ist verschieden. Im allgemeinen liegt es plan-
konvex an der Kernmembran, es kann auch rund, dreieckig, diskusförmig und
unregelmäßig sein (MOORE u. BARR 1954). Die Größe beträgt zwischen 0,8 und
1,1 μ, sie wechselt etwas mit der Zellart. Nebennierenrinden- und Schilddrüsen-
epithelzellen haben die größten Kernkörperchen, mit Ausnahme der Nervenzellen
liegen sie meist an der Kernmembran. Das Geschlechtschromatin färbt sich mit
basischen Farbstoffen, also mit Hämatoxylin, Kresylviolett, Thionin, Fuchsin
u. a., es ist feulgenpositiv, d. h. es enthält Desoxyribonucleinsäure. In normalen
diploiden weiblichen Zellen ist 1 vorhanden, in normalen tetraploiden Zellen, also
z. B. in den Leberzellen des Menschen, stellen sich 2 dar. Wenn in einem Gewebe
mehr als ein Chromatinkörper gefunden wird, in dem die Kerne normalerweise
diploid sind, dann darf auf eine anormale Chromosomenzusammensetzung ge-
schlossen werden (BARR 1961).

In der Praxis verwendet man die Zellen der Schleimhäute (Mund, Vagina,
Rectum, Blase, Urethra). Das Chromatinkörperchen in den Mundepithelien stellt
sich am schlechtesten dar, es ist hier flacher und seltener als in anderen Epithelien.
Zwischen normalen Frauen bestehen in der Darstellbarkeit in den Mundepithelien
erhebliche individuelle Unterschiede, so daß man für die Kontrollfärbung immer
auf eine Frau mit bekannten Chromatinzahlen zurückgreifen muß.

In der Routinediagnostik verwendet man am einfachsten Schleimhautzellen
des Mundes, die 1—2 Std nach Lutschen einer Penicillintablette mit einem ge-
schliffenen Objektträger entnommen werden, andere Epithelien gewinnt man durch
Absaugen. Durch das Penicillin wird der Abstrich bakterienfrei, so daß eine große
Fehlerquelle wegfällt (OVERZIER 1961). Die Kerne dürfen in keiner Phase der
Färbung schrumpfen. Der Abstrich wird daher sofort, also noch feucht, in einer
Mischung von 96—99%igem Äthylalkohol und Äther zu gleichen Teilen fixiert. Nach
1—2 Std — längeres Fixieren schadet nicht — werden die Objektträger über 80-,
70-, 60-, 50%igen Alkohol in destilliertes Wasser gebracht, wobei die Präparate
je 5 min in den einzelnen Gläsern bleiben. Ohne zu trocknen, erfolgt Färbung mit
1%igem Kresylechtviolett, Hämatoxylin Harris oder Thionin (3—5 min). Eine
leichte Säurehydrolyse, wie sie KLINGER und LUDWIG (1957) empfehlen, akzen-
tuiert das Geschlechtschromatin und entfärbt eventuell noch vorhandene Bak-
terien. Für die Diagnostik dürfen nur ganz platt und einzeln liegende Zellen mit
großem Kern verwendet werden. Man zählt nur die an der Kernmembran
liegenden Körperchen, obwohl das Chromozenter bei Schleimhautzellen im
Inneren liegen kann. Bei jeder Färbung läuft eine Kontrolle einer Frau mit be-
kannter Zahl von Chromatinkörperchen mit (vgl. Abb. 44). Die normale Schwankungsbreite der Frau liegt zwischen 10 und 75% positive Zellen (BARR 1961).
Beim Mann können bis in 3% der Zellen ähnliche Chromatinverdichtungen vorhanden sein.

Der Geschlechtsdimorphismus läßt sich auch an den neutrophilen Leukocyten
des peripheren Blutes feststellen (DAVIDSON u. SMITH 1954). Die der weiblichen
Individuen tragen wie Trommelschlegel aussehende, sich intensiv färbende Anhängsel mit einem Kopf von 1,4—1,6 μ im Durchmesser, der mit dem Kern durch

einen feinen, zwirnähnlichen Hals verbunden ist. Auch die Granulocyten von Männern können trommelschlegelähnliche Anhängsel haben, aber nie mehr als 1 auf 1000 Neutrophile, außerdem sind diese nicht tropfenförmig, sondern abgeflacht, eckig und kantig, es fehlt auch der typische kleine Spalt zwischen Anhängsel und Kern. Bei der normalen Frau findet man die Trommelschlegel im Verhältnis 1:36. Linksverschiebung verringert ihre Zahl, Rechtsverschiebung vermehrt sie.

Die Bestimmung des chromosomalen Geschlechtes mit Hilfe der Segmentkernigen entspricht grundsätzlich dem Ergebnis anderer Gewebe. Nur beim echten Klinefelter-Syndrom kann die Zahl der Anhängsel seltener sein, als man nach dem positiven Ergebnis der Schleimhautzellen annehmen sollte. Die Ursache hierfür ist nicht klargestellt.

Über die Häufigkeit der Anomalien des Geschlechtschromosoms hat man noch keine abschließenden Kenntnisse. Seit 1959 werden wohl an einzelnen Frauenkliniken sämtliche Neugeborene mit Hilfe des Schleimhautabstriches untersucht, doch ist die Gesamtzahl der Untersuchten, die außerdem eine gewisse Auslese darstellen, noch nicht groß genug. MOORE berichtet 1959 aus Winnipeg bei 1911 männlichen Neugeborenen über 5 chromatinpositive, BERGEMANN 1960 aus Bern bei 1890 Untersuchten über 4 positive und McLEAN u. Mitarb. 1961 aus Edinburgh bei 3000 Untersuchten über 9 positive. Bei einer Gesamtzahl von etwa 6800 entfallen auf 1000 männliche Neugeborene 2,65 chromatinpositive.

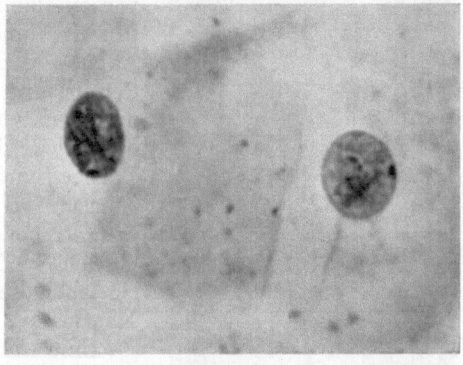

Abb. 44. Chromatinpositive Zellen der Wangenschleimhaut rechts bei 3 Uhr, links bei 6 Uhr (1200fach)

Bei Mädchengeburten sind Anomalien seltener. So fand MOORE unter 1800 neugeborenen Mädchen keine Abwegigkeit, BERGEMANN unter 1838 einen Fall mit einem negativen Geschlechtschromatin im Mundepithel und im Blutausstrich.

Bei minderbegabten Kindern sind Chromosomenanomalien häufiger (s. bei Klinefelter-Syndrom).

Im folgenden werden nur die Krankheitsbilder, die mit einem Hypoandrogenismus einhergehen, eingehender besprochen, während die auf die Kanälchen beschränkten Fehlbildungen und die echten und Pseudohermaphroditen nur kurz erwähnt werden. Ihre ausführliche Darstellung erfolgt in Band III.

III. Gonadendysgenesie mit Anomalien der Geschlechtschromosomen

1. Gonadendysgenesie mit Monosomie von X (Ullrich-Turner Syndrom)

Ursprünglich war ULLRICH (1930, 1949), BONNEVIE (1934, 1940), ROSSI und CAFLISCH bei Kindern beiderlei Geschlechtes eine Häufung multipler Abartungen aufgefallen, die die verschiedensten Organe betrafen. Wesentliche Charakteristica waren eine Flügelhaut am Hals, das sog. Pterygium colli, eine doppelseitige Ptose, Facialisschwäche, hoher Gaumen, angewachsene Ohrläppchen, sehr kleine Mamillen, untersetzter Wuchs (bei ULLRICH), Flossenhaut der Ellbeugen und der Kniekehlen, Hyperteleorismus mit Epikanthus, Hypoplasie der Brust, Impressiones digitatae, Ödeme an den Füßen und am Handrücken (bei ROSSI). ULLRICH (1930, 1949) faßte 40 weibliche und 9 männliche, ROSSI und CAFLISCH später 115 weibliche und 67 männliche Kinder mit solchen Abartungen zusammen. Unabhängig davon hatten schon vorher einige Pathologen, Chirurgen und Gynäkologen als Zufallsbefunde eine Dysplasie der Keimdrüsen bei minderwüchsigen Mädchen und Frauen mit hypoplastischem, aber normal weiblich gebildetem äußeren und inneren Genitale als Gonadenaplasie beschrieben (RÖSSLE u. WALLART 1930, OLIVER, SCHURMANN). PICK sammelte diese, vorwiegend in der deutschen Literatur veröffentlichten Fälle 1937 und fügte zwei eigene hinzu (Abb. 45).

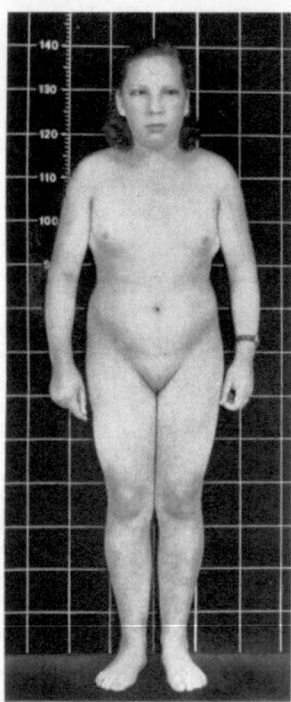

1938 hat dann TURNER sieben Mädchen mit Pterygium colli, Cubitus valgus, Minderwuchs und primärer Amenorrhoe zu dem nach ihm genannten Syndrom zusammengefaßt. VARNEY u. Mitarb., ALBRIGHT u. Mitarb. berichteten 1942 über eine Erhöhung der Gonadotropinausscheidung und bewiesen damit, daß die Keimdrüseninsuffizienz eine primäre und nicht Folge einer Erkrankung der Adenohypophyse ist. Von da an wurde von allen Seiten eine große Zahl von Mädchen und Frauen mit rudimentären Keimdrüsen, Minderwuchs und multiplen Abartungen beschrieben. Die Benennung Turner-Syndrom hat sich für Fälle mit Gonadendysgenesie und Minderwuchs weitgehend durchgesetzt. POLANI benennt Fälle ohne Gonadendysgenesie als Ullrich-Syndrom. Historisch gesehen ist dies unrichtig, aber die Gonadendysgenesie mit Monosomie von X verlangt eine eigene Bezeichnung.

Eine Erklärung brachte die Möglichkeit der Bestimmung des *chromosomalen Geschlechtes* der Träger dieser Anomalie nach BARR (1954), die gleichzeitig und unabhängig voneinander von WILKINS und FLEISCHMANN (1944b), POLANI u. Mitarb. (1954), DECOURT u. Mitarb. (1945) vorgenommen wurde. Dabei ergab sich, daß bei einem hohen Prozentsatz dieser Menschen das Geschlechtskörperchen des Zellkerns fehlt. Von 103 Patienten, die NELSON (1956) untersuchte, gehörten 87, von 667, die LENZ (1959c) aus der Literatur zusammenstellte 512 dem männlichen Typ an. Unter den chromatinpositiven befinden sich vorwiegend solche mit normaler Körpergröße und fehlenden oder nur einzelnen Mißbildungen. Das chromatinnegative Ullrich-Turner-Syndrom erschien eine Zeitlang als kryptogenetischer männlicher Zwitter mit rudimentären Hoden. Zur Erklärung des weiblichen Genitales bezog man sich auf die Untersuchungen von JOST (s. Entwicklung), daß sich bei Fehlen funktionierender Hoden während der ersten Embryonalwochen inneres und äußeres Genitale trotz des männlichen chromosomalen Geschlechtes vollständig in weiblicher Form ausbildet (JOST 1953) (s. Entwicklung). Auch diese Deutung war keine endgültige. Chromosomenanalysen beim Ullrich-Turner-Syndrom (FORD 1959c, FRACCARO 1959, STEWART 1959) ergaben, daß die Träger dieser Anomalie statt 46 Chromosomen nur 45 besitzen. Das fehlende Chromosom ist höchstwahrscheinlich ein Geschlechtschromosom, so daß nur ein einziges X-Chromosom vorhanden ist, während das zweite X- bzw. das Y-Chromosom fehlen. Das chromatinnegative Ullrich-Turner-Syndrom mit weiblichem Genitale

Abb. 45. 22jähriges Mädchen. Ullrich-Turner-Syndrom. Negatives Kernchromatin besitzt also kein männliches Kerngeschlecht (XY), sondern es handelt sich um eine genetische Aberration mit der Chromosomenformel X0. Durch diesen Befund ist das negative Geschlechtschromatin erklärt, die Keimdrüsen sind Rudimente von Ovarien.

Die wesentlichen Charakteristica des Turner-Syndroms sind:

1. Eine Dysgenesie der Keimdrüsen, die meist einem völligen Funktionsausfall gleichkommt. Innere und äußere Genitalorgane sind normal weiblich gebildet, aber stark unterentwickelt. Es besteht eine primäre Amenorrhoe, die Entwicklung der sekundären weiblichen Geschlechtsmerkmale unterbleibt oder ist mangelhaft.

2. Eine Häufung kongenitaler Anomalien, die vielen Kranken ein ganz charakteristisches Gepräge gibt.

3. Ein vom innersekretorischen System unabhängiger Minderwuchs.

4. Ein chromatinnegatives Verhalten der Mehrzahl der untersuchbaren Körperzellen. bedingt durch eine X0 Chromosomenkonstitution.

Eigentliche *Gonaden* fehlen. an ihrer Stelle liegen unscheinbare, fibröse Körper, die man als sog. Keimplatten bezeichnet — vestigial streaks —, die aus einem kernreichen Bindegewebe bestehen, das dem Stroma des normalen Ovars nahesteht und in den schweren Formen keine Spur von Follikeln, Eizellen oder Tubuli seminiferi erkennen läßt. In den tieferen Schichten können hyperplastische Zellkomplexe, die an die sympathicotropen Zellen von BERGER oder an Hiluszellen erinnern. vorhanden sein. Sowohl im Stroma als auch im Hilusgebiet finden sich Reste der Wolffschen Gänge und des Mesonephron (WILKINS u. FLEISCHMANN 1944b, DEL CASTILLO u. Mitarb. 1957, PHILIPP 1952). Die Keimdrüsenrudimente sind weder eindeutig als Ovar noch als Hoden anzusprechen, obwohl manche Autoren das kernreiche Bindegewebe mit dem Stroma des Ovars gleichsetzen. Die seltenen Fälle mit positivem Chromatinmuster können denselben histologischen Befund zeigen wie die mit negativem (HOFFENBERG).

Mit wachsender Erfahrung kamen Fälle mit negativem Geschlechtschromatin hinzu, deren Genitale etwas weiter entwickelt war, die spärliche Menstruationsblutungen hatten, eine gewisse Achsel- und Schambehaarung und eine mäßige Entwicklung der Brust aufwiesen. Hier enthält das Keimdrüsenrudiment eine Tunica albuginea, Primodialfollikel, Follikelcysten und atrophische Follikel. Zahl und Entwicklung der Follikel ist verschieden und entspricht nicht immer dem körperlichen Entwicklungsgrad, aber die Keimdrüsenrudimente sind eindeutig als primitive Ovarien gekennzeichnet (RUSSEL u. Mitarb. 1955, KERKHOF und STOLTE 1956, HOFFENBERG 1951, KLOTZ 1958, 1959, HUTCHINS 1959, OLIVERT).

Nach dem histologischen Befund ist es schwierig, ja unmöglich, die Grenze zu den Fällen mit Ovarhypoplasie zu ziehen, die außer einem Hypogonadismus keine weiteren Anomalien aufweisen. Der Befund an den Keimdrüsen allein kann nicht als maßgebendes Einteilungsprinzip angesehen werden. Wenn man statt der alle Möglichkeiten einschließenden Bezeichnung Turner-Syndrom den Krankheitsbegriff auf den histologischen Befund an den Rudimenten abstellt und dabei den Begriff „Gonadendysgenesie" so eng faßt wie HAUSER, der darunter nur die extremen Fälle mit Keimleisten ohne Keimzellen versteht, dann fällt ein großer Teil der Fälle, die sonst alle Zeichen des typischen Turner-Syndroms einschließlich der Chromosomenanomalie aufweist, weg. Die normal weibliche Ausbildung des Gangsystems mit Tuben, Uterus, Vagina, weiblichem äußeren Genitale mit unterentwickelten großen Labien bedarf in den Fällen mit X0-Chromosomenkonstitution oder dem Mosaik X0/XX keine weitere Erklärung, da die rudimentären Keimdrüsen rudimentäre Ovarien sind. Schwieriger ist die Deutung der Fälle mit chromatinnegativen Kernen und XY-Konstitution — Fall HARDEN-STUART — mit weiblichem Genitale und hypoplastischem Ovar. FORD nimmt hier ein defektes Y-Chromosom an, das die Ausbildung einer männlichen Gonade gegen das X-Chromosom, im Gegensatz zum normalen Y-Chromosom nicht erzwingt. Das weibliche innere Gangsystem zeigt, daß trotz der XY-Formel auch in den ersten Wochen der Embryonalentwicklung kein funktionierendes Hodengewebe vorhanden war.

Die Art der *Anomalien* ist unübersehbar. Eine umfassende Darstellung haben OVERZIER (1961) und MIDULLA (1955) gegeben. Sie betreffen die Haut, die Muskulatur, das knöcherne Skelet, das Herz- und Gefäßsystem, den Respirationstrakt, das Urogenitalsystem, das Nervensystem und die Sinnesorgane. Sie finden sich in den vielen Organen und Systemen, scheinen gänzlich wahllos miteinander kombiniert, so daß sie weder einer bestimmten embryonalen Entwicklungsperiode noch einem bestimmten embryonalen Gewebe zugeschrieben werden können. Den Urologen interessiert, daß die Hufeisenniere, die Beckenniere, Doppelung der Nierenbecken mit Ureter bifidus zu den häufigeren Anomalien gehören, während Hydronephrosen mit Hydroureter selten sind.

Vielfach wird angegeben, daß die Fälle ohne Anomalien häufiger seien als früher angenommen wurde. Solche Ansichten kommen durch das verschieden zusammengesetzte Krankengut der einzelnen Disziplinen zustande. Der Kinderkliniker kann dieses Syndrom nur vermuten und erkennen, wenn Mißbildungen vorhanden sind, zum Endokrinologen werden die Mädchen meist wegen des mangelhaften Wachstums und der gänzlich fehlenden Entwicklung gebracht, der Gynäkologe dagegen wird wegen der Amenorrhoe oder der Sterilität konsultiert, jeder sieht also ein anders ausgewähltes Krankengut. Außerdem können Organanomalien nur bei ausgedehnter röntgenologischer Untersuchung *aller* in Frage kommender Organe ausgeschlossen werden. Je zahlreicher die Mißbildungen sind, um so sicherer kann man klinisch die Zuordnung zum Ullrich-Turner-Syndrom vornehmen, fehlen sie, dann genügen Kriterium 4 und 1.

Es ist nicht klargestellt, ob das fehlende Y-Chromosom die Entstehung der Anomalien begünstigt (FORD 1959c). Für diese Ansicht spricht die Beobachtung, daß Zahl und Schwere der Defekte bei der einfachen Gonadendysgenesie mit weiblichem Kernchromatin (XX) beträchtlich seltener ist als bei den chromatinnegativen. Auf der anderen Seite kommen auch bei den negativen Fälle ohne Anomalien vor, außerdem beobachtet man dieselben Defekte beim Mann mit normaler XY-Konstitution und nur geringgradigem Defekt der Hodenentwicklung (männliches Turner-Syndrom) und endlich bei Menschen ohne jede genitale Mißbildung. Das fehlende Y-Chromosom kann nicht die einzige Ursache der zahlreichen Fehlentwicklungen sein, sein Fehlen erleichtert aber offenbar das Manifestwerden anderer Chromosomendefekte, wobei die Beschränkung auf Anomalien der Gewebestruktur und das Fehlen von Stoffwechselanomalien, also von Enzymdefekten jeglicher Art, auffällt.

Der *Kleinwuchs* ist neben der Gonadendysgenesie die häufigste Anomalie. Alle hormonalen Deutungen — Mangel an Ovarialhormon, an Androgenen der Nebennierenrinde, an Wachstumshormon — können mit guten Gründen widerlegt werden, man braucht nur die normal, zum Teil hochwüchsige Frau mit Gonadendysgenesie, Keimplatten, positivem Geschlechtschromatin und XX-Konstitution, die dieselben hormonalen Abwegigkeiten hat wie das Turner-Syndrom — keine Eigenproduktion von Sexualhormonen, dauernd stark erhöhte Bildung der hypophysären Gonadotropine — dagegen halten. Der Mangel an Sexualhormonen verstärkt aber das ungenügende Wachstum der Epiphysen und die Verzögerung der Reifung des Skeletsystems, so daß unbehandelt aus einem Kleinwuchs ein Zwergwuchs, aus einem Minderwuchs ein Kleinwuchs wird. Trotzdem überrascht die gute, wenn auch verzögerte Entwicklung des Skelets ohne Sexualhormon, das bei Jugendlichen männlichen Geschlechts mit schwerem Hypogonadismus erheblich stärker retardiert ist. Frühzeitige Behandlung mit anabolen Steroiden bis zum 13. Lebensjahr, mit Oestrogenen und anabolen Hormonen ab dem 13. Lebensjahr, kann bei konsequenter Therapie im Laufe von Jahren einen Gewinn von 8—18 cm bringen und zeigt dann erst die wahre Körpergröße. Der Minderwuchs kann neben der Gonadendysgenesie oder Hypoplasie die einzige Anomalie sein.

Ein weiteres Charakteristicum, das bis jetzt als wesentlich für die Diagnose des Turner-Syndroms angesehen wurde, ist das Fehlen des *Geschlechtschromatins* in den Kernen der verschiedenen Gewebe. Beim größten Teil der Untersuchten wurden in der Gewebekultur 45 Chromosomen mit einer Geschlechtschromosomenkonstitution von X0 festgestellt (FORD 1959c, FRACCARO u. Mitarb. 1960a, 1961, TJIO u. Mitarb., STEWART 1959, JACOBS u. Mitarb. 1959a, FERGUSON-SMITH u.a.). Diese X0-Monosomie gilt gegenwärtig als typisch für das Ullrich-Turner-Syndrom.

Schon 1957 berichteten DANON und SACHS, daß sich unter den Fällen mit positivem Geschlechtschromatin einige mit einer abnorm geringen Zahl von chromatinpositiven Zellen im Vergleich zum normal weiblichen Verhalten befinden. Heute hat man erkannt, daß das Geschlechtschromatin in verschiedener Form vorliegen kann und daß seine genaue Untersuchung für die Deutung der Befunde der Chromosomenkulturen sehr wichtig ist. Von der Gruppe der geschlechtschromatinpositiven Fälle muß eine in ihrer Größe nicht genau bekannte Zahl mit wesentlich geringerer Häufigkeit des Körperchens als bei der normalen Frau — nur 10—20% positive Kerne — abgetrennt werden. In solchen Fällen wurde in den Zellkulturen ein *Mosaik* von X0- und XX-Chromosomen gefunden (FORD u. Mitarb. 1960). Neben dem X0/XX-Mosaik wurde auch X0/XY und X0/XYY beobachtet. JACOBS u. Mitarb. (1961) untersuchten kleinwüchsige, chromatinnegative Frauen mit primärer Amenorrhoe und Pterygium und fanden in 3 von 13 ein Chromosomenmosaik, das zweimal aus X0- und XY-Zellen und einmal aus X0- und XYY-Zellen bestand. Früher schon hatten HARNDEN und STUART über eine Frau mit primärer Amenorrhoe ohne sonstige Anomalien mit negativem Kernchromatin berichtet, die eine Chromosomenformel XY aufwies. In diesen Fällen soll das Y-Chromosom geschädigt sein, da nach allen Erfahrungen ein normales Y-Chromosom die Entwicklung der Gonaden in männlicher Richtung garantiert.

Neben dieser Mosaikstruktur der Gewebe werden laufend neue Besonderheiten entdeckt, deren Einordnung noch Schwierigkeiten macht. GRUMBACH u. Mitarb. (1960) finden bei einem typischen Ullrich-Turner-Syndrom mit positivem Geschlechtschromatin in den Zellen des Knochemarkes und der Haut nur 45 Chromosomen und die Chromosomenkonstitution X0. Ob hier das X-Chromosom einen heteropyknotisch färbbaren Anteil besitzt und deshalb darstellbar wird, ist unklar. FRACCARO u. Mitarb. (1960a) fanden bei drei Fällen mit Keimdrüsenrudimenten und positivem, abnorm großem Geschlechtschromatin wohl die Chromosomenkonstitution XX, aber eines der beiden X-Chromosome war abnorm groß, es handelt sich wahrscheinlich dabei um ein Isochromosom, also um eine pathologische Teilung der X-Chromosomen in horizontaler Ebene. Unter den Fällen von JACOBS (1961) befindet sich eine Frau mit Minderwuchs, ohne sonstige Anomalien, primärer Amenorrhoe und genitaler Hypoplasie und einem abnorm kleinen Geschlechtschromatinkörperchen. Die Chromosomenuntersuchung ergab 46 Chromosomen, ein normales X-Chromosom und ein zweites, besonders kleines metazentrisches Chromosom, das die Autoren als unvollständiges X-Chromosom deuten. Die Entstehung der Mosaike wird noch diskutiert. FORD (1960) nimmt an, daß sie durch Störungen der Chromosomenverteilung während der ersten

Zellteilungen des Zygoten entstehen *(developmental mosaicism)*. Der Zeitpunkt dieser somatischen Non-Disjunktionen ist wahrscheinlich verschieden. Liegt sie früh, dann ist der Anteil der abweichenden Zellen groß, liegt sie spät, dann ist das Mosaik nur auf ein bestimmtes Gewebe oder einen Körperteil beschränkt. Ford (1960) hält es für wahrscheinlich, daß beim Mosaik XX/X0 der XX-Kern aus einem X0-Kern entsteht, da eine XX-Zelle in einem X0-Embryo mehr Vorteile zu wachsen und sich auszubreiten hat als eine X0-Zelle. Kranke mit dem Mosaik X0 und XX könnten demnach als einfache somatische Abarten des typischen Turner-Syndroms mit der Chromosomenkonstitution X0 angesehen werden.

Für die Deutung der Genese der Gonadendysgenesie muß man die Fälle heranziehen, bei denen als einziges Symptom eine primäre Amenorrhoe und schwere sexuelle Hypoplasie mit dem histologischen Befund der Keimplatten festgestellt wurde. Diese sonst normal gebildeten, normal großen Frauen haben nach der Untersuchung von Jacobs u. Mitarb. (1961) in zwei histologisch untersuchten Fällen eine normale XX-Konstitution und ein normales Geschlechtschromatin im Kern. Dies bedeutet, daß auch bei normal geformten XX-Chromosomen die Entwicklung der weiblichen Gonade ausbleiben kann. Bei den Fällen mit einem Chromosomenmosaik nehmen Jacobs u. Mitarb. (1961) an, daß die Entwicklung der Gonaden von der in der primitiven Gonade vorherrschenden Stammlinie abhängig ist. Es ist denkbar, daß die XX- und chromatinpositiven Keimplattenträgerinnen in den Gonaden doch ein Mosaik besitzen oder daß das zweite X-Chromosom wohl morphologisch, aber nicht funktionell „normal" ist. Bevor Chromosomenbestimmungen im Keimdrüsengewebe selbst nicht vorliegen, kann die Frage der nicht chromosomal bedingten Keimdrüsendysgenesie nicht entschieden werden.

Die Zuordnung zum Ullrich-Turner-Syndrom ist leicht, wenn das Vollbild der Erkrankung vorliegt, d. h. wenn alle unter 1—4 genannten Kriterien zutreffen. Die Zuordnung darf auch erfolgen, wenn bis auf den Minderwuchs Anomalien fehlen oder normale Körpergröße mit und ohne sonstige Anomalien vorhanden ist, aber eine Kümmerform bzw. eine schwere Hypoplasie der Keimdrüsen vorliegt und das Geschlechtschromatin fehlt. Chromatinnegatives Verhalten ist aber keine absolute Voraussetzung. Fälle mit einem Mosaik von X0-XX-Zellen sind wahrscheinlich echte X0-Zygoten. Eine geringe Zahl von chromatinpositiven Kernen widerspricht der Zuordnung daher nicht, ebensowenig abnorm kleine Geschlechtschromatinkörperchen, die Ausdruck eines Defektes des X-Chromosoms sein können. Voraussetzung der Zuordnung ist aber die Anomalie der XX-Chromosomen.

Phänotypisch sind die Patienten im allgemeinen leicht am Fehlen der sekundären Geschlechtsmerkmale, den kleinen Mamillen, dem Minderwuchs, und an zahlreichen, beim einfachen Betrachten auffallenden Anomalien, wie kurzem breiten Hals, Andeutung eines Pterygiums, angewachsenen Ohrläppchen, Turmschädel, Schielen, Epicanthus, abnorm kurze Hände oder Füße, zu erkennen, so daß die eingehendere Analyse nur noch die Vermutungsdiagnose bestätigen kann.

Ein Teil der Kranken bietet Besonderheiten. So berichten Wilkins und Fleischmann schon 1944 über ein Mädchen mit einer mäßigen Entwicklung der Brust. Solche Beobachtungen sind in der Folge wiederholt gemacht worden und auch in unserem Krankengut vertreten (Hoffenberg 1957, Lisser 1947, Varney 1942, Wilkins 1944). Bei der histologischen Gewebsuntersuchung sind die Milchgänge bei einem Teil der Fälle entwickelt, bei der Mehrzahl handelt es sich um reine Fettanhäufung.

Eine mäßige Entwicklung der Genital- und Achselbehaarung ist nicht selten, ohne daß die 17-Ketosteroidausscheidung erhöht ist. Die vermehrte Behaarung ist manchmal verbunden mit einer Hypertrophie der Klitoris (GREENBLATT 1956, GORDAN 1955, MEYER 1925). Die histologische Untersuchung der Gonaden- rudimente einiger Fälle dieser Art ergab größere Massen von leydigzellartigen Zellen, die wahrscheinlich hypertrophen Hiluszellen entsprechen. Bei zwei eigenen bildete sich die Klitorishypertrophie nach Verabreichung von Oestrogenen, die eine Normalisierung der erhöhten Gonadotropinausscheidung im Urin zur Folge hatte, zurück, so daß die Hypertrophie der Hiluszellen wahrscheinlich durch die vermehrte Produktion der hypophysären Gonadotropine zustande kommt.

Neben der Verzögerung des Epiphysenschlusses kommt zusätzlich noch eine deutlich ausgeprägte Osteoporose vor, wie sie ALBRIGHT (1942) und WILKINS (1944a) schon erwähnen. Bei Jugendlichen konnten wir eine nennenswerte Osteoporose nicht feststellen, jedoch war sie bei zwei Frauen mit 40 und 42 Jahren erheblich ausgeprägt.

Auch eine Weiterentwicklung in Richtung des Hermaphroditismus verus ist beobachtet. DEL CASTELLO und ARGONZ (1957) beschrieben eine chromatin- negative Frau mit Gonadendysgenesie, die mehrmals menstruiert hatte, eine geringe Brustentwicklung zeigte, bei der die Genitalfalten sowohl einige Follikel enthielten, zum Teil mit luteinisierten Theca-Zellen als auch Nester von unreifen Tubuli seminiferi. Hier waren sowohl Mark- als auch Rindenanteile der Gonaden in differenzierterer Form vorhanden. Die Keimdrüse unterschied sich von der- jenigen eines echten Hermaphroditen nur bezüglich des Grades der Entwicklung des Gewebes.

Ebenso kommen Übergangsformen von Gonadendysgenesie zum männlichen Pseudohermaphroditen vor. GRUMBACH u. Mitarb. (1955) beschrieben ein $8^{1}/_{2}$jähriges Mädchen mit Minderwuchs und negativem Chromatinverhalten, dessen wahres Geschlecht wegen eines hypospaden Phallus unklar war. Bei der Laparatomie fand sich links ein Gonadenrudiment ohne spezifische Zellelemente, eine hypoplastische Tube und ein blind endender rudimentärer Uterus, rechts ein unreifer Hoden mit wenigen ganz unreifen Kanälchen, die einige Spermatogonien enthielten, eingebettet in ein undifferenziertes Stroma. Daran schloß sich ein Vas deferens an. Links also ein Rudiment wie beim klassischen Turner-Syndrom, das auch in den Embryonalmonaten funktionslos gewesen war, rechts ein Hoden- rudiment, das, wie die Anlage eines Vas deferens und des hypospaden Phallus zeigt, in den ersten Entwicklungswochen hormonal aktiv gewesen sein mußte. Einen ähnlichen Fall mit männlichem Kernchromatin beschrieben JONES und SCOTT (1958). Ein $2^{1}/_{2}$jähriges Kind mit Phallus, Labien und Vagina hatte links ein weibliches Gangsystem mit Keimdrüsenrudiment, rechts ein Hodenrudiment mit männlichem Gangsystem.

Befunde der *Hormonuntersuchungen:*
Die meisten Autoren berichten über erniedrigte 17-Ketosteroidausscheidung, ein Teil über tief normal, wenige über erhöhte 17-Ketosteroidwerte. Setzt man die 17-Ketosteroidausscheidung zur Körperoberfläche in Beziehung, dann liegen unsere eigenen Werte an 20 Kranken achtmal im Normbereich, zwölfmal wenig unter der physiologischen Schwankungsbreite. Bei der fraktionierten Auftrennung der 17-Ketosteroide ist besonders Ätiocholanolon erniedrigt.

Der wichtigste Befund, der zugleich die Diagnose der primären Keimdrüsen- insuffizienz sichert, ist die erhöhte Ausscheidung der Uringonadotropine. In allen Fällen mit schwerem Hypogonadismus sind sie stark vermehrt, wenn hypo- plastische Ovarien vorliegen, können sie normal sein, da das hypoplastische Organ noch so viel Oestrogene produziert, daß die normale Hemmung der Hypophyse zustande kommt.

Die *Behandlung* ist eine symptomatische. Bei jugendlichen Menschen mit noch offenen Epiphysenfugen erreicht man mit anabolen Steroiden, die man bis zum 12.—14. Lebensjahr allein gibt, eine deutliche Anregung des Längenwachstums. Nach dem 15. Lebensjahr fügt man kleine Mengen von Oestrogenen hinzu, um die Entwicklung in weiblicher Richtung anzuregen. 17 cm war der größte Gewinn bei einer Zwölfjährigen bei dreijähriger konsequenter Behandlung, 17—20jährige können aber auch noch um 1—6 cm wachsen. Mit der Gabe größerer Oestrogendosen ist man solange zurückhaltend, so lange die offenen Fugen noch die Möglichkeit des Wachstums anzeigen. Oestrogendosen, die die primären und sekundären Geschlechtsorgane zur Entwicklung bringen, bedingen gleichzeitig den vorzeitigen Epiphysenschluß und verhindern den Gewinn, den die Anabolica oder auch Testosteron dem Kranken bringen.

Ist die Möglichkeit der Wachstumssteigerung ausgeschöpft, dann wird die Oestrogendosis erhöht. Man gibt sie in den ersten Monaten laufend, bis der Uterus eine etwa normale Größe erreicht hat, später mit Unterbrechungen alle 3 Wochen für 8—10 Tage, um den Kranken durch die eintretende Abbruchsblutung das Gefühl einer normalen Frau zu geben. Jetzt entwicklen sich die sekundären weiblichen Geschlechtsmerkmale, also Achsel- und Schambehaarung, die Brust, die weibliche Körperkontur, so daß mit Ausnahme des Minderwuchses nichts mehr an die schwere Anomalie erinnert. Trotz eingehender Aufklärung über das Wesen der Störung erlebten wir dreimal (von 20), daß die Betreffenden heirateten, angeblich mit normaler vita sexualis.

2. Gonadendysgenesie mit Trisomie von XXY
(Echtes Klinefelter-Syndrom)

Klinefelter; Reifenstein und Albright beschrieben 1942 eine besondere Form eines hypergonadotropen Hypogonadismus. Dieser ist vollständig in bezug auf die Funktion der Kanälchen, unvollständig in bezug auf die Funktion der Leydigzellen. Wichtige Befunde waren die erhöhte Gonadotropinausscheidung, wodurch die periphere Ursache der Keimdrüseninsuffizienz bewiesen werden konnte und eine doppelseitige Gynäkomastie, die eine pathologische Hormonbildung nahelegten. Bei den neun Fällen der Autoren war die frühere Entwicklung normal abgelaufen, die Keimdrüsen descendiert, in der Vorgeschichte bestand kein Anhalt für eine Orchitis, Mumps oder andere Infektionskrankheiten. Die Gynäkomastie war doppelseitig und wurde zum erstenmal 1—6 Jahre nach Beginn der Pubertät bemerkt. Das Wachstum der Brust hielt mehrere Jahre an, um dann stationär zu bleiben. Die Gynäkomastie war in sieben Fällen recht beträchtlich. Die Keimdrüsen maßen $1,5 \times 1,0 \times 0,5$ cm und waren normal in Konsistenz und Empfindlichkeit. In allen Fällen bestand eine Azoospermie. Acht von den neun hatten gut entwickelte akzessorische Geschlechtsorgane. Nur bei einem war die Funktion der Leydigzellen deutlich vermindert, die anderen boten nur geringe Erscheinungen eines Eunuchoidismus. Bei einem 21jährigen waren die Epiphysen von Radius und Ulna noch offen, die Spannweite überschritt aber bei allen die Körpergröße.

Die histologische Untersuchung des Hodengewebes zeigte verschiedene Grade von tubulären Schäden, bestehend in mehr oder weniger weitgehender Hyalinisierung und Verlust der Spermiogenese. Die Leydigzellen waren zahlreich und normal geformt.

Solche Beobachtungen sind auch schon vorher vereinzelt niedergelegt worden (Berblinger 1934). In der Folgezeit haben Heller und Nelson (1945), Howard u. Mitarb. (1950), McCullach (1948c) und viele andere eine große Zahl ähnlicher

Fälle beobachtet. Das wesentliche histologische Charakteristicum, das alle verbindet, ist die weitgehende Sklerohyalinose der Kanälchen und eine Vermehrung der interstitiellen Zellen. Die Fälle von HELLER und NELSON (1945), HOWARD u. Mitarb. (1950) u. a. waren im klinischen Bild variabler, so daß man eine eunuchoide Gruppe von einer weitgehend normalen abtrennte. Erstere sind weder groß noch klein, die Spannweite übertrifft die Körpergröße aber deutlich. Gynäkomastie ist kein hervorstechendes Zeichen. Das äußere Genitale ist infantil oder unterentwickelt, die Stimme hoch, Bartwuchs fehlt ganz oder weitgehend, Behaarung ist feminin, die Muskelentwicklung schlecht, die 17-Ketosteroidausscheidung etwas erniedrigt. Neben diesem schweren Eunuchoidismus gibt es alle Übergänge zu den oben genannten beinahe normalen. Bei genauer Betrachtung boten aber alle unsere eigenen Fälle, auch die mit normal ausgebildeten sekundären Geschlechtsorganen, feminine Züge in der Behaarung, der Fettverteilung, in den Gesichtszügen und geringe eunuchoide Körperproportionen (vgl. Abb. 51 und 52). Das Syndrom kann auch ohne Gynäkomastie und mit deutlichem Hypogonadismus einhergehen. Das klinische Bild des Hypogonadismus, das histologische Aussehen der Leydigzellen, die Höhe der 17-Ketosteroid- und der Gonadotropinausscheidung stehen in keinem rechten Verhältnis zueinander.

Bald wurden dann Stimmen laut, die die Einheitlichkeit der Gruppe der Dysgenesie der Kanälchen in Zweifel zogen (NELSON 1956, GRUMBACH 1957), teils wegen abweichender histologischer Befunde, wobei besonders das Ausmaß der Hyalinisierung, die Größe der Kanälchen, die Masse der Zwischenzellen und eine Bindegewebsvermehrung im Interstitium zu einer Teilung des Syndroms anregten. Es fiel auf, daß das histologische Bild bei sporadischen Einzelfällen und bei familiärem Auftreten, bei der Dystrophia myotonica, beim kryptorchen Hoden, bei Folgezuständen der Orchitis nach Mumps, Lepra, Tuberkulose oder Traumen ähnlich sein konnte.

Die Bestimmung des Geschlechtschromatins (PLUNKETT u. BARR 1956, BRADBURY u. Mitarb. 1956, WITSCHI 1956, NELSON 1956) eröffnete neue Perspektiven. Der weitaus größere Teil der beobachteten Fälle verhält sich in den Zellkernen von Haut, Schleimhaut, den Leydig- und Sertolizellen, weniger häufig an den Leukocyten (BARR u. Mitarb. 1950) positiv, d.h. das Kernmuster gleicht dem einer normalen Frau (PLUNKETT 1956, VAGUE 1956, GRUMBACH 1957, ACHENBACH 1957, NOWAKOWSKI 1957a). Bei 184 Untersuchten waren 106 chromatinpositiv, 28 negativ (NELSON 1956). Damit war eine völlig neue Deutung und andere Einteilung notwendig geworden. NELSON (1956) u. a. trennten das echte vom falschen Klinefelter-Syndrom ab. Das echte Klinefelter-Syndrom umfaßt nur die chromatinpositive Gruppe. Das falsche Klinefelter-Syndrom wurde auch als „Hodenatrophie mit schwerer tubulärer Hyalinisierung und Fibrosierung" (NELSON 1956) oder als „primäre Kanälchenfibrose" bezeichnet (s. S. 851).

Der Defekt wird im allgemeinen nicht vor der Pubertät erkannt. Die meisten Patienten kommen zwischen dem 16. und dem 40. Lebensjahr zur Beobachtung. Viele suchen wegen Kinderlosigkeit zum erstenmal den Arzt auf.

Wie erwähnt, reicht das Aussehen der Träger der Anomalie vom praktisch normal gebildeten bis zum ausgesprochen eunuchoiden Individuum. Als einzige Zeichen der innersekretorischen Unterwertigkeit der Gonaden kann eine schwache oder fehlende Körperbehaarung bei horizontaler Schamhaargrenze, schwacher Bart- und Körperbehaarung vorhanden sein. Muskulatur, Achselbehaarung, äußeres Genitale, Prostata sind in solchen Fällen wohlgebildet. Bei der größeren Zahl findet man aber bei genauer Betrachtung doch Zeichen eines Hypogonadismus wie schlecht entwickelte Skeletmuskulatur, Überwiegen der Spannbreite der Arme über die Körpergröße, Überwiegen der Beckenbreite über Schulterbreite, schlechten Bartwuchs, herabgesetzte Sekundärbehaarung, Pelzmütze des Kopfhaars, höhere Stimme, X-Beine, angedeutete weibliche Fettverteilung am Rumpf, einen kleineren Penis und kleine Prostata. Heller u. Nelson (1945) u. a. fügten dieser größten Gruppe mit leichtem Eunuchoidismus noch eine dritte mit schwerem Hypoleydigismus ohne Gynäkomastie hinzu. Hier ist das äußere Genitale ausgesprochen infantil, Genital-, Sekundär- und Bartbehaarung stark herabgesetzt, die Stimme hoch, der Epiphysenschluß verzögert. Die Körpergröße kann bei den leichteren und schweren eunuchoiden Formen übergroß sein, die anderen sind weder groß noch klein. Die schweren Eunuchoiden altern früh, ein echtes Klimakterium virile soll schon zwischen dem 30.—40. Lebensjahr eintreten. Libido und Potenz wird in den beiden ersten Gruppen als noch normal angegeben, bei der eunuchoiden Gruppe ist sie stark herabgesetzt, aber nicht aufgehoben. Die Menge des Ejaculates ist auch in diesen Fällen ein gutes Maß der androgenen Leistung des Hodens. Die Azoospermie ist praktisch obligat, obwohl einige seltene Fälle mit einzelnen Spermatozoen im Ejaculat beschrieben sind (Munro).

Die *Häufigkeit* wird verschieden angegeben. Prader (1958b) errechnet auf 1000 normale Männer 1 Klinefelter-Syndrom. Moore (1959) fand unter 1911 männlichen Neugeborenen 5 positive, das entspricht 1 auf 400 bei einer nicht ausgewählten Bevölkerungsgruppe. 3% aller Männer, die wegen Sterilität eine Klinik aufsuchen, leiden an der Anomalie (Biskind u. Mitarb.).

Familiäres Vorkommen wurde früher angenommen, es betrifft aber nur die chromnegativen Fälle. Ein eineiiges Zwillingspaar haben Grumbach u. Mitarb. (1957) beschrieben, auch unser Beobachtungsgut umfaßt ein solches Paar. Das Alter der Mütter der Patienten liegt höher als der Durchschnitt der Bevölkerung, aber bei weitem nicht so hoch wie beim Mongolismus (Lenz 1959a). Anomalien anderer Organe scheinen etwas häufiger als beim Bevölkerungsdurchschnitt. Erst in den letzten Jahren stellte man bei einem Teil der Träger *Intelligenzdefekte*, von leichtem Schwachsinn bis zu Debilität, fest (Zublin 1953, Pasqualini 1957, Prader 1958a). 20 der 40 Fälle von Nowakowski (1958) sind mehr oder weniger stark schwachsinnig. Bei unseren 22 sind es nur fünf, zwei studieren. Vor der Pubertät erleichtert ein leichter Schwachsinn die Diagnosestellung. Unter 336 *Hilfsschülern* entdeckten Prader u. Mitarb. (1958a) acht chromatinpositive mit männlichem Genitale, das sind 2,4%. Von anderer Seite wird diese große Koinzidenz nicht bestätigt. Je größer die Zahl der Untersuchten, um so niedriger wird die prozentuale Häufigkeit. Israelson u. Taylor entdeckten unter 1928 Jungen in den Schulen für „educationally subnormal children" eines bestimmten Londoner Bezirkes, die sich aus 81% der Gesamtbevölkerung des Distriktes rekrutierten, nur sieben Chromatinpositive = 0,45%. Werden in Anstalten untergebrachte *Debile männlichen Geschlechtes* herangezogen, so ergeben sich nach den zusammengefaßten Untersuchungen von Ferguson-Smith, Barr, Mosier u. Mitarb. und McLean u. Mitarb. auf 1000 Untersuchte 8,1 Fälle mit einem einzigen Geschlechtschromatinkörperchen und 1,4 Fälle mit zwei und mehr Kernkörperchen. Die Untersuchungen von McLean u. Mitarb. sind deshalb besonders interessant, weil sie bei ihren 28 pathologischen Fällen Chromosomenanalysen durchführten. Dabei ergab sich 17mal eine XXY-Konstitution (6,5 auf 1000), 4mal eine XXXY-Konstitution (1,5 auf 1000), 2mal eine XXYY-Konstitution (0,8 auf 1000) und 5mal (1,5 auf 1000) ein Mosaik verschiedener Art.

Die Vergleichszahlen bei 1907 untersuchten *weiblichen* minderbegabten *Kindern* sind 9 Anomalien der Kernchromatinkörperchen und zwar fanden die Autoren 8mal (4,2 auf 1000) 2 Geschlechtskörperchen und nur 1mal (0,53 auf 1000) fehlte es. Die Fälle mit gedoppeltem Geschlechtschromatin verteilen sich auf

XXX 7mal, ein Mosaik von XXX und XX 1mal. Der chromatinnegative Fall
hatte eine X0-Konstitution (McLean).

Hodenbefund. Die Hoden sind deutlich kleiner als normal, vielfach sind sie nur
bohnengroß. Der Gewebsverlust geht auf Kosten der Kanälchen. Die Konsistenz
ist nicht immer derb und fest, die Druckempfindlichkeit oft herabgesetzt. Nach
der Pubertät besteht das charakteristische Bild in der völligen Hyalinisierung von
mehr als 70% der Kanälchen. Der sklerosierende Prozeß betrifft sowohl die Basalmembran als auch die Tunica propria, letztere in stärkerem Maße. Die elastischen
Fasern sind vermindert und gegen die Peripherie gedrängt, während die kollagenen
an Dicke und Zahl zunehmen. Dazwischen wird hyalines Material eingelagert, so

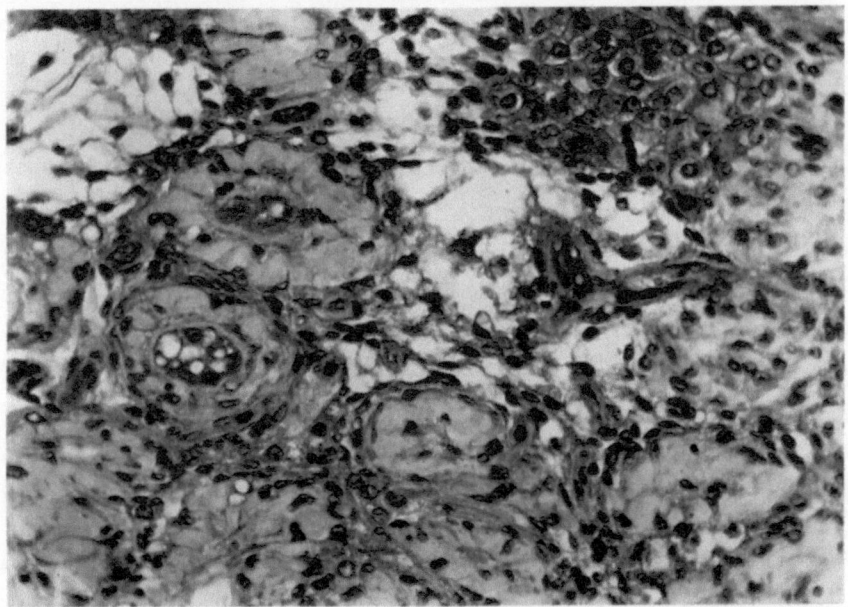

Abb. 46. Biopsie von Fall G. O.: Sehr kleine, meist völlig hyalinisierte Kanälchen, einzelne mit Sertolizellen.
Vermehrung des intertubulären Bindegewebes und Wucherung. Gut differenzierte Leydigzellen.
(Hämatoxylin-Eosin, 300fach)

daß das Endergebnis eine völlige Sklerosierung ist (Heller u. Nelson 1945).
Das hyaline Material färbt sich mit Eosin rot, die Amyloidreaktionen sind negativ.
In den völlig sklerosierten Tubuli sind die Sertolizellen untergegangen, man sieht
nur noch Kanälchenschatten (Abb. 46). In einem kleinen Teil der Kanälchen ist
die Sklerosierung geringer ausgeprägt oder fehlt ganz (Abb. 47 und 48). De la
Balze u. Mitarb. (1952) und Tonutti (1960) unterscheiden drei Schweregrade
der Kanälchenveränderung. Basalmembran und Tunica propria sind etwas verbreitert, die retikulären und kollagenen Fasern sind vermehrt. Der Sertolibelag
ist erhalten, daneben finden sich indifferente Zellen oder Spermiogonien (Stufe I
von Tonutti 1960). In Stufe II ist eine Verdichtung des Bindegewebes in den
mittleren Lagen der Tunica propria zu bemerken. In den äußeren Randzonen
erscheinen die Fibrocyten hypertrophisch und vermehrt. Zur Basalmembran hin
sind die inneren Bindegewebslagen in hyaliner Umwandlung begriffen. Die dritte
Stufe führt zu einer vollständigen Umwandlung der Tunica propria in eine hyaline
amorphe Masse, so daß nur noch Kanälchenschatten vorhanden sind. Gelegentlich
sieht man an einzelnen Stellen Tubuli mit vollständiger Spermiogenese (Harrer
1958, Ferguson-Smith 1959, Munro 1929, Tonutti 1960 u.a.). Nelson (1956)

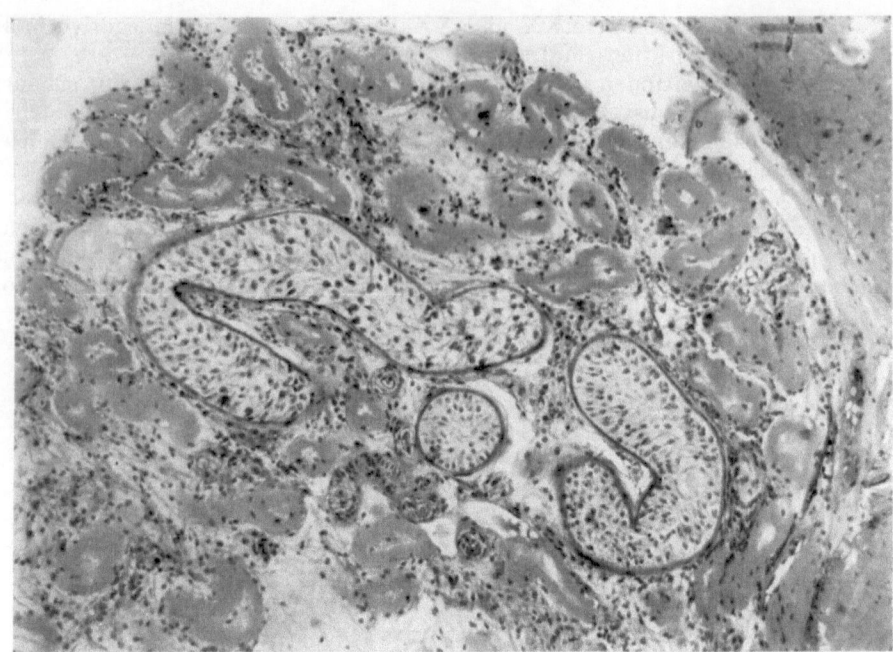

Abb. 47. H. L. Echtes Klinefelter-Syndrom. Die Kanälchen des ganzen Präparates sind gleichmäßig verödet, dazwischen liegen zwei mit mäßig verdickter Tunica propria, die von Sertolizellen ausgefüllt sind. Zwischengewebe locker mit kleineren Komplexen wenig entfalteter Leydigzellen. (Hopa, 120fach)

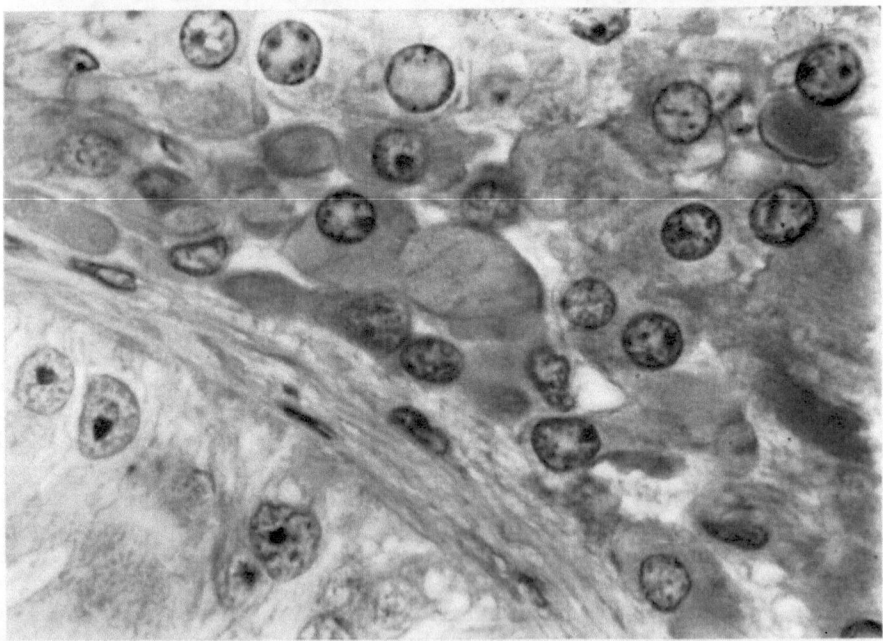

Abb. 48. Ausschnitt von echtem Klinefelter-Syndrom. Gut differenzierte Leydigzellen, einige chromatinpositiv. Kanälchenwand an dieser Stelle wenig verdickt, Sertolizellen erhalten. (Hämatoxylin-Eosin, 1200fach)

beobachtete bei 49 chromatinpositiven Fällen nur zweimal Spermiogonien in weniger sklerosierten Kanälchen, dreimal einige primäre Spermiocyten und einmal

Spermatiden. Man muß bedenken, daß der Befund der kleinen Probeexcision nur einen unvollständigen Einblick gibt. Alle Fälle von NELSON (1956), bei denen eine vollständige Spermiogenese vorhanden war, waren im Kernchromatin männlich. Die Mehrzahl der Kanälchen hat einen sehr kleinen Durchmesser im Gegensatz zu den größeren und einheitlicheren Tubuli der erworbenen Schäden (NELSON 1956).

Die *Leydigzellen* sind hyperplastisch. Nach ihrer Verteilung kann man noduläre bzw. adenomartige Bildungen und eine mehr disseminierte Vermehrung unterscheiden (Abb. 49 und 50). Auf das einzelne Gesichtsfeld bezogen sind sie vermehrt. Ob die Vermehrung eine absolute oder infolge der mangelhaften Anlage

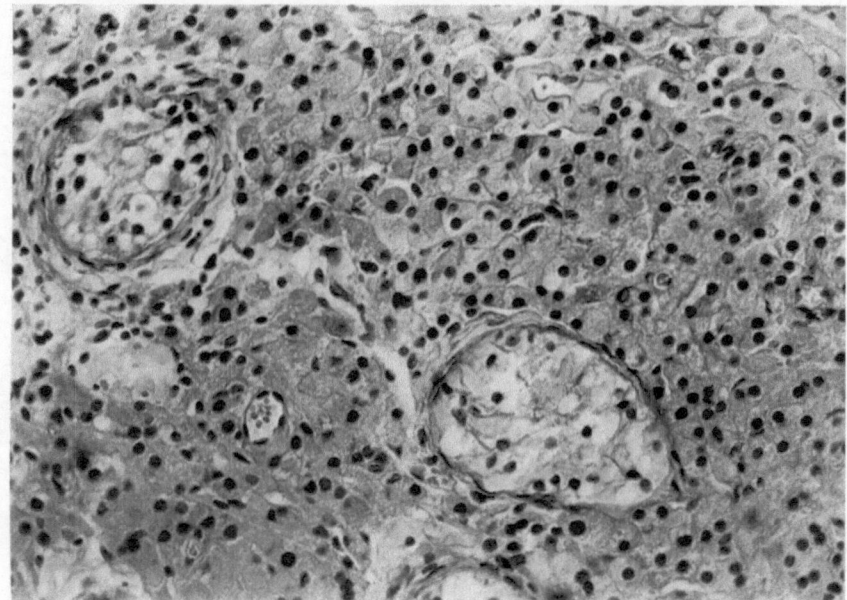

Abb. 49. Leberzellähnliche Leydigzellhyperplasie bei echtem Klinefelter-Syndrom. (Hämatoxylin-Eosin, 300fach)

der Kanälchen nur eine relative ist, ist noch nicht eindeutig geklärt. Die Zellen selbst erscheinen vielfach unreif. Sie sind gewöhnlich ovoid, polyedrisch oder fibrocytenartig und wechseln in der Größe zwischen 14 und $25\,\mu$ im Durchmesser.

TONUTTI (1960) unterscheidet drei Zelltypen. Bei der disseminierten Zellverteilung ist der epitheloide Charakter der Zwischenzellen noch zu erkennen, sie haben jedoch ihre typische polygonale Form verloren, sind mehr oder weniger rund oder länglich in Abstufungen bis zu fibrocytenähnlichen Elementen. Die Kerne sind klein und rund, färben sich stark, sind ohne besondere Chromatinzeichnung und häufig ohne sichtbare Nucleolen. Das Cytoplasma läßt das Bild der sekretorisch aktiven Zelle vermissen.

Der zweite Zelltyp findet sich in den nodulären Ansammlungen. Runde bis ovale strukturreiche Kerne liegen in Zelleibern, die zum Teil eine typische zonale Gliederung des Protoplasmas erkennen lassen. Andere wiederum zeigen aufgeblähte und vacuolisierte Plasmaleiber.

Einen dritten Zelltyp stellen solche Elemente dar, bei denen normal erscheinende Kerne in einem kleinen homogenen, stark färbbaren acidophilen Plasmaleib gelegen sind. Nach TONUTTI (1960) spricht das Bild für eine gonadotrope Stimulierung, es gibt jedoch keine Aufschlüsse über die inkretorische Aktivität dieser Leydigzellen.

DE LA BALZE u. Mitarb. (1952) untersuchten die interstitiellen Zellen und die Bildung von fibrillären Elementen eingehender. Sie finden in typischen Fällen eine progressive Sklerose, eine sog. fibroblastische Involution der Leydigzellen und sprechen von einer Dissoziation der Morphologie und der Funktion, indem die Hyperplasie dieser Zellen mit ihrer Unterfunktion kontrastiert. Sie glauben eine örtliche Beziehung herstellen zu können zwischen dem Ausmaß der Hyalinisierung und der Funktion der Leydigzellen. Die Hyalinisierung ist um so geringer, je

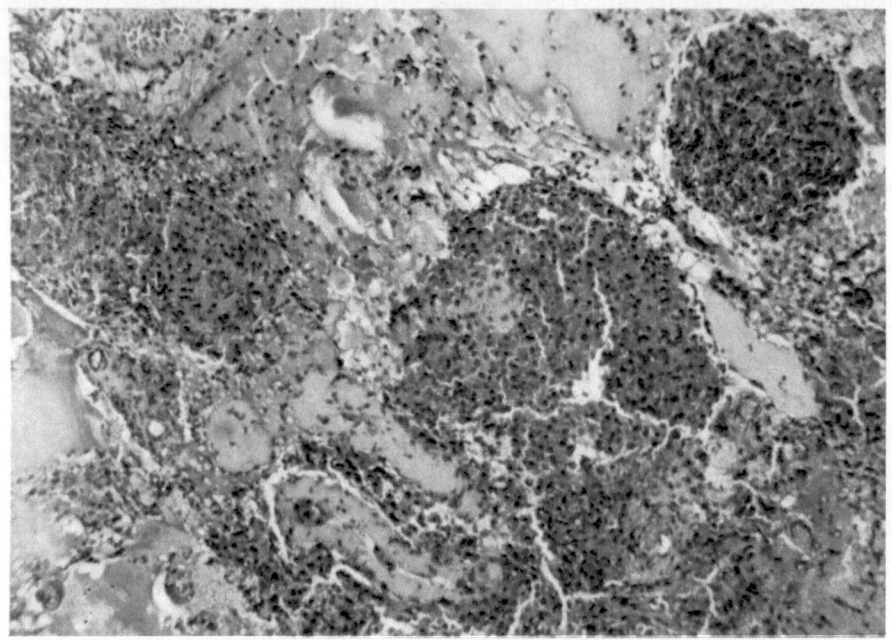

Abb. 50. Echtes Klinefelter-Syndrom. Nur noch Kanälchenschatten. Interstitium ausgefüllt von großen Paketen von Leydigzellen, die wie zusammenhängende epitheliale Gewebskomplexe imponieren.
(Hämatoxylin-Eosin, 120fach)

besser die Funktion der Leydigzellen histochemisch erscheint, je besser also die Androgenbildung an Ort und Stelle ist.

GRUMBACH (1957) macht darauf aufmerksam, daß große und kleine Kanälchen bei beiden Arten vorhanden sein können. Beim echten Klinefelter-Syndrom besteht eine Art Hiatus, indem inmitten von regulären großen Kanälchen sehr kleine fibrosierte ohne intermediäre Stadien eingestreut liegen.

Verklumpung der Leydigzellen und Pseudoadenombildungen fand er bei sechs der acht echten Formen und bei zwei von acht mit männlichem Kernmuster.

Bei der *falschen* Form können die Leydigzellen ebenfalls hyperplastisch und vermehrt sein, seltener sind sie aber in Haufen angeordnet, sie zeigen nur geringe Degenerationsmerkmale.

Es war lange strittig, ob die Kanälchenfibrose sich erst um die Zeit der Pubertät entwickelt oder angeboren ist. Neuerdings konnten PRADER u. SIEBEMANN (1958a) zwei Kinder im Alter von 11 und 13 Jahren untersuchen, die bei einer Reihenuntersuchung durch einen gewissen femininen Habitus und durch ein weibliches Kernchromatin aufgefallen sind, beide waren chromatinpositiv. Das Genitale war bei beiden normal entwickelt. Histologisch fanden sich bei dem jüngeren zahlreiche zartwandige Kanälchen, die noch zu größeren Feldern geordnet waren. Der Durchmesser betrug im Durchschnitt 62 μ. Die Kanälchen werden von unreifen Zellen mit ovalären Kernen ausgekleidet. Dazwischen liegen große, typische Spermatogonien mit runden, großen Kernen, eine Reifung der Keimzellen ist nicht feststellbar, Leydigzellen fehlen.

Im zweiten Fall, dem etwas älteren Kind, schwankt der Kanälchendurchmesser zwischen 50 und 90 μ. Die Wandung ist nur an einzelnen Kanälchen geringfügig hyalin verdickt, einzelne Tubuli sind vollständig hyalin verödet. Die übrigen weisen absolut intakte Wandungen auf. Elastische Fasern sind nicht nachweisbar. In den größeren Kanälchenzellen ist eine deutliche Reifung der Sertolizellen festzustellen. Nur ganz selten findet man in einzelnen Schnitten eine Spermatogonie, das Bild erinnert an die Keimzellaplasie von DEL CASTILLO (1957).

Ähnliche Beobachtungen bestätigen, daß die Tubulussklerose beim echten Klinefelter-Syndrom erst zur Zeit der Pubertät einsetzt. Die so charakteristischen histologischen Befunde des Erwachsenen sind erst Folge der Einwirkung der Gonadotropine, erst dann manifestiert sich die defekte Entwicklungspotenz. BUNGE und BRADBURY (1956), FERGUSON-SMITH (1959) fanden bei jugendlichen chromatinpositiven Fällen in den Stützzellen der Kanälchen einzelne unreife Gonien.

Die *Gynäkomastie*, anfänglich als integrierender Bestand des Syndroms angesehen, ist häufig nur gering ausgeprägt und fehlt nicht selten ganz. Von unseren zwölf Kranken mit Klinefelter-Syndrom hatten sechs eine deutliche Vergrößerung des Drüsenkörpers, der links und rechts verschieden stark entwickelt sein kann, die Sekretion fehlt. Bei Fettsüchtigen ist es manchmal schwer, eine echte Vergrößerung des Drüsenkörpers von der reinen Fettanhäufung abzutrennen. Die Mammae beginnen um die Zeit der Pubertät zu wachsen und vergrößern sich in Schüben.

Histologisch finden sich alveolare Strukturen, Hyperplasien der Milchgänge, Vermehrung des intra- und interlobulären Bindegewebes.. Die Proliferation des Epithels tritt gegenüber der starken Vermehrung und Verdichtung des interlobulären Bindegewebes in den Hintergrund. Das Epithel der Milchgänge ist etwas höher als normal. Das Überwiegen der Bindegewebsreaktion steht in Gegensatz zu den Befunden nach Stilboestrolgabe. Die Ursache der Gynäkomastie ist nicht geklärt. KLINEFELTER u. Mitarb. (1942) diskutieren das Zusammenwirken des hypothetischen Inhibins mit den androgenen Hormonen des Hodens, andere eine Vermehrung des luteotropen Hormons und der Oestrogene.

Autoptische Befunde. BURT u. Mitarb. (1954) sammelten aus der Literatur 21 autoptisch untersuchte Fälle und fügten einen eigenen Fall hinzu. 28% dieser Kranken hatten eine Gynäkomastie, 28% wiesen große Schilddrüsen auf, 38% zeigten hyperplastische Nebennieren, in drei Fällen fanden sich Rindenknötchen über 1 cm im Durchmesser. Dieser ketztere Befund ist bemerkenswert, da bei routinemäßig durchgeführten Autopsien in 9000 Fällen nur bei 1,45% solche benigne Rindenadenome festgestellt werden konnten. Es scheint, daß sowohl die Schilddrüse als auch die Nebennieren in einem höheren Prozentsatz als für gewöhnlich an der Hyperplasie der innersekretorischen Organe beim Klinefelter-Syndrom teilnehmen. Die histologische Untersuchung der Hypophyse ergab eine beträchtliche Vermehrung der schiff-positiven amphophilen Zellen.

Laboratoriumsuntersuchungen. Eine der wichtigsten Befunde ist die Erhöhung der *Gonadotropinausscheidung.* Die Werte schwanken etwas von Kranken zu Kranken, KLINEFELTER (1942) selbst findet die Ausscheidung immer höher als normal. Auch in unseren Fällen war die Gonadotropinausscheidung beträchtlich erhöht (über 96 ME). Ob auch normale Werte vorkommen, ist nicht sicher entschieden. Es wird angenommen, daß mehr Follikelreifungshormon und weniger Luteinisierungshormon produziert wird.

Die Ausscheidung der *17-Ketosteroide* ist bei den Kranken mit geringem oder fehlendem Eunuchoidismus normal, vermindert nur bei schweren Formen des Hypogonadismus. Bei diesem liegen die Werte um $1/3$—$1/4$ niedriger als bei den gleichaltrigen Kontrollen. Bei der fraktionierten Auftrennung der 17-Ketosteroide in sechs Fraktionen ergeben sich keine Unterschiede gegenüber Gesunden.

Es ist nicht entschieden, ob das Verhältnis von *Androgenen zu Oestrogenen*, die beide in den Leydigzellen gebildet werden, von der Norm abweicht. Die genaue Bestimmung der Oestrogene begegnet immer noch großen Schwierigkeiten, so daß selbst aus letzter Zeit keine eindeutigen Untersuchungsergebnisse berichtet wurden. Früher gaben HELLER und NELSON (1945) an, daß Kranke vom eunuchoiden Typ ohne Gynäkomastie unternormale Mengen von Oestrogen ausscheiden, während solche mit guter Entwicklung der Brust normale Mengen ausscheiden. Der Einwand, daß eine höhere Oestrogenproduktion mit der erhöhten Gonadotropinausscheidung nicht vereinbar sei, bedarf der Überprüfung, nachdem HOHLWEG (1953b) feststellte, daß sich bei langdauernder Gabe von Oestrogen in kleiner Dosis als Folge der veränderten Einstellung des Sexualzentrums die Gonadotropinausscheidung normal erhalten kann.

Verhalten der Chromosomen. Das *Kerngeschlecht* der echten Klinefelter-Kranken ist vom weiblichen Typ, also chromatinpositiv. Bei der Festlegung der Chromatinbefunde ergibt die Untersuchung der Schleimhäute, der Haut und der Leydigzellen eindeutige Ergebnisse, während Blutausstriche manchmal nicht sicher eingeordnet werden können, da ganz typische Drumstick fehlen (PLUNKETT 1956, DAVIDSON 1954, WIEDEMANN 1957, NOVAKOWSKI 1958). Das Vorkommen einer Rot-Grün-Schwäche in drei von 34 Patienten, wie es NOVAKOWSKI u. Mitarb. (1958) festgestellt haben, war einer der ersten Hinweise dafür, daß das echte Klinefelter-Syndrom nicht einfach genetisch weiblich sein kann. In den letzten Jahren konnte die Chromosomenkonstitution einer Reihe Kranker untersucht werden (JACOBS u. STRONG 1959a, FORD 1959a). Dabei zeigte sich, daß diese Patienten statt 46 47 Chromosomen haben. Das überzählige Chromosom ist ein zweites X-Chromosom. Reduplikation des X-Chromosom ist wahrscheinlich das Ergebnis des Nichtauseinandertretens (Non-disjumtion) der Geschlechtschromosome während der meiotischen Teilung. Eine mütterliche Keimzelle besitzt dann schon zwei X-Chromosome und erhält vom Vater zusätzlich noch ein Y-Chromosom, eine väterliche schon ein X- und ein Y-Chromosom und erhält von der Mutter noch ein X-Chromosom, so daß die Genformel XXY resultiert. Die Chromosomenanomalie ist Voraussetzung für die Diagnose echter Klinefelter.

Das Vorkommen von Farbenblindheit bei Trägern des Syndroms ist ein Hinweis, daß die Non-disjunction vorwiegend die mütterliche Eizelle betrifft. Wenn beide Elternteile farbentüchtig sind, dann kann die fehlende Chromosomenteilung nur während der zweiten meiotischen Teilung erfolgt sein. Die schematische Darstellung von FERGUSON-SMITH (Abb. 43) gibt die möglichen Störungen der Chromosomenverteilung wieder.

Neben diesem typischen Verhalten der Chromosomen beim Klinefelter-Syndrom wurden vier weitere Varianten beschrieben. In wenigen Einzelfällen fand sich die Chromosomenkonstitution XXXY (FERGUSON-SMITH u. Mitarb.. CARR u. Mitarb.), XXYY (MULDAL und OCKEY; CARR u. Mitarb.), XXXXY (FRACCARO u. Mitarb., ANDERS u. Mitarb., MILLER u. Mitarb., FRASER u. Mitarb.) und ein Mosaik von XXY/XY-Zellen (FORD u. Mitarb.. CROOKE u. Mitarb.). Die Fälle mit mehr als zwei X-Chromosomen sind bei der Untersuchung der Zellkerne der Schleimhäute an einem doppelten bzw. dreifachen Chromatinkörperchen zu vermuten. Die Entstehung dieser Anomalien ist nicht geklärt, man diskutiert eine Non-disjunction in der ersten und in der zweiten *meiotischen* Teilung der Eizelle, wodurch ein XXXX-Ei entstehen kann, das von einem Y-Spermium befruchtet wird, oder daß sich in einem befruchteten XXY-Ei, das durch Non-disjunction in einem der Elternpaare entstanden ist, bei der nachfolgenden *mitotischen* Teilung wieder durch Non-disjunction 4 X-Chromosome und 1 Y-Chromosom auf eine Zelle und 1 Y-Chromosom auf die andere Zelle verteilt. Da die Y-Zelle nicht lebensfähig ist, entwickeln sich nur die XXXY-Zellen weiter. Der XXXY- und XXXXY-Status kann als extremere Variante des normalen XXY-Klinefelter-Types angesehen werden.

In dem Fall von MILLER (XXXXY) handelt es sich um einen 21jährigen Hypogonaden mit Körpergröße 164 cm und multiplen Anomalien des Skeletsystems, Gaumenspalte, Strabismus und stark herabgesetzter Intelligenz, stark erniedrigten 17-Ketosteroidwerten bei normaler FRH-Ausscheidung im Urin. Er stammt aus einer Familie, in der bei einer Schwester des Vaters und bei einer Tochter einer anderen Schwester des Vaters echte Mongolen mit Trisomie von 21 vorgekommen sind. Das Kernchromatin fiel dadurch auf, daß in 14% der Zellen drei Körperchen vorhanden waren. Der Fall von FRACCARO u. Mitarb. war ein siebenjähriger Junge mit unterentwickeltem und gespaltenem Scrotum, in dem beidseits eine erbsgroße Masse tastbar war. Die histologische Untersuchung der rechten Keimdrüse ergab einen Hoden mit großen Bindegewebsmassen und wenigen erhaltenen Kanälchen, die undifferenzierte Zellen, ähnlich unreifen Sertolizellen, enthielten, Keimzellen waren nicht vorhanden. Andere Kanälchen waren völlig verödet, Leydigzellen waren nicht vorhanden. An sonstigen Anomalien fand sich ein offener Ductus arteriosus, ein beidseitiger Epikanthus und ein angedeuteter Turmschädel. Auch bei dem 8$\frac{1}{2}$jährigen Jungen von FRASER u. Mitarb. war das Scrotum unterentwickelt, die Testes nicht deszendiert. Die Hoden lagen im kleinen Becken, Vas deferens und Epididymis waren normal entwickelt. Histologisch sah man nur sehr spärlich Kanälchen ohne Keimzellen. Der debile Junge hatte multiple Knochenanomalien, vergrößerte und tiefe Sella turcica, beidseitige Coxa valga, proximales Radius- und Ulnarende waren deformiert, links mit Sinostose, zahlreiche abnorme Ossifikationszentren im Bereich der Handknochen.

Die Fälle mit mehr als zwei X-Chromosomen sind debil oder geistig unterentwickelt, die mit 4 X-Chromosomen haben zusätzlich zahlreiche Skeletanomalitäten. Es ist fraglich, ob diese Defekte etwas mit den überzähligen X-Chromosomen zu tun haben, da ähnliche Mißbildungen auch bei anderen schweren Chromosomendefekten auftreten können.

Beim Menschen bestimmt offenbar das Y-Chromosom die Entwicklung der Keimdrüse in männlicher Richtung, selbst bei Überwiegen des weiblichen Anteiles mit 2, 3 und 4 X-Chromosomen. Trotz der wenigen Fälle, die bis jetzt chromosomal untersucht sind, hat es den Anschein, daß die Schwere des Hodendefektes mit der Zahl der X-Chromosomen zunimmt.

Die Zahl der Zellen mit atypischen Chromosomen ist nicht ganz einheitlich. Im Falle ANDERS u. Mitarb. zeigte wohl die größte Zahl der Zellen 4 X-Chromosomen, ein kleiner Teil aber auch 3, zwei Zellen sogar 5. In 10% der Mitosen war das Y-Chromosom nicht nachweisbar. NOVAKOWSKI u. Mitarb. (1960) finden in neun von 13 durch Kulturen aus Hautbiopsien untersuchter Klinefelter-Syndrome ebenfalls wechselnde Chromosomenzahlen. Der größte Teil der Metaphasen hatte 47 Chromosomen (XXY), es fanden sich aber auch Abweichungen nach oben und unten, meist 46 und 48, aber auch 45 und zweimal 49 Chromosomen. Von einem echten Mosaik kann man nur sprechen, wenn, wie in den Fällen von FORD u.

Mitarb., Crooke u. Mitarb., etwa ein gleicher Prozentsatz einer genügend großen Zellzahl verschiedene Chromosomenzahlen aufweist.

Inzwischen wurden auch eine Reihe gonadal männlicher, geschlechtschromatin-negativer, sog. *falsche Klinefelter-Syndrome* untersucht. Kulturen ergaben normale Chromosomenzahlen und einen normalen XY-Geschlechtschromosomentyp (Court Brown 1960).

Heute ist man geneigt, die fehlende Entwicklungspotenz des normal angelegten Hodens dem abnormen Geschlechtschromosomensatz zuzuschreiben, die überzähligen X-Chromosome sollen einen hemmenden Einfluß auf die normale Entwicklung der Kanälchen haben. Die analoge Gewebsstruktur des „falschen" Klinefelter mit normalem Geschlechtschromosomensatz läßt Zweifel an ihrer alleinigen Bedeutung aufkommen und macht zum mindesten deutlich, daß Entwicklungsstörungen der Keimdrüsen nicht nur chromosomal bedingt sind, sondern auch andere Ursachen haben können, wobei besonders die von Witschi erarbeiteten Möglichkeiten diskutiert werden müssen.

Tonutti (1960) interpretiert die pathologischen Ereignisse folgendermaßen: Die präpuberale Größe der hyalinisierten Kanälchen zeigt, daß ein Defekt vorliegt, der die normale Differenzierung und Entfaltung des Samenepithels behindert. Hinzu kommt, daß die aus derselben Ursache heraus geschädigten Zwischenzellen selbst unter der Wirkung der erhöhten Gonadotropine keine normale Aktivität aufnehmen. Diese mangelnde inkretorische Leistung wirkt sich in zweifacher Richtung aus. Sie bedingt eine ungenügende Entwicklung der sekundären Geschlechtsmerkmale und verstärkt die Veränderungen am Tubulusapparat, und zwar indirekt über die insuffiziente androgene Kontaktwirkung auf die Tubuluswand. Die Veränderungen im Hodenbild werden um so tiefgreifender und massiver, je länger der Sekretionsausfall zurückliegt und je älter der Patient geworden ist. Nach dieser Auslegung spielt die Zwischenzellschädigung mit eine besondere Rolle. Eine Dysharmonie der Hormonsynthese erscheint bei diesen stark hyperplastischen Leydigzellen mit dem klinischen Bild des Hypoandrogenismus sehr wahrscheinlich, wobei neben dem vermehrten Anfall wenig wirksamer Vorstufen und deren Abbauprodukten auch mit der Bildung von Oestrogenen zu rechnen ist.

Eine kausale *Behandlung* ist nicht möglich. Die Träger der Anomalie bleiben steril. Nur wenn ein stärkerer Eunuchoidismus vorhanden ist, kommt die Dauertherapie mit Testosteron in Frage. Es ist interessant, daß unter hohen Dosen Choriongonadotropin (dreimal 5000 E/Woche) vorübergehend ein Ansteigen der 17-Ketosteroide und der Oestrogene eintreten kann (Leach 1957). Selbst so hyperaktive Leydigzellen sind noch zu einer Mehrarbeit fähig.

Zwei Beipiele sollen zur Erläuterung dienen:

Fall 6. H. L., 22jährig.

Der 22jährige hat sich als Kind normal entwickelt. Keine besonderen Krankheiten. In der Schule angeblich immer unter den größten. Mäßige Schulleistungen, viel Sport. Mit 13 Jahren beginnende Pubesbehaarung, Achselhaare zeigten sich erst mit 16 Jahren, blieben immer spärlich, kein Bartwuchs, auch Körperbehaarung dürftig. Bis zum 21. Lebensjahr noch gewachsen. Soweit er sich zurückerinnert, sind die Hoden nie größer gewesen wie jetzt.

Im Alter von 13 Jahren entwickelte er zum erstenmal masochistische Züge. Er befand sich damals in einem Waisenhaus und prügelte sich öfters mit anderen Kindern. Hier empfand er zum erstenmal Schläge als angenehm. Später betrieb er das Boxen, weil er nicht genug Prügel bekommen konnte. Im 15. Lebensjahr hat er sich während eines Streites mit seinem Vater zum erstenmal mit dem Rasiermesser am Brustkorb eine Wunde beigebracht, um diesem zu imponieren. Dabei merkte er, daß dieser Vorgang mit Lustgefühlen verbunden war. In den folgenden Jahren verletzte er sich wiederholt mit Rasiermessern oder Rasierklingen, trotz intensiver psychotherapeutischer Behandlung keine Änderung.

176 cm, Oberlänge 82 cm, Unterlänge 94 cm. Kräftig gebaut. Muskulatur ordentlich entwickelt, aber weiche Körperformen ohne deutliches Muskelrelief. Etwas feminine Anhäufung des Fettpolsters, besonders um die Hüften, keine Gynäkomastie, leichte X-Beine.

Genitale: Penis 6,7 cm, normal pigmentiert. Scrotum etwas kurz, wenig faltenreich, normal pigmentiert, Hoden an normaler Stelle, beide kleinbohnengroß, flach, fest und derb, rechter 2,2 : 1,25 cm, linker 2,1 : 1,2 cm. Prostata pfennigstückgroß, flach, kaum zu fühlen, weich (vgl. Abb. 51 a u. b).

17-Ketosteroide: 4,6, 8,6, 5,8 mg/24 Std.

Uringonadotropine mehr als 384 MUE.

Skeletsystem: Radius- und Ulna-Epiphysenlinie noch erkennbar. Fingerskelet normal entwickelt.

Darmbeinapophyse noch nicht verknöchert. An der Brustwirbelsäule sind die Randleisten noch ausgebildet.

Chromatin: Mundschleimhaut positiv.

Hodenbiopsie (Prof. TONUTTI): Die Tubuli sind vollkommen verödet, so daß das ganze Präparat von einem ziemlich gleichmäßigen Kanälchenschatten erfüllt ist. An einer Stelle zwei Anschnitte eines Kanälchens, dessen ganzes Lumen mit Sertolizellen erfüllt ist. Das Zwischengewebe besteht aus Klumpen und Ballen von Leydigzellen mit unterschiedlichem Entfaltungszustand. Verhältnismäßig wenig Zellen zeigen ein helles Plasma und feine Granulationen, die meisten weisen ein dunkelgefärbtes, dichtes Plasma, zum Teil mit reichlichen Pigmenteinschlüssen auf. Zum überwiegenden Teil ist das Zwischengewebe verhältnismäßig locker gebaut und enthält größere und kleinere Komplexe von Leydigzellen (vgl. Abb. 47).

Fall 7. G. O., geb. 23. 9. 26, Steinhauer.

Wird vom Arzt geschickt wegen mäßigem Hypogonadismus.

Früher nicht ernstlich krank.

Die Entwicklung hat erst mit 16 bis 17 Jahren eingesetzt, mit 18 bis 20 sind die Schamhaare erst richtig gewachsen, Körperbehaarung immer dürftig, Achsel- und Schambehaarung jetzt normal entwickelt, praktisch keine Bartbehaarung. Seit 5 Jahren verheiratet, normale Libido und Potenz; keine Kinder.

Der Kranke hat einen *Zwillingsbruder*, der ihm völlig gleicht. Auch dieser ist seit mehreren Jahren kinderlos verheiratet; habe denselben schlechten Haar- und Bartwuchs wie er. Eine Schwester ist normal entwickelt, verheiratet, hat Kinder.

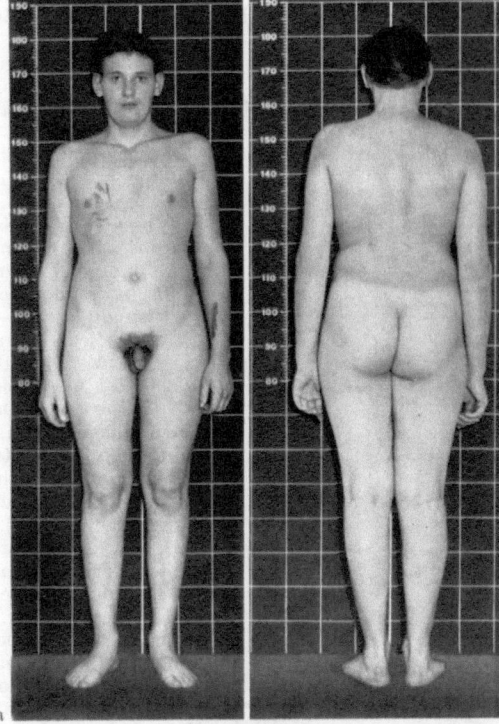

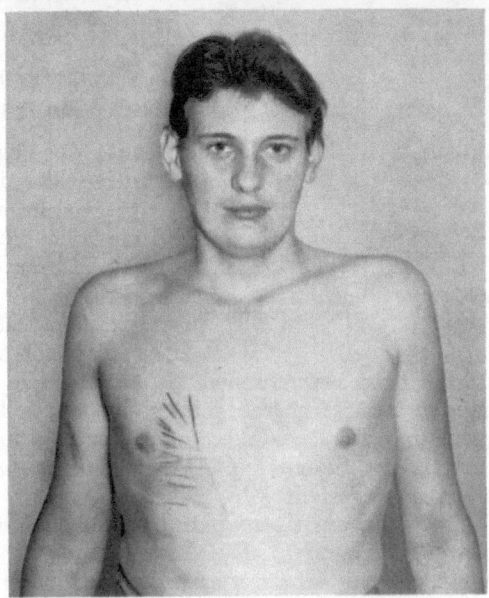

Abb. 51 a u. b. H. L., 23jährig, echtes Klinefelter-Syndrom, Masochismus, zahlreiche Reste von älteren und frischeren Verletzungen auf Brust und Oberarmen

Untersuchung 1957: Größe 182 cm, Oberlänge 88 cm, Unterlänge 94 cm. Gewicht 79,5 kg. Gut entwickelte Muskulatur, etwas pastöser Habitus mit weichen Körperkonturen (vgl. Abb. 52).

Gynäkomastie. Zweimarkstückgroße flache Drüsenkörper.

Behaarung: An Kinn und Oberlippe 10—20 Härchen, sonst völlig bartloses Gesicht. Achselbehaarung: Nur 30—40 mäßig lange Haare, Schambehaarung normal, Körperbehaarung dürftig.

Genitale: Beide Hoden etwa kirschgroß, flach, Konsistenz etwas weicher als normal.

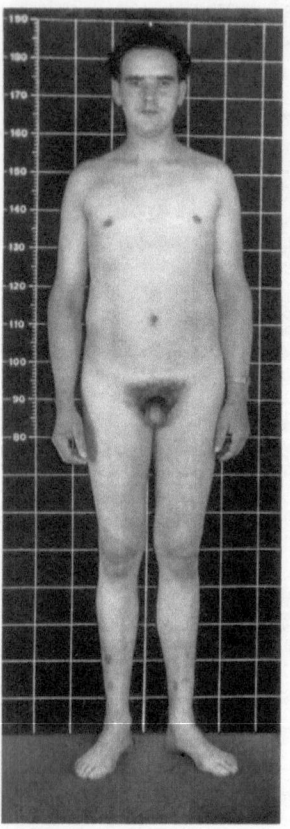

Abb. 52.   33 jähriger Kranker, G. O. Echtes Klinefelter-Syndrom

Penis normal entwickelt. Prostata: kleinkastaniengroß, fest, deutlich gelappt.

Gonadotropinausscheidung 192 ME, mehrmals positiv.

Spermatogramm: keine Spermien.

Mundschleimhaut: chromatinpositiv.

Funktion der Nebennierenrinde normal.

Grundumsatz —2%.

Jodspeicherung nach 6 Std 63%, nach 24 Std 72%.

Biopsie: sehr kleine Kanälchen, die zum größten Teil vollständig hyalinisiert sind. Dazwischen liegen andere, ebenfalls mit kleinem Durchmesser, die noch einen Zellbesatz von Sertolizellen tragen. Ganz vereinzelt finden sich in solchen Kanälchen Spermatogonien. Vermehrung des intertubulären Bindegewebes, mächtige Wucherung der Zwischenzellen, die teilweise gut differenziert sind und sich scharf voneinander abgrenzen (Abb. 46).

Nach diesen Befunden handelt es sich bei dem Kranken um ein echtes Klinefelter-Syndrom.

Der gleichaltrige *Bruder* war am 11. 4. 57 zusammen mit dem Patienten hier. Beide können nicht voneinander unterschieden werden. Der Bruder hat dieselbe Form und Ausprägung eines Hypogonadismus. Gleiche Behaarung, gleiche Körperkontur. Penis normal entwickelt, beide Hoden nur kleinkirschgroß, Prostata kastaniengroß. Einbestellt zur genaueren Untersuchung, doch verunglückte er am 22. 4. 57 tödlich.

IV. Hermaphroditismus und Pseudohermaphroditismus (testiculäre Feminisierung)

Nach der gegenwärtigen Auffassung sind die Mißbildungen der inneren und äußeren Genitalorgane des Hermaphroditismus durch eine frühembryonale Störung der inkretorischen Gonadenfunktion hervorgerufen. Durch die mangelhafte Wirkung der Induktoren bleibt die Entwicklung der Gangsysteme vorzeitig stehen. Die frühembryonale endokrine Insuffizienz kann sich später wieder vollständig ausgleichen, so daß beim erwachsenen Menschen keine Zeichen eines Hypogonadismus vorhanden sind. Insofern gehört eine kurze Besprechung des Hermaphroditismus verus und des Pseudohermaphroditismus masculinus hierher. Ob die hormonale Insuffizienz die einzige Ursache der Genitalmißbildung darstellt, ist aber noch nicht sichergestellt.

Beim echten Hermaphroditismus sind sowohl ovarielles als auch testiculäres Gewebe vorhanden. Die Entwicklung der Müllerschen und Wolffschen Gänge hängt von der Art der vorhandenen Gonade ab. Die Ausbildung des äußeren und inneren Genitales gleicht der des männlichen und weiblichen Pseudohermaphroditismus. OVERZIER hat eine neue Einteilung der einzelnen Typen vorgenommen, die sich auf fünf Grundtypen beschränkt und die die früheren, schwer verständlichen Klassifizierungen ersetzt. Auf seine neueste Zusammenstellung, die 146 seit 1900 veröffentlichte Fälle umfaßt, sei besonders hingewiesen, ebenso auf das

Buch: „Hermaphroditismus" von Jones und Scott. Der Nachweis von Eierstock
und Hodengewebe, die getrennt oder in einem sog. Ovotestis liegen, kann nur
durch die histologische Untersuchung erfolgen. Die Gonaden selbst zeigen histologisch alle Reifegrade von der hochgradigen Hypoplasie bis zum spermien-
produzierenden Hoden bzw. zum reifen Ovar. Die innersekretorische Funktion
ist auch beim Erwachsenen selten vollwertig.

Genetisch handelt es sich um männliche oder um weibliche Individuen. Der
größere Teil der untersuchten Fälle ist chromatinpositiv. Chromosomenuntersuchungen liegen bis jetzt von zehn Fällen vor. Dabei ergab sich sechsmal eine
normale XX-Konstitution, einmal ein Mosaik von XX/XXX und zweimal ein
Mosaik von X0/XY, einmal ein Mosaik XX/XY. Die Entwicklung von testiculärem Gewebe bei einem XX-Individuum sucht man durch die Annahme
eines Mosaikes von XX- und XY-Zellen in den Gonaden zu erklären, eine
Annahme, die der Bestätigung bedarf. Das starke Überwiegen der normalen
XX-Konstitution beim echten Hermaphroditismus macht (Waxmann) wahrscheinlich, daß sich Hodengewebe auch bei Fehlen des Y-Chromosoms entwickeln
kann (Harnden und Jacobs 1961).

Pseudohermaphroditismus masculinus, testiculäre Feminisierung. Der männliche Pseudohermaphrodit hat ein chromosomal männliches Geschlecht mit männlicher Chromosomenkonstitution XY, negativem Kernchromatin, ein gonadales
männliches Geschlecht und besitzt männliche Keimdrüsen. Die Geschlechtsorgane sind aber gemischt männlich und weiblich oder rein weiblich ausgebildet. In
den extremsten Fällen bleibt der Hoden im Abdomen liegen und verliert schon vor
Ende der zehnten Woche die Kontrolle über die Differenzierung des Gangsystems.
Innere und äußere Genitalorgane erhalten dann wie beim Ullrich-Turner-Syndrom
eine rein weibliche Form, es wird dann nicht einmal eine Epididymis oder ein
Rudiment des Ductus deferens gebildet. Meist ist die induktive Kraft des Hodens
jedoch weniger stark herabgesetzt, häufig auch erst in den späteren Stadien der
Entwicklung. Folge davon ist, daß alle Übergänge der Entwicklung zwischen
weiblicher und männlicher Differenzierung, also von der „Frau mit Hoden" bis
zum anatomisch normalen Mann mit einfacher Hypospadie und normal deszendierten Hoden zu beobachten sind. Als wichtigstes Stigma bleibt ein Phallus
vom klitoralen Typ (Einzelheiten s. bei Jones und Scott; Overzier). Die
Ursache dieser Mißbildungen ist nicht sichergestellt. Auf Grund der Jostschen Versuche (s. Entwicklung) nimmt man an, daß die mangelnde Ausbildung des männlichen Gangsystems durch einen mehr oder weniger weitgehenden Defekt der
Androgenbildung des embryonalen Hodens bedingt ist, ein Defekt, der sich mit
der Pubertät wieder ausgleichen kann. Die andere Möglichkeit ist, daß die Leydigzellen während der embryonalen Entwicklungsperiode mehr Oestrogene als
Androgene produzieren. Witschi nimmt an, daß von der Mutter irgendein
Agens auf den Fet übertragen wird, das mit der normalen Hodenfunktion
interferiert, so daß die embryonale Androgenproduktion nicht zur Wirkung
kommen kann.

Fälle mit männlichem äußeren Genitale sind häufiger als solche mit vorwiegend
weiblichem, das innere Genitale ist dann stärker in Richtung der weiblichen
Adnexe verändert. Die *Hoden,* die meist in der Bauchhöhle liegen, sind stark
verändert und erheblich verkleinert. Die Kanälchenwand besteht vorwiegend aus
Sertolizellen, das Keimepithel fehlt meist vollständig, doch sind einige Fälle mit
Spermatogonien und Spermatocyten, ausnahmsweise sogar mit reifen Spermatozoen beschrieben worden. Im Interstitium ist das Bindegewebe stark vermehrt,
reife Leydigzellen sind selten anzutreffen. Die Ausscheidung der 17-Ketosteroide
ist normal, die Oestrogene sind wenig untersucht, in einigen Fällen waren sie

vermehrt, dagegen wird die Gonadotropinausscheidung im Urin fast regelmäßig vermehrt gefunden.

Eine merkwürdige Form des Pseudohermaphroditismus masculinus ist die *testiculäre Feminisierung*. Nach PRADER versteht man darunter eine Form der Intersexualität mit rein weiblichem äußeren Genitale mit Vagina bei fehlendem Uterus und Adnexen, weiblicher Brustentwicklung, weiblichem Körperbau und chromosomal und gonadal männlichem Geschlecht. Andere Bezeichnungen sind *„hairless woman with testis"* (WILKINS), männliche Intersexform mit rein weiblichen Genitalorganen und Habitus (HAUSER).

Das äußere Genitale ist meist normal weiblich entwickelt, die angelegte Vagina endet blind, der Uterus fehlt. Von den Gonaden ziehen Stränge bis zum Ende der Vagina hinter die Blase, die als Ligamente beschrieben werden.

Die *Gonaden* liegen häufig in Inguinalhernien (60%) und werden bei der Operation zufällig entdeckt, in 19% in den großen Labien, in 21% im Abdomen. Sie bestehen aus Hodengewebe und zeigen enge lumenlose Kanälchen, die in ihrer Entwicklung einem fetalen oder frühkindlichen Hoden entsprechen (SNIFFEN 1950). Bei der Mehrzahl der Fälle konnten Sertolizellen unterschieden werden, bei einzelnen jedoch nur undifferenzierte Zellen. Charakteristisch ist das vollständige Fehlen von Spermatogonien, wobei nicht bekannt ist, ob die Gonien nicht einwandern oder sekundär zugrunde gehen. Die Zwischenzellen sind gut ausgebildet, oft überreichlich entwickelt und manchmal sogar adenomartig gewuchert. Das intertubuläre Bindegewebe ist vermehrt, während die Verdickung der Basalmembran mit Hyalinisierung an den einzelnen Kanälchen verschieden stark ausgeprägt ist. Verhältnismäßig häufig finden sich tubuläre Adenome, sog. Picksche Adenome, die als Begleitsymptom von Fehlbildungen gelten.

Das überraschendste ist der normal weibliche Körperbau mit typischer Fettverteilung und gut entwickelten Mammae. Werden die Hoden vor der Pubertät entfernt, dann bleibt ihre Entwicklung aus (HAIN u. SCHOFIELD 1947). Bei den typischen Fällen fehlt die Körper- und Sexualbehaarung ganz, was WILKINS (1957) veranlaßte, diese Menschen als „haarlose Frauen mit Hoden" zu benennen. Bei einem kleinen Teil sind die Pubes etwas entwickelt. Die Stimme bleibt weiblich hoch und ungebrochen. Bei einem eigenen Fall war das äußere Genitale weiblich, die Stimme hoch, die Körperproportion weiblich, Achsel- und Schambehaarung mäßig entwickelt, es fehlten die Mamae jedoch vollständig, die Mamillen waren viril. Im Hoden bestand links das Bild der schweren Sklerohyalinose der Kanälchen mit Leydigzellhyperplasie, rechts hatte sich ein Seminom entwickelt. Geschlechtschromatin negativ, Chromosomenanalyse XY. Die „Frauen" verhalten sich in Psyche und Sexualität rein weiblich. Das Syndrom wird immer durch klinisch gesunde Frauen übertragen und betrifft nur *chromosomal* und gonadal *männliche* Individuen. Die Vererbung erfolgt nach PRADER durch ein recessivgeschlechtsgebundenes Gen oder ein Autosom, das eine Androgenresistenz bedingen soll.

Hormonuntersuchungen. Bis jetzt sind nur wenige Untersuchungen mit ausreichender Methodik durchgeführt worden. Im allgemeinen wird die Ausscheidung der Oestrogene gegenüber der normalen Frau als erniedrigt, gegenüber dem normalen Mann als erhöht angegeben (KESSLER 1959, SCHREINER 1959, WILKINS 1957, HAUSER 1957a und b). Der Vaginalabstrich zeigt eine verminderte Oestrogeneinwirkung (STANGE 1957, HAUSER 1957a und b). Die 17-Ketosteroidausscheidung ist im allgemeinen normal, einzelne berichten über erhöhte Werte, die chromatographische Auftrennung zeigt keine Bevorzugung einer Fraktion. Die Ausscheidung der Gonadotropine wird meist als leicht erhöht angegeben.

WILKINS u. v. a. nehmen als *Ursache* für diese Anomalie eine Resistenz der Gewebe gegenüber den im Hoden produzierten Androgenen an. Die Erfolgsorgane, also Haarfollikel, Larynx, Wolffsche Gänge, äußeres Genitale und Klitoris sprechen auf die in normaler Menge produzierten Androgene nicht an, während sich der Uterus und die anderen weiblichen Adnexe zurückbilden. Die vermehrt entwickelte Brust und die weiblichen Körperkonturen zeigen nicht nur ein normales Ansprechen auf Oestrogene, sondern auch die Oestrogenproduktion des Hodens an. Andere diskutieren als Ursache eine früh intrauterin einsetzende Hodeninsuffizienz. Die embryonale Hodenfunktion soll die Entwicklung der oberen Teile der Müllerschen Gänge in geringem Maße hemmen (Uterus und eventuell Teile der Vagina), sie ist aber zu schwach, um die Wolffschen Gänge zur Entwicklung zu bringen. Die Körperzellen enthalten kein Geschlechtschromatin. In wenigen bis jetzt durchgeführten Chromosomenuntersuchungen fand sich eine *normale X Y-Konstitution* (LENNOX 1959, JACOBS 1959 b).

V. Morphologie und Klinik der Gonadendysgenesie
1. Anorchie

Nach den experimentellen Untersuchungen von JOST (1947 a) an Kaninchen entwickelt sich bei genetisch männlichen Embryonen nach frühzeitiger Zerstörung beider Keimdrüsen ein weibliches inneres und äußeres Genitale. Eine Bestätigung dieser experimentellen Befunde für den Menschen scheint das Ullrich-Turner-Syndrom gebracht zu haben, wobei sich als Folge der rudimentären funktionslosen Gonadenanlage ein normal weibliches inneres und äußeres Genitale ausbildet. Wie oben ausgeführt, wurde in den bis jetzt vollständig untersuchten Fällen meist eine Monosomie der Geschlechtschromosomen (X0) oder ein Mosaik von X0 und XX gefunden, während die wenigen Fälle mit XY eine Minderwertigkeit des Y-Chromosoms nahelegen.

Unter dem Begriff Anorchie faßte man bis jetzt Kranke mit schwerem Hypogonadismus zusammen, bei denen die Revision des Scrotums bzw. des Retroperitonealraumes wohl Reste des Wolffschen Ganges, ein Vas deferens und Reste der Epididymis ergeben hat, bei ausgedehnter Revision des Retroperitonealraumes Rudimente der Hoden aber nicht festgestellt werden konnten. Diese Kranken bezeichneten HELLER u. Mitarb. (1943) rein nach dem klinischen Bild als *präpuberale funktionelle Kastraten".* OVERZIER (1956 b) anerkennt diese Auffassung nicht, da die fehlende Hodenanlage eine andere anatomische Ausprägung der Genitalgänge zur Folge habe. Er beschreibt zwei Geschwister, die im Alter von 10 und 13 bzw. 12 und 15 Jahren untersucht wurden. Beide sind als Mädchen erzogen, beide haben ein männliches Kernchromatin. Die Ältere ist knabenhaft muskulös gebaut, die Jüngere noch kindlich unbestimmt. Die 15jährige hat einen Anflug von Schambehaarung, jedoch noch keine Achselbehaarung. Brustentwicklung fehlt, Mamillen unauffällig. Äußeres Genitale: penisähnliches Gebilde von 2 cm bzw. 1,5 cm Länge mit zurückstreifbarem Praeputium und einem Innenteil ohne Glans. Von der Basis der Glans aus führt eine doppelte Raphe über den etwa 5—7 cm langen Damm. Es ist äußerlich weder eine Vagina noch ein Scrotum zu erkennen. Mit Hilfe der Röntgendarstellung wird ein Sinus urogenitalis ausgeschlossen, es stellt sich nur eine gebogene Harnröhre dar. Bei der digitalen Untersuchung kann eine Prostata nicht nachgewiesen werden. Sonstige Anomalien, besonders solche wie sie beim Turner-Syndrom vorkommen, fehlen.

Bei der Laparotomie fehlen Uterus, Tuben, Ovarien, ebenso Vagina, Hoden oder Hodenrudimente. Beidseits findet sich oberhalb der Linea inominata, kranial der normalen Insertionsstelle des Ligamentum infund. pel. und lateral des Ureters ein kaum erbsgroßes, etwa 20 mm langes, 3 mm dickes Gebilde, das rechts abgetragen wird. Die histologische Untersuchung ergibt einen muskulären Kanal mit wenigen niedrigen Schleimhautfalten aus einfachem Cylinderepithel, ähnlich einer fetalen Tube. Daneben läßt sich ein gut entwickeltes Epoophoron darstellen. Zwei Drittel desselben besteht aus zahlreichen gewundenen, mit kubischem Epithel ausgekleideten Kanälchen, in deren Wand einige zirkuläre Muskelfasern eingelagert sind. Das letzte Drittel enthält einen vielfach gewundenen Gang mit einreihigem hohem Cylinderepithel ausgekleidet, das seinem Aussehen nach eine auffallende Ähnlichkeit mit dem Ductus epididymidis erkennen läßt. Die zuerst genannten Kanälchen entsprechen den Ductuli efferentes des Nebenhodens, das letzte Drittel dem Körper und dem Schwanz des Nebenhodens, also dem stark gewundenen Wolffschen Gang (Urnierengang). Die Ausscheidung der Gonadotropine beträgt bei der Älteren 19,2 MEU, bei der Jüngeren 38,4 MEU. Philip (1956) konnte einen ähnlichen Fall beschreiben. Ein weiblicher Agonadismus dieser Art ist bis jetzt nicht bekannt.

Das Besondere dieser beiden Fälle ist das gleichzeitige Vorhandensein von Resten der Wolffschen und der Müllerschen Gänge, ein Befund, der bislang bei keinem Fall erhoben worden ist. Overzier (1956b) baut darauf seine Theorie der Initial- und Dauerinduktion auf. Er nimmt an, daß von der sich bildenden männlichen oder weiblichen Keimdrüse ein Initialimpuls nicht hormonaler Art zur Entwicklung des Gangsystems ausgeht. Fehlt dieser Initialimpuls — z.B. wenn keine Keimdrüse angelegt ist —, dann bleibt die Entwicklung des Gangsystems auf frühembryonaler Stufe stehen. Die Ausbildung des Wolffschen und des Müllerschen Ganges in der embryonalen Periode ist nach Overzier also an das Vorhandensein einer funktionierenden Keimdrüse gebunden. Ist die Entwicklung des Gangsystems abgelaufen, dann erfolgt die weitere Differenzierung in männlicher Richtung, wenn männliche Gonaden einen Dauerimpuls auf die Differenzierung ausüben oder in weiblicher Richtung, wenn männliche Gonaden fehlen, also bei weiblichen oder bei frühkastrierten männlichen Individuen.

Die Theorie der Initialinduktion der Keimdrüsen ist bis jetzt experimentell nicht bewiesen, die der Dauerinduktion durch die Jostschen Experimente belegt. Jost (1947a) ist der Ansicht, daß ein 20 Tage alter Kaninchenembryo, bei dem Wolffsche und Müllersche Gänge ausgebildet sind, die letzteren gerade den Urogenitalsinus erreicht haben, eigentlich überhaupt keinen Genitaltrakt besitzt, da sich der Urogenitalsinus, der Wolffsche und der Müllersche Gang in Verbindung mit dem frühen exkretorischen System entwickeln. Es erhebt sich die Frage, ob die rudimentäre Entwicklung in den beiden Overzierschen Fällen nicht eine von der fehlenden Keimdrüsenanlage unabhängige Mißbildung darstellt. Die rudimentäre Ausbildung des äußeren Genitales mit dem hohen geschlossenen Damm, der männlichen Harnröhre entspricht nicht den Ergebnissen der Jostschen Experimente, das äußere Genitale müßte weiblich sein.

Einen auch histologisch ganz untersuchten Fall eines 27 cm langen menschlichen Feten ohne Keimdrüsenanlage hat Meyer (1925) beschrieben. Es fehlten Nieren, Keimdrüsen, Harnleiter, Nebenhoden und Vas defferens völlig, es war aber ein normal gebildeter Penis und ein normales Scrotum vorhanden, die Prostata war angelegt. Die Mißbildung ist in diesem Falle noch ausgedehnter als in dem Overzierschen, es fehlen auch die Rudimente der Gangsysteme. während wiederum den Jostschen Experimenten widersprechend das äußere Genitale normal männlich entwickelt war. Auch in den Fällen von Kretschmer (1949) — neugeborenes Kind — und im Falle Hepburn (1949) fehlen Hoden und Gänge, während Penis und Scrotum männlich ausgebildet waren.

2. Funktioneller präpuberaler Kastrat

Eine wesentlich größere Gruppe von Anorchien fassen HELLER; NELSON und ROTH (1943) unter dem Begriff des funktionellen präpuberalen Kastraten zusammen. Hierher gehören die von COUNSELLER und WALKER (1933) zusammengestellten elf Fälle und die Fälle 4 und 6 von HELLER u. Mitarb. Ein kleiner Teil ist postmortal untersucht, die meisten wurden bei der operativen Revision wegen Kryptorchismus erfaßt, wobei Scrotum, der Inguinalkanal und der retroperitoneale Raum abgesucht wurde. Hierbei fand man blind im Scrotum oder in der Inguinalgegend endende Samenstränge, eine schlecht ausgebildete Epididymis, Reste des Wolffschen Ganges, während Reste von Keimdrüsengewebe nur ganz selten nachgewiesen werden können.

Unbehandelt besteht klinisch ein vollständiger Defekt der Androgenproduktion, wie z. B. bei dem 20jährigen, 173,5 cm großen Kranken von WILDBOLZ (1917) mit 4 cm langem Penis, kleinem Scrotum, fehlender Prostata, fehlender Achsel-, Scham- und Gesichtsbehaarung. Beim Erwachsenen entspricht das Genitale einem 6—8jährigen, Achsel- und Schambehaarung sind ganz dürftig, Muskulatur schlecht entwickelt, die Prostata ist palpatorisch nicht feststellbar und auch sonst finden sich alle Zeichen eines präpuberalen Eunuchoidismus.

Die Körpergröße ist meist normal, selten besteht ein Hochwuchs, manche sind etwas klein. In allen Fällen hat das *Skelet* eunuchoide Proportionen mit der charakteristischen Überlänge der Spannweite gegenüber der Körpergröße. Die Reifung des Skeletsystems ist verzögert, doch tritt im Alter von etwa 25—30 Jahren doch der Epiphysenschluß ein.

Ein wichtiger Befund ist die *erhöhte Ausscheidung der Gonadotropine*, wobei bei der differenzierten Testung sowohl FSH als auch das ICSH vermehrt ausgeschieden wird. Die 17-Ketosteroidausscheidung lieg an der unteren Grenze des Normalen. Die Verabreichung von Choriongonadotropin, auch in hohen Dosen, erhöht die Ausscheidung der Androgene und Oestrogene nicht, sie hat auch keinen Einfluß auf die Sexualreifung.

Im Scrotum tastet man bei einem Teil der Fälle beidseits etwa erbsgroße, weiche Stränge, die sich bei der Probeexcision als Reste der Epididymis bzw. des Ductus deferens erweisen. Auch bei weiterer Suche im Leistenkanal und im Retroperitonealraum, die in einigen der veröffentlichten Fälle außerordentlich gründlich durchgeführt worden ist, ließ sich Hodengewebe nicht nachweisen. Bei anderen ist das Scrotum völlig leer, dann endet der Ductus deferens schon im Leistenkanal.

Nach der gegenwärtigen Anschauung nimmt man an, daß in diesen Fällen der Hoden embryonal angelegt war und auch Wirkstoffe produzierte — Rückbildung der Müllerschen Gänge, Ausbildung des Ductus deferens, Prostata, männliches äußeres Genitale seien ein Beweis dafür —, später aber zugrunde ging. Ungeklärt und merkwürdig ist allerdings, daß man gar keine Reste des embryonal funktiontätigen Hodens feststellen kann, ist er in diesen Fällen vielleicht doch nicht angelegt? Bei vier eigenen Fällen war das Geschlechtschromatin der Mundschleimhaut negativ.

Es sei an die komplizierten Vorgänge beim Descensus der Keimdrüsen erinnert. Während des sechsten Embryonalmonats nimmt das Rete testis Verbindung mit den Ductuli efferentes auf. Diese vereinigten sich mit der aus dem Wolffschen Gang stammenden Epididymis. Bleibt die Vereinigung aus, dann entsteht ein Hoden ohne Ausführungsgänge, der dann an Ort und Stelle liegenbleibt, da das Gubernaculum testis an die Wolffschen Gänge und nicht an den Hoden angeheftet ist. Es deszendieren also nur die Epididymis und Vasa deferentia. Kranke mit den Zeichen einer gewissen Androgenproduktion — geringe Sekundärbehaarung, tastbare Prostata — gehören morphologisch zur nächsten Gruppe, klinisch werden sie meist dem Kryptorchismus mit Hypogonadismus zugeordnet.

3. Schwere Hodenhypoplasie

Neben diesen offensichtlichen frühembryonalen Entwicklungsstörungen der Gonaden wurde in den letzten Jahren auch über schwere und leichtere Formen angeborener Defekte des exkretorischen und inkretorischen Hodenanteils berichtet. Ein von Sohval und Soffer (1952) beschriebener Fall sei kurz angeführt, da er die ganze Problematik widerspiegelt.

Es handelt sich um einen 23jährigen jungen Mann mit elf gesunden Geschwistern, mit einem schweren präpuberalen Hypogonadismus, $1^1/_4$ cm langer Penis, normaler Lage der Urethra, rudimentärem Scrotum, beidseitigem Kryptorchismus ohne Hernien, nicht palpabler Prostata, keine Gynäkomastie, keine Retinadegeneration, Farbsehen normal, *Anosmie*, dabei aber eine chronische Pansinusitis. Grundumsatz —8%, Hb 14 g-%. *Gonadotropine* nach Klinefelter 30 MEU negativ bei zweimaliger Untersuchung. 17-Ketosteroide 3,2 mg.

Bei der chirurgischen Exploration findet man rechts am oberen Eingang des Inguinalkanals ein kleines, gelbes Knötchen, 5 mm Durchmesser, das entfernt wird. Die linke Seite wird nicht freigelegt.

Bei der histologischen Untersuchung stellen sich ganz kleine unreife Kanälchen mit einem mittleren Durchmesser von 40 μ ohne Lumen dar. Auf einer normalen Basalmembran liegt eine einzellige Schicht undifferenzierter Zellen, die durch einen runden oder ovalen Kern mit feinen und groben Chromatingranula und einer deutlichen Kernmembran charakterisiert sind. Das Cytoplasma ist schlecht abgegrenzt. Weder Spermatogonien noch Sertolizellen können identifiziert werden. Im intertubulären Gewebe keine Fibrose, keine Reste einer Entzündung, Leydigzellen nicht zu erkennen.

Die Autoren diskutieren die einzelnen Möglichkeiten und schließen eine Schädigung durch die abnorme Lage der Keimdrüse aus, da beim Kryptorchismus im Alter von 23 Jahren entweder Sertolizellen und die ersten Stadien der Spermatogenese nachweisbar sind, oder aber eine fortschreitende Fibrosierung und bindegewebige Umwandlung des Interstitiums und der Kanälchenwand vorliegt. Das Bild des nichtstimulierten Hodens, wie er bei Ausfall der Gonadotropinproduktion der Adenohypophyse gefunden wird, zeigt nicht diese schwere Unterentwicklung. Hierbei bleibt wohl die Reifung der Sertoli- und der Leydigzellen aus, aber Spermatogonien sind feststellbar. Auch die abnorme Kleinheit von 0,5 cm Durchmesser spricht gegen den einfachen idiopathischen hypogonadotropen Eunuchoidismus. Sohval u. Mitarb. (1952) deuten den Befund als Entwicklungsstörung, die alle drei cellulären Anteile des Hodens betrifft, so daß nur rudimentäre Kanälchen gebildet werden, die primitive, undifferenzierte Zellen enthalten.

Wenn es sich um einen einfachen primären Hodendefekt handelt, müßte man erwarten, daß die Gonadotropine im Alter von 23 Jahren wenigstens feststellbar sind, bei dieser schweren Unterentwicklung der Kanälchen müßten sie stark erhöht sein. Die Ursache der fehlenden Gonadotropinerhöhung konnte nicht geklärt werden und so bleibt die Frage offen, inwieweit die mangelnde Gonadotropinbildung vielleicht schon in den entscheidenden ersten Embryonalwochen zu der hochgradigen Unreife des Hodens beigetragen hat.

Wir konnten ähnliche Beobachtungen machen:
Fall 8. G. S., 34jähriger Mann. Nie ernstlich krank gewesen. Etwa vom 10. Lebensjahr ab
im Wachstum zurückgeblieben, Pubertät blieb aus, körperlich immer schwächlich mit Neigung
zu Adipositas. Mehrmalige Untersuchungen. 154 cm, 43 kg, eunuchoide Proportionen, sieht
aus wie 18jähriger, Extremitäten grazil, Hohlfußbildung beiderseits, Kyphoskoliose, Cubitus
valgus, Synostose der ersten und zweiten Rippe rechts, Lobus venae azygos, keinerlei Behaarung, kindlich hohe Stimme. Genitale: Penis 2,5 cm, Hoden erbsgroß, weich, Prostata
nicht tastbar. 17-Ketosteroide 4,2—5,3 mg. Gonadotropine bei 24 MEU negativ. Grundumsatz —6%, Hb 88%, reichlich Kreatinin im Urin. Neurologisch o.B. Sella normal, Augen
o.B. Skelet: Entwicklungszustand und Epiphysenfugen wie bei 18jährigem, Osteoporose.
Diagnose: hypogonadotroper Hypogonadismus. Behand-
lung: wöchentlich dreimal 1000 E Choriongonadotropin
über 4 Monate, keine Änderung (Abb. 53).

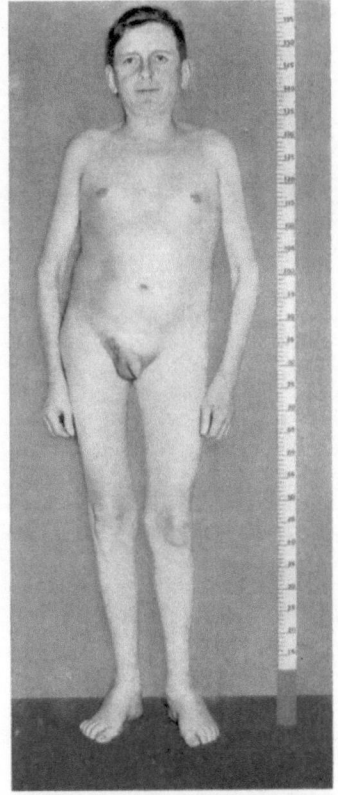

Mit 38 Jahren: Größe 157,8 cm, Oberlänge 67,8 cm,
Unterlänge 90 cm. Gewicht 50,4 kg. Schwerer präpuberaler Eunuchoidismus, keinerlei Behaarung, dürftige
Muskulatur, kindliches Genitale, erbsgroße Hoden, Prostata wie früher. Epiphysen der Extremitätenknochen
noch offen (Abb. 54). Farbentüchtig, Geruchssinn normal.
Chromatinnegativ. Grundumsatz —6%, 17-Ketosteroide
4,9—6,1 mg. Porter-Silberchromogen 5,8—7,4 mg, unter 10, ACTH-Anstieg auf 18,2 mg. Gonadotropine bei
24 MEU (Alkoholpräcipitation) mehrmals negativ. Probeexcision rechts: Kanälchen sehr klein, ausgekleidet von
gleichförmigen unreifen Zellen mit runden oder ovalen
Kernen, in 1—3 Schichten, keine Spermatogonien, keine
Sertolizellen, Wand ganz zart, lockeres Zwischengewebe
mit Fibrocyten und Fibroblasten ohne Leydigzellen,
Bild der kompakten Kanälchen (vgl. Abb. 55).
Choriongonadotropin: 5 Wochen lang dreimal 1500 E
je Woche. Keine Änderung der 17-Ketosteroide.
Danach jetzt neunjährige Dauerbehandlung mit De-
pottestosteronen. Penis beinahe normal groß, Sexual-
funktionen normal, Prostata kleinkastaniengroß, erheblich verbesserte Muskulatur, geringe Scham- und Achselbehaarung, im Gesicht nur Flaum, keine Glatzenbildung.
Hodengewebe wie zu Anfang.

Fall 9. W. B., 42jährig.
Lernte erst mit 5 Jahren sprechen und besuchte mit
8 Jahren die Hilfsschule. War immer der Kleinste. Da er
sich mit 16 Jahren noch nicht entwickelte, erste ärztliche
Untersuchung. Dabei fiel ein schwerer Hypogonadismus
auf. Die deszendierten Hoden waren nur kleinerbsgroß
und weich. Mehrjährige Hormonbehandlung — Art
nicht bekannt — brachte keine Besserung. Der debile
Junge kam vorübergehend in eine Anstalt. Er arbeitet

Abb. 53. S. G., 35jähriger Mann mit
schwerer Hodenhypoplasie (Fall 8)

seit dem 20. Lebensjahr als Spulenausträger in einer
Spinnerei.
Größe 153,5 cm, Oberlänge 71,5 cm, Unterlänge 82 cm, Spannweite 163 cm. Dys-
plastischer Habitus, Kyphose der Brustwirbelsäule mit leichter Skoliose, Schrägstellung des
Beckens. Pastöses Gesicht mit groben Runzeln, trockene Haut, fehlende Rumpf- und
Extremitätenbehaarung. Debilität. (Abb. 56.)
Genitale: Penis 4,5 × 2,0 cm, Hoden rechts kleinbohnen-, links erbsgroß, ganz weich,
Prostata nicht sicher feststellbar. Scham- und Achselbehaarung fehlen, Oberlippe und Kinn
nur Lanugobehaarung.
17-Ketosteroide 4,18; 5,4 mg, 40 E Depot-ACTH: Anstieg auf 7,5 mg, Abfall der Eosino-
philen 100%.
Urin: Gonadotropin 24 E, negativ, 135 E mg.
Grundumsatz +8%, Jodspeicherung 45%, 62% (8 und 24 Std), Hb 14,2 g-%.
Serumeiweiß 6 g-%, geringe α_2-Vermehrung.
Calcium 9,6 mg-%, Phosphor 3,1 mg-%, Phosphatase: sauer 0,42, alkalisch 1,56 mm
Mol E.
Skelet: Schädel seitlich: Kalkgehalt und Feinstruktur regelrecht, Cavum sellae nach
Form und Größe regelrecht, Kalkeinlagerungen in der normal liegenden Epiphyse.

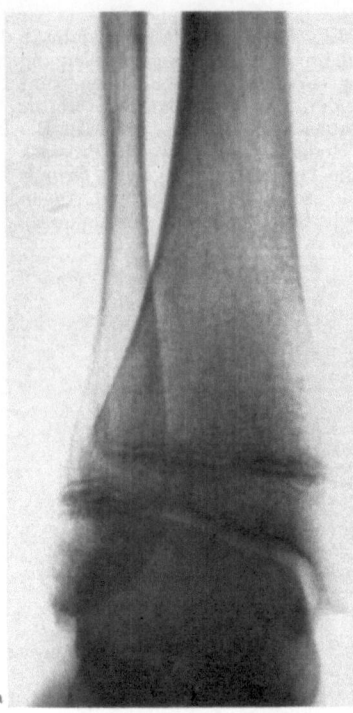

Wirbelsäule: Vermehrter Rundrücken der Brustwirbelsäule, deutliche spondylotische Randzacken, Verschmälerung einzelner Wirbelkörper und Zwischenwirbelscheiben im Bereich der Brustwirbelsäule, im Scheitelpunkt der Kyphose wellig konfigurierte Grund- und Deckplatten.

Halswirbelsäule: Erweiterung des oberen Cervicalkanales.

Lendenwirbelsäule: Die obere Vorderkante des 1. und 4. Lendenwirbels ist stark abgeschrägt (Aufbaustörung), fehlender Bogenschluß am 5. Lendenwirbel, mäßige Osteoporose der gesamten Lendenwirbelsäule.

Kalkgehalt des übrigen Skelets ebenfalls mäßig vermindert. Sklerosierungslinien der ehemaligen Epiphysenlinien an Femur und Tibia beidseits.

Chromatinkörper der Mundepithelien negativ.

Hodenbiopsie (rechts) nach achtwöchiger Gabe von zweimal 1500 HCG/Woche: Hoden, Nebenhoden und Ductus deferens vorhanden. Epithel des Nebenhodens regelrecht gebildet. Die Kanälchen des Hodens sind sehr klein und ohne Lumen, die Wand ist zart und besetzt von undifferenzierten Zellen mit dichten Kernen ohne Nucleolen, weder Sertolizellen noch Spermatogonien sind erkennbar. Das Zwischengewebe ist derbfaserig und enthält trotz der vorausgegangenen Choriongonadotropinbehandlung nur undifferenzierte Bindegewebszellen. Es besteht also das Bild der schweren Hodenhypoplasie (Abb. 57).

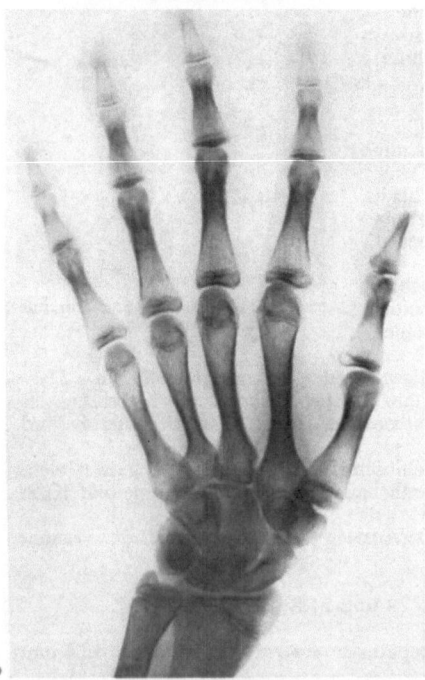

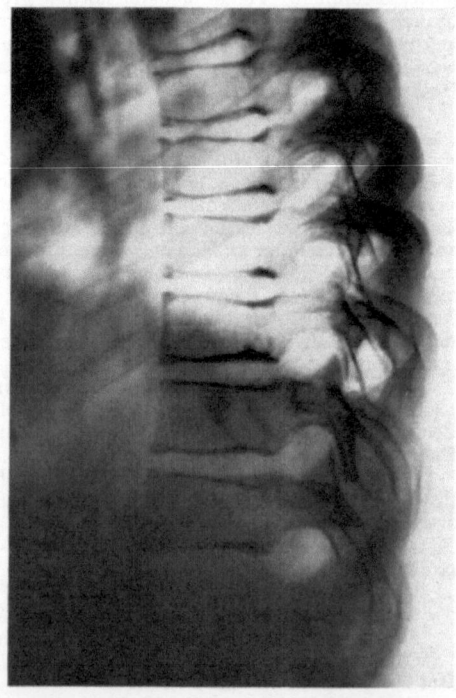

Abb. 54 a u. b. Skelet von Patient 8, 31jährig, mit schwerem primärem (?) Eunuchismus. Offene Epiphysenfugen an Hand, Skelet *und* Unterschenkeln, niedrige Wirbelkörper mit noch nicht verknöcherter Randleiste

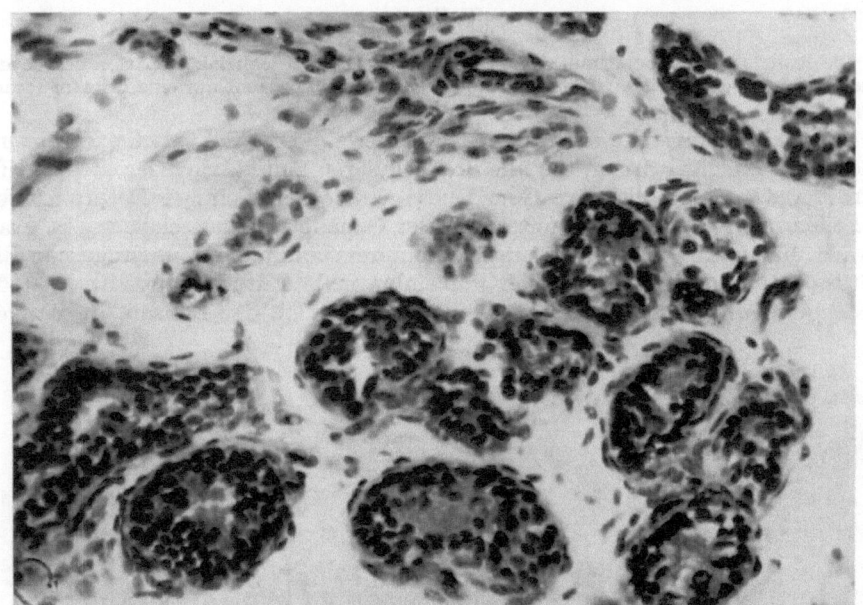

Abb. 55. Biopsie von Fall 8. Tubuli stark verkleinert, nur unreife Zellen in ein bis drei Zellschichten, keine Spermatogonien. Kanälchenwand zart. Interstitium: lockeres Bindegewebe mit Fibrocyten und Fibroblasten, keine Leydigzellen. Bild der kompakten Tubuli seminiferi. (Hämatoxylin-Eosin, 300fach)

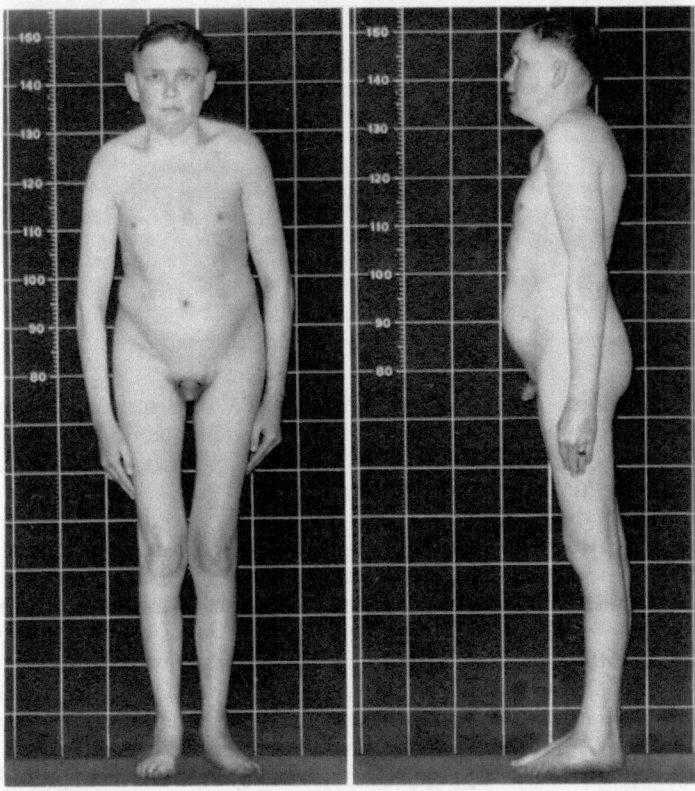

Abb. 56. Hodenbiopsie eines 42jährigen Debilen mit schwerem präpuberalem Eunuchismus, normal gebildetem Genitale, chromatinnegativen Epithelzellen. Nach 8wöchiger Behandlung mit Choriongonadotropin (zweimal 1500 E) besteht das Zwischengewebe aus einem faserreichen Bindegewebe ohne Leydigzellen, die kleinen Kanälchen nur aus undifferenzierten Zellen. Vergrößerung (Gison, 230fach) (Fall 9)

Die erfolglose Hormonbehandlung früher und das Fehlen jeglicher Reaktion der Leydigzellen auf eine achtwöchige HCG-Therapie erwecken den Verdacht auf eine primäre Hodendysgenesie.

Die Einordnung dieser Fälle ist schwierig. Die Sohvalsche Auffassung einer Entwicklungsstörung, die alle drei cellulären Anteile des Gewebes betrifft, wurde erwähnt. Die primäre Gonadendysgenesie als alleiniger Defekt ist aber in Fällen mit fehlender oder unternormaler Gonadotropinausscheidung in Frage gestellt, da sie in Wirklichkeit stark erhöht sein müßte. Das anatomische Bild läßt wohl vermuten, daß es sich um embryonale Entwicklungsstörungen des Hodengewebes handelt, aber es ist nicht bekannt, ob der schwere hypophysär

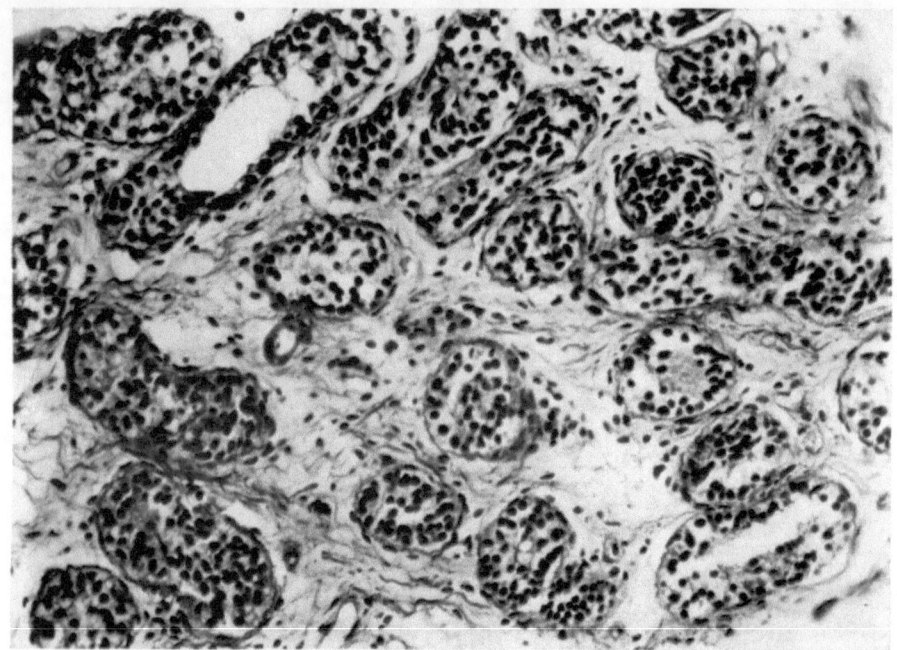

Abb. 57. 42jähriger Mann mit primärem Eunuchismus. Dysplastischer Habitus, Debilität, Skeletanomalien (Fall 9)

bedingte Eunuchismus nicht dasselbe anatomische Bild haben kann, wenn der Ausfall des Gonadotropins sehr früh erfolgt oder wenn das mütterliche Choriongonadotropin während der embryonalen Entwicklung unwirksam ist. Ich rechne diese Fälle zum sekundären Eunuchismus.

Klinisch haben diese Kranken einen schweren präpuberalen Eunuchismus. Das Fehlschlagen der Gonadotropinbehandlung gehört mit zur Diagnose. Der Defekt betrifft sowohl das Kanälchenepithel als auch die Leydigzellen. Bei den wenigen Fällen, die in der Literatur niedergelegt sind, waren meistens noch Mißbildungen anderer Organe vorhanden, so daß sie teilweise den verschiedenen Syndromen zugeordnet wurden. Sie finden sich unter dem männlichen Turner-Syndrom, dem Kallmann-Syndrom, dem Laurence-Moon-Biedl-Syndrom u. ä. Die normale Bildung des Gangsystems macht wahrscheinlich, daß Leydigzellen in den ersten Embryonalwochen Hormone produziert haben.

Neben dieser schweren Hypoplasie, die das gesamte Hodengewebe gleichförmig betrifft, gibt es eine *zweite Gruppe*, bei der in einem Hoden ganz verschiedene Schweregrade der Entwicklungsstörung anzutreffen sind. Man sieht hier ganz kleine Kanälchen, die mit einem unreifen, nicht differenzierbaren

Zellbesatz ausgekleidet sind neben anderen, etwas größeren, die nur Sertolizellen enthalten, und eine dritte Gruppe, die die Zeichen einer schweren Reifungsstörung des Samenepithels bieten. In wieder anderen kann die Spermatogenese bis zu den reifen Formen fortschreiten. Häufig sind einzelne Kanälchen mehr oder weniger stark fibrosiert, im Interstitium finden sich entweder nur Bindegewebszellen, oder spärlich, wenig entwickelte Leydigzellen, die, wie der präpuberale Eunuchoidismus der Kranken zeigt, eine unzureichende Menge von Sexualhormonen bilden. Die Gonadotropinausscheidung ist normal oder erhöht. Solche Befunde werden besonders beim Kryptorchismus, beim männlichen Pseudohermaphroditismus, seltener auch im normal deszendierten Hoden erhoben. Minderwertig ist nicht nur die Anlage des Kanälchenepithels, sondern auch die der Leydigzellen.

Ein typischer Fall dieser Art wurde von SOHVAL (1956) beschrieben. Es handelt sich dabei um einen 58jährigen Mann mit schwerem Eunuchoidismus, Gynäkomastie und erhöhter Gonadotropinausscheidung im Urin. Im Hoden fanden sich ganz verschiedene Schweregrade einer tubulären Fibrose. Viele Kanälchen waren sehr klein und völlig obliteriert, andere mit mäßiger Fibrose enthielten undifferenzierte Zellen und Spermatogonien, in größeren mit geringer Fibrose waren die Sertolizellen differenziert, während die Keimzellen fehlten. Im Interstitium sah man nur Bindegewebszellen, keine Leydigzellen.

Eine ähnliche Beobachtung berichten SWYER und HUGHESDON (1954). 24jähriger Mann mit geistiger und seelischer Unterentwicklung ohne zusätzliche Defektbildungen. Der Kranke hatte eunuchoide Körperproportionen, spärliche Achsel- und Schambehaarung, eine geringe Gynäkomastie, Penis normal groß, beide Hoden sehr klein und weich, Prostata nicht sicher zu tasten. Mäßige Erhöhung der Gonadotropinausscheidung. Histologisch zeigte das Hodengewebe drei verschiedene Entwicklungsstadien. Ein Teil der Kanälchen bot das Bild der Keimzellaplasie, ein anderer Teil war völlig hyalinisiert, als dritte Gruppe fanden sich Kanälchen mit aktiver Spermatogenese bis zu den Spermatozoen, die Leydigzellen waren trotz der vermehrten Gonadotropinproduktion spärlich entwickelt und produzierten nach dem klinischen Bild zu urteilen ungenügende Hormonmengen.

4. Tubulusdysgenesie mit Sklerohyalinose

Unter dem Begriff des „falschen Klinefelter-Syndroms" wird eine inhomogene Gruppe von Kranken zusammengefaßt, die anatomisch den Befund einer Kanälchenfibrose bei normalen oder hyperplastischen Leydigzellen zeigen, eine Azoospermie haben, vermehrt Gonadotropine ausscheiden und sich im Kernchromatin negativ verhalten. Bei 134 Fällen, die als Klinefelter-Syndrom diagnostiziert waren, fanden NELSON u. Mitarb. 106 mit positivem und 28 mit negativem Kernchromatin. Das falsche Klinefelter-Syndrom wird vielfach als erworbener Schaden aufgefaßt, wobei eine schleichend verlaufende Orchitis die häufigste Ursache sein soll (NELSON 1951 b).

Es gibt eine Gruppe, die sich klinisch vom echten Klinefelter-Syndrom nicht unterscheidet. Die Kranken haben die Zeichen eines mehr oder weniger starken präpuberalen Eunuchoidismus, kleine Hoden bzw. Oligospermie, Gynäkomastie und teilweise defekte Anlagen anderer Organe. In der Vorgeschichte erfährt man nichts über eine früher durchgemachte Orchitis. Da der unreife, nicht durch die Gonadotropine stimulierte Hoden gegenüber exogenen Schäden, insbesondere gegenüber der Ansiedelung von Erregern oder deren Toxinen unempfindlich ist, müßten diese Infektionen mit der Pubertät oder kurz danach aufgetreten sein.

Nur eine schwere Orchitis kann aber das Hodengewebe so stark zerstören, daß die restlichen Leydigzellen nicht mehr zur normalen Androgenproduktion ausreichen, daß also ein Hypogonadismus entsteht. Diese Fälle kann man aber nach dem histologischen Bild abtrennen. Der präpuberale Eunuchoidismus dieser Kranken spricht dafür, daß es sich um einen angeborenen Defekt mit Minderwertigkeit der Leydigzellen handelt.

Man hat auf gewebliche Unterschiede zwischen dem echten und dem falschen Klinefelter-Syndrom hingewiesen (Nelson 1951 b). Der Durchmesser der Kanäl-

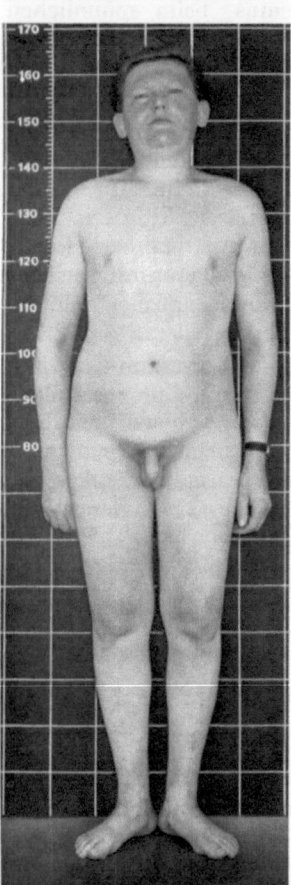

chen ist beim falschen Klinefelter-Syndrom im allgemeinen größer, eine größere Zahl von Kanälchen ist zartwandig, enthält Sertolizellen und häufiger reifere Formen der Spermiogenese. Grundsätzliche Unterschiede liegen aber nicht vor und im Einzelfall ist es unmöglich, an Hand eines Präparates den chromatinpositiven vom chromatinnegativen abzutrennen (Tonutti 1960).

Wichtig ist das familiäre Vorkommen. Reiffenstein hat 1947 eine aus Syrien stammende Familie beschrieben, bei der in zwei Generationen von zehn männlichen Mitgliedern neun das Bild des „Klinefelter-Syndroms" boten. Sieben der neun Kranken hatten eine Gynäkomastie, einige eine Hypospadie. Die Biopsie ergab dieselben Veränderungen wie beim echten Klinefelter-Syndrom. Einer nachträglichen Mitteilung zufolge war das Kerngeschlecht in diesen Fällen männlich. Auch die beiden unter dem Turner-Syndrom angeführten Geschwister von Sohval und Soffer (1953) muß man hier erwähnen. Nelson und Heller (1951 b) berichten über drei Geschwisterpaare dieser Art.

Endlich sei daran erinnert, daß das gewebliche Hodenbild des Klinefelter-Syndroms auch bei Erbkrankheiten, die häufig mit einem Hypogonadismus kombiniert sind wie dem Laurence-Moon-Biedl-Syndrom, dem Werner-Syndrom und der Dystrophia myotonica vorkommen kann.

Daß das anatomische Bild des „falschen Klinefelter-Syndroms" auch bei erworbenen Schädigungen entstehen kann, ist an anderer Stelle betont. Für einen angeborenen Defekt spricht im Einzelfalle das

Abb. 58. M. J. Falsches Klinefelter-Syndrom mit präpuberalem Eunuchoidismus

familiäre Vorkommen, die Kombination mit Mißbildungen anderer Organe und ein präpuberaler Eunuchoidismus. Es handelt sich um eine besonders schwere Form der Kanälchendysgenesie, die von einer Leydigzellinsuffizienz begleitet ist. Als Ursache kommen die früher für das echte Klinefelter-Syndrom diskutierten frühembryonalen Entwicklungsstörungen in Betracht, also eine Minderwertigkeit der Keimzellen, die vorzeitig zugrunde gehen und nur einzelne Kanälchen besiedeln, oder eine Entwicklungsschwäche des Cölomepithels, aus dem der Markanteil der embryonalen Gonade entsteht (Witschi 1951). Die Zahl der Geschlechtschromosomen war bei den untersuchten Fällen normal. Ob das Y-Chromosom aber defekte Gene trägt, konnte noch nicht ausgeschlossen werden.

Als Beispiel sei folgender Fall wiedergegeben:

Fall 10. M. J., 35jährig.

An Kinderkrankheiten kann er sich nicht erinnern. Angeblich zu normaler Zeit gehen gelernt. In der Schule war er bis zur Schulentlassung immer der Kleinste, nicht wiederholt. Schon von früher Jugend an mußte er in der Landwirtschaft mithelfen, lernte als Schuhmacher, arbeitet aber jetzt als Elektroschweißer.

Hat sich erst nach dem 16. Lebensjahr langsam entwickelt, beide Hoden immer klein gewesen, ist bis 25 Jahre noch gewachsen, Libido mit 20 Jahren. Seit 6 Jahren kinderlos verheiratet. Unter Testosteron besseres subjektives Befinden.

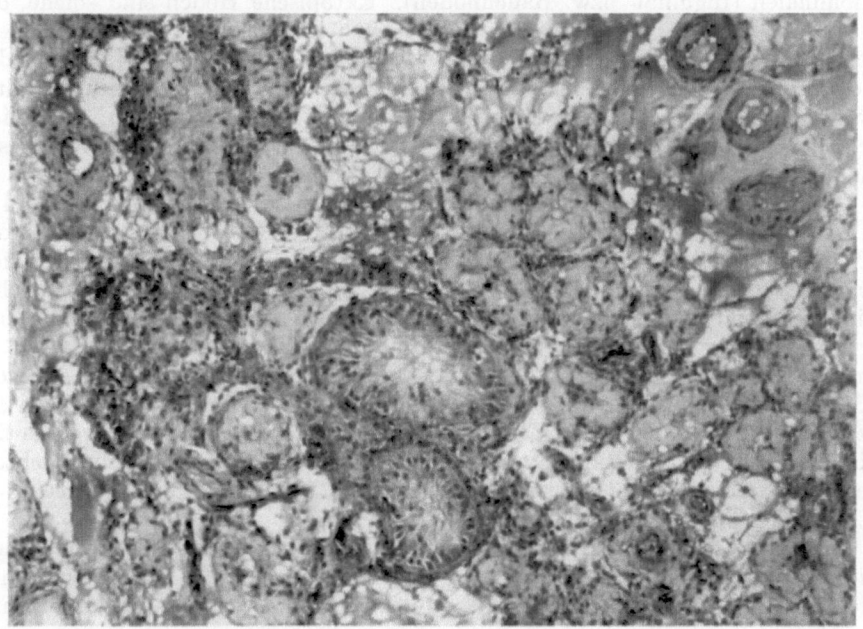

Abb. 59. Biopsie von Fall 10. Kanälchen sehr klein und zum größten Teil völlig hyalinisiert, in einzelnen Sertolizellen und Spermatogonien. Wucherung der Leydigzellen. (Hämatoxylin-Eosin, 300fach)

Familie: Vater war 170 cm, Mutter nur 145 cm groß. Drei Geschwister leben und sind gesund, alle sind verheiratet und haben Kinder.

162 cm, 64 kg. Leichte Adipositas mit gleichmäßiger Verteilung des Fettes, gedrungene Gestalt, kräftig. Keine Bartbehaarung, spärliche Lanugobehaarung an der Oberlippe, ebenso am Oberarm, ganz vereinzelt am Unterarm, keine Behaarung an Ober- und Unterschenkel, Brust, Rücken, Bauch, in der Axilla wenige 2—3 cm lange Haare. Die Schambehaarung ist sehr spärlich. Weiches Kopfhaar.

Penis 7 cm, beide Hoden bohnengroß, flach, wenig druckschmerzhaft. Prostata: V-förmig angeordnete Lappen von Dattelkerngröße (Abb. 58).

Knochensystem: noch angedeutet offene Epiphysenlinien an Hand und Darmbeinkamm. An der ganzen Wirbelsäule strähnige Osteoporose.

Mundepithel: chromatinnegativ.

Hormonuntersuchungen: Gonadotropine 192 MEU positiv.

17-Ketosteroide 11,8, 5,9 mg.

Porter-Silberchromogene 8,05, 9,3 unter 20 E ACTH intramuskulär; Anstieg auf 11,9 mg in 24 Std.

Abfall der Eosinophilen nach 4 Std auf —91%.

Grundumsatz —5%.

Insulin 2 E intravenös: leichter Schwindel.

Jodspeicherung: nach 6 Std 91%, nach 24 Std 91%.

Biopsie (Prof. TONUTTI): Kanälchen sehr klein, der größte Teil ist vollständig sklero-hyalinisiert, einzelne enthalten Sertolizellen und Spermatogonien. Das intertubuläre Bindegewebe ist nicht wesentlich vermehrt. Die Kanälchen sind von teilweise mächtigen Paketen von Leydigzellen, die in der Nähe der nicht hyalinisierten Kanälchen gut differenziert sind, umgeben. Das Bindegewebe ist nur wenig vermehrt (Abb. 59).

Mäßig ausgeprägter Hypogonadismus, histologisch das Bild der schweren Tubulus-dysgenesie bei negativem Kernchromatin, „falscher Klinefelter".

5. Kryptorchismus

Bleibt die Gonade auf dem normalen Descensusweg liegen ohne das Scrotum zu erreichen, dann spricht man vom Kryptorchismus, dem inguinalen bzw. dem abdominalen (Inguinal- bzw. Bauchhoden). Ektopische Hoden sind solche, die an anormaler Stelle liegen. Davon zu unterscheiden ist der retraktile Hoden, auch als Wanderhoden oder Pseudo-Kryptorchismus bezeichnet. Hier liegt der Hoden im Scrotum, wird aber auf die geringsten Reize, z.B. Berührung, Kälte, psychische Erregung, sofort in den offenen Inguinalkanal hochgezogen. Bezüglich der anatomischen Verhältnisse sei auf den Beitrag von Williams, Bd. XV dieses Handbuches, verwiesen.

Die Häufigkeit wird verschieden angegeben, sie schwankt zwischen 1 und 14% bei *Neugeborenen*, im Mittel 4% [1% Colbi (1950), 10% Charny (1956b), Bishop, 14% Deming, 4% Scorer]. Bei 419 geistig normalen *Schulkindern* findet sich der echte Kryptorchismus in 2,6%, der Pseudokryptorchismus in 6,7%, bei Geistesschwachen ist die Häufigkeit 5,5 bzw. 7,3% (de Medeiros). Um die Zeit der *Pubertät* sind es noch etwa 2% (Bishop), beim *Erwachsenen* noch 0,2—0,7% (Charny 1956b, Winterstein, Bishop, Scorer). Aus diesen Zahlen geht hervor, daß der kryptorche Hoden häufig noch spontan tiefertritt. In 10% (Winter-stein) bis 30% (Wilkins u. Cara 1954) ist der Kryptorchismus doppelseitig, er ist bei Geschwistern (Brimblecombe) und bei eineiigen Zwillingen beobachtet. Die große Statistik von Gross und Jewett mit 1022 Fällen zeigt ihn rechts in 44%, links in 30%, doppelseitig in 26%.

Die Anlage der Keimdrüse befindet sich in der Lumbalregion. Gegen Ende des dritten uterinen Monats wandert sie in die Inguinalgegend, im vierten Monat wird der Eingang des Inguinalkanals erreicht. Im siebten Fetalmonat beginnt der Abstieg durch den Leistenkanal mit einer Ausstülpung des Peritoneums. Der endgültige Eintritt in das Scrotum erfolgt nicht vor dem achten bis neunten Monat. Bei Frühgeburten ist daher die Häufigkeit des Kryptorchismus viel größer als bei zu normaler Zeit geborenen Kindern. Beim Abstieg spielt das Gubernaculum testis als Leitseil eine wichtige Rolle. Das Tiefertreten des Hodens erfolgt wahrscheinlich mit Hilfe der Bauchpresse. Fehlt der Hauptstrang des Gubernaculum, dann kann der Hoden durch einen der Nebenstränge aus der normalen Gleitbahn abgelenkt werden und in die Dammregion, die Schenkel-region oder gegen die Peniswurzel verlagert werden (Ectopia testis).

Eine einheitliche Erklärung für den Kryptorchismus gibt es nicht. In Betracht kommen mechanische, endokrine Faktoren und anlagebedingte Unterentwick-lung (Charny 1957a).

Mechanische Hindernisse können bestehen in einem verschlossenen oder zu engen Inguinalring, in peritonealen Adhäsionen im Bereich des Inguinalkanals, in einem zu kurzen Gubernaculum, in abnorm kurzen Gefäßen und zu kurzem Samenstrang u.ä. Der Kryptorchismus ist dann häufig einseitig. Die verschie-denen anatomischen Hindernisse lassen sich meist erst bei der Operation auf-klären.

Die Rolle der *hormonalen Faktoren* ist nicht sichergestellt. Smith (1930) hat als erster bei Ratten gezeigt, das Hypophysektomie im jugendlichen Alter das Tiefertreten des Hodens verhindert. Umgekehrt kann man durch Verabreichung von Choriongonadotropin oder von Androgenen bei Tieren ein vorzeitiges Tiefertreten auslösen (ENGLE 1932, ZONDEK 1929, SHAPIRO, HAMILTON 1936). Die unter der Wirkung des Choriongonadotropins gebildeten oder zugeführten Androgene führen zu einem Wachstum der Epididymis, des M. Cremaster, zu einer Entwicklung des Scrotums, sie verlängern auch die Bänder und Gefäße (HAMILTON 1936). Beim Menschen sind die Leydigzellen während der embryonalen Entwicklung teilweise entfaltet, so daß der fehlende Descensus auf der mangelnden Aktivierung durch die Hypophyse beruhen kann, dies wird besonders beim doppelseitigen diskutiert.

Neuerdings mehren sich die Angaben über *Defekte der Hodenanlage.* Der dysplastische Hoden spricht auf die Gonadotropine nicht an und bleibt deshalb auf dem Weg zum Hoden liegen.

a) Histologie

Die Spermiogenese ist bei den meisten Säugern abhängig von einer relativ kühlen Umgebungstemperatur, wie sie im Scrotum garantiert ist. Auch beim Menschen hat die um 1,5—2,0⁰ niedrigere Scrotaltemperatur entscheidende Bedeutung. Setzt man Hoden auch nur für kurze Zeit einer erhöhten Temperatur aus, dann können Reifungsstörungen auftreten. MCLOED und HOTCHISS beobachteten erhebliche Oligospermien bei sechs freiwilligen Männern, die 30 min lokal Diathermie von 43⁰ erhalten hatten. NELSON (1951a) wiederholte und erweiterte die Versuche von MOORE u. KOCH (1927) und verlagerte die Hoden von ausgewachsenen Ratten verschieden lange Zeit in die Bauchhöhle zurück. Längeres Verweilen der Hoden in der Bauchhöhle führt zu einem progressiven Verlust aller spermiogenen Zellen einschließlich der Spermatogonien. Vier Monate nach der Einbringung in die Bauchhöhle enthalten nur noch 50% der Tubuli Spermatogonien. Irreparable Schäden treten nach einer Retention von 7 Monaten auf. Die Fähigkeit zur Erholung hängt ab von der Zahl der noch Spermatogonien enthaltenden Kanälchen. Wie frühere Untersucher, findet NELSON (1951a), daß die reifen Spermatozoen, die Spermatiden und die sekundären Spermatocyten am empfindlichsten gegenüber der Wärmeschädigung sind.

NELSON (1951a) verglich kryptorche Hoden mit normalen desselben Lebensalters. Bei Kindern von 1—6 Jahren ergaben sich keine sicheren Unterschiede. Bei 6—11jährigen ist die Zahl der Spermatogonien etwas vermindert, der Durchmesser der Kanälchen etwas kleiner. Sertoli- und Leydigzellen befinden sich in Reifung. Bei 12- und 13jährigen sind Leydigzellen in genügender Menge vorhanden, die Zahl der Spermatogonien ist aber eindeutig geringer, primäre Spermatocyten sind selten, die Kanälchen sind schmäler und es besteht eine leichte peritubuläre Fibrose. Je älter die Jungen werden, um so größer werden die Unterschiede. Die Spermatogonien sind beträchtlich vermindert, eine peritubuläre Fibrose ist praktisch immer vorhanden, während Sertolizellen und Leydigzellen normal sind. Bei der postpuberalen Gruppe ist die Fibrose ausgedehnt, Keimzellen fehlen, während die Leydigzellen normal und nicht zahlreicher sind.

DE LA BALZE u. Mitarb. (1960) untersuchten sieben 10- und 13jährige mit einseitigem, mechanisch bedingtem Kryptorchismus und verglichen den Befund mit den normal deszendierten Hoden der anderen Seite. Der Kanälchendurchmesser ist kleiner und im Samenepithel sind die Spermatogonien und reiferen Formen weniger zahlreich. Stärkere morphologische Abnormitäten des Samenepithels finden sich nur bei einer Schädigung der Kanälchenwand. Die Differenzierung des Zwischengewebes bleibt gegenüber dem normalen zurück. Fibroblasten, aus denen sich die Leydigzellen entwickeln, sind seltener, involvierte und stark vacuolisierte Formen dagegen häufiger. Die Zeichen eines angeborenen Defektes fehlen.

Andere erheben grundsätzlich dieselben Befunde, nur daß Robinson und Engle eine mögliche Entwicklungsstörung schon ab dem 5. Lebensjahr, Charny (1957a) erst ab dem zehnten datieren. Die anatomischen Abweichungen sind gering, ihre Deutung nicht einheitlich.

Etwa vom 10.—13. Lebensjahr ab kommt die Entwicklungshemmung jedoch deutlich zum Ausdruck. Das Wachstum und die Differenzierung des Kanälchens bleibt zurück, die Zahl der Spermatogonien nimmt ab, die Sertolizellen differenzieren sich noch normal. Anfangs ist auch die Wand zart und ohne pathologische Veränderung, aber verschieden rasch fortschreitend verschwinden die Spermatogonien, die Kanälchenwand verdickt sich, die Sertolizellen gehen unter, bis nur noch eine vollständige Sklerohyalinose übrig ist. Selten ist die Degeneration der Kanälchen in allen Teilen gleichweit fortgeschritten. Im Zwischengewebe vermehren sich die Fibrocyten und die kollagenen Fasern, die Leydigzellen erleiden Schädigungen. Der Endzustand besteht in einer völligen Sklerohyalinose der Kanälchen und einer Degeneration des Zwischengewebes, wobei atypische Leydigzellen knotenförmig wuchern und schwere degenerative Veränderungen zeigen können (pericelluläre Hyalinose) (Záhór).

Der präpuberale Hoden ist gegen Schäden verhältnismäßig resistent. Da aber schon ab dem 6. Lebensjahr normalerweise Zeichen der beginnenden Reifung feststellbar sind, von diesem Zeitpunkt an also Entwicklungsstörungen auftreten können, wird vereinzelt die Forderung erhoben, die Behandlung nicht wie früher vor der Pubertät, also dem 10.—12. Lebensjahr zu beginnen, sondern schon um das 6. Lebensjahr. Nur dann sei das natürliche Wachstum des Keimepithels gewährleistet.

Der Ablauf ist also ein progressiver. Mit dem Untergang der Spermatogonien hört die Spermiogenese auf und jeder spätere Aufbau des Samenepithels nach Verlagerung in das Scrotum ist von hier ab ausgeschlossen.

Die Verhältnisse werden durch das Hinzutreten von anlagebedingten Schäden des Keimepithels kompliziert. Charny (1957a) gibt bei 30 bioptisch untersuchten Kryptorchen 20% an, Sohval (1954) findet bei 17 von 33 jenseits des puberalen Alters eine Unreife der Kanälchen vom präpuberalen Typ. Die Tubuli des einzelnen Organs haben unterschiedliche Durchmesser, die unreifen sind ohne Lumen und enthalten nur undifferenzierte Zellen, keine Sertolizellen, die reifen zeigen mehrere Zellagen. Sie beschreiben kompakte Kanälchen, die von undifferenzierten Zellen ausgefüllt sind und dem testiculären Adenom von Pick gleichen. Bei einem kleinen Teil fehlen die Spermatogonien oder es besteht der schwerste Grad der Dysgenesie mit Fehlen der Spermatogonien, der Sertoli- und Leydigzellen (Sohval 1954). Solche rudimentären Strukturen können bei ein- und doppelseitigem Kryptorchismus vorkommen. In diesen Fällen ist die innersekretorische Leistung der Leydigzellen häufig eine ungenügende, so daß Zeichen eines präpuberalen Eunuchoidismus vorhanden sind. Ein Beispiel dieser Art gibt Fall 11. Neben der unterschiedlichen Entwicklung der Kanälchen zeigt das Protoplasma der Leydigzellen Veränderungen, die ein Ausdruck ihrer ungenügenden Funktion sein können.

Fall 11. A. M., 20jährig.
Mit 6 Jahren Operation doppelseitiger Leistenhernien, dabei sei auch ein beidseitiger Leistenhoden operiert worden, der linke blieb deszendiert, der rechte war bald wieder in der Leiste verschwunden.
In der Schule gute Leistungen, auch im Sport. Schon mit 7 Jahren dicker als seine Kameraden, war aber immer einer der Größeren seiner Klasse.

Erst mit 16—18 Jahren Wachstum der Sekundärbehaarung und Stimmbruch. Rasiert sich heute nur alle 6—8 Tage. Adipositas, besonders des Stammes, rundliches Gesicht, Stiernacken, Doppelkinn, fettreiche Mammae, jedoch kein Drüsenkörper tastbar. Muskulatur kräftig, aber nicht konturgebend. Behaarung: Kopfhaar glatt und dicht, wenig Bartbehaarung an Kinn, etwas mehr an Oberlippe, in beiden Achselhöhlen reichlich bis 3 cm lange Haare. Brust nicht behaart, an beiden Mamillen je drei 1—2 cm lnge schwarze Haare. Ausreichende Pubesbehaarung.

Größe 180,5 cm, Oberlänge 80,5 cm, Unterlänge 100 cm, Spannweite 186 cm, Oberlänge/Unterlänge = 0,8.

Genitale: Penis 5,3/3,5 cm, Phimose. Hoden rechts nicht zu tasten, bei starkem Pressen glaubt man am äußeren Leistenring ein haselnußgroßes weiches Organ zu fühlen, die Beurteilung ist jedoch wegen der Adipositas unsicher. Hoden links 4,2/2,2 cm, fest, druckempfindlich. Prostata V-förmig, jeder Lappen nur etwa kirschkerngroß, weich, schlecht abgrenzbar. Ejaculat 1,2 cm³, 0,8 Mill. Spermien, davon nur 25% normal geformt und gut beweglich. Kernchromatin des Wangenschleimhautepithels männlich.

Grundumsatz +3%. 17-Ketosteroide 12,7 mg; 13,7 mg; 15,1 mg.

Biopsie aus dem deszendierten linken Hoden (TONUTTI): Die Tubuli sind von unterschiedlicher Größe. Teilweise sehr klein mit scharf begrenztem Lumen, teilweise annähernd normal groß. Die Wand ist durchweg mäßig verdickt. In den meisten Kanälchen finden sich alle Stadien der Spermiogenese bis zu den reifen Spermien, starke Desquamation. Die kleinen Kanälchen enthalten teilweise nur Sertolizellen, teilweise auch die ersten Stufen der Spermiogenese.

Das Zwischengewebe ist auffallend locker und enthält reichlich Komplexe von epitheloiden Leydigzellen verschiedener Größe. Ihr Kern ist rund, das Cytoplasma färbt sich ungemein stark an. Vielfach erscheint es undurchsichtig, homogen lackfarben, Granulierung fehlt. Im Zwischengewebe reichlich stark anfärbbare Gewebsflüssigkeit (vgl. Abb. 60 und 61).

In seltenen Fällen ergibt die chirurgische Exploration keinerlei Hodengewebe, selbst bei Absuchung des retroperitonealen Raumes (funktioneller präpuberaler Eunuchoidismus). Auch das echte Klinefelter-Syndrom kann mit einem doppelseitigen Kryptorchismus kombiniert sein.

Angeborene Schäden des Keimepithels sind offenbar häufiger als man bisher angenommen hat. Ein solches Epithel entwickelt sich dann auch nach erfolgtem Descensus nicht normal. Hinzu kommt, daß beim einseitigen Kryptorchismus auch der deszendierte kontralaterale Hoden verhältnismäßig häufig Defekte aufweist (NELSON 1953b). HANSEN (1949) berichtet, daß 11 von 35 Untersuchten infertil waren.

Sterilität mit Azoo- und Oligospermie ist ein unverhältnismäßig häufiges Spätsymptom des behandelten und unbehandelten ein- und doppelseitigen Kryptorchismus.

Wie erwähnt, bleiben die Leydigzellen im allgemeinen erhalten, so daß auch bei doppelseitigem Kryptorchismus ein Eunuchoidismus fehlt. Die Ausprägung der sekundären Geschlechtsmerkmale, Libido und Potenz sind daher nicht gestört. Die Pubertät tritt oft verspätet ein, so daß in den Körperproportionen eunuchoide Züge vorhanden sind, während die Sekundärbehaarung und Genitalentwicklung ganz aufholt. Auch die Pseudodystrophie ist häufig. Leichtere Formen des Hypogonadismus sind aber im späteren Leben beim doppelseitigen Kryptorchismus nicht ganz selten. ENGBERG (1948, 1949), der alle Kryptorche Kopenhagens zwischen 6 und 30 Jahren untersuchte, findet die *17-Ketosteroidausscheidung* bei doppelseitigem Kryptorchismus etwas vermindert. Zwischen Operierten und Nichtoperierten fand er keinen Unterschied. Die Oestrogenausscheidung war dagegen nur in 10% herabgesetzt. Bei einseitigem Kryptorchismus ist die Steroidausscheidung normal. Leichtere und schwerere Formen der angeborenen Hodenhypoplasie gehen häufig mit ein- oder doppelseitigem Kryptorchismus einher. In diesen Fällen bestehen ausgeprägte Zeichen des präpuberalen Hypogonadismus. Wichtig ist die erhöhte *Ausscheidung an Gonadotropinen* bei doppelseitigem Kryptorchismus. Sie beginnt nach der Pubertät, bleibt dauernd erhalten und kann so hoch wie beim Kastraten sein.

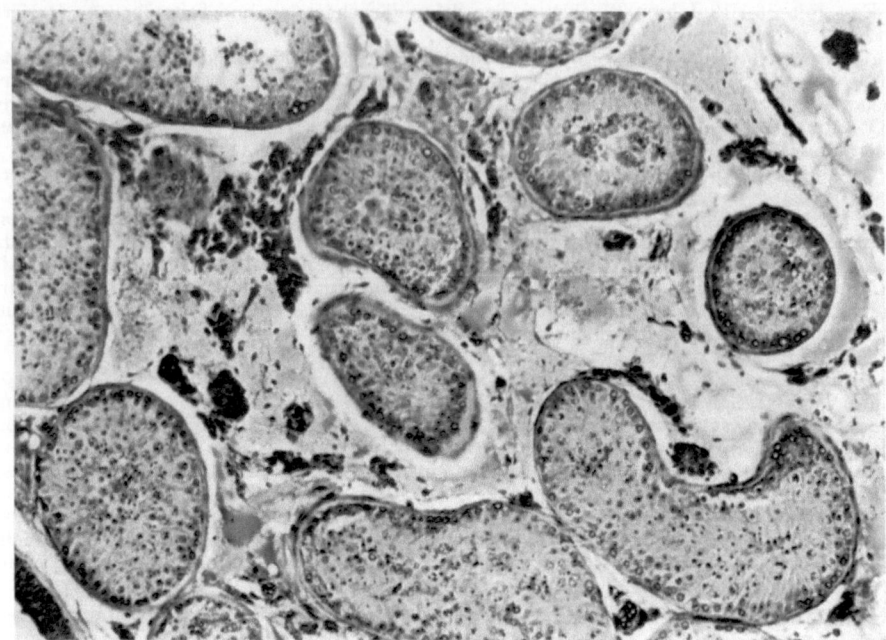

Abb. 60

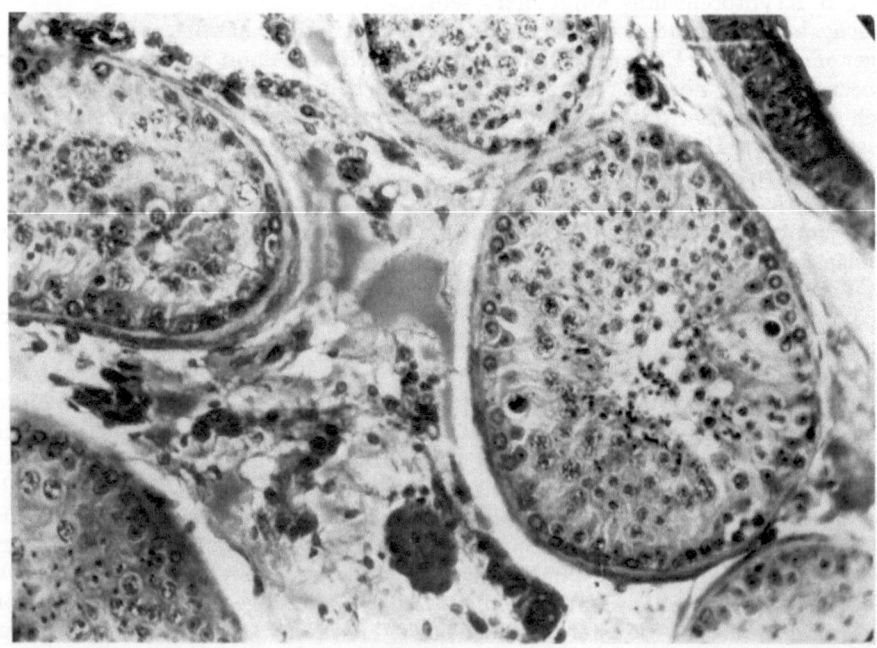

Abb. 61

Abb. 60 und 61. Fall 11. Hodenbild eines 20jährigen, der mit 6 Jahren wegen doppelseitigem Kryptorchismus operiert wurde und jetzt einen leichten präpuberalen Eunuchoidismus und eine Oligospermie hat. Hypospermiogenese, Tubuluswand mäßig verdickt, reichlich Leydigzellen, vielfach mit homogen lackfarbigem Cytoplasma ohne Granulation (b), stark anfärbbare Gewebsflüssigkeit im Zwischengewebe. Dieser Befund erinnert an die pericelluläre Hyalinose. Vergrößerung Abb. 60 Hämatoxylin-Eosin, 135fach; Vergrößerung Abb. 61 Hämatoxylin-Eosin, 265fach

ENGBERG (1949) findet die Erhöhung bei 16 von 23, NOWAKOWSKI (1957a) bei 15 von 21. Ursache ist der Untergang der Kanälchen. Bei einseitigem Kryptorchismus fanden wir bei normalem kontralateralem Hoden immer normale Werte. Eine erhöhte Gonadotropinausscheidung beweist beim doppelseitigen und einseitigen Kryptorchismus eine erhebliche Schädigung der Kanälchen und die Erfolglosigkeit einer hormonalen Therapie.

Die *Diagnose* ist im allgemeinen nicht schwierig. Wenn man im Liegen keine Hoden im Scrotum tastet, dann läßt man den Kranken etwas in die Hocke gehen und etwas pressen. Der hochgezogene Hoden wird dann gut tastbar. Auch die Untersuchung im warmen Bade bewährt sich. Manchmal tastet man den Hoden im unteren Ende des Leistenkanals, aus dem er durch Streichen wohl in das Scrotum gebracht werden kann, von wo er sich aber sofort wieder zurückzieht. Dieser dauernd hochgezogene Wanderhoden ist in seiner Entwicklung ebenfalls gefährdet, da ebenfalls eine erhöhte Temperatur auf das Samenepithel einwirkt. Die Kombination mit Leistenhernien ist beim reinen chirurgischen Krankengut groß (bis 90%) (GROSS u. JEWETT). Beim einseitigen Kryptorchismus ist der betreffende Scrotumteil weniger gut ausgebildet. Die Ursache der Unterentwicklung ist keine hormonale, sondern der fehlende mechanische Reiz des normalliegenden Hodens. Bei Tieren kann das Wachstum des Scrotums durch Fremdkörper angeregt werden. Die häufigsten Fehldiagnosen werden bei fettsüchtigen Kindern gestellt, bei denen die Hoden oft etwas hochgezogen sind und im Fett des oberen Scrotums liegen. Besonders bei retardierter Entwicklung muß man nach den kleinen, weichen Hoden richtig suchen.

b) Tumorentstehung

Die Angaben über die Häufigkeit von Hodentumoren im kryptorchen Hoden sind nicht einheitlich. In der bekannten Übersicht von GILBERT und HAMILTON (1940) mit 7000 malignen Hodengeschwülsten wird angegeben, daß 11% davon im kryptorchen Hoden aufgetreten sind. Je nachdem, wie hoch das Vorkommen des kryptorchen Hoden von den einzelnen Autoren angesetzt wird (0,1% MARSHALL, 4,7% COLEY) hat man errechnet, daß der Tumorbefall des retinierten Hoden 10—55mal häufiger ist als der des normal gelagerten. Bei der Seltenheit der Hodengeschwülste überhaupt (0,58% aller bösartigen Geschwülste) und der beschränkten Zahl retinierter Hoden der erwachsenen Bevölkerung haftet allen Statistiken der Makel der kleinen Zahl an. Obwohl beweisende Zahlen noch nicht vorliegen, sprechen sich immer mehr Chirurgen und Urologen für die Entfernung des retinierten Hoden aus (PATTON u. Mitarb.; LINKE u. Mitarb.; BÖHMINGHAUS u. a.).

Von großer Bedeutung ist die Feststellung, daß in ehemals kryptorchen Hoden Tumoren auch nach Verlagerung in das Scrotum auftreten können (CHARNY u. WOLGIN 1956b). Man vermutet daher mit Recht, daß Anlagedefekte der dysgenetischen Drüse neben der dauernden Einwirkung des hohen Gonadotropintiters eine wesentliche Voraussetzung für die Tumorentwicklung sind.

Selbst bei normalliegenden Hoden erfolgt die Diagnosestellung eines Tumors häufig recht spät. Sie ist praktisch unmöglich beim ektopischen Hoden. Hier wird man erst durch die eingetretene Metastasierung, durch ein Tumorpaket um die Aorta auf die Möglichkeit einer malignen Hodengeschwulst aufmerksam gemacht. Erfahrene Chirurgen empfehlen daher beim Erwachsenen die prophylaktische Entfernung des nicht deszendierten Hodens. Es muß aber das Ziel sein, jeden vor der Pubertät nicht deszendierten Hoden operativ in das Scrotum zu verlagern, damit eine eventuelle Geschwulstentwicklung frühzeitig erfaßt werden kann. Mit der Orchektomie sei man beim doppelseitigen Kryptorchismus zurückhaltend, da die innersekretorische Leistung immer noch recht beträchtlich sein kann.

c) Behandlung

Der Zeitpunkt des Behandlungsbeginnes ist nicht einheitlich. Diejenigen Untersucher, die der Auffassung sind, daß die normale Entwicklung des Hodens nicht erst mit der Pubertät einsetzt, sondern schon im 5.—6. Lebensjahr beginnt, treten für die Frühbehandlung ein. Einigkeit herrscht darin, daß der Behandlungsbeginn unbedingt vor der Pubertät, also vor dem 10. Lebensjahr liegen muß. CHARNY und WOLGIN (1956b) schlagen die Zeit vor dem 10. Lebensjahr vor, da sie bis dahin keine irreversiblen Schädigungen feststellen konnten, ROBINSON und ENGLE beginnen im 4.—5., HINMAN im 6., NELSON (1934) empfiehlt das 5.—7., BISHOP das 7.—10., HANSEN (1946) das 12.—14. Lebensjahr. Die meisten Autoren haben aber wegen der später zu besprechenden schlechten Behandlungsergebnisse den Beginn der Behandlung einige Jahre vorverlegt und beginnen zwischen dem 6. und 9. Lebensjahr.

Die eigentliche Domäne der *hormonalen Behandlung* ist der doppelseitige Kryptorchismus. CERENEA erreichte in 72% der Fälle den Descensus. Beim einseitigen sind die Erfolge weniger günstig, aber auch hier werden zwischen 40 und 50% Erfolge berichtet (CERENEA, BIERICH).

Da eine primäre Dysplasie nicht ohne bioptische Untersuchung diagnostiziert werden kann, beginnt man die Behandlung grundsätzlich mit *Choriongonadotropin*. Die Art der Verabreichung wird verschieden gehandhabt. Die meisten geben das Hormon in ein- oder mehrmaligen Kuren von vier- bis achtwöchiger Dauer, andere behandeln intensiv gleichmäßig weiter bis zum Eintritt des Erfolge.

Man sollte in jedem Falle sowohl beim einseitigen als auch beim doppelseitigen Kryptorchismus durch die Untersuchung der 17-Ketosteroide und der Oestrogene im Urin, die Reaktionsfähigkeit der Leydigzellen verfolgen. Wir geben in den ersten 5 Tagen eine Testdosis von 500 E täglich, wenn diese unbeantwortet bleibt, in den nächsten 5—10 Tagen 1500 E täglich. Man kann auf diese Weise ungefähr die notwendige Gesamtdosis errechnen.

In der Praxis richtet man sich bezüglich der Dosierung nach den klinischen Symptomen der Androgenwirkung. Als erstes Zeichen sieht man eine Schwellung und Rötung des Scrotum, dann folgt eine Dickenzunahme der Peniswurzel, später eine Längenzunahme des Penis. Beim einseitigen Kryptorchismus erhöht sich die Konsistenz des deszendierten Hoden, er nimmt auch an Größe zu, beim doppelseitigen muß man sich rein nach den Auswirkungen der Androgene richten. Ein Mißerfolg der hormonalen Behandlung darf nicht angenommen werden, bevor nicht die Pubesbehaarung sichtbar wird.

Bei der ersten Kur gibt man zwischen 6—12000 E im gesamten, pro Woche dreimal 1000—1500 E. Es ist besser, die Gesamtdosis in etwas kürzerer Zeit zu geben, als sie über einen längeren Zeitraum zu verzetteln. Tritt der Hoden mit der ersten Kur tiefer, dann darf man mit Wahrscheinlichkeit eine normale Weiterentwicklung bei Fortsetzung der Behandlung annehmen. Schlägt die erste Kur fehl, dann kann man einen zweiten Versuch machen (6—8 Wochen mit einer höheren Dosierung, 12000—20000 E). Nicht selten sieht man, wie die Hoden mit jeder Kur im Leistenkanal etwas tiefer treten.

Die Bestimmung des richtigen Zeitpunktes des operativen Eingriffes ist recht schwierig. Sind die Zeichen der Reifung während ein- oder mehrmaliger Kuren deutlich, ohne daß ein Descensus eingetreten ist, dann schließt man die Orchidopexie oder die Verlagerung des Hodens in das Scrotum direkt an eine hormonale

Kur an. Die Ansicht, daß die Hormonbehandlung den Hoden beweglicher macht, den Leistenkanal weitet, Bänder und Gefäße verlängert und die Mobilisierung beträchtlich erleichtert, wird nicht allgemein anerkannt (WILLIAMS).

Die Erfolge der hormonalen Behandlung werden besonders von chirurgischer Seite skeptisch beurteilt. Man sagt, daß der Descensus nur bei dem Kranken erreicht wird, bei dem er um die Zeit der Pubertät doch noch spontan erfolgen würde (THOMPSON und HECKEL 1939). Das mag in manchen Fällen zutreffen, aber man muß den vor der Pubertät erreichten Descensus in jedem Fall als Erfolg buchen, da er zu einem Zeitpunkt eingetreten ist, in dem eine dauernde Schädigung noch nicht gegeben ist. Insofern haben die Erfolgsangaben von 60—90% einzelner Autoren durchaus ihre Berechtigung.

Auch heute steht man manchmal noch vor der Entscheidung, ob man einen 12—15jährigen, der sich schon in der Pubertät befindet, noch hormonal behandeln oder gleich der Orchidopexie zuführen soll. Beim doppelseitigen Kryptorchismus verläuft die Pubertät nicht selten protrahiert und es bleibt verhältnismäßig lange ein leichter Hypogonadismus bestehen. Obwohl in solchen Fällen eine anlagemäßige Minderwertigkeit wahrscheinlich ist, erreicht man mit hochdosierten Kuren (dreimal 3000 E pro Woche, 4—6 Wochen gegeben) doch immer wieder den Descensus. Offenbar reichen in solchen Fällen die endogen gebildeten Gonadotropine nicht ganz aus, um die etwas minderwertigen Leydigzellen genügend anzuregen.

Von einigen wird bei einer höher dosierten und wiederholten Behandlung mit Choriongonadotropin eine Schädigung des deszendierten normalen Hodens befürchtet. Bei Kindern über 12 Jahren, bei denen die Pubertät schon spontan begonnen hat, ist dies durchaus möglich, da die Gonadotropinbildung des Hypophysenvorderlappens durch die künstliche Anregung der Leydigzellen wieder abgestoppt wird und sich das etwas entwickelte Samenepithel durch den Wegfall der FSH-Einwirkung wieder zurückbildet. Es ist aber unwahrscheinlich, daß dadurch eine dauernde Schädigung hervorgerufen wird, mit großer Wahrscheinlichkeit ist sie wie beim Erwachsenen nur vorübergehender Natur und gleicht sich nach Wiederaufnahme der Eigenproduktion wieder von alleine aus.

Die Frage der Verabreichung von *Testosteron* und seiner Derivate ist umstritten. Diese Hormone werden von vielen vor der Pubertät in der Behandlung ganz abgelehnt. Man vergißt aber, daß auch das Choriongonadotropin nicht direkt, sondern nur über die Bildung der Androgene in den Leydigzellen wirksam wird und daß diese Androgenproduktion ihrerseits ebenfalls die Hypophyse hemmen kann. Die Konzentrationsunterschiede zwischen dem endogen gebildeten und parenteral verabreichten sind aber recht beträchtlich. Die unterschiedlichen Hormonkonzentrationen, die bei der Behandlung mit HCG bzw. mit Testosteron lokal im Hoden und in den benachbarten Geweben erreicht werden, fallen ebenfalls ins Gewicht. Vor der Pubertät kann die Testosterontherapie des Kryptorchismus nicht empfohlen werden.

Die Beurteilung der *Orchidopexie* muß ausgehen von den Spätresultaten, wobei die normale Lage, Größe und Konsistenz des Organs nicht allein entscheidend sind, sondern auch die normale Funktion, geprüft mit Untersuchung des Ejaculats, der Gonadotropinausscheidung und wenn irgend möglich mit Biopsie, herangezogen werden muß.

Bei der Harmlosigkeit der Probeexcision sollte grundsätzlich jede Descensusoperation mit einer *Biopsie* verbunden werden. Die Zahl der verwertbaren Nachuntersuchungen ist heute noch verhältnismäßig klein, die meisten Operationen sind nach der gegenwärtigen Auffassung zu spät — nach dem 10. Lebensjahr — durchgeführt worden. Hansen (1946) verglich 9 unbehandelte und 25 operierte *doppelseitige* Kryptorche. Die Nichtoperierten hatten alle eine Aspermie, von den 25 Operierten hatten 14 eine Aspermie, 4 eine schwere, 5 eine leichte Oligospermie und nur 2 normale Spermienzahlen. Von 36 *einseitig* Operierten hatten nur 40% ein normales Ejaculat. Gegenüber dem nichtoperierten (35 Fälle) einseitigen Kryptorchismus ergab sich kein signifikanter Unterschied. Nowakowski (1959) konnte 33 im Alter von 10—33 Jahren *doppelseitig* Operierte nach mehreren Jahren nachuntersuchen. Von 24 war bei 3 kein Ejaculat zu gewinnen (Hypogonadismus), 17 hatten eine Aspermie, 4 eine Oligospermie, 5 die Zeichen eines Hypogonaden, bei 11 war die Prostata geschwunden, bei 14 von 30 die Gonadotropinausscheidung deutlich erhöht. Bei einseitig Operierten fand sich einmal eine Aspermie, siebenmal Oligospermie und nur sechsmal normale Spermienzahlen. Ähnlich schlecht sind die Ergebnisse der Nachuntersuchung von Raboch und Záhor (1955). Von 34 doppelseitig Operierten hatten 17 eine Aspermie, 11 eine Oligospermie. Bei sieben bioptisch untersuchten Fällen, die nach dem 14. Lebensjahr operiert waren, bestanden schwerste degenerative Veränderungen, bei zwei frühzeitig Operierten waren die Kanälchen praktisch normal. Nowakowski (1959) konnte in seinen Fällen keinen wesentlichen Einfluß des Operationsalters feststellen. Die Statistiken von McCollum (1935) und Gross und Jewett (1956) sind dagegen günstiger, doch sind die Befunde des Ejaculates bei doppelseitig Operierten auch nur in etwa $^1/_3$ der Fälle normal ausgefallen. Nelson (1951b) konnte sieben Kranke, die im Alter von 5—12 Jahren operiert waren, nach 13—22 Jahren bioptisch untersuchen. Bei zwei fand sich eine völlige Fibrose, wahrscheinlich als Folge einer gestörten Blutversorgung durch den Eingriff, bei drei enthielten viele Kanälchen keine Keimzellen und waren schwer fibrosiert, bei den übrigen zwei war der Befund praktisch normal.

Bayle (1957) fand in 68% von 198 doppelseitig Operierten eine Azoospermie, aber nur bei 23,6% von 93 einseitig Operierten. Seine Beobachtungen zeigen auch eine deutliche Abhängigkeit vom Lebensalter, in dem die Orchidopexie vorgenommen wurde. Vor der Pubertät Operierte haben in 30%, nach der Pubertät Operierte nur in 13,5% erhaltene Spermiogenese. In der Statistik von Weyeneth (1956) sind die Fälle von doppelseitigem Kryptorchismus mit normaler Spermienzahl alle vor dem 8. Lebensjahr operiert, bei Bayle 8 von 16 sogar vor dem 6. Lebensjahr.

Bezüglich des operativen Eingriffes stimmt die hohe Zahl der postoperativen Hodenatrophie sehr bedenklich [Hansen (1949) 11,6%; Blum (1943) 14%; Bayle (1947) 30%; Charny (1957a) 35%]. Ursache ist die Störung bzw. Unterbrechung der Blutversorgung. Die Orchidopexie ist ein sehr delikater Eingriff und erfordert große Erfahrung. Die Gefäße sind sehr fein, brüchig und oft nicht sichtbar. Die Blutversorgung muß unter allen Umständen intakt bleiben, da das Samenepithel gegenüber Störungen der Blutversorgung sehr empfindlich ist. Bei schweren Störungen kann auch das Interstitium völlig bindegewebig umgewandelt werden. Man spricht dann von der *Fibrosis testis*.

6. Einfache Tubulusdysgenesie ohne endokrine Störung

a) Keimzellaplasie

Diese Bezeichnung wurde zum erstenmal 1947 von Engle auf Kanälchen angewandt, in denen alle Zellen der spermatogenetischen Reihe fehlten. Solche Kanälchen sieht man in einem kleinen Prozentsatz auch im Hoden des Gesunden.

Del Castillo, Trabucco und de la Balze beschrieben 1947 das völlige Fehlen des Samenepithels als Keimzellaplasie, ein Syndrom, das nach ihnen benannt und später in zahlreichen Fällen beobachtet wurde (HELLER u. NELSON 1951, HOWARD 1950, SNIFFEN 1950, TONUTTI 1960). Der Durchmesser der Kanälchen ist etwas kleiner als normal, Basalmembran und Tunica propria sind nicht verdickt und nicht sklerosiert. Die Kanälchen enthalten eine große Zahl von normal aussehenden Sertolizellen, die eng aneinandergereiht liegen. Zellen der spermatogenetischen Reihe fehlen. Das intertubuläre Gewebe hat ein normales Aussehen, zeigt keine Reste von Entzündungen, keine Sklerose, keine peritubuläre Fibrose und keine Gefäßveränderungen. Die Leydigzellen sind an Zahl und Aussehen normal.

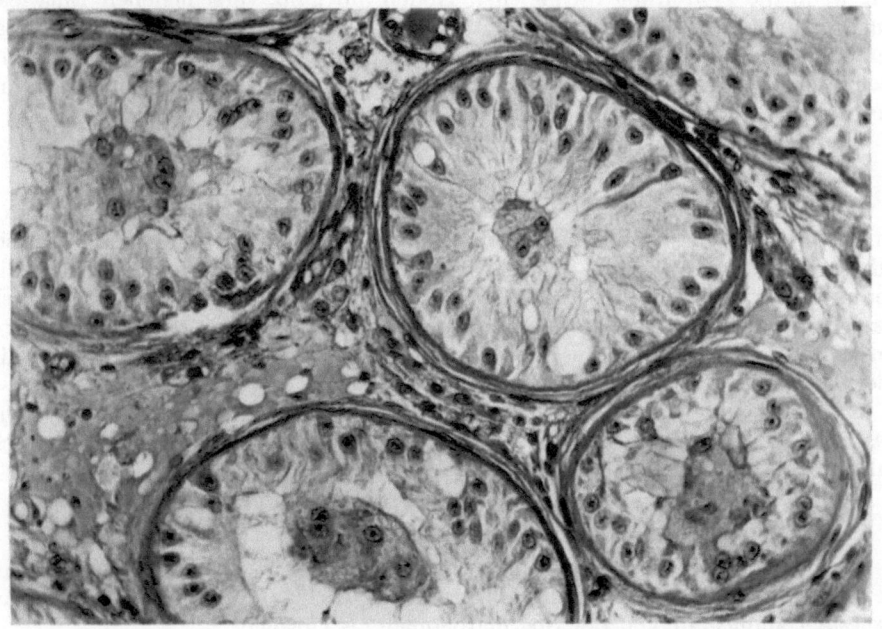

Abb. 62. 25jähriger. Keine Vorkrankheiten. Azoospermie. „Sertoli cells only", Kanälchen stark verkleinert, beträchtliche Wandverdickung. Depopulation bis auf Sertolizellen, Leydigzellen normal. (Hämatoxylin-Eosin, 300fach)

In zwei von 18 Fällen konnte HOWARD (1950) in einzelnen Kanälchen eine aktive Spermatozoenbildung beobachten. Zwischen einer ganzen Serie von Kanälchen mit dem typischen Befund taucht unvermutet eines mit fortschreitender Spermiogenese auf. Im klinischen Bild bestehen keine Zeichen eines Hypogonadismus, die Gonadotropinausscheidung wird normal oder etwas erhöht angegeben (DEL CASTILLO 1947, HOWARD 1950, NELSON u. HELLER 1951 b). Als Ursache nimmt man an, daß die primitiven Gonien nicht in das Keimfeld einwandern (DEL CASTILLO 1947) oder hier frühzeitig zugrunde gehen (NELSON). Man lernte erst allmählich, daß die Depopulation bis auf den Sertolizellbelag auch die Folge von exogenen Schäden der verschiedensten Art sein kann. Hierbei ist der Sertolizellbelag im allgemeinen unterschiedlich ausgebildet, er zeigt wechselnde Zellhöhen, verwaschene Zellgrenzen, eckige Kernformen mit pyknotischem Aussehen (TONUTTI 1960) (vgl. Abb. 62). Eine sichere Abtrennung von den angeborenen Defekten ist aber nicht immer möglich. Die häufigsten Ursachen sind die Einwirkung von Röntgenstrahlen bzw. radioaktiven Strahlen, die Verabreichung von Cytostatica in hoher Dosis und die Einwirkung abnorm hoher Körpertemperatur auf den Hoden. Neben der isolierten Schädigung der

Keimzellen wird auch eine Funktionsstörung der Sertolizellen, die mit der gewöhnlichen histochemischen Technik nicht darstellbar ist, als Ursache diskutiert. Die Sertolizellen — sagt man — sind nicht imstande, das Samenepithel zu ernähren.

Während man schon beim Fehlen des Samenepithels nicht sicher unterscheiden kann, ob es sich im Einzelfalle um eine Aplasie oder um eine Depopulation handelt, wird die Trennung zwischen angeborenen Reifungsstörungen und erworbenen Schäden unmöglich, je mehr man sich den nur auf einer *Störung der Zellteilungsvorgänge* beruhenden Abweichungen des Samenepithels zuwendet. Nur wenn die Zellreifung im gleichen Hoden auf ganz verschiedenen Entwicklungsstufen stehen bleibt, also ein buntes Bild vorhanden ist und wenn Anhaltspunkte für eine exogene Schädigung fehlen, kann man eine Dysgenesie vermuten, aber nie beweisen. Diese Menschen kommen wegen Infertilität zur Untersuchung und haben keine Zeichen eines Androgenmangels. Man unterscheidet:

b) Spermiogenese-Stop

Den *Spermiogenese-Stop* (germinal cell arrest). Hier kommt die Spermatogenese über eine bestimmte Entwicklungsphase nicht hinaus, meistens bleibt sie auf der Stufe der primären Spermatocyten stehen. Anstatt daß die Kerne die Reduktionsteilung eingehen, zerfallen sie, werden pyknotisch oder teilen sich bizarr unter der Bildung von mehrkernigen Zellen. Das histologische Bild wird durch die zahlreichen Spermatocyten beherrscht, spätere Stadien fehlen, die Spermatogonien sind unauffällig.

Seltener bleibt die Reifung auf der Stufe der Spermatogonien stehen. Hier sieht man im normal erscheinenden Sertolizellverband nur Spermatogonien, die sich teilen, aber nicht zu Spermatocyten heranwachsen.

c) Hypospermatogenese

Bei der *Hypospermatogenese* sind alle Stadien der Entwicklung vorhanden, die Gesamtzahl ist aber gleichmäßig vermindert. Man vermutet eine herabgesetzte Teilungsfähigkeit der Spermatogonien als Ursache.

VI. Klinische Syndrome
1. Männliches Ullrich-Turner-Syndrom

Wie beim weiblichen Ullrich-Turner-Syndrom erwähnt, fand Ullrich unter seinen 49 Fällen mit verschiedenen Mißbildungen neun phänotypisch männliche. Rossi u. Mitarb. stellten später neben 115 phänotypisch weiblichen, 67 männliche Kinder mit multiplen Abartungen zusammen, die unter dem Typ des Status Bonnevie-Ullrich-Rossi-Kaflisch bei Pädiatern schon lange geläufig waren. Der Begriff des männlichen Turner-Syndroms wurde erst eingeführt, nachdem allmählich der Status Bonnevie-Ullrich auch beim Erwachsenen auffiel und die Mißbildungen des phänotypisch weiblichen Ullrich-Turner-Syndroms auch beim männlichen Individuum „entdeckt" wurden. Die Priorität gehört den Pädiatern. Nur die von ihnen beschriebenen Anomalien erlauben die Aufstellung dieses Syndroms beim Erwachsenen. Das Epitheton „Turner" bedeutet eine zusätzliche Gonadendysgenesie, die häufig nur den Kanälchenapparat betrifft und von den Pädiatern naturgemäß nicht festgestellt werden konnte, Chromosomenanomalien fehlen.

Über den ersten Fall beim Erwachsenen berichtete Flavell 1943. Prunty u. Mitarb. konnten 1953 acht, Halonen 1956 elf, Fraccaro u. Mitarb. 1961 17 Fälle aus der Literatur zusammenstellen. In der letzten Zeit sind einige neue hinzugekommen, wir haben drei Fälle in 6 Jahren gesehen. Der Hypoandrogenismus ist kein obligates Symptom, ein Teil der beschriebenen Fälle gehört noch dem Jugendalter an, beim Erwachsenen besteht Azoo- bzw. Oligospermie. Nur wenige Fälle sind bioptisch untersucht (FLAVELL 1943, GREENBLATT u. NIEBURGS 1948, RYAN u. MCCULLAGH 1946, SOHVAL u. SOFFER 1952), so daß man noch keine endgültige Aussage über Art und Ausmaß des Gonadendefektes machen kann. Am häufigsten findet sich das Bild der unvollständigen Reifung des Keimepithels, teilweise auch eine minderwertige Ausbildung des Zwischengewebes, über dessen Funktion das klinische Bild besseren Aufschluß gibt als die Histologie. Zwei von SOHVAL und SOFFER (1953) beschriebene Fälle werden als besonderer Typus angesprochen. Es handelt sich dabei um zwei Brüder von 36 und 47 Jahren, die beide minderwüchsig waren, von denen der jüngere nur mäßige, der ältere deutliche Zeichen eines Hypogonadismus bot. Beide hatten eine Gynäkomastie und stark erhöhte Gonadotropinausscheidung. Der jüngere wies zahlreiche Anomalien am Skeletsystem, besonders an der Wirbelsäule, der ältere nur eine kurze erste Rippe und eine Fusion der ersten mit der zweiten auf. Beide hatten einen Diabetes mellitus. Kernchromatin männlich. Hoden 1,5 cm größte Länge. Beide Fälle hatten zwei ganz verschiedene Kanälchentypen im selben Organ. Die größere Zahl war im Durchmesser kleiner als normal, lag dicht aneinander, Basalmembran und Tunica propria waren nicht verdickt, die Wand war mit normal aussehenden Sertolizellen ausgekleidet. Weniger häufig ist ein zweiter Typ mit kompletter Sklerohyalinose ohne epitheliale Zellen und Lumen. Der Kranke mit den geringen Zeichen des Hypogonadismus hatte ein normales Interstitium mit spärlichen Leydigzellen, der mit dem schwereren Hypogonadismus stark gewebsartig gewucherte Leydigzellen wie beim Klinefelter-Syndrom.

Das Charakteristische dieser Fälle ist das Nebeneinander von völligem Fehlen der Keimzellen und Sklerosierung einzelner Kanälchen. Zusammen mit den anderen Mißbildungen und dem familiären Vorkommen nehmen die Autoren einen angeborenen Defekt an. MCCULLAGH (1948c) findet eine tubuläre Hypoplasie, keine sicheren Leydigzellen bei normaler Gonadotropinausscheidung, GREENBLATT und NIEBURGHS eine tubuläre Hypoplasie bei reichlich Leydigzellen und normaler Gonadotropinausscheidung, REFORZO-MEMBRIVES ein Bild wie bei einem zehnjährigen mit den ersten Stadien der sich entwickelnden Spermiogenese, HALLONEN eine einfache Hypoplasie des Keimepithels mit unreifen Spermien, normalen Sertolizellen, spärlichen Leydigzellen, REINER und GRNJA spärliche Kanälchen mit großen Massen degenerierter Spermiogonien, BECKER nur wenige Spermiogonien und Präspermatiden, FACCARO u. Mitarb. Kanälchen mit verkleinertem Durchmesser, leichter Wandsklerose, Sertolizellen, keine Spermiogonien, also das Bild der „Sertoly cells only“. 5—10% der Kanälchen war oblieteriert. Leydigzellen wohl entwickelt mit relativer Hyperplasie, aber ohne Klumpenbildung. Zwei eigene Fälle mit Minderwuchs, Anomalien des Skelets wie Synostose der Rippen, Blockwirbelbildung im Bereich der Brustwirbelsäule, fehlendem Bogenschluß von L 5, Verkürzung der Metakarpale 4 der Hand, Hufeisennieren, Lobus venae azygos, zeigten histologisch verschiedene Bilder. Bei dem einen bestanden die kleinen Kanälchen nur aus normal gebildeten Sertolizellen, die Kanälchenwand war nicht verdickt, das Zwischengewebe enthielt eine normale Zahl und normal gebildete Leydigzellen. Beim anderen waren die Kanälchen unterschiedlich groß, aber durchweg verkleinert, die Wand stark verdickt, ein kleiner Teil war völlig hyalinisiert, die anderen enthielten vorwiegend Sertolizellen und nur selten wenige Spermatocyten. Das lockere Zwischengewebe zeigte reichlich gut differenzierte Zwischenzellen, in einzelnen Partien waren sie adenomartig gewuchert und verklumpt (vgl. Abb. 63 und 64).

Im allgemeinen ist der Defekt der Kanälchen viel stärker ausgeprägt als der der Leydigzellen. Die Einordnung eines Falles in die Gruppe des männlichen Ullrich-Turner-Syndroms kann nicht auf Grund des histologischen Befundes, sondern nur auf Grund zusätzlicher Mißbildungen anderer Organe erfolgen, wie sie für das Ullrich-Turner-Syndrom des weiblichen Geschlechts charakteristisch sind, also besonders Minderwuchs, Pterygium colli, Schwimmhäute, Cubitus valgus, Genu

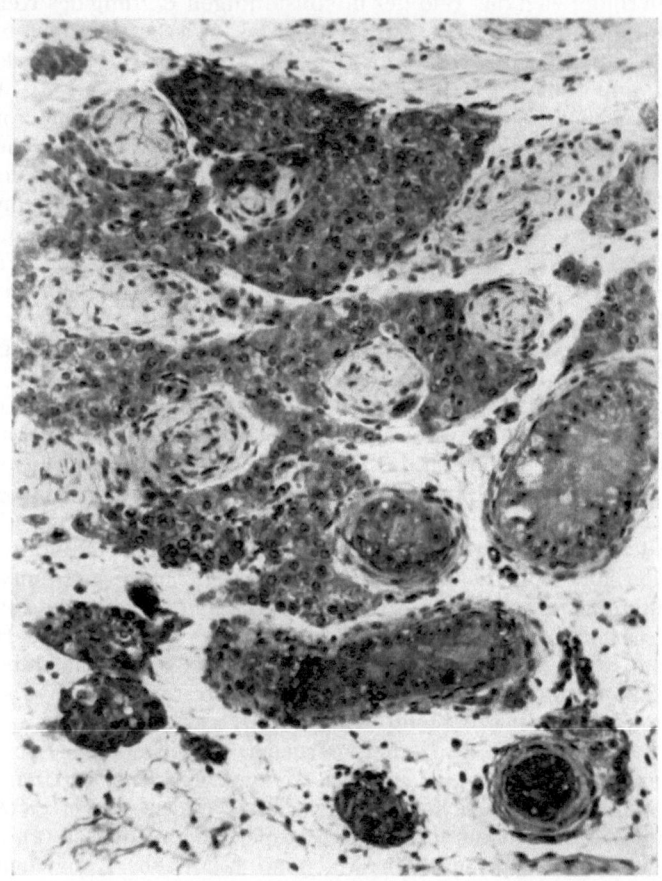

Abb. 63. Hodenbild eines 34jährigen Mannes mit Ullrich-Turner-Syndrom. Ein kleiner Teil der Kanälchen war völlig hyalinisiert, das Zwischengewebe darum herum stark gewuchert. Vergrößerung Hämatoxylin-Eosin, 230fach

valgum, Kyphoskoliose, Poly- und Syndaktylie, Zahndefekte, verschiedenartige Mißbildungen des Skeletsystems, Gefäßanomalien, angeborene Herzfehler u. ä. (s. S. 821). Man sollte niemals von einem männlichen Turner-Syndrom, sondern nur von einem Ullrich-Turner-Syndrom sprechen. Die meisten Erwachsenen sind minderwüchsig (155—168 cm) aber nicht ausgesprochen kleinwüchsig wie das weibliche Turner-Syndrom. Fälle ohne Hypogonadismus und ohne Kanälchen-dysgenesie gehören zum Status Bonnevie-Ullrich-Kaflisch und nicht zum Ullrich-Turner-Syndrom. Über ihre Häufigkeit beim Erwachsenen ist wenig bekannt, wahrscheinlich überwiegen sie die Fälle mit Hodendysgenesie.

Die Gonadotropinausscheidung verhält sich nicht einheitlich, sie scheint vom Grad der Zerstörung des Kanälchenepithels abhängig. Die einfache Keimzell-aplasie kann mit normalen Gonadotropinwerten einhergehen, die Ausscheidung erhöht sich erst, wenn eine größere Zahl von Kanälchen ganz zugrunde gegangen ist. Da man aus den kleinen, zur histologischen Untersuchung entnommenen Stückchen die Gesamtgestalt des Hodens nicht beurteilen kann, ist die größte Zurückhaltung in der Verallgemeinerung und Deutung der Befunde entgegen der gegenwärtig gültigen „feed back"-Theorie geboten.

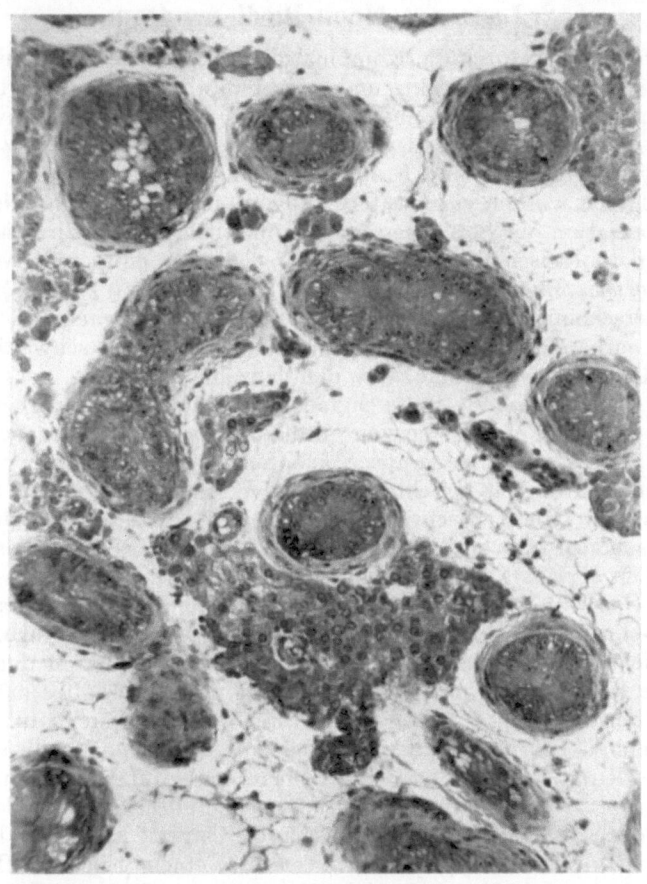

Abb. 64. Hodenbild eines 34jährigen Mannes mit Ullrich-Turner-Syndrom. Stark verkleinerte Kanälchen mit verdickter Wand, die nur Sertolizellen enthalten, lockeres Zwischengewebe mit reichlich Leydigzellen. Vergrößerung Hämatoxylin-Eosin, 230fach

In allen untersuchten Fällen ist das *Geschlechtschromatin* in der Schleimhaut und in den Leukocyten negativ. In einigen Fällen wurde auch die Chromosomenzahl untersucht und mit 46 normal gefunden, wobei ein normales X- und Y-Chromosom vorhanden sind (FRACCARO u. Mitarb. 1961). Die Abtrennung dieser Fälle gegenüber anderen Formen der Gonadendysgenesie ist unsicher. FRACCARO u. Mitarb. (1961) schlagen beim männlichen Ullrich-Turner-Syndrom den Begriff der *„testiculären germinalen Dysgenesie"* vor, da bei den meisten bis jetzt histologisch untersuchten Fällen nur das Keimepithel von der Mißbildung betroffen war, während die übrigen Anteile des Hodengewebes normal schienen. Leichte Zeichen eines Hypoandrogenismus sind jedoch nicht selten (zwei eigene Fälle), selbst schwere kommen vor, wie die Sohvalschen Fälle zeigen. Wir ziehen die Bezeichnung männliches Ullrich-Turner-Syndrom vor und nehmen nur solche Kranke auf, die neben einer Dysgenesie der Kanälchen mit und ohne klinische Zeichen eines präpuberalen Eunuchoidismus noch angeborene Miß-bildungen an anderen Organen aufweisen, wie sie für das Ullrich-Turner-Syndrom des weiblichen Geschlechts charakteristisch sind.

2. Laurence-Moon-Biedl-Syndrom

Dieses Syndrom ist durch die Kombination von Fettsucht, Retinitis pigmen-tosa, Polydaktylie, geistige Defekte und Hypogenitalismus charakterisiert.

LAURENCE und MOON beschrieben 1866 drei Brüder und eine Schwester einer Familie mit Adipositas, Retinitis pigmentosa und Schwachsinn, BARDET fügte 1920 die Polydaktylie hinzu und BIEDL 1922 den Hypogenitalismus.

In der Folgezeit wurden viele weitere Fälle mitgeteilt, doch sind die Ansichten über die Lokalisation der Störungen nicht einheitlich, da verhältnismäßig wenig verwertbare pathologisch-anatomische Untersuchungen mitgeteilt wurden. Die unvollständige Ausprägung des Syndroms ($1/4$ aller Fälle, WARKANY), wobei nur einzelne Teilerscheinungen wie eine Adipositas, ein Schwachsinn, ein Hypo-genitalismus vorhanden sind, machen die Beurteilung noch schwieriger, da die Wertigkeit der Einzelsymptome von den einzelnen Autoren verschieden be-stimmt wird. Fälle ohne Retinitis pigmentosa sollten nicht hierher gerechnet werden. Es sind auch eine Reihe von Mißbildungen anderer Organe wie Ptose, Kyphoskoliose, Glaukom, Nystagmus, angeborene Herzfehler, angeborener Hydro-cephalus, Ataxie, Taubheit berichtet (SORSBY u. Mitarb., WARKANY u. Mitarb.). Vier der fünf von ROTH beschriebenen Fälle hatten keine typische Retinitis pigmentosa, sondern eine einfache Atrophie. Das gehäufte Vorkommen in ein-zelnen Familien spricht für eine Erbkrankheit, wobei neuerdings ein recessives, autosomales Gen mit wechselnder Penetranz angenommen wird, das Entwick-lungsstörungen an verschiedenen Geweben auslöst (OETTLÉ u. Mitarb.).

Die Ähnlichkeit der Fettsucht und des Hypogonadismus mit dem Fröhlich-Syndrom, die Kombination mit geistigen Defekten, das verhältnismäßig häufige Vorkommen der Polydypsie legten schon immer den Verdacht auf eine hypo-physär-diencephale Störung, die die Fettsucht und den Hypogonadismus erklären würden, nahe (ROTH). FRANCKE machte 1950 als erster auf einen primären Defekt der Keimdrüsen aufmerksam und beschrieb einen Fall mit dem typischen histo-logischen Bild des Klinefelter-Syndroms. Auch OETTLÉ u. Mitarb. kommen zu der Auffassung, daß der Hypogonadismus durch einen primären Hodendefekt und nicht durch eine Schädigung der Adenohypophyse bedingt ist. Im Oettleschen Fall war das Zwischengewebe normal entwickelt, die Kanälchenwand etwas verdickt ($4-8\,\mu$), die Wand besetzt von normalen Sertolizellen, während das Samenepithel bis auf zwei Kanälchen, die einzelne normale, Spermatogonien ent-hielten, fehlte. Neben der Keimzellaplasie von Typ des Del Castillo-Syndroms zeigen andere auch Reifungsstörungen, wobei die Entwicklung der Samenzellen auf der Höhe der Spermatogonien stehen bleibt, während das Zwischengewebe normal entwickelt ist (ANDERSON, ROSS u. Mitarb.). In anderen Fällen wiederum fehlen die Zeichen eines Hypogonadismus ganz, Interstitium und Kanälchen sind normal entwickelt (McGULLAGH u. Mitarb. 1957, ROTH). OETTLÉ macht auch auf die besondere Häufung des ein- und beidseitigen Kryptorchismus (42%) und auf das Vorkommen einseitig atrophischer Hoden in 13% der Bellschen Zusammen-stellung aufmerksam.

Die wenigen autoptischen Befunde des Hypothalamus und der Hypophyse bestätigen die zentrale Genese des Hypogonadismus nur in einem Fall. In drei anderen war die Hypophyse normal, ebenso in einem eigenen, dreimal fand sich eine Vermehrung der Basophilen, nur einmal war der Vorderlappen durch eine epitheliale Cyste ersetzt. Auffällige Befunde am Zwischenhirn fehlen (OETTLÉ).

In der Mehrzahl der Fälle handelt es sich beim Laurence-Moon-Biedl-Syndrom offenbar um eine primäre Dysgenesie der Gonaden, selten um einen zentralen Defekt der Gonadotropinproduktion. Wie schwierig die Entscheidung sein kann, zeigt nachstehende eigene Beobachtung.

Fall 12. R. M., 19jähriger Junge, Aufnahme 18. 11. 59.

Einziges Kind. Hat sich in der Jugend normal entwickelt, war immer ein schlechter Schüler, neigt seit dem 14. Lebensjahr zu Erkältungskrankheiten, klagt seit 3 Jahren über zunehmende Atemnot, seit einem Jahr über starkes Hautjucken.

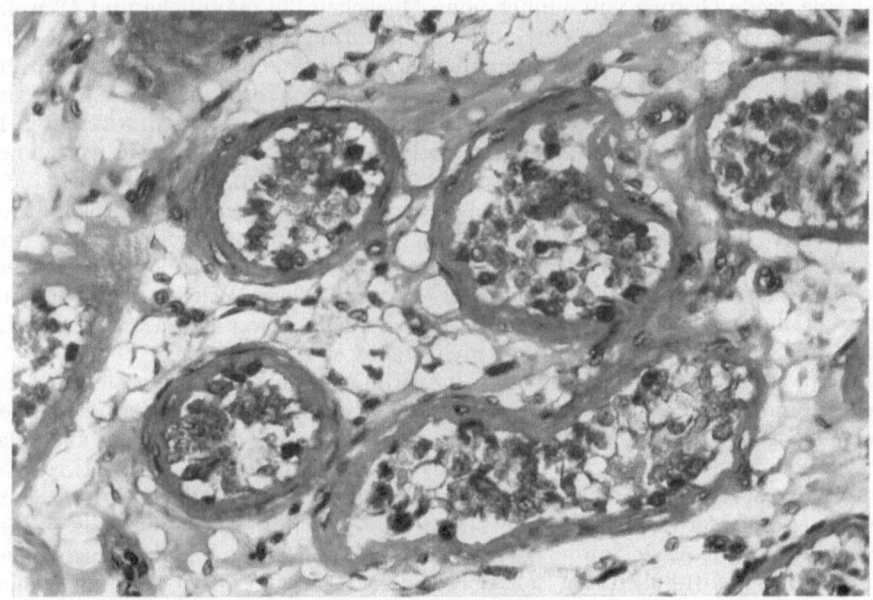

Abb. 65. 21jährig. Laurence-Moon-Biedl-Syndrom. Kanälchen: Kleiner Durchmesser ohne Lumen, Wand beträchtlich verdickt durch Hyalinablagerung, Samenepithel undifferenziert, einzelne Spermatogonien und Spermatocyten. Zwischengewebe faserarm, weder reife noch unreife Leydigzellen sicher nachweisbar. (Ilopa, 300fach) (Fall 12)

156 cm, 58 kg Gewicht. Körperlich und geistig weit zurückgebliebener Junge, mäßige Fettanhäufung am Rumpf und im Gesicht. Die Entwicklung des äußeren Genitale entspricht einem 12jährigen, die Hoden sind deszendiert, 1,5:1 cm groß, von weicher Konsistenz, ganz spärliche Scham- und Achselbehaarung, fehlende Körper- und Bartbehaarung. Im Augenhintergrund das typische Bild einer *ausgedehnten Retinitis pigmentosa* beidseits.

Die weitere Untersuchung deckt eine Urämie mit Hochdruck auf, RR um 170/130 mm Hg, Proteinurie 0,6⁰/₀₀, Harnstoff 340 mg-%, Anämie von 63%, 17-Ketosteroide 1,5—2,2 mg, Porter-Silberchromogene 1,1—2,09 mg, Gonadotropine nicht nachweisbar. Jodspeicherung der Schilddrüse nach 6 Std 15, nach 24 Std 36%. Der Kranke stirbt an der Urämie.

Anatomisch (Pathologisches Institut der Universität Tübingen) finden sich an den Nieren die Zeichen einer fortgeschrittenen arteriolo-sklerotischen Schrumpfniere mit völliger Verödung der Glomerula. Leber: Zeichen einer chronischen Stauung. Gehirn: an mehreren Stellen untersucht, grobe Struktur unauffällig, in den Marklagern kleinste perivasculäre Ringblutungen. Gebiet des Zwischenhirns, des Hypophysenstiels und der Hypophyse makroskopisch unauffällig. Mikroskopisch in der Adenohypophyse gewisse Vermehrung der Basophilen und chromophoben Anteile ohne Überschreitung des normalen Maßes.

Hoden: kleiner Kanälchendurchmesser, kein Lumen. Die Wand ist teilweise durch Ablagerung von hyalinen Massen beträchtlich verdickt, während der Faseranteil nicht vermehrt erscheint. Samenepithel größtenteils undifferenziert, in einzelnen Kanälchen lassen sich Spermatogonien und vermutlich Vorstadien von Spermatocyten erster Ordnung unterscheiden. Im verhältnismäßig faserarmen Zwischengewebe sind reife Leydigzellen nicht zu erkennen, auch unreife Formen können nicht mit Sicherheit identifiziert werden (vgl. Abb. 65).

Es findet sich das Bild eines präpuberalen Hodens, in dem einzelne Kanälchen, und zwar die mit verdickter Wand, bereits eine geringe puberale Entfaltung durchgemacht zu haben scheinen. Die Pubertätsentwicklung war hier offenbar eben im Begriffe einzutreten, als die Niereninsuffizienz hinzutrat und nicht nur die Entwicklung verhinderte, sondern durch Unterbrechung der Gonadotropinproduktion regressive Veränderungen an den Kanälchen auslöste. Also sekundärer Hypogonadismus nicht infolge eines angeborenen Defektes, sondern als Folge einer Niereninsuffizienz.

3. Weidenreich-Kallmann-Syndrom

Bei einer weiteren Gruppe eines familiären Hypogonadismus ist die Ursache des Defektes noch nicht geklärt. KALLMANN, SCHÖNFELD und BARRERA sammelten 1944 eine große Gruppe von eunuchoiden Menschen (36 männliche und 12 weibliche). In drei Familien war eine auffällige Häufung mit elf Männern und einer Frau vorhanden, wobei Organanomalien wie Anosmie, Farbenblindheit, Synkinesien und Schwachsinn diese Fälle als etwas Besonderes abgrenzte. Auf das Zusammentreffen von Eunuchoidismus und Anosmie hat WEIDENREICH 1914 schon hingewiesen, DE MORSIER sammelte 1955 31 Fälle von Anosmie, von denen 50% einen Hypogonadismus aufwiesen. ALTMANN, KÖHNE, NOWAKOWSKI (1959) haben neue Fälle beschrieben. Die von Geburt an vorhandene Anosmie soll durch einen Defekt im Olfactoriumsystem bedingt sein. Der Eunuchoidismus ist präpuberaler Art, die Kranken haben ausgesprochen eunuchoide Skeletproportionen, eine hohe Stimme, kindliches Genitale, sehr spärliche Behaarung. Nur ganz wenige Fälle sind hormonal durchuntersucht. Im Fall von NOWAKOWSKI (1959) waren mit 25 Jahren Gonadotropine nicht nachweisbar.

Es ist nicht klar, ob es sich um eine primäre Gonadendysgenesie oder um einen sekundären Hypogonadismus handelt. Histologisch findet sich am Hoden eine hochgradige Reifungshemmung, die sowohl die Leydigzellen als auch das Kanälchenepithel betrifft und vielfach als sekundär angesehen wird (ALTMANN, KÖHNE, NOWAKOWSKI 1959). Rechnet man aber den Fall von SOHVAL und SOFFER (1952) hierher: 23jährig mit Anosmie bei chronischer Sinusitis — der weniger als 30 E Gonadotropine im Urin hatte und bei dem die kleinen Kanälchen nur von einer undifferenzierten Zellart besiedelt waren (s. S. 846) —, dann scheint ein primärer Bildungsdefekt des Hodens mit Fehlen der Spermatogonien, der Sertoli- und Leydigzellen vorzuliegen. Auch im Köhneschen Fall waren die Kanälchenepithelien ganz undifferenziert, das Zwischengewebe bestand nur aus zellarmen Bindegewebszügen. KÖHNE gibt eine eingehende Untersuchung der Hypophyse und des Zwischenhirns. Letzteres war in Serienschnitten unauffällig, dagegen zeigte die Hypophyse eine beträchtliche Vermehrung der Basophilen, wie sie beim primären Hypogonadismus vorkommt. NOWAKOWSKI (1959) erwähnt das besonders schlechte Ansprechen des Weidenreich-Kallmann-Syndroms auf HCG, auch ein im Sinne der primären Dysgenesie verwertbares Symptom. Differentialdiagnostisch muß man erwähnen, daß auch suprasellläre Tumoren den Olfactorius schädigen können.

4. Rothmund- bzw. Werner-Syndrom

Das *Rothmund-Syndrom* und das Werner-Syndrom sind angeborene Defekte, die von TOURAINE als erbliche Zustände mit Hautatrophien und vorzeitiger Vergreisung zusammengefaßt wurden. Die klinische Abtrennung ist unsicher, man findet Hautdegenerationen von eigentümlicher Marmorierung und Gefäßerweiterungen, doppelseitigen Katarakt, vorzeitiges Ergrauen der Haare, Glatzenbildung, auch bei Frauen, so daß Perücken getragen werden müssen, Atrophie der Nägel, Störungen der Zahnentwicklung, Intelligenzdefekte, juvenile Arteriosklerose, Fistelstimme, psychische Störungen. Manchmal ist auch die Ossifikation gestört, ein Teil bleibt kleinwüchsig, die Knochen zeigen eine umschriebene Osteosklerose, aber auch Osteoporose.

Das *Werner-Syndrom* zeigt mehr Hautveränderungen im Sinne der Poikilodermie oder der Sklerodermie. Ein Teil der Fälle hat einen schweren Hypogonadismus, dessen Genese nicht klar ist. Im Falle BROUWER handelte es sich um eine primäre Form mit erhöhter Gonadotropinausscheidung, Leydigzellhyperplasie, Kanälchenfibrose und Gynäkomastie.

5. Dystrophia myotonica

Zur klassischen Ausprägung dieser Krankheit gehören neben der Myopathie ein Katarakt, Pigmentdegeneration der Netzhaut, Haarausfall, Intelligenzminderung, auch eine langsam fortschreitende Hodenatrophie, wobei im Anfang nur die Zeichen des Kanälchenschwundes, in den Endstadien aber auch die Symptome eines Hypoandrogenismus vorhanden sind. Ein Drittel der Kranken bleibt ledig oder kinderlos. Das Manifestationsalter der Parentalgeneration liegt bei 50,5 Jahren, der Filialgeneration bei 27,4 Jahren (KLEIN). Man nimmt eine autosomale dominante Vererbung mit verschieden starker Penetranz an. Erst nach dem 30. Lebensjahr nehmen Libido und Potenz ab, die Sekundärbehaarung an Rumpf und Extremitäten geht zurück, Achsel- und Schambehaarung, Bartwuchs schwinden, die Prostata verkleinert sich erheblich. Die 17-Ketosteroidausscheidung fanden wir in vier Fällen stark erniedrigt, wahrscheinlich mehr als Folge des schweren Muskelschwundes und weniger als Folge des Hypoandrogenismus. Häufig entwickelt sich eine Gynäkomastie. Der erste Hinweis, daß es sich um eine primäre Form eines Hypogonadismus handelt, stammt von NADLER u. Mitarb. Sie berichteten über zwei Brüder mit fortgeschrittener Atrophie und Hyalinisierung der Kanälchen und völligem Defekt der Spermatogenese. Die Leydigzellen traten in einzelnen Gebieten stark hervor, in anderen waren sie schlecht entwickelt. Beide Brustdrüsen waren vergrößert, die Gonadotropinausscheidung vermehrt, so daß kein Zweifel an der primären Keimdrüsenatrophie bestand. Solche Fälle wurden später von HOWARD u. Mitarb. (1950), von BENDA und BIX, TONUTTI, OVERZIER u. LINDEN (1956b), NOWAKOWSKI (1957a) u.a. beschrieben.

Der Kanälchenschaden ist verschieden schwer, er ist im wesentlichen abhängig von der Dauer und Schwere der Krankheit. Bei den leichten Formen findet man nur eine Hypospermiogenese mit einzelnen sklerosierten Kanälchen bei normal aussehenden Leydigzellen. Je mehr die Krankheit fortschreitet, um so schwerer wird auch der Grad der Kanälchensklerosierung. Beim Vollbild sieht man nur noch Kanälchenschatten. Der Kanälchendurchmesser ist im allgemeinen deutlich größer als beim echten Klinelfelter-Syndrom. Die Leydigzellen verhalten sich verschieden. Meist sind sie normal oder nur wenig vermehrt, nicht ganz selten aber auch diffus vermehrt, hyperplastisch, knotenförmig wuchernd (BENDA u. BIXBY, GILBERT-DREYFUS 1954, GÖBEL u. Mitarb. 1958, KAPPAS u. Mitarb., NADLER u. Mitarb., PERLOFF u. Mitarb., TIMME). Bei vier eigenen Fällen bestand keine enge Beziehung zwischen der Schwere der Muskelatrophie und der Ausdehnung der Kanälchenfibrosierung, eher zu der Dauer der Erkrankung.

Die Ursache der Hodenatrophie ist nicht bekannt, man nimmt wohl meist eine der Muskelatrophie gleichgeschaltete Erkrankung an, doch muß die Möglichkeit einer Kanälchenschädigung durch pathologische Muskelabbauprodukte offengelassen werden. Verabreichung von Vitamin E, Glykokoll und Aminosäuren hat keinen Einfluß auf die Hodenschädigung. Testosteron bringt nur eine symptomatische Besserung.

VII. Behandlung

Wirkungsdauer und Wirkungsintensität der verschiedenen Testosteronester ist abhängig von der Geschwindigkeit ihrer Resorption, Inaktivierung und Ausscheidung (s. S. 725).

Die Hauptindikation für die Verwendung des Testosterons ist der *primäre Hypogonadismus*. Die Dosierung muß verschieden gehandhabt werden, je nachdem, ob es sich um den präpuberalen Eunuchismus eines Jugendlichenoder eines Erwachsenen handelt. Aus Experimenten beim Tier und aus Beobachtungen beim Menschen weiß man, daß die Gewebe um die Zeit der natürlichen Pubertät am empfindlichsten gegen Testosteron sind. Bis zum 17. Lebensjahr beginnt man daher beim präpuberalen Eunuchismus mit einer verhältnismäßig kleinen Dosis. Wir geben dreimal 25 mg Testosteronpropionat intramuskulär pro Woche, oder 50 mg Isobutyrat alle 14 Tage oder 100 mg Oenanthat alle 3 Wochen. Im Alter zwischen 18 und 22 Jahren wird die Dosis verdoppelt. Bei der richtigen Dosierung rötet sich nach 3—4 Wochen das Scrotum, die Haut wird dicker und fängt an, sich zu runzeln. Weitere 3—4 Wochen später fängt der Penis an zu wachsen, wobei sich zuerst die Wurzel verdickt, gleichzeitig sprossen die Pubes. Bei Jugendlichen bis zum 16. Lebensjahr soll man den Ablauf der Pubertät nicht zusammenraffen, sondern ungefähr die natürlichen zeitlichen Verhältnisse, um 2—4 Jahre verschoben, nachahmen. Über 16 Jahre schadet eine raschere Entwicklung beim Normalwüchsigen nicht.

Nach 2—3jähriger Behandlung stellt sich ein junger Mann vor, der den Pubertätswachstumsstoß hinter sich hat, dessen Penis, Scrotum, Pubes- und Achselbehaarung praktisch normal entwickelt sind, der aber immer noch die eunuchoide Verteilung des Fettes zeigt und dessen Muskeln schlecht ausgeprägt sind. Die Stimme ist noch nicht normal tief, der Bartwuchs noch dürftig, das Knochensystem reifer, aber die Epiphysenfugen sind noch weit offen. In dieser Phase, die der eine früher, der andere später erreicht, ist zur Komplettierung der Reifung die Dosis weiter zu erhöhen.

Kommen die Kranken erst im Alter über 22 Jahre mit dem Bild des präpuberalen Eunuchismus oder Eunuchoidismus zur Behandlung, dann wählt man die Dosis von Anfang an hoch, 50 mg Testosteronisobutyrat alle Woche oder 250—300 mg Testosteronoenanthat alle 3—4 Wochen. Sowohl die Entwicklung der Genitalorgane, als auch die Reifung des Gewebes verläuft in diesen Fällen protrahierter. Trotz konsequenter Fortführung der Therapie erreicht man die volle Reifung nicht mehr.

Die Durchführung der Behandlung ist nicht einfach. Bei zu hoher Dosierung treten schon vor einer nennenswerten Entwicklung des Genitale unangenehme, schmerzhafte Erektionen auf, die sich bis zum Priapismus steigern. Sedativa bessern, stören aber die Berufsausübung. Ältere Menschen haben sich manchmal an ihren Zustand so gewöhnt, daß ihnen jede Änderung unangenehm ist. Viele Kranke werden nachlässig, sobald sie ein Stadium des körperlichen Wohlbefindens und der Entwicklung erreicht haben, in dem sie nicht mehr auffallen. Da die feste Bindung an eine Partnerin scheitert und auch nicht empfohlen werden kann, genügt den Kranken ein Zustand, in dem sie äußerlich nicht mehr auffallen. Bei Menschen mit normaler Intelligenz und ohne sonstige Gebrechen muß man aber die Behandlung zu Ende führen, denn nur dann ist die volle Entwicklung der Muskulatur, des Knochensystems, der geistigen Leistung und der Psyche, die dem Einzelnen mitgegeben ist, gewährleistet. Hierbei wird die damit verbundene Intensivierung der Sexualität als störend empfunden. Wahrscheinlich kann man in Zukunft mit Erfolg die mehr anabol wirkenden Derivate des

Testosteron einsetzen und kombiniert behandeln. Bei unvollständiger Behandlung entwickeln sich im jugendlichen Alter verhältnismäßig häufig Belastungsschäden, wie die Perthes- oder Scheuermannsche Erkrankung, starke X-Beine, Plattfüße, beim Erwachsenen eine vorzeitige Osteoporose, vorzeitiger Muskelschwund und sonstige für das Alter charakteristische Gewebsatrophien.

In der Praxis wird die Dosierung vielfach zu niedrig gewählt, da man eine zu rasche sexuelle Entwicklung und den vorzeitigen Epiphysenschluß befürchtet. Bei normal großen Jugendlichen über 16 Jahre schadet auch die zu hoch gewählte Dosis nicht. Der Wachstumsstoß der Pubertät, künstlich ausgelöst durch die Testosteronbehandlung, scheint Voraussetzung zu sein für die Reifungsvorgänge, die zum Epiphysenschluß führen (TONUTTI). Man kann aus diesem Grunde auch den abnormen Hochwuchs eines Jugendlichen durch eine intensive Testosteronbehandlung nicht abstoppen!

Komplizierter sind die Verhältnisse bei Minderwüchsigen, die zugleich im Knochenreifungsalter erheblich zurückgeblieben sind (hypophysärer Zwerg- und Minderwuchs). Es ist nicht bekannt geworden, daß eine zu intensive Behandlung die Reifung überstürzt, das Epiphysenwachstum behindert und einen vorzeitigen Epiphysenschluß auslöst. Wahrscheinlich erfolgt auch in diesen Fällen, wie TONUTTI u. Mitarb. (1960) annehmen, der normal große Wachstumsstoß der Pubertät, aber nach unseren Erfahrungen langsamer und erst nach intensiver hochdosierter Behandlung. Erst wenn die volle Ausprägung der männlichen Körperform erreicht ist, wird die Hormondosis auf die *Erhaltungsdosis* reduziert. Wie beim *postpuberalen Kastraten*, der durch Krankheit oder Unfall im Erwachsenenalter beide Gonaden verloren hat, braucht man zur Erhaltung des Entwickelten weniger Hormon. In diesen Fällen können auch die oral verabreichbaren Präparate mit Erfolg Verwendung finden. Man gibt: 50 mg Testosteronisobutyrat alle 2—4 Wochen, 100—150 mg Testosteronoenanthat alle 4 Wochen, Methyltestosteron per os 20—40 mg in unterteilten Dosen täglich, Fluoxymestinon 5—10 mg per os täglich. Wenn man die Erhaltung der Gewebstrophik, der geistigen und körperlichen Leistung als Maß verwenden kann, kommt man mit kleineren Dosen aus, als wenn die Normalisierung von Libido und Potenz verlangt wird. Bei der starken individuellen Verschiedenheit dieser Lebensäußerungen können sie nie als alleiniges Maß verwendet werden. Ein objektiver Wertmesser ist bis 50 Jahre die Größe der Prostata. Zur Feineinstellung eignet sich die Messung der Ejaculatmenge und des Fructosegehaltes. Der gut eingestellte erwachsene Kastrat kann ein völlig normales Leben führen. Seine körperliche Leistungsfähigkeit ist unbehindert, seine geistige voll erhalten. Aus der Kindheit stammende psychische Hemmungen werden durch das gestärkte Selbstbewußtsein meist überwunden. Seelische Abnormitäten sind häufiger als bei den sich zu normaler Zeit Entwickelnden, aber man ist immer wieder erstaunt, wie gering die bleibenden Schäden einer um Jahre verspäteten Pubertät bei unkomplizierten und natürlich empfindenden Menschen sind.

VIII. Exogene Schäden

Exogene Schäden können sich in verschiedener Weise auf den Hoden auswirken. Als empfindlichster Teil reagiert das Samenepithel als erstes. Man findet alle Zeichen der *desorganisierten Reifung*, des *Reifungsstopps*, der *Depopulation* der Kanälchen bis auf die Sertolizellen. Fortschreitende Depopulation bedingt eine geringe Abnahme des Innendurchmessers der Kanälchen, dadurch verkürzen sich die Fasern der Wand, so daß diese selbst etwas dicker wird. Damit ist die Möglichkeit von Diffusionsstörungen gegeben, die nun ihrerseits wieder ungünstig auf die Funktion des Kanälchenepithels wirkt. Es ist möglich, daß auf diese Weise ein nur für kurze Zeit einwirkender Schaden das Keimepithel für dauernd schädigt. Das Zwischengewebe bleibt normal, keine Hypertrophie der Leydigzellen.

Mit Ausnahme einer Oligo- bzw. Azoospermie hat diese einfache Keimepithelschädigung keine Rückwirkung auf den Gesamtorganismus. Gonadotropine sind normal.

In einzelnen Fällen von *Strahlenschädigungen*, in denen die Kanälchen nur noch von Sertolizellen ausgekleidet waren, sieht man intertubulär die ersten Wucherungen der Leydigzellen. Dies ist ein Hinweis darauf, daß als Folge der Keimepithelschädigung eine Vermehrung der Gonadotropinproduktion eingetreten ist. Im allgemeinen sind die Leydigzellen bei alleinigem Fehlen des Samenepithels nicht hypertroph oder hyperplastisch, es gibt aber Ausnahmen, besonders nach Entzündungen und traumatischer Schädigung. Fehlen in weiten Bezirken auch die Sertolizellen, dann ist die Leydigzellhyperplasie zusammen mit der *Sklerohyalinose der Kanälchenwand* ein regelmäßiger Befund. Die Ursache dieser fortschreitenden Tubulusdegeneration ist nicht sicher bekannt, wahrscheinlich ist sie nicht einheitlich.

Die Bedeutung der Sertolizellen als primärer Faktor für die bindegewebige Wandverdickung hat besonders Sniffen u. Mitarb. (1951) hervorgehoben. In der Tat hat man den Eindruck, daß immer dann, wenn die Sertolizellen morphologisch degenerative Veränderungen zeigen und ihre normale histochemische Färbbarkeit verlieren, auch Veränderungen der Kanälchenwand auftreten. Daß die Sertolizellen für die Ernährung der inneren Kanälchenwand Bedeutung haben ist wahrscheinlich, eine Funktionsstörung trifft daher sowohl das Samenepithel als auch die Kanälchenwand. Der zweite wichtige Faktor ist der Gefäß-Bindegewebsapparat. Störung der Diffusion durch entzündliche Vorgänge im Interstitium oder schlechte Blutversorgung als Folge von Gefäßprozessen oder Innervationsstörungen führt ebenfalls zu Wandverdickung und Untergang des Samenepithels (Heller u. Nelson 1945).

Bei gleichmäßiger Verteilung der Sklerosierung ist die Gonadotropinausscheidung immer stark vermehrt. Hyperplasie der Leydigzellen, die sich in Haufen und Klumpen anordnen können, ist die Folge. Klinisch sind beide Hoden verkleinert, es besteht eine Oligo- oder Azoospermie, häufig eine Gynäkomastie, aber Zeichen eines Androgenmangels sind selten. Es ist nicht geklärt, ob hiefür die Verminderung der Gesamtgewebsmasse des Hodens die einzige Ursache ist, oder ob sich die hyperplastischen Leydigzellen erschöpfen und degenerieren.

Die dritte Form der Hodenschädigung ist anatomisch durch die *Fibrosis testis* charakterisiert. Hier ist der gesamte Hoden oder große Teile bindegewebig umgewandelt. Häufig, aber nicht immer, erkennt man im Bindegewebe noch stark veränderte Kanälchen eingelagert. Diese Fibrosis testis geht meist auf die Unterbrechung der Hauptgefäße zurück, kann aber auch Folge von traumatischen Schäden oder schweren Entzündungen sein.

Das klinische Bild hängt von der noch erhaltenen Restfunktion des Hodens ab. Im allgemeinen besteht ein Hypogonadismus erheblichen Ausmaßes. Die Gonadotropinausscheidung ist erhöht, die Vergrößerung der Brustdrüse häufig.

1. Kastration

Nur noch bei Geschwülsten und Verletzungen kommt es vor, daß beide Hoden entfernt werden müssen. Die einseitige Kastration führt bei den Säugern zu einer innersekretorisch voll ausreichenden kompensatorischen Hypertrophie des verbleibenden Hodens. Entfernt man einen Hoden ganz und nimmt vom zweiten noch einen großen Teil weg, dann reicht ein verhältnismäßig kleines Gewebsstück für die Funktion aus. Beim Hahn genügen z. B. 0,3 g Gewebe, um den entwickelten Kamm zu erhalten, sogar ein Gewebsstückchen von 0,027 g läßt noch eine geringe Wirkung erkennen. Das verbliebene Hodengewebe wächst, die interstitiellen Zellen nehmen das Aussehen von sehr aktiven Zellen an. Die innersekretorischen Funktionsreserven eines normalen Hodengewebes scheinen recht beträchtlich zu sein.

Auch beim Menschen ist die Entfernung eines Hodens und die weitgehende des zweiten ohne Folgen für die Ausprägung der sekundären Geschlechtsmerkmale, Voraussetzung ist aber ein normales Hodengewebe, das zur Hyperplasie fähig ist, andernfalls entwickelt sich ein postpuberaler Eunuchoidismus.

2. Verletzungen und Operationen

Schädigungen des Hodengewebes sind am häufigsten nach operativen Eingriffen im Bereich des Inguinalkanals, besonders bei Operationen des Kryptorchismus oder von Hernien. Es ist nicht nur die direkte Unterbindung der Gefäße, wie sie beim Kleinkind häufig vorkommt, sondern die gewollte straffe Verengerung der Bruchpforte beim Erwachsenen, die zur Minderdurchblutung des Hodens mit sekundärer Atrophie führt. Von chirurgischer Seite wird die Häufigkeit der Fibrosis testis nach lege artis durchgeführten Hernienoperationen mit bis 3,5% angegeben!

Örtliche Traumen sind in ihren Folgen schwer zu beurteilen. Im allgemeinen müssen schwerere Quetschungen, Gefäßzerreißungen oder intratesticuläre Hämatome vorhanden gewesen sein, wenn eine Hodenatrophie traumatisch bedingt sein soll. Entscheidend ist immer nur der histologische Befund, meist mit dem Bild der Fibrosis testis, seltener mit dem der schweren Tubulusdegeneration. Während man früher die Meinung vertrat, daß traumatische Hodenblutungen bei Steißgeburten keine Schädigungen hinterlassen (OBERNDORFER), mehren sich andersartige Beobachtungen. NOWAKOWSKI (1959) berichtet über einen sehr eindrucksvollen Fall.

Der Kranke kam als 22jähriger Mann mit den Zeichen eines präpuberalen Eunuchoidismus mit beidseitiger Hodenatrophie und Aspermie zur Untersuchung. Die Biopsie ergab normal große, vom Keimepithel völlig entblößte Samenkanälchen, die nur von Sertolizellen ausgekleidet waren. Intertubulär exzessive Proliferation der Leydigzellen, Gonadotropine im Urin erhöht. Man konnte erfahren, daß bei der Geburt, die in Steißlage erfolgt war, ein ausgedehntes Hämatom des Scrotums und beider Hoden vorgelegen hat, das Kind war damals photographiert worden.

Die Hodengefäße nehmen auch an Gefäßerkrankungen des Gesamtorganismus teil, besonders bei der Arteriosklerose und der Panarteriitis. Dadurch bedingte Durchblutungsstörungen schädigen vorwiegend die Kanälchen, während Androgenmangelerscheinungen selten sind.

Folgendes Beispiel sei gegeben:

Fall 13. G. Sch., 38jährig.
Eltern und sechs Geschwister angeblich gesund.
E. A.: Mit 12 Jahren Diphtherie, mit 14 Jahren Blutvergiftung, mit 15 Jahren Mumps, mit 16 Jahren Prellung am linken Bein.
Normal entwickelt. 22jährig *beidseitige Leistenbruchoperation.* Von da an langsam abnehmende Libido und Potenz, seit etwa dem 30. Lebensjahr braucht er sich nicht mehr zu rasieren. Seither öfters hohes Fieber mit Bronchitis.
164 cm, 61,3 kg. Oberlänge 84 cm, Unterlänge 80 cm.

Schlaffe, welke Haut, zahlreiche Runzeln im Gesicht. Kein Bart, schlecht entwickelte Achselbehaarung, mäßige Schambehaarung mit horizontaler Begrenzung, praktisch keine Körperbehaarung. Prostata markstückgroß, ganz flach. Erhebliche Gynäkomastie. Skelet: erhebliche Osteoporose der Wirbelsäule.

Genitale: Penis 7 cm lang, normal dick. Hoden beidseits knapp mandelgroß, ganz weich. Prostata kleinkastaniengroß, aber ganz flach.

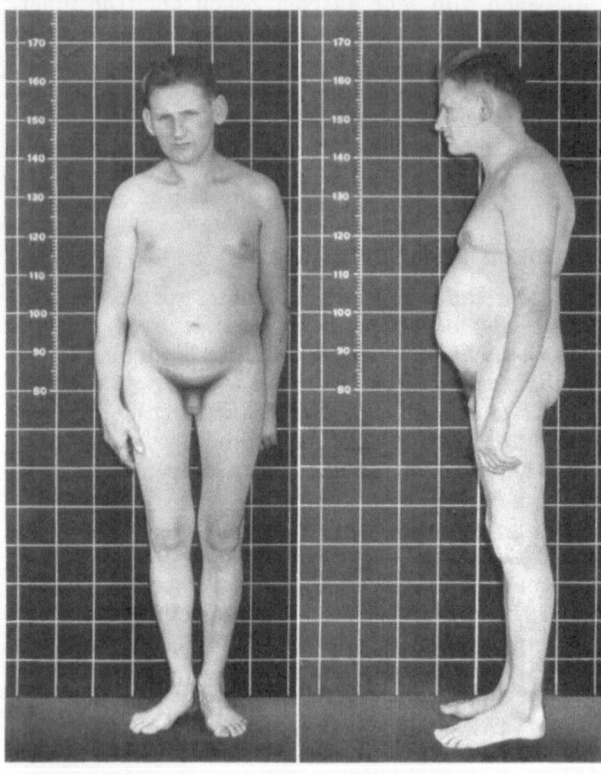

17-Ketosteroid-Urin: 5,3, 4,5, 7,2. Nach fünftägiger Gabe von 3000 E Chorion-gonadotropin kein Anstieg. Porter - Silberchromogene 5,7, 6,3, 7,2 mg, unter ACTH intravenös E 8 Std 21,9 mg. Abfall der Eosinophilen um 90%.

Grundumsatz —5%. Jod-speicherung: 6 Std 48%, 24 Std 62%.

Uringonadotropine > 96 MEU.

Hodenbiopsie: zeigt voll-kommen verödetes Gewebe, es finden sich lediglich Binde-gewebsmassen, in denen weder Kanälchen noch Zwischen-zellen auszumachen sind, ein zweites Biopsiestückchen zeigt Nebenhodenkanälchen. Fibrosis testis ?

Chromosomales Geschlecht: Blutausstrich auf 500 Seg-mentkernige nur 4 Drum-stick, Wangenschleimhaut chromatinnegativ.

Wahrscheinlich ist bei der doppelseitigen Leisten-bruchoperation eine artifi-zielle Gefäßunterbrechung er-folgt, als deren Folge beide Hoden bindegewebig umge-wandelt wurden. Klinisch das Bild des postpuberalen Eunuchoidismus (Abb. 66).

Abb. 66. 38jähriger Mann mit beidseitiger Fibrosis testis nach beid-seitiger Hernienoperation. Normale Körperproportionen, Gynäkomastie, Rundrücken infolge vorzeitiger Osteoporose (Fall 13)

3. Entzündung, physikalische Schäden, Querschnittslähmung u. a.

Beim Erwachsenen sind es besonders die Paroditis epidemica und die Brucel-losen, die eine ein- und doppelseitige Orchitis hervorrufen, während die Besiedelung des Hodengewebes beim Typhus, Paratyphus, dem Fleckfieber selten ist. Tuber-kulose, Gonorrhoe und Syphilis können heute so frühzeitig bekämpft werden, daß schwerere Zerstörungen des Hodengewebes nicht mehr vorkommen.

Nur etwa 10% der Kranken, die eine Mumps-Orchitis durchmachen, zeigen später eine beidseitige Hodenatrophie mit inkretorischer Insuffizienz. Den patho-logisch-anatomischen Ablauf der Mumps-Orchitis haben CHARNY und MERANZE (1947) ausführlich beschrieben.

Die Entzündung ergreift sowohl die Kanälchen als auch das Interstitium. Die am stärksten betroffenen Kanälchen gehen in der Entzündung unter, das Inter-stitium, in dem reichlich Fibrin abgelagert wird, ist durchsetzt von entzündlichen Zellen, die Leydigzellen sind normal. Nach 14 Tagen geht die celluläre Infiltration zurück, viele Kanälchen sind bis auf den Sertolizellbelag entvölkert, im Inter-stitium besteht noch eine dichte Ansammlung von Entzündungszellen. Nach dem

21. Tag gibt die *fleckförmige Verteilung* von atrophischen Kanälchen und von solchen, in denen die Spermiogenese wieder aufgenommen wird, dem Bild das charakteristische Gepräge. Die vom Entzündungsprozeß verschont gebliebenen erholen sich wieder, die geschädigten gehen zugrunde. Das Interstitium bleibt im allgemeinen unbeteiligt. Bei verbreiteter Schädigung der Kanälchen entstehen hyperplastische Zellgruppen und auch adenomartige Wucherungen der Leydigzellen, so daß das anatomische Bild dem der schweren Tubulusdegeneration gleicht. Androgenmangelerscheinungen sind sehr selten, kommen aber bei Zerstörung größerer Gewebsteile vor. Die wesentlichste Folge der Mumps-Orchitis ist die Oligo- bzw. Azoospermie bei atrophischen Hoden.

MARBERGER und NELSON (1957) nehmen eine blande und schleichend verlaufende Orchitis als häufigste Ursache des falschen Klinefelter-Syndroms, der idiopathischen Tubulusdegeneration an. Das ist nach dem anatomischen Endzustand. den eine Orchitis hinterlassen kann, sehr wohl möglich. Ein Teil dieser Kranken geht aber mit einem Androgenmangelsyndrom einher, das den Beginn vor die Pubertät legt. Nun ist aber die Orchitis beim Kind etwas außerordentlich seltenes, so daß die Einbeziehung der „idiopathischen Tubulusdegeneration" mit *präpuberalem* Eunuchoidismus in die Gruppe der Entzündungsfolgen problematisch ist. Dagegen kann die „idiopathische Tubulusdegeneration mit *postpuberalem* Eunuchoidismus" sehr wohl hierhergehören.

Verschiedene *physikalische Schäden* führen meist nur zu einer Beeinträchtigung des Samenepithels, wobei die schwerste Form die Depopulation bis auf den Sertolizellbelag darstellt. Die Ursache dieser Schäden sind: längerdauernde hochfieberhafte Erkrankungen, Erhöhung der Hodentemperatur durch das Tragen enger Beinkleider, durch Arbeit bei hoher Außentemperatur, besonders an Schmelzöfen mit intensiver Strahlungswärme (NELSON 1953 b) u. ä. Die Leydigzellen werden dadurch nicht beeinträchtigt.

Dasselbe gilt für die Exposition gegen α-, β- und γ-Strahlen. Auch hier erfolgt im allgemeinen nur eine Depopulation bis auf die Sertolizellen, während Wandverdickungen der Kanälchen und irreparable Schädigung der Leydigzellen ausbleiben.

Neuerdings wurden auch bei hochdosierter Behandlung mit Cytostatica schwere Reifungsstörungen des Samenepithels beschrieben (NELSON 1953 b).

Die Veränderungen bei *Querschnittslähmung* beschränken sich ebenfalls auf das Kanälchenepithel. BORS u. Mitarb. finden bei 34 Fällen 22mal den Befund der einfachen Hypospermiogenese, dreimal eine Reifungshemmung, siebenmal eine tubuläre Fibrose, elfmal einen normalen Befund. Das Interstitium war immer normal, es bestand keine Hyperplasie der Leydigzellen. Die Hodenschädigung ist um so ausgedehnter, je höher der Sitz der Querschnittslähmung liegt. In einzelnen Fällen wurde aber bei ausgedehnterer tubulärer Fibrose eine Hyperplasie der Zwischenzellen beschrieben. Die häufig begleitende Gynäkomastie kann Folge einer zusätzlichen Leberschädigung oder Folge der Kanälchenatrophie sein. Innersekretorische Ausfälle fehlen. Als Ursache vermuten BORS u. Mitarb. eine lokale Hyperämie und Hyperthermie, die als Folge der Unterbrechung des Sympathicus eintritt.

Früher hat man angenommen, daß die *Unterbindung der Ausführungsgänge* eine Zerstörung des Keimepithels nach sich zieht. Bei seinen Verjüngungsversuchen durch Unterbindung der Ductus deferentes glaubte STEINACH nach einer gewissen Zeit eine Hyperplasie der Leydigzellen feststellen zu können. Genauere Beobachtungen beim Menschen nach Obliteration der Epididymis durch Gonorrhoe und Tuberkulose, nach Unterbindung der Vasa deferentes haben keine Änderung der innersekretorischen Funktion des Hodens ergeben. Der

Hoden bleibt normal groß. Selbst bei jahrelanger Atresie der Ausführungsgänge sind die histologischen Veränderungen an den Kanälchen nur geringfügig. In den meisten Fällen sieht man eine aktive Spermatogenese, Spermatozoen werden in normalen Mengen produziert. Geringe Erweiterung der Kanälchen, geringe Kompression des interstitiellen Gewebes, mäßige Verminderung der Spermatogenese mit und ohne Verdickung der Tunica propria, umschriebene Kanälchenatrophie und interstitielle Fibrose. sind so inkonstast, daß sie nicht als Folge der Verlegung angesehen werden können. Dagegen ist die Desquamation einer ungewöhnlich großen Zahl von Spermatocyten, Spermatiden und Spermatozoen in das Kanälchenlumen ein häufiger Befund. Die Leydigzellen zeigen weder qualitative noch quantitative Veränderungen (SNIFFEN u. Mitarb. 1950).

IX. Keimdrüse im Alter

Die geweblichen Veränderungen des Hodens im Alter werden nicht einheitlich beschrieben. Dies liegt zum Teil an dem unterschiedlichen Krankengut, das der einzelne bearbeiten konnte — ein Großteil der Betreffenden ist an akuten oder chronischen Krankheiten gestorben —, zum anderen an der Schwierigkeit, die der Verwendung von Leichenmaterial für eine einwandfreie histologische Untersuchung entgegensteht.

Größe und Gewicht verändern sich nur wenig (RÖSSLE u. Mitarb. 1932). Faßt man z.B. die Altersgruppen von 16 und 49 und 50—90 Jahren zusammen, dann sind die mittleren Hodengewichte praktisch gleich. Trennt man aber nach dem histologischen Befund der Aktivität der Spermiogenese, dann ergibt sich ein Unterschied von 21,5 gegenüber 19,7 g. Das Hodengewicht nimmt im Alter also nur ab, wenn deutliche Veränderungen an den Kanälchen vorhanden sind (OLESEN 1948).

1. Histologie

Der einzige *histologische Befund*, den STIEVE (1921) beim Altershoden regelmäßig erheben konnte, war eine Verdickung der Tunica propria. Eine geringe Abnahme des Kanälchendurchmessers, eine Verminderung der Aktivität der Spermiogenese, eine Zunahme degenerierender Samenzellen sind aber Veränderungen, die an einem größeren Beobachtungsgut regelmäßig zu erheben sind (CLARA 1930, GÖGL 1957, ROMEIS 1926, SPANGARO 1902).

Schon SPANGARO (1902) hat den *einfach senilen* Hoden vom *atrophisch-senilen* unterschieden. Bei normalen senilen Hoden findet sich nach TONUTTI ein allgemeines Nachlassen der spermiogenetischen und auch der inkretorischen Aktivität. Im Hodenbild hebt sich dabei kein Bauelement vor dem anderen besonders hervor. Beim atrophischen senilen Hoden hingegen stehen neben Veränderungen am Gefäßapparat des Interstitiums vor allem die Veränderungen der Tubuluswand im Vordergrund, die sich unter dem Bilde der Sklerohyalinose äußern und sich frühzeitig auf den Kanälcheninhalt auswirken. Das Samenepithel reagiert am raschesten und schnellsten auf die Beeinträchtigung der Ernährungsverhältnisse. Stärkere Grade führen zur Entvölkerung (Depopulation) bis auf den Sertolizellbelag, zu einer Verkleinerung der Kanälchen und zu einer relativen Wandverdickung. Letztlich können auch die Sertolizellen zugrunde gehen, so daß das Bild der totalen Sklerohyalinose zustande kommt.

In der Altersgruppe über 90 Jahren sind die Kanälchenveränderungen meist ausgesprochen (BÜRGI u. HEDINGER 1959), der Querschnitt ist mit 160—230 μ gegenüber 200—260 μ des normalen deutlich verringert, in der Mehrzahl der Untersuchten (12 von 16) zeigten sich fleckförmig angeordnete Bezirke mit total sklerosierten Samenkanälchen neben fast normalen. Drei von 16 hatten eine totale Atrophie mit diffuser Sklerohyalinose und nur bei einem war der Aufbau der Kanälchen praktisch normal (Bürgi u. Hedinger 1959).

In den letzten Jahren wurden besonders die Leydigzellen eingehender untersucht. Tillinger (1957) findet bei der Untersuchung von 227 Hoden der verschiedenen Altersgruppen, daß die relative Zahl der Leydigzellen, bezogen auf die Kanälchen zwischen dem 20. und 30. Lebensjahr, einen Gipfel erreicht, um von da an progressiv abzunehmen. Es besteht eine auffällige Parallele zwischen dieser Abnahme und dem Rückgang der 17-Ketosteroidausscheidung mit zunehmendem Lebensalter. Andere sprechen dagegen von einer Vermehrung (Kasai). Auch Bürgi und Hedinger finden die relative Zahl der Leydigzellen bei über 90jährigen eher vermehrt, es können sogar herdförmige Wucherungen vorhanden sein. Die Größe der Leydigzellen nimmt im allgemeinen ab (Clara), der Lipoidgehalt ist zwischen 20 und 30 Jahren am größten und sinkt im Alter (Lynch).

Nowakowski und Schmidt (1948) verwenden den Fructosegehalt des Spermas als Maß für die Leydigzellfunktion und finden bei Patienten, deren Spermien sowohl hinsichtlich der Quantität als auch der Qualität normal waren, eine kontinuierliche Abnahme mit zunehmendem Lebensalter. Zwischen 20 und 30 Jahren liegen die Mittelwerte bei 2800 γ/cm³ Ejaculat, sie sinken auf 800 γ zwischen dem 60. und 70. Lebensjahr. Auch der Gesamtfructosegehalt des Ejaculates nimmt ab, in 50% der im 6. Lebensjahrzehnt stehenden Männer ist er signifikant reduziert (Nowakowski u. Schmidt).

2. Klimakterium virile

Unter dem Klimakterium virile versteht man einen Symptomenkomplex neurovegetativer Erscheinungen, die beim Mann meist um das 50. Lebensjahr auftreten und mit einem Androgenmangel in Beziehung gebracht werden. Der Rückgang der Leydigzellfunktion erfolgt normalerweise so langsam, daß keine Erscheinungen auftreten. Beim Klimakterium virile soll die Abnahme der androgenen Aktivität rasch eintreten, nur dann treten Symptome auf.

Die Existenz dieses Symptomenkomplexes und seine Deutung als Androgenmangel wird von vielen mit Recht in Zweifel gezogen.

Die Symptome sind ähnlich denen der Menopause der Frau: Nervosität, abnehmendes Konzentrationsvermögen, rasche geistige und körperliche Ermüdbarkeit, Schlaflosigkeit, Schwitzen, Frieren, Tachykardie, Herzklopfen, Schwindel, Parästhesien, depressive Stimmungsschwankungen, Reizbarkeit, Versagen im Beruf, Abnahme von Libido und Potenz.

Der Beginn liegt zwischen dem 41.—64. Jahr (Werner 1939). Betroffen sind besonders schon vorher vegetativ Labile und Angehörige geistiger Berufe. Der Zusammenhang dieser Symptome mit einem rasch einsetzenden Androgenmangel ist bis heute noch nicht erbracht, obwohl man seit langem versucht, das Syndrom auf eine objektive Grundlage zu stellen (Heller u. Myers 1944a). McCullagh (1940) fand bei 23 Männern mit den charakteristischen Symptomen eine beträchtliche Erhöhung der Gonadotropinausscheidung im Urin, in acht Fällen bioptisch abnorme Leydigzellen. Im allgemeinen ist das Biopsiebild wenig charakteristisch (Tonutti u. Mitarb. 1960). Wenn auch eine erhöhte Gonadotropinausscheidung nicht als entscheidendes diagnostisches Kriterium gelten darf, so gibt ihr Vorhandensein doch einen wichtigen ätiologischen Hinweis. In diesen Fällen findet sich häufig auch eine Gynäkomastie. Objektive Symptome eines Androgenmangels fehlen bei 40—50jährigen so gut wie immer und gerade Menschen dieses Alters leiden am stärksten. Die 17-Ketosteroidausscheidung liegt meist an der unteren Grenze der Norm, so daß sie nicht beweiskräftig ist. Ob sich die Bestimmung des Fructosegehaltes des Spermas als Maß der abnehmenden Leydigzellfunktion in der Objektivierung des männlichen Klimakteriums bewähren wird, bleibt abzuwarten. NOWAKOWSKI und SCHMIDT (1948) beobachteten häufige Klagen über leicht depressive Erscheinungen, Nachlassen des Gedächtnisses und der Konzentrationsfähigkeit, Schlafstörungen sowie Potenzstörungen, wenn der Fructosegehalt um 50% gegenüber dem jüngerer Jahrgänge abgesunken war.

Die Abnahme der Leistung der Leydigzellen ist im Alter ein physiologischer Vorgang. Der objektive Nachweis dieser Minderleistung über dem 50. Lebensjahr kann daher zur Diagnosestellung nicht sicher verwendet werden. Nur wenn ein krasser Unterschied zur gleichen Altersgruppe vorhanden ist, kann man sich auf das Ergebnis stützen.

Vielfach läßt sich die Diagnose durch objektive Unterlagen nicht sichern, so daß man zu einem Behandlungsversuch mit Testosteron gezwungen ist. Man überzeuge sich vorher, daß keine Kontraindikationen gegen die Testosteronverabreichung bestehen, insbesondere muß durch eine rectale Untersuchung das Vorliegen von malignen Erkrankungen der Prostata ausgeschlossen werden. Auch Ödeme, kardiale Dekompensation, Hochdruck, schwere Arteriosklerose müssen Berücksichtigung finden.

Man gibt 25 mg Testosteronpropionat 4—5mal pro Woche für 2 Wochen. Tritt in dieser Zeit keine wesentliche Besserung ein, dann ist die Diagnose eines männlichen Klimakteriums praktisch ausgeschlossen. Auf der anderen Seite ist das Ansprechen auf die Behandlung nicht ohne weiteres für die Diagnose zu verwerten, da auch psychoneurotische Patienten auf Testosteron nicht ganz selten günstig reagieren. Bei ihnen ist jedoch die Wirkung meist nur eine vorübergehende, so daß ein bleibender Erfolg sehr für ein Klimakterium virile spricht.

Die Ergebnisse der Testosteronbehandlung werden von vielen als gut angegeben (WERNER 1939, HELLER u. MYERS 1944a, SCHATTMANN). Meine eigenen Erfahrungen sind nicht so günstig. Völliges Verschwinden der Symptome ist selten, Rezidive häufig, auch Behandlung mit Placebos kann einen Therapieerfolg erhalten. Hydrotherapeutische Maßnahmen leisten Wertvolles. Auch bei längerer Testosterontherapie braucht man nach den Beobachtungen von LESSER u. Mitarb. die Aktivierung eines möglichen Prostatacarcinoms nicht zu fürchten. Eine endgültige Beurteilung dieser Frage ist allerdings noch nicht möglich.

Literatur

ACHENBACH, W., u. W. ERNST: Beitrag zur Problematik des Klinefelter-Syndroms. Klin. Wschr. **35**, 380 (1957). — AITHEN, E. H., and J. R. K. PREEDY: The estimation of oestrone, oestradiol-17 β and oestriol in human urine by gradient elution partition chromatography. Biochem. J. **62**, 15 (1956). — ALBERT, A.: Human urinary gonadotropin. Recent Progr. Hormone Res. **12**, 227 (1956). — ALBERT, A., and J. DERNER: Studies on the biologic characterization of human gonadotropins. J. clin. Endocr. **20**, 859 (1960). — ALBERT, A., and S. KELLY: Studies on biologic characterization of human gonadotropins. J. clin. Endocr. **18**, 1067 (1958a). — ALBERT, A., S. KELLY, L. SILVER and J. KOBI: Extraction and purificaion of human pituitary gonadotropin. J. clin. Endocr. **18**, 6 (1958b). — ALBERT, A., J. KOBI, J. LEIFERMAN and J. DERNER: Purification of pituitary gonadotropin from urine of normal men. J. clin. Endocr. **21**, 1 (1961). — ALBERT, A., and E. ROSENBERG: Assay of human pituitary gonadotropin from male and postmenopausal urine. J. clin. Endocr. **19**, 127 (1959). — ALBERT, A., L. O. UNDERDAHL, L. F. GREENE and N. LORENZ: Male hypogonadism. I. The normal testis. Proc. Mayo Clin. **28**, 409 (1953). — ALBRIGHT, F.: The effect of hormones on osteogenesis in man. Recent Progr. Hormone Res. **1**, 293 (1947). — Zit. nach E. C. REIFENSTEIN, Steroid hormones and the aging sheleton. In: Hormone und Psyche, S. 172. Berlin-Göttingen-Heidelberg: Springer 1958. — ALBRIGHT, F., E. BLOOMBERG and P. H.

SMITH: Post-menopausal osteoporosis. Trans. Ass. Amer. Phycns 55, 289 (1940). — ALBRIGHT, F., A. M. BUTTLER, A. O. HAMPTON and P. SMITH: Syndrome characerized by osteitis fibrosa disseminata, areas of pigmentation and endocrine dysfunction with precocious puberty in females. New Engl. J. Med. 216, 727 (1937). — ALBRIGHT, F., W. PARSON and E. BLOOMBERG: Cushings's syndrome interpreted as hyperadrenocorticism leading to hypergluconeogenesis: Results of treatment with testosterone propionate. J. clin. Endocr. 1, 375 (1941). — ALBRIGHT, F., P. H. SMITH and R. FRASER: A syndrome characterized by primary ovarian insufficiency and decreased stature, a report of 11 cases with a digression on hormone control of axillary and pubic hair. Amer. J. med. Sci. 204, 625 (1942). — ALLEN, W. M.: Physiology of the corpus luteum. Amer. J. Physiol. 107, 207 (1934). — ALLEN, W. M., and O. WINTERSTEINER: Crystalline progestin. J. biol. Chem. 107, 321 (1934). — ALTMANN, F.: Über Eunuchoidimus. Virchows Arch. path. Anat. 276, 455 (1930). — ANDERS, J. G., A. PRADER, E. HANSCHTECK, K. SCHÄRER, R. E. SIEBENMANN u. R. HELLER: Multiples Sex-Chromatin und komplexes chromosomales Mosaik bei einem Knaben mit Idiotie und multiplen Mißbildungen. Helv. paediat. Acta 15, 515 (1960). — ANDERSEN, N. L.: The Lawrence-Moon-Biedl-syndrome: Case report with complete autopsy. J. clin. Endocr. 1, 905 (1941). — ANLIKER, R., O. ROHR u. M. MARTI: Über den Nachweis von Testosteron in einem virilisierenden Nebennierenrindentumor. Helv. chim. Acta 39, 1100 (1956). — APOSTOLAKIS, M., A. JOHN and D. LORAINE: Renal clearance of pituitary gonadotropins in postmenopausal woman. J. clin. Endocr. 20, 1437 (1960). — ASCHHEIM, S., u. B. ZONDEK: Hypophysenvorderlappenhormon und Ovarialhormon im Harn von Schwangeren. Klin. Wschr. 6, 1322 (1927). — ASCHNER, B.: Über die Beziehungen zwischen Hypophysis und Genitale. Arch. Gynäk. 97, 200 (1912). — ASLEV, J., u. H. REINWEIN: Über das familiäre Vorkommen des sogenannten Ullrich-Turner-Syndroms. Dtsch. med. Wschr. 1958, 601. — ASTWOOD, E. B.: The regulation of corpus luteum function by hypophyseal luteotrophin. Endocrinology 28, 309 (1941).
  BABINSKI, M. J.: Tumeur du corps pituitaire sans acromégalie et avec. Arret developement des organes genetiaux. Rev. neurol. 8, 531 (1900). — BAGG, H. J.: Factors involved in experimental productuion of teratoma testis in the fowl. Occasional publications of the Amer. Ann. Advanc. Sci. 4, 92 (1937). — BAGGETT, B., L. L. ENGEL, L. BALDERAS, G. LANMAN, K. SAVARD and J. DORFMAN: Conversion of C^{14}-testosterone to C^{14}-estrogenic steroids by endocrine tissues. Endocrinology 64, 600 (1959). — BAGGETT, B., L. L. ENGEL, K. SAVARD and R. J. DORFMAN: The conversion of testosterone-3-C^{14} to C^{14}-estradiol-17 β by human ovarian tissue. J. biol. Chem. 221, 931 (1956). — BAHN, R. C., N. LORENZ, W. A. BENNET and A. ALBERT: Gonadotropins of the pituitary gland and the urine of the adult human female. Endocrinology 52, 135 (1953). — Gonadotropins of the pituitary of postmenopausal woman. Endocrinology 53, 455 (1953). — BAHNER, F., u. G. SCHWARZ: Experimentelle Pubertas praecox bei Ratten durch Testosteron. Acta endocr. (Kbh.) 30, 574 (1959). — BAHNER, F., G. SCHWARZ, D. G. HARNDEN, P. A. JACOBS, H. A. HIENZ and K. WALTER: A fertile female with X0 sex chromosome constitution. Lancet 1960 II, 100. — BAILEY, P.: Die Funktion der Hypophysis cerebri. Ergebn. Physiol. 20, 162 (1922). — Die Hirngeschwülste. Stuttgart: Ferdinand Enke 1951. — BAILEY, P., and F. BREMER: Experimental diabetes insipidus and genital atrophy. Endocrinology 5, 761 (1921). — BALZE, F. A. DE LA: Puberal maturation of the normal human testis. A histologic study. J. clin. Endocr. 20, 266 (1960). — BALZE, F. A. DE LA, F. C. ARRILAGA, J. JRAZA and R. E. MANCINI: Klinefelter's syndrome: A study of 5 cases. J. clin. Endocr. 12, 1426 (1952). — BALZE, F. A. DE LA, G. E. BUR, SCARPA-SMITH and J. JRAZU: Elastic fibers in the tunica propria of normal and pathologic human testes. J. clin. Endocr. 14, 626 (1954a). — BALZE, F. A. DE LA, R. E. MANCINI, G. E. BUR and J. IRAZU: Morphologic and histochemical changes produced by estrogens on adult human testes. Fertil. and Steril. 5, 421 (1954b). — BANSI, H. W.: Neue Ziele der „Hormon"-Behandlung. Med. Klin. 14, 1 (1959). — BARDET, G.: Sur un syndrome d'obésité congénitale avec polydactylie et rétinite pigmentaire. Thèse de Paris (Le grand) 470, 107, 1920. — BARR, M. L.: In interim note on the application of the skin biopsy test of chromosomal sex to hermaphrodites. Surg. Gynec. Obstet. 99, 184 (1954). — Das Geschlechtschromatin. In: Die Intersexualität. Von C. OVERZIER, S. 50. Stuttgart: Georg Thieme 1961. — BARR, M. L., and E. G. BERTRAM: A morphological distinction between neurones of the male and female, and the behaviour of the nucleolar satellite during accelerated nucleoprotein synthesis. Nature (Lond.) 163, 676 (1949). — BARR, M. L., L. F. BERTRAM and H. A. LINDSAY: The morphology of the nerve cell nucleus, according to sex. Anat. Rec. 107, 283 (1950). — BARR, M. L., E. L. SHAVER, D. H. CARR and E. R. PLUNKETT: Males and females with two chromatin bodies in buccal mucosa cell nuclei. J. ment. bific. Res. 3, 78 (1959). — BARR, R. W., and S. C. SOMMERS: Quantitative study of effect of thyrotropin on thyroidal secretion rate in euthyroid and thyrotoxic subjects. J. clin. Endocr. 17, 1017 (1957). — BARTTER, F. C., F. ALBRIGHT, A. P. FORBES, A. LEAF, E. DEMPSEY and E. CARROLL: The effects of adrenocorticotropic hormone and cortisone in the adrenogenital syndrome associated with congenital adrenal hyperplasia: an attempt to explain and correct its disordered hormonal pattern. J. clin.

Invest. **30**, 237 (1951). — BARTTER, F. C., R. C. SNIFFEN, F. A. SIMMONS, F. ALBRIGHT and R. P. HOWARD: Effects of chorionic gonadotropin (APL) in male "eunuchoidism with low follicle stimulating hormone": aqueous solution versus oil and beeswax suspension. J. clin. Endocr. **12**, 1532 (1952). — BAUER, H. G.: Endocrine and other manifestations of hypothalamic disease. J. clin. Endocr. **14**, 13 (1954). — BAYLE, H.: Le traitement chirurgical des cryptorchidies. La Fonction Endocrine du Testicule, p. 453. Paris: Masson & Cie. 1957. — BEALL, D.: The isolation of α-oestradiol and oestrone from horse testes. Biochem. J. **34**, 1293 (1940). — BEER, C. T., and T. F. GALLAGHER: Excretion of estrogen metabolites by humans. I. The fate small doses of estrone and estradiol-17β. J. biol. Chem. **214**, 335 (1955). — BENDA, C. E., and E. M. BIXBY: Urinary excretion of 17-ketosteroide in various conditions of oligophrenia. J. clin. Endocr. **7**, 503 (1947). — BENOIT, J., and J. ASSENMACHER: The control by visible rediations of the gonadotropic activity of the duck hypophysis. Recent Progr. Hormone Res. **15**, 143 (1959). — BERBLINGER, W.: Pathologie und pathologische Morphologie der Hypophyse des Menschen. In Handbuch der inneren Sekretion von M. HIRSCH, Bd. 1, S. 910. Leipzig: Kabitzsch 1932. — Hypophysenveränderungen bei schweren Atrophien und Fibrosen der Hoden. Endokrinologie **14**, 73 (1934). — Ist die Pars tuberalis der Hypophyse gonadotorop wirksam? Endokrinologie **23**, 251 (1941). — Die Kastrationshypophyse des Menschen unter Sexualhormonbehandlung. Endokrinologie **25**, 16 (1942). — BERDINELLI, W.: Hermaphroditismus verus lateralis. Acta endocr. (Kbh.) **9**, 297 (1952). — BERGMANN, E.: Geschlechtschromatinbestimmungen am Neugeborenen. Schweiz. med. Wschr. **10**, 292 (1961). — BERTHOLD, A. A.: Transplantation der Hoden. Arch. Anat. Physiol. wiss. Med. **42** (1849). — BERTRONG, M., W. E. GOODWIN and W. W. SCOTT: Estrogen production by the testis. J. clin. Endocr. **9**, 579 (1949). — BIBEN, R. L., and G. S. GORDAN: Familial hypogonadotropic eunuchoidism. J. clin. Endocr. **15**, 931 (1955). — BIDDULPH, C.: The effect of testosterone propionate on gonadal development and gonadotropic hormone secretion in young male rats. Anat. Rec. **73**, 447 (1939). — BIEDL, A.: Ein Geschwisterpaar mit adipös-genitaler Dystrophie. Dtsch. med. Wschr. **48**, 1630 (1922. — BIERICH, J. R.: Hypophysärer Zwergwuchs bei Kindern. Medizinische **1957**, 1375. — BIGGART, J. H.: Hypophysis of human castrate. Bull. Johns Hopk. Hosp. **54**, 157 (1934). — BIRKE, G.: The 17-ketosteroid excretion in cirrhosis of the liver and epidemic hepatitis. Acta med. scand. Suppl. **53**, 285 (1953). — BIRKE, G., E. DICZFALUSY, C. FRANKSSON, J. HELLSTRÖM, S. HULTBERG, L. O. PLANTIN and A. WESTMAN: In A. R. CURRIE (Edit.), Endocrine aspects of breat cancer, p. 213. Edinburgh: Livingstone 1958. — BISKIND, G. R., and M. A. MEYER: Inactivation of estrone in normal male rabbits. Proc. Soc. exp. Biol. (N.Y.) **53**, 91 (1943). — BISHOP, P. H., D. P. v. MEURS, D. R. C. WILLCOX and D. ARNOLD: Interstitial-cell tumours of the testis in a child, report of a case and a review of the literature. Brit. med. J. **1960 I**, 238. — BLIVAISS, B. B., R. O. HANSON, R. E. ROSENZWEIG and H. KUTUZOW: Effects of progesterone on the induction of leydig-cell tumors with estrogen in strain a mice. J. clin. Endocr. **15**, 875 (1955). — BLOCH, E., R. J. DORFMAN and G. PINCUS: Conversion of acetate to C 19 steroids by human adrenal gland slices. J. biol. Chem. **224**, 737 (1957). — BOGDANOVE, E. M., and N. S. HALMI: Effects of hypothalamic lesions and subsequent propylthiouracil treatment of pituitary structure and function in the rat. Endocrinology **53**, 274 (1953). — BONGIOVANNI, A. M.: In vitro hydroxylation of steroids by whole adrenal homogenates of beef, normal man, and patients with the adrenogenital syndrome. J. clin. Invest. **37**, 1342 (1958). — BONGIOVANNI, A. M., and W. EBERLEIN: The renal clearance of neutral 17-ketosteroids in man. J. clin. Endocr. **17**, 238 (1957). — BONGIOVANNI, A. M., W. R. EBERLEIN, J. D. SMITH and A. J. McPADDEN: The urinary excretion of three C-21 methyl corticosteroids in the AGS. J. clin. Endocr. **19**, 1608 (1959). — BONNEVIE, K.: Embryological analysis of genemanifestation in little and bagg's abnormal mouse tribe. J. exp. Zool. **67**, 443 (1934). — Manifestierung des m^{bl}-Gens in der Entwicklung der Little- und Baggschen Blasenmäuse. In Handbuch der Erbbiologie des Menschen von G. JUST, Bd. 1, S. 127. Berlin: Springer 1940. — BONSER, G. M., and J. M. ROBSON: Effects of prolonged oestrogen administration upon male mice. J. Path. Bact. **51**, 9 (1940). — BORS, E., E. T. ENGLE, R. C. ROSENQUIST and V. H. HOLLIGER: Fertility in paraplegic males. J. clin. Endocr. **10**, 381 (1950). — BOTTOMLEY, A. C., and S. J. FOLLEY: The effect of androgenic substances on the growth of the teat and mammary gland in the immature male guinea-pig. Proc. roy. Soc. **126**, 224 (1938a). — The effect of high doses of androgenic substances on the weights of the testes accessory reproductive organs and endocrine glands of young male guineapigs. J. Physiol. (Lond.) **94**, 26 (1938b). — BOUIN, M. M. P., et P. ANCEL: Sur les cellules interstitielles du testicule des mammifères et leur signification. C.R. Soc. Biol. (Paris) **55**, 1397 (1903). — BRADBURY, J. T., W. E. BROWN and L. A. GRAY: Maintenance of corpus luteum and physiologic actions of progesterone. Recent Progr. Hormone Res. **5**, 151 (1950). — BRADBURY, J. T., R. G. JUNGE and R. A. BOCCABELLA: Chromatin test in Klinefelter's syndrome. J. clin. Endocr. **16**, 689 (1956). — BRADLOW, H. L., and T. F. GALLAGHER: Metabolism of 11β-hydroxy-Δ4-androstene-3,17-dione in congenital adrenal hyperplasia. J. clin. Endocr. **19**, 12, 1575 (1959). — BRADY, R. O.:

Biosynthesis of radioactive testosterone in vitro. J. biol. Chem. **193**, 145 (1951). — BREIT, A., u. A. HIRSCHAUER: Röntgenbestrahlung des Hypophysentumors durch Pendeltechnik. Strahlentherapie **98**, 398 (1955). — BREUEMAN, W. R.: The effect of gonadal hormones alone and in combination with pregnant mare serum on the pituitary, gonad, and comb of white leghorn cockerles. Anat. Rec. **117**, 533 (1953). — BREUER, H., W. NOCHE and J. M. BAYER: Effect of ACTH and cortisone on the urinary oestrogens in oophorectomized and postmenopausal women with mammary mized and postmenopausal woman with mammary cancer. Acta endocr. (Kbh.) Suppl. **38**, 69 (1958). — BRIMBLECOMBE, S. L.: Bilateral cryptorchidism in three brothers. Brit. med. J. **1946 I**, 526. — BRINCK-JOHNSEN, T., and K. EIK-NES: Effect of human chronic gonadotropin on the secretion of testosterone and 4-androstene-3,17-dione by the canine testis. Endocrinology **61**, 676 (1957). — BRISSAUD, E.: L'infantilisme vrai. Nouv. Iconogr. Salpèt. **20**, 1 (1907). — BROOKHART, J. M., F. L. DEY and S. W. RANSON: The abolition of mating behavior by hypothalamic lesions in guinea pigs. Endocrinology **28**, 561 (1941). — BROUWER, K.: Het syndrom van Werner. Ned. T. Geneesk. **1955**, 2056. — BROWN, J. B.: A chemical method for the determination of oestriol, oestrone and oestradiol in human urine. Biochem. J. **60**, 185 (1955). — The relationship between urinary oestrogens and oestrogens produced in the body. Lancet **1956 I**, 704. — BROWN, W. E., J. T. BRADBURY and E. JUNGCK: The effect of estrogens and other steroids on the pituitary gonadotrophins in woman. Amer. J. Obstet. Gynec. **65**, 733 (1953). — BRUM, N., A. LAGUARDIA and F. A. SAEZ: A study on sex chromatin. Texas Rep. Biol. Med. **17**, 73 (1959). — BUCHHOLZ, R.: Untersuchungen über die Beeinflussung der Gonadotropinausscheidung beim Menschen durch Keimdrüsenhormone. Geburtsh. u. Frauenheilk. **19**, 851 (1959). — BÜRGI, H., u. CH. HEDINGER: Histologische Hodenveränderungen im hohen Alter. Schweiz. med. Wschr. **47**, 1236 (1959). — BULBROOK, R. D., F. C. GREENWOOD, G. J. HADFIELD and E. F. SCOWEN: Adrenalectomy in breast cancer. Brit. med. J. **11**, 12 (1958a). — BULBROOK, R. D., and P. C. WILLIAMS: In A. R. CURRIE (Edit.), Endocrine aspects of breat cancer, p. 181. Edinburgh: Livingstone 1958b. — BUNGE, R. G., and J. T. BRADBURY: Genetic sex: chromatin test versus gonadal histology. J. clin. Endocr. **16**, 1117 (1956). — BURROWS, H.: Biological actions of sex hormones. New York: Univ. Press. Cambridge University Press 1945. — Biological action of sex hormones. London: Cambridge University Press 1949. — BURT, A. S., L. REINER, R. B. COHEN and R. C. SNIFFEN: Klinefelter's syndrome: report of an autopsy, with particular reference to the histology and histochemistry of the endocrine glands. J. clin. Endocr. **14**, 719 (1954). — BUSTAMENTE, M., H. SPATZ u. E. WEISSCHEDEL: Die Bedeutung des Tuber cinereum des Zwischenhirns für das Zustandekommen der Geschlechtsreifung. Dtsch. med. Wschr. **1942**, 289. — BUTENANDT, A.: Über „Progynon", ein kristallisiertes weibliches Sexualhormon. Naturwissenschaften **17**, 879 (1929). — Über die chemische Untersuchung der Sexualhormone. Z. angew. Chem. **44**, 905 (1931). — BUTENANDT, A., u. H. DANNENBAUM: Isolierung eines neuen physiologisch unwirksamen Sterinderivates am Männerharn, seine Verknüpfung mit Dehydroandrosteron und Androsteron. Hoppe-Seylers Z. physiol. Chem. **229**, 192 (1934a). — BUTENANDT, A., u. H. KUDZUS: Über Androstendion, einen hochwirksamen männlichen Prägnenstoff. Hoppe-Seylers Z. physiol. Chem. **237**, 75 (1935). — BUTENANDT, A., U. WESTPHAL u. H. COBLER: Über einen Abbau des Stigmasterins zu corpusluteumwirksamen Stoffen, ein Beitrag zur Konstitution des Corpus luteum-Hormons. Ber. dtsch. Ges. inn. Med. **67**, 1611, 2085 (1934b). — BUTLER, G. C., and G. F. MARRIAN: The isolation of pregnane-3,17, 20-triol from the urine of women showing the AGS. J. biol. Chem. **119**, 565 (1937). — BUTLER, A. M., N. B. TALBOT, MAC LACHLAN, J. E. APPLETON and M. A. LINTON: Effect of testosterone propionate on losses incident to inadequate dietary intake. J. clin. Endocr. **5**, 327 (1945). — BUTT, W. R.: Studies on urinary gonadotrophins after fractionation by tricalcium phosphate. J. Endocr. **13**, 167 (1956). — BYRNES, W. W., and R. K. MEYER: The inhibition of gonadotrophic hormone secretion by physiological doses of estrogen. Endocrinology **48**, 133 (1951).

CAHILL, G. F., and J. N. ROBINSON: Androgenic symptom tumors of the adrenal cortex in children: a report of four cases. J. Urol. (Baltimore) **61**, 680 (1949). — CAHILL, G. F., M. M. MELICOW and H. H. DARBY: Adrenal cortical tumors. Surg. Gynec. Obstet. **74**, 281 (1942). — CALLOW, N. H., R. K. CALLOW and C. W. EMMENS: Colorimetric determination of substances containing the grouping —CH$_2 \cdot$CO— in urine extracts as an indication of androgen content. Biochem. J. **32**, 1312 (1938). — 17-ketosteroid, androgen and oestrogen excretion in urine of cases of gonadal or adrenal cortical deficiency. J. Endocr. **2**, 88 (1940). — CAMUS, J., et G. C. R. ROUSSY: Hypophysectomie et polyurie experiméntales. C. R. Soc. Biol. (Paris) **75**, 483 (1913). — CAROLL, W. A.: Malignancy in cryptorchism. J. Urol. (Baltimore) **61**, 396 (1949). — CARTER, A. C., E. J. COHEN and E. SHORR: Androgens in woman. Vitam. and Horm. **5**, 317 (1947). — CASTILLO, E. B. DEL, et J. ARGONZ: Syndrome de l'ovaire rudimentaire. Ann. Endocr. (Paris) **12**, 121 (1951). — CASTILLO, E. B. DEL, et A. PINTO: Action de l'œstrone et de la testosterone sur l'appareil genital masculin. C. R. Soc. Biol (Paris) **129**, 868 (1938). — CASTILLO, E. B. DEL, and A. TRABUCCO: A syndrome of testicular insufficiency characterized by the complete absence of leydig cells disturbance of germinal epithelium and decreased urinary gonadotrophins. Acta endocr. (Kbh.) 12, 8 (1953). — CASTILLO, E. B. DEL, A. TRABUCCO and F. A. DE LA BALZE: Syndrome produced by absence of the germinal epithelium without impairment of the sertoli or leydig cells. J. clin. Endocr. 7, 493 (1947). — CASTILLO, E. G. DEL, and J. ARGONZ: Syndrome of rudimentary gonad. Acta endocr. (Kbh.) 24, 379 (1957). — CATCHPOLE, H. R., and W. W. GREULICH: Excretion of gonadotropic hormone by prepuberal and adolescent girls. Amer. J. Physiol. 129, 331 (1940). — CATCHPOLE, H. R., W. W. GREULICH and R. T. SOLLEN-BERGER: Urinary excretion of follicle stimulating hormone in young and adolescent boys. Amer. J. Physiol. 123, 32 (1938). — CATCHPOLE, H. R., and J. B. HAMILTON: Suppression of pituitary gonadotropic function by testosterone propionate. Amer. J. Physiol. 126, 459 (1939). — CATCHPOLE, H. R., J. B. HAMILTON and G. R. HUBERT: Effect of male hormone therapy on urinary gonadotropins in man. J. clin. Endocr. 2, 181 (1942). — CENDRON, J., P. CANLORBE, P. BORNICHE et J. PUJOL: Les cryptorchidies. In: La Fonction Endocrine du Testicule, p. 295. Paris: Masson & Cie. 1957. — CERENEA, R.: Zur Hormonbehandlung des Kryptorchismus. Hippokrates (Stuttgart) 22, 241 (1951). — CHANG, E., and T. L. DAO: Vortrag Amer. Endocrin. Ges., Atlantic City, 1959. — CHARNY, C. W.: Testicular biopsy. J. Amer. med. Ass. 115, 1429 (1940). — Equine gonadotropin in male infertility. Amer. J. med. Sci. 207, 519 (1944). — Treatment of male infertility with large doses of testosterone. J. Amer. med. Ass. 160, 98 (1956a). — In W. WOLGIN, Cryptorchidism. London: Cassell & Co. Ltd. 1957b. — Anomalies du développement morphologique du testicule dans la puberté et la pré-puberté. In: La Fonction Endocrine du Testicule, p. 439. Paris: Masson & Cie. 1957c. — The use of androgens for human spermatogenesis. Fertil. and Steril. 10, 557 (1959). — CHARNY, C. W., and D. R. MERANZE: Testicular biopsy. Surg. Gynec. Obstet. 74, 836 (1942). — CHARNY, C. W., and W. WOLGIN: The management of cryptorchism. Surg. Gynec. Obstet. 102, 177 (1956b). — Cryptorchism. New York: Paul B. Hoeber 1957a. — CHU, E. H. Y., and N. H. GILES: Human chromosome complements in normal somatic cells in culture. Amer. J. human. Genet. 11, 63 (1959). — CLARA, M.: Untersuchungen an Hodenzwischenzellen bei einigen Haussäugetieren. Z. mikr.-anat. Forsch. 20, 51 (1930). — CLARINGBOLD, P. J., and L. MARTIN: The mitogenic action of oestrogens in the vaginal epithelium of the ovariectomized mouse. J. Endocr. 20, 173 (1960). — CLAUBERG, C.: Der biologische Test für das Corpus luteum-Hormon. Klin. Wschr. 1930 II, 2004. — COLBY, F. H.: Essential urology. Baltimore: Williams & Wilkins Company 1950. — COLE, H., and G. HART: The potency of blood serum of mavrs in progressive stages of pregnancy in effecting the sexual maturity of the immature rat. Amer. J. Physiol. 93, 57 (1930). — COLLIP, J. B., H. PELYE and D. THOMSON: Gonad-stimulating hormones in hypophysectomized animals. Nature (Lond.) 131, 56 (1933). — Committee on Clinical Endocrinology: Proposed standard method of 17-ketosteroid determination. Lancet 1951 II, 585. — CONRAD, K.: Der Konstitutionstypus als genetisches Problem. Berlin: Springer 1941. — CONTI, C., V. MARESCOTTI e A. FABRINI: Ipogonadismo leydigiano postpuberale. Folia endocr. (Pisa) 141, 164 (1952). — COOK, C. D., R. E. GROSS, B. H. LANDING and A. S. ZYGMUNTOWICZ: Interstitial cell tumor of the testis. J. clin. Endocr. 12, 725 (1952). — COPPEDGE, R. L., and A. SEGALOFF: Urinary prolactin excretion in man. J. clin. Endocr. 11, 465 (1951). — COREY, E. L.: The effect of cortico-adrenal extract injection on the estrons cycle of the rat. Amer. J. Physiol. 105, 24 (1933). — Comparative effects of progesterone and corticoadrenal extracts on normal, adrenalectomized and other animals. Amer. J. Physiol. 132, 446 (1941). — COREY, E. L., and S. W. BRITTON: The ovarion cycle and the adrenal glands. Amer. J. Physiol. 107, 207 (1934). — COX, R. I., and M. FINKELSTEIN: Pregnane-3α,17α,20α-triol and pregnane-3α,17α,20α-triol-11-one excretion by patients with adrenocortical dysfunction. J. clin. Invest. 36, 1726 (1957). — COTTMAN, J. R., and F. C. KOCH: The effect of testosterone propionate on induced creatinuria in rats. J. biol. Chem. 135, 519 (1940). — COUSELLER, V. S., and M. A. WALKER: Congenital absence of testes (anorchia). Ann. Surg. 98, 104 (1933). — COURRIER, R., et G. GROS: Action de la folliculine chez le singe male impubère, modification des annexes. C. R. Soc. Biol. (Paris) 118, 686 (1935). — COURT-BROWN, W. M., P. A. JACOBS and R. DOLL: Interpretation of chromosome counts made on bone-marrow cells. Lancet 1960 I, 160. — CURRIE, A. R., and J. B. DEKANSKI: Gonadotrophins and prolactin in human pituitary glands. Acta endocr. (Kbh.) 36, 185 (1961).

DALGAARD, J. B., and F. HESSELBERG: Interstitial cell tumors of the testis. Acta path. microbiol. scand. 41, 219 (1957). — DANON, M., and L. SACHS: Sex chromosomes and human sexual development. Lancet 1957 II, 20. — DAVID, K., E. DINGEMANSE, J. FREUD u. E. LAQUEUR: Über krystallinisches männliches Hormon aus Hoden (Testosteron), wirksamer als aus Harn oder aus Cholesterin bereitetes Androsteron. Hoppe-Seylers Z. physiol. Chem. 233, 281 (1935). — DAVID, K., J. FREUD and S. E. DE JOUGH: Conditions of hypertrophy of seminal vesicles in rats. Biochem. J. 28, 1360 (1934). — DAVIDSON, R., P. KOETS, W. G. SNOW and L. G. GABRIELSON: Excretion of 17-ketosteroids in ankylosing spondylarthritis and in rheumatoid arthritis. A preliminary report. J. clin. Endocr. 7, 201 (1947). — DAVIDSON,

W. M., and D. R. Smith: A morphological sex difference in the polymorphonuclear neutrophil leucocytes. Brit. med. J. 1954 II, 6. — Davidson, W. M.: Inherited variations in leucocytes. Brit. med. Bull. 17, 3 (1961). — Deanesly, R.: Adrenal cortex differences in male and female mice. Nature (Lond.) 141, 79 (1938). — Deanesly, R., and A. S. Parkes: Oestrogenic action of compounds of the androsterone testosterone series. Brit. med. J. 1936 I, 257. — Decker, K., u. H. Lauter: Behandlungsergebnisse bei Hypophysengeschwülsten. Dtsch. med. Wschr. 12, 468 (1960). — Decomt, L., W. de Sasso, E. Chiorboli e J. M. Fernandes: Sobre o sexo genetico nas pacients con sindrome de Turner. Rev. Ass. méd. bras. 1, 203 (1954). — Deming, C. L.: The evaluation of hormonal therapy in cryptorchidism. J. Urol. (Baltimore) 68, 354 (1952). — Deulofeu, V., u. J. Ferrari: Krystallisiertes α-Follikelhormon aus Hengstharn. Hoppe-Seylers Z. physiol. Chem. 226, 192 (1934). — Dey, F. L.: Evidence of hypothalamic control of hypophyseal gonadotropic functions in the female guinea pigs. Endocrinology 33, 75 (1943). — Failure to induce ovulation in constant estrons guinea pigs. Proc. Soc. exp. Biol. (N.Y.) 52, 312 (1943). — Dey, F. L., C. R. Leininger and S. W. Ranson: Effect of hypophysial lesion on mating behavior in female guinea pig. Endocrinology 30, 232 (1942). — Diczfalusy, E.: Chorionic gonadotrophin and oestrogens in the human placenta. Acta endocr. (Kbh.) Suppl. 12, XII (1953). — Characterization of the oestrogens in human semen. Acta endocr. (Kbh.) 15, 317 (1954). — Diczfalusy, E. G. Birke, C. Franksson, J. Hellström, S. Hultberg, L. O. Plantin and A. Westman: In A. R. Currie (Edit.), Endocrine aspects of breast cancer, p. 186. Edinburgh: Livingstone 1958. — Diczfalusy, E., and O. Cassmer: Urinary 17-ketosteroids following administration of long-acting testosterone esters. J. clin. Endocr. 21, 271 (1961 b). — Diczfalusy, E., u. Ch. Lauritzen: Oestrogene beim Menschen, S. 78. Berlin-Göttingen-Heidelberg: Springer 1961. — Diczfalusy, E., K. G. Tillinger and A. Westman: Studies on oestrogen metabolism in new-born boys. Acta endocr. (Kbh.) 26, 303 (1957). — Diczfalusy, E., and A. Westman: Urinary excretion of natural oestrogens in oophorectomized woman treated with polyoestradiol phosphate (PEP). Acta endocr. (Kbh.) 21, 321 (1956). — Diepen, K.: Vergleichende anatomische Untersuchungen über das Hypophysen-Hypothalamus-System bei Amphibien und Reptilien. Verh. Anat. Ges. (50. Tagg) S. 79, 1952. — Dingemanse, E., H. Borchart and E. Laqueur: Capon comb growth-promoting substances ("male hormones") in human urine of males and females of varying ages. Biochem. J. 31, 500 (1937). — Dingemanse, E., Huisin't Veld and B. M. de Laat: Clinical method for the chromatographic colorimetric determination of urinary 17-ketosteroids. J. clin. Endocr. 6, 535 (1946). — Dirscherl, W., u. U. Dardenne: Spaltung von Seroidhormonestern durch menschliche und tierische Organe. Biochem. Z. 325, 195 (1954). — Dixon, F. J., and R. A. Moore: Tumors of the male sex organs. In: Atlas of Tumor Pathology, Sect. VIII, Fasc. 32, p. 48. 1952. — Dörner, G., u. W. Hohlweg: Über den „Overproduktion-Effekt" des Hodens nach Abbruch einer längeren Gonadotropinbehandlung. Endokrinologie 36, 40 (1958). — Doisy, E. A., C. D. Veler and S. A. Thayer: Folliculin from urine of pregnant women. Amer. J. Physiol. 90, 329 (1929). — Domm, L. V.: Observations concerning anterior pituitary-gonadal interrelations in the fowl. Cold Spr. Harb. Symp. quant. Biol. 5, 241 (1937). — Dorbriner, K., S. Lieberman and C. P. Rhoads: Studies in steroid metabolism. J. biol. Chem. 172, 241 (1948). — Dorff, G. B.: Rapid growth in height produced by chorionic gonadotrophin in dwarfed infantile identical twins. J. clin. Endocr. 1, 940 (1941). — Dorfman, R. I., and J. B. Hamilton: The urinary excretion of estrogenic substances after the administration of testosterone propionate. Endocrinology 25, 33 (1939). — Dorfman, R. J.: Biochemistry of androgens. In: The Hormons, edit. by G. Pincus and K. V. Thimann. New York: Academic Press Inc. 1948. — Comments on the metabolism of steroid hormones. Cancer Res. 17, 535 (1957). — Metabolism of androgens. Proc. fourth intern. Congr. Biochemistry, Vienna 1958, vol. IV, p. 175. — Dorfman, R. J., and R. H. Shipley: Androgens, biochemistry, physiology and clinical significance. New York: John Wiley & Sons 1956. — Drehter, J. J., S. Pearson, E. Bartczak and T. H. Mc Gavack: A rapid method for the determination of total urinary 17-ketosteroids. J. clin. Endocr. 7, 795 (1947). — Driggs, M., u. H. Spatz: Pubertas praecox bei einer hyperplastischen Mißbildung des Tuber cinereum. Virchows Arch. path. Anat. 305, 567 (1939). — Dubois, K. P., K. W. Cochran and M. M. Zerwig: Influence of sex hormones on citrate synthesis in liver. Proc. Soc. exp. Biol. (N.Y.) 78, 452 (1951). — Dyke, D. C. van, M. E. Simpson, C. H. Li and H. M. Evans: Suroival in the circulation of the growth and adrenocorticotrophic hormones as evidenced by parabiosis. Amer. J. Physiol. 163, 297 (1950a). — Dyke, H. B. van, B. F. Chow, R. O. Greep and A. Rothen: The isolation of a protein from the pars neutralis of the ox pituitary with constant oxytocic, pressor and diuresis inhibiting activities. J. Pharmacol. exp. Ther. 74, 190 (1942). — Dyke, H. B. van, and T. Shedlovsky: Follicle stimulating hormones of the anterior pituitary of the sheep and the hog. Endocrinology 46, 563 (1950b).
       Eberlein, W. R., and A. M. Bongiocanni: Plasma and urinary corticosteroids in the hypertensive form of congenital adrenal hyperplasia. J. biol. Chem. 223, 85 (1956). —

Steroid metabolism in the "salt-losing" form of congenital adrenal hyperplasia. J. clin. Invest. **37**, 889 (1958). — Eik-Nes, K. B., G. W. Oertel, R. Nimer and F. H. Tyler: Effect of human chorionic gonadotropin on plasma concentrations of 17-hydroxycortico-steroids, dehydroepiandrosterone and androsterone in man. J. clin. Endocr. **19**, 1405 (1959). — Elert, R.: Direkte und indirekte Oestrogenwirkung auf die männliche Keimdrüse. In: Fünftes Sympos. Dtsch. Ges. Endokrin. März 1957 v. H. Nowakowski, S. 328. Berlin-Göttingen-Heidelberg: Springer 1958. — Emmens, C. W., and R. J. Cox: Dimethylstilb-oestrol as an oestrogen inhibitor. J. Endocr. **17**, 265 (1958). — Emmens, C. W., R. J. Cox and L. Martin: Oestrogeninhibitors of the stilboestrol series. J. Endocr. **18**, 372 (1959). — Oestrogeninhibition by steroids and other substances. J. Endocr. **20**, 198 (1960). — Engberg, H.: Testis endocrine funktion ved kryptorchisme. Kopenhagen: E. Munksgaard 1948. — Investigations on the endocrine function of the testicle in cryptorchidism. Proc. roy. Soc. Med. **42**, 652 (1949). — Engbring, N. H., and W. W. Engstrom: Effects of estrogen and testosterone on circulating thyroid hormone. J. clin. Endocr. **19**, 783 (1959). — Engel, L. L., R. I. Dorfman and A. R. Abarbanel: Neutral steroids in urine of patient with ovarian eutcoma, of ovary. J. clin. Endocr. **13**, 903 (1953). — Engle, E. T.: Effect of daily transplants of anterior lobe from gonadectomized rats on immature test animals. Amer. J. Physiol. **88**, 101 (1929). — Experimentally induced descent of the testis in the macacus monkey by hormones from the anterior pituitary and pregnancy urine. Endocrinology **16**, 513 (1932). — Sex and internal secretion. p. 1003. Baltimore: Williams & Wilkins Company 1939. — Testis biopsy in infertility. J. Urol. (Baltimore) **57**, 789 (1947). — Atypical cytology in testis biopsies. J. Urol. (Baltimore) **62**, 694 (1949). — Endocrine aspects of infertility in the male. In: Progr. Clin. Endocrinology, edit. by S. Soskin. New York: Grune & Stratton 1950. — Cowdry's problems of ageing (Lansing, ed.), p. 708. Baltimore: Williams & Wilkins Company 1952. — Erdheim, J. S.: Über Hypophysengangsgeschwülste und Hirnchole-steatome. Akad. Wiss. Wien, Abt. III **113**, 537 (1904). — Evans, H. M., u. M. E. Simpson: A comparison of anterior hypophyseal implants from normal and gonadectomized animals with reference to their capacity of stimulate the immature ovary. Amer. J. Physiol. **89**, 371 (1929). — Physiology of the gonadotropins, chap. VI, in: The hormones. II. (G. Pincus and K. V. Thiman). New York: Acad. Press 1950. — Evans, H. M., M. E. Simpson and R. I. Pencharz: Detection of mammotropin in the urine of lactating women. Proc. Soc. exp. Biol. (N.Y.) **32**, 1048 (1935). — Evans, T. N., and G. M. Riley: Pseudohermaphroditism, a clinical problem. Obstet. and Gynec. **2**, 363 (1953). — Everett, J. W.: Luteotrophic function of autografts of the rat hypophysis. Endocrinology **54**, 685 (1954). — The time of release of ovulating hormone from the rat hypophysis. Endocrinology **58**, 580 (1956).

Federman, D. D., J. Robbins and J. E. Rall: Effects of methyltestosterone on thyroid function, thyroxine metabolism, and thyroxinebinding protein. J. clin. Invest. **37**, 1024 (1958). — Feldman, E. B., and A. C. Carter: Endocrinologic and metabolic effects of 17α-methyl-19-nortestosterone in women. J. clin. Endocr. **20**, 843 (1960). — Ferguson-Smith, M. A.: Chromatin-positive Klinefelter's syndrome (primary microorchidism). Lancet **1958 I**, 928. — The prepuberal testicular lesion in chromatin-positive Klinefelter's syndrome (primary micro-orchidism) as seen in mentally handicapped children. Lancet **1959 I**, 219. — Ferguson-Smith, M. A., and A. W. Johnston: Chromosome abnormalities in certain diseases of man. Ann. intern. Med. **53**, 359 (1960a). — Ferguson-Smith, M. A., A. W. Johnston and S. D. Handmaker: Primary amentia and microorchidism associated with an XXXXY sexchromo-some constitution. Lancet **1960 II b**, 184. — Ferguson-Smith, M. A., B. Lennox, W. S. Malk and J. S. S. Stewart: Klinefelter's syndrome: frequency and testicular morphology in relation to nuclear sex. Lancet **1957 II**, 167. — Fevold, H. L., F. L. Hisaw, A. Hellbaum and R. Hertz: The gonad stimulating and the luteinizing humanes on the anterior lab of the hypophysis. Amer. J. Physiol. **97**, 291 (1931). — Finerty, J. C.: Parabiosis in physiological studies. Physiol. Rev. **32**, 277 (1952). — Finkelstein, M., and S. S. Goldzieher: A test for qualitative and quantitative estimation of pregnane-3α, 17α, 20α-triol-11-one in urine and its significance in adrenal disturbances. J. clin. Endocr. **17**, 1063 (1957). — Finkelstein, M., and J. Schoenberger: Urinary steroids in 10 cases of adrenal carcinoma, with special reference to pregnane-3α, 17α, 20α-triol-11-one. J. clin. Endocr. **19**, 608 (1959). — Flavell, G.: Webbing of the neck, with Turner's syndrome in the male. Brit. J. Surg. **31**, 150 (1943). — Forbes, A. P.: La deuxième hormone testiculaire. La fonction endocrine du testicule, p. 109. Paris: Masson & Cie. 1957. — Ford, C. E.: Human cytogenetics: its present place and future possibilities. Amer. J. hum. Genet. **12**, 104 (1960). — Die Zytogenese der Inter-sexualität des Menschen. In: Die Intersexualität. Von C. Overzier, S. 90. Stuttgart: Georg Thieme 1961. — Human cytogenetics. Brit. med. Bull. **17**, 3 (1961). — Ford, C. E., K. W. Jones, O. J. Miller, U. Mittwoch, L. S. Penrose, M. Ridler and A. Shapiro: The chromosomes in a patient showing both mongolism and the Klinefelter syndrome. Lancet **1959 I b**, 709. — Ford, C. E., K. W. Jones, P. E. Polani, J. C. de Almeida and J. H. Briggs: A sex-chromosome anomaly in a case of gonadal dysgenesis (Turner's syndrome).

Lancet **1959** I c, 711. — FORD, C. E., P. E. POLANI, J. H. BRIGGS and P. M. F. BISHOP: A presumptive human XXY/XX mosaic. Nature (Lond.) **183**, 1030 (1959a). — FORDYCE A. D., and W. H. EVANS: Suprarenal virilism. Quart. J. Med. **22**, 557 (1929). — Foss, G. L., and L. SIMPSON: Oral methyltestosterone and jaundice. Brit. med. J. **1959** II, 259. — FOTHER-BY, K.: The isolation of 3β-hydroxy-Δ5-steroids from the urine of normal men. Biochem. J. **69**, 596 (1958). — FRACCARO, M., C. A. GEMZELL and J. LINDSTEN: Plasma level of growth hormone and chromosome complement in four patients with gonadal dysgenesis (Turner's syndrome). Acta endocr. (Kbh.) **34**, 496 (1960a). — FRACCARO, M., D. JKKOS, J. LINDSTEN, R. LUFT and K. G. TILLINGER: Testicular germinal dysgenesis (male Turner's syndrome). Acta endocr. (Kbh.) **36**, 98 (1961). — FRACCARO, M., K. KAIJSER and J. LINDSTEN: A child with 49 chromosomes. Lancet **1960** II b, 890. — The chromosomes of man. Lancet **1959** I, 886. — FRACCARO, M., and J. LINDSTEN: A child with 49 chromosomes. Lancet **1960** II c, 1303. — FRÄNKEL, L., u. E. FELS: Neue Beobachtungen über Wirkung und Wert der Sexualhormonpräparate. Dtsch. med. Wschr. **2**, 2156 (1927). — FRANCKE, C.: The gonads in the Laurence-Moon-Biedl-Syndrome. J. Urol. (Baltimore) **57**, 427 (1947). — The gonads in the Laurence-Moon-Biedl-Syndrome. J. clin. Endocr. **10**, 108 (1950). — FRANK, R. T.: A suggested test for functional cortical adrenal tumor. Proc. Soc. exp. Biol. (N.Y.) **31**, 1204 (1933). — FRANK, R. T., M. L. FRANK, R. G. GUSTAVSON and W. W. WEYERTS: Demonstration of the female sex hormone in the circulating blood. J. Amer. med. Ass. **85**, 510 (1925). — FRANK, R. T., and U. J. SALMON: Effect of administration of estrogenic factor upon hypophyseal hyperactivity in the menopause. Proc. Soc. exp. Biol. (N.Y.) **33**, 311 (1935). — FRASER, R. W., A. P. FORBES, A. ALBRIGHT, H. SULKOWITCH and E. C. REIFENSTEIN: Colorimetric assay of 17-ketosteroids in urine. J. clin. Endocr. **1**, 234 (1941). — FRIEDEMAN, N. B., and R. A. MOORE: Tumors of testis: Milit. Surg. **99**, 573 (1946). — FRIEDGOOD, H. B., and A. D. DAWSON: Physiological significance and morphology of the carmine cell in the cat's anterior pituitary. Endocrinology **26**, 1022 (1940). — FRÖHLICH, A.: Ein Fall von Tumor der Hypophysis cerebri ohne Akromegalie. Wien. klin. Rdschr. **15**, 883 (1901). — FUKUSHIMA, D. K., H. L. BRADLOW, L. HELLMAN and T. F. GALLAGHER: Further studies of 21-deoxyhydrocortisone-4-C¹⁴ in man. J. clin. Endocr. **19**, 393 (1959). — FUKUSHIMA, D. K., and T. F. GALLAGHER: Steroid isolation studies in congenital adrenal hyperplasia. J. biol. Chem. **229**, 85 (1957).

GALLAGHER, T. F.: On alterations in adrenal function, especially with adrenocortical carcinoma. Cancer Res. **17**, 520 (1957b). — Experimental studies of adrenal hyperfunction in man. Proc. fourth intern. Congr. Biochemistry, Vienna 1958, vol. IV, p. 143. — GALLAGHER, T. F., L. BRADLOW, D. K. FUKUSHIMA and CH. T. BEER: Studies of the metabolites of isotopic steroid hormones in man. Recent Progr. Hormone Res. **9**, 411 (1954). — GALLAGHER, T. F., and D. K. FUKUSHIMA: Steroid isolation studies in congenital adrenal hyperplasia. J. biol. Chem. **229**, 85 (1957a). — GALLAGHER, T. F., D. H. PETERSON, R. I. DORFMAN, A. T. KENYON and F. C. KOCH: Daily urinary excretion of estrogenic and androgenic substances by normal men and woman. J. clin. Invest. **16**, 695 (1937). — GANS, E.: The ICSH-content of serum of intact and gonadectomized rats and of rats treated with sex hormones. Acta endocr. (Kbh.) **32**, 373 (1953). — The FSH-content of serum of intact and of gonadectomized rats and of rats treated with sex hormones. Acta endocr. (Kbh.) **32**, 363 (1959). — GARDINER-HILL, H., and J. S. RICHARDSON: Macrogenitosomia praecox in one of twin boys without demonstrable pathological lesion. StThom. Hosp. Rep. **4**, 35 (1939). — GARDNER, W. U.: Hypertrophy of interstitial cells in the testes of mice receiving estrogenic hormones. Anat. Rec. **68**, 339 (1937). — Studies on steroid hormones in experimental carcinogenesie. Recent Progr. Hormone Res. **1** (1947). — GAUPP, G. R.: Die histologischen Befunde und bisherigen Erfahrungen über die Zwischenhirnsekretion des Menschen. Z. ges. Neurol. Psychiat. **154**, 314 (1935). — GEMZELL, C. A.: Demonstration of growth hormone in human plasma. J. clin. Endocr. **19**, 1049 (1959). — GEMZELL, C. A., E. DICZFALUSY and G. TILLINGER: Clinical effect of human pituitary follicle-stimulating hormone (FSH). J. clin. Endocr. **18**, 1333 (1958). — GEMZELL, C. A., and G. NOTTER: Effects of androgens on plasma levels of 17-hydroxycorticosteroids. J. clin. Endocr. **16**, 483 (1956). — GERMAN, E., H. HOROWITZ, R. W. VANDE, and R. M. TORACK: Leydig-cell tumor of the ovary: case report and review. J. clin. Endocr. **21**, 91 (1961). — GILBERT, J. B.: Studies in malignant testis tumors. J. Urol. (Baltimore) **46**, 740 (1941). — GILBERT, J. B., and J. B. HAMILTON: Studies in malignant testis tumors, incidence and nature of tumors in ectopic testes. Surg. Gynec. Obstet. **71**, 731 (1940). — Incidence and nature of tumors in ectopic testes. Surg. Gynec. Obstet. **70**, 731 (1940). — GILBERT-DREYFUS, J., C. SAVOIE et J. SEBAOUN: Les impubérismes gonadiques et gonadotrophiques. In: La fonction endocrine du testicule, S. 335. Paris: Masson & Cie. 1957. — GILBERT-DREYFUS, J., M. ZARA, J. C. SAVOIE et P. LUMBROSO: Dystrophia myotonica. Ann. Endocr. (Paris) **15**, 477 (1954). — GLASS, S. J.: Doppelseitiger Kryptorchismus bei eineiigen Zwillingen. J. clin. Endocr. **6**, 797 (1946). — GÖBEL, P., F. HENI u. A. D'ADDABBO: Eine Methode zur papierchromatographischen Trennung und quantitativ-kolorimetrischen

Bestimmung der 17-Ketosteroide im Urin. Hoppe-Seylers Z. physiol. Chem. 311, 201 (1958). — GÖGL, H., u. F. LANG: Geschlechtsorgane. In Lehrbuch der speziellen pathologischen Anatomie von G. KAUFMANN, Bd. II, Teil 1. Berlin: W. de Gruyter 1957. — GOLDZIEHER, J.: The fluorescence reactions of steroids. Analyt. Chem. 26, 853 (1954). — GOLDZIEHER, M.: The endocrine glands. New York 1939. — GOLDZIEHER, M., and J. W. GOLDZIEHER: The male climacteric and the postclimacteric state. Geriatrics 8, 1 (1953). — GOODWIN, W. E., P. L. SCARDINO and W. W. SCOTT: A true hermaphrodite. J. Urol. (Baltimore) 71, 748 (1954). — GORDAN, G. S., E. W. OVERSTREET, H. F. TRAUT and G. A. WINCH: A syndrome of gonadal dysgenesis: a variety of ovarian agenesis with androgenic manifestations. J. clin. Endocr. 15, 1 (1955). — GORDON, M. B., and E. M. FIELDS: Effect of chorionic gonadotrophin and male sex hormone on height increase and bone development. J. clin. Endocr. 2, 715 (1942). — GRAHAM, M. A.: Detection of the sex of cat embryos from nuclear morphology in the embryonic membrane. Nature (Lond.) 173, 310 (1954). — GRAHAM, M. A., and M. L. BARR: A sex difference in the morphology of metabolic nuclei in somatic cells of the cat. Anat. Rec. 112, 709 (1952). — GREENBLATT, R. B., W. E. BARFIELD, E. C. JUNGCK and A. W. RAY: Induction of ovulation with MRL/41. J. Amer. med. Ass. 178, 101 (1961). — GREENBLATT, R. B., N. CARMONA and L. HIGDON: Gonadal dysgenesis with androgenic manifestations in the fall eunuchoid female. J. clin. Endocr. 16, 235 (1956). — GREENBLATT, R. B., and H. E. NIEBURGS: Turner's syndrome. J. clin. Endocr. 8, 993 (1948). — GREEP, R. O.: Effects of a digested pituitary extract on reproductive tract of hypophysectomized adult male rats. Proc. Soc. exp. Biol. (N.Y.) 42, 454 (1939). — GREEP, R. O., and R. J. BARNETT: The effect of pituitary stalk-secretion on the reproductive organs of female rats. Endocrinology 49, 172 (1951). — GREEP, R. O., and J. C. JONES: Steroid control of pituitary jones. Recent Progr. Hormone Res. 5, 197 (1950). — GREER, M. A.: Evidence of hypothalamic control of the pituitary release of thyrotrophin. Proc. Soc. exp. Biol. (N.Y.) 77, 603 (1951). — GREULICH, W. W., and T. H. BURFORD: Testicular tumors associated with mamary, prostatic and other changes in cryptorchid dogs. Amer. J. Cancer 28, 496 (1936). — GREULICH, W. W., R. J. DORFMAN, H. R. CATCHPOLE, C. J. SOLOMAN and C. S. CULOTTA: Somatic and endocrine studies of puberal and adolescent boys. Soc. Res. Child Develop. 7, 3 (1942). — GREULICH, W. W., and S. J. PYLE: Radiographic atlas of skeletal development of the hand and wrist. Stanford: Stanford University Press 1950. — GROSS, R. E., and T. C. JEWETT: Surgical experiences from 1222 operations for undescended testis. J. Amer. med. Ass. 160, 634 (1956). — GRUMBACH, M. M., and M. L. BARR: Cytologic tests of chromosomal sex in relation to sexual anomalies in man. Recent Progr. Hormone Res. 14, 255 (1958). — GRUMBACH, M. M., W. A. BLANC and E. T. ENGLE: Sex chromatin pattern in seminiferous tubule dysgenesis and other testicular disorders: relationship to true hermaphrodism and to Klinefelter's syndrome. J. clin. Endocr. 17, 703 (1957). — GRUMBACH, M. M., A. MORISHIMA and E. H. Y. CHU: On the sex chromatin and the sex chromosomes in sexual anomalies in man: relation to origin of the sex chromatin. In: Proc. I. Internat. Congr. Endocr., Kopenhagen, 1960. — GRUMBACH, M. M., J. J. VAN WYK and L. WILKINS: Chromosomal sex in gonadal dysgenesis (ovarian agenesis) relationship to male pseudohermaphrodism and theories of human sex differentiation. J. clin. Endocr. 15, 1161 (1955) — GRUMBRECHT, P., u. A. LOESER: Künstliche Brunststoffe. Naunyn-Schmiedeberg's Arch. exp. Path. Pharmak. 193, 34 (1939). — GUINET, P.: Les anomalies du sinus urogénital. La fonction endocrine du testicule, p. 276. Paris: Masson & Cie. 1957. — GUINET, P., J. MATHIEU et J. TATIN: Etude histologique de l'ovaire dans un cas de syndrome de Turner. Ann. Endocr. (Paris) 15, 499 (1954).

HÄUSSLER, E. P.: Über das Vorkommen von α-Follikelhormon (3-Oxy-17-keto-1,3,5-oestratrien) im Hengsturin. Helv. chim. Acta 17, 531 (1934). — HAIN, A. M.: The constitutional type of precocious puberty. J. clin. Endocr. 7, 171 (1947a). — HAIN, A. M., and J. E. SCHOFIELD: A case of intersexuality. A clinical and hormonal study. J. Obstet. Gynaec. Brit. Emp. 54, 97 (1947b). — HAJASHIDA, T., and CH. H. LI: A comparative immunological study of pituitary growth hormone from various species. Endocrinology 65, 944 (1959). — HAMBURGER, C.: Normal urinary excretion of neutral 17-ketosteroids with special reference to age and sex variations. Acta endocr. (Kbh.) 1, 19 (1948). — The assay of gonadotrophic hormones a survey. Acta endocr. (Kbh.), Suppl. 31, 59 (1957). — HAMBURGER, C., and E. GODTFREDSEN: Excretion of androgenic substances and gonadotrophin in cases of malignant tumors of testes. Acta path. microbiol. scand. 18, 485 (1941). — HAMBURGER, C., and S. KAALE: Testosterone treatment and 17-ketosteroid excretion. Acta endocr. (Kbh.) 2, 257 (1949). — HAMILTON, J. B.: The effects of male hormone upon the descent of the testis. Anat. Rec. 70, 534 (1936). — Action of male sex hormone with and without estrin in the female rat. Proc. Soc. exp. Biol. (N.Y.) 37, 361 (1937). — The role of testicular secretions as indicated by the effects of castration in man and by studies of pathological conditions and the short lifespan anociated with maleness. Recent Progr. Hormone Res. 3, 280 (1948b). — Androgenic activity per milligram of colorimetrically measured KS in urine. J. clin. Endocr. **14**, 452 (1954). — HAMILTON, J. B., R. J. DORFMAN and G. HUBERT: Androgenic and estrogenic substances in normal of eunuchoid and castrate men. J. Lab. clin. Med. **27**, 917 (1942). — HAMILTON, H. B., u. J. B. HAMILTON: Ageing in apparently normal men. I. Urinary titers of ketosteroids and of α-hydroxy and β-hydroxy ketosteroids. J. clin. Endocr. **8**, 433 (1948a). — HANHART, E.: Über heredodegenerativen Zwergwuchs mit Dystrophia adiposo-genitalis. Arch. Klaus-Stift. Vererb.-Forsch. **1**, 182 (1925). — HANSEMANN, D.: Über die sogenannten Zwischenzellen des Hodens und deren Bedeutung bei pathologischen Veränderungen. Virchows Arch. path. Anat. **142**, 538 (1895). — HANSEN, T. S.: Fertility in operatively treated and untreated cryptorchism. Acta chir. scand. **94**, 117 (1946). — HARNDEN, D. G., and P. A. JACOBS: Cytogenetics of abnormal sexual development in man. Brit. Med. Bull. **17**, 206 (1961). — HARRER, G.: Kasuistischer Beitrag zur Pathogenese des Klinefelter - Syndroms. Wien. klin. Wschr. **1958**, 280. — HARRIS, G. W.: Neural control of pituitary gland. Physiol. Rev. **28**, 139 (1948). — HARRIS, G. W., and D. JACOBSOHN: Functional hypophyseal grafts. Ciba Found. Coll. Endocrinol. **4**, 115 (1952). — HARRIS, G. W., and R. T. JOHNSON: Regeneration of the hypophyseal portal vessels, after secretion of the hypophyseal stalk in the monkey (Macacus rhesus). Nature (Lond.) **165**, 819 (1950). — HARRIS, G. W., and D. F. PFLEWS: Hypernephroma with virilism in child of 3 years. Canad. med. Ass. J. **23**, 244 (1930). — HARRIS, M. M., E. BRAND and L. E. HINSIE: Studies of the urinary secretion of gonadal stimulating substance in neutral patients. Amer. J. Psychiat. **91**, 1239 (1935). — HAUSER, G. A., M. KELLER, TH. KOLLER, R. WENNER u. F. GEOOR: Testikuläre Feminisierung bei Erwachsenen. Schweiz. med. Wschr. **87**, 1573 (1957a). — HAUSER, G. A., M. KELLER u. R. WENNER: Gonadendysgenesie. In IV. Sympos. Dtsch. Ges. Endokrinol., S. 207. Berlin-Göttingen-Heidelberg: Springer 1957b. — HEARD, R. D. H., P. H. JELLINEK and V. J. O'DONNELL: Biogenesis of the estrogens: The conversion of testosterone-4-C¹⁴-estrone in the pregnant mare. Endocrinology **57**, 200 (1955). — HECHTER, O., and G. PINCUS: Introduction to mechanism of corticosteroid action in disease processes. Ann. N.Y. Acad. Soc. **56**, 623 (1953). — HECHTER, O., A. ZAFFARON, R. JACOBSEN, H. LEVY, R. JEANLOZ, V. SCHENKER and G. PINCUS: The nature and the biogenesis of the adrenal secretory product. Recent Progr. Hormone Res. **6**, 215 (1951). — HECKEL, N. J.: The influence of testosterone-propionate upon benign prostatic hypertrophy and spermatogenesis: a clinical and pathological study in the human. J. Urol. (Baltimore) **43**, 286 (1940). — HECKEL, N. J., and J. H. McDONALD: The rebound phenomena of the spermatogenic activity of the human testis following the administration of testosterone propionate. Fertil. and Steril. **3**, 49 (1952). — HEDINGER, CH., u. D. HÜRZELER: Hypopituitarismus bei Dystopie des Hypophysenhinterlappens. Acta endocr. (Kbh.) **14**, 170 (1953). — HEINKE, E., u. E. TONUTTI: Studien zur Wirkung des Testosterons auf die spermiogenetische Aktivität des Hodens bei Oligospermie. Dtsch. med. Wschr. **1**, 81 (1956). — HELLER, A. L., and R. A. SHIPLEY: Endocrine studies in aging. J. clin. Endocr. **11**, 945 (1951). — HELLER, C. G.: Steroid control of pituitary function. Recent Progr. Hormone Res. **5**, 260 (1950). — HELLER, C. G., R. E. CHANDLER and G. B. MYERS: Effect of small and large doses of diethylstilbestrol upon menopausal symptoms, vaginal smear and urinary gonadotropins in 23 ovarectomized women. J. clin. Endocr. **4**, 109 (1944b). — HELLER, C. G., and E. J. HELLER: Gonadotropic hormone: clinical application of extraction methods for assay purposes. Endocrinology **24**, 319 (1939). — HELLER, C. G., and G. B. MYERS: Male climacteric, its symptomatology, diagnosis and treatment. J. Amer. med. Ass. **126**, 472 (1944a). — HELLER, C. G., and W. O. NELSON: Hyalinization of seminiferons tubules associated with normal or failing leydig-cell-function. J. clin. Endocr. **5**, 1 (1945). — The testis in human hypogonadism. Recent Progr. Hormone Res. **3**, 229 (1948a). — Classification of male hypogonadism. J. clin. Endocr. **8**, 345 (1948b). — HELLER, C. G., W. O. NELSON, J. C. HILL, E. HENDERSON, W. O. MADDOCK and E. C. JUNGCK: The effect of testosterone administration upon the human testis. J. clin. Endocr. **10**, 816 (1950). — HELLER, C. G., W. O. NELSON, W. O. MADDOCK, E. C. JUNGCK, C. A. PAULSEN and G. E. MORTIMORE: Effect of testosterone upon the human testis. J. clin. Invest. **30**, 648 (1951). — HELLER, C. G., W. O. NELSON and A. A. ROTH: Anorchism. J. clin. Endocr. **3**, 573 (1943). — HELLMAN, L., H. L. BRADLOW, B. ZUMOFF, D. K. FUKUSHIMA and T. F. GALLAGHER: Thyroid-androgen interrelations and the hypocholesteremic effect of androsterone. J. clin. Endocr. **19**, 936 (1959). — HENCH, P. S., E. C. KENDAL, C. H. SLOCUM and H. F. POLLEY: The effect of a hormone of the adrenal cortex (17-hydroxy-11-dehydrocorticosterone (Compound E) and of pituitary adrenocorticotropic hormone on rheumatoid arthritis; preliminary report. Proc. Mayo Clin. **24**, 181 (1949). — HENDERSON, E., and M. WEINBERG: Endocrine review—Methylandrostenediol. J. clin. Endocr. **11**, 641 (1951). — HENI, F.: Das Morgagni-Turner-Syndrom. Klin. Wschr. **29**, 75 (1951). — Primäre Atrophie der Keimdrüsen des Mannes. Klin. Wschr. **1952**, 741. — HENI, F., u. P. GÖBEL: Der Wert der papierchromatographischen Trennung der 17-Ketosteroide im Urin für die Differentialdiagnose der Überfunktion der Nebennierenrinde. Verh. dtsch. Ges. inn. Med. **64**,

166 (1958). — HENI, F., u. H. MAST: Hypophysentransplantation. In 4. Symp. der Dtsch. Ges. für Endokrinologie 1956. Berlin-Göttingen-Heidelberg: Springer 1957. — HEPBURN, H. R.: Anorchism. J. Urol. (Baltimore) 62, 65 (1949). — HERLANT, M.: Study of the pituitary body with the periodic acid-Schiff-reaction. Nature (Lond.) 164, 703 (1949). — HERR, M. E., J. A. HOGG and R. H. LEVIN: Synthesis of potent oral anabolic-androgenic steroids. J. Amer. chem. Soc. 78, 500 (1956). — HERMANN, W. L., F. BUCKNER and A. BASKIN: Interstitial-cell tumor of the testis with gynecomastia. J. clin. Endocr. 18, 834 (1958). — HERTZ, R., J. K. CROMER and B. B. WESTFALL: A case of ovarian agenesis with normal urinary gonadotropin titer. J. clin. Endocr. 10, 610 (1950). — HERSHBERGER, L. G., E. G. SHIPLEY and R. K. MEYER: Myotrophic activity of 19-nortestosterone and other steroids determined by modified levator ani muscle method. Proc. Soc. exp. Biol. (N.Y.) 83, 175 (1953). — HETHERINGTON, A. W., and S. W. RANSON: Experimental hypothalamico hypophyseal obesity in the rat. Proc. Soc. exp. Biol. (N.Y.) 41, 465 (1939). — HIBBIT, L. L., W. R. STARNES and S. R. HILL: Studies in man on testicular and adrenal response to adreno-corticotropin and human chorionic gonadotropin. J. clin. Endocr. 18, 1315 (1958). — HIGGINS, G. A., W. E. BROWNLEE and F. E. MANZ: Feminizing tumors of the adrenal cortex. Amer. Surg. 22, 56 (1956). — HILL, R. T.: Ovaries secrete male hormone. Endocrinology 21, 633 (1937). — HILLARP, N. A.: Studies on the localization of hypothalamic centres controlling the gonadotrophic function of the hypophysis. Acta endocr. (Kbh.) 4, 87 (1949). — HILLARP, N. A., S. M. MCCANN, L. M. SCHREINER, E. ROSEMBERG, D. M. K. RIOCH and E. ANDERSON: Alterations of adrenal cortical and ovarian activity following hypothalamic lesions. Endocrinology 57, 44 (1955). — HINMAN, F.: Optimum time for orchiopexy in cryptorchidism. Fertil. and Steril. 6, 206 (1955). — HOAGLAND, C. L., H. GILDER and R. E. SHANK: The synthesis storage and excretion of creatine creatinine, and glycocyanine of certain hormones on these processes. J. exp. Med. 81, 423 (1945). — HOFFENBERG, R., and W. P. U. JACKSON: Gonadal dysgenesis in normal looking females. Brit. med. J. 1957 I, 1281. — HOHLWEG, W.: Veränderungen des HVL und des Ovariums nach Behandlung mit großen Dosen von Follikelhormon. Klin. Wschr. 1934, 92. — Über die Hemmung der Oestrusfraktion durch Vitamin A-Überdosierung. Klin. Wschr. 1951, 193. — Die Hormone der Keimdrüsen. In SEITZ-AMREICH, Biologie und Pathologie des Weibes. Wien: Urban & Schwarzenberg 1952. — Endokrinologie des Krebses. Aus den Abh. der Dtsch. Akad. Wiss. Nr 1, 1953a (Probleme der Krebsforschung und Krebsbekämpfung). — Die Desensibilisierung des Hypophysenzwischenhirnsystems. Vortr. der Berliner Gynäkolog. Ges. 1953b. — Die Adaptation des Hypophysenzwischenhirnsystems an Keimdrüsenhormone bei langdauernder Zufuhr. Aus: Zweites Sympos. Dtsch. Ges. Endokrin., März 1954, S. 156. Berlin-Göttingen-Heidelberg: Springer 1955. — Über die Bedeutung der Regulation der peripheren Hormondrüsen im Hinblick auf eine praktische Hormontherapie. Dtsch. Gesundh.-Wes. 11, 245 (1956). — HOHLWEG, W., u. A. CHAMORRO: Über die luteinisierende Wirkung des Follikelhormons durch Beeinflussung der luteogenen Hypophysenvorderlappen-sekretion. Klin. Wschr. 16, 196 (1937). — HOHLWEG, W., u. M. DOHRN: Die Beziehung zwischen Hypophysenvorderlappen und Keimdrüsen. Klin. Wschr. 1932, 233. — HOHLWEG, W., u. H. ZAHLER: Über die Wirkung der Einpflanzung von Testosteron in den Hoden infantiler und hypophysektomierter Ratten. Z. Ges. inn. Med. 1, 42 (1946). — HOLLANDER, F., R. FRANK and E. KLEMPNER: A dosage response equation for androgen assay by the chick comb method. Proc. Soc. exp. Biol. (N.Y.) 46, 1 (1941). — HOMBURGER, F., S. C. KASDON and W. H. FISHMAN: Methylandrostenediol: A non-virilizing derivative of testosterone in metastatic cancer of the breast. Proc. Soc. exp. Biol. (N.Y.) 74, 162 (1950). — HOOFT, C., K. DIERICKS and P. CIETERS: Brain tumor and precocious puberty. Maandschr. Kindergeneesk. 12, 87 u. franz. Zus.fass. 95 (1943). — HOOKER, C. W.: The biology of the interstitial cells of the testis. Recent Progr. Hormone Res. 3, 173 (1948). — HOOKER, C. W., and TH. R. FORBES: A bio-assay for minute amounts of progesterone. Endocrinology 41, 158 (1947). — HOOKER, C. W., W. O. GARDNER and C. A. PFEIFFER: Testicular tumors in mice receiving estrogens. J. Amer. med. Ass. 115, 443 (1940). — HORN, E. H.: Nutritional and hormonal influences upon reproductive maturation, organ weights and histochemistry of the immature male rat. Endocrinology 57, 399 (1955). — HORNSTEIN, D.: Puberaler FSH-Mangel. Klin. Wschr. 37, 105 (1959). — HORSTMANN, P.: The function of the endocrine glands in diabetes mellitus. Acta endocr. (Kbh.) 2, 379 (1949). — HOTCHKISS, R. S.: Testicular biopsy in sterility in the male. Bull. N.Y. Acad. Med. 18, 600 (1942). — Fertility in men. Philadelphia: J. B. Lippincott Company 1944. — HOUSSAY, B. A., et E. HUG: Action de l'hypophyse sur la croissance. C.R. Soc. Biol. (Paris) 85, 1215 (1921). — HOWARD, R. P., R. C. SNIFFEN, F. A. SIMMONDS and F. ALBRIGHT: Testicular deficiency: A clinical and pathological study. J. clin. Endocr. 10, 121 (1950). — HUBBLE, O.: The endocrine orchestra. Brit. med. J. 1961, 225. — HÜBENER, H. E.: Die physiologische Funktion der Nebennierenrindenhormone als Enzyminduktion. Dtsch. med. Wschr. 87, 438 (1962). — HUFFMAN, L. F.: Interstitial cell tumor of the testicle: report of a case. J. Urol. (Baltimore) 45, 692 (1941). —

HUGGINS, CH., and PH. J. CLARK: Quantitative studies of prostatic secretion. II. The effect of castration and of estrogen injection of the normal and the hyperplastic prostate glands of dogs. J. exp. Med. 72, 747 (1940). — HUGGINS, C., and C. V. HODGES: The effect of castration, of estrogen and of androgen injection on serum phosphatases in metastatic carcinoma of the prostate. Cancer Res. 1, 293 (1941). — HUGGINS, C., and P. V. MOULDER: Estrogen production by sertoli cell tumors of the testis. Cancer Res. 5, 510 (1945). — HUMPHREY, G. F., and T. MANN: Citric acid in semen. Nature (Lond.) 161, 352 (1948). — Studies on metabolism of semen. Biochem. J. 44, 97 (1949). — HUNT, V. C., and J. W. BUDD: Gynecomastia associated with interstitial cell tumor of the testicle. J. Urol. (Baltimore) 42, 1242 (1939). — HURXTHAL, L. M.: Sublingual use of testosterone in seven cases of hypogonadism: report of 3 congenital eunuchoids occurring in one family. J. clin. Endocr. 3, 551 (1943). — HUTCHINS, J. J.: Complete sex reversal: A case report. J. clin. Endocr. 19, 375 (1959). — HUTCHINS, J. J., R. F. ESCAMILLA, W. C. DEAMER and CH. H. LI: Metabolic changes produced by human growth hormone (Li) in a pituitary. J. clin. Endocr. 19, 759 (1949). — HYDE, P. M., W. H. ELLIOTT, E. A. DOISY and E. A. DOISY: Synthesis and metabolic studies of 17-methyl-C^{14}-testosterone. J. biol. Chem. 208, 521 (1954a). — HYDE, P. M., W. H. ELLIOTT, E. A. DOISY and E. A. DOISY: Synthesis and metabolic studies of 17α-methyl-C^{14}-Δ5-androstene-3β,17β-diol. J. biol. Chem. 207, 287 (1954b).

ISELSTÖGER, H., u. A. RETT: Zur Bedeutung der quantitativen Hormonanalyse in der Kinderheilkunde. Wien. med. Wschr. 103, 611 (1953).

JACOBS, P. A., A. G. BAIHIE, W. M. C. BROWN, H. FORREST, J. R. ROY, J. S. S. STEWART and B. LENNOX: Chromosomal sex in the syndrome of testicular feminisation. Lancet 1959 I b, 591. — JACOBS, P. A., A. G. BAIKIE, W. M. C. BROWN and J. A. STRONG: The somatic chromosomes in mongolism. Lancet 1959 I c, 710. — JACOBS, P. A., D. G. HARNDEN, K. E. BUCTATON, W. M. C. BROWN, M. J. KING, J. A. MCBRIDE, T. N. MCGREGOR and N. McLEAN: Cytogenetic studies in primary amenorrhoea. Lancet 1961 I, 1183. — JACOBS, P. A., and J. A. STRONG: A case of human intersexuality having a possible XXY sex determining mechanism. Nature (Lond.) 183, 302 (1959a). — JACOBSON, B. D.: Zit. nach H. SIMMER, Hormonbehandlung während der Schwangerschaft als Ursache eines Pseudohermaphroditismus femininus externus Neugeborener. Dtsch. med. Wschr. 4, 173 (1961). — JAGIELLO, G., and J. D. ATWELL: Prevalence of testicular feminisation. Lancet 1962 I, 329. — JAILER, J. W.: Effect of testosterone propionate on creatinuria of experimental hyperthyroidism in male and female monkeys. Endocrinology 29, 89 (1941). — Fluorometric method for clinical determination of estrone and estradiol. J. clin. Endocr. 8, 564 (1948). — JAILER, J., J. J. GOLD, R. VANDE-WIELER and S. LIEBERMAN: 17α-hydroxyprogesterone and 21-desoxyhydrocortisone, their metabolism and possible role in congenital adrenal virilism. J. clin. Invest. 34, 1639 (1955). — JAILER, J. W., J. J. GOLD and E. Z. WALLACE: Evaluation of "Cortisone Test" as diagnostic aid in differentiating adrenal hyperplasia from adrenal neoplasia. Amer. J. Med. 3, 340 (1954). — JAILER, J. W., and J. H. LEATHEM: Antigonadotropic substances in man following treatment with pregnant mare serum. Proc. Soc. exp. Biol. (N.Y.) 45, 506 (1940). — JAKOBSEN, H. D.: The influence of oestrogenic hormones on prostate. Oestrogenic reactions in the human prostate after artificial hormone administration, in the normal human prostate at birth and in cases of senile hyperplasia of the prostate. Acta path. microbiol. scand. 29, 419 (1951). — JAOUDÉ, F. A., E. E. BAULIEN et M. F. JAYLE: Fractionnement par chromatographic sur papier des 17-cetosteroides neutres urinaires au cours de l'hyperplasie virilisante congenitale corticosurrenale. Acta endocr. (Kbh.) 26, 30 (1957). — JAYLE, M. F., and O. ERÉPY: The excretion and measurement of urinary phenolsteroids. Ciba Found. Coll. Endocrinol. 2, 84 (1952). — JOHNSEN, S. G.: Fractionation of urinary 17-ketosteroids. Acta endocr. (Kbh.) 21, 127 (1956). — JOLLY, H.: Sexual precocity. Oxford: Blackwell Scientific Publ. 1955a. — Sexual precocity. Springfield, Ill.: Ch. C. Thomas 1955b. — JONES, H. W., and G. E. S. JONES: The gynecological aspects of adrenal hyperplasia and allied disords. Amer. J. Obstet. Gynec. 68, 1330 (1954). — JONES, H. W., and W. W. SCOTT: Hermaphroditism, genital anomalies and related endocrine disorders. Baltimore: Williams & Wilkins Company 1958. — JONES, M. S., and T. N. MCGREGOR: Inhibitory effect of follicular hormone on the anterior pituitary in humans. Lancet 1936 II, 974. — JOST, A.: The age factor in the castration of male rabbit fetuses. C.R. Soc. Biol. (Paris) 140, 121 (1947a). — Recherches sur la différenciation sexuelle de l'embryo de lapin. I. Introduction et embryologie génitale normale. Arch. Anat. micr. Morph. exp. 36, 151 (1947b). — Problems of fetal endocrinology: the gonadal and hypophyseal hormones. Recent Progr. Hormone Res. 8, 379 (1953). — Die Wirkung der Sexualhormone beim Embryo. In: Fermente, Hormone, Vitamine (R. AMMON u. W. DIRSCHERL). Stuttgart: Georg Thieme 1960. — JUNGCK, E. C., W. O. MADDOCK, C. G. HELLER and W. O. NELSON: Antihormone formation complicating pituitary gonadotropin therapy in infertile men. J. clin. Endocr. 9, 355 (1949). — JUNGCK, E. C., F. A. POMER, R. E. STILES and J. H. GRAHAM: Interstitial-cell tumors of the testis in children. New Engl. J. Med. 250, 233 (1954).

KALLMANN, F. J., W. A. SCHOENFELD and S. E. BARRERA: The genetic aspects of primary eunuchoidism. Amer. J. ment. Defic. 48, 203 (1944). — KAPPAS, A., A. T. MILHORAT, C. P. RHOADS and T. F. GALLAGHER: Dystrophia myotonica. Amer. J. phys. Med. 34, 303 (1955). — KARNS, W. M.: The treatment of male infertility with estrogenic substance. J. Urol. (Baltimore) 75, 852 (1956). — KASAI, K.: Über die Zwischenzellen des Hodens. Virchows Arch. path. Anat. 194, 1 (1908). — KAUFMANN, C.: Echte menstruelle Blutung bei kastrierten Frauen nach Zufuhr von Follikel- und Corpus luteum-Hormon. Zbl. Gynäk. 57, 42 (1933). — KELLIE, A. E., and A. P. WADE: The analysis of urinary 17-oxo-steroids by gradient elution. Biochem. J. 66, 196 (1957). — KENNEDY, B. J., D. M. TIBBETS and J. T. NATHANSON: Effects of intensive sex steroid hormone therapy in advanced breast cancer. J. Amer. med. Ass. 152, 1135 (1953b). — KENNEDY, B. J., D. M. TIBBETS, J. T. NATHANSON and J. B. AUB: Hypercalcaemia, complication of hormone therapy of advanced breast cancer. Cancer Res. 13, 445 (1953a). — KESSLER, A.: Über totale testikuläre Feminisierung. Geburtsh. u. Frauenheilk. 19. 31 (1959). — KIMMIG, J.: Fertilität des Mannes und Fragen der künstlichen Insemination. Z. Urol., Sonderbd. Hamburger Kongreßber. 1955 der Dtsch. Ges. Urologie. — KINCL, F. A., H. J. RINGOLD and R. J. DORFMAN: Pituitary gonadotropin inhibition by subcutaneously administered steroids. Acta endocr. (Kbh.) 36, 83 (1961). — KINSELL, J. W.: Spermatogenesis in a "panhypopituitary" eunuchoid as the result of testosterone therapy. J. Clin. Endocr. 7, 781 (1947). — KLEIN, J.: Dystrophia myotonica. Génét. Hum. Suppl. 7 (1958). — KLINEFELTER, H. F., F. ALBRIGHT and G. C. GRISWOLD: Experience with a quantitative test for normal or decreased amounts of follicle stimulating hormone in the urine in endocrinological diagnosis. J. clin. Endocr. 3, 529 (1943). — KLINEFELTER, H. F., E. C. REIFENSTEIN and F. ALBRIGHT: Syndrome characterized by gynecomastia, aspermatogenesis without a-leydigism, and increased excretions of follicle-stimulating hormone. J. clin. Endocr. 2, 615 (1942). — KLOTZ, H. P., H. CHEMÈNES et P. MANVAIS: Le syndrôme «ovaires non fonctionnels. Infantilisme génitale et sexe chromosomique mâle». Sem. Hôp. Paris 35, 3230 (1959). — KLOTZ, H. P., H. CHEMÈNES, J. NATHAN-KAHN et M. ROBEL-TUTIN: Aplasie des petites lèvres, infantilisme génital et sclérose ovarienne chez des femmes présentant un sexe génétique mâle. Ann. Endocr. (Paris) 19, 751 (1958). — KNOWLTON, K., A. T. KENYON, J. SANDIFORD, G. LOTWIN and R. FRICHER: Comparative study of metabolic effects of estradiol benzoate and testosterone propionate in man. J. clin. Endocr. 2, 671 (1942). — KOCH, W., E. HEIM u. J. ESCHWEILER: Der Einfluß der Geschlechtshormone auf die Muskulatur. Acta endocr. (Kbh.) 16, 369 (1954). — KOCHAKIAN, C. D.: Testosterone and testosterone acetate and protein and energy metabolism of castrate dogs. Endocrinology 21, 750 (1937). — Protein anabolic effects of steroid hormones. Vitam. and Horm. 4, 255 (1946). — The effect of castration on the weight and composition of the muscles of the guinea pig. Endocrinology 58, 315 (1956b). — Metabolism of androgens by tissue enzymes. Proc. fourth intern. Congr. Biochemistry, Vienna 1958 IV, p. 196. — KOCHAKIAN, CH. D., and B. R. ENDAHL: Influence of androgens on transaminase activities of different tissues. Amer. J. Physiol. 186, 460 (1956a). — KOCHAKIAN, D. C., B. R. ENDAHL and H. D. HALL: Anginase activity of the salivary gland and its regulation by androgens. Proc. Soc. exp. Biol. (N.Y.) 89, 289 (1955). — KÖHNE, G.: Die Beziehung des angeborenen Olfaktorumdefekts zum primären Eunuchoidismus des Mannes. Virchows Arch. path. Anat. 314, 345 (1947). — KOHLER, H. G.: Thalidomide and congenital abnormalities. Lancet 1962 I, 326. — KORENCHERSKY, V., and M. DENNISON: The effect of oestrone on normal and castrated male rats. Biochem. J. 28, 1474 (1934). — KORENCHERSKY, V., and K. HALL: Prolonged injections of male sex hormones into normal and senile male rats. Brit. med. J. 1939 I, 4. — KORY, R. C., M. H. BRADLEY, R. W. WATSON, R. CALLAHAN and B. J. PETERS: A six-month evaluation of an anabolic drug, norethandrolone, in in underweight persons. Amer. J. Med. 26, 243 (1959). — KORY, R. C., R. N. WATSON, M. H. BRADLEY and B. J. PETERS: A six-months evaluation of an anabolic drug, norethandrone, in chronically underweight individuals. J. clin. Invest. 36, 907 (1957). — KOWALEWSKI, K., and R. T. MORRISON: The effects of certain androgenic steroids on the uptake of radiosulphor in a healing fractured bone in the rat. Canad. J. Biochem. 35, 771 (1957). — KRABBE, K.: Early synostosis of the epiphyses, with dwarfism in pubertas praecox. Endocrinology 3, 459 (1919). — KRABBE, K. H.: La sclérose tubéreuse du cerveau. Encéphale 17, 281 (1922). — KRAYENBÜHL, H., u. U. ZOLLINGER: Malignes metastasierendes Pinealcytom mit dem klinischen Bild der Dystrophia adiposo-genitalis. Operationsmortalität beim Hypophysentumor. Schweiz. Arch. Neurol. Psychiat. 51, 77 (1943). — KRETSCHMER, E.: Zit. nach H. R. HEPBURN, Anorchism. J. Urol. (Baltimore) 62, 65 (1949).

LACASSAGNE, A.: Métaplasie épidermoide de la prostate provoquée, chez la souris, par des injections répétées de fortes doses de folliculine. C. R. Soc. Biol. (Paris) 113, 590 (1933). — Mesure de l'action des hormones sexuelles sur la glande sousmaxillaire de la souris. C. R. Soc. Biol. (Paris) 133, 227 (1940a). — Réaction de la glande sousmaxillaire à l'hormone mâle chez la souris et le rat. C. R. Soc. Biol. (Paris) 133, 539 (1940b). — LAMAR, C. P.:

Climacteric in aging men. J. Amer. med. Ass. 118, 458 (1942). — LANDAU, R. L.: Hypogonadism with spermatogenesis; a case report. J. clin. Endocr. 13, 510 (1953). — LANDAU, R. L., and M. L. LAVES: Urinary pregnanetriol of testicular origin. J. clin. Endocr. 19, 1399 (1959). — LANGECKER, H.: Die Metaboliten im menschlichen Harn nach Verabreichung von 17α-Aethinyl-19-nortestosteron (Noraethisteron). Acta endocr. (Kbh.) 37, 14 (1961). — LANGE-COSACK, H.: Pubertas praecox. Dtsch. Z. Nervenheilk. 162, 235 (1950). — Verschiedene Gruppen der hypothalamischen Pubertas praecox (2. Mitt.). Dtsch. Z. Nervenheilk. 168, 237 (1952). — LAQUEUR, E.: Männliches und weibliches Hormon. Schweiz. med. Wschr. 1, 1041 (1935). — Effects of testosterone propionate in immature and adult female rats. Endocrinology 30, 93 (1942). — LAQUEUR, E., E. DINGEMANSE, P. C. HART u. S. E. DE JONGH: Über das Vorkommen weiblichen Sexualhormons (Menhormon) im Harn von Männern. Klin. Wschr. 6, 1859 (1927). — LAQUEUR, E., S. E. DE JONGH and S. ZUCHERMANN: Zit. in H. J. JAKOBSEN, The influence of oestrogenic hormones on prostate. Oestrogenic reaction in the human prostate after artificial hormone administration, in the normal human prostate at birth and in case of senile hyperplasia of the prostate. Acta path. microbiol. scand. 29, 419 (1951). — LAROCHE, G., H. SIMONNET et E. BOMPARD: Contribution à l'étude de l'élimination urinaire des corps oestrogènes après injection d'hormones sexuelles. C.R. Soc. Biol. (Paris) 130, 521 (1939). — LARON, Z.: Effectiveness of fluoxymesterone on linear growth and weight in children with growth retardation and underweight. Acta endocr. (Kbh.) 36, 541 (1961). — LAURENCE, J. Z., and R. C. MOON: Four cases of retinitis pigmentosa occurring in the same family and accompanied by general imperfections of development. Ophthal. Rev. 2, 32 (1866). — LEACH, R. B., W. O. MADDOCK, J. TOKUYAMA, C. A. PAULSEN and W. O. NELSON: Clinical studies of testicular hormone produktion. Recent Progr. Hormone Res. 12, 377 (1956). — LEACH, R. B., W. O. MADDACK, C. A. PAULSEN, J. LANMAN and W. O. NELSON: Correction of androgen deficiency in Klinefelter's syndrome by chronic gonadotrophin treatment. J. Lab. clin. Med. 50, 925 (1957). — LEATHEM, J. H.: Hormones and protein nutrition. Recent Progr. Hormone Res. 14, 141 (1958). — LEATHEM, J. H., and A. E. RAKOFF: Equine pituitary gonadotrophin and antihormone formation. Endocrinology 40, 454 (1947). — Studies on antihormone specificity with particular reference to gonadotropic therapy in the female. J. clin. Endocr. 8, 262 (1948). — LEDERER, J.: Le testicule du cirrhotique. In: La fonction endocrine du testicule, p. 373. Paris: Masson & Cie. 1917. — LENNOX, B.: Chromosomal sex in the syndrome of testicular feminisation. Lancet 1959 II, 277, 591. — LENZ, W.: Klinik und Therapie genetisch bedingter Störungen. Dtsch. med. Wschr. 84, 10 (1959c). — LENZ, W., H. NOWAKOWSKI, A. PRADER u. C. SCHIRREN: Die Ätiologie des Klinefelters. Schweiz. med. Wschr. 1959 a, 727. — LENZ, W., u. B. W. ORT: Das Wachstum von Hamburger Schülern in den Jahren 1877—1957. Medizinische 1959 b, 2265. — LESSER, M. A., S. N. VOSE and G. M. DIXEY: Effect of testosterone propionate on the prostate gland of patients over 45. J. clin. Endocr. 15, 297 (1955). — LEWIS, L. G.: Testis tumors. Advanc. Surg. 2, 419 (1949). — LI, C. H.: Bioassay of growth hormone. Ciba Found. Coll. Endocrinol. 5, 115 (1953). — LI, C. H., M. E. SIMPSON and H. M. EVANS: Isolation of pituitary follicle-stimulating hormone (FSH). Science 109, 445 (1949). — LIEBERMAN, S., and K. DORBRINER: The isolation of pregnandiol-3,17-one-20 from human urine. J. biol. Chem. 161, 269 (1945). — LIEBERMAN, S., K. DORBRINER, B. R. HILL, L. F. FIESER and C. P. RHOADS: Studies in steroid metabolism. J. biol. Chem. 172, 263 (1948). — LIEBERMAN, S., H. J. TAGNON and P. SCHULMAN: The in vitro metabolism of estrogens by the liver studies by means of a colorimetric method. J. clin. Invest. 31, 341 (1952). — LIEBERMAN, S., and R. VAN DER WIELE: Dehydroisoandrosterone, its origin and importance as a precursor of urinary 17-ketosteroids. In: Biochemistry of steroids. Proc. fourth intern. Congr. Biochem. vol. IV, p. 153. London: Pergamon Press 1959. — LINDNER, H. R.: Androgens in the bovine testis and spermatic vein blood. Nature (Lond.) 183, 1605 (1959). — LINKE, C. A., and J. A. KIEFER: Occurrence of testis tumor in undescendet testes. J. Urol. (Baltimore) 82, 347 (1959). — LINSER, P.: Über die Beziehungen zwischen Nebennieren und Körperwachstum, besonders Riesenwuchs. Bruns' Beitr. klin. Chir. 37, 282 (1903). — LISSER, H.: Successful removal of adrenal cortical tumors causing sexual precocity in boy 5 years old. Trans. Ass. Amer. Phycns 48, 224 (1933). — LISSER, H., L. E. CURTIS, R. F. ESCAMILLA and M. B. GOLDBERG: The syndrome of congenitally apleastic ovaries with sexual infantilism, high urinary gonadotropins, short stature and other congenital abnormalities. J. clin. Endocr. 7, 665 (1957). — LISTER, S. C., G. H. LUND and R. O. STAFFORD: Androgenic and myotrophic properties of orally administered 9-fluors-11-oxymethyltestosterones. Endocrinology 58, 781 (1956). — LLOYD, C. W., E. C. HUGHES, M. L. EVA and J. LOBOTSKY: The urinary excretion of chronic gonadotropin by human females following parenteral administration of aqueous of beeswax solutions. J. clin. Endocr. 3, 268 (1949a). — LLOYD, C. W., M. MORLEY, K. MORROW, J. LOBOTSKY and E. C. HUGHES: Estimation of urinary gonadotropin of the nonpregnant human by the mouse uterine weight and ovarian hyperemia responses. J. clin. Endocr. 9, 636 (1949 b). — LLOYD, C. W., and R. H. WILLIAMS: Endocrine changes associated with Laennec's cirrhosis of liver. Amer. J. med. Sci. 4, 315 (1948). — LOESER, A., u. K. MIKULICZ: Inaktivierung gonadotroper Wirkstoffe durch Lithospermum officinale. Klin. Wschr. 1955, 1017. — LOEWE, S., u. H. E. VOSS: Gewinnung, Eigenschaften und Testierung eines männlichen Sexualhormons. S.-B. Akad. Wiss. Wien, math.-nat. Kl. 29, 20 (1928). — Der Stand der Erfassung des männlichen Sexualhormons (Androkinins). Klin. Wschr. 1930, 481. — LORAIN, J. A.: Zit. nach P. HORSTMANN, Bioassay of pituitary and placental gonadotropins in relation to clinical problems in man. Vitam. and Horm. 14, 305 (1956). — LUCAS, W. M., W. F. WHITMORE and C. D. WEST: Identification of testosterone in human spermatic vein blood. J. clin. Endocr. 17, 465 (1957). — LUDWIG, D. J.: The effect of androgen on spermatogenesis. Endocrinology 46, 453 (1950). — LÜHRS, W., u. G. P. WILDNER: Beitrag zur Hyperkalzämie bei ossalen Metastasen des Mammakarzinoms. Dtsch. Gesundh.-Wes. 11, 609 (1956). — LURIE, C. A., and J. HERTZMAN: Linear growth and epiphyseal closures. Effect of treatment with chorionic gonadotrophin. J. clin. Endocr. 1, 717 (1941). — LYNCH, K. M., and W. W. SCOTT: The sertoli cells as related to age of man and experimental alterations of the pituitary gonad axis in the animal. Fertil. and Steril. 3, 35 (1952). — LYNGBYE, J., and E. F. MOGENSEN: Oestrogen metabolism in women with cirrhosis of the liver. Acta endocr. (Kbh.) 36, 350 (1961). — LYNN, W. S., and R. H. BROWN: The conversion of progesterone to androgens by testes. J. biol. Chem. 232, 1015 (1958).

MACLEOD, J., and R. S. HOTCHKISS: The effect of hyperpyrexia upon spermatozoa counts in men. Endocrinology 28, 780 (1941). — MADDOCK, W. O.: Antihormone formation complicating pituitary gonadotropin therapy in infertile men. J. clin. Endocr. 19, 213 (1949). — MADDOCK, W. O., and C. G. HELLER: Dichotomy between hypophyseal content and amount of circulating gonadotrophins during starvation. Proc. Soc. exp. Biol. (N.Y.) 66, 595 (1947). — MADDOCK, W. O., and W. O. NELSON: The effects of chorionic gonadotropin in adult men: increased estrogen and 17-ketosteroid excretion, gynecomastia. Leydig cell stimulation and seminiferons tubule damage. J. clin. Endocr. 12, 985 (1952). — MAINZER, F.: NNR-Syndrom mit arterieller Hypertension. Acta med. scand. 87, 50 (1935). — MANCINI, R. E., D. BRANDES, A. PORTELA, J. JZQUIERDO and P. KIRSCHBAUM: Autoradiography and histochemical study of the coch's com in normal and hormonally treated birds. Endocrinology 67, 430 (1960). — MANCINI, R. E., J. NOLAZCO and F. A. DE LA BALZE: Histochemical study of normal adult human testis. Anat. Rec. 114, 127 (1952). — MANN, T.: Studies on the metabolism of semen. Biochem. J. 40, 481 (1946). — The biochemistry of semen. London: Methuen & Co., Ltd. 1954. — MANN, T., and N. PARSON: Effect of testicular hormone on the formation of seminal fructose. Nature (Lond.) 160, 294 (1947). — MARBERGER, E., u. W. O. NELSON: Geschlechtsbestimmung am Zellkern bei geschlechtlichen Anomalien, mit besonderer Berücksichtigung des Klinefelter-Syndroms. Endokrinologie 35. 9 (1957). — MARBURG, O.: Die Klinik der Zirbeldrüsenerkrankungen. Ergebn. inn. Med, Kinderheilk. 10, 146 (1913). — MARQUAND, H. S. LE: Congenital hypogonadotrophic hypogonadism in five members of a family, three brothers and two sisters. Proc. roy. Soc. Med. 47, 442 (1954). — MARQUARDT, G. H., and CH. J. FISHER: Effect of anabolic steroids on liver function tests and creatine excretion. J. Amer. med. Ass. 175, 851 (1961). — MARRIAN, G. F.: Some aspects of progesteron metabolism. Recent Progr. Hormone Res. 4, 3 (1949). — The urinary estrogens and their quantitative determination. Cancer (Philad) 10, 704(1957). — MARRIAN, G. F., and A. S. PARKES: The effect of anterior pituitary preparations administered during diatary anoestrus. Proc. roy. Soc. 105, 248 (1929). — MARTI, M.: Die chromatographische Trennung und Bestimmung der 17-Ketosteroide im Urin. Helv. med. Acta 18, 215 (1951). — MARTI, M., u. A. HEUSSER: Über das hormonal aktive Prinzip eines feminisierenden Hodentumors. Helv. chim. Acta 37, 327 (1954). — MARTIN, J. D.: A highly sensitive assay for oestrogens. Nature (Lond.) 181, 620 (1958a). — MARTIN, J. D., and J. H. MILLS: The effects of pregnancy on adrenal steroid metabolism. Clin. Sci. 17, 137 (1958b). — MARTIN, M. M., and L. WILKINS: Pituitary dwarfism: diagnosis and treatment. J. clin. Endocr. 18, 679 (1958). — MARTIN, S. J.: Effect of certain endocrine secretions on the X-zone of the adrenal cortex of the mouse. Proc. Soc. exp. Biol. (N.Y.) 28, 41 (1930). — MASON, H. L., and W. W. ENGSTROM: The 17-ketosteroids: their origin, determination and significance. Physiol. Rev. 30, 321 (1950). — MASON, H. L., and E. L. KEPLER: Isolation of steroids from the urine of patients with adrenal cortical tumors and adrenal cortical hyperplasia: a new 17-ketosteroide, androstane-3,11-diol-17-one. J. biol. Chem. 161, 235 (1945). — Urinary steroids isolated after administration of dehydroisoandrosterone to human subjects. J. biol. Chem. 167, 73 (1947). — MASON, K. E., and J. M. WOLFE: The physiological activity of the hypophyses of rats under various experimental conditions. Anat. Rec. 45, 232 (1930). — MASSON, G.: Spermatogenetic activity of various steroids. Amer. J. med. Sci. 209, 324 (1945). —. MASSON, R.: Etude sur le séminome. Rev. canad. Biol. 5, 361 (1946). — MASTERS, W. H., and M. H. GRODY: Estrogen-androgen substitution therapy in the aged female. II. Clinical response. Obstet. and Gynec. 2, 139 (1953). — MAZER, M., and C. MAZER: The effects of testosterone propionate on the ovariectomized mature rat. Endocrinology **26**, 662 (1940). — McArthur, J. W.: The identification of pituitary interstitial cell stimulating hormone in human urine. Endocrinology **50**, 304 (1952a). — The bioassay of pituitary interstitial cell stimulating hormone (ICSH) in human urine: preliminary report. J. clin. Endocr. **12**, 914 (1952b). — McCann, S. M.: Effect of hypothalamic lesions on adrenal cortical response to stress. Amer. J. Physiol. **171**, 746 (1952). — McCollum, D.: Clinical study of the spermatogenesis of undescended testicles. Arch. Surg. (Chicago) **31**, 290 (1935). — McCullagh, E. P.: Testicular dysfunction. Bull. N.Y. Acad. Med. **24**, 341 (1948a). — Sex hormone deficiencies some clinical considerations. Recent Progr. Hormone Res. **2**, 295 (1948b). — McCullagh, E. P., J. C. Beck and C. A. Schaffenburg: A syndrome of eunuchoidism with spermatogenesis, normal urinary FSH and low or normal ICSH ("fertile eunuchs"). J. clin. Endocr. **13**, 489 (1953). — McCullagh, E. P., and F. J. Hruby: Testis-pituitary interrelationship. J. clin. Endocr. **19**, 113 (1949). — McCullagh, E. P., and A. E. Leiser: Turner's syndrome and Laurence-Moon-Biedl-syndrome in siblings. J. clin. Endocr. **17**, 985 (1957). — McCullagh, E. P., and F. J. McGurl: Effects of testosterone propionate on epiphyseal closure, sodium and chloride balance and on sperm counts. Endocrinology **26**, 377 (1940). — McCullagh, E. P., H. S. Rosenberg and N. Norman: Tumor of the tuber cinereum with precocious puberty: case report with hormone assays. J. clin. Endocr. **20**, 1286 (1960). — McCullagh, E. P., R. W. Schneider, W. Bowman and M. B. Smith: Adrenal and testicular deficiency. J. clin. Endocr. **8**, 275 (1948c). — McCullagh, E. P., W. T. Sirridge and H. W. McIntosh: Gametogenic failure with high urinary gonadotropin (FSH). J. clin. Endocr. **10**, 1533 (1950). — McCullagh, E. P., and E. L. Walsh: Experimental hypertrophy and atrophy of the prostate gland. Endocrinology **19**, 466 (1935). — McLean, N., J. M. Mitchell, D. G. Harnden, J. Williams, P. Jacobs, K. Buckton, A. G. Baikie, W. M. C. Brown, J. A. McBride, J. A. Strong, H. G. Close and D. C. Jones: A survey of sex-chromosome abnormalities among 4514 mental defectives. Lancet **1962 I**, 293. — Medeiros, B. de, N. Botelko y F. Fernandes: Alguns comentários sobre uma centena de casos de criptorquidia. Rev. ibér. Endocr. **4**, 331 (1957). — Melicow, M. M., J. N. Robinson, W. Ivers and L. K. Rainsford: Interstitial cell tumors of testis. J. Urol. (Baltimore) **62**, 672 (1949). — Meyer, A. S.: Conversion of 19-hydroxy-Δ4-androstene-3,7-dione to estrone by endocrine tissue. Biochim. biophys. Acta **17**, 441 (1955). — Meyer, J. E.: Pubertas praecox. Arch. Psychiat. Nervenkr. **118**, 378 (1948). — Meyer, R.: Zum Mangel der Geschlechtsdrüsen mit und ohne zwittrige Erscheinungen. Virchows Arch. path. Anat. **255**, 33 (1925). — Meyer, R. K.: Influence of oestrin in gonad-stimulating complex of anterior pituitary of castrated male and female rats. Endocrinology **16**, 655 (1932). — Meyer, R. K., S. L. Leonard, F. L. Hisaw and S. J. Martin: Effect of eostrin on gonad stimulating power of hypophysis. Proc. Soc. exp. Biol. (N.Y.) **27**, 702 (1930). — Midulla, M.: La sindrome dello pterygium e la disgenesia delle gonadi. Pediat. int. (Roma) **5**, 1 (1955). — Migeon, C. L., and L. J. Gardner: Urinary estrogens (measured fluorometrically and biologically) in hyperadrenocorticism: influence of cortisone, compound F, compound B and ACTH. J. clin. Endocr. **12**, 1513 (1952). — Migeon, C. J., A. R. Keller, B. Lawrence and T. H. Shepard: Dehydroepiandrosterone and androsterone levels in human plasma. Effect of age and sex; day-to-day and diurnal variation. J. clin. Endocr. **17**, 1051 (1957). — Migeon, C. J., P. E. Wall and J. Bertrand: Some aspects of the metabolism of 16-C14-estrone in normal individuals. J. clin. Invest. **38**, 619 (1959). — Miller, O. J., W. R. Berg, R. D. Schmickel and W. Tretter: A family with an XXXXY male, a leukaemic male, and two 21-trisomic mongoloid females. Lancet **1961 II**, 78. — Mills, J. H.: The transport state of steroid hormones. In: ed. P. C. Williams and C. R. Austin, p. 81. Cambridge: Cambridge University press 1961. Cell mechanisms in hormone production and action. — Moore, C. R.: The behavior of the testis in transplantation, experimental cryptorchidism, vasectomy, scrotal insulation and heat application. Endocrinology **8**, 493 (1924). — Moore, C. R., T. F. Gallagher and F. C. Koch: The effects of extracts of testis in correcting the castrated condition in the fowl and in the mammal. Endocrinology **13**, 367 (1929). — Moore, C. R., and D. Price: Gonad hormone functions and the reciprocal influence between gonads and hypophysis with its bearing on the problem of sex hormone antagonism. Amer. J. Anat. **50**, 13 (1932). — Some effects of synthetically prepared male hormone (androsterone) in the rat. Endocrinology **21**, 313 (1937). — Some effects of testosterone and testosterone-propionate in the rat. Anat. Rec. **71**, 59 (1958). — Moore, K. L.: Sex reversal in newborn babys. Lancet **1959 I**, 217. — Moore, K. L., and M. L. Barr: Morphology of the nerve cell nucleus in mammals, with special reference to the sex chromatin. J. comp. Neurol. **98**, 213 (1953). — Nuclear morphology, according to sex, in human tissue. Acta anat. (Basel) **21**, 197 (1954). — Smears from the oral mucosa in the defection of chromosomal sex. Lancet **1955 II**, 57. — Moricard, R.: Posologic pondérale de l'hormonothérapie androgénique et gonadotrophique. In: La fonction endocrine du testicule, p. 480. Paris: Masson & Cie. 1957. — Morsier, G. de: Etudes sur les dysraphies crânio encéphaliques. Arch. suisse neurol. **74**, 309 (1955). — Mortimore, G. E., C. A. Paulsen and C. G. Heller:

The effect of steroids and lactone derivates on hypophyseal gonadotropin content. Endocrinology 48, 143 (1951). — Mottram, J. C., and W. Cramer: Effect of exposure to radium on metabolism and tumor growth in the rat and special effects on testis and pituitary. Quart. J. exp. Physiol. 13, 209 (1923). — Mudal, S., and C. H. Ockey: The "double male": A new chromosome constitution in Klinefelter's syndrome. Lancet 1960 II, 492. — Deletion of Y chromosome in a family with muscular dystrophy and hypospadias. Brit. med. J. 1962 I, 291. — Mueller, A. M., R. J. Dorfman and E. L. Sevringhaus: Metabolism of the steroid hormones: The isolation of an androgen from human urine containing an 11-oxygen substitution in the steroid ring. Endocrinology 38, 19 (1946). — Mueller, G. C.: A discussion of the mechanism of action of steroid hormones. Cancer Res. 17, 490 (1957). — Munro, S. S.: Über einen Fall von Eunuchoidismus. Z. menschl. Vererb.- u. Konstit.-Lehre 14, 401 (1929). — Murlin, J. R., C. D. Kochakian, C. L. Spurr and R. A. Harvey: Influence of androgens on the growth and metastasis of the brown-pearce epithelioma. Arch. Path. (Chicago) 28, 777 (1939).

Nadler, C. S., W. A. Steiger, M. Troncelleti and T. M. Ducant: Dystrophia myotonica. J. clin. Endocr. 10, 630 (1950). — Nalbandor, A. F., and L. Card: Effect of FSH and LH upon the ovaries of immature chicks and lowproducing hens. Endocrinology 38, 71 (1946). — Nathanson, J. T.: Studies on the etiology of human breast disease. I. Urinary excretion of FSH, estrogens and 17-ketosteroids in adolescent mastitis of males. J. clin. Endocr. 2, 311 (1942). — Nathanson, J. T., and J. C. Aub: Excretion of sex hormones in abnormalities of puberty. J. clin. Endocr. 3, 321 (1943). — Nathanson, J. T., and L. E. Towne: The urinary excretion of estrogens, androgens and FSH following the administration of testosterone to human female castrates. Endocrinology 25, 754 (1939). — Nathanson, J. T., L. E. Towne and J. C. Aub: Normal excretion of sex hormones in childhood. Endocrinology 28, 851 (1941). — Nathanson, J. T., and H. Wilson: Factors affecting colorimetric urinary 17-ketosteroid determination. Endocrinology 33, 189 (1943 a). — Nation, E. F., H. A. Edmondsen and R. W. Hammack: Interstitial cell tumors of testis. Arch. Surg. (Chicago) 48, 415 (1944). — Neher, R., P. Oesaulles, E. Vischer, P. Weiland u. A. Wettstein: Isolierung, Konstitution und Synthese eines neuen Steroids aus Nebennieren. Helv. chim. Acta 41, 1667 (1958). — Nelson, D. H., and L. T. Samuels: A method for the determination of 17-hydroxycorticosteroids in blood: 17-hydroxycorticosterone in the peripheral circulation. J. clin. Endocr. 12, 519 (1952). — Nelson, W. O.: Effect of gonadotropic hormone injections upon hypophysis and sex-accessories of experimental cryptorchid rats. Proc. Soc. exp. Biol. (N.Y.) 31, 1192 (1934). — Some factors involved in the control of the gametogenic and endocrine functions of the testis. Cold Spr. Harb. Symp. quant. Biol. 5, 123 (1927). — Testicular morphology in eunuchoidal and infertile man. Fertil. and Steril. 1, 477 (1950). — Mammalian spermatogenesis: Effect of experimental cryptorchidism in the rat and non-descent of the testis in man. Recent Progr. Hormone Res. 6, 29 (1951). — Interpretation of testicular biopsy. J. Amer. med. Ass. 151, 449 (1953a). — Some problems of testicular function. J. Urol. (Baltimore) 69, 325 (1953b). — Sex differences in human nuclei with particular reference to the "Klinefelter syndrom", gonadal agenesie and other types of hermaphroditism. Acta endocr. (Kbh.) 23, 227 (1956). — Nelson, W. O., and C. G. Heller: Diseases of the reproductive system. Ann. Rev. Med. 2, 179 (1951). — Nelson, W. O., and C. G. Merckel: Effects of androgenic substances in the female rat. Proc. Soc. exp. Biol. (N.Y.) 36, 823 (1937). — Nelson, W. O., and S. J. Segal: Genetic, developmental and hormonal aspects of gonadal dysgenesis and sex inversion in man. J. clin. Endocr. 17, 737 (1957). — Nesbit, R. M., and W. C. Baum: Endocrine control of prostatic carcinoma. J. Amer. med. Ass. 143, 1317 (1950). — Nielsen, R. L., R. V. Sniffen, F. A. Simmons, F. Albright and H. Henneman: Prolonged human chorionic gonadotropin therapy in male "eunuchoidism with low FSH". J. clin. Endocr. 16, 968 (1956). — Nikolowski, E.: Persönliche Mitteilung. — Novak, E.: The constitutional type of female precocious puberty with a report of 9 cases. Amer. J. Obstet. 47, 20 (1944). — Nowakowski, H.: Zur Auslösung der Ovulation durch elektrische Reizung des Hypothalamus beim Kaninchen und ihre Beeinflussung durch Rückenmarksdurchschneidung. Acta neuroveg. (Wien) 1, 13 (1950). — Störungen der Keimdrüsenfunktion beim Manne. In Handbuch der medizinischen Sexualforschung (H. Giese). Stuttgart: Ferdinand Enke 1954. — Diagnosis and therapy of male hypogonadism. Acta endocr. (Kbh.) 31, 117 (1957). — Der Hypogonadismus im Knaben- und Mannesalter. Ergebn. inn. Med. Kinderheilk. 12, 219 (1959). — Nowakowski, H., u. G. Assmann: Die Therapie des idiopathischen hypophysären Kleinwuchses mit Choriongonadotropin. In: 4. Symp. Dtsch. Ges. Endokrinologie. Berlin-Göttingen-Heidelberg: Springer 1957. — Nowakowski, H., W. Lenz, S. Bergman u. J. Reitaler: Chromosomenbefunde beim echten Klinefelter-Syndrom. Acta endocr. (Kbh.) 34, 483 (1960). — Nowakowski, H., W. Lenz u. J. Parade: Diskrepanz zwischen Chromatinbefund und chromosomalem Geschlecht beim Klinefelter-Syndrom. Klin. Wschr. 1958a, 683. — Nowakowski, H., u. J. Parada: Klinische Erfahrungen mit 19-Nortestosteron-phenylpropionat. Dtsch. med.

Wschr. **34**, 1421 (1958b). — NOWAKOWSKI, H., u. L. PÜSCHEL: Zit. nach A. JORES, Die Nebennieren und ihre Krankheiten. In Handbuch der inneren Medizin, Bd. VII/1, S. 256. Berlin-Göttingen-Heidelberg: Springer 1955. — NOWAKOWSKI, H., u. H. SCHMIDT: Das Altern der männlichen Keimdrüsen. In: Hormone und Psyche, S. 207. Berlin-Göttingen-Heidelberg: Springer 1948.

OBERDISSE, K.: Die partielle Vorderlappeninsuffizienz. In 4. Symp. Dtsch. Ges. Endokrinologie, S. 40. Berlin-Göttingen-Heidelberg: Springer 1957. — OBERNDORFER, S.: Die inneren männlichen Geschlechtsorgane. In Handbuch der speziellen pathologischen Anatomie, Bd. VI/3, S. 427. Berlin: Springer 1931. — OERTEL, G. W., S. P. WEISS and K. B. EIK-NES: Determination of progesterone in human blood plasma. J. clin. Endocr. **19**, 213 (1959). — OETTLÉ, A. G., D. RABINOWITZ and H. C. SEFTEL: The Laurence-Moon-syndrom with germinal aplasia of the teatis. J. clin. Endocr. **20**, 683 (1960). — OHNO, S., and S. MAKINO: The single-x nature of sex chromatin in man. Lancet **1961 I**, 78. — OLESEN, H.: Morphologiske Sperma- og Testis-undersogelser. Copenhagen: Munksgaard 1948. — OLIVER, J.: Über den angeborenen Mangel beider Eierstöcke. Frankfurt. Z. Path. **29**, 477 (1923). — OSTER, H.: Die Reifeentwicklung unserer Jugend. In: Deutsche Nachkriegskinder (C. COEPER, W. HAGER u. H. THOMAE). Stuttgart: Georg Thieme 1954. — OVERZIER, C.: Idiopathischer sekundärer Hypogonadismus. 4. Symp. Dtsch. Ges. Endokrinologie. Berlin-Göttingen-Heidelberg: Springer 1956. — Klinik der Störungen der embryonalen Geschlechtsdifferenzierung. Verh. dtsch. Kongr. inn. Med. **64**, 425 (1958a). — Klinik der Störungen der embryonalen Geschlechtsdifferenz. Verh. dtsch. Ges. inn. Med. **64**, 448 (1958b). — Die Intersexualität. Stuttgart: Georg Thieme 1961. — OVERZIER, C., u. H. LINDEN: Anorchismus. Gynaecologia (Basel) **142**, 215 (1956).

P'AN, S. Y., H. B. VAN DYKE, H. KANNITZ and C. A. SLANETZ: Effect of vitamin-E deficiency on amount of gonadotropin in the anterior pituitary of rats. Proc. Soc. exp. Biol. (N.Y.) **72**, 523 (1949). — PAPANICOLAOU, G. N., H. S. RIPLEY and E. SHORR: Suppressive action of testosterone propionate on menstruation and its effect on vaginal mears. Endocrinology **24**, 339 (1939). — PAPANICOLAOU, G. N., and E. SHORR: The action of ovarian follicular hormone in the menopause, as indicated by vaginal smears. Amer. J. Obstet. Gynec. **31**, 806 (1936). — PARKES, A., and S. ZUCKERMAN: Experimental hyperplasia of the prostate. Lancet **1935 I**, 925. — Ovarian responses to testosterone propionate. J. Physiol. (Lond.) **93**, 16 (1938). — PARKES-WEBER, F.: Cutaneou striae, purpura, high blood pressure, amenorrhea, and obesity of type sometimes connected with cortical tumor of adrenal glands. Brit. J. Derm. **38**, 1 (1926). — PASQUALINI, R.Q.: Hypoandrogenic syndrome with normal spermatogenesis. J. clin. Endocr. **13**, 128 (1953). — PASQUALINI, R. Q., G. VIDAL and G. E. BUR: Psychopathology of Klinefelter's syndrome. Review of 31 cases. Lancet **1957 II**, 164. — PATTON, J. F., D. N. SEITZMANN and P. A. ZONE: Diagnosis and treatment of testicular tumors. Amer. J. Surg. **99**, 525 (1960). — PEARLMAN, W. H.: Circulating steroid hormone levels in relation to steroid hormone production. Ciba Found. Coll. Endocrinol. **11**, 233 (1957). — PEDERSEN-BJERGAARD, K.: Titrierung von Oestrin und gonadotropem Hormon im Harn. Zbl. Gynäk. **60**, 372 (1936). — PEDERSEN-BJERGAARD, K., and M. TENNESEN: Oestrogenic, androgenic and gonadotrophic substances in the urine of normal women. Acta endocr. (Kbh.) **1**, 38 (1948). — PEETERS, F., M. VAN ROY u. H. OEYEN: Ovulationsunterdrückung durch Prostagene. Geburtsh. u. Frauenheilk. **20**, 12, 1306 (1960). — PENDL, C., u. A. SCHERLACHER: Pubertas praecox (Hypernephrom der Leber). Z. Kinderheilk. **4**, 269 (1950). — PERLMAN, P. L.: The functional significance of testis cholesterol in the rat: effects of hypophysectomy and cryptorchidism. Endocrinology **46**, 341 (1950). — PERLMAN, R. M.: Spermatogenesis following the administration of androgen and gonadotrophin in a case of eunuchoidism. J. clin. Endocr. **9**, 163 (1949). — PERLOFF, W. H., K. B. CONGER and L. M. LEVY: Female pseudohermaphrodism; 2 unusual cases. J. clin. Endocr. **13**, 783 (1953).— PERSSON, B. H.: Zit. in: Östrogene beim Menschen von E. DICZFALUSY u. CH. LAURITZEN. Berlin-Göttingen-Heidelberg: Springer 1961. — PFEIFFER, K.: Röntgenbefunde behandelter Knochenmetastasen des Mammakarzinoms unter besonderer Berücksichtigung einer kombinierten Behandlung mit Röntgenstrahlen und Sexualhormonen. Strahlentherapie **103**, 257 (1957). — PHILIPP, E.: Fünf durch Laparatomie sichergestellte Fälle von Fehlen der weiblichen Keimdrüsen. Dtsch. med. Wschr. **1952**, 1209. — Die Fehlbildungen der Keimdrüsen. Dtsch. med. Wschr. **1956**, 1298. — PHOENIX, C. H., R. W. GOY, A. A. GERALL and W. C. YOUNG: Organizing action of prenatally administered testosterone propionate in the tissues mediating mating behavior in the female guinea pig. Endocrinology **65**, 369 (1959). — PINCUS, G.: Studies of the role of the adrenal cortex in the stress of human subjects. Recent Progr. Hormone Res. **1**, 123 (1947). — The physiology of ovarian and testis hormones. In: The hormones, vol. 3. New York: Acad. Press, Inc. 1955. — PINCUS, G., R. J. DORFMAN, L. P. ROMANOFF, B. L. RUBIN, E. BLOCH, J. CARLO and H. FREEMAN: Steroid metabolism in aging men and women. Recent Progr. Hormone Res. **11**, 307 (1955). — PINCUS, G., A. E. RAKOFF, E. M. COHN and H. J. TUMEN: Hormonal studies in patients with chronic liver disease. Gastroenterology **19**, 735 (1951). — PICK, G.: Über den angeborenen Eierstocksmangel. Beitr. path. Anat. **98**, 218 (1937). — PICK, L.: Über Adenome der männlichen und weiblichen Keimdrüse bei Hermaphroditismus verus und spurius nebst Bemerkungen über das endometriumähnliche Adenom am inneren weiblichen Genitale. Klin. Wschr. **42**, 502 (1905). — PLUM, P.: Spermatogenesis in a eunuchoid man after 4 years of hormone therapy. Acta med. scand. **115**, 36 (1943). — PLUNKETT, E. R., and M. L. BARR: Testicular dysgenesis affecting the seminiferous tubules principally, with chromatinpositive nuclei. Lancet **1956 II**, 853. — POLANI, P. E.: Turner's syndrome and allied conditions. Clinical features and chromosome abnormalities. Brit. med. Bull. **17**, 201 (1961). — POLANI, P. E., P. M. F. BISHOP, M. A. FERGUSON-SMITH, B. LENNOX, J. STEWART and A. PRADER: Colom vision studies and the X-chromosome constitution of patients with Klinefelter's syndrome. Nature (Lond.) **102**, 1092 (1958). — POLANI, P. E., W. F. HUNTER and B. LENNOX: Chromosomal sex in Turner's syndrome with coarctation of the aorta. Lancet **1954 II**, 120. — POWELL, T. D.: Value of correlating hormonal tests with histologic sections in tumor of testis. J. Urol. (Baltimore) **39**, 522 (1938). — PRADER, A.: Diagnose und Therapie des hypophysären Zwergwuchses im Kindesalter. Schweiz. med. Wschr. **84**, 375 (1954). — Gonadendysgenesie (Gonadenagenesie, Ovaragenesie, Turner-Syndrom). In: Klinik der inneren Sekretion, S. 668. Berlin-Göttingen-Heidelberg: Springer 1957. — PRADER, A., J. SCHNEIDER, J. M. FRANCES and W. ZÜBLIN: Frequency of the true (chromatinpositive) Klinefelter's syndrome. Lancet **1958 I**, 968. — PRADER, A., u. R. E. SIEBENMANN: Das echte Klinefelter-Syndrom vor der Pubertät. Schweiz. med. Wschr. **1958**, 607. — PRISEL, A.: Die Mißbildungen der männlichen Geschlechtsorgane. In Handbuch der speziellen pathologischen Anatomie und Histologie, Bd. VI. Berlin: Springer 1931. — PRUNTY, F. T. G., R. R. McSWINEY and B. E. CLAYTON: Primary gonadal insufficiency in a girl and a boy. J. clin. Endocr. **13**, 1480 (1953).

RABINOWITZ, J. L.: The biosynthesis of radioactive β-hydroxyisovaleric acid in rat liver. Amer. chem. Soc. **77**, 1295 (1955). — RABOCH, J., and J. SIPOVÁ: The mental level in 47 cases of true Klinefelter's syndrome. Acta endocr. (Kbh.) **36**, 404 (1961). — RABOCH, J., u. Z. ZÁHOR: Über die Fertilität von Männern mit Kryptorchismus. Schweiz. med. Wschr. **1955**, 1196. — RANDOLPH, P. W., A. J. LOSTROH, R. GRATTAROLA, P. G. SQUIRE and CH. H. LI: Effect of ovine interstitial cell-stimulating hormone on spermatogenesis in the hypophysectomized mouse. Endocrinology **65**, 433 (1959). — RAPAPORT, E., M. Z. GOLDBERG, G. S. GORDAN and F. HINMAN: Mortality in surgically treated adrenocortical tumors, review of cases reported for 20 years periods, 1930—1949. Postgrad. med. **11**, 325 (1952). — RAVERA, P.: Banti syndrome (fibrocongestive splenomegaly). Arch. intern. Med. **66**, 879 (1940). — Splenoportal renous obstruction without splenomegaly. Arch. intern. Med. **72**, 786 (1943). — RAYNAUD, A., et M. FRILLEY: Destruction des glandes génitales de l'embryon de souris par une irradiation au moyen des rayon X, 13 J. Ann. Endocr. (Paris) **8**, 400 (1947). — REES, G. P. VAN: Influence of steroid sex hormones on the FSH-release by rat hypophyses in vitro. Acta endocr. (Kbh.) **36**, 485 (1961). — REFARZO-MEMBRIVES, J., A. TRABUCCO and G. A. ESCARDÓ: A case of rudimentary testes, delayed growth and congenital malformations. Turner's syndrom in a male. J. clin. Endocr. **9**, 1333 (1949). — REICHERT, F. L.: The results of replacement therapy in an hypophysectomized puppy: four months of treatment with daily pituitary heterotransplants. Endocrinology **12**, 451 (1928). — REIFENSTEIN, E. C.: Besondere Wirkung der Depotpräparate des Testosterons auf die Natrium-, Phosphor- und Calziumretention beim Kastraten. In: Hormone und Psyche, S. 161. Berlin-Göttingen-Heidelberg: Springer 1958. — REILLY, W. A., H. LISSER and J. HINMAN: Pseudo-sexual-precocity, adrenal cortical syndrome in pre-adolescent girls. Endocrinology **24**, 91 (1939). — REYNOLDS, S. R. M.: The effect of oestrine on the uterine fistula during pseudopregnancy. Amer. J. Physiol. **98**, 230 (1931). — RIDDLE, O., R. W. BATES and E. L. LAHR: Prolactin induces brovdiness in fowl. Amer. J. Physiol. **111**, 352 (1935). — ROBERTS, S., and C. M. SZEGO: Steroid interaction in the metabolism of reproductive target organs. Physiol. Rev. **33**, 593 (1953a). — The influence of steroids on uterine respiration and glycolysis. J. biol. Chem. **201**, 21 (1953b). — ROBERTSON, M. E., M. STIEFEL and J. C. LAIDLAW: The influence of estrogen on the secretion disposition and biologic activity of cortisol. J. clin. Endocr. **19**, 1381 (1959). — ROBINSON, J. N., and E. T. ENGLE: Some observations on cryptorchid testis. J. Urol. (Baltimore) **71**, 726 (1954). — ROBSON, J. M.: Quantitative data on the inhibition of oestrus by testosterone, progesterone, and certain other compounds. J. Physiol. (Lond.) **92**, 371 (1938). — ROMEIS, B.: Hoden, samenableitende Organe und accessorische Geschlechtsdrüsen. In Handbuch der normalen und pathologischen Physiologie, Bd. 14, S. 693. Berlin: Springer 1926. — Über ein beinahe acht Jahre altes Hodentransplantat mit erhaltener inkretorischer Funktion. Klin. Wschr. **12**, 1640 (1933). — Einfluß der Androgene auf den weiblichen Genitalapparat. Anat. Anz. **57**, Suppl. **75**, 207 (1944). — ROSEMBERG, E.: Urinary gonadotropin excretion measured by the mouse uterine response, employing estrone as the standard reference material. J. clin.

Endocr. **20**, 306 (1960 b). — Rosemberg, E., F. X. Dufault, E. Bloch, E. Budnitz, P. Butler and J. Brem: The effects of progressive reduction of sodium intake on adrenal steroid excretion and electrolyte balance in a case of congenital adrenal hyperplasia of the saltlosing type. J. clin. Endocr. **20**, 214 (1960a). — Rosenman, R. H., M. Friedman and S. O. Byers: The effect of upon the hepatic synthesis of cholesterol. Endocrinology **51**, 142 (1952). — Rössle, R., u. F. Roulet: Maß und Zahl in der Pathologie. Berlin: Springer 1932. — Rössle, R., u. J. Wallart: Der angeborene Mangel der Eierstöcke und seine grundsätzliche Bedeutung für die Theorie der Geschlechtsbestimmung. Beitr. path. Anat. **84**, 401 (1930). — Ross, C. F., L. Crome and D. Y. Mackenzie: The Laurence-Moon-Biedl syndrome. J. Path. Bact. **72**, 161 (1956). — Rossi, E., et A. Caflisch: Le syndrome du pterygium status Bonnevie-Ullrich, dystrophia brevicolli congenita, syndrome de Turner et arthromyodysplasia congenita. Helv. paediat. Acta **6**, 119 (1951). — Roth, A. A.: Familial eunuchoidism: the Laurence-Moon-Biedl syndrome. J. Urol. (Baltimore) **57**, 427 (1947). — Rowlands, J. W., and E. P. Sharply-Schafer: Effect of oestradiol benzoate on amount of gonadotropin found in pituitary gland and urine of post menopausal women. Brit. med. J. **1940 I**, 205. — Rowlands, J. W., and A. W. Spence: Production of antigonadotrophic activity in man by injection of extract of pregnant males serum. Brit. med. J. **1939 II**, 947. — Rowlands, R. P., G. W. Nicholson and F. Parkes-Weber: Growth of left testicle with precocious sexual and bodily development. Guy's Hosp. Rep. **79**, 401 (1929). — Roy, G. V. Le: The medical sequelae of the atomic bomb explosion. J. Amer. med. Ass. **134**, 1143 (1947). — Royer, P., et J. Rivron: La précocité isosexuelle du garcon. In: La fonction endocrine du testicule. Paris: Masson & Cie. 1957. — Rubinstein, H. S., and A. A. Kurland: The effect of testosterone propionate on the rat testis. Endocrinology **28**, 495 (1941). — Rush, H. P., J. B. Bilderback and D. Slocum: Pubertas praecox (macrogenitosomia). Endocrinology **21**, 404 (1937). — Ruzicka, L., M. W. Goldberg u. H. Brüngger: Über die Gewinnung von 3-Chlor- und 3-Oxy-ätioallocholanon-(17). Synthese einer Verbindung von den Eigenschaften des Testikelhormons. Helv. chim. Acta **17**, 1389 (1934). — Ruzicka, L., M. W. Goldberg u. H. R. Rosenberg: Herstellung des 17-Methyl-testosterons und anderer Androsten- und Androstenderivate. Zusammenhänge zwischen chemischer Konstitution und männlicher Hormonwirkung. Helv. chim. Acta **18**, 1487 (1935). — Ruzicka, L., u. V. Prelog: Untersuchungen von Extrakten. Helv. chim. Acta **26**, 975 (1943). — Ryan, E. J., and E. P. McCullagh: Congenital hypogonadism in the male. Proc. centr. clin. Res. **19**, 43 (1946). — Ryan, K. J., and L. L. Engel: The interconversion of estrone and estradiol-17β by rat liver slices. Endocrinology **52**, 277 (1953).

Salmon, U. J.: Effect of testosterone propionate upon gonadotropic hormone excretion and vaginal smears of human female castrate. Proc. Soc. exp. Biol. (N.Y.) **37**, 488 (1937). — Samuels, L. T.: The metabolism of androgens by tissues. Recent Progr. Hormone Res. **4**, 65 (1949). — Discussion of Dr. Gallagher's paper. Cancer Res. **17**, 530 (1957). — In Discussion in W. Dirschel: Einwirkung von Steroidhormonen auf Enzyme und Enzymsysteme. Proc. fourth intern. Congr. Biochem. Vienna 1958 IV, S. 123. — Sand, K., and H. Okkels: Histological variability of the testis from normal and sexual-abnormal castrated men. Endokrinologie **19**, 369 (1938). — Sandberg, A. A., and W. R. Slaunwhite: Studies on phenolic steroids in human subjects. II. The metabolic fate and hepatobiliary euteric circulation of C 14-estrone and C 14-estradiol in woman. J. clin. Invest. **36**, 1266 (1957). — J. clin. Invest. **38**, 1290 (1959). — Sandblom, Philip: Precocious sexual development produced by an interstitial cell tumor of the testis. Acta endocr. (Kbh.) **1**, 107 (1948). — Saunders, F. L., and V. A. Drill: The myotrophic and androgenic effects of 17-ethyl-19-nortestosterone and related compounds. Endocrinology **58**, 567 (1956). — Savard, K., K. Andrec, L. Brooksbank, C. Reyneri and R. J. Dorfman: The biosynthesis of estrone and progesterone in the pregnant mare. J. biol. Chem. **231**, 765 (1958). — Savard, K., and J. W. Goldzieher: Biosynthesis of steroids in stallion testis tissue. Endocrinology **66**, 617 (1960). — Savard, K., M. Gut, R. J. Dorfman, J. L. Gabrilove and L. J. Soffer: Formation of androgens by human arrhenoblastoma tissue in vitro. J. clin. Endocr. **21**, 170 (1961). — Savard, K. R., J. Dorfman, B. Baggett and L. L. Engel: Biosynthesis of androgens from progesterone by human testicular tissue in vitro. J. clin. Endocr. **16**, 12, 1629 (1956). — Savard, K. R., I. Dorfman and E. Pontasse: Biogenesis of androgens in the human testis. J. clin. Endocr. **12**, 935 (1952). — Sawyer, C. H.: Rhinencephalic involvement in pituitary activation by intraventricular histamine in the rabbit under nembutal anesthesia. Amer. J. Physiol. **180**, 37 (1955). — Schattmann, K.: Perlinguale Testoviron-Medikation bei Alterskrankheiten. Ärztl. Wschr. 1950, 615. — Schiller, J., and G. Pincus: The fate of α-estradiol and of estriol injected into a human male subject. Arch. Biochem. **2**, 317 (1946). — Schmalz, A.: Über einen Fall von Hirntumor mit Pubertas praecox. Beitr. path. Anat. **73**, 168 (1925). — Schmidt, H.: Die Suprarenal-Genital-Syndrome (Kraus). Virchows Arch. path. Anat. **251**, 8 (1924). — Schmidt, G. W., u. E. Tonutti: Pseudopubertas praecox und unvollständige Pubertas praecox bei einem

Leydig-Zell-Tumor des Hodens. Helv. paediatr. Acta 11, 436 (1956). — Schmidt-Voigt, J.: Das Körperbild im Reifungsalter. Ergebn. inn. Med. Kinderheilk. 64, 995 (1945). — Schmith, G. V., O. W. Smith, S. Schiller and B. S. Brookline: Clinical experiments in relation to the excretion of the estrogens. Amer. J. Obstet. Gynec. 44, 606 (1942). — Schoeller, W., M. Dohrn u. W. Hohlweg: Die Überlegenheit des weiblichen Hormons in seiner Wirkung auf die männliche und weibliche Kastratenhypophyse gegenüber männlichen Hormonen. Klin. Wschr. 1936, 1907. — Schönenberg, H., K. Hollstein u. W. Kosenow: Das klinische Bild und das chromosomale Geschlecht der Gonadendysgenesie an Hand von 15 eigenen Beobachtungen. Z. Kinderheilk. 79, 383 (1957). — Schonfeld, W. A.: Primary and secondary sexual characteristics. Amer. J. Dis. Child. 65, 535 (1943). — Schuchardt, E.: Zur quantitativen Beurteilung menschlicher Hodenbiopsien. In 1. Symp. Dtsch. Ges. Endokrinologie, Febr./März 1953, S. 159. Berlin-Göttingen-Heidelberg: Springer 1955. — Schürmann, P.: Über einen Fall von allgemeinem Infantilismus, bedingt durch beiderseitigen Eierstocksmangel. Virchows Arch. path. Anat. 263, 649 (1927). — Schreiner, W. E.: Über eine hereditäre Form von Pseudohermaphroditismus masculinus („testikuläre Feminisierung"). Geburtsh. u. Frauenheilk. 19, 1110 (1959). — Scorer, C. G.: Descent of the testicle in the first year of life. Brit. J. Urol. 27, 374 (1955). — Scott, W. W., and C. Vermeulen: Studies on prostatic cancer. J. clin. Endocr. 2, 450 (1942). — Seckel, H. P.: II. Six examples of precocious sexual development. Amer. J. Dis. Child. 79, 278 (1950). — Seckel, H. P., W. W. Scott and E. P. Benditt: I. Six examples of precocious sexual development. Amer. J. Dis. Child. 78, 484 (1949). — Seeman, A., et R. T. Saracino: Contribution à l'étude de la formation d'androgenes par l'ovaire. Acta endocr. (Kbh.) 37, 31 (1961). — Segaloff, A., D. Gordon, R. A. Carabasi, B. N. Horwitt, J. V. Schlosser and P. J. Murison: Hormonal therapy in cancer of the breast. Cancer (Philad.) 7, 758 (1954). — Segaloff, A., and S. L. Steelman: The human gonadotropins. Recent Progr. Hormone Res. 15, 127 (1959). — Selye, H., and S. Albert: The effect of various steroids in intact male rats. Amer. J. med. Sci. 204, 876 (1942). — Selye, H., and S. Friedman: The action of various steroid hormones on the testis. Endocrinology 28, 129 (1941). — Selye, H., and S. Renaud: On the anticatabolic and anticalcinatic effects of 17-ethyl-19-nortestosterone. Amer. J. med. Sci. 235, 1 (1958). — Shapiro, B.: Kann man mit Hypophysenvorderlappen den unterentwickelten männlichen Genitalapparat beim Menschen zum Wachstum anregen? Dtsch. med. Wschr. 56, 1605 (1930). — Shay, H., J. Gershon-Cohen, K. E. Paschkis and S. S. Fels: Inhibition and stimulating of testes in rats treated with testosterone propionate. Endocrinology 28, 485 (1941). — Shorr, E., G. N. Papanicolaou and B. F. Stimmel: Neutralization of ovarian follicular hormone in women by simultaneous administration of male sex hormone. Proc. Soc. exp. Biol. (N.Y.) 38, 759 (1938). — Siebke, H.: Ergebnisse von Mengenbestimmungen des Sexualhormons. Zbl. Gynäk. 53, 2450 (1929). — Sigrist, E.: Über drei Fälle von genuiner und einen Fall von cerebraler Pubertas praecox. Ann. paediat. (Basel) 155, 84 (1940). — Simmer, H.: Hormonbehandlung während der Schwangerschaft als Ursache eines Pseudohermaphroditismus femininus externus Neugeborener. Dtsch. med. Wschr. 4, 173 (1961). — Simmons, F. A.: Correlation of testicular biopsy material with semen analysis in male infertility. Ann. N.Y. Acad. Sci. 55, 643 (1952). — Simmons, F. A., and R. Sniffen: Testicular biopsy in sterile male. West. J. Surg. 55, 508 (1947). — Simpson, M. E., C. H. Li and H. M. Evans: Sensitivity of the reproductive system of hypophysectomized 40 days male rats to gonadotropic substances. Endocrinology 35, 96 (1944). — Simpson, M. E., C. H. Li and H. M. Evans: Synergism between pituitary follicle stimulating hormone (FSH) and human chorionic gonadotrophin. Endocrinology 48, 370 (1951). — Simpson, S. L., and C. A. Joll: Feminization in a male adult with carcinoma of the adrenal cortex. Endocrinology 22, 595 (1938). — Slaunwhite, W. R., and L. T. Samuels: Progesterone as a precursor of testicular androgens. J. biol. Chem. 220, 341 (1956). — Slotta, K. H., H. Ruschig u. E. Fels: Schwangerschaftshormon I und II. Hoppe-Seylers Z. physiol. Chem. 228, 207 (1934). — Smith, E. P.: Ablation and transplantation of the hypophysis in the rat. Anat. Rec. 32, 221 (1926). — Smith, O. W., and G. V. Smith: Endocrinology and related phenomena of the human menstrual cycle. Recent Progr. Hormone Res. 1, 239 (1952). — Smith, P. E.: Hypophysectomy and a replacement therapy in the rat. Amer. J. Anat. 45, 205 (1930). — Smith, P. S.: Maintenance and restoration of spermatogenesis in hypophysectomized rhesus monkeys by androgen administration. Yale J. Biol. Med. 17, 281 (1944). — Sniffen, R. C.: Histology of the normal and abnormal testis at puberty. Ann. N.Y. Acad. Sci. 55, 609 (1952). — Sniffen, R. C., R. P. Howard and F. A. Simmons: The testis. Abnormalities of spermatogenesis atresia of the excretory ducts. Arch. Path. (Chicago) 50, 285 (1950a). — The normal testis. Arch. Path. (Chicago) 50, 259 (1950b). — The testis. III. Absence of germinal cells, sclerosing tubular degeneration "male climacteric." Arch. Path. (Chicago) 51, 293 (1951). — Sobel, E. H., C. S. Raymond, K. V. Quinn and N. B. Talbot: The use of methyltestosterone to stimulate growth: relative influence on skeletal maturation and linear growth. J. clin.

Endocr. **16**, 241 (1956). — Sobel, F. H., R. C. Sniffen and W. B. Talbot: Use of testicular biopsies in the differential diagnosis of precocious puberty. Pediatrics **8**, 701 (1951). — Sohval, A. R.: Testicular dysgenesis as an etiologic factor in cryptorchidism. J. Urol. (Baltimore) **72**, 693 (1954). — In L. J. Soffer: Diseases of endocrine glands. Edit. by H. Kimpton, p. 535. London 1956. — Sohval, A. R., and L. J. Soffer: Congenital testicular deficiency. J. clin. Endocr. **12**, 1229 (1952). — Congenital familial testicular deficiency. Amer. J. Med. **14**, 328 (1953). — Solomon, S. S., J. T. Lauman and S. Lieberman: The biosynthesis of Δ^4-androstendione and 17α-hydroxyprogesterone from progesterone by surviving human fetal adrenals. J. biol. Chem. **233**, 1084 (1958). — Solomon, S. S., R. van de Wiele and S. Lieberman: The "in vitro" synthesis of 17α-hydroxyprogesterone and Δ^4-androstene-3,17-dione from progesterone by bovine ovarian tissue. J. Amer. chem. Soc. **78**, 5453 (1956). — The in vitro synthesis of 17α-hydroxyprogesterone and Δ^4-androstene-3,17-dione from progesterone by bovine ovarian tissue. J. clin. Endocr. **61**, 171 (1961). — Somerford, A. E.: A case of interstitial cell tumour of the testis in a boy of eleven years. Brit. J. Urol. **13**, 13 (1941). — Sorsby, A., H. Avery and E. A. Cockayne: Obesity, hypo genitalism, mental, retardation, polydactyl, and retinal pigmentation. Quart. J. Med. **8**, 51 (1939). — Soulairac, A., et M. L. Soulairac: Modifications du comportement sexuel et du tractus génital du rat male après lésions hypothalamiques. C. R. Soc. Biol. (Paris) **150**, 1097 (1956). — Spangaro, S.: Über die histologischen Veränderungen des Hodens, Nebenhodens und Samenleiters von Geburt bis zum Greisenalter, mit besonderer Berücksichtigung der Hodenatrophie, des elastischen Gewebes und des Vorkommens von Kristallen im Hoden. Anat. H. **18**, 593 (1902). — Spatz, B.: Hypothalamic of precocious puberty. Dtsch. med. Wschr. **2**, 1929 (1956). — Spatz, H.: Das Hypophysen-Hypothalamus-System in Hinsicht auf die zentrale Steuerung der Sexualfunktion. In 1. Symp. Dtsch. Ges. Endokrinologie, 1953. Berlin-Göttingen-Heidelberg: Springer 1955. — Spencer, H., B. Kabakow, J. Samachson and D. Laszlo: Metabolic effects of mytatrienediol in man. J. clin. Endocr. **19**, 1581 (1959). — Stange, H. H., K. Rumphorst u. K. W. Schaumkell: Turner-Syndrom mit Vermännlichungserscheinungen. Zbl. Gynäk. **79**, 1281 (1957). — Steinach, E., u. H. Kun: Die entwicklungsmechanische Bedeutung der Hypophysis als Aktivator der Keimdrüseninkretion. Med. Klin. **24**, 524 (1928). — Steinach, E., H. Kun u. O. Peczenik: Beiträge zur Analyse der Sexualhormonwirkungen. Wien. klin. Wschr. **49**, 899 (1936). — Sternberg, J., and E. Pascoc-Dawson: Studies on the mechanism of the catabolic action of estrogens. Rev. canad. Biol. **18**, 23 (1959). — Stewart, C. A.: Interstitial cell tumor of the testes with hypergenitalism in child of 5 years. Amer. J. Cancer **26**, 144 (1936). — Stieve, H.: Entwicklung, Bau und Bedeutung der Keimdrüsenzwischenzellen. Ergebn. Anat. Entwickl.-Gesch. **23**, 1 (1921). — Stokes, P. E., M. Horwith, T. G. Pennington and B. Clarkson: 17α-Ethyl-19-nortestosterone as an anabolic agent and its effect on creatine metabolism and vaginal cytology in humans. Metabolism **8**, 5, 709 (1959). — Strauss, J., and A. M. Kligman: Androgenic effects of a progestional compound, 17α-ethynyl-19-nortestosterone (norlutin) on the human sebaceous gland. J. clin. Endocr. **21**, 218 (1961). — Stutte, H.: Pubertas praecox. In: Die Sexualität des Menschen. Stuttgart: Ferdinand Enke 1954. — Suchowsky, G. K., u. K. Junkmann: Experimentelle Untersuchungen an anabolen Steroiden. 8. Symp. Dtsch. Ges. Endokrinologie München 1961. — Sveringhaus, A. E.: Anterior hypophyseal cytology in relation to the reproductive hormones. In: Sex and Internal Secretions, p. 1045. Baltimore: Williams & Wilkins Company 1939. — Swyer, A. J., J. S. Berger, H. M. Gordon and D. Laszlo: Hypercalcaemia in osteolytic metastatic cancer of the breast. Amer. J. Med. **8**, 724 (1950). — Swyer, G. J.: Hormone assays in normal and abnormal pregnancies. Brit. med. J. **1952 I**, 619. — Gonadal dysgenesis. Brit. med. J. **1957 I**, 1421. — Swyer, G. J., and P. E. Hughesdon: A misleading testicular biopsy. In: Studies on Fertility, edit. by R. G. Harrison, p. 29. London 1954. — Szego, C. M., and S. Roberts: Nature of circulating estrogens. Fed. Proc. **5**, 103 (1946). — Steroid action and interaction in uterine metabolism. Recent Progr. Hormone Res. **8**, 419 (1953).

Talbot, N., and E. Sobel: Certain factors with influence the rate of growth and the duration of growth of children. Recent Progr. Hormone Res. **1**, 355 (1947). — Taubert, M., u. O. Weller: Chromatographische Gonadotropingewinnung. Klin. Wschr. **1956**, 84. — Taupitz, A.: Vergleichende Untersuchungen über die Nebenwirkungen der Östrogen-Therapie bei Anwendung verschiedener Hormonformen an Prostata-Karzinom und Prostata-Adenom-Patienten. Medizinische **1959**, 18. — Taupitz, A., E. Taupitz u. K. Otaguro: Tierexperimentelle Untersuchungen über die Leberverträglichkeit oestrogener Substanzen. Endokrinologie **39**, 5 (1960). — Taylor, F. B.: Histochemical changes in the ovaries of hormone and experimentally treated rats. Acta endocr. (Kbh.) **36**, 361 (1961). — Teilum, G.: Gonocytoma. Homologous ovarian and testicular tumors. Acta path. microbiol. scand. **23**, 242 (1946). — Thamdrup, E.: Macrogenitosomia caused by interstitial cell tumour of the testis a case in a $7^1/_2$-year old boy. Acta paediat. (Uppsala) **42**, 369 (1953). — Thompson, W. O., and H. J. HECKEL: Undescended testes. Present status of glandular therapy. J. Amer. med. Ass. 112, 397 (1939). — Treatment of pituitary dwarfism with chorionic gonadotropin and male sex hormone: end results. J. clin. Endocr. 4, 206 (1944). — THORN, G. W., and G. A. HARROP: The sodium retaining effect of the sex hormones. Science 40, 86 (1937). — TILLINGER, K. G.: Testicular morphology. Acta endocr. (Kbh.) Suppl. 30 (1957). — TIMME, W.: Dystrophia myotonica. Arch. intern. Med. 19, 79 (1917). — TÖNNIS, W., W. MÜLLER u. H. BRILMAYER: Zur Problematik der „mixed types" der Hypophysenadenome. Acta endocr. (Kbh.) 13, 227 (1953). — TOKUYAMA, J., R. B. LEACH, S. SHEINFELD and W. O. MADDOCK: Depression of gonadotropin excretion as a method for assay of estrogens in human subjects. J. clin. Endocr. 14, 5 (1954). — TONUTTI, E.: Zur Histophysiologie der Leydig-schen Zwischenzellen des Rattenhodens. Z. Zellforsch. 32, 495 (1943). — Vitaminmangel — Hypogonadismus. Z. ges. exp. Med. 114, 336 (1945). — Experimentelles zum Problem der Toxinwirkung auf zelluläre Substrate. Pharmazie 4, 441 (1949). — Normale Anatomie der endokrinen Drüsen und endokrinen Regulation. In E. KAUFMANN, Lehrbuch der spe-ziellen pathologischen Anatomie, Bd. I, S. 1285. Berlin: W. de Gruyter 1955a. — Über die Strukturelemente des Hodens und ihr Verhalten unter experimentellen Bedingungen. In 1. Symp. Dtsch. Ges. Endokrinologie, Febr./März 1953, S. 146. Berlin-Göttingen-Heidel-berg: Springer 1955b. — Die Keimdrüsen. In E. KAUFMANN u. M. STAEMMLER, Lehrbuch der speziellen pathologischen Anatomie, Bd. I, S. 1306. Berlin: W. de Gruyter 1956. — TONUTTI, E., F. BAHNER u. E. MUSCHKE: Die Veränderungen der Nebennierenrinde der Maus nach Hypophysektomie und nach ACTH-Behandlung, quantitativ betrachtet am Verhalten der Zellvolumina. Endokrinologie 31, 266 (1954). — TONUTTI, E., u. S. FETZER: Über Entwicklung und Differenzierung der glandotrop gesteuerten inkretorischen Gewebe beim Menschen. In 3. Symp. Dtsch. Ges. Endokrinologie. Berlin-Göttingen-Heidelberg: Springer 1956. — TONUTTI, E., O. WELLER, E. SCHUCHARDT u. E. HEINKE: Die männliche Keimdrüse. Stuttgart: Georg Thieme 1960. — TOURAINE, E.: Les états héréditaires d'atro-phies cutanées avec sénescence prématurée. Ann. Derm. Syph. (Paris) 79, 446 (1952). — TURNER, C. D.: General Endocrinology. Philadelphia: W. B. Saunders & Company 1948. — TURNER, H. T.: A syndrome of infantilism, congenital webbed neck and cubitus valgus. Endocrinology 23, 566 (1938). — TWOMBLY, G. H.: Relationship of hormones to testicular tumors. Endocrinology of neoplastic diseases. New York: Oxford Univ. Press 1947. — Hormonally active tumors of the testis. In: Progress in Clin. Endocr. Edit. by S. SOSKIN. New York: Grune & Stratton 1950. — TWOMBLY, G. H., D. MEISEL and A. P. STOUT: Leydig-cell tumors induced experimentally in the rat. Cancer (Philad.) 2, 884 (1949). — TYLER, E. T.: Norethinedrone in clinical anti-fertility studies. Acta endocr. (Kbh.) 35, Suppl. 51, 933 (1960). — TYLER, E. T., and H. J. OLSON: Fertility promoting and inhibiting effects of new steroid hormonal substances. J. Amer. med. Ass. 169, 1843 (1959). – TYLER, F. H., and G. J. PERKOFF: Dystrophia myotonica. Arch. intern. Med. 88, 175 (1951).

ULLRICH, O.: Über typische Kombinationsbilder multipler Abartungen. Z. Kinderheilk. 49, 271 (1930). — Turner's syndrome and status Bonnevie-Ullrich. Amer. J. human Genet. 1, 179 (1949). — UMIKER, W.: Interstitial cell hyperplasia in association with testicular tumors: a study of its relationship to urinary gonadotropins, testicular atrophy and histo-logical type of tumor. J. Urol. (Baltimore) 72, 895 (1954).

VAGUE, J.: La différenciation sexuelle humaine. Paris: Masson & Cie. 1953. — VAGUE, J., D. PICARD, G. VITRY, G. TAVIER et G. MILLER: Nouvelles remarques sur la chromatine sexuelle. Ann. Endocr. (Paris) 17, 857 (1956). — VARNEY, R. F., A. T. KENYON and F. C. KOCH: An association of short stature, retarded sexual development and high urinary titer in women. J. clin. Endocr. 2, 137 (1942). — VENNING, E. H., L. G. JOHNSON and B. ROSE: Proceedings of the second clinical ACTH conference, p. 91 (J. R. MOTE, ed.). New York: Blakiston Co. 1951. — VENNING, E. H., C. J. PATTEE, F. McCALL and J. S. BROWNE: Effect of cortisone in excretion of 17-ketosteroids in adrenal tumors. J. clin. Endocr. 12, 1409 (1952). — VENNING, E. H., P. G. WEIL and J. S. BROWNE: Excretion of sodium pregnanediol glucuronidate in the AGS. J. biol. Chem. 107, 128 (1939). — VOEGT, H., u. O. WELLER: Die Funktion der männlichen Keimdrüse und der Nebennierenrinde bei akuter Hepatitis und bei Lebercirrhose. Dtsch. med. Wschr. 1959, 1093.

WAGENEN, G. van: The effect of oestrin on the urogenital tract of the male monkey. Anat. Rec. 63, 387 (1935). — WAGENSEIL, F.: Beiträge zur Kenntnis der Kastrationsfolgen und des Eunuchoidismus beim Mann. Z. Morph. Anthrop. 26, 264 (1927). — Chinesische Eunuchen. Z. Morph. Anthrop. 32, 415 (1933). — WALKER, G.: A special function discovered in a glandular structure hitherto supposed to from a part of the prostate gland in rats and guinea-pigs. Bull. Johns Hopk. Hosp 21, 182 (1910). — WALLACH, S., H. BROWN, E. ENG-LERT and K. EIK-NES: Adrenocortical carcinoma with gynecomastia. J. clin. Endocr. 17, 945 (1957). — WALSH, E. L., W. K. CUYLER and D. R. McCULLAGH: The physiologic main-tenance of the male sex glands. Amer. J. Physiol. 107, 508 (1934). — WARKANY, J., C. S. FRAUENBERGER and A. G. MITCHELL: Heredofamilial deviations. Laurence-Moon-Biedl-syndrome. Amer. J. Dis. Child. **53**, 455 (1937). — WARREN, F. L.: Urinary 17-ketosteroids in diagnosis of adrenal cortical tumors. Cancer Res. **5**, 49 (1945). — WARREN, S., and K. W. OLSHAUSEN: Interstitial cell growths of testicle. Amer. J. Path. **19**, 307 (1943). — WAXMAN, S. H., V. C. KELLEY, S. M. GARTLER and B. BURT: Chromosome complement in a true hermaphrodite. Lancet 1962 I, 161. — WEIDENREICH, D.: Über partiellen Riechlappendefekt und Eunuchoidismus beim Menschen. Z. Morph. Anthrop. **18**, 157, (1914). — WEINBERGER, L. M., and F. C. GRANT: Precocious puberty and tumors of the hypothalamus. Arch. intern. Med. **67**, 762 (1941). — WELLER, O.: Untersuchungen über die Wirkung des Choriongonadotropins. Ärztl. Forsch. **7**, 280 (1953). — WERBIN, H., and G. V. LE ROY: Cholesterol — a precursor of tetrahydrocortisone in man. J. Amer. chem. Soc. **76**, 5260 (1954). — Cholesterol — a precursor of tetrahydrocortisone (THF) and 11-ketoetiocholanolone in man. Fed. Proc. **14**, 303 (1955). — WERNER, A. A.: Male climacteric. J. Amer. med. Ass. **112**, 1441 (1939). — WERNER, A. A., H. L. SPECTOR, A. E. VITT, W. L. ROSS and W. A. ANDERSON: Pubertas praecox in a six-year old boy produced by a tumor of the testis, probably of interstitial cell origin. J. clin. Endocr. **2**, 527 (1942). — WERNER, C. W.: Über Katarakt in Verbindung mit Sklerodermie. Inaug.-Diss. Kiel, 1904. — WERNER, S. C.: Failure of gonadotropic function of the rat hypophysis during chronic inanition. Proc. Soc. exp. Biol. (N.Y.) **41**, 101 (1939). — Spermatogenesis and apparent fertility in a eunuchoid male in the eleventh year of androgen therapy. J. clin. Endocr. **11**, 612 (1951). — WEST, C., B. DAMAST and O. H. PEARSON: Urinary estrogen excretion in Cushing's syndrome. J. clin. Endocr. **18**, 15 (1958). — WEST, CH. D., B. L. DAMAST, S. D. SANO and O. H. PEARSON: Conversation of testosterone to estrogens in castrated, adrenalectomized human females. J. biol. Chem. **218**, 409 (1956). — WESTMAN, A., D. JACOBSOHN u. N. HILLARP: Über die Bedeutung des Hypophysenzwischenhirnsystems für die Produktion gonadotroper Hormone. Mschr. Geburtsh. Gynäk. **16**, 225 (1943). — WEYENETH, R.: Quand fant-il opérer un testicule ectopique? Rev. méd. Suisse rom. **76**, 654 (1956). — WHEDON, G. D., and E. SHORR: Metabolic studies in paralytic acute anterior poliomyelitis. IV. Effects of testosterone propionate and estradiol benzoate on calcium, phosphorus, nitrogen, creatine and electrolyte metabolism. J. clin. Invest. **36**, 995 (1957). — WIEDEMANN, H. R., M. TOLKSDORF u. H. ROMATOWSKI: Ergebnisse hämatologischer Kerngeschlechts-Diagnosen bei Intersexen und sonstigen Anomalien auf dem Gebiet der Sexualentwicklung. Ärztl. Wschr. 1957, 857. — WIENER, M., CH. J. LUPU and E. J. PLOTZ: Metabolism of 17α-hydroxy-progesterone-4-C^{14}-17α-caproate by homogenates of rat liver and human placenta. Acta endocr. (Kbh.) **36**, 511 (1961). — WILDBOLZ, H.: Anorchism. Korresp.-Bl. schweiz. Ärz. **42**, 1307 (1917). — WILDER, V. M.: Kreatinurie beim Jugendlichen und Kastraten. Arch. Biochem. **42**, 69 (1953). — WILKINS, L.: Feminizing adrenal tumor causing gynecomastia in boy of 5 years contrasted with virilizing tumor in 5 year old girl, classification of 70 cases of adrenal tumor in children according to their hormonal manifestation and review of 11 cases of feminizing adrenal tumor in adults. J. clin. Endocr. **8**, 111 (1948). — The diagnosis and treatment of endocrine disorders in childhood and adolescence. Springfield, Ill.: Ch. C. Thomas 1950. — The diagnosis and treatment of endocrine disorders in childhood and adolescence. Springfield, Ill.: Ch. C. Thomas 1957. — WILKINS, L., and J. CARA: Further studies on the treatment of congenital adrenal hyperplasia with cortisone. J. clin. Endocr. **14**, 287 (1954). — WILKINS, L., J. F. CRIGLER, S. H. SILVERMAN, L. J. GARDNER and C. J. MIGEON: Further studies on the treatment of congenital adrenal hyperplasia with cortisone. J. clin. Endocr. **12**, 1015 (1952). — WILKINS, L., and W. FLEISCHMANN: Sexual infantilism in females. J. clin. Endocr. **4**, 306 (1944a). — Ovarian agenesis, pathology, associated clinical symptoms and the bearing on the theories of sex differentiation. J. clin. Endocr. **4**, 357 (1944b). — WILKINS, L., W. FLEISCHMANN and J. E. HOWARD: Creatinuria induced by methyl testosterone in the treatment of dwarfed boys and girls. Bull. Johns Hopk. Hosp. **69**, 493 (1941). — WILKINS, L., and M. M. RAVITCH: Adrenocortical tumor arising in the liver of three year old boy with signs of virilism and Cushing's syndrome. Pediatrics 9, 671 (1952). — WILLIAMS, R. G.: Studies of living interstitial cells and pieces of seminiferous tubules in autogenous grafts of testis. Amer. J. Anat. **86**, 343 (1950). — WINTERSTEIN, O.: Über den Kryptorchismus. Chirurg 24, 433 (1953). — WITSCHI, E.: Embryogenesis of the adrenal and the reproductive glands. Recent Progr. Hormone Res. **6**, 1 (1951). — WITSCHI, E., and W. T. LEVINE: Oestrus in hypophysectomised rats parabiotically connected with castrates. Proc. Soc. exp. Biol. (N.Y.) **32**, 101 (1934). — WITSCHI, E., W. O. NELSON and S. J. SEGAL: Genetic, developmental and hormonal aspects of gonadal dysgenesis and sex inversion in man. J. clin. Endocr. **17**, 737 (1957). — WITSCHI, E., u. J. M. OPITZ: Grundlagen der Intersexualität. In: Die Intersexualität (C. OVERZIER), S. 17. Stuttgart: Georg Thieme 1961. — WOOTEN, E., M. M. NELSON, M. E. SIMPSON and H. M. EVANS: Effect of pyridoxine deficiency on the gonadotrophic content of the anterior pituitary in the rat. Endocrinology 1, 59 (1955). — WOTIZ, H. H., J. W. DAVIS, H. M. LEMON and M. GUT: Studies in steroid metabolism. J. biol. Chem. **222**, 487 (1956). — WOTIZ, H. H., H. M. LEMON and P. MARCUS: Determination of urinary 11-oxygenated 17-ketogenic steroids. J. clin. Endocr. 17, 116 (1957). — Wynn, V., J. Landon and E. Kawerau: Studies of hepatic function during methandienone therapy. Lancet 1961 I, 69.

Zahler, H.: Über die Wirkung verschiedener Gaben von Androgen auf den Rattenhoden. Virchows Arch. path. Anat. 312, 138 (1944). — Záhôr, Z., u. J. Raboch: Ein Beitrag zum Problem der Hodenbiopsie bei Kryptorchismus unter besonderer Berücksichtigung des Optimalalters für die Orchidopexie. Schweiz. med. Wschr. 1956, 311. — Zander, J.: Progesteron in menschlichem Blut und Geweben. I. Progesteron im peripheren venösen Blut der Frau. Klin. Wschr. 33, 697 (1955). — Steroids in the human ovary. J. biol. Chem. 232, 117 (1958). — Zander, J., u. A. Münstermann: Weitere Untersuchungen über Progesteron in menschlichem Blut und Geweben. Klin. Wschr. 1954, 894. — Zanow, M. X., P. L. Munson and W. T. Salter: A comparison of androgens determined chemically and 17-ketosteroids determined chemically in urine (normal and abnormal). J. clin. Endocr. 10, 692 (1950). — Zenzen, G., u. A. de Mas: Zum Stand der Androgen-Depotbehandlung im gynäkologischen Anwendungsbereich. Med. Wschr. 12, 593 (1958). — Zimmermann, W.: Chemische Bestimmungsmethoden von Steroidhormonen in Körperflüssigkeiten. Berlin-Göttingen-Heidelberg: Springer 1955. — Zondek, B.: Weitere Untersuchungen zur Darstellung, Biologie und Klinik des Hypophysenvorderlappenhormons (Prolan). Zbl. Gynäk. 53, 834 (1929). — Über das Schicksal des Follikelhormons (Follikulin) im Organismus. Skand. Arch. Physiol. 70, 133 (1934). — Zondek, B., u. S. Aschheim: Hypophysenvorderlappen und Ovarium. (Beziehungen der endokrinen Drüsen zur Ovarialfunktion.) Arch. Gynäk. 130, 1 (1927). — Zondek, B., u. H. Euler: Follikulinausscheidung im Harn des Kindes, der Frau und des Mannes. Skand. Arch. Physiol. 67, 259 (1934). — Zondek, H.: Die Krankheiten der endokrinen Drüsen. Berlin 1926. — Zubirán, S., u. F. Gomez-Mont: Endokrine Störungen bei chronischer Unterernährung. Vitam. and Horm. 11, 97 (1953). — Zublin, W.: Psychology of the Klinefelter's syndrome. Acta endocr. (Kbh.) 14, 137 (1953). — Zuckerman, S.: Inhibition of menstruation and ovulation by means of testosterone propionate. Lancet 1937 I, 676. — Zuckerman, S., and T. McKeawn: The canine prostate in relation to normal and abnormal testicular changes. J. Path. Bact. 46, 7 (1938b). — Zuckerman, S., and A. S. Parkes: The effect of male hormone on a mature castrated rhesus monkey. J. Anat. (Lond.) 72, 277 (1938a).

Namenverzeichnis — Author-Index —
Index alphabétiques des noms d'auteurs

Die *kursiv* gesetzten Seitenzahlen beziehen sich auf die Literaturverzeichnisse
Page numbers in *italics* refer to the references
Les nombres en caractères *italiques* reportent aux index bibliographiques

Sachverzeichnis — Subject Index — Table analytique des matières

Die *kursiven* Seitenzahlen weisen auf ausführliche Besprechungen im Text hin.
The numbers printed in *italics* refer to detailed descriptions in the text.
Les chiffres imorimés en *italique* indiquent la page ou le sujet est traité en détails.